T0385135

The Shoulder

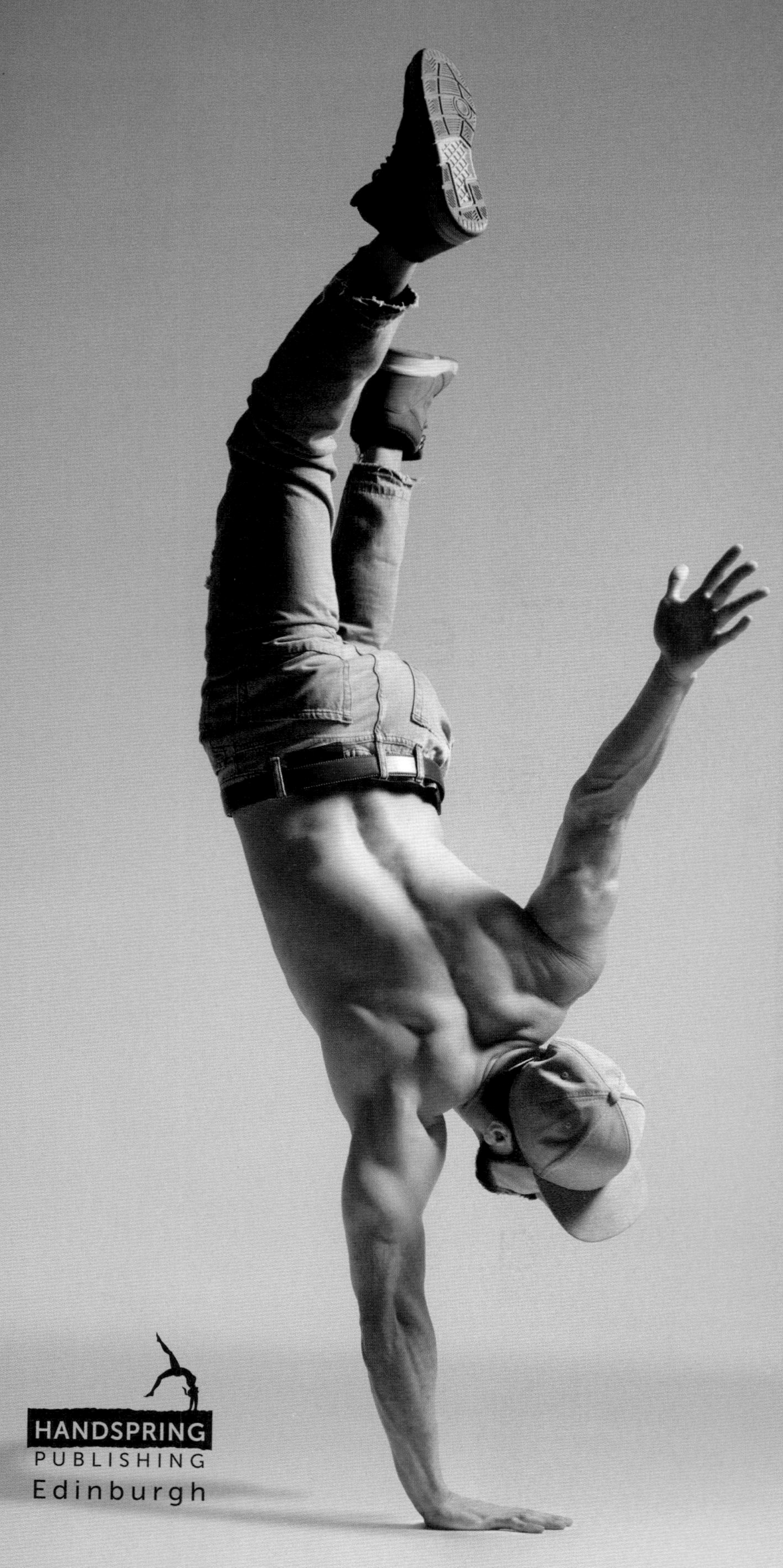

HANDSPRING
PUBLISHING
Edinburgh

The Shoulder

Theory and Practice

Editors
Jeremy Lewis
César Fernández-de-las-Peñas

Forewords
Wilbour Kelsick
Clare Ardern and Karim Khan

The Old Manse, Fountainhall,
Edinburgh
EH34 5EY, Scotland
Tel: +44 1875 341 859
Website: www.handspringpublishing.com

First published 2022 in the United Kingdom by Handspring Publishing Limited

ISBN 978-1-913426-17-0
ISBN (Kindle eBook) 978-1-913426-18-7

British Library Cataloguing in Publication Data
A catalogue record for this book is available from the British Library
Library of Congress Cataloging in Publication Data
A catalog record for this book is available from the Library of Congress

Notice
Neither the Publisher nor the Authors assume any responsibility for any loss or injury and/or damage to persons or property arising out of or relating to any use of the material contained in this book. It is the responsibility of the treating practitioner, relying on independent expertise and knowledge of the patient, to determine the best treatment and method of application for the patient.
All reasonable efforts have been made to obtain copyright clearance for illustrations in the book for which the authors or publishers do not own the rights. If you believe that one of your illustrations has been used without such clearance, please contact the publishers and we will ensure that appropriate credit is given in the next reprint.

This book is a guide for personal exploration and is in no way meant to substitute for any type of medical advice – allopathic, Western, Eastern, Indian. It can complement a healing protocol. Ultimately all movement ideas are to be visited with gentleness allowing your body responses and related sensations to guide you.

Commissioning Editor Mary Law
Project Manager Morven Dean
Copy Editor Susan Stuart
Designer Bruce Hogarth
Typesetter Ditech, India
Indexer Aptara, India

Book printed in Great Britain by Bell and Bain Ltd, Glasgow

The Publisher's
policy is to use
paper manufactured
from sustainable forests

Contents

Contents *continued*

Contents *continued*

About the editors

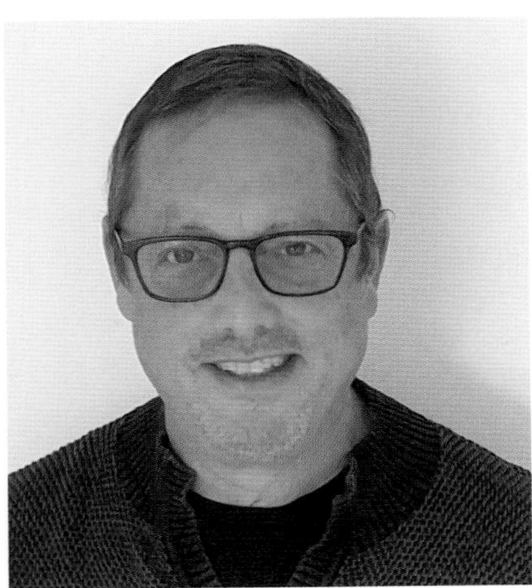

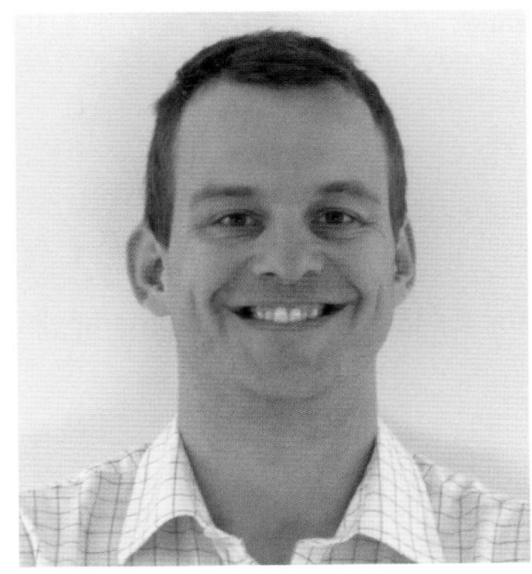

Jeremy Lewis PhD FCSP is a consultant physiotherapist in the Central London Community Health Care Trust (UK National Health Service) and is also Professor of Musculoskeletal Research at the University of Limerick in the Republic of Ireland. He was born in New Zealand, trained in Australia, and lived there for some time before moving to the UK. Jeremy is acknowledged as an eminent clinician in his profession and has been awarded a Fellowship of the Chartered Society of Physiotherapy, the highest award the CSP can offer. His clinical practice and research have focused on musculoskeletal conditions involving the shoulder. He has also completed an MSc (musculoskeletal physiotherapy), and has postgraduate diplomas in sports physiotherapy, and biomechanics. He is qualified as an Independent (non-medical) Prescriber, and as an MSK sonographer, and uses these skills to perform ultrasound-guided shoulder injections, to complement his clinical practice.

Jeremy is frequently invited to present keynote lectures and has taught over 500 international workshops in over 50 countries and territories. He has appeared on TV news programs and his work has been picked up in newspapers and through other media outlets. He has presented podcasts, seminars, and webinars discussing shoulder problems.

Jeremy works both clinically and in the academic world and has authored more than 250 publications including contributions to both books and journals. He is a member of the editorial team for *Grieve's Modern Musculoskeletal Therapy* and a special features editor for the *Journal of Orthopedic and Sports Physical Therapy (JOSPT).* He has challenged many aspects of clinical practice and his suggestions for change have been widely adopted internationally. His main areas of research interest are rotator cuff-related shoulder pain, frozen shoulder, injection therapy, rehabilitation, virtual reality, self-management, healthcare sustainability, and behavioral change. He also writes about the medicalization of normality, and the need to reframe musculoskeletal practice. In addition to his own research, Jeremy supervises PhD and MSc students around the world.

César Fernández-de-las-Peñas PT, PhD, DrMedSci is full professor and practicing clinician at Universidad Rey Juan Carlos, Madrid, Spain. He received a bachelor degree in physical therapy from Universidad Rey Juan Carlos and a PhD and the Doctoral Master of Sciences from Aalborg University in Denmark. He has published around 550 peer-reviewed articles and is the first-named author of approximately 250. His research activities are concentrated on the neuroscience of pain. Specific research areas have been on pain and assessment of pain in volunteers and chronic pain patients. The main focus is on human clinical chronic pain research. César is the main editor of 10 textbooks on manual therapy for chronic musculoskeletal pain including *Temporomandibular Disorders*, also published by Handspring Publishing. He is one of the editors of the third edition of *Travell, Simons & Simons' Myofascial Pain and Dysfunction: The Trigger Point Manual* published in 2019. He combines his research activity with clinical practice as the Head of the Division of Physical Therapy Department, University Physical Therapy Clinic at Universidad Rey Juan Carlos, Madrid.

Contributors

Caroline Alexander PhD, MSc, MMACP, MCSP, HPCP
Lead Clinical Academic for Therapies
Imperial College Healthcare NHS Trust;
Adjunct Reader
Department of Surgery & Cancer
Imperial College London
London, UK

Ben Ashworth MSc (S&C), MSc (Physiotherapy), BSc (Hons), ASCC
Director
Athletic Shoulder Ltd
London, UK;
Director of Performance
AC Sparta Prague
Prague, Czech Republic

Martin Asker PhD, DN, CST
Head of Handball Research Group
Department of Health Promotion Science
Sophiahemmet University
Stockholm, Sweden;
Research and Development Director
Scandinavian College of Naprapathic Manual Medicine
Stockholm, Sweden

Panos Barlas BSc (Hons), PDD, DPhil, LicAc
Lecturer
School of Allied Health Professions
Keele University
Keele, UK

Joletta Belton MSc
Cofounder
Endless Possibilities Initiative
Fraser, Colorado, USA

Joel Bialosky PT, PhD
Clinical Associate Professor
University of Florida Department of Physical Therapy
Brooks Rehabilitation-College of Public Health and Health Professions Research Collaboration
Gainesville, Florida, USA

Christine Bilsborough Smith MSc (Physiotherapy), MCSP, PGCert (MSK Sonography)
Consultant Physiotherapist
Musculoskeletal Therapies
Central London Community Healthcare NHS Trust
Finchley Memorial Hospital
London, UK

Craig Boettcher PhD, Titled Sports Physiotherapist, BASc (Physiotherapy)
Honorary Associate
University of Sydney
Faculty of Medicine and Health;
Director
Regent Street Physiotherapy;
Consultant Physiotherapist
Swimming Australia
New Lambton, NSW, Australia

Sarah Boyd BSc (Hons) Physiotherapy
Clinical Lead of Musculoskeletal Physiotherapy
Musculoskeletal Physiotherapy Outpatients
Imperial College Healthcare Trust
St Mary's Hospital London
London, UK

Niamh Brady MPhty, BSc (Hons)
Lecturer in Anatomy
Department of Anatomy and Neuroscience
University College Cork, Ireland;
Director
Evolve Health Physiotherapy and Rehabilitation Clinic
Co. Cork, Ireland

Graham Burne MSc (Advanced Physiotherapy), BSc (Physiotherapy), BSc (Sports Science), PGCert (Musculoskeletal Ultrasound)
Advanced Practice Physiotherapist
Musculoskeletal Assessment Triage and Treatment Service (MCATTS)
Guy's & St Thomas' NHS Foundation Trust
London, UK

Angela Cadogan PhD (Musculoskeletal Diagnostics), M.Sports Physio, PGCert (Sport & Exercise), Dip MT, Dip Phys
Specialist Physiotherapist (Musculoskeletal)
Advance Physiotherapy
Christchurch, New Zealand;
Orthopaedic Outpatients Department
Canterbury District Health Board
Christchurch, New Zealand

Rachel Chester PhD, MSc, MCSP, MMACP
Lecturer in Physiotherapy
University of East Anglia;
Physiotherapist
University of East Anglia Sportspark
Norwich, UK

Joshua A Cleland PT, PhD, FAPTA
Director, Research and Faculty Development
Professor, Doctor of Physical Therapy Program
Tufts University School of Medicine
Boston, Massachusetts, USA

Chad Cook PT, PhD, FAPTA
Program Director, Interim Chief, Professor in Orthopaedic Surgery
Department of Orthopaedics
Duke University School of Medicine
Durham, North Carolina, USA

Tim Cook MSc (Advanced Neuromusculoskeletal Physiotherapy), BSc (Hons) Physiotherapy
Advanced Practice MSK Physiotherapist
Department of Physiotherapy
Sussex Community NHS Foundation Trust
Bognor Regis War Memorial Hospital
Bognor Regis, UK;
Senior Lecturer
Department of Physiotherapy
Institute of Sport
University of Chichester
Chichester, UK

Ann Cools PT, PhD
Associate Professor
Department of Rehabilitation Sciences
Universiteit Gent
Gent, Belgium

Michel Coppieters PT, PhD
Menzies Foundation Professor of Allied Health Research
Griffith University
Brisbane and Gold Coast Campuses
Queensland, Australia

Thomas Cosker MB BCh, MSc FRCS (Tr & Orth), FAS
Consultant Orthopaedic Oncology Surgeon and Director of Human Anatomy
University of Oxford
Oxford, UK

Mike Cummings MB ChB, DipMedAc
Medical Director
British Medical Acupuncture Society;
Honorary Clinical Specialist
Royal London Hospital for Integrated Medicine
London, UK

Liesbet de Baets PT, PhD
Pain in Motion Research Group
Department of Physiotherapy;
Human Physiology and Anatomy
Faculty of Physical Education & Physiotherapy
Vrije Universiteit Brussel
Brussels, Belgium

Benjamin JF Dean FRCS(Orth), DPhil
Senior Research Fellow
Nuffield Department of Orthopaedics, Rheumatology and Musculoskeletal Sciences
University of Oxford
Oxford, UK

Beate Dejaco PT, MSc
Physiotherapist and Manual Therapist
Sports Medical Centre Papendal
Arnhem, The Netherlands;
Lecturer
Master Program Musculoskeletal Therapy
HAN, University of Applied Sciences
Nijmegen, The Netherlands

Ruth Delaney MB BCh, MMedSc, FRCS, FFSEM
Consultant Shoulder Surgeon
Beacon Hospital and Sports Surgery Clinic
Dublin, Ireland;
Associate Professor
Orthopaedic Surgery
University College Dublin
Dublin, Ireland

François Desmeules PT, PhD
Head of Programs and Associate Professor
Advanced Practice Physiotherapy Programs
School of Rehabilitation
Faculty of Medicine
University of Montreal;
Montreal, Quebec, Canada
Investigator
FRQ-S Research Scholar
Orthopaedic Clinical Research Unit
Centre de Recherche de l'Hôpital Maisonneuve-Rosemont (CRHMR)
Montreal, Quebec, Canada

Baljinder Singh Dhinsa MBBS, FRCSEd (T&O), MSc, MFSTEd
Consultant Trauma and Orthopaedic Surgeon
William Harvey Hospital
Ashford, UK

Marc-Olivier Dubé M.PT
Physiotherapist
Physio Interactive – Clinique Cortx
Quebec, Canada

Jessica Dukes MSc (Advanced Physiotherapy), BSc (Physiotherapy)
Advanced Physiotherapy Practitioner
Integrated Pain and Spinal Service
Berkshire Healthcare NHS Foundation Trust
West Berkshire, UK

Uzo Ehiogu MSc, BSc (Physio), BSc (App Exercise Science), MMACP
Consultant
Rehabilitation & Physical Preparation
Inside Edge Physiotherapy
Birmingham, UK;
Clinical Teaching Fellow
Royal Orthopaedic Hospital NHS Foundation Trust
Birmingham, UK;
Honorary Clinical Lecturer
College of Medical & Dental Sciences
Birmingham University Medical School
Birmingham, UK;
Visiting Fellow
The Centre for Human Performance, Musculoskeletal & Orthopaedic Sports Medicine and Performance in Extreme Environments
Leeds Beckett University
Leeds, UK

Kathryn Fahy MSc, BSc, MISCP (Shoulder)
TA Anatomy, MSK Clinical Specialist
Allied Health
University of Limerick
Limerick, Ireland

Edel Fanning BSc (Physiotherapy), MSc (Advanced Musculoskeletal Physiotherapy)
Shoulder Physiotherapist
Sports Surgery Clinic
Dublin, Ireland

Laura Finucane MSc, FCSP, FMACP
Consultant Physiotherapist
Sussex MSK Partnership
Brighton, UK

Lennard Funk BSc (Physiotherapy), MSc (Orth Engin), FRCS (Tr&Orth), FFSEM (UK)
Consultant Orthopaedic Surgeon
Wrightington Upper Limb Unit
Wrightington Hospital
Wigan, UK

Rochelle Furtado BSc, MSc, MPT
Student and Research Assistant
Health and Rehabilitation Sciences
Western University
London, Canada

Olivier Gagey MD, PhD
Emeritus Professor
University of Paris-Saclay
Orsay, France

Alessandra N Garcia PT, PhD
Assistant Professor
College of Pharmacy & Health Sciences
Doctor of Physical Therapy Program
Campbell University
Lillington, North Carolina, USA

Jo Gibson MCSP, Grad Dip Phys, MSc (Adv Pract)
Clinical Specialist Physiotherapist
Liverpool University Hospitals NHS Foundation Trust;
Consultant Physiotherapist
West Kirby Physiotherapy
Wirral, UK

Karen Ginn PhD, MHPEd, GDManipTher
Professor of Musculoskeletal Anatomy
Faculty of Medicine & Health
University of Sydney
Sydney, Australia

Angela Spontelli Gisselman PT, PhD, DPT, OCS
Assistant Professor
Doctor of Physical Therapy Program
Tufts University
Phoenix, Arizona, USA

Rodney Green BSc (Hons) DipEd, MSc, PhD
Past President, Australian & New Zealand Association of Clinical Anatomists;
Adjunct Associate Professor in Human Anatomy
Department of Pharmacy and Biomedical Sciences
La Trobe University
Melbourne, Australia

Derek Griffin BSc, PhD
Clinical Specialist Physiotherapist
Bon Secours Hospital Tralee
Tralee, Ireland

Kevin Hall MSc, NIHR Academy Member
Advanced Physiotherapy Practitioner
Physiotherapy Outpatient Department
University Hospitals Sussex NHS Foundation Trust
Shoreham-by-Sea, UK

Toby Hall FACP, PhD, MSc, PGDip Manip Ther
Specialist Musculoskeletal Physiotherapist;
Adjunct Associate Professor
Curtin School of Allied Health
Curtin University;
Director, Manual Concepts
Perth, Australia

Eric Hegedus PT, DPT, PhD, MHSc
Orthopaedic Certified Specialist;
Professor, Physical Therapy Program
Tufts University School of Medicine
Boston, Massachusetts, USA

Alastair Hepburn BSc, PhD, FRCP
Consultant Rheumatologist
Department of Rheumatology
Western Sussex Hospitals NHS Foundation Trust
Worthing, UK

Danielle Hollis BPhty (Hons), BHlthSc
Physiotherapist
University Academic School of Allied Health Sciences
Griffin University and Australian Catholic University
Brisbane, Australia

Ian Horsley PhD, MSc, MCSP, CSCS
Technical Lead Physiotherapist
English Institute of Sport;
Clinical Director, Back In Action Rehabilitation
Wakefield, UK

Balraj Jagdev MBChB, BSc, MRCS
Specialist Registrar
Trauma and Orthopaedics
Leicester Royal Infirmary
Leicester, UK

Anju Jaggi BSc (Hons) Physiotherapy
Consultant Physiotherapist
Shoulder & Elbow Unit
Royal National Orthopaedic Hospital NHS Trust
Stanmore, UK

Mark Jones CertPT, BS(Psych), Grad Dip (Advanced Manipulative Therapy), MAppSc (Manipulative Physiotherapy)
Lecturer in Physiotherapy
Allied Health & Human Performance Academic Unit
University of South Australia
Adelaide, Australia

Rhiannon Joslin BSc (Physiotherapy)
Specialist Paediatric Physiotherapist
Paediatric Chronic Pain Team
University Hospitals Sussex NHS Foundation Trust;
Physiotherapy Lecturer
University of Southampton
Southampton, UK

Gwendolen Jull MPhty, PhD, FACP
Emeritus Professor in Physiotherapy
School of Health and Rehabilitation Sciences
The University of Queensland
Brisbane, Australia

Roger Kerry PhD
Associate Professor
School of Health Sciences
University of Nottingham
Nottingham, UK

Tony Kochhar MSc, FRCS (Tr & Orth)
Consultant Orthopaedic Surgeon
Visiting Professor
Faculty of Sports Science
University of Greenwich
London, UK

William King BSc (Hons) Physiotherapy, MSc (Manipulative Physiotherapy), MRes, HCPC, MCSP, MMACP
Advanced Physiotherapy Practitioner
Musculoskeletal Service
Sussex Community NHS Foundation Trust
Bognor Regis, UK

Simon Lafrance PT, MSc
Physiotherapist
School of Rehabilitation, Faculty of Medicine
Université de Montréal
Montreal, Quebec, Canada

Simon Lambert BSc, FRCS, FRCSEdOrth
Consultant Orthopaedic Surgeon
Department of Trauma and Orthopaedics
University College London Hospital
London, UK

Neil Langridge DClinP, MSc, BSc (Hons), FCSP, FMACP
Consultant Physiotherapist
Department of Musculoskeletal Services
Southern Health NHS Foundation Trust
Lymington, Hants, UK

Dana Lewis MBBS, BSc, MRCP
Specialist Haematology Registrar
Department of Haematology
Hammersmith Hospital – Imperial College Healthcare NHS Trust
London, UK

Keren Lewis BMBS, BMedSci
Foundation Year 3 Medical Doctor
Royal Free London NHS Foundation Trust
London, UK

Maya Lewis BSc (Accounting and Finance), BSc (Midwifery)
Midwife
Maternity Unit
Kingston Hospital NHS Foundation Trust
Kingston-upon-Thames, London, UK

Stephen Loftus PhD
Associate Professor
Department of Foundational Medical Studies
Oakland University William Beaumont School of Medicine
Rochester, Michigan, USA

Matthew Low MSc, BSc, MMACP, MCSP
Consultant Physiotherapist
Therapy Outpatient Department
Christchurch Hospital
University Hospitals Dorset Foundation NHS Trust
Dorset, UK

Jonathan Lucas MBChB
Academic Clinical Fellow in General Practice
School of Medicine
Keele University
Keele, UK

Greg Lynch Dip Phty, Dip MT, Dip MDT
Senior Physiotherapist
Inform Physiotherapy Ltd
Wellington, New Zealand

Joy MacDermid PT, PhD, FCAHS, FRSC
Distinguished University Professor
Fellow – Canadian Academy of Health Sciences
Fellow – Royal Society of Canada
Physical Therapy and Surgery
University of Western Ontario
London, Ontario, Canada

Michael Mansfield MSc, BSc (Hons), HCPC, MCSP, MMACP, FHEA
Lecturer Musculoskeletal Physiotherapy
School of Sport, Exercise and Rehabilitation Sciences
University of Birmingham
Edgbaston, Birmingham, UK

Lorenzo Masci MBBS, FACSP
Consultant, Sports and Exercise Medicine
OneWelbeck Sports Medicine
London, UK

Jenny McConnell AM, FACP, BAppSci (Physiotherapy), Grad Dip (Man Ther), MBiomedE
Practice Principal
McConnell Physiotherapy Group
Mosman, NSW, Australia

Karen McCreesh PhD, MSc (Manip Ther), BSc (Physiotherapy)
Senior Lecturer
School of Allied Health
University of Limerick;
Senior Lecturer
Ageing Research Centre
Health Research Institute
University of Limerick
Limerick, Ireland

Jillian McDowell MPNZ, Dip Phys, Reg Physio Acup, PGCert Sports Med, Dip MT, Cred MDT, MPhty, MCTA
International Chair
Mulligan Concept Teachers Association;
President, Physiotherapy Acupuncture Association of New Zealand;
Director, Prohealth Physiotherapy Ltd
Queenstown, New Zealand

Sally McLaine BA Appl Sci (Physiotherapy), PhD
APA Sports Physiotherapist
Physiotas Launceston
Launceston, Tasmania, Australia

Mira Meeus PT, PhD
Full Professor
University of Antwerp & Ghent University
Departments of Rehabilitation Sciences and Physiotherapy
Ghent, Belgium

Christopher Mercer FMACP, FCSP, MSc, Grad Dip Phys, PGCert (Clin Ed)
Consultant Physiotherapist
Physiotherapy Department
Western Sussex Hospitals NHS Trust
Sussex, UK

Brian Mulligan FNZSP (Hon), Dip MT
Mulligan Concept Founder
Auckland, New Zealand

Margie Olds PhD, MSc, BPhty
Physiotherapy Specialist
Auckland Shoulder Clinic
Auckland, New Zealand

Shaun O'Leary BPhty (Hons), MPhty (Musculoskeletal), PhD, FACP
Associate Professor in Physiotherapy (Clinical Academic)
Physiotherapy Department
University of Queensland/Royal Brisbane and Women's Hospital
Brisbane, Australia

Kieran O'Sullivan PhD, M Manip Ther, BPhysio
Senior Lecturer
School of Allied Health
University of Limerick
Limerick, Ireland

Peter O'Sullivan Dip Physio, Grad Dip Manip Ther, PhD, FACP
John Curtin Distinguished Professor
Specialist Musculoskeletal Physiotherapist
School of Allied Health
Curtin University
Perth, WA, Australia

Yemi Pearse BM, BCh, MA (Oxon), FRCS (Orth)
Consultant Orthopaedic Surgeon and Department Lead
Department of Trauma and Orthopaedics
St George's Hospital
London, UK

Tamar Pincus BSc, MSc, MPhil, PhD
Professor in Health Psychology
Department of Psychology
Royal Holloway University of London
Surrey, UK

Jared Powell DPhty, BExsc/BBus
Physiotherapist
Faculty of Health Sciences and Medicine
Bond University
Robina, QLD, Australia

Shelly Prosko PT, C-IAYT
Physiotherapist, Yoga Therapist
www.physioyoga.ca
Alberta, Canada

Raja Bhaskara Rajasekaran MS, DNB, FNB
Clinical Fellow & Girdlestone Scholar
Oxford Sarcoma Service
Oxford University Hospitals
NHS Foundation Trust
Oxford, UK

Gajan Rajeswaran MBBS, FRCR, PGCME
Consultant Musculoskeletal Radiologist
OneWelbeck Imaging & Diagnostics
London, UK

Eleanor Richardson MSc (Advanced Musculoskeletal Physiotherapy Practice), PGDip (Orthopaedic Medicine), BSc (Hons) Physiotherapy
Clinical Shoulder Specialist
Physiotherapy Department
BMI The Alexandra Hospital
Cheadle, Manchester, UK

Richard Rosedale PT, Dip MDT
International Director of Education
McKenzie Institute International
Coldstream, Ontario, Canada

Jean-Sébastien Roy PT, PhD
Full Professor
Department of Rehabilitation
Faculty of Medicine, Université Laval;
Researcher, Center for Interdisciplinary Research in Rehabilitation and Social Integration
Université Laval
Quebec City, Quebec, Canada

Paul Salamh PT, DPT, PhD
Assistant Professor
Krannert School of Physical Therapy
College of Health Sciences
University of Indianapolis
Indianapolis, Indiana, USA

Emma Salt Grad Dip (Physiotherapy), MSc (Musculoskeletal Physiotherapy), PhD
Consultant Physiotherapist
University Hospitals of Derby and Burton NHS Foundation Trust;
Fellow, National Institute for Health and Care Excellence;
Honorary Research Physiotherapist
Keele University
Keele, UK

Fiona Sandford PhD Physiotherapy, MSc (Upper Limb Rehabilitation), BSc Physiotherapy
Consultant Physiotherapist
Clinical Lead
Hand Therapy & Hand Unit Co-Lead
Guy's & St Thomas' Foundation NHS Trust
London, UK

Martin Scott MSc (Health Services Research), PGDip (Assessment & Treatment of the Shoulder), BSc (Hons) Physiotherapy
Clinical Specialist Physiotherapist
Physiotherapy Department
Nottingham University Hospitals NHS Trust
Nottingham, UK

Amee L Seitz PT, DPT, PhD
Associate Professor
Department of Physical Therapy & Human Movement Sciences
Feinberg School of Medicine
Northwestern University
Chicago, Illinois, USA

Mitchell Simpson MD, BPhysio (Hons)
Paediatric Basic Physician Trainee
Department of General Medicine
The Royal Children's Hospital
Melbourne, Australia

Gisela Sole BSc (Physio), MSc (Med) Exercise Science, PhD
Associate Professor
School of Physiotherapy
University of Otago
Dunedin, New Zealand

Lonnie Soloff BSci (Exercise Science), PT, ATC, DPT
Vice President
Medical Services
Cleveland Indians Baseball
Cleveland, Ohio, USA

Gareth Stephens BSc (Hons), MSc
Clinical Research Physiotherapist
Physiotherapy Department
The Royal Orthopaedic Hospital
Birmingham, UK

Mike Stewart MSc, BSc (Hons), MCSP, SRP, PGCert (Clin Ed)
Physiotherapist, Educator & Researcher
Know Pain Ltd
Kent, UK

Filip Struyf PT, MSc, PhD
Professor in Rehabilitation Sciences and Physiotherapy
University of Antwerp
Antwerp, Belgium

Alan J Taylor MCSP, MSc
Assistant Professor
Physiotherapy & Rehabilitation Sciences, School of Health Sciences
University of Nottingham
Nottingham, UK

Duncan Tennent FRCS(Orth)
Consultant Orthopaedic Surgeon
St. George's Hospital NHS Trust;
Professor of Orthopaedic Education
St. George's University of London
London, UK

Danielle van der Windt PhD
Professor of Primary Care Epidemiology
School of Medicine
Keele University
Newcastle-under-Lyme, UK

Hubert van Griensven PhD, MSc(Pain), BSc, DipAc
Physiotherapist and Acupuncturist;
Senior Lecturer
School of Health and Social Work
University of Hertfordshire
Hatfield, UK

Bill Vicenzino PhD, MSc, Grad Dip Sports Phty, BPhty
Chair in Sports Physiotherapy
University of Queensland
Brisbane, QLD, Australia

Sanjay Vijayanathan MRCP, FRCR
Consultant Radiologist
Lead for Musculoskeletal Imaging
Radiology
Guy's and St Thomas' NHS Foundation Trust
London, UK

Lennard Voogt PhD, PT
Research Centre for Healthcare Innovations and Department of Physiotherapy Studies
Rotterdam University of Applies Sciences
Rotterdam, The Netherlands;
Pain in Motion Research Group (PAIN)
Department of Physiotherapy, Human Physiology and Anatomy
Faculty of Physical Education and Physiotherapy
Vrije Universiteit Brussel
Brussels, Belgium

Helen Walker PhD, B App Sc Physio, Grad Dip App Sc Sports Physio
APA Sports Physiotherapist
Principal
Physio4athletes;
Consultant Physiotherapist Swimming Australia
Melbourne, VIC, Australia

Craig Wassinger PT, PhD
Associate Professor
Department of Physical Therapy
East Tennessee State University
Johnson City, Tennessee, USA

Grant Watson Dip Phys, Adv Dip Phys, Dip MDT, Dip MT, NZSP
Consultant Physiotherapist
Mohua Rehabilitation
Collingwood Health Centre
Collingwood, Golden Bay, New Zealand

Tim Watson PhD, BSc (Hons), FCSP
Professor of Physiotherapy
University of Hertfordshire
Hatfield, UK

Rod Whiteley PhD, FACP
Assistant Director, Rehabilitation Department
Aspetar Sports Medicine Hospital
Doha, Qatar

Stuart Wildman BSc (Hons) Physiotherapy, MSc (Advanced Neuromusculoskeletal Physiotherapy), PGCert (Musculoskeletal Sonography), PG Dip (Society of Orthopaedic Medicine Diploma)
Advanced Physiotherapy Practitioner and Consultant Musculoskeletal Sonographer
Royal Surrey County Hospital NHS Foundation Trust
Guildford, Surrey, UK

Chris Worsfold MSc, AFHEA
The Tonbridge Clinic
Tonbridge, UK

Foreword by Wilbour Kelsick

Producing a book to address shoulder pain and dysfunction is a daunting task. However, Jeremy and César tackled this project with an enlightened passion which shines through the entire manuscript. Treatment or management of shoulder issues are not mutually exclusive events in musculoskeletal medicine. The editors approached their project with this false dichotomy at the forefront, reflecting their plan for the pragmatic content and organization of their book.

The shoulder is one of the most complex and versatile joints in the human body. Its integration with the hand is one of the physical features that makes humans unique in the animal kingdom. Its functional capacity depends on a wide range of motion, and, at the same time, it needs to exhibit its own stability to create the precision of motion needed for the hand. This functional feature of the shoulder is a perfect example of dynamic stability where there is contradictory dance between stability and mobility to create motion that exhibits integrity and efficiency. It is this contradictory dance (maintaining stability while maximizing mobility) which gives the shoulder its unique complexity and at the same time makes it susceptible to injury and chronic dysfunction.

Shoulder dysfunction and pain is ubiquitous and one of the most challenging musculoskeletal conditions to manage because of its complex functional architecture. Practitioners who manage patients with shoulder dysfunction need no convincing of the need for a unified source which provides the evidence-based knowledge in anatomy, physiology, biomechanics, psychosocial interplay, and integrative management strategies to treat shoulder dysfunction. Understanding shoulder dysfunctional etiologies from such a prospective will enable clinicians and students to engage in a more holistic approach to manage shoulder problems. Proficient holistic examination, diagnostics, and treatment protocols are paramount in managing shoulder dysfunction and pain. In this book, the editors provide the necessary tools to holistically manage shoulder dysfunction.

Jeremy and César were on a mission to deliver a comprehensive, cogent, and practical textbook and they have accomplished it. Based on their life stories as learned practitioners, what evolved is a transdisciplinary manuscript that includes both the basic theory necessary to understand the normal and pathological dysfunction, and the evidence-based tools for evaluating and clinically managing shoulder dysfunction. The text provides exceptional and convincing scientific literature references to inform, guide, and clarify for the reader the supporting evidence underlying the contributors' theses.

This book is timely in this era when conventional management of chronic musculoskeletal pain by opioid-based analgesic medication is under tremendous scrutiny worldwide because of its addictive and lethal effects on chronic pain patients. The contributors to the book highlight the awareness that there are other pain management options like alternative care, and biopsychosocial and environmental considerations, which should be considered in managing patients with chronic shoulder dysfunction and pain.

From a functional anatomical prospective, the shoulder complex has the most degrees of freedom in the body. Its overall function depends on the force transmission links to the upper, mid- and lower body structures. Its entire integrity of movement is about cooperation and coordination to support its complex and precise function in human activity. The editors' strategy in creating this text, including an impressive array of experts in shoulder dysfunction and pain management, strongly mirrors the theme of cooperation and coordination.

Managing shoulder pain and dysfunction is not an easy clinical task. However, having a reliable and pragmatic source of evidence-based clinical knowledge is paramount for practitioners working in this field. Knowing the editors' backgrounds attests to my opinion that this book was methodically designed so the information is reader friendly. The information presented has incredible clarity and is well- researched with up-to-date references. The text is beautifully illustrated with diagrams, tables, "clinical tip" boxes, focus points, skills for communicating with patients, and photographs of treatment and examination techniques, all of which facilitate comprehension of the core message. The virtual reality approach headline in Chapter 30 and future access to a website for additional knowledge resources are superb and pertinent added features. No matter what is your field of expertise in musculoskeletal medicine, there is something in this book for you. It is an invaluable resource for clinicians and students whose aim is to deliver optimum care to the patient. I am honoured by the invitation to write the foreword for this manuscript. I highly recommend this book.

Wilbour Kelsick DC, BSc, FRCCSS(C), FRCCRS(C)

Clinical Director

Maxfit Movement Institute Inc.

Port Moody, Canada;

Team Practitioner,

Canadian Olympic Track and Field Team

Port Moody, Canada, January 2022

Foreword by Clare Ardern and Karim Khan

When a new book arrives, it is an exciting time. The community senses the need, appreciates the authority of the authors, and the buzz begins: "Have you seen the new shoulder book by Lewis and Fernández-de-las-Peñez?" This excitement begins as a murmur among co-authors and reviewers for they have seen the drafts, and quickly overflows to the true shoulder aficionados (pre-orders). The early adopters are next to discover the buzz; hot on their heels are the clinical and research communities. In the 2020s, the buzz skips and whoops around the world – amplified by social media. In *The Shoulder: Theory and Practice*, the buzz will be about at least four features.

Feature number 1: This book is comprehensive. Whereas the leading sports medicine texts cover shoulder pain in one chapter or at best a section with a few chapters, we now have four parts, 43 chapters and more than 700 quality pages.

Feature number 2: Written by whom? By the best: 116 of the world's leading shoulder authorities. Imagine the buzz at the shoulderpalooza when this who's-who of the shoulder meet in person.

Feature number 3: The patient focus. Let's be honest – *Gray's Anatomy* wasn't patient-focused and neither were the foundation texts in physiotherapy that are now in their fourth editions and beyond. Kudos Drs Lewis and Fernández-de-las-Peñez for walking the walk (if we are permitted a lower limb metaphor?!). The book begins with patient stories: Chapter 1 – boom! The raison d'être. But it's not "one (chapter) and done". You will find thoughtful discussion of the biopsychosocial model, a chapter on communicating with people who have shoulder pain, and a focus on specific sports in rehabilitation. All underscore the authors' commitment to improving patients' lives – not merely "outcomes".

Feature number 4: The humility the authors bring to their work. Authority and humility. It sounds paradoxical but it's not. Authority that results from hard work – knowing the literature, having done the research, and pouring it into one's clinical work. All 115 authors reflect and share lifetimes of wisdom, and an essential humility that underpins all health care. There is humility in the prefaces from both editors, especially where they acknowledge that "As you read this book you will appreciate how much knowledge we still require to better inform our practice so as to help those experiencing shoulder symptoms."

It takes a village to raise a child. A cliché or an aphorism? Never mind semantics – the expression came to our minds because this new book – this new life among textbooks – was nurtured by a passionate, caring, and wise community. And as with any new life, the world is the better for it. We (health professionals, researchers, patients, citizens) are stronger together and this author community – superbly led by Drs Lewis and Fernández-de-las-Peñez – deserves our gratitude.

Clare L Ardern BPhysio (Hons), PhD
Senior researcher,
Centre for Hip Health & Mobility
University of British Columbia.
Editor-in-Chief, Journal of Orthopaedic & Sports Physical Therapy

Vancouver, Canada, January 2022

Karim M Khan MD, PhD, MBA
Professor,
University of British Columbia;
Scientific Director
Canadian Institutes of Health Research – Institute of Musculoskeletal Health and Arthritis (CIHR-IMHA)
Co-author, Brukner and Khan's Clinical Sports Medicine

Vancouver, Canada, January 2022

Preface and Acknowledgments by Jeremy Lewis

Shoulder pain can be frightening, is commonly disabling, and when persistent, life-changing. The purpose of this book is to make some sense of how the shoulder works, what goes wrong, and for clinicians, what can we do to help those seeking care. At all times the focus remains on the most important person in healthcare – the patient.

I love medical history, and some of the books I most treasure in my personal library are over 100 years old. It is fascinating to read literature that describes what was state-of-the-art a century ago and earlier. One hundred years from now our understanding of shoulder function, assessment and treatment will be vastly different than it is today and will be informed by patients' experiences, new research knowledge and clinical practice. I thank the future researchers who will add to our knowledge in the years to come, as I thank those current and past, who have informed the content of this textbook. As you read this book you will appreciate how much knowledge we still require to better inform our practice so as to help those experiencing shoulder symptoms.

This book was written during the SARS-CoV-2 pandemic. Many lives have been lost, families devastated, and for many, the way we live our lives has changed dramatically. It has given us all an opportunity to reflect, and as always in human history, to hope for better times. Personally, I lost family members and friends to COVID-19 and am still experiencing the effects of long (haul) covid, but I am thankful the symptoms are steadily improving. The lead authors of the chapters and their co-authors have all worked tirelessly to produce this book during the pandemic. In the circumstances, it was a real challenge for me to edit chapters and make suggestions to the contributors, especially as we relied on their good faith, and more so as they volunteered their precious time during this terrible period in history. I am indebted to each of them and offer all of them my warmest and most heartfelt thanks. Wholehearted thanks also to the publishers, copyeditors, artists, and everyone at Handspring Publishing for their support, guidance, and advice. What a privilege to work on this project with you César – thank you. "It takes a village" to put a book together.

This book is intended to be a source of learning and I hope that its pages will soon be well-thumbed, filled with colored sticky notes, and used as a basis for discussion with colleagues and to support clinical practice.

Online resources

Many of the chapter authors have signposted readers to websites for pictures, videos, and supplementary resources. To facilitate this, I have dedicated a section on my website, www.drjeremylewis.com (Resources section) where chapter by chapter the websites and other resources are listed.

Dedication

I would like to dedicate this book to my loved ones and dearest friends, and to all those who have inspired me. You have helped make me who I am, a better version of myself than I could have ever made myself.

May your heart always be joyful. May your song always be sung.

Bob Dylan – Nobel Prize Laureate

Jeremy Lewis

Wellington, Melbourne, and London

June 2021

Preface and Acknowledgments by César Fernández-de-las-Peñas

The shoulder is a fascinating region, both anatomically and biomechanically. When symptomatic it is frequently associated with substantial morbidity, and the management of that morbidity is a challenge for clinicians. The treatment of shoulder conditions continues to evolve, especially with increased recognition that, like back pain, symptoms are not only due to mechanical dysfunction, but are also associated with psychological and social factors. Appreciating this management of shoulder conditions has shifted from a bio-only approach to one which is more holistic and biopsychosocial. To reflect this change, this book adopts a patient-centered, biopsychosocial approach to management. We also know that the environment in which the patient lives influences both access to healthcare and outcomes, and we consider this as well.

Exercise is probably the best, safest, and most appropriate therapeutic option to manage most shoulder conditions. It is also associated with other important health benefits, but even though there may be related benefits, exercise does not meaningfully reduce shoulder disability for everyone. By itself it is not enough and must be provided with appropriate education underpinned by a strong therapeutic alliance. We also know that addressing lifestyle factors is essential, and there are conditions, or phases of conditions, where injections and surgery outperform exercise, and sometimes it is best not to "intervene," but take a watch and wait approach. We also understand that clinicians' experiences and patients' values and beliefs must not be undervalued in the management of musculoskeletal shoulder conditions.

Appreciating this complexity, we were inspired to bring together clinicians and researchers from around the world and from many disciplines to provide a comprehensive synthesis of the diverse approaches to assessing and treating people seeking solutions for their shoulder problems. We recognize that we do not have all the answers to all the questions relating to assessment and management of the shoulder, and because of this we have taken an approach that combines research evidence and expert opinion to produce an evidence-informed approach to assessment and management.

We hope this textbook will become a valued resource for clinicians worldwide, informing and contributing to uniting practitioners, and ultimately benefiting people living with shoulder pain and related symptoms. As with this edition, we hope that future editions will be informed by evolving research and knowledge, and that the book will continue to be a solid foundation for all those involved in managing shoulder conditions.

After many years working with patients with persistent shoulder pain and athletes with shoulder problems, I received an invitation from Handspring Publishing to put together a definitive shoulder textbook. Once we had agreed on the need for this book, it took only a second to decide that my colleague and friend, Jeremy Lewis, should be *the* person to lead on this ambitious project. In the beginning, neither Jeremy nor I realized how many people would enthusiastically volunteer and agree to participate: they all said "It's time for this textbook."

First, I would like to thank Jeremy, who has dedicated and focused much of his clinical and research career on helping people experiencing shoulder symptoms. He would be the first person to say he has not always got it right and there is a long way to go, but he remains dedicated to this cause.

Secondly, an enormous thank you to all the co-authors, the clinicians, and researchers who have so skillfully contributed to these pages.

Thirdly, thank you to the people living with shoulder pain who have contributed directly as co-authors to this textbook and who have inspired us to do better in our clinics. Next, thank you to Handspring Publishing for your professionalism, support, and enthusiasm and for entrusting us with this project.

Lastly, we recognize our families, friends, and colleagues. We realize that our professional activities – clinical practice, teaching, supervising, writing, researching – often take us away. We are forever indebted to your understanding and support for our endeavors.

César Fernández-de-las-Peñas

Madrid, Spain

June 2021

Part 1
Musculoskeletal shoulder problems

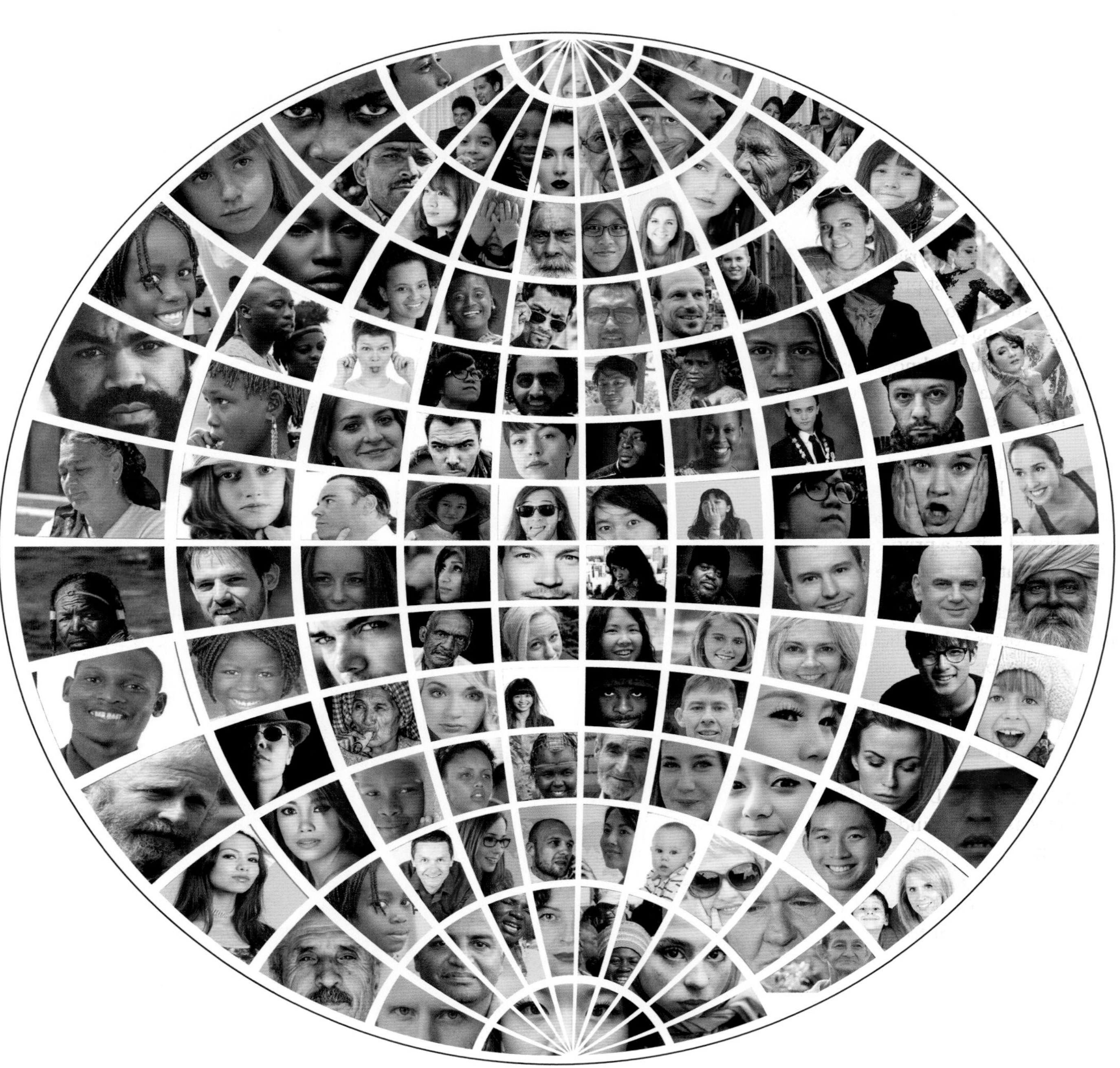

Our stories: living with shoulder pain

1

Jeremy Lewis

One of the many reasons for writing this book was to bring the collective knowledge and skills of internationally renowned experts together to produce a synthesis of contemporary knowledge relating to musculoskeletal problems involving the shoulder. To achieve this aim, the authors will present how and why the shoulder does what it does, why things go wrong, make suggestions for assessment and management, and will help answer the question, "Why does my shoulder hurt?" The book will discuss the global burden of shoulder pain, identify ongoing uncertainties and challenges, and discuss new advances.

Another of the myriad aims of this book is to support practitioners with a clinical interest in this area to do what they do best: provide best practice, reduce disability, and enable the person seeking care to return to the highest level of function possible, aiming to exceed the patient's expectations. However, there is one higher purpose, and to achieve that aim we must unconditionally recognize that the most important person in healthcare is not the clinician, but the person seeking care. In doing so we must acknowledge that the lived experience, fears and concerns, beliefs, and aspirations of the person in front of us are crucial for that individual. And the only way to understand any of that is to listen carefully to the individual's story, which is the focus of this first chapter.

People who have lived with shoulder pain in the past or are currently living with shoulder pain are the authors of this chapter. By hearing their stories, we can reflect on how we listen and communicate with members of our communities who have decided they require care for the shoulder symptoms they are experiencing. I am indebted to those who have contributed – it is a privilege to read their accounts. They are trying to help us be better versions of ourselves, to ensure past communication errors are not taken forwards.

To protect anonymity some names have been changed, and editing has been kept to a minimum to ensure it is the patients' voices we are hearing. I would like to thank everyone who sent in their personal story, although space did not permit all to be published.

Zana Hakimi, Iran

Before moving to London [UK] I was a scientist, but my passion was body building. I had won many international competitions. Each year I would do the fire-fighting physical examination and my record for pull-ups was 58. Then a few years ago I developed right shoulder pain, it didn't go away, and I went to see top specialists and had an MRI scan. The doctors told me I had an extra bone in my shoulder that was pressing on the tendon, and that if I kept exercising my tendon would tear and I may not be able to use my arm. Surgery was recommended to remove the bone. I talk to my father a lot, I respect his advice, he said he knew people after surgery who were no better off and sometimes worse. I didn't know what to do. In my head all I could see was this sharp piece of extra bone digging into my tendon. My fear would be my tendon would snap and I not only wouldn't be able to lift my arm, but I would lose muscle definition because there would be no muscle to strengthen, and I would never be able to compete again.

My world had collapsed. For more than two years I didn't lift my arm out to the side to protect it, the pain had become unbearable, especially at night, I couldn't even pull my trousers up, my girlfriend would help me, I couldn't do anything. None of the treatments I was offered made any sense; people told me (and I also saw on the Internet) that injections make tendons worse, so that wasn't an option; surgery may not work, and physiotherapy [physical therapy] would only push the tendon into the sharp bone and cause more damage. I looked in the mirror and didn't recognize the person in front of me – the person who used to have great [muscle] definition and won international competitions was now fat and incapable of even getting dressed.

Desperate, I decided to try one more time. This time it was different, I wasn't told I have to exercise my muscles to get them strong again, and I wasn't made to push my arm to cause more [tendon] damage. We started with talking – we actually went for a walk together outside. I cried when I was asked, "What is it like living with this pain?" Treatment started with very gentle movements, my shoulder was held in a position that took some pain away. This was a breakthrough moment for me, my pain could change, and in this position, I was asked to throw and catch a very light ball against the wall in the clinic. I was using my shoulder again.

Five months later I still feel pain from time to time, but in my culture, we call it "far" pain: pain that I don't think about, pain that is far away from me, it doesn't bother me and it doesn't stop me doing what I want to do. I am now exercising maybe harder than I ever have. I did 60 pull-ups. I have just won an international competition. I ask myself how is it possible that I can do this with the extra bone still there? My father gives me energy, I think this treatment did, too.

Jennifer Truscott, New Zealand

I am a retired nurse, aged 72, and live on my own. In November 2019 I was playing a competitive game of croquet when I experienced intense pain in my right shoulder after a long hard shot. I continued to play with some difficulty, and we actually won the game and the competition. Croquet is a game that requires mental and physical input, and it was proving to be an enjoyable experience in my retirement. But this was the last game I played due to the pain, and the worry that I may further injure my shoulder.

I went to see my GP [primary care/family doctor] regarding my shoulder injury and his first comment was, "Yes, looks like you have torn the rotator cuff, surgery is not an option as you are over 70, and it will probably take at least a year to heal." He actually was right, but it was not what I really wanted to hear. As I was going away for Christmas, he offered to do an injection in the shoulder. I agreed, but he did not get the right spot and it made no difference to the pain.

I asked about physio [physical therapy] and he referred me to a local physiotherapist. In New Zealand if you have an injury, this is partially covered by ACC [Accident Compensation Corporation, the governmental no-fault healthcare payment scheme]. The person I was referred to was not very helpful, I was just another number to her so I stopped going.

In January 2020 I went back to my GP as I was still severely restricted in what I could do and was only averaging 1–2 hours' sleep a night. He sent me for an ultrasound and X-ray of my shoulder. The conclusion was I had a partial thickness tear, diffuse tendinosis, and the bursa was thickened with fluid present. X-ray was normal. One week after the ultrasound I saw a radiologist, and had an injection under ultrasound guidance into the subacromial bursa. The effect of this only lasted two weeks.

In March 2020 I reinjured my shoulder by doing a very simple thing – changing a duvet cover and tossing it in the air to get it in the right places. I went back to my GP and was referred for another ultrasound. This now showed that I had a full thickness partial width anterior and mid tendon tear. On the same day I got this result, a radiologist gave me another injection in the shoulder. Once again, this only helped reduce the pain for about two weeks.

Two weeks later I phoned the GP and said I was not coping with the pain due to severe sleep deprivation and I was not able to do my usual activities to maintain my independence. I remember yelling at him and saying that sleep deprivation was used as a torture during the war. He increased my anti-inflammatories, I started taking these at night and this was helpful. I started on paracetamol [acetaminophen/Tylenol] and codeine, but as these had little or no effect on night pain, I stopped them.

In April 2020, nearly six months after the original injury, I saw a shoulder specialist. He said the tear was very small and it would be technically difficult with the size of the instruments to repair it arthroscopically. He also said that current research is now showing that physiotherapy [physical therapy] gives as good a result in the same length of time as surgery for rotator cuff tears. He suggested referring me to a physiotherapist specialist who has a PhD in shoulder issues. He said he had worked with her and was confident she would be able to help me. The three visits to the orthopedic surgeon and six visits to the physiotherapist were covered by the ACC at no charge to me.

This was the best thing that had happened to me since the injury in November. The physiotherapist listened to me and made suggestions for my daily activities that would help decrease the pain. Simple things, like how I could avoid heavy lifting that caused pain. For example, I have a pellet fire and the bags of pellets come in 15 kg [33 lbs] bags – she suggested dividing the bags into three buckets, not two as I was doing. Or when I'm boiling the jug for a cup of tea, only putting in enough water for one cup, not filling the jug. Asking for help from family and friends as usually I don't like to do this. Only doing small amounts of gardening at a time – I have a large garden and gardening was one of the things that was causing my shoulder to become swollen.

We tried different exercises until we sorted out what exercises worked best for me. Massage was also very good in the short term for relieving pain. We talked about positions in bed so I could hopefully get longer periods of sleep. I cannot sleep on either side as even sleeping on my good side with a supporting pillow causes pain. Eventually I found that sleeping upright with 4–5 pillows works best for me. Lack of sleep due to pain has been my main problem: 1–2 hours' sleep a night for the first 4–5 months post injury, and even now over 12 months later, 5 hours' sleep in one go is a fantastic sleep.

I always wake in pain and usually get up and start the day. I read lots of books to fill in time until I meet friends for walks on the beach. My recovery has been very up and down, and I continue to hope that one day all my shoulder pain will be gone. I haven't tried playing croquet again as I am scared that I could cause a further tear and be back at the beginning again. I always felt I had a good tolerance of pain, but sleep deprivation due to constant pain is another story.

Jean-Paul Thivierge, Canada

During the winter of 2007 I fell on black ice, and tore the rotator cuff tendons of my left shoulder. In December 2008 I fell again, this time in the snow, with the tearing of tendons of the rotator cuff of my right shoulder. In August 2009, an ultrasound of both shoulders confirmed complete tears of rotator cuff tendons [on both sides]. I had a cortisone shot, before the first repair surgery. Around 2010, I had orthopedic surgery for a rotator cuff repair – successful but not easy. Following the right shoulder surgery, there were no symptoms, everything was fine. On August 13, 2019 I woke up with intense pain in my neck and shoulder blade on the right side. [Another ultrasound scan confirmed] a full thickness tear of the tendons of the supraspinatus, infraspinatus, and subscapularis muscles, with atrophy of these muscles and edema of the supraspinatus and infraspinatus muscles, and to a lesser extent of the subscapularis.

In October 2019, I met a new orthopedic surgeon specializing in shoulders, offering the option of a total reverse shoulder arthroplasty [TRSA] for the right shoulder. Then I consulted with a private physiotherapist and was offered some general exercises for both shoulders. I had the TRSA surgery on March 9, 2020. Quite a chance three days before the first severe containment of the COVID-19 pandemic. Around two weeks postoperatively, visits to the outpatient physiotherapy clinic began with a physiotherapist who had expertise in the shoulder. From that moment on, a dozen regular appointments followed for education, exercise proposals, and evaluation of progress in range of motion and strength. However, I still can't scratch my back with my right hand, my arm can move backwards, but I can't bend my elbow to place my hand higher behind my back. Also, it is difficult for me to reach the top of the right thigh. However, I manage to put my hand on my head.

At the end of October 2020, seven months postoperatively, I had the last assessment of the condition of my right shoulder by the physiotherapist. Then X-rays were taken, and I met with the orthopedic surgeon to make sure the prosthesis was stable. In the end, everything is within the norms considering my age, the type of surgery, and my good health.

In my opinion, everything has been done well to optimize my chances of becoming independent again with a functional right arm. I can imagine that, considering my age of 76, muscle mass does not return as at 45. However, all things considered, this operation allows me to be functional, quite autonomous, for more than 80% of my daily activities. I made some easy adjustments in my closets and kitchen for everyday needs. When I need help with actions that require more strength, I can get it from my relatives and good neighbors.

As I am right-handed and have always been very good with my hands, it is very constraining and frustrating to have to hesitate and be slower and less agile in carrying out my manual tasks. I have done all kinds of sports, expert alpine skiing, competitive sailing on catamarans, cycling, ice hockey, etc. Now, I can barely raise my arms higher than my shoulders; often I have to ask for help to access objects placed higher. I am also limited to doing things lower than shoulder height because my left rotator cuff tendons are also torn. I must learn to cope with this. I consider that I will have to get used to it and develop alternative means and techniques. Thank you to the Quebec public health system.

May (16), UK

Everything happened and changed fast. I remember sitting in the car after school and sneezing: something cracked, and my shoulder fell and looked deformed. That is when it all started. I slowly began to lose control of my shoulder and the pain became unbearable. I found myself avoiding doing things I had been doing all my life. As a teenager, independence is an important part of growing up. Yet I found myself struggling to brush my hair, clean my teeth, even sometimes dressing. Having to ask for help all the time for the most mundane things got to me, I felt vulnerable.

I was surrounded by a constant panic of my teachers, my friends, and my family. This led to me being on a constant high alert, as the simplest movement would make my shoulder dislocated. For a while I could not even lift my arm above my head. I could no longer write, sleep, eat without my shoulder dislocating. My shoulder was out of place more than it was in place, and the pain grew as time passed. During school I could not keep up with the workload. I was constantly being sent home or going to hospital with a cold, blue, unresponsive hand.

The dislocations reached the point where I simply was unable to relocate it. I suffered with shooting, throbbing, stabbing pains, and pins and needles which were relentless. The pain changed my personality, as did the lack of sleep. I became withdrawn, isolating myself for fear of being hurt. Friendships broke. I developed unhealthy coping mechanisms (dissociation) which still affects me today. I was referred to a more specialist hospital and a diagnosis was given. I went on to spend two weeks in hospital receiving physiotherapy and occupational therapy. This has helped me cope better and adjust how I tackle tasks.

However, this was not the end of it or a magic cure. Still to this day my arm and hand go numb, my skin looks like corned beef. The muscles in my chest go into spasms and harden over time, and my shoulder blade no longer sits in position. I must take the knowledge given and apply it by retraining my muscles how to work, and learn how to deal with muscle spasms by relaxing the muscles to prevent this. I have had to relearn how to do simple things such as cleaning my teeth, washing my hair, and writing.

I am still learning, but with the help of a local pain specialist team I am beginning to understand that my emotions affect my dislocations and muscle spasms. With their help I no longer live on painkillers, and understand that regaining my physical strength will decrease the dislocations. I have good days and bad days and I am now able to keep my shoulder in longer. I am beginning to get back into more physical activities. But in conclusion I still hurt.

Ted Dreisinger, USA

It began with little notice, as these things often do. If it were prose, one might say it was alliterative – irresistibly, insidiously, idiopathic. But it wasn't prose, it was my right shoulder, and with the speed of an advancing glacier, I developed capsulitis.

In the beginning, range of motion slowly was reduced, but I ignored it because it had little functional impact. A swimmer at the time, the alarm sounded loudly when I could no longer complete a crawl stroke with my right arm – pain and obstruction to movement. I was prescribed exercises, which I did diligently for months, but they made no impact on my shoulder. I was also advised to do very specific end-range stretching exercises. As with the strengthening exercises, there was some slight relief with only minor and unsatisfactory functional gains.

I decided to "heal myself" and to take treatment into my own hands. I combined both previous models (strengthening and end-range movement) in an aggressive, twice-a-week regime.

The exercises:

1. Straight arm static hang from a bar with bodyweight for 90 seconds, followed by pulsed (single set, 25 reps) loading in the same position.

2. Anterior, static internal medial flexion against external rotation of trunk for 90 seconds, followed by pulsed loading (single set, 25 reps) in the same position.
3. Posterior, static internal medial flexion against internal rotation of the trunk, followed by pulsed loading in the same position.

These exercises were twice repeated in each session and were excruciatingly painful. However, within two months, the shoulder had full pain-free range with a return to normal functional activity.

Mark Watson, UK

I don't know where to start really. My first procedure (a [Bankart] repair) was undertaken privately in 2007 (when I was 43), which as far as I can remember went quite smoothly. Although the outcome wasn't as good as [the surgeon had] led me to believe it would be, the repair did last seven years.

My shoulder started playing up again in 2015, giving me the same if not more severe pain than I had in 2007, so I went to see my GP who referred me to [an orthopedic surgeon] in the NHS [National Health Service]. The referral took about four months to materialize. I felt very reassured by [the surgeon] as his manner was very engaging and thorough, so I was full of hope that things would be resolved, and I would get my life back on track as I am a keen sportsman.

After this procedure (a second [Bankart] repair and a SLAP repair) and despite weekly NHS and privately funded physio [physical therapy], my shoulder movement was becoming more and more limited; even more of a problem, the daily pain was increasing making daily life very uncomfortable and limited.

After about 12 months I had my final consultation with the surgeon who decided to give me a painkilling injection to see how the shoulder reacted, followed by arthroscopy to release/remove any scar tissue. The injection worked well for about six weeks which was a great relief, but when I went back to see him, he totally changed his mind about the arthroscopy and told me to live with my shoulder as it was, and to go back and see him when I was 60 and he would give me a new shoulder! This was devastating.

I then became very disillusioned with the whole process so decided to go back to my GP to discuss the matter. He suggested that I pay privately to get a second opinion, which I did at the local hospital, and this is where things got silly. Initially, I saw [another orthopedic surgeon] who arranged a variety of tests but was unable to come to a diagnosis, so he referred me to his colleague [another orthopedic surgeon] who was at best very dismissive. When I asked if he would put me on his private list so I could shorten the waiting time, he refused, saying that he would only operate on the NHS so as to limit his responsibility if the outcome was poor, which didn't fill me with much confidence.

[Another orthopedic surgeon] performed a capsular release privately, which despite my initial confidence, left me with the same level of pain and lack of movement. I have since had a second capsular release [with another orthopedic surgeon] and am waiting for an Ostinil [sodium hyaluronate] injection as my final throw of the dice before having to have a total shoulder replacement. My overall feelings are disappointment as I have wasted four years of my life and a fair amount of money and energy trying to find the best course of treatment, which now thanks to COVID-19, I feel is quite unlikely.

Tim McGary, USA

I injured my right shoulder at the campus of the university for which I work. I was walking on a flagstone sidewalk and had to make a sharp right turn due to construction. I slipped and fell directly onto my shoulder as if I had been tackled. I reported the fall to my employer and completed the standard workplace injury reports. The next day I was examined by a doctor in Employee Health, had an X-ray, and was given a sling for the weekend and told to ice it and rest, to be re-examined after the swelling subsided.

After the next examination, I was prescribed physical therapy [PT] through Employee Health. My pain level was high, and PT was primarily focused on range of motion stretches. I was re-examined after series of PT, reporting continuation of pain and range of motion restrictions. I was prescribed another set of PT through Employee Health. Additionally, I had difficulty seeing the same doctor through Employee Health and became concerned about consistency of care.

During the second round of PT, the therapist told me he believed there was a structural issue that needed further tests. I expressed this to the Employee Health doctor and asked if I could see a shoulder specialist. The decision was first to do more PT. After the therapist continued to express concern, I was referred to a shoulder surgeon. All of this took place between December 2018 to June 2019.

Upon examination, the first prescription was an X-ray-guided injection. The result of this treatment provided no relief, and I had to go back to Employee Health before seeing the shoulder specialist again. It took me asking for an MRI to be ordered and completed before my next appointment with the shoulder surgeon in late July 2019. And the delays in Employee Health's approval process caused the MRI not to be scheduled until the very last opportunity.

The MRI arthrogram revealed three complex tears of the labrum, including one at the connection of the bicep tendon. The shoulder surgeon told me my MRI "lit up like a Christmas tree." At that point I wondered why it took so long to get an MRI. What could or should I have said in my previous interactions that would have motivated the Employee Health doctors to order an MRI? How much more quickly could I have had my shoulder repaired?

I had surgery in August 2019, with weeks of immobilization and loss of work time after it. The tear at the bicep tendon was not repaired, rather the tendon was detached and reattached, while the other two tears were repaired. I received extensive PT through Sports Sciences PT rather than Employee Health, throughout the fall-winter of 2019–20. I was told progress would be slow, yet steady. I was told to expect full recovery to take a year. I prepared myself and practiced patience, yet as we got into the spring, some clicking, clunking, and catching persisted while pain was subsiding.

Then COVID hit the southeastern US in March 2020, and everything shut down. Employee Health cancelled all of my follow-up appointments. My PT went to telehealth, and while my therapist was encouraging and thorough in providing exercises I should do, it did not replace having her work with my shoulder directly or observe me doing exercises and motions to determine the best course of actions. Telehealth with the surgeon was even worse, as the first two attempts for follow-up appointments failed due to technology issues.

Still, I felt I was making some progress, and was cleared to try to do some activities, like catching a baseball (I am left-handed) while coaching my Little League team and swinging a golf club. Because golf was a permitted exercise activity during COVID, I worked up to playing weekly during the summer, and the shoulder felt good for this underhanded motion. Yet when coaching baseball in the spring, and then summer after pausing due to COVID, it felt difficult trying to catch a baseball over my head or with arm outstretched to the side. In the fall of 2020, I reported both the positives about my golf swing and the negatives about catching a baseball to my surgeon, who ordered an MRI to investigate. The MRI results did not indicate any additional issues, so the doctor offered encouragement, an injection, and more PT, with a follow-up in December 2020.

The injections did little to offer relief for more than an initial time period, and while I definitely felt that my strength was improving with PT, I continued to have pain at rest and while running, and experienced the clicking, clunking, and catching feelings with overhead and extended motions throughout fall 2020. I had the follow-up with the surgeon in December 2020, who, after listening to my frustration that I continue to have pain at rest, which prevents me from falling asleep, wakes me up, and increases when I run, and that I also feel the clicking, clunking, and catching in my overhead and extended motions, suggested another surgery to investigate because the MRI didn't indicate the symptoms that I described and that were found during my exam. I have agreed to the second surgery because I want answers, and hope this will offer a better long-term prognosis, and because I would prefer to be recovering during a time when I am working remotely.

I wonder, still, about the disjointed nature of my care: from how long it took for Employee Health to order an MRI or refer me to a specialist in 2019, to how much COVID impacted normal patterns or decision-making for determining appropriate treatments and procedures. None of that is clear to me, nor do I expect it can be being outside the medical field. Yet, I know something has continued to be wrong with my shoulder for a long period, and I wonder again, as I did in 2019, what could or should I have said to motivate more aggressive or different treatment for a more efficient result and resolution. And now, my case continues, remaining inconclusive.

Philip Jones, South Africa

I couldn't believe my ears. The physio [physical therapist] actually said these words: "We don't use those [passive] treatments anymore" [referring to a hands-on shoulder procedure that had been offered a few years previously]. I just asked how can a treatment be passive if it helps me become more active?

Olwyn Kelly, Ireland

My journey began back when my 21-year-old son was a toddler, and unlike my oldest son who ran off as soon as he could walk and never came back again, this one wanted to go everywhere on my hip. He'd look up and say "uppy mummy" with arms outstretched, and I always picked him up and put him on my left hip and did everything I had to do with my right hand while he watched.

I noticed a raised hardness on the left shoulder and pain all around the area. I went to several "quacks" who massaged it. Eventually I went to my doctor who gave me anti-inflammatories and sent me for an MRI as there was a distinctive lump. I don't know where my copy of the report is now as I've since changed doctors, or what exactly it showed. I began the journey of going to several physios [physical therapists] for various massages, dry needling and exercises, and every time it would flare up.

I continued my usual routine doing gym, swimming, yoga, and walks. I'm fairly active and don't sit down for long. My usual routine would have always been some form of exercise every morning, with yoga one night a week. Every so often [the pain] would flare up and I'd go to an osteopath who seemed to settle it for a bit again. Really it was in the background all the time. Around nine years ago I found an interventional radiologist who injected into the area using an MRI to assist. This seemed to settle it for a bit and last year I was thinking of trying that again. I went to [...] who thought the problem was in my neck and sent me to a physio for neck strengthening exercises. I had MRIs for shoulder and neck there, too.

I've never been too comfortable doing much overhead gym work and eventually shied away from that. I went to a spin circuit class for years and loved it, but I stopped that as I felt some exercises were aggravating the situation. I always thought I had way less shoulder strength than the other women at any of the weight training classes I had tried, but didn't stick to.

I started doing reformer Pilates at a place run by physios with all the classes physio led. I felt they knew my story, so it should be OK. One of them suggested another physio, who did shockwave therapy. He insisted on a color MRI being done, but I'm not sure what was written on the report.

A colleague identified a possible dead nerve area in the supraspinatus muscle. Anyway, that physio continued with shockwave therapy for another few sessions. He then gathered a few people together with shoulder injuries and ran a class of strengthening exercises for us. Did I feel any benefit? I'm not sure exactly. He said he saw an improvement in strength but I'm not sure.

I mentioned my problem by chance in the pool one night to a yoga teacher who said she'd had a problem for years and had made an appointment with [...]. I was dubious as I'd seen so many physios. Anyway, I said I'd give it one last shot and I couldn't believe the interest he took. He got me back a second time at no extra charge to take videos of my movement, and sent them to [an orthopedic surgeon] who he said was an expert at complex shoulder issues. I saw her and she took another MRI, and confirmed white-out of supraspinatus muscle. I am now waiting for nerve conduction studies. I think I'm stuck with shoulder difficulty for life at this point.

Panos Barlas, Australia

In November 2020 I fell off a chair I was standing on at home (then in the UK). I sustained an avulsion fracture of my right greater tuberosity. I was quickly seen in hospital and received good care. In January 2021 I had my final appointment with the hospital shoulder specialist: identification of a neck of humerus fracture, as well as greater tuberosity fracture; rotator cuff tendons are intact and the fracture appears stable. No further intervention required, except physiotherapy [physical therapy] and patience.

It had been a few years since I was a patient with a serious enough condition to warrant hospital appointments. As soon as I suffered the injury, I wanted to believe that it was just a bad sprain, no (long-term) damage done, and that I would walk away from this. But, as soon as I realized things were a bit more serious than I thought, a million thoughts were in my head. I am an active outdoorsman, walk my dogs, cut my own firewood, extract game from the woods, carve wood... I had visions of me not being able to do any of this. No one had asked what the fracture meant to me. The medical care I received was top notch, they could do no more than what they did already, yet the impact of the fracture to me, as a person, was not a priority at this point.

But what this experience left me with were lessons I should have learned a long time ago. Patients are anxious. I am. I still don't know whether I'll ever enjoy the same freedom of my right shoulder I had before. Understanding the impact of disease on the person may not change clinical pathways but goes a long way to reassuring that the condition is taken seriously. There are aspects of care that as a patient, I came to understand are lacking. My fracture could not have had better care. The same can't be said about the person with the fracture. I have been guilty of this as a clinician. For me it's another back, another knee, another neck...for my patient it is a national emergency.

Elaine Saunders, UK

I am 53, I have a frozen shoulder. The pain was really bad, it is getting a bit better now, but I can't move my arm properly and it still really hurts. No one at home or work understood the pain I was in. For a few days they helped me. Then I felt at home they were getting frustrated at how slow I was, and that I wasn't able to do what I normally do round the house. At work I had a few comments like, "You haven't had surgery or a break, why can't you do your job?" I think they thought I was making a story up or being lazy. I've worked there for ages. They know that's not true.

Worse has been the night pain – it's agony, I'm exhausted and can't think straight. Worse still have been the [doctors] I've spoken with; everyone [has] given me a different thing to do to treat this – massage, exercises, injections, surgery, "just wait until it goes away" – doesn't anyone know what's best to take the pain away? Why did they go to school, didn't they learn anything? Can you imagine being told to just wait? It's like you have a broken leg and they don't help you, and someone says, "Just wait, we won't do anything, it will get better". Has no one ever had this problem and knows how painful it is? I wish they could have it for a day, then they would help me more.

Joletta Belton, USA

Joletta is a co-author of Chapter 11: Communicating with people experiencing shoulder pain. The powerful words that follow are hers. They do not relate to a shoulder problem, but they very easily could. Her words have frequently been expressed by people whose individual journey through the healthcare system seeking care for shoulder problems has involved multiple nonsurgical interventions, multiple injections, surgery, and revision surgery.

I felt as though my concerns were never addressed, that I was never really heard. The solution was always more strength, more stability, more exercise. But I was a firefighter when I got hurt. I was the strongest and fittest I'd ever been in my life. I worked out and ran most days of the week. Strength and stability were not my issues, yet they were the focus of much of my care.

Evolution of the human shoulder and upper limb function

2

Jeremy Lewis, Rod Whiteley

Introduction

Humans throw with incredible speed, accuracy, and power. During a baseball pitch the shoulder moves through an arc of 80° in 30 milliseconds: this results in the shoulder moving at approximately 9000°/second, generating ball speeds up to 170 km/hour (106 mph). High-speed throwing requires energy to be transferred from the lower limbs, as well as energy stored in the muscles and tendons that accelerate the humerus, especially pectoralis major,[26] to be rapidly released. Energy is stored in pectoralis major when it is stretched, such as the cocking position of throwing (shoulder abduction and horizontal extension, also known as horizontal abduction). Many sports such as tennis, cricket, volleyball, handball, and basketball involve similar actions. Javelin and shot-put as well as grandparents throwing frisbees or balls with their grandchildren also involve similar requirements, energy transfer from the lower limbs, and energy storage and release from shoulder muscles. The role of lower limb energy transfer is discussed in detail in Chapter 4, and the biomechanics and rehabilitation of throwing in Chapter 38. For now, the bigger questions are: why do modern humans (*Homo sapiens*) throw, and why do we throw with such power and accuracy?

Although the exact timeline and lineage are still being debated, the answer to the question of throwing lies in the fossil records. The original purpose of throwing was likely defense from predators. Throwing leaves, sticks and stones would provide defense from bigger, stronger, faster predators. Over time, throwing gave our ancestors not only a means of defense but also a method for predation that provided another evolutionary advantage: consumption of higher calorific food derived from meat, which resulted in stronger bones, bigger bodies, and larger brains.

Hitting a soccer ball-sized target from 15 meters (16.5 yards) requires an opposable thumb for such a precise motor skill, and a release timing accuracy in the order of 1/1600th of a second.[3]

While the shoulder generates the highest rotational angular velocity in the proximal kinetic chain, the thumb is integral to throwing by contributing to object stabilization, from cocking position to release, and directional precision of the projectile at release. A single neuron can't discharge with 1/1600th of a second accuracy, and neuronal pools combine to give greater precision. Increasing the neuronal pool to throw powerfully and precisely requires a bigger brain, specifically in an area above the lateral sulcus in the left hemisphere. Consumption of higher calorific food provided this.

Hemispheric symmetry implied that an evolutionary increase in the size of the left hemisphere allowed humans to develop other higher functions in the right hemisphere, including Broca's area – crucial for subsequent language development. Throwing not only predates language, it possibly facilitated the bigger brain capacity that language required. The association between enhanced throwing and higher cognition has been identified recently in chimpanzee populations.[8] Modern-day chimpanzees that throw more skillfully than their contemporaries demonstrate significantly better communication skills and have more white matter in the Broca's area homologue.[8] The hypothesis being that throwing and the concomitant increase in size of both hemispheres in the brain was the evolutionary step to enable higher levels of communication. The debate as to whether throwing drove the development of language, or if language was the driver for throwing, remains unresolved and controversial. However, the argument that language has a less immediate impact on survival, whereas throwing provides greater certainty in "the plain devoid of fruit but abundant with rabbits",[3] is compelling.

Homo sapiens and *Homo neanderthalensis* (Neanderthals) probably split from a common ancestor about 600,000 years ago[4] with both species moving from Africa into Europe. Not only did Neanderthals walk like us,[6] live sophisticated lives, produce art[11,28] and jewelry,[34] participate in burial rituals,[21] construct artifacts deep in caves, and make use of fire,[29] they were probably substantially stronger[7] than the *Homo sapiens* they inhabited the planet with. We co-existed (with some interbreeding[13]), for approximately 100,000 years, with recent suggestions that a long-fought war between the two groups ensued[18] as we competed for space and resources.

This begs the question: how could the weaker *Homo sapiens* have triumphed over these strong, sophisticated pack hunters? Skeletal remains suggest that Neanderthals fought large animals at a close proximity.[2] Hunting at a distance, a skill only humans (and archerfish) demonstrate, enhances survival and is undoubtedly safer than combat at close range.

Throwing was probably a decisive factor in the likely clashes between humans and Neanderthals. Our ability to throw probably lead to the extinction of the Neanderthals.

Fashioning available resources such as stones into cutting and hunting tools required our ancestors to have the necessary cognitive and manipulative skills. The tools would be crafted within the visual field and then used for a variety of purposes by the increasingly mobile upper limbs. Initially it was thought that *Homo habilis* (Latin for "handy" or "able person"), was the first of our ancestors to use tools around 2.3 to 2.4 million years ago. However, cut marks in animal bones that date around 1 million years earlier (3.39 million years ago) suggest earlier hominins such as *Australopithecus afarensis* may have started crafting simple hand tools. The most famous example of *Australopithecus* (southern ape) *afarensis* is affectionately nicknamed Lucy, and her fossil remains were found in the Afar region in Ethiopia in 1974. She is displayed at the National Museum of Ethiopia in Addis Ababa, and replicas of her skeleton are found in museums around the world. Lucy and her contemporaries possibly consumed a wide range of foods, including fruit, leaves and meat. The varied diet meant there was always something to eat. Lucy was capable of upright stance and bipedal gait but probably only for relatively short distances. Her ability to stand freed her upper limbs and started the journey to human throwing.

The development of bipedal posture and a versatile upper limb

Modern human bipedalism and the multifunctionality of the modern human upper limb has been the response to evolutionary demands. The replacement of the tropical rainforests in Africa with grassland savannah 4 million years ago may have provided *Australopithecus afarensis* an evolutionary stimulus to stand, to observe for predators, and throw for defense and possibly hunting. *Australopithecus afarensis* may have lived in one familiar habitat and this may have enhanced survival by decreasing infant mortality. Another advantage of an upper limb that wasn't required for locomotion would enable food, once found, to be carried back to the core locality.[19,20] Being able to carry would allow *Australopithecus afarensis* to range further for food. Standing upright and bipedal gait would also have reduced the need for hydration. Being upright would reduce thermal stress by exposing a smaller surface area of the body to the sun and this possibly reduced daily water requirements from 2.5 to 1.5 liters, with an associated benefit of being able to range further for food.[31] This enabled migration from the fruit-filled shade of the jungle through the savannah by a combination of reduced hydration requirements, and being able to throw and prey on grazing animals.[3]

Advanced manipulative skills have been critical for the evolutionary success of *Homo sapiens*. Although the first recognizable tools, such as stones for cutting and hunting may date back more than 3 million years, use of advanced tools appeared much later.[10] This further supports the argument that the evolutionary development of an upper limb not essential for weight bearing was initially functional for throwing (for protection on the grassland savannah and predation) and carrying (food transport). The ability to throw with high speed dates back approximately 2 million years.[24] Another potential form of protection afforded by two "freed" hands may have been the ability to bang rocks together to frighten predators. This behavior is used today by black-striped (bearded) capuchin monkeys (*Sapajus libidinosus*).[22] These monkeys appear to be the first non-ape primates to use rocks as tools for cracking nuts. They are capable of bipedal gait for short distances which also enables them to use their upper limbs for carrying fruit and stones.[22]

Why homo sapiens can throw and manipulate tools, and chimpanzees can climb

Clearly *Homo sapiens* (modern humans) can climb and throw, as can chimpanzees (*Pan troglodytes*), but each species has evolved biomechanical attributes that favor the superiority of one of these functions over the other. This section presents the biomechanical differences between modern humans and other primates, and then discusses how the differences relate to function.

Anatomical variations and the impact on function

Modern humans exhibit both similarities and differences to our evolutionary ancestors, and to modern-day primates. Humans and chimpanzees can throw and both can climb, but clearly each species excels at one function to a greater extent than the other. Chimpanzees are evolutionarily the species closest to modern humans. They use leaves, twigs and sticks to forage for food, and they have been observed to use stones as hammers and anvils to crack open nuts.[14] Chimpanzees have been documented throwing stones and sticks in aggressive acts and possibly for rituals and communication.[14] Despite their strength, chimpanzees don't throw to hunt or defend. They demonstrate throwing speeds similar to 5-year-old human children of approximately 30 km/hour (20 miles/hour). From a distance of less than 2 meters (6.6 feet), wild chimpanzees have been reported to hit a target on only 5 attempts from 44 throws.[5]

The first rib of early hominoids articulated with the seventh cervical and first thoracic vertebra, whereas the hominid *Australopithecus afarensis* demonstrated an articulation between the first rib and first thoracic vertebra. The single vertebral articulation was an important evolutionary step towards throwing, as it allowed the upper limb to be freed from the constraints of quadrupedal locomotion.[23] Modern humans have evolved a barrel shaped chest; *Australopithecus afarensis*, like modern-day chimpanzees, had a more conical (triangular) shaped chest, and being conical the scapula is placed in an upwardly rotated position on the thorax (Figure 2.1). The scapula of *Australopithecus afarensis* appears to be more like modern apes than modern humans – in addition to the upwardly rotated scapular placement, the glenoid fossa faces more superiorly than modern humans (Figure 2.2). As the glenoid fossa provides a base of support to the humeral head, the upwardly rotated scapula and the superiorly facing glenoid fossa are perfectly designed for climbing and brachiating (arboreal locomotion), and less well designed for throwing and manipulating tools inside the visual field.[9,17,30]

Human evolution has resulted in a larger infrascapular fossa, and a suprascapular fossa that has remained static in size. This has resulted in larger infraspinatus and teres minor, allowing these muscles to work more effectively as external rotators and humeral head depressors.[27] The clavicle has elongated, and the coracoid and acromial processes have enlarged. The deltoid has concomitantly enlarged with the larger acromion and its insertion has migrated more distally. This may have resulted in two beneficial attributes for throwers: the first by allowing the arm to work as a more efficient third-class lever system during abduction, with the second occurring when the glenohumeral joint is positioned to throw. Contraction of the deltoid would facilitate compression of the humerus into the glenoid fossa, facilitating glenohumeral stabilization while the pectoralis major and latissimus dorsi accelerates the humerus, aided by the rotator cuff. After the object has left the hand, the larger posterior rotator cuff muscles can then work eccentrically to slow the humerus.[1,17]

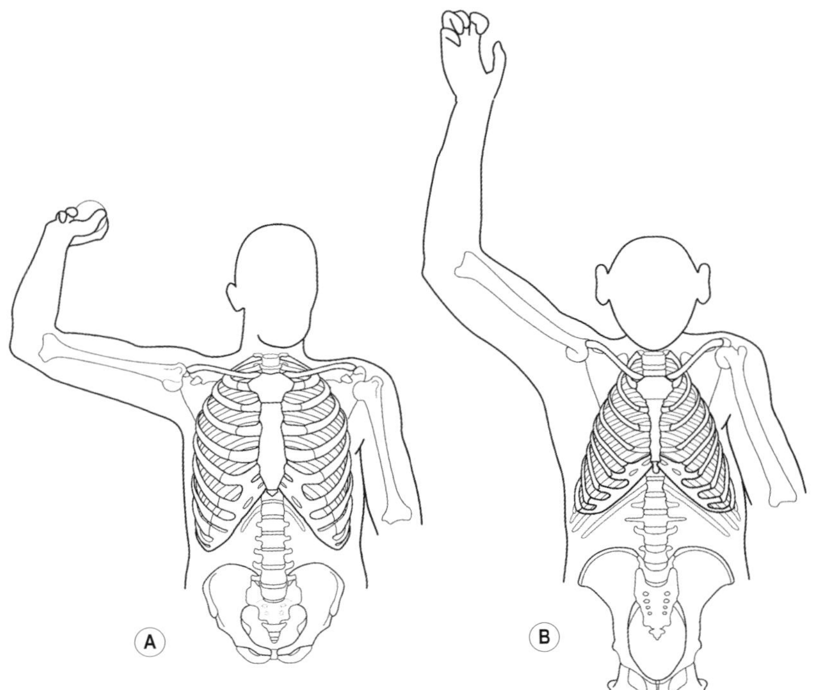

FIGURE 2.1

Comparison between *Homo sapiens* (modern human) and *Pan troglodytes* (chimpanzee) thorax, scapular position, and upper limb function. The *Pan* scapula (right) sits in a more upwardly rotated position because of the conically shaped rib cage. This is ideal for climbing and arboreal locomotion (brachiating). The scapula is less upwardly rotated in modern humans (left) due to the more barrel shaped thorax which places the glenohumeral joint in an ideal position for high-speed throwing and manipulating tools within the visual field.

(Illustrations © Vicky Earle, Medical Illustrator.)

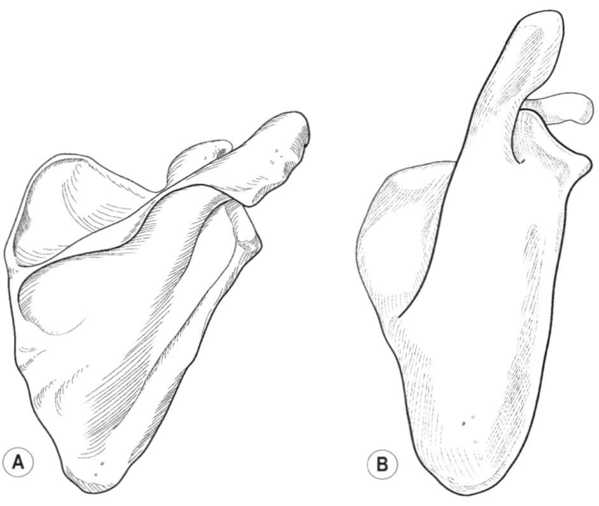

FIGURE 2.2

Comparison between modern human and chimpanzee scapular and acromial shape and glenoid fossa orientation. The scapula is broader in *Homo sapiens* (modern human, left) than *Pan troglodytes* (chimpanzee, right). The evolutionary enlargement of the intrascapular fossa in *Homo* has allowed for a concomitant enlargement in infraspinatus and teres minor, which have evolved as large and powerful muscles. Acromial shape in *Pan* permits sustained upper limb elevation and arboreal locomotion (brachiation). In *Homo* the glenoid fossa faces laterally. This is ideal for powerful throwing and positioning the hands in the visual field to use and manipulate tools. The orientation of the glenoid fossa in *Pan* is superior. This provides an excellent base of support for the humeral head when the upper limb is used in an elevated position.

(Illustrations © Vicky Earle, Medical Illustrator.)

The humeral head has enlarged and become more globular, permitting more mobility. Medial torsion of the humeral head, as detailed in Figure 2.3, is the axis made by the head of the humerus and the mediolateral axis of the elbow.[15] The torsion has enabled the humeral head to maintain contact with the glenoid fossa during extremes of shoulder external rotation required for powerful throwing.[32,33] Torsion has also enabled the elbow to flex and extend in the sagittal and not frontal plane for the purposes of manipulating tools in the visual field.[15] Crucially for throwing, humeral torsion permits a greater absolute range of shoulder external rotation and is associated with enhanced throwing velocity.[25] To forcefully throw (long distances, high speeds), the release trajectory needs to be above horizontal. In powerful throwing, this happens by accelerating from stationary at the point of maximal external rotation up to the point of release (maximum velocity).

In skilled baseball pitchers, the shoulder moves from approximately 175° of shoulder external rotation (late cocking) to release at approximately 90° of external rotation. The 90° of rotation occurring from late cocking to ball release takes approximately 30 to 60 milliseconds, with a concomitant shoulder velocity of approximately 7000–9000°/second. Although rare, ball speeds approaching 170km/h (106 mph) have been recorded, implying the ball reaches home plate in under 400 milliseconds, around the same speed it takes for the eyes to blink. The longest baseball throw is reported to be 136 meters (almost 446 feet), and the farthest recorded unaided throw is 427.2 meters (1401.5 feet) with a boomerang in Australia.

Chimpanzees can't throw hard enough to kill, or probably even injure. Human history provides evidence of the effectiveness of throwing. In the Middle Ages, the crossbow was possibly the equivalent to today's cruise missiles. In 1139, Pope Innocent II condemned it as "deathly and hateful to God and unfit to be used among Christians." Nonetheless it proved no match for the Guanches of the Canary Islands, as they hurled stones to break shields and the arms holding them. In the 15th century CE, Canary Islanders repelled a Portuguese landing party by throwing stones that felt like "a bolt from a crossbow". In the 18th and 19th centuries, Australian aboriginals "cut to pieces by a shower of stones, picked up and hurled with a force and precision that must be seen to be believed" colonial invaders armed with rifles, muskets, and swords (https://www.abc.net.au/radionational/programs/ockhamsrazor/throwing-and-human-evolution/5759974).

Similarly to modern apes, *Australopithecus afarensis* demonstrated forearm and hindlimb bone lengths and muscle masses in reverse proportions to humans. A significant evolutionary change in modern humans has been the shortening of the forearms. This evolutionary adaption has permitted greater dexterity enabling tools to be manipulated in the visual field. It has also resulted in better control and precision when throwing.[17] The sacrifice has been a loss of sustained and powerful overhead activities – brachiating and climbing. In contrast, orangutans weighing up to 90 kg (198 lb) spend 80% of their time in trees, have arms that are 50% longer than their legs,

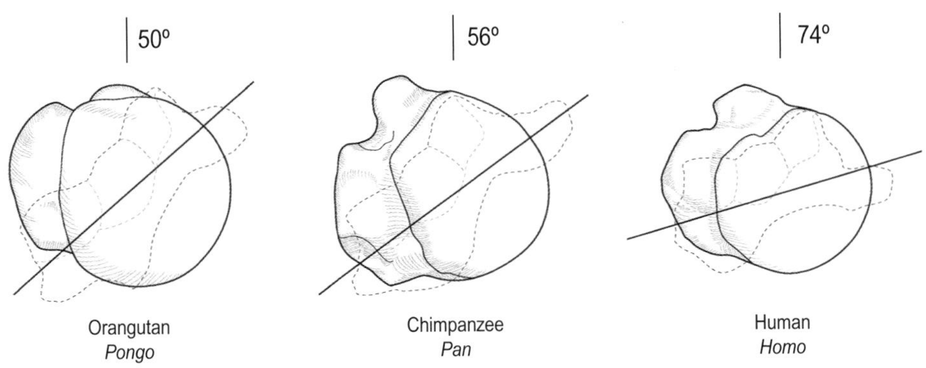

FIGURE 2.3

Illustration of the average amount of humeral torsion across orangutan (*Pongo* spp.), chimpanzee (*Pan troglodytes*), and modern human (*Homo sapiens*). In each image the proximal end of the humerus is "standardized" by placing the long axis of the proximal epiphysis horizontally, i.e., the glenohumeral joint is in the same position in all three images. The amount of twist along the long axis of the humerus is then measured by the angle that the distal epicondylar axis (dashed outline) makes. For the humerus on the right, with the glenohumeral joint in the same position, the human will apparently have 74° of shoulder external rotation, whereas the orangutan will have 50°. The "extra" 24° of external rotation is the difference in the amount of twist along the long axis of the humerus. The additional humeral torsion in humans permits a greater absolute range of shoulder external rotation and is essential for high speed throwing.

(Image adapted from Krahl.[12] Illustrations © Vicky Earle, Medical Illustrator.)

more triangular shaped thoraxes, and upwardly rotated scapulae – perfect adaptions for brachiating, hanging, and arboreal living. Another adaption for arboreal locomotion exhibited by chimpanzees is an upward flare on the lateral end of the clavicle. This upward flare is not observed in *Homo sapiens*; further evidence for a shoulder primarily evolved for throwing and manipulating tools, rather than for prolonged overhead activities.

Conclusion

Having a scapula positioned on the posterior chest wall and a lateral facing glenoid fossa, a lateral facing acromion, rotator cuff muscles and tendon that merge with the strong fibrous capsule, a relatively small suprascapular fossa, and a relatively flat clavicle without an upward flare on the lateral border implies that modern humans are born to throw, and manipulate tools within the visual field. The anatomy suggests that prolonged activities in elevation, such as climbing and brachiating as expertly demonstrated by chimpanzees and orangutans, are less well suited to modern day humans. This is supported by research that has demonstrated that prolonged activities in elevation are a risk factor for developing shoulder pain in humans.[16]

Evolution has endowed modern humans with a shoulder with an extensive range of movement, that, when combined with elbow movement, enables the hand to perform myriad functions. Although the human shoulder girdle is capable of impressive ranges of movement, commonplace in many sporting and vocational pursuits, there are many features that suggest the modern human shoulder is less well adapted for use in an elevated position. This is supported by the origin and insertion and functional capability of pectoralis major, which is perfectly adapted for energy storage and release at around 90° of shoulder abduction.[26]

The evolutionary success of the genus *Homo sapiens* has been the development of an upper limb not essential for perpetual weight bearing. A stable and mobile scapula providing a base of support for the humeral head has permitted powerful and accurate throwing and manipulation of tools within the visual field. Throwing was essential for protection and hunting, and carrying was necessary to transport food; the use of the freed upper limbs for the manipulation of advanced tools came much later in our evolutionary development. The modern human shoulder permits participation in an unparallel array of sporting, cultural and vocational activities, many of which will be explored throughout the chapters of this textbook.

References

1. Ashton EH, Oxnard CE. Functional adaptions in the primate shoulder girdle. Proceedings of the Zoological Society of London. 1964;142:49-66.
2. Berger TD, Trinkaus E. Patterns of trauma among the Neandertals. Journal of Archaeological Science. 1995;22:841-852.
3. Calvin WH. The Throwing Madonna: Essays on The Brain. New York: McGraw-Hill; 1983.
4. Chan EKF, Timmermann A, Baldi BF, et al. Human origins in a southern African palaeo-wetland and first migrations. Nature. 2019;575:185-189.
5. Darlington PJ, Jr. Group selection, altruism, reinforcement, and throwing in human evolution. Proc Natl Acad Sci U S A. 1975;72:3748-3752.
6. Haeusler M, Trinkaus E, Fornai C, et al. Morphology, pathology, and the vertebral posture of the La Chapelle-aux-Saints Neandertal. Proc Natl Acad Sci U S A. 2019;116:4923-4927.
7. Helmuth H. Body height, body mass and surface area of the Neanderthals. Z Morphol Anthropol. 1998;82:1-12.
8. Hopkins WD, Russell JL, Schaeffer JA. The neural and cognitive correlates of aimed throwing in chimpanzees: a magnetic resonance image and behavioural study on a unique form of social tool use. Philos Trans R Soc Lond B Biol Sci. 2012;367:37-47.
9. Hunt KD. The evolution of human bipedality: ecology and functional morphology. Journal of Human Evolution. 1994;26:183-202.
10. Isaac G, Leakey REF. Human Ancestors: Readings from “Scientific American.” San Francisco: Freeman; 1979.
11. Jaubert J, Verheyden S, Genty D, et al. Early Neanderthal constructions deep in Bruniquel Cave in southwestern France. Nature. 2016;534:111-114.
12. Krahl VE. The torsion of the humerus: its localization, cause and duration in man. Am J Anat. 1947;80:275-319.
13. Krings M, Stone A, Schmitz RW, Krainitzki H, Stoneking M, Paabo S. Neandertal DNA sequences and the origin of modern humans. Cell. 1997;90:19-30.
14. Kuhl HS, Kalan AK, Arandjelovic M, et al. Chimpanzee accumulative stone throwing. Sci Rep. 2016;6:22219.
15. Larson SG. Subscapularis function in gibbons and chimpanzees: implications for interpretation of humeral head torsion in hominoids. Am J Phys Anthropol. 1988;76:449-462.
16. Leong HT, Fu SC, He X, Oh JH, Yamamoto N, Hang S. Risk factors for rotator cuff tendinopathy: a systematic review and meta-analysis. J Rehabil Med. 2019;51:627-637.
17. Lewis J, Green A, Yizhat Z, Pennington D. Subacromial impingement syndrome: has evolution failed us? Physiotherapy. 2001;87:191-198.
18. Longrich NR. Were other humans the first victims of the sixth mass extinction? 2019. Available at: https://phys.org/news/2019-11-humans-victims-sixth-mass-extinction.html.
19. Lovejoy CO. Evolution of human walking. Sci Am. 1988;259:118-125.
20. Lovejoy CO. The origin of man. Science. 1981;211:341-350.
21. Maureille B, Vandermeersch B. Les sépultures néandertaliennes. In: Vandermeersch B, Maureille B, eds. Les Néandertaliens, Biologie et Cultures. Comité des travaux historiques et scientifiques (CTHS), Paris; 2007:311-322.
22. Moura AC. Stone banging by wild capuchin monkeys: an unusual auditory display. Folia Primatol (Basel). 2007;78:36-45.
23. Ohman JC. The first rib of hominoids. Am J Phys Anthropol. 1986;70:209-229.
24. Roach KE, Budiman-Mak E, Songsiridej N, Lertratanakul Y. Development of a shoulder pain and disability index. Arthritis Care Res. 1991;4:143-149.
25. Roach NT, Lieberman DE, Gill TJ, 4th, Palmer WE, Gill TJ, 3rd. The effect of humeral torsion on rotational range of motion in the shoulder and throwing performance. J Anat. 2012;220:293-301.
26. Roach NT, Venkadesan M, Rainbow MJ, Lieberman DE. Elastic energy storage in the shoulder and the evolution of high-speed throwing in Homo. Nature. 2013;498:483-486.
27. Roberts D. Structure and Function of the Primate Scapula. New York: Academic Press; 1974.
28. Rodríguez-Vidal J, d’Errico F, Pacheco FG, et al. A rock engraving made by Neanderthals in Gibraltar. Proceedings of the National Academy of Sciences. 2014;111:13301-13306.
29. Roebroeks W, Villa P. On the earliest evidence for habitual use of fire in Europe. Proceedings of the National Academy of Sciences. 2011;108:5209-5214.
30. Stern JT, Jr., Susman RL. The locomotor anatomy of Australopithecus afarensis. Am J Phys Anthropol. 1983;60:279-317.
31. Wheeler PE. The influence of stature and body form on hominid energy and water budgets; a comparison of Australopithecus and early Homo physiques. J Hum Evol. 1993;24:13-28.
32. Whiteley R, Adams R, Ginn K, Nicholson L. Playing level achieved, throwing history, and humeral torsion in Masters baseball players. J Sports Sci. 2010;28:1223-1232.
33. Yamamoto N, Itoi E, Minagawa H, et al. Why is the humeral retroversion of throwing athletes greater in dominant shoulders than in nondominant shoulders? J Shoulder Elbow Surg. 2006;15:571-575.
34. Zilhão J, Angelucci DE, Badal-García E, et al. Symbolic use of marine shells and mineral pigments by Iberian Neandertals. Proceedings of the National Academy of Sciences. 2010;107:1023-1028.

The burden of shoulder pain and disability

3

Danielle van der Windt, Jonathan Lucas, Eric Hegedus, Jeremy Lewis

Introduction

Shoulder pain and associated disability is common, and a frequent reason for consultation in primary care and referral for specialist care. The pain and disability associated with musculoskeletal shoulder conditions often has a detrimental impact on individuals and their families, affecting sleep, social interaction, daily functioning, and the ability to work. It also places a substantial burden on healthcare systems and providers. In a random sample of 540 adults living in New Zealand, Taylor[58] reported that shoulder pain was the most common musculoskeletal problem for participants over the age of 65. They reported that for some people, the experience of musculoskeletal pain was associated with impaired quality of life that was comparable to people living with complicated diabetes mellitus, chronic liver disease requiring transplantation, and terminal cancer, demonstrating the impact of shoulder pain in people's lives. The purpose of this chapter is to synthesize the current literature to better understand the burden of shoulder pain and disability.

Defining shoulder pain and disability

An individual's experience of shoulder pain may range from short-term episodes with limited impact on daily life, to persistent symptoms associated with concomitant physical and psychological features and high levels of disability. The definition of "shoulder pain" used in epidemiological research has varied in terms of: 1) the anatomical description of the shoulder region; 2) the assumed pathoanatomical cause of the pain; and 3) specification of the severity, duration or impact of shoulder pain. Additionally, patient perception of the source of symptoms may differ, due to the varied, often changing, and nonspecific locations at which the symptoms are felt. In short, there are different ways to define and classify shoulder pain (referred to as *case definition*), and a wide range of definitions have been used across research studies.

Pope et al[49] demonstrated how different definitions can result in different estimates of the prevalence and burden of shoulder pain in the community. In a community-based survey, they used various questions and body diagrams to ask respondents about the presence of shoulder pain and disability. The use of these different ways of defining shoulder pain resulted in widely varying estimates (between 20% and 51%) of the prevalence of (disabling) shoulder pain. It will, therefore, be important to agree on a definition of shoulder pain for epidemiological research, similar to what has been proposed for low back pain.[16]

In order to more fully appreciate the impact of shoulder pain on the individual and society, the definition needs to be clarified through use of relevant dimensions (duration, location, type of pain); estimations of physical and psychological impact on the individual; and appreciation of the impact on society and healthcare. Acknowledging the absence of an agreed-upon case definition, we aim to offer a summary of the burden and impact of painful shoulder conditions in the community and primary care, as reported by survey participants or recorded by primary care professionals during routine consultations. We further aim to summarize the quality and magnitude of evidence for the burden of shoulder pain across the globe, highlighting areas of concern and gaps in our knowledge.

The Global Burden of Disease

The Global Burden of Disease (GBD) Study has been the most comprehensive collaboration to date to estimate summary measures of global population health, generating repeated measures of the prevalence and impact of a wide range of health conditions (291 diseases and injuries) in 195 countries and territories from 1990 to 2017.[7,52] The latest iteration of the GBD Study estimated there were globally 1.3 billion people with current musculoskeletal disorders (95% uncertainty interval 1.2 to 1.4) and more than 120,000 deaths due to these conditions in 2017. The prevalence rate of musculoskeletal disorders was higher in females and increased with age in both sexes. The prevalence was greatest for low back pain (36.8%) followed by "other musculoskeletal disorders" (21.5%), osteoarthritis (19.3%), neck pain (18.4%), gout (2.6%) and rheumatoid arthritis (1.3%).[52]

The results of the GBD study have been instrumental to demonstrate the impact of musculoskeletal conditions globally, especially for low back pain which was identified as the greatest contributor to disability worldwide, contributing more than 10% of total years lost due to disability.[7,66] Prevalence and burden of musculoskeletal conditions in terms of years lived with disability is greatest in high income countries (Western Europe, North America), but shows a faster increase in eastern Mediterranean countries[44] and in eastern and western sub-Saharan countries[66] compared with the rest of the world.

Shoulder pain is generally considered the third most common musculoskeletal pain condition after low back pain and osteoarthritis, but its prevalence and burden are not yet specifically reported in the GBD study. Included as part of "other musculoskeletal conditions", disability adjusted life years increased from an estimated 20.6 million in 1990 to 30.9 million in 2010.[57] Reliable estimates of the global burden of shoulder pain would require a similar process as was undertaken for low back pain in 2010, with the involvement of an expert group to develop valid case definitions, functional health states, and disability weights that adequately reflect the impact of shoulder pain in people and society. For low back pain, a series of comprehensive systematic reviews were undertaken to obtain data to derive the burden estimates, which highlighted a lack of data from many regions in the world, wide heterogeneity between included studies, and lack of information on the impact of pain on broader aspects of life, such as social participation and well-being.[28] We expect that very similar, and much wider, gaps in evidence are present for shoulder pain.

Incidence and prevalence of shoulder pain and disability

For this chapter, we reviewed studies reporting on the epidemiology of shoulder pain in the community or primary care. We included observational studies reporting on the incidence or prevalence of shoulder pain in a sample of at least 100 people. We selected studies using a case definition that focused on the shoulder, excluding studies investigating neck–upper limb pain.

Characteristics and results of the 30 studies included in this scoping review are summarized in Table 3.1. Fourteen studies were conducted in Europe; 9 in Asia; 3 in Australia; 2 in the Middle East/North Africa; and 2 in South America. Apart from 5 studies investigating the epidemiology of shoulder pain in primary care, all studies were community-based cross-sectional surveys. Case definitions varied, focusing on shoulder pain only or also including stiffness or swelling, as did definitions of incidence or prevalence period, which ranged from point prevalence (5 studies) to life-time prevalence (1 study). Eleven studies were conducted as part of a project funded by the World Health Organization (WHO-ILAR), using similar methods to investigate the burden of musculoskeletal conditions in the community across several countries. In the Community Oriented Program for Control of Rheumatic Diseases (COPCORD) studies, shoulder pain was defined as pain, stiffness or swelling of the shoulder in the past 7 days. Most studies (21 out of 30) used face to face questionnaires or telephone interviews to collect data on shoulder pain; 5 used postal questionnaires, and 4 extracted information from primary care records.

Community-based studies

Estimates of prevalence or incidence of shoulder pain were extracted or estimated from each study along with 95% confidence interval.[27] In the 15 studies that reported on current shoulder pain or pain in the past 7 days, prevalence estimates ranged between 2.5% and 37.6%. Estimates from 9 studies using longer prevalence periods (1 month to 1 year) ranged between 15.9% and 55.2%. The forest plot in Figure 3.1 presents estimates of the prevalence of shoulder pain for men and women separately, generally showing higher prevalence rates in women, consistent with other musculoskeletal pain conditions, with differences up to 15%. The heat map (Figure 3.2) highlights the absence of evidence for the prevalence of shoulder pain for many geographical regions but shows higher prevalence rates in Western European countries, reflecting findings for low back pain and musculoskeletal disorders more broadly from the GBD study. Only one study, conducted in Kuwait, investigated the incidence of shoulder pain in the community by contacting participants by telephone every two weeks, estimating the cumulative incidence of new pain, stiffness or swelling in the shoulder at 11.4 per 1000 over the course of a year.[1]

Primary care

Studies investigating the incidence or prevalence of shoulder pain in primary care were all conducted in the United Kingdom or the Netherlands, and reported lower estimates, reflecting that most people with shoulder pain will not seek healthcare for their shoulder pain. Estimates of the incidence of shoulder pain in primary care varied between 11.2

Table 3.1 Summary of design and results of studies reporting on the prevalence and/or incidence of shoulder pain in the community or primary care

Study	Country	Sample size (at risk population)	Ascertainment method	Case definition	Prevalence or incidence	Prevalence or incidence estimate (95% CI)
Community-based studies						
Vindigni et al[64]	Australia (Aboriginal)	189	Face-to-face questionnaire	Shoulder pain, ache or discomfort	Point prevalence	9.52% (5.34–13.71)
Chard et al[9]	United Kingdom	644	Face-to-face questionnaire	Current pain in shoulder	Point prevalence	26.4% (22.99–29.80)
van Schaardenburg et al[62]	Netherlands	105	Face-to-face questionnaire and physical examination	Current pain in shoulder	Point prevalence	25.71% (17.35–34.07)
Picavet et al[48]	Netherlands	3664	Postal questionnaire	Shoulder pain	Point prevalence	20.91% (19.6–22.2)
Ihlebaek et al[29]	Norway	1240	Postal questionnaire	Shoulder pain	Point prevalence	37.58% (34.88–40.28)
Davatchi et al[15]	Iran	19786	Face-to-face questionnaire	Pain, stiffness or swelling in shoulder	7 days prevalence	15.6% (15.1–16.1)
Sandoughi et al[53]	Iran	2100	Face-to-face questionnaire	Pain, stiffness or swelling in shoulder	7 days prevalence	22.26% (20.48–24.04)
Chaaya et al[8]	Lebanon	3530	Face-to-face questionnaire	Pain, stiffness or swelling in shoulder	7 days prevalence	14.31% (13.1–15.5)
Joshi et al[31]	India	8145	Face-to-face questionnaire	Pain, stiffness or swelling in shoulder	7 days prevalence	2.49% (2.21–2.91)
Davatchi et al[14]	Iran	10291	Face-to-face questionnaire	Pain, stiffness or swelling in shoulder	7 days prevalence	14.5% (13.5–15.6)
Haq et al[23]	Bangladesh	5211	Face-to-face questionnaire	Pain, stiffness or swelling in shoulder	7 days prevalence	9.88% (8.73–11.04)
Dai et al[12]	China	6584	Face-to-face questionnaire	Any pain, tenderness, swelling, or stiffness in any bone, joint or muscle in the shoulder	7 days prevalence	7.0% (6.4–7.6)
Minaur et al[43]	Australia (Aboriginal)	847	Face-to-face questionnaire	Any pain, tenderness, swelling, or stiffness in any bone, joint or muscle in the shoulder	7 days prevalence	8.85% (6.94–10.77)
Granados et al[20]	Venezuela	3973	Face-to-face questionnaire	Pain, stiffness or swelling in shoulder	7 days prevalence	6.02% (5.2–6.8)
Davatchi et al[13]	Iran	1565	Telephone and self-report questionnaire	Pain, stiffness or swelling in shoulder	7 days prevalence	22.68% (19.0–26.4)
Bingefors et al[5]	Sweden	4506	Postal questionnaire	Shoulder pain assessed by self-report in 2 weeks prior to questionnaire	14 days prevalence	20.99% (19.81–22.18)
Pope et al[49]	United Kingdom	232 312	Face-to-face interview	Shoulder pain	1-month prevalence	44.83% (38.0–51.0)

(Continued)

Table 3.1 *(Continued)*

Study	Country	Sample size (at risk population)	Ascertainment method	Case definition	Prevalence or incidence	Prevalence or incidence estimate (95% CI)
			Postal questionnaire	Shoulder pain	1-month prevalence	34.29% (29.0–40.0)
Ben Ayed et al 2019[3]	Tunisia	1221	Face-to-face questionnaire	Ache, pain, discomfort, numbness in shoulder	1-month prevalence	43% (39.07–46.92)
Urwin et al[59]	United Kingdom	5752	Postal questionnaire	Shoulder pain	1-month prevalence	15.99% (15.05–16.94)
Choi et al[11]	Republic of Korea	1576	Face-to-face questionnaire	Pain caused by activities of daily living including work activities that continued for over a week in the previous year or at least once every month at a severe or extremely severe level	1-year prevalence	16.88% (15.03–18.73)
Meroni et al[42]	Italy	302	Face-to-face questionnaire	Ache, pain, discomfort, numbness in shoulder	1-year prevalence	25.5% (20.58–30.41)
Bento et al[4]	Brazil	600	Face-to-face questionnaire	Pain located at a restricted area in or around the shoulder complex	1-year prevalence	24% (20.3–27.5)
Engebretsen et al[18]	Norway	2722	Postal questionnaire (1990)	Localized shoulder pain – excluded pain in nearby regions	1-year prevalence	46.73% (44.9–48.6)
		2890	(1994)		1-year prevalence	48.65% (46.8–50.2)
		3325	(2004)		1-year prevalence	55.22% (53.5–56.9)
Hill et al[26]	Australia	3488	Face-to-face questionnaire and interviews	Ever had pain or aching in the shoulder at rest or when moving, on most days for at least a month and ever had stiffness in the shoulder when getting out of bed in the morning on most days for at least a month	Lifetime prevalence	18.41% (14.48–22.33)
Al-Awadhi et al[1]	Kuwait	3341	Telephone questionnaire (every two weeks)	Pain, stiffness or swelling in the shoulder	1-year cumulative incidence	11.4 per 1000 per year (0.79–1.49)
Primary care studies						
Van der Windt et al[60]	Netherlands	35150	GPs recorded cases during consultation (face-to-face)	Consultation for shoulder complaints as recorded by GP	1-year cumulative incidence	11.2 per 1000 per year (10.1–12.3)

(Continued)

Table 3.1 ***(Continued)***

Study	Country	Sample size (at risk population)	Ascertainment method	Case definition	Prevalence or incidence	Prevalence or incidence estimate (95% CI)
Bot et al[6]	Netherlands	375899	Primary care electronic health records	Coded primary care consultations for shoulder symptoms or conditions (ICPC codes)	1-year incidence rate	11.6 per 1000 person-years (11.2–11.9)
Linsell et al[39]	United Kingdom	658469	Primary care electronic health records	Coded primary care consultations for shoulder pain or shoulder conditions (Read codes)	1-year prevalence Cumulative incidence	2.36% (2.32–2.40) 14.7 per 1000 per year (14.4–15.0)
Jordan et al[30]	United Kingdom	100758	Primary care electronic health records	Coded primary care consultations for shoulder pain or shoulder conditions (Read codes)	1-year prevalence	19.9 per 1000 per year (19.1–20.7)
Greving et al[21]	Netherlands	Average annual population: 30000	Primary care electronic health records, average follow-up 4.3 years	Coded primary care consultations for shoulder symptoms or conditions (ICPC codes)	1-year prevalence Incidence rate	41.2 to 48.4 per 1000 person-years 29.3 per 1000 person-years (28.48–30.04)

and 29.3 per 1000 per year, indicating between 1% and 3% of adults consult their primary care doctor (GP) for shoulder pain over the course of a year.

It is important to note the sources of bias in the studies from which prevalence and incidence data were extracted. Risk of bias in each study was assessed using the checklist for prevalence studies developed by Hoy et al.[28] Figure 3.3 shows that the main limitation of studies was the fact that the target population was often not representative of the national population, meaning those who were eligible and invited to the study were different from their national peers. For example, many studies were conducted in a single city, or in a specific subgroup of the population such as women or older people only. Interpretation of the results is further complicated by variability between studies in the prevalence period, which ranged from current pain to lifetime prevalence, with most studies asking participants retrospectively about their experience of shoulder pain. The ascertainment method generally was a musculoskeletal pain questionnaire, either sent by post or used as part of an interview, and in some studies followed by a clinical assessment, with results likely to vary in terms of response rates and outcomes.

The case definition was generally considered to be acceptable, but was not uniform across the included studies, ranging from a simple question, "Did you have pain in your shoulder during the past 12 months?",[48] to more specific case definitions, such as used by Hill et al[26]: "ever had pain or aching in their shoulder at rest or when moving, on most days for at least a month and if they had ever had stiffness in their shoulder when getting out of bed in the morning on most days for at least a month"; or Choi et al[11]: "pain caused by activities of daily living including work activities that continued for over a week in the previous year or at least once every month at a severe or extremely severe level according to the National Institute for Occupational Safety and Health (NIOSH) criteria." Finally, the results of studies using primary care consultation records[6,21,30,39] depend on the likelihood of patients to consult for their painful shoulder and the quality of primary care coding.

The bottom line is that evidence regarding the burden of shoulder pain appears to be lacking from many geographical regions, including Africa, Eastern Europe, Asia, and America. There are substantial gaps in our knowledge in terms of the global population prevalence and incidence of shoulder pain, and our understanding of sources of

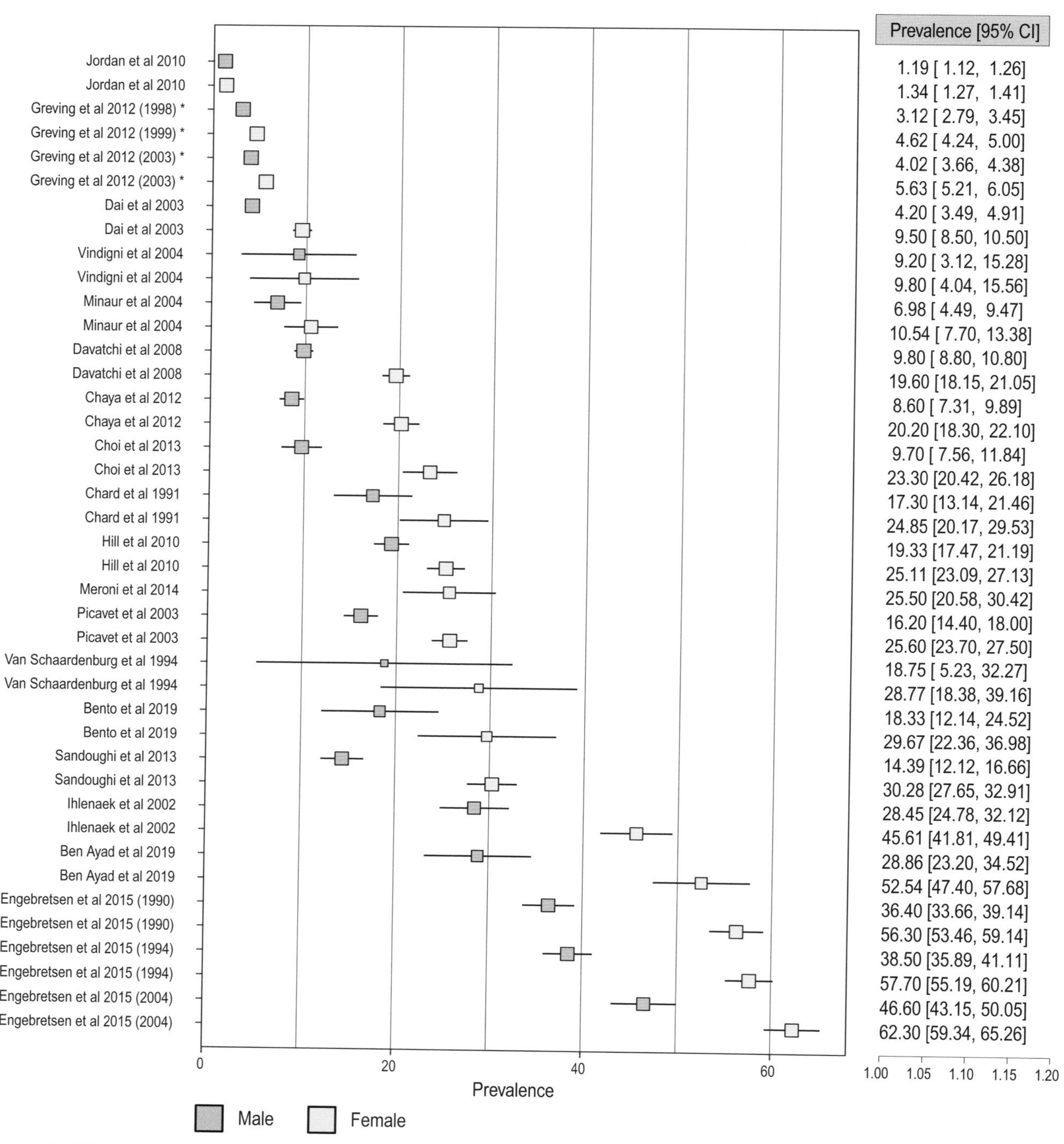

FIGURE 3.1

Forest plot presenting estimates for men and women of the prevalence of shoulder pain in community settings and two primary care studies.[21,30] CI, confidence interval.

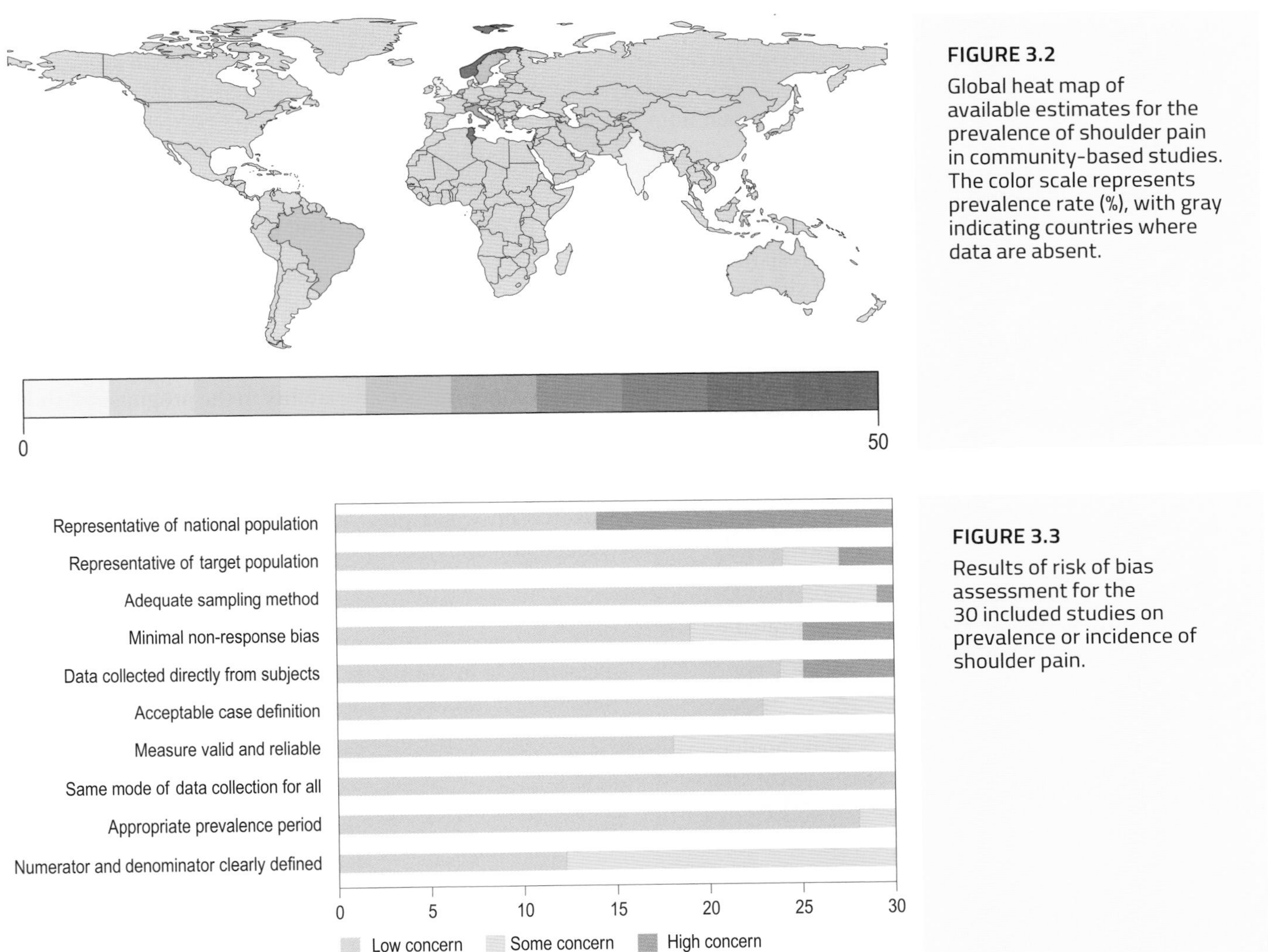

FIGURE 3.2

Global heat map of available estimates for the prevalence of shoulder pain in community-based studies. The color scale represents prevalence rate (%), with gray indicating countries where data are absent.

FIGURE 3.3

Results of risk of bias assessment for the 30 included studies on prevalence or incidence of shoulder pain.

variability such as deprivation, urban versus rural communities, ethnicity, or access to care. Regardless, the evidence shows that a substantial proportion of adults, estimated between 15% and 50%, experience an episode of shoulder pain over the course of a year, which may affect their ability to work, lead to loss of productivity, and healthcare costs.

Economic burden of shoulder pain and disability

Despite the varying case definitions and estimates of prevalence, we know that many people will be afflicted with musculoskeletal-related shoulder pain in their lifetime. What is lacking is an estimate of the economic burden associated with shoulder pain. Finding and synthesizing data on the healthcare costs and productivity loss due to shoulder pain is difficult for many reasons. Estimates of economic burden vary significantly based on countries and their individual healthcare systems; providers and their approach to care (imaging, surgery, physiotherapy, medication, time off work); employers and their compensation system; and patients and their individuality with regard to biopsychosocial factors. In addition, economic burden may be viewed through different lenses: work-related costs, healthcare utilization, or cost of illness. Despite this complexity, the universal truths seem to be that: 1) a minority of patients with persisting symptoms require a majority of the resources; 2) we are not yet clearly able to identify these people early in their episode of shoulder pain; and 3) estimates of the costs of shoulder pain are especially high when the costs related to time off work and decreased productivity at work are taken into account.[35,41,47,65] What follows is a compendium of available evidence.

One of the oft-cited studies of the economic burden of shoulder pain[35] found, in the Netherlands, that 12% of the people experiencing shoulder pain were responsible for 74% of the total costs, mostly as a result of sick leave from paid work. Annual costs of shoulder pain were estimated to be €345 million (US $410 million) per year in primary healthcare in the Netherlands (using tariffs in 2001). A similar study focusing on healthcare utilization was conducted in Jyväskylä (Finland), using data from a cohort study of 128 people presenting with shoulder pain in two community-based health centers in 2007–2008. The average direct costs associated with the treatment of shoulder pain were estimated at €543 (US $645) per patient per year.[47] A third (37%) of the individuals did not incur costs after the index visit, and a total of 15% of the patients generated 69% of the total costs (>€1,000/patient, >US $1,190/patient) during the one year following the first consultation, with surgery incurring the highest costs. On the west coast of Sweden, the mean annual total cost for patients with shoulder pain in primary healthcare (physiotherapist/physical therapist or GP) was estimated at €4,139 (US $4,923) per patient based on tariffs in 2009.[65] The costs for secondary care for this group were estimated at €22,475 (US $26,732). Fifty percent of patient cases closed in 6 weeks and 16% remained in the healthcare system for more than 6 months, and 2% went on to have surgery. The 35% who went directly to physiotherapy/physical therapy had higher physiotherapy/physical therapy costs but lower healthcare and total costs. Eighty-four percent of total costs were due to sick leave from work.[65]

A Spanish Health Service study found that in 5035 cases of shoulder pain, the total cost of physiotherapy/physical therapy was €1,581,356 (US $1,880,944) with 31.6% or €432,901 (US $514,914) spent on evidence-based (exercise and manual) therapies, and the rest being spent on interventions with evidence of no effect, or where the evidence is inconclusive or unknown.[55] In addition to ineffective treatments adding to economic burden, so do inefficiencies in the healthcare system. An Australian study conducted in patients on the waiting list for an orthopedic consult found that the cost of healthcare and domestic support was AU $7,563 (US $5,833) per patient annually. When missed work or decreased productivity at work were included in cost estimates, the economic burden ranged between AU $13,885 (US $10,711) and AU $22,378 (US $17,262) annually.[41]

Prognosis of shoulder pain and disability

The health economic studies described above demonstrated a wide variability in healthcare utilization among people with shoulder pain, with a minority (12–15%) of those presenting in primary care incurring 70–75% of the costs. These findings reflect a variability in the prognosis of shoulder pain that has been highlighted in several longitudinal studies. Many people with shoulder pain will experience a reduction of pain within a few weeks after onset, but 40–50% of people presenting in primary care report persistent pain and disability 6–12 months after their first consultation.[34–37,45,54] Shoulder pain intensity has been reported to reduce from a mean score of approximately 5.2 points (SD 2.2) on a 0–10 numerical rating scale at the time of presentation in healthcare, to between 1.7 (SD 2.8)[36] and 3.2 (SD 2.7)[25] points at 12 months follow-up. The large standard deviation reflects the high individual variability in the level of pain one year after first presentation.

Shoulder pain prognosis can be influenced by many factors: increasing age, lower educational level, longer symptom duration, previous episodes, higher disability scores, and multisite pain increasing the likelihood of persistent shoulder pain.[17,32,36,46] Evidence for the role of psychological and social factors is less clear, and often based on cross-sectional data. Results from prospective research vary depending on healthcare setting (primary/secondary care), shoulder pain diagnosis or definition, and treatment received, but evidence indicates that fear-avoidance beliefs, pain catastrophizing, poor outcome expectations, low self-efficacy, depressive symptoms, and aspects of the psychosocial work environment (e.g., high job strain, low supervisor/co-worker support) are associated with an unfavorable long-term outcome.[10,19,33,36,46,50,51,56]

Several studies have combined prognostic factors into multivariable prediction models aiming to identify patients at increased risk of poor outcome,[10,34,36,63] yet few of these models have been validated, and their predictive performance and usefulness in routine clinical practice has been questioned.[61] Therefore, despite evidence for prognostic value of a range of factors, it is not yet clear which combination of prognostic factors can optimally discriminate between patients at high versus low risk of poor outcome, and which prognostic factors (moderators) can help to identify those patients who may benefit most from specific treatment options, including advice and education, exercise, corticosteroid injection, or more invasive and costly interventions such as surgery.

So far, these prognostic models have not taken the changing nature of symptoms into account, and only use prognostic information collected at a single point in time, often soon after first presentation, to predict outcome. We know, however, that many people experience substantial reduction in symptoms during the first six weeks after onset, or in research after baseline measurements, and this short-term change in pain or disability may be highly predictive of long-term outcome.[40] Incorporating monitoring of early response to treatment in the assessment of individuals with shoulder pain is likely to provide information regarding long-term prognosis, and better guidance regarding decisions for further treatment. Finally, little is known about the pathways that may explain a favorable or poor outcome in patients with shoulder pain.

Generating evidence regarding the role of modifiable prognostic factors (mediators), including lifestyle (e.g., physical activity), comorbidity (e.g., diabetes or metabolic risk factors), or psychological factors (e.g., symptoms of depression, fear-avoidance behavior) along these pathways may allow the identification of targets for improved advice and treatment of people with shoulder pain. There is little evidence for diagnostic information to explain variability in the course and prognosis of shoulder pain. Traditionally, painful shoulder conditions are classified based on the anatomical (bony or soft tissue) structures assumed to be the origin of symptoms, including glenohumeral and acromioclavicular joints, subacromial structures including the rotator cuff, or the cervical/thoracic spine. Information from clinical history, physical examination, and diagnostic imaging (ultrasound, MRI, X-ray) may be used to assess the severity and possible origin of shoulder problems, but empirical evidence for the reproducibility or validity of these classifications is limited (e.g., Lenza et al[38]). Systematic reviews of physical examination tests (e.g., Hanchard et al,[22] Alqunaee et al,[2] Hegedus et al[24]) have highlighted diversity in performance and interpretation of these tests, poor diagnostic accuracy (pooled estimates of sensitivity <0.75, specificity <0.60) and, more importantly, lack of evidence as to which combination of symptoms and signs is most accurate in predicting patient outcome and response to treatment.

Diagnostic classification may provide information that is important for clinical decision-making, however, in patients with shoulder pain, this assumption has been challenged by a lack of evidence. Importantly, factors other than the assumed (anatomical) source of the shoulder condition are likely to influence patient outcome. Incorporating such prognostic information may provide an alternative framework for clinical practice that embraces a holistic view of patients presenting with shoulder pain, and incorporates a wide range of information to predict future patient outcomes and guide decisions regarding advice, treatment, and referral.

Summary and implications

Compared to low back pain and other musculoskeletal conditions (e.g., osteoarthritis, osteoporosis, inflammatory arthritis), evidence regarding the burden of shoulder pain and disability is limited. Most research has been carried out in high income countries, providing little insight into the societal impact of painful shoulder conditions in low- and middle-income countries. Research into the incidence, prevalence, and economic impact of shoulder pain would benefit from the use of agreed upon and validated case definitions for shoulder pain and disability, but what seems likely is that shoulder pain ranks with low back and arthritis with regard to prevalence and cost. Consistent use of such case definitions will make it possible to assess, describe, and compare the impact and burden of shoulder pain across geographical regions, healthcare settings, and relevant subgroups in order to inform policymakers regarding healthcare needs and provision in populations of interest.

The impact and burden of shoulder pain on individuals, healthcare and society is strongly influenced by prognosis. Research has highlighted large variability in overall prognosis, with 40–50% of people experiencing persistent pain and impact on everyday life at 6–12 months after first presenting with shoulder pain in healthcare. Early identification of those at high risk of persistent problems might help to target treatment to those who need it the most, while offering reassurance and advice to people likely to recover quickly from an episode of shoulder pain. This requires high-quality evidence of prognostic (biological, psychological, social) factors associated with the future course and impact of shoulder pain, and with patients' response to treatment.

There are still substantial gaps in evidence, and although many factors have been proposed to be associated with outcome in people with shoulder pain, information regarding their predictive performance is limited. This means that there is uncertainty regarding the accuracy of predictions when trying to identify vulnerable (high risk) subgroups, or when predicting the risk of persistent pain and disability, or benefit (or harm) from specific treatments in individuals presenting with shoulder pain. These are important questions to address in future research in order to contribute to a better understanding of the impact of shoulder pain in the community, improve outcomes for those with high healthcare needs, and ensure optimal and efficient use of healthcare resources.

References

1. Al-Awadhi AM, Olusi SO, Al-Saeid K, et al. Incidence of musculoskeletal pain in adult Kuwaitis using the validated Arabic version of the WHO-ILAR COPCORD core questionnaire. Annals of Saudi Medicine. 2005;25:459-462.
2. Alqunaee M, Galvin R, Fahey T. Diagnostic accuracy of clinical tests for subacromial impingement syndrome: a systematic review and meta-analysis. Archives of Physical Medicine and Rehabilitation. 2012;93:229-236.
3. Ben Ayed H, Yaich S, Trigui M, et al. Prevalence, risk factors and outcomes of neck, shoulders and low-back pain in secondary-school children. Journal of Research in Health Sciences. 2019;19:e00440.
4. Bento TPF, Genebra CVdS, Cornélio GP, et al. Prevalence and factors associated with shoulder pain in the general population: a cross-sectional study. Fisioterapia e Pesquisa. 2019;26:401-406.
5. Bingefors K, Isacson D. Epidemiology, co-morbidity, and impact on health-related quality of life of self-reported headache and musculoskeletal pain–a gender perspective. European Journal of Pain. 2004;8:435-450.
6. Bot SD, Van der Waal J, Terwee C, et al. Incidence and prevalence of complaints of the neck and upper extremity in general practice. Annals of the Rheumatic Diseases. 2005;64:118-123.
7. Buchbinder R, Blyth FM, March LM, Brooks P, Woolf AD, Hoy DG. Placing the global burden of low back pain in context. Best Practice & Research Clinical Rheumatology. 2013;27:575-589.
8. Chaaya M, Slim ZN, Habib RR, et al. High burden of rheumatic diseases in Lebanon: a COPCORD study. International Journal of Rheumatic Diseases. 2012;15:136-143.
9. Chard M, Hazleman R, Hazleman B, King R, Reiss B. Shoulder disorders in the elderly: a community survey. Arthritis & Rheumatism: Official Journal of the American College of Rheumatology. 1991;34:766-769.
10. Chester R, Jerosch-Herold C, Lewis J, Shepstone L. Psychological factors are associated with the outcome of physiotherapy for people with shoulder pain: a multicentre longitudinal cohort study. British Journal of Sports Medicine. 2018;52:269-275.
11. Choi K, Park J-H, Cheong H-K. Prevalence of musculoskeletal symptoms related with activities of daily living and contributing factors in Korean adults. Journal of Preventive Medicine and Public Health. 2013;46:39.
12. Dai S-M, Han X-H, Zhao D-B, Shi Y-Q, Liu Y, Meng J-M. Prevalence of rheumatic symptoms, rheumatoid arthritis, ankylosing spondylitis, and gout in Shanghai, China: a COPCORD study. The Journal of Rheumatology. 2003;30:2245-2251.
13. Davatchi F, Banihashemi AT, Gholami J, et al. The prevalence of musculoskeletal complaints in a rural area in Iran: a WHO-ILAR COPCORD study (stage 1, rural study) in Iran. Clinical Rheumatology. 2009;28:1267-1274.
14. Davatchi F, Jamshidi A-R, Banihashemi AT, et al. WHO-ILAR COPCORD study (stage 1, urban study) in Iran. The Journal of Rheumatology. 2008;35:1384-1390.
15. Davatchi F, Sandoughi M, Moghimi N, et al. Epidemiology of rheumatic diseases in Iran from analysis of four COPCORD studies. International Journal of Rheumatic Diseases. 2016;19:1056-1062.
16. De Vet HC, Heymans MW, Dunn KM, et al. Episodes of low back pain: a proposal for uniform definitions to be used in research. Spine. 2002;27:2409-2416.
17. Engebretsen K, Grotle M, Bautz-Holter E, Ekeberg OM, Brox JI. Predictors of shoulder pain and disability index (SPADI) and work status after 1 year in patients with subacromial shoulder pain. BMC Musculoskeletal Disorders. 2010;11:1-9.
18. Engebretsen KB, Grotle M, Natvig B. Patterns of shoulder pain during a 14-year follow-up: results from a longitudinal population study in Norway. Shoulder & Elbow. 2015;7:49-59.
19. George SZ, Parr JJ, Wallace MR, et al. Inflammatory genes and psychological factors predict induced shoulder pain phenotype. Medicine and Science in Sports and Exercise. 2014;46:1871.
20. Granados Y, Cedeño L, Rosillo C, et al. Prevalence of musculoskeletal disorders and rheumatic diseases in an urban community in Monagas State, Venezuela: a COPCORD study. Clinical Rheumatology. 2015;34:871-877.
21. Greving K, Dorrestijn O, Winters J, et al. Incidence, prevalence, and consultation rates of shoulder complaints in general practice. Scandinavian Journal of Rheumatology. 2012;41:150-155.

22. Hanchard NC, Lenza M, Handoll HH, Takwoingi Y. Physical tests for shoulder impingements and local lesions of bursa, tendon or labrum that may accompany impingement. Cochrane Database of Systematic Reviews. 2013(4):CD007427.

23. Haq SA, Darmawan J, Islam MN, et al. Prevalence of rheumatic diseases and associated outcomes in rural and urban communities in Bangladesh: a COPCORD study. The Journal of Rheumatology. 2005;32:348-353.

24. Hegedus EJ, Goode AP, Cook CE, et al. Which physical examination tests provide clinicians with the most value when examining the shoulder? Update of a systematic review with meta-analysis of individual tests. British Journal of Sports Medicine. 2012;46:964-978.

25. Henschke N, Ostelo RW, Terwee CB, van der Windt DA. Identifying generic predictors of outcome in patients presenting to primary care with nonspinal musculoskeletal pain. Arthritis Care & Research. 2012;64:1217-1224.

26. Hill CL, Gill TK, Shanahan E, Taylor AW. Prevalence and correlates of shoulder pain and stiffness in a population-based study: the North West Adelaide Health Study. International Journal of Rheumatic Diseases. 2010;13:215-222.

27. Hoy D, Bain C, Williams G, et al. A systematic review of the global prevalence of low back pain. Arthritis & Rheumatism. 2012;64:2028-2037.

28. Hoy DG, Smith E, Cross M, et al. Reflecting on the global burden of musculoskeletal conditions: lessons learnt from the Global Burden of Disease 2010 Study and the next steps forward. Annals of the Rheumatic Diseases. 2015;74:4-7.

29. Ihlebæk C, Eriksen HR, Ursin H. Prevalence of subjective health complaints (SHC) in Norway. Scandinavian Journal of Public Health. 2002;30:20-29.

30. Jordan KP, Kadam UT, Hayward R, Porcheret M, Young C, Croft P. Annual consultation prevalence of regional musculoskeletal problems in primary care: an observational study. BMC Musculoskeletal Disorders. 2010;11:1-10.

31. Joshi VL, Chopra A. Is there an urban-rural divide? Population surveys of rheumatic musculoskeletal disorders in the Pune region of India using the COPCORD Bhigwan model. The Journal of Rheumatology. 2009;36:614-622.

32. Keijsers E, Feleus A, Miedema HS, Koes BW, Bierma-Zeinstra SM. Psychosocial factors predicted nonrecovery in both specific and nonspecific diagnoses at arm, neck, and shoulder. Journal of Clinical Epidemiology. 2010;63:1370-1379.

33. Kromer TO, Sieben JM, de Bie RA, Bastiaenen CH. Influence of fear-avoidance beliefs on disability in patients with subacromial shoulder pain in primary care: a secondary analysis. Physical Therapy. 2014;94:1775-1784.

34. Kuijpers T, van der Windt D, Boeke JPA, et al. Clinical prediction rules for the prognosis of shoulder pain in general practice. Pain. 2006;120:276-285.

35. Kuijpers T, van Tulder MW, van der Heijden GJ, Bouter LM, van der Windt DA. Costs of shoulder pain in primary care consulters: a prospective cohort study in The Netherlands. BMC Musculoskeletal Disorders. 2006;7:1-8.

36. Laslett M, Steele M, Hing W, McNair P, Cadogan A. Shoulder pain in primary care–part 2: predictors of clinical outcome to 12 months. Journal of Rehabilitation Medicine. 2015;47:66-71.

37. Laslett M, Steele M, Hing W, McNair P, Cadogan A. Shoulder pain patients in primary care–part 1: Clinical outcomes over 12 months following standardized diagnostic workup, corticosteroid injections, and community-based care. Journal of Rehabilitation Medicine. 2014;46:898-907.

38. Lenza M, Buchbinder R, Takwoingi Y, Johnston RV, Hanchard NC, Faloppa F. Magnetic resonance imaging, magnetic resonance arthrography and ultrasonography for assessing rotator cuff tears in people with shoulder pain for whom surgery is being considered. Cochrane Database of Systematic Reviews. 2013(9):CD009020.

39. Linsell L, Dawson J, Zondervan K, et al. Prevalence and incidence of adults consulting for shoulder conditions in UK primary care; patterns of diagnosis and referral. Rheumatology. 2006;45:215-221.

40. Mansell G, Jordan K, Peat G, et al. Brief pain re-assessment provided more accurate prognosis than baseline information for low-back or shoulder pain. BMC Musculoskeletal Disorders. 2017;18:1-11.

41. Marks D, Comans T, Bisset L, Thomas M, Scuffham PA. Shoulder pain cost-of-illness in patients referred for public orthopaedic care in Australia. Australian Health Review. 2019;43:540-548.

42. Meroni R, Scelsi M, Boria P, Sansone V. Shoulder disorders in female working-age population: a cross sectional study. BMC Musculoskeletal Disorders. 2014;15:1-7.

43. Minaur N, Sawyers S, Parker J, Darmawan J. Rheumatic disease in an Australian Aboriginal community in North Queensland, Australia. A WHO-ILAR COPCORD survey. The Journal of Rheumatology. 2004;31:965-972.

44. Moradi-Lakeh M, Forouzanfar MH, Vollset SE, et al. Burden of musculoskeletal disorders in the Eastern Mediterranean Region, 1990–2013: findings from the Global Burden of Disease Study 2013. Annals of the Rheumatic Diseases. 2017;76:1365-1373.

45. Nørregaard J, Jacobsen S, Kristensen JH. A narrative review on classification of pain conditions of the upper extremities. Scandinavian Journal of Rehabilitation Medicine. 1999;31:153-164.

46. O'Doherty L, Masters S, Mitchell GK, Yelland M. Acute shoulder pain in primary care: an observational study. Australian Family Physician. 2007;36:473.

47. Paloneva J, Koskela S, Kautiainen H, Vanhala M, Kiviranta I. Consumption of medical resources and outcome of shoulder disorders in primary health care consulters. BMC Musculoskeletal Disorders. 2013;14:1-7.

48. Picavet H, Schouten J. Musculoskeletal pain in the Netherlands: prevalences, consequences and risk groups, the DMC3-study. Pain. 2003;102:167-178.

49. Pope DP, Croft PR, Pritchard CM, Silman AJ. Prevalence of shoulder pain in the community: the influence of case definition. Annals of the Rheumatic Diseases. 1997;56:308-312.

50. Rasmussen-Barr E, Grooten WJA, Hallqvist J, Holm LW, Skillgate E. Are job strain and sleep disturbances prognostic factors for low-back pain? A cohort study of a general population of working age in Sweden. J Rehabil Med. 2017;49:591-597.

51. Roh YH, Lee BK, Noh JH, Oh JH, Gong HS, Baek GH. Effect of depressive symptoms on perceived disability in patients with chronic shoulder pain. Archives of Orthopaedic and Trauma Surgery. 2012;132:1251-1257.

52. Safiri S, Kolahi A-A, Cross M, et al. Prevalence, deaths and disability adjusted

life years (DALYs) due to musculoskeletal disorders for 195 countries and territories 1990-2017. Arthritis Rheumatology. 2021;73(4):702-714.

53. Sandoughi M, Zakeri Z, Tehrani Banihashemi A, et al. Prevalence of musculoskeletal disorders in southeastern Iran: a WHO-ILAR COPCORD study (stage 1, urban study). International Journal of Rheumatic Diseases. 2013;16:509-517.

54. Schellingerhout JM, Verhagen AP, Thomas S, Koes BW. Lack of uniformity in diagnostic labeling of shoulder pain: time for a different approach. Manual Therapy. 2008;13:478-483.

55. Serrano-Aguilar P, Kovacs FM, Cabrera-Hernández JM, Ramos-Goñi JM, García-Pérez L. Avoidable costs of physical treatments for chronic back, neck and shoulder pain within the Spanish National Health Service: a cross-sectional study. BMC Musculoskeletal Disorders. 2011;12:1-10.

56. Sindhu BS, Lehman LA, Tarima S, et al. Influence of fear-avoidance beliefs on functional status outcomes for people with musculoskeletal conditions of the shoulder. American Physical Therapy Association. 2012;92(8):992-1005.

57. Smith E, Hoy DG, Cross M, et al. The global burden of other musculoskeletal disorders: estimates from the Global Burden of Disease 2010 study. Ann Rheum Dis. 2014;73:1462-1469.

58. Taylor W. Musculoskeletal pain in the adult New Zealand population: prevalence and impact. N Z Med J. 2005;118:U1629.

59. Urwin M, Symmons D, Allison T, et al. Estimating the burden of musculoskeletal disorders in the community: the comparative prevalence of symptoms at different anatomical sites, and the relation to social deprivation. Annals of the Rheumatic Diseases. 1998;57:649-655.

60. Van der Windt D, Koes BW, de Jong BA, Bouter LM. Shoulder disorders in general practice: incidence, patient characteristics, and management. Annals of the Rheumatic Diseases. 1995;54:959-964.

61. van Oort L, Verhagen A, Koes B, de Vet R, Anema H, Heymans M. Evaluation of the usefulness of 2 prediction models of clinical prediction models in physical therapy: a qualitative process evaluation. Journal of Manipulative and Physiological Therapeutics. 2014;37:334-341.

62. van Schaardenburg D, Van den Brande K, Ligthart GJ, Breedveld FC, Hazes J. Musculoskeletal disorders and disability in persons aged 85 and over: a community survey. Annals of the Rheumatic Diseases. 1994;53:807-811.

63. Vergouw D, Heymans MW, de Vet HC, van der Windt DA, van der Horst HE. Prediction of persistent shoulder pain in general practice: comparing clinical consensus from a Delphi procedure with a statistical scoring system. BMC Family Practice. 2011;12:1-10.

64. Vindigni D, Griffen D, Perkins J, Da Costa C, Parkinson L. Prevalence of musculoskeletal conditions, associated pain and disability and the barriers to managing these conditions in a rural, Australian Aboriginal community. Rural and Remote Health. 2004;4:1.

65. Virta L, Joranger P, Brox JI, Eriksson R. Costs of shoulder pain and resource use in primary health care: a cost-of-illness study in Sweden. BMC Musculoskeletal Disorders. 2012;13:1-11.

66. Wu A, March L, Zheng X, et al. Global low back pain prevalence and years lived with disability from 1990 to 2017: estimates from the Global Burden of Disease Study 2017. Annals of Translational Medicine. 2020;8(6):299.

Shoulder anatomy and function

4

Karen Ginn, Rodney Green, Eleanor Richardson, Olivier Gagey

Introduction

The upper limb functions to facilitate efficient and effective use of the hand for personal, vocational, social, and sporting activities. To be effective the hand must be appropriately located in space and it is the role of the shoulder to provide the large range of movement required to position the hand for the myriad functional tasks it is capable of performing.[90] The functional and, therefore, clinical importance of the musculoskeletal structures that comprise the shoulder region is determined by this requirement to maximize range of movement for the hand. As mobility and stability of joints are opposing concepts, greater freedom of movement comes at the expense of structural stability, and this is true of the glenohumeral joint.[113]

The glenohumeral joint is classified as a ball and socket articulation, and the multidirectional range of motion available at the joint is made possible because of the structure of the bony articular surfaces, labrum, joint capsule and ligaments that offer minimal passive restraint to movement except at the extremes of range of motion.[67] The substantial range of motion available at the shoulder is possible because of synchronous movement of the bones that make up the glenohumeral joint, the humerus and scapula, as well as the clavicle and the thoracic spine. The modifications to the bony and fibrous structures of the glenohumeral joint and the reliance on movement of both the humerus and the scapula to achieve the large movement range required to position the hand for maximal function results in an unparalleled reliance on muscles to maintain functional stability at the shoulder.

To explore the relative functional and therefore clinical importance of the anatomical structures that comprise the shoulder region, this chapter has been divided into two sections. The first explores the contribution of each structure to facilitating maximum shoulder mobility and, the second, the contribution of each structure to shoulder region stability. Within each section the structures making a greater relative contribution to shoulder mobility or stability are discussed first, with contribution from additional structures discussed in decreasing order of functional significance. The final section discusses the shoulder as an integral and sequential part of the whole musculoskeletal system.

Anatomical features facilitating maximum range of shoulder region motion

Shoulder (pectoral) girdle movement

The shoulder girdle provides the bony link between the upper limb and the axial skeleton via the glenohumeral and sternoclavicular joints. It consists of the scapula and clavicle and the intervening articulation – the acromioclavicular joint. Full range of movement at the shoulder can only be achieved by significant contribution from the humerus and the bones of the shoulder girdle, particularly the scapula.[50] Because the humeral head is approximately three times larger than the glenoid fossa,[114] coordinated movement of the scapula with the humerus is required to position the glenoid fossa. This maintains the ball and socket configuration at the glenohumeral joint to achieve full range shoulder movement, and also maintains the mechanical advantage of many shoulder muscles, including the rotator cuff muscles.[58, 67]

Scapular movement occurs because the fascia covering the adjacent layers of muscles between the scapula and the thorax facilitates gliding and sliding movements. Anatomically, six scapular movements are traditionally described: upward (lateral) rotation – movement causing glenoid fossa to face increasingly upwards; downward (medial) rotation – movement causing glenoid fossa to face downwards; protraction – lateral movement forward around chest wall; retraction – medial movement toward vertebral column; elevation – upward movement toward head; depression – downward movement toward feet. However, these movements do not occur independently and all scapular movements involve some degree of movement in all planes.[113] Furthermore, the scapula tilts anteriorly and posteriorly around an axis located at the scapular spine.[65]

Scapular upward and downward rotation are the major contributors to maintain optimal mechanical articular surface alignment through shoulder range of motion. Scapular movement also situates the scapulohumeral muscles (deltoid, rotator cuff, teres major) into mechanically advantageous positions to perform their roles at the glenohumeral joint.[58] During routine upper limb elevation, scapular motion follows a pattern of progressive upward rotation, posterior tilt and highly variable protraction and retraction, in the coronal, sagittal and scapular planes.[65] There is considerable variation in the position and movement (kinematics) of the scapula. There is no one ideal scapular resting position or movement pattern and reported differences in both represent a range of normal. Combined with the fact that few clinical tests assessing scapular kinematics have shown acceptable inter-rater reliability, it is a challenge clinically to determine when observed variations representing aberrant scapular positioning and movement, known as scapular dyskinesis, are present.[130] Interestingly, scapular upward and downward rotation is not possible independent of movement of the humerus, and this emphasizes the intimate functional relationship between scapular and humeral movement to produce full range shoulder movement.

Scapular movements are always accompanied by movement of the clavicle at the clavicular joints which are classified as multiaxial, plane, synovial joints. The range of scapular movement is increased by movements at the sternoclavicular joint and the acromioclavicular joint that allow the acromion, and hence the scapula, anteroposterior gliding and rotation on the clavicle.[1] Movement is facilitated at both the sternoclavicular and acromioclavicular joints by the presence of relatively loose joint capsules and fibrocartilaginous intra-articular discs which improve the congruency of the articular surfaces and provide some cushioning (shock absorption) from forces transmitted along the clavicle from upper trapezius activity and from the upper limb[46,52,113] (Figures 4.1 and 4.2).

Movements of the clavicle are described in the same terms as scapular movements. Elevation, depression, protraction, and retraction are produced by direct muscle action on the clavicle about a fulcrum that passes through the costoclavicular ligament, an exceptionally strong ligament attaching from the inferior, medial surface of the clavicle to the first costal cartilage (Figure 4.1). Axial rotation occurs about the longitudinal axis of the clavicle and is entirely passive, being produced by the coracoclavicular ligament, an extremely powerful ligament situated medial to the acromioclavicular joint anchoring the lateral end of the clavicle to the coracoid process of the scapula. It consists of two parts: the posteromedial conoid ligament and the anterolateral trapezoid ligament (Figure 4.2).

Mechanically the clavicle acts as a strut and by articulating with the acromion holds the scapula away from the trunk.

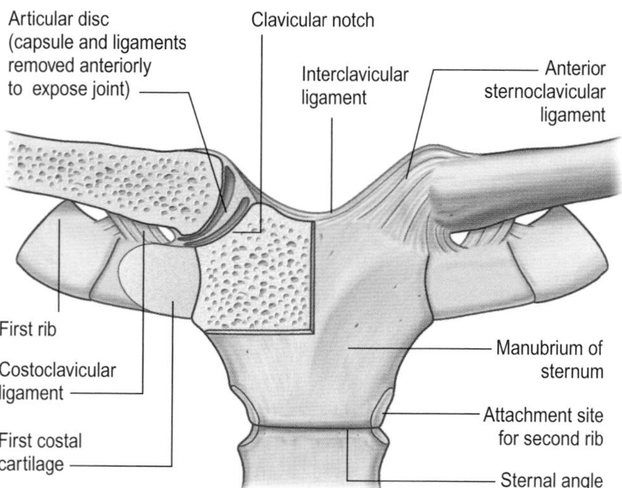

FIGURE 4.1

Anterior view of the sternoclavicular joints, sternum, sternal articulation of the first rib, and surrounding anatomical structures.

(Reproduced with permission from Drake R, Vogl AW, Mitchell A. Gray's Anatomy for Students, 4th edition. Elsevier; 2019.)

One advantage of this mechanism is to increase the available range of shoulder and upper limb movement.[113] Full shoulder range of motion is dependent on the synchronized movement of the humerus, scapula, and clavicle, and is called scapulohumeral rhythm.[113] The scapula contributes 30–40% of the total movement at the shoulder region,[59,70] and the synchronized contribution from humerus and scapula during upper limb elevation occurs simultaneously, except in the initial 25–30° when most, and often all, of the movement occurs at the glenohumeral joint.[1,94] Although characteristic for each individual, scapular movement during the initial phase is irregular and is referred to as the setting phase, as the axioscapular muscles prepare to move the scapula.[49] For every 15° of elevation after this initial setting phase, humeral movement is said to be 10° and scapular movement 5°,[49] although significant variation occurs and is related to factors such as speed of movement and muscle fatigue.[80]

Upward rotation of the scapula is accompanied at first by movement at the sternoclavicular joint to enable elevation of the lateral end of the clavicle. Sternoclavicular movement is almost complete by 90° elevation of the limb.[1] Elevation of the lateral end of the clavicle tenses the conoid part of the coracoclavicular ligament which then produces

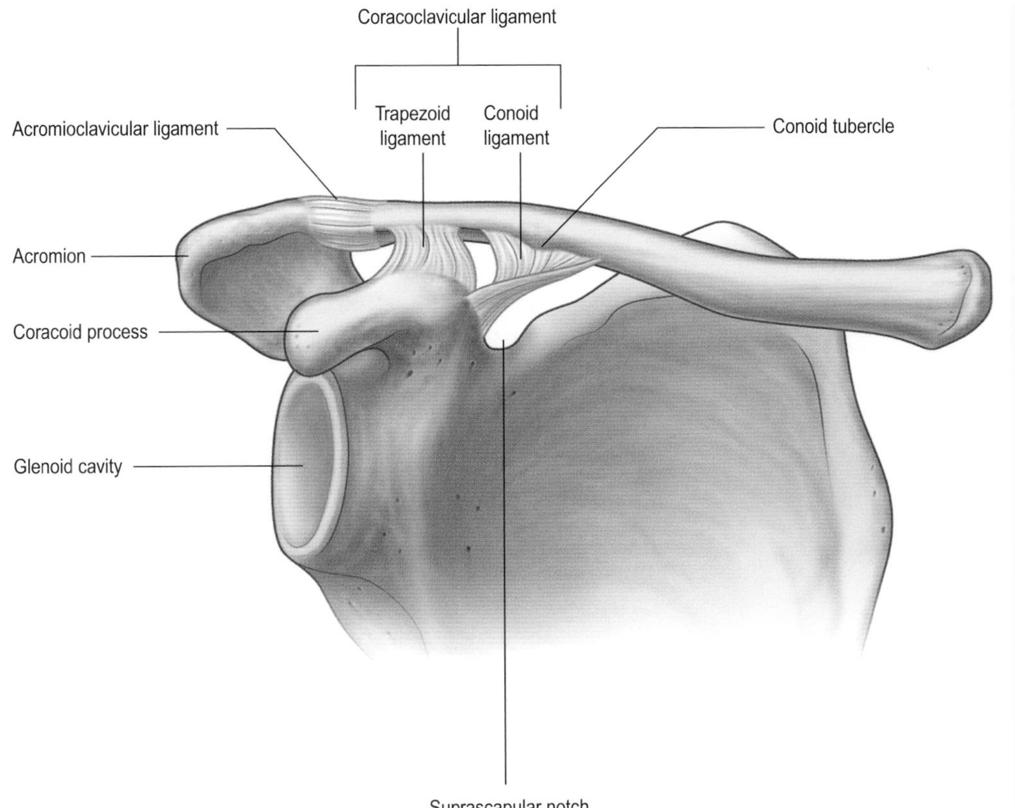

FIGURE 4.2
Anterior view of the upper aspect of a right scapula detailing the glenoid fossa, acromion, coracoid process, acromioclavicular joint, and coracoclavicular ligament.

(Reproduced with permission from Drake R, Vogl AW, Mitchell A. Gray's Anatomy for Students, 4th edition. Elsevier; 2019.)

approximately 30° of posterior rotation of the clavicle at the clavicular joints, initially occurring at the sternoclavicular joint with contribution from the acromioclavicular joint in the final stages of elevation.[49] One of the clinical implications of this relationship between scapular and clavicular movement is that clavicular joint pain and/or dysfunction, not associated with direct trauma to the clavicular joints, may reflect an abnormal scapular contribution to upper limb elevation disrupting this normal kinematic relationship between the scapula and the clavicle.

Muscles

The position and orientation of a muscle relative to a joint determines the plane and direction of movement it can produce at that joint. At the glenohumeral joint, these factors create a moment arm around the joint center of rotation to produce each movement as follows: abductors lie superior, adductors lie inferior, flexors lie anteriorly, extensors lie posteriorly, medial rotators lie horizontal or oblique and insert anteriorly, and external rotators lie horizontal or oblique and insert posteriorly. A summary of the actions of the shoulder muscles, i.e., the movement(s) produced when each muscle shortens (contracts concentrically), is detailed in Table 4.1,[113] with the muscle position and orientation illustrated in Figures 4.3 to 4.7. The extent to which a muscle is responsible for producing an action will depend on the size of the muscle, the size of the moment arm to produce that movement, and the position of the shoulder when the movement is initiated. For example, supraspinatus is superior to the joint (Figure 4.7) and therefore, potentially produces glenohumeral abduction, but because of its small size and short moment arm its contribution is small relative to deltoid which is much larger and has a longer moment arm.

Most shoulder muscles are of parallel form, and this arrangement of muscle fibers promotes the attainment of large ranges of movement. One notable exception is deltoid. While the muscle fibers in the lateral portion of deltoid extend the length of the muscle allowing it to produce large abduction range of motion, the fibers in the majority of the

Table 4.1 Muscles producing movements at glenohumeral joint and movements of the scapula

Shoulder action	Muscles responsible
Glenohumeral abduction	Deltoid Supraspinatus
Glenohumeral adduction	Pectoralis major, sternal head Latissimus dorsi Teres major Coracobrachialis
Glenohumeral flexion	Pectoralis major, clavicular head Deltoid, anterior fibers Coracobrachialis Biceps brachii
Glenohumeral extension	Latissimus dorsi Teres major Deltoid, posterior fibers Pectoralis major, sternal head Triceps brachii, long head
Glenohumeral internal (medial) rotation	Subscapularis Teres major Latissimus dorsi Pectoralis major Deltoid, anterior fibers
Glenohumeral external (lateral) rotation	Infraspinatus Supraspinatus[13,61,79,99,103] Teres minor Deltoid, posterior fibers
Scapular upward (lateral) rotation	Trapezius, upper and lower fibers Serratus anterior
Scapular downward (medial) rotation	Rhomboid major Rhomboid minor Pectoralis minor Levator scapulae
Scapular elevation	Trapezius, upper fibers Levator scapulae
Scapular depression	Trapezius, lower fibers Pectoralis minor
Scapular protraction	Serratus anterior Pectoralis minor
Scapular retraction	Rhomboid major Rhomboid minor Trapezius, middle fibers

muscle belly are of pennate form, aligned obliquely to the line of pull – a form which is better adapted to producing powerful contractions.[68]

To achieve full range shoulder movement both the humerus and the scapula must move. Therefore, the muscles responsible for producing full range shoulder movements, the mover muscles, include muscles that move the humerus and the scapula. Full range shoulder abduction in the scapular plane involves abduction and external rotation of the humerus, and upward rotation of the scapula. External rotation of the humerus is essential to avoid abutment of the greater tubercle of the humerus against the coracoacromial arch. Consequently, the agonist/mover muscles for full range abduction in the scapular plane include the humeral abductor (deltoid), the scapular upward rotators (trapezius and serratus anterior) and the external rotators of the humerus (infraspinatus, supraspinatus, teres minor, posterior deltoid). These muscles will be the mover muscles for full range abduction working concentrically as they raise the arm into abduction, and working eccentrically as they slowly lower the arm back to the side. Difficulty performing full range shoulder movement, therefore, may be the result of dysfunction in the mover roles of humeral abductors, humeral external rotators, and/or scapular upward rotators.

All shoulder movements require coordination of the appropriate mover muscles. For example, full range shoulder flexion in the sagittal plane requires flexion and external rotation of the humerus and upward rotation of the scapula. Both the clavicular head of pectoralis major and anterior fibers of deltoid can flex the humerus but not in the sagittal plane. The clavicular head of pectoralis major will flex and adduct the humerus, while anterior fibers of deltoid will flex and abduct the humerus. For the clavicular head of pectoralis major and anterior deltoid to function as movers to produce flexion of the humerus in the sagittal plane, they also function to cancel out these unwanted adduction and abduction humeral movements, i.e., they must also function as synergists.

Similarly, scapular rotation is achieved by coordinated activity in axioscapular muscles as no single axioscapular

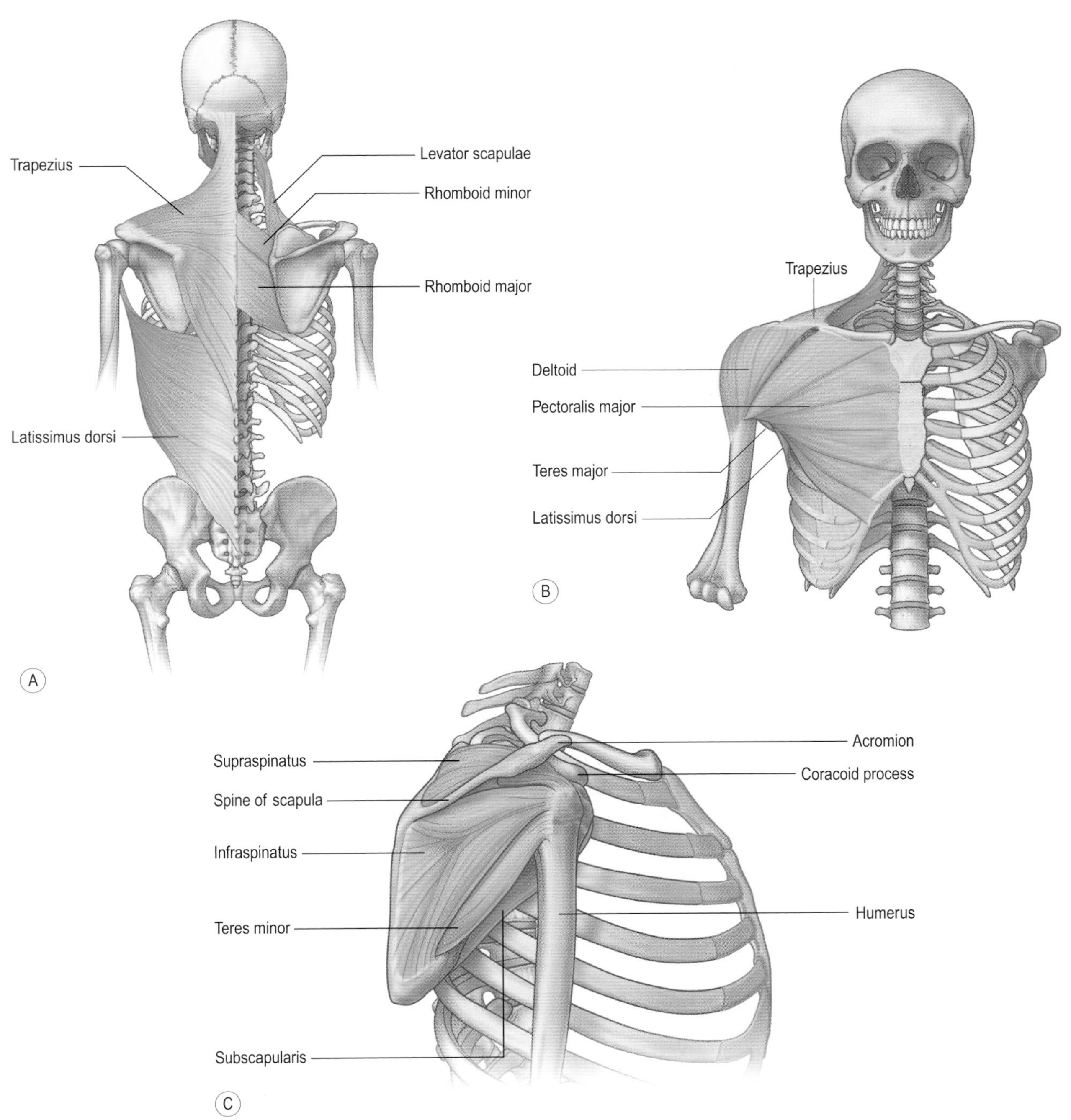

FIGURE 4.3
Shoulder muscles: posterior (A), anterior (B), and lateral (C).
(Reproduced with permission from Drake R, Vogl AW, Mitchell A. Gray's Anatomy for Students, 4th edition. Elsevier; 2019.)

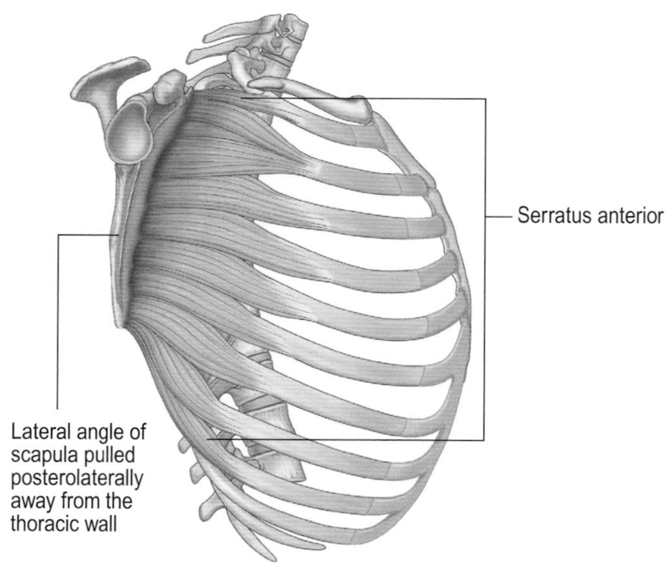

FIGURE 4.4
Lateral view of serratus anterior.
(Reproduced with permission from Drake R, Vogl AW, Mitchell A. Gray's Anatomy for Students, 4th edition. Elsevier; 2019.)

muscle has an action to only produce scapular rotation.[113] Coordinated muscle forces to produce movement are termed a muscular force couple.[49] The upward rotation scapular force couple consists of forces generated by upper trapezius pulling superomedially on the lateral clavicle, by lower trapezius pulling inferomedially on the medial end of the spine of the scapula, and by serratus anterior pulling anterolaterally on the inferior angle of the scapula[5] (Figure 4.8).

For trapezius and serratus anterior to function as movers to produce upward rotation of the scapula they also must function as synergists to cancel out unwanted scapular movements. Lower trapezius has to cancel out scapular elevation due to contraction of upper trapezius, and likewise, upper trapezius needs to cancel out scapular depression due to contraction of lower trapezius. Similarly, middle trapezius (or other scapular retractors) need to cancel out unwanted scapular protraction created by contraction of serratus anterior. The axioscapular muscle coordination required to produce scapular upward rotation not only requires the mover muscles for upward rotation to contract simultaneously to produce appropriate forces on the scapula, but also to function as synergists contracting with the appropriate force to cancel out the unwanted scapular elevation, depression, and protraction that the mover muscles will otherwise produce. Similarly, contraction of the downward rotators of the scapula (rhomboid major and minor) will also produce scapular retraction requiring coordinated, synergist activity of scapular protractors, e.g., serratus anterior, to counterbalance and thus prevent this unwanted scapular movement. Abnormal scapular movement (scapular dyskinesis) may result from alteration in the timing of recruitment of the muscles that rotate the scapula as well as strength imbalances in the components of the scapular rotary force couples.

The rotator cuff muscles attach from the blade of the scapula to insert on the greater (supraspinatus, infraspinatus, and teres minor) and lesser (subscapularis) tubercles of the humerus (Figures 4.3, 4.5 and 4.6). By way of their attachment to the mobile scapula, the rotator cuff muscles, together with the other scapulohumeral muscles (deltoid and teres major), maintain optimal mechanical alignment throughout shoulder range of motion to perform their various functional roles.

Findings from cadaveric studies have confirmed that the insertions of the four rotator cuff muscles are more variable than often described.[82,120] Not only do their tendons tightly fuse with the lateral part of the fibrous joint capsule on its superior (supraspinatus), posterior (infraspinatus and teres minor) and anterior (subscapularis) aspects, but they also fuse with each other.[19,20] The supraspinatus and infraspinatus tendons join approximately 15 mm (0.6 in) from their insertions onto the humerus, infraspinatus and teres minor tendons join just proximal to the musculotendinous junction, and supraspinatus and subscapularis fuse to form a sheath that surrounds the long head of biceps brachii tendon at the proximal end of the bicipital groove.[20] In addition, the rotator cable, a semicircular thickening of the shoulder joint capsule between the tubercles of the humerus, interweaves between and connects the supraspinatus and infraspinatus tendons.[16,20,95]

These structural features of the distal attachments of the rotator cuff tendons have been described as stress-shielding mechanisms, to improve the resistance of the rotator cuff tendons to failure under load by distributing tension in any one of the rotator cuff muscles over a wide area.[16,20]

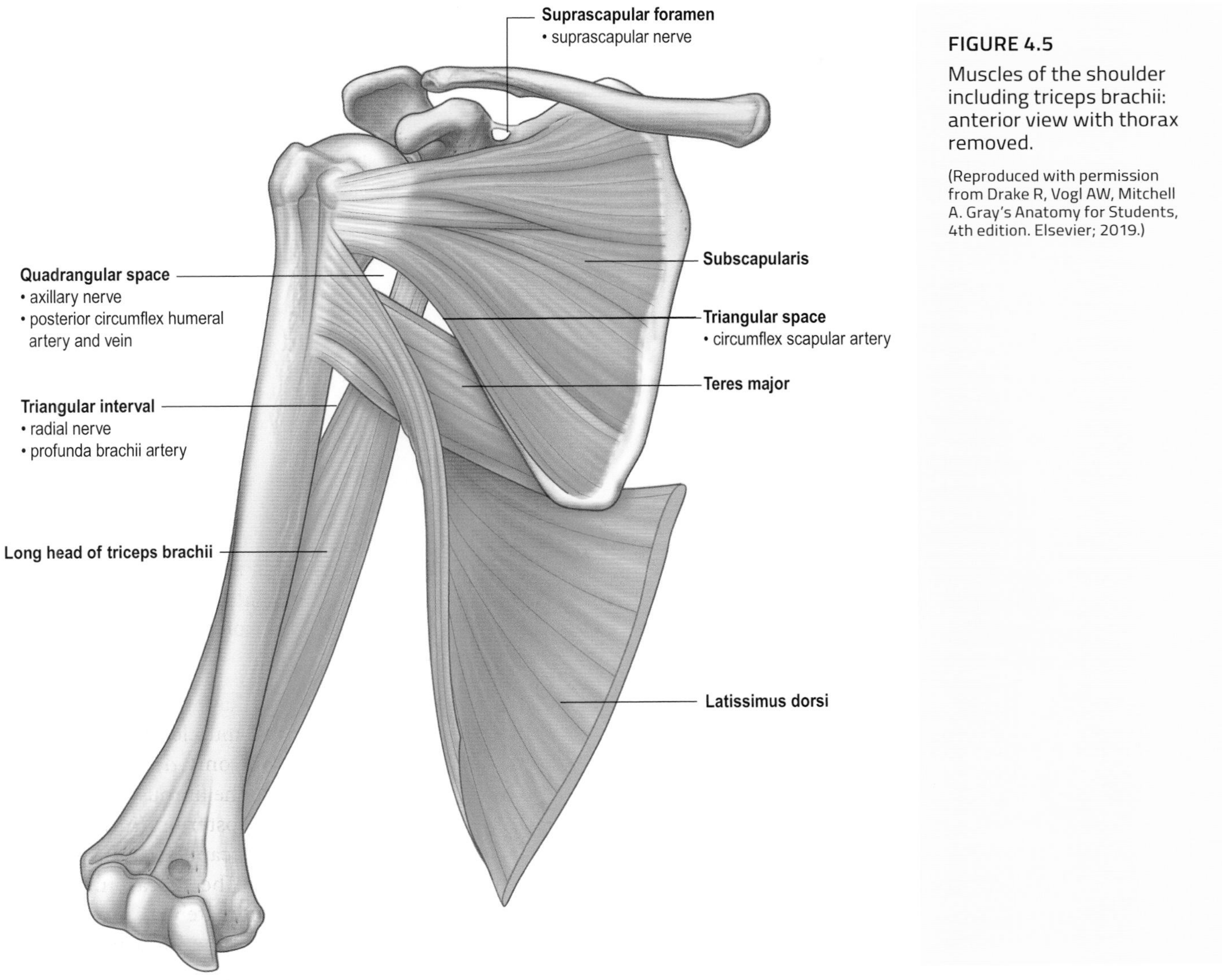

FIGURE 4.5
Muscles of the shoulder including triceps brachii: anterior view with thorax removed.

(Reproduced with permission from Drake R, Vogl AW, Mitchell A. Gray's Anatomy for Students, 4th edition. Elsevier; 2019.)

The structural integration of tendons of the rotator cuff with each other may also provide a mechanical contribution facilitating coordination between the rotator cuff muscles, and may explain why shoulder movement is still possible in the presence of rotator cuff tendon tears lateral to these fibrous interconnections.

Detailed understanding of rotator cuff muscle function has been obtained from studies based on cadaveric dissection, often combined with medical imaging,[12,111,120,131] electromyography (EMG), [25,44,62,97,102,126] and simulated models based on cadaveric work, motion analysis systems, and EMG.[3,11,26] Interpretation of these studies needs to recognize potential limitations; for example, cadaveric studies may simulate the line of force of a muscle that has multiple segments as a single line of force and, like computer models, are theoretical rather than data from a living person. Similarly, electromyographic activity of a muscle during a particular movement does not mean that the muscle produces that movement, as it may be active in another functional role, e.g., as a stabilizer or a synergist.

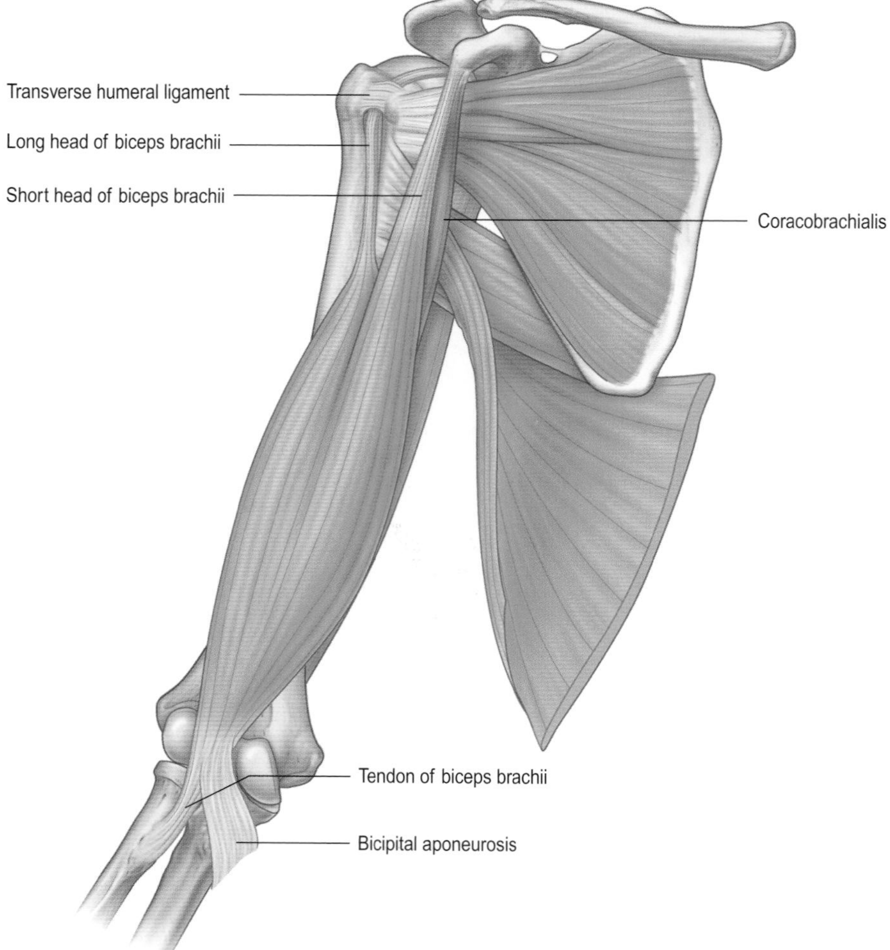

FIGURE 4.6

Muscles of the shoulder: anterior view with thorax removed.

(Reproduced with permission from Drake R, Vogl AW, Mitchell A. Gray's Anatomy for Students, 4th edition. Elsevier; 2019.)

The commonly held belief that supraspinatus "initiates" abduction has long been rejected[53,121] and this has been confirmed by EMG studies that show while supraspinatus is active before movement occurs, it is not active earlier than middle deltoid, infraspinatus or the scapular upwards rotators.[99,126] Multiple EMG studies indicate that supraspinatus has a primary action to externally rotate the humerus.[13,24,62,79,103] It shares this action with the other parts of the rotator cuff that attach to the posterior/dorsal aspect of the scapular blade, i.e., infraspinatus[13,36,47,97] and teres minor.[26,97] As traditionally described in anatomy textbooks, recent EMG evidence supports the action of subscapularis, which attaches to the anterior/ventral aspect of the scapular blade, as an internal rotator of the shoulder.[38]

Cadaveric studies have identified the presence of an anterior and posterior segment in supraspinatus based on fiber orientation.[120] The presence of these segments, in addition to the fusing of the supraspinatus tendon with the infraspinatus tendon posteriorly and the subscapularis tendon anteriorly, suggests that the posterior segments are more likely to contribute to the known role of supraspinatus as an external rotator of the shoulder.[13,96] The anterior portion may act as a shoulder internal rotator.[120]

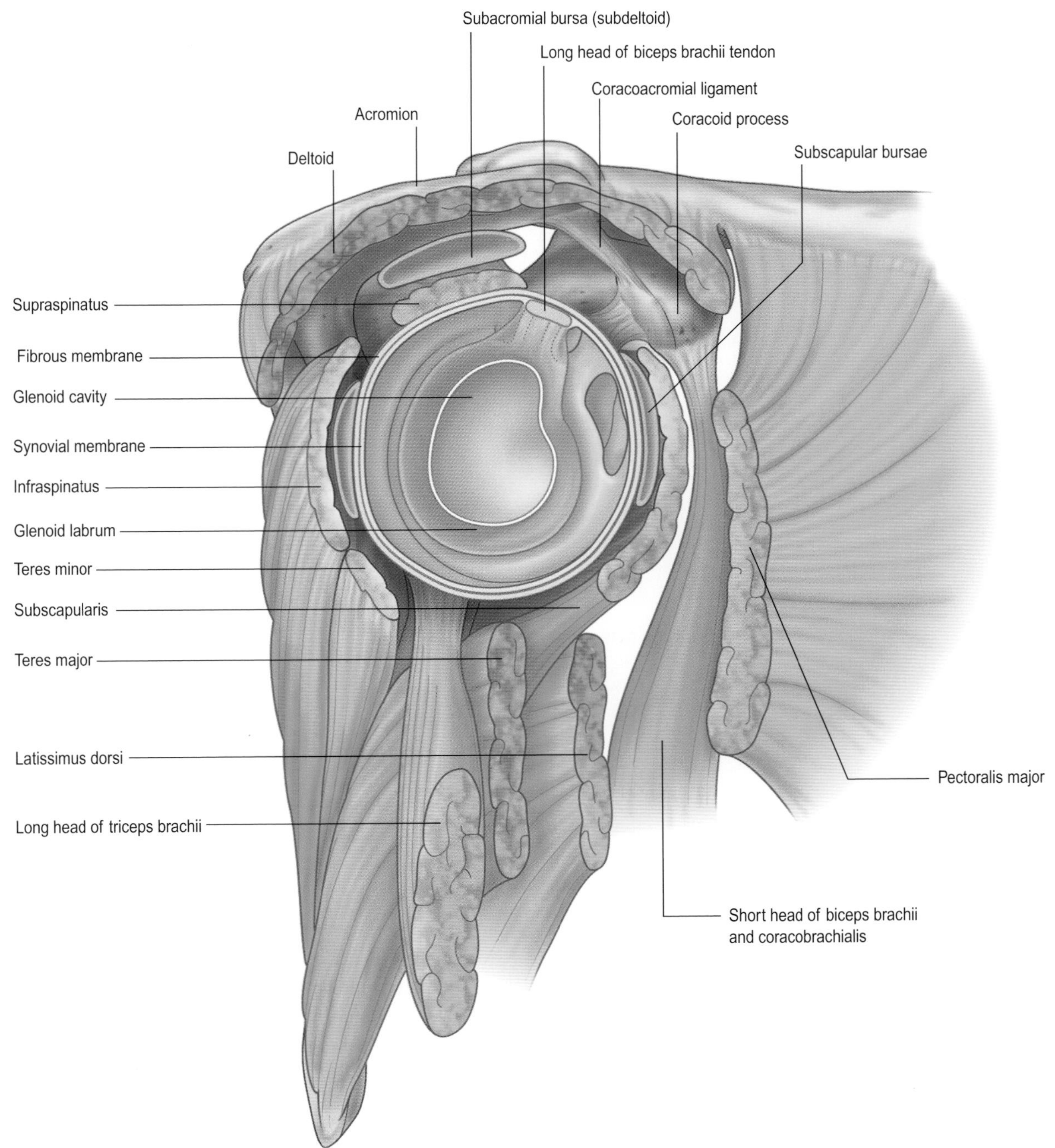

FIGURE 4.7

Lateral view of the right glenohumeral joint with humerus removed.

(Reproduced with permission from Drake R, Vogl AW, Mitchell A. Gray's Anatomy for Students, 4th edition. Elsevier; 2019.)

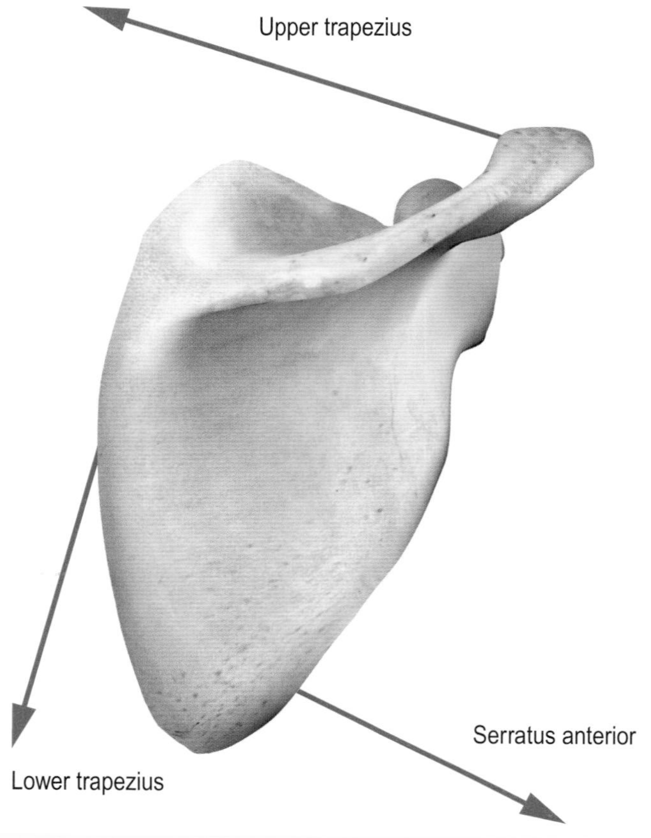

FIGURE 4.8
Muscular force couple producing upward rotation of the scapula.

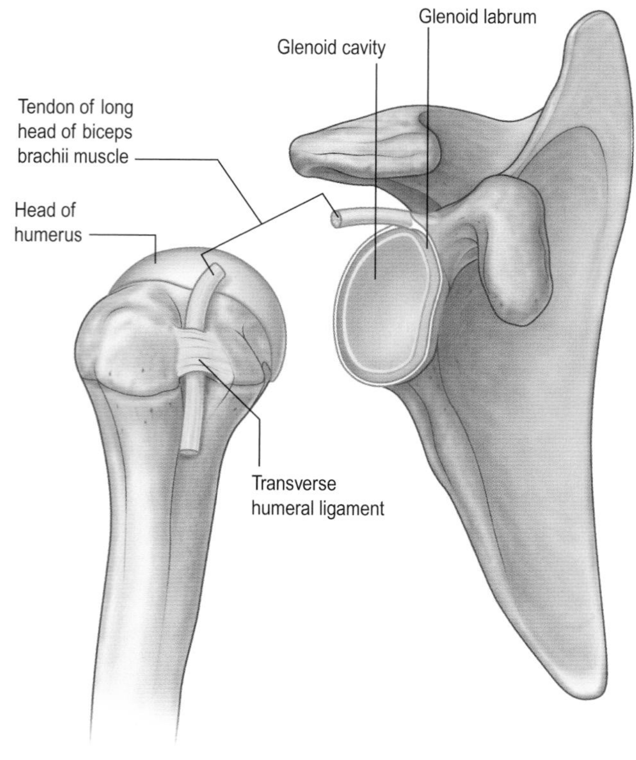

FIGURE 4.9
The humeral head and glenoid cavity.
(Reproduced with permission from Drake R, Vogl AW, Mitchell A. Gray's Anatomy for Students, 4th edition. Elsevier; 2019.)

Glenohumeral articular surfaces and glenoid labrum

The articular surfaces of the glenohumeral joint, the head of the humerus and the glenoid fossa of the scapula, facilitate large range of motion because they afford minimal bony constraint (Figures 4.7 and 4.9). The humeral head is spherical in shape with a surface area of approximately three times that of the glenoid fossa[114] (Figure 4.9). The pear-shaped glenoid fossa is very shallow with a maximum concavity of 2.5 mm (0.1 in) along its anteroposterior axis and 4.5 mm (0.2 in) along its superior–inferior axis.[46] The humeral head and glenoid fossa are reciprocally curved and typically described as being incongruent on account of their differences in size and shape.[116] With only a small proportion of the humeral head (approximately 30%) in contact with the glenoid fossa in any shoulder joint position, the articular surfaces offer minimal restraint to shoulder movement.

The humeral head has a retroverted orientation of approximately 30°, i.e., it is rotated posteriorly 30° with respect to the humeral condyles inferiorly.[72] This structure improves congruency with the anteriorly oriented glenoid due to the position of the scapula around the thoracic wall and thus facilitates shoulder movement.[69] There is considerable variation in the orientation of the humeral head,[91] and an increase in retroversion of the humeral head has been associated with a shift in the range of transverse plane

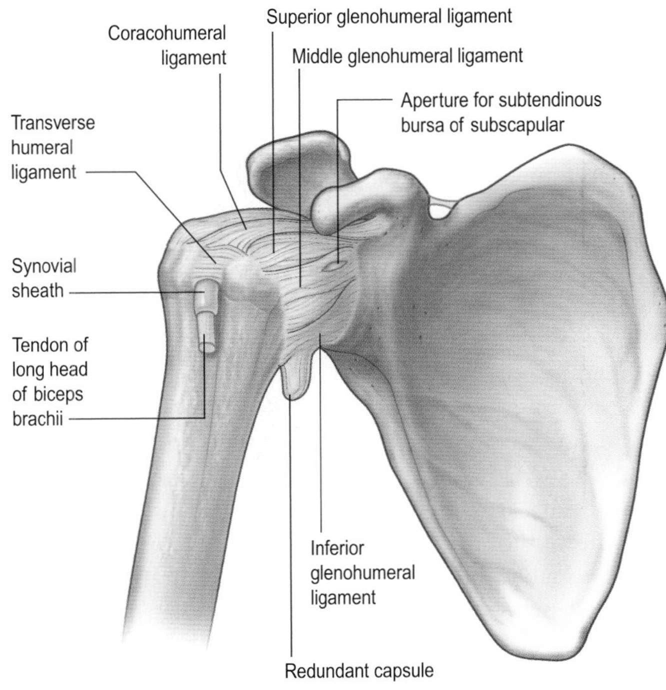

FIGURE 4.10

Anterior view of capsule of the glenohumeral joint.

(Reproduced with permission from Drake R, Vogl AW, Mitchell A. Gray's Anatomy for Students, 4th edition. Elsevier; 2019.)

movement to favor external over internal rotation in the dominant limb of overhead athletic populations.[91,98] It has been suggested that absence of increased retroversion in the dominant limb of throwing athletes may lead to shoulder pain[91] (see Chapter 38).

The glenoid labrum is largely made up of circumferential fibrous connective tissue of the same kind as the joint capsule and forms a ring around the bony glenoid fossa (see Figure 4.9).[45,84] The attachments of the labrum are variable with a generally looser superior attachment and a more substantive attachment to the glenoid inferiorly.[23] Consistent with this stronger attachment to the glenoid articular cartilage inferiorly, the inferior labrum contains some fibrocartilage.[23,45] The superior labrum attaches via the long head of biceps brachii tendon to the supraglenoid tubercle of the scapula and, like the anterior parts of the labrum, often exhibits firmer attachment to the joint capsule than to the glenoid fossa itself.[23] The appearance of the glenoid labrum varies in relation to movement, disappearing anteriorly with full external rotation and posteriorly with full internal rotation, leading some authors to conclude that it is a redundant fold of shoulder capsular tissue.[84] As such, its function may be to facilitate shoulder mobility by protecting the rim of bony glenoid fossa from damage.

The glenohumeral joint is typically described as a ball and socket joint with three degrees of freedom.[116] However, this description has been extended by others to include three degrees of rotatory motion and three degrees of translatory motion.[69] The most studied movement of the shoulder is elevation in a variety of planes: abduction in the coronal plane, abduction in the scapular plane, or flexion in the sagittal plane with instantaneous centers of rotation typically being identified within the ball of the head of the humerus.[94] The substantial difference in size of the articular surfaces means that as the humerus is elevated it rolls superiorly on the glenoid fossa (rotatory movement produced by deltoid), but slides inferiorly (translatory movement produced by inferior muscles of the rotator cuff) to maintain contact with the much smaller glenoid fossa and avoid impingement on the coracoacromial arch.[69] A similar model exists to control anterior–posterior translation of the humeral head during flexion and extension movements. For example, contraction of anterior deltoid to produce flexion will also produce an anterior translation that needs to be tethered by contraction of the posteriorly located rotator cuff muscles such as infraspinatus and supraspinatus.[125]

A pattern of the humeral head rolling superiorly and sliding inferiorly with elevation of the humeral instantaneous center of rotation during abduction is consistent with reported articular contact patterns of the glenoid and humeral head in a cadaveric model. The humeral head rests on the inferior glenoid in the dependent position and then progressively moves superiorly and possibly posteriorly, with maximal contact areas being achieved at approximately 120° of abduction.[115] The contact zone on the humeral head moves from the inferior to superior aspect of the articular surface during the same movements.[115]

Glenohumeral joint capsule and ligaments

The glenohumeral joint capsule, a loose cylindrical sleeve between the articular surfaces, facilitates shoulder mobility because of its laxity[113] (Figure 4.10). With the humeral head being able to translate approximately 2 cm (0.8 in) in anteroposterior directions on the glenoid fossa without damage to the capsule, laxity is a significant feature of the normal glenohumeral joint.[28]

The capsule extends from outside the glenoid labrum anteriorly and inferiorly, and from the labrum superiorly and posteriorly to the anatomical neck of the humerus, except inferiorly where it extends for more than 1 cm (0.4 in) onto the medial humeral shaft[113] (Figure 4.10). It is very thin posteroinferiorly (<1 mm, <0.04 in) and thickest in the rotator interval between subscapularis and supraspinatus (>2 mm, >0.1 in).[19] Approximately 35% of the portion of the capsule adjacent to the humeral tubercles receives tightly adhered insertions from the rotator cuff muscles.[19] In addition, the capsule is reinforced anterosuperiorly by inconsistent thickenings called the glenohumeral ligaments, superiorly where the coracohumeral ligament blends with the capsule, and laterally by a thickening between the humeral tubercles termed the transverse humeral ligament (Figure 4.10).

Consistent with the need for large ranges of movement, the shoulder joint has relatively few ligaments to restrict motion. Only the coracohumeral and glenohumeral ligaments connect the articulating bones and are therefore capable of restraining normal physiological movement. In addition, the glenohumeral ligaments vary considerably in size and location, are seldom prominent and are sometimes absent.[84,117]

Two consistent openings in the fibrous joint capsule connect the shoulder joint cavity to the subscapular bursa anteriorly and, at the upper end of the intertubercular groove, to the synovial sheath surrounding the tendon of the long head of biceps brachii. A third opening into the infraspinatus bursa is sometimes present posteriorly.[113] These connections enable the flow of synovial fluid between the shoulder joint cavity and surrounding synovial structures. As a result, an inflammatory response initiated at the glenohumeral joint associated with an increase in synovial fluid and accumulation of inflammatory cells, could track into these bursae or into the bicipital sheath. The common clinical finding of tenderness in the bicipital groove associated with painful shoulder dysfunction, therefore, may not represent local pathology of the long head of biceps brachii but rather be a consequence of glenohumeral joint pathology due to other causes.

Bursae

The glenohumeral joint contains numerous bursae, pockets lined by synovial membrane that facilitate movement of adjacent structures where pressure or friction may occur. While the most substantial of these is the subacromial or subdeltoid bursa, there are others including the subscapular, coracobrachial and subcoracoid bursae. Descriptions of these bursae suggest that they may be variable in both presence and structure, but there are only limited studies that have described these bursae in detail.[55] The large subacromial bursa has a roof attached to the deep surface of the acromion process, the coracoacromial ligament and the deltoid, and a floor attached to the rotator cuff insertions, particularly the supraspinatus, and the proximal end of the humerus. It is therefore located at the point of maximal reflection of deltoid,[30] and facilitates the movement of the proximal humerus under the contracting deltoid muscle. It also serves to protect structures in the subacromial space from damage in the event of superior migration of the humeral head. The subacromial bursa is known to contain nociceptive nerve endings[48,122] but the presence of mechanoreceptors is less certain.[55] Pain associated with subacromial bursopathy has the potential to detrimentally affect shoulder muscle function by limiting force production or interfering with normal muscle recruitment patterns.[37]

Anatomical features facilitating shoulder region stability

Glenohumeral joint muscles

Rotator cuff

Cadaveric, biomechanical modelling, and EMG evidence indicates that the rotator cuff muscles contribute to functional shoulder joint stability via two related mechanisms. Firstly, they compress the head into the glenoid fossa to limit humeral head translation, the so-called concavity compression stabilizing mechanism.[46,72,83,116] This role is supported by findings from cadaveric studies that have confirmed the moment arms of rotator cuff muscles are shorter than other prime movers for most glenohumeral movements,[2,7] resulting in their ability to produce significant compressive forces.[108] Computer modelling also indicates that supraspinatus, infraspinatus and subscapularis have a greater stabilizing role at the glenohumeral joint than the global muscles,[3] and that supraspinatus has a significant role in glenohumeral compression during lifting tasks.[11]

Secondly, the rotator cuff muscles function to stabilize the glenohumeral joint by counterbalancing/tethering potential humeral head translation created by muscles moving the humerus, i.e., the rotator cuff muscles coordinate with muscles moving the humerus in muscular force couples to maintain functional glenohumeral joint stability.[12,97,111,125,128,131] The role of the rotator cuff in preventing deltoid from superiorly translating the humeral head during glenohumeral abduction was proposed more than 80 years ago.[8,50,89,111] This theory contends that during abduction from the pendant position, deltoid contraction will initially produce an upward force which, if unopposed, will tend to slide the humeral head superiorly, jamming it against the coracoacromial arch. The four rotator cuff muscles provide a coordinated, synchronized, downward as well as medial force during the initial phase of abduction to counteract this superior shearing force, to create a stable fulcrum about which abduction can occur. [50,89,111,133]

Early radiographic studies provided some evidence to support the potential destabilizing effect of deltoid contraction on the humeral head in the initial stages of shoulder abduction. While people with shoulder pathology were more variable, people without symptoms demonstrated an initial superior movement of the instantaneous center of rotation during the first 30–60° of abduction, followed by a relatively constant position throughout the remainder of the range of abduction.[94] This superior movement of the humeral head is presumed to relate to the action of deltoid.[93] This is also likely to explain results reported with living participants completing isometric contractions through the range of abduction with joint positions recorded using magnetic resonance imaging techniques, whereby an isometric contraction at 0° abduction showed a more superiorly located head of humerus.[107]

Evidence to support stabilizing roles for the rotator cuff muscles during abduction has been provided by both cadaveric and EMG studies. Decreasing simulated rotator cuff muscle forces in cadaveric models resulted in increases in humeral head translation in superior,[111,128] anterosuperior,[131] and anterior[12] directions. Cadaveric models also showed that reduction in the simulated force of rotator cuff muscles reduced anterior and posterior translation of the humeral head in response to externally applied forces[131] and that, while supraspinatus may assist with glenohumeral joint compression during abduction, it does not reduce subacromial impingement, with this role being attributed to the lower fibers of the rotator cuff.[132]

Stabilizing roles of lower segments of the rotator cuff are also confirmed by EMG studies, particularly when multiple segments of muscles are examined using separate electrodes. The oblique lower segments of both subscapularis and infraspinatus are more involved than their transverse upper segments in limiting superior migration of the humeral head during abduction.[47] However, despite the relatively inferior location of teres minor, it does not have the same stabilizing role to prevent superior migration of the humeral head as lower subscapularis or infraspinatus.[97] This may relate to the fact that teres minor has a less oblique line of pull than lower infraspinatus, due to a higher origin on the lateral border of the scapula and a lower insertion on the lower facet of the greater tubercle of the humerus.

Electromyographic studies confirm that the rotator cuff muscles also provide dynamic anteroposterior glenohumeral joint stability during flexion and extension via a muscular force couple mechanism. However, in contrast to their role in abduction where the rotator cuff muscles contribute in equal proportions[100] in providing dynamic anteroposterior stability, the rotator cuff muscles work in a direction-specific manner.[62,97,124] In adults without shoulder symptoms, the rotator cuff muscles that attach to the posterior surface of the scapula (supraspinatus, infraspinatus and teres minor) are significantly more active than the anteriorly located subscapularis during dynamic glenohumeral flexion, and during externally applied anterior translation of the humeral head confirmed by real time ultrasound.[97,124] In contrast, during dynamic glenohumeral extension and passive posterior translation of the humeral head, subscapularis is activated at significantly higher levels than supraspinatus, infraspinatus and teres minor.[97,124] Contrary to common clinical belief, these results indicate that it is the posterior rotator cuff muscles (supraspinatus, infraspinatus and teres minor) that maintain anterior glenohumeral joint stability by counterbalancing potential anterior humeral head translation created by contraction of flexor muscles. Conversely, subscapularis, the anterior rotator cuff, functions in a force couple with glenohumeral extensors to maintain posterior glenohumeral stability, by preventing potential posterior humeral head translation associated with extensor muscle activity.[124]

The preceding evidence indicates that, during glenohumeral abduction, flexion and extension, functional glenohumeral stability is achieved by a balance between potential destabilizing translation forces created by muscles moving the humerus, and tethering forces generated by the rotator cuff muscles to counterbalance potential humeral head translation. The highly synchronous recruitment patterns between the muscles producing glenohumeral abduction, flexion and extension, and rotator cuff muscles confirmed by EMG studies, provide further evidence to support a model of functional glenohumeral joint stability based on a balance of muscle forces on the humeral head.[100,124] Subacromial impingement and anteroposterior instability at the glenohumeral joint, therefore, may be the result of abnormal recruitment and/or abnormal recruitment timing of the rotator cuff muscles as well as strength and/or length deficits. A recent EMG study has provided preliminary evidence that people with persistent shoulder pain who demonstrated signs of instability and/or impingement have greater variability in the relative timing of infraspinatus and supraspinatus recruitment compared to healthy participants.[37]

In contrast to glenohumeral abduction, flexion and extension, the rotator cuff muscles appear to play a minor stabilizing role during glenohumeral adduction. During maximal isometric shoulder adduction tasks, EMG studies indicate that the rotator cuff muscles are only recruited at minimal to low levels.[102] This low rotator cuff activity may be explained by the line of pull and balanced arrangement of the glenohumeral adductor muscles (sternal head of pectoralis major anteriorly, and latissimus dorsi and teres major posteriorly) which enables them to produce compression forces and not translational forces on the humeral head as they produce adduction.

Deltoid

In contrast to the view that rotator cuff muscle activity is required to prevent deltoid from superiorly gliding the humeral head during abduction, an alternative theory has been proposed. This theory contends that instead of pulling the humerus upward, deltoid contraction will push the humeral head downward.[10] Taking into account that the deltoid wraps around the upper end of the humerus, and that when contracted, the deltoid muscle belly becomes a semi-rigid body able to interact with the underlying structures, it has been contended that deltoid will apply a downwardly oriented force to the upper end of the humerus. This force would then counteract the upward-oriented force applied by the deltoid at the level of its humeral attachment.[10] In this theoretical model, deltoid would thus be functioning as both a mover and a stabilizer during the initial stages of glenohumeral abduction.

As the humerus moves through abduction range of motion, the pull of deltoid changes from one that potentially creates an upward force on the humeral head in the early stages of abduction, to one that compresses the humeral head into the glenoid fossa, thus contributing to dynamically stabilizing the glenohumeral joint.[13] It is interesting to note that a baseball pitch, the fastest throwing motion that the shoulder can perform, is executed with the shoulder at 90° abduction, a position in which the deltoid, one of the strongest glenohumeral muscles, can provide dynamic joint stability, while the rotator cuff muscles function to accelerate and decelerate the pitch.[29,39]

Biceps brachii

The long head of biceps brachii typically attaches to both the supraglenoid tubercle and the superior part of the glenoid labrum prior to traversing the glenohumeral joint cavity, to emerge in the anterior arm via the bicipital groove (Figure 4.6). This intracapsular course means that it has a very short moment arm thus limiting its ability to produce movements at the glenohumeral joint, but it is commonly believed to have a role in stabilizing this joint.[63] Cadaveric studies have suggested that biceps brachii may provide this stabilizing role via increased torsional rigidity but disagree as to whether this is in the lower[87] or upper part[32] of the glenohumeral joint range. However, as biceps brachii is a multi-joint muscle, the ability to influence the glenohumeral joint depends on the position of the elbow and radioulnar joints over which it also passes. Biceps brachii will be shortened when the elbow is flexed and the radioulnar joints are supinated, rendering it actively insufficient, i.e., its ability to provide force at the glenohumeral joint is decreased when it is shortened over the elbow and radioulnar joints.

While not a direct impact on glenohumeral stability, the attachment of biceps brachii to the superior labrum has been exploited as the basis for numerous clinical tests to assess superior labral tears, albeit with limited clinical accuracy.[81]

The lack of diagnostic accuracy of these clinical tests probably reflects the relatively loose superior attachment of the glenoid labrum and the fact that any passive tension applied to the distal biceps tendon is dissipated in the extensible belly of the muscle.[40]

Axioscapular muscles

The scapula plays an important role as the base for attachment of the scapulohumeral muscles (deltoid, rotator cuff muscles and teres major; Figures 4.3, 4.5 and 4.6). To enable the scapulohumeral muscles to effectively produce torque at, and dynamically stabilize, the glenohumeral joint, the axioscapular muscles must contract to dynamically stabilize the scapula to prevent contraction of the scapulohumeral muscles from moving the scapula.[58] As biceps brachii and the long head of triceps brachii also attach to the scapula, axioscapular muscles will be required to dynamically stabilize the scapula during contraction of these muscles as well (Figures 4.5 and 4.6). During full range abduction in the scapular plane performed under low, medium and high load conditions, strong correlations have been demonstrated between the activation patterns of scapulohumeral (middle deltoid, infraspinatus and subscapularis) and axioscapular muscles (upper and lower trapezius, serratus anterior and rhomboid major).[101] This result indicates that as middle deltoid and rotator cuff activity increase, similar increases occur in all the axioscapular muscles examined. As increased load on the arm does not directly increase load on the scapula, the role of axioscapular muscles to produce the scapular upward rotation torque required during shoulder abduction cannot explain the increased activity in the scapular upward rotators with increases in abduction load. In addition, as rhomboid major is a downward rotator of the scapula, it cannot be functioning to upwardly rotate the scapula in the abduction task examined.[88]

A stabilizer function for the axioscapular muscles can explain the strong correlation reported between the activation patterns of axioscapular and scapulohumeral muscles.[101] As middle deltoid, infraspinatus and subscapularis increase their activation levels with increasing abduction load, they exert an increased lateral pull on the scapula necessitating a corresponding increase in axioscapular muscle activation levels to counterbalance this destabilizing force on the scapula. The results from this study suggest that the stabilizing function of axioscapular muscles is not direction specific. Increasing load during full range abduction in the scapular plane resulted in similar increases in activation levels in both upward and downward rotators of the scapula which were strongly correlated.[101]

The stabilizer function of the axioscapular muscles requires them to contract with the appropriate force, at the correct time, to prevent scapulohumeral muscles from displacing the scapula. To improve the important stabilizer function of axioscapular muscles, exercises that train the axioscapular muscles to react to the potentially destabilizing forces created by scapulohumeral muscles are required. Given the strong correlation between the recruitment pattern of axioscapular and scapulohumeral muscles, functionally specific, graduated strengthening of axioscapular muscles could be achieved by gradually increasing activity in scapulohumeral muscles, by either increasing activity in individual muscles or increasing the number of active scapulohumeral muscles.

Clavicular joint structures

Passive joint structures are responsible for providing most of the stability at the sternoclavicular and acromioclavicular joints. Elevation of the clavicle is limited by the extremely strong costoclavicular and coracoclavicular ligaments (Figures 4.1 and 4.2). The vertically placed intra-articular disc in the sternoclavicular joint, attaches to the joint capsule and divides the joint into two separate cavities (Figure 4.1). Mechanically this disc may also contribute to limiting clavicular elevation, and subclavius, a muscle located between the clavicle and the first rib, provides a dynamic element to protect these passive structures from damage under high stress conditions (Figure 4.1). The intra-articular disc also limits depression of the clavicle but ultimately, depression is limited by contact with the first rib and/or the coracoid process of the scapula.

Protraction and retraction are limited by the costoclavicular, coracoclavicular, and the anterior and posterior sternoclavicular ligaments which attach from the medial end of the clavicle to the manubrium of the sternum anteriorly, and posteriorly to the sternoclavicular joint (Figures 4.1 and 4.2). The costoclavicular ligament is composed of an anterior and a posterior layer usually separated by a bursa and situated at right angles to each other. The anterior fibers of the costoclavicular ligament, the conoid part of the coracoclavicular ligament, and the anterior sternoclavicular ligament limit protraction. The posterior fibers of the costoclavicular ligament, the trapezoid part of the coracoclavicular ligament, and the posterior sternoclavicular ligament limit retraction. In addition, the coracoclavicular ligament, especially the trapezoid part, prevents the acromion from being carried medially under the lateral end of the clavicle when forces are applied at the glenohumeral joint due to a fall on the point of the shoulder, or an outstretched upper limb.[113]

Glenohumeral joint articular surfaces and glenoid labrum

The glenoid fossa constitutes only one-third of the articular surface of the humeral head.[106,114] However, congruency and stability are enhanced, as the curvatures of the articular surfaces become similar when the articular cartilage is considered.[114] The relative size of the glenoid versus humeral head can be expressed as the glenohumeral index, and this index is much lower for the transverse compared to the vertical dimensions of the two articular surfaces at the glenohumeral joint.[106] This greater incongruity in the transverse plane suggests that muscular control of anterior and posterior translation is critical to glenohumeral stability and this is supported by reports that lower forces are required for dislocation in these directions as compared to superior and inferior directions.[67]

The glenoid labrum increases the depth of the glenoid socket by approximately 50%, resulting in a superior inferior depth of 9 mm (0.4 in) and anteroposterior depth of 5 mm (0.2 in).[46] By creating a glenoid socket of significantly greater depth than the bony glenoid fossa, the glenoid labrum makes a contribution to glenohumeral joint stability by increasing the contact area between the articular surfaces to resist humeral head translation.[46,114] The recent finding of mechanoreceptors in the glenoid labrum able to register changes in tension and compression, indicates that it contributes to glenohumeral joint dynamic stability by providing proprioceptive feedback regarding humeral head position in addition to its mechanical constraint role.[129]

Glenohumeral joint capsule and ligaments

The role of the glenohumeral joint capsule as a mechanical stabilizing structure for the shoulder is minimal because of its laxity. However, in the sections where the shoulder capsule is reinforced by rotator cuff tendons or ligaments, its capacity to act as a mechanical restraint is increased. Due to the tightly adhered insertions of the rotator cuff muscles into the capsule, contraction of these muscles tighten the lax capsule preventing it and its synovial lining from becoming trapped between the articular surfaces during movement.[113]

Most of the ligaments of the glenohumeral joint can function as partial restraints to physiological movement, but only at the extremes of shoulder motion.[78] The three glenohumeral ligaments (superior, middle, and inferior), are thickenings of the anterior capsule which are seldom prominent and sometimes absent, suggesting that they have limited mechanical functional significance[33,84] (see Figure 4.10). When present, cadaveric studies indicate that all glenohumeral ligaments limit external rotation. The superior glenohumeral ligament contributes more in the adducted position, with increasing contribution from the middle and inferior ligaments as abduction range increases.[84,123]

The coracohumeral ligament is a broad band of inconsistent size, that extends from the lateral coracoid process to the anatomical neck of the humerus in the region of the greater and lesser tubercles, and the intervening transverse humeral ligament[113] (Figure 4.10). As it passes laterally it blends with the joint capsule, the tendon of supraspinatus superiorly, and the tendon of subscapularis and the superior glenohumeral ligament inferiorly.[33] As the glenoid cavity is oriented slightly superiorly by 4–10.5° at rest, the coracohumeral ligament can prevent lateral, and therefore, inferior translation of the humeral head.[71] It also limits external rotation of the humerus between 0° and 60° of abduction.[6,33]

Finally, the transverse humeral ligament, previously thought to be a thickening of the glenohumeral joint capsule, has been shown to consist of tendinous fibers of subscapularis and pectoralis major (Figure 4.10). It functions as a retinaculum preventing bowstringing of the long head of biceps brachii, and plays no direct mechanical restraint function at the glenohumeral joint.[73]

The coracoacromial ligament is a strong triangular band not directly associated with the glenohumeral joint. Together with the coracoid and acromion processes, it forms a fibro-osseous band above the humeral head,[113] and functions to prevent superior dislocation of the humeral head. The coracoacromial arch, however, cannot prevent superior migration (subluxation) of the humeral head on the glenoid fossa, resulting in malalignment of the glenohumeral joint articular surfaces and impingement of structures in the subacromial space. In addition, the coracoacromial ligament has a role to dissipate large forces on the coracoid process, derived from contraction of the muscles that attach to the coracoid process (short head of biceps brachii, pectoralis minor and coracobrachialis), to the acromion process.[35]

Despite the limited mechanical restraint provided to the glenohumeral joint by its capsule and ligaments, these structures may play a significant role in providing shoulder joint stability via neuromuscular feedback mechanisms. The significant numbers of mechanoreceptors present in the glenohumeral joint capsule and ligaments indicate that these structures can provide proprioceptive input to inform the coordination of muscles to dynamically stabilize the glenohumeral joint.[41,51,122,129]

The role of the kinetic chain in shoulder function

It has been clearly demonstrated that the shoulder complex works as an integral and sequential part of the whole musculoskeletal system and does not function in isolation.[18,21,56,77,110,127] Consequently, shoulder rehabilitation needs to be multifaceted, with optimal function requiring local, sensorimotor and biomechanical integrity, as well as contributions from distant body segments of the kinetic chain.[18,56,110]

The term kinetic chain refers to the task-specific sequence of activation from one body segment to another during movement.[18,56] An efficient kinetic chain will generate, summate and permit efficient mechanical energy transfer during functional tasks.[18,77] A partial or complete compromise at any “link” within the kinetic chain has the potential to detrimentally affect the transfer of force along the segments.[18,56,77] This may necessitate an increase in contribution from other “links” within the chain to accommodate the reduction in transferred force.[18,77] To maintain the same speed, power and duration of activity, the increased contribution from the link(s) compensating for the reduced force may be subject to a load that exceeds their physiological capacity, and this in turn may lead to symptoms at that link or series of links. This has been postulated as a predisposing factor, increasing injury risk and symptoms at the shoulder in overhead athletes. Increasing evidence supports the relevance of kinetic chain deficits in the pathogenesis of shoulder injury and symptoms.[4,9,18,31,58,64,92,105,109]

The leg and the trunk provide 50–55% of the total kinetic energy required during upper limb force generation by providing rotational momentum.[77] Several studies have highlighted lumbopelvic–hip stability and gluteal muscle activation as essential requirements for efficient upper limb function during baseball pitching.[15,17,60,66] Reduced hip abduction strength, range of motion, and lower limb muscle length increase the risk of shoulder and elbow injury in throwing athletes.[4,9,18,31,64,92,105,109] Martin et al.[77] compared energy flow from the trunk to the shoulder between injured and non-injured expert tennis players. They reported that suboptimal energy from the trunk during the tennis serve results in decreased ball velocity and a concomitant increase in upper limb joint kinetics. The shoulder, elbow, and wrist absorbed more energy than did the joints of uninjured players. Martin et al.[77] concluded that suboptimal energy flow is a likely mechanism of overuse injuries in the upper limb, including the shoulder. Overhead athletes sustaining a lower limb injury are at an increased risk of developing shoulder pain.[66]

These findings highlight the importance of the whole kinetic chain in relation to optimal shoulder function, as well as the possible relevance of incorporating both local and global musculoskeletal assessments into the clinical examination. Suboptimal kinetic chain performance is not only linked to an increased risk of upper limb injury,[4,9,18,31,64,92,105,109] but directly to suboptimal upper limb performance.[15,17,34,77] Lower limb peak power has been found to be the primary determinant of throwing velocity in elite handball players, and a significant correlation has been found between maximum velocity and volume of the lower limb during elite javelin throwing performance. Consequently, strength and peak power of both the upper and lower limbs are acknowledged to be strongly associated with optimal performance in overhead sports,[15,17,43] and the throwing motion is increasingly recognized as a reflection of the power output obtained from a series of integrated whole body movements rather than an isolated movement pattern[43] (see Chapter 38).

As a result of the increased understanding of the impact of the kinetic chain on shoulder function, there is an increasing trend to include exercises that target the re-establishment of optimal segmental activation and energy transfer when rehabilitating people with musculoskeletal shoulder conditions.[18,21,77] Using the available biomechanical and electromyographic data, those recommending incorporating the lower extremity and trunk do so as a way to mimic more functional kinetic chain sequencing occurring during many daily tasks.[18,21,56,76,110,127] Due to altered global muscle activation patterns observed in some people with shoulder injuries,[18,21,56,127] proponents of kinetic chain exercises as part of shoulder rehabilitation programs do so, suggesting that isolated shoulder exercises may not address the reason for onset, and perpetuation of symptoms.

Including the kinetic chain in shoulder rehabilitation has been advocated by expert clinicians for well over a decade but remains poorly understood and researched.[18,21,56,76,110,127] Despite the numerous theoretical frameworks[18,21,56,76,110,127] and increasing evidence,[27,42,54,57,74,75,85,86,104,112,118,119,134] there is no consensus or certainty if preferential effects exist when taking a more global kinetic chain approach over an isolated exercise approach in the rehabilitation of the shoulder. For example, Borms et al.[14] found that incorporating the kinetic chain during shoulder elevation did not increase serratus anterior muscle activity in people without symptoms, but did increase upper trapezius muscle activity, which then resulted in an "unfavorable" upper trapezius to serratus anterior activity ratio. An expert commentary by Cools et al.[22] reiterated these findings, citing a paucity of evidence to guide clinical practice. As highlighted in Chapter 10, we are faced with many clinical uncertainties, including definitive evidence to support the contention that incorporating kinetic chain exercises is a superior approach than only including local isolated shoulder exercises.

A recent systematic review comparing muscle activity levels between shoulder rehabilitation exercises that integrated the kinetic chain and those that did not in people without symptoms, concluded that involving the kinetic chain may increase axioscapular muscle activity levels, may result in more favorable upper trapezius to lower trapezius activity level ratios, and may reduce the demands on infraspinatus.[104] Consistent evidence favored lower quadrant weight transference methods such as stepping, over commonly advocated kinetic chain integration strategies such as squatting, for eliciting these potentially clinically favorable outcomes in axioscapular muscle activity.[104]

In studies where no significant difference in axioscapular muscle activity was reported between exercises involving the kinetic chain and those that did not, the kinetic chain exercises did not involve fluid weight transference through the lower quadrant. This systematic review evaluated the effect of adding kinetic chain components to shoulder rehabilitation regimes in healthy subjects, as the majority of research has been conducted in this group. It remains to be seen what effect integrating kinetic chain exercises into shoulder rehabilitation for those experiencing symptoms has on shoulder muscle activity levels, ratios and most importantly, symptoms.

References

1. Standring S. Gray's Anatomy: The Anatomical Basis of Clinical Practice, 42nd edition. London: Elsevier; 2020.
2. Ackland DC, Pak P, Richardson M, Pandy MG. Moment arms of the muscles crossing the anatomical shoulder. J Anat. 2008;213:383-390.
3. Ameln DJD, Chadwick EK, Blana D, Murgia A. The stabilizing function of superficial shoulder muscles changes between single-plane elevation and reaching tasks. IEEE T Bio-Med Eng. 2019;66:564-572.
4. Andersson H, Bahr R, Clarsen B, Myklebust G. Preventing overuse shoulder injuries among throwing athletes: a cluster-randomised controlled trial in 660 elite handball players. Br J Sports Med. 2017;51:1073-1080.
5. Bagg S, Forrest W. Electromyographic study of the scapular rotators during arm abduction in the scapular plane. Am J Phys Med. 1986;65:111-123.
6. Basmajian JV, Bazant FJ. Factors preventing downward dislocation of the adducted shoulder joint: an electromyographic and morphological study. J Bone Jt Surg 1959;41A:1182-1186.
7. Bassett RW, Browne AO, Morrey BF, An KN. Glenohumeral muscle force and moment mechanics in a position of shoulder instability. J Biomech. 1990;23:405-415.
8. Bassett RW, Browne AO, Morrey BF, An KN. Glenohumeral muscle force and moment mechanics in a position of shoulder instability. J Biomech. 1990;23:405-415.
9. Beckett M, Hannon M, Ropiak C, Gerona C, Mohr K, Limpisvasti O. Clinical assessment of scapula and hip joint function in preadolescent and adolescent baseball players. Am J Sports Med. 2014;42:2502-2509.
10. Billuart F, Gagey O, Skalli W, Mitton D. Biomechanics of the deltoideus. Surg Radiol Anat. 2006;28:76-81.
11. Blache Y, Begon M, Michaud B, Desmoulins L, Allard P, Dal Maso F. Muscle function in glenohumeral joint stability during lifting task. PLOS ONE. 2017;12:e0189406.

12. Blasier RB, Guldberg RE, Rothman ED. Anterior shoulder stability: contributions of rotator cuff forces and the capsular ligaments in a cadaver model. J Sh Elbow Surg. 1992;1:140-150.

13. Boettcher CE, Cathers I, Ginn KA. The role of shoulder muscles is task specific. J Sc Med Sport. 2010;13:651-656.

14. Borms D, Maenhout A, Cools A. Incorporation of the kinetic chain into shoulder elevation exercises: does it affect scapular muscle activity? J Athl Train. 2020;55:343-349.

15. Bouhlel E, Chelly M, Tabka Z, Shephard R. Relationships between maximal anaerobic power of the arms and legs and javelin performance. J Sports Med Phys Fitness. 2007;47:141-146.

16. Burkhart SS, Esch JC, Jolson RS. The rotator crescent and rotator cable: an anatomic description of the shoulder's "suspension bridge". Arthroscopy. 1993;9:611-616.

17. Chelly M, Herassi S, Shephard R. Relationship between power and strength of the upper and lower limb muscles and throwing velocity in male handball players. J Strength Cond Res. 2010;24:1480-1487.

18. Chu S, Jeyabalan P, Kibler W, Press J. The kinetic chain revisited: new concepts on throwing mechanics and injury. PM & R. 2016;8:S69-S77.

19. Clark J, Sidles J, Matsen F. The relationship of the glenohumeral joint capsule to the rotator cuff. Clin Orthop. 1990;254:29-34.

20. Clark JM, Harryman DT. Tendons, ligaments, and capsule of the rotator cuff. Gross and microscopic anatomy. J Bone Jt Surg 1992;74A:713-725.

21. Cools A, Johansson F, Borms D, Maenhout A. Prevention of shoulder injuries in overhead athletes: a science-based approach. Braz J Phys Ther. 2015;19:331-339.

22. Cools A, Maenhout A, Vanderstukken F, Decleve P, Johansson F, Borms D. The challenge of the sporting shoulder: from injury prevention through sport-specific rehabilitation toward return to play. Ann Phys Rehabil Med. 2020; 101384.

23. Cooper DE, Arnoczky SP, O'Brien SJ, Warren RF, DiCarlo E, Allen AA. Anatomy, histology, and vascularity of the glenoid labrum. An anatomical study. J Bone Jt Surg. 1992;74A:46-52.

24. Dark A, Ginn KA, Halaki M. Shoulder muscle recruitment patterns during commonly used rotator cuff exercises: an electromyographic study. Physical Therapy. 2007;87:1039-1046.

25. David G, Magarey ME, Jones MA, Dvir Z, Turker KS, Sharpe M. EMG and strength correlates of selected shoulder muscles during rotations of the glenohumeral joint. Clin Biomech. 2000;15:95-102.

26. de Castro M, Ribeiro D, Forte F, de Toledo J, Krug R, Loss J. Estimated force and moment of shoulder external rotation muscles: differences between transverse and sagittal planes. 2012;28:701.

27. De Mey K, Dannels L, Cagnie B, Bosch L, Filer J, Cools A. Kinetic chain influences on upper and lower trapezius muscle activation during eight variations of a scapular retraction exercise in overhead athletes. J Sc Med Sport. 2013;16:65-70.

28. Debski R, Sakane M, Woo S, Wong E, Fu F, Warner J. Contribution of the passive properties of the rotator cuff to glenohumeral stability during anterior-posterior loading. J Orthop Res. 1999;17:769-776.

29. Dillman C, Fleisig G, Andrews J. Biomechanics of pitching with emphasis upon shoulder kinematics. J Orthop Sports Phys Ther. 1993;18:402-408.

30. Duranthon L, Gagey O. Anatomy and function of the subdeltoid bursa. Surg Radiol Anat. 2001;23:23-25.

31. Endo Y, Sakamoto M. Correlation of shoulder and elbow injuries with muscle tightness, core stability and balance by longitudinal measurements in junior high school baseball players. Phys Ther. 2014;26:689-693.

32. Eshuis R, De Gast A. Role of the long head of the biceps brachii muscle in axial humeral rotation control. Clin Anat. 2012;25:737-745.

33. Ferrari DA. Capsular ligaments of the shoulder: anatomical and functional study of the anterior superior capsule. Am J Sports Med. 1990;18:20-24.

34. Gabbett T, Jenkins D, Abernethy B. Correlates of tackling ability in high-performance rugby league players. J Strength Cond Res. 2011;25:72-79.

35. Gallino M, B Battiston GA, Terragnoli F. Coracoacromial ligament: a comparative arthroscopic and anatomic study. Arthroscopy. 1995;11:564-567.

36. Gaudet S, Tremblay J, Begon M. Muscle recruitment patterns of the subscapularis, serratus anterior and other shoulder girdle muscles during isokinetic internal and external rotations. J Sports Sci. 2018;36:985-993.

37. Ginn KA, Cathers I, Boettcher C, Halaki M. Analysis of phase can detect differences in muscle recruitment between subjects with and without shoulder pain. J Electromyogr Kinesiol. doi.org/10.1016/j.jelekin.2021.102621

38. Ginn KA, Reed D, Jones C, Downes A, Cathers I, Halaki M. Is subscapularis recruited in a similar manner during shoulder internal rotation exercises and belly press and lift off tests? J Sc Med Sport. 2017;20:566-571.

39. Gowan I, Jobe F, Tibone J, Perry J, Moynes D. A comparative electromyographic analysis of the shoulder during pitching. Am J Sports Med. 1987;15:586-590.

40. Green R, Taylor N, Mirkovic M, Perrott M. An evaluation of the anatomical basis of the O'Brien active compression test for superior labral anterior and posterior (SLAP) lesions. J Sh Elbow Surg. 2008;17:165-171.

41. Guanche C, Noble J, Solomonow M, Wink C. Periarticular neural elements in the shoulder joint. Orthopedics. 1999;22:615-617.

42. Hardwick D, Beebe J, McDonnell M, Lance C. A comparison of serratus anterior muscle activation during a wall slide exercise and other traditional exercises. J Orthop Sports Phys Ther. 2006;36:903-910.

43. Hawley J, Williams M, Vickovic M, Hancock P. Muscle power predicts freestyle swimming performance. Br J Sports Med. 1992;26:151-156.

44. Hess SA, Richardson C, Darnell R, Friis P, Lisle D, Myers P. Timing of rotator cuff activation during shoulder external rotation in throwers with and without symptoms of pain. J Orthop Sports Phys Ther. 2005;35:812-820.

45. Hill A, Hoerning E, Brook K, et al. Collagenous microstructure of the glenoid labrum and biceps anchor. J Anat. 2008;212:853-862.

46. Howell S, Galinat B. The glenoid–labral socket: A constrained articular surface. Clin Orthop. 1989;243:122-125.

47. Hughes PC, Green RA, Taylor NF. Isolation of infraspinatus in clinical test positions. J Sc Med Sport. 2014;17:256-260.

48. Ide K, Shirai Y, Ito H, Ito H. Sensory nerve supply in human sub-acromial bursa. J Shoulder Elbow Surg. 1996;5:371-382.

49. Inman V, Saunders J, Abbott L. Observations on the function of the shoulder joint. J Bone Jt Surg. 1944;26:1-31.

50. Inman VT, Saunders JdM, Abbott LC. Observations on the function of the shoulder joint. J Bone Jt Surg 1944;26:1-30.

51. Jerosch J, Castrol W. Proprioceptive function of the glenohumeral joint. Acta Orthop Scand. 1996;67:9-10.

52. Johnson G, Bogduk N, Nowitzke A, House D. Anatomy and actions of the trapezius muscle. Clin Biomech. 1994;9:44-50.

53. Kapandji I. The Physiology of the Joints. Vol. 1: Upper Limb. 5th edition. Edinburgh: Churchill Livingstone; 1982.

54. Kaur N, Bhanot K, Brody L, Birdges J, Berry D, Ode J. Effects of lower extremity and trunk muscles recruitment on serratus anterior muscle activation in healthy male adults. Int J Sports Phys Ther. 2014;9:924-937.

55. Kennedy M, Nicholson H, Woodley S. Clinical anatomy of the subacromial and related shoulder bursae: a review of the literature. Clin Anat. 2017;30:213-226.

56. Kibler B, McMullen J, Uhl T. Shoulder rehabilitation strategies, guidelines and practice. Oper Tech Sports Med. 2000;8:258-267.

57. Kibler B, Sciascia A, Uhl T, Tambay N, Cunningham T. Electromyogrpahic analysis of specific exercises for scapular control in early phases of shoulder rehabilitation. Am J Sports Med. 2008;36:1789-1798.

58. Kibler W. The role of the scapula in athletic shoulder function. Am J Sports Med. 1998;26:325-337.

59. Kibler W, Ludewig P, McClure P, Michener L, Bak K, Sciascia A. Clinical implications of scapular dyskinesis in shoulder injury: the 2013 consensus statement from the "Scapular Summit". Br J Sports Med. 2013;47:877-885.

60. Kibler W, Press J, Sciasia A. The role of core stability in athletic function. Sports Med. 2006;36:189-198.

61. Kronberg M, Nemeth G, Brostrom L-A. Muscle activity and co-ordination in the normal shoulder. Clin Orthop. 1990;257:76-85.

62. Kronberg M, Nemeth G, Brostrom L-A. Muscle activity and coordination in the normal shoulder: an electromyographic study. Clin Orthop. 1990;257:76-85.

63. Landin D, Thompson M, Jackson M. Actions of the biceps brachii at the shoulder: a review. J Clin Med Res. 2017;9:667-670.

64. Laudner K, Wong R, Onuki T, Lynall R, Meister K. The relationship between clinically measured hip rotational motion and shoulder biomechanics during the pitching motion. J Sc Med Sport. 2015;18:581-584.

65. Lefevre-Colau M-M, Nguyen C, Palazzo C, et al. Recent advances in kinematics of the shoulder complex in healthy people. Ann Phys Rehabil Med. 2018;61:56-59.

66. Lintner D, Noonan T, Kibler W. Injury patterns and biomechanics of the athlete's shoulder. Clin Sports Med. 2008;27:527-551.

67. Lippitt S, Matsen F. Mechanisms of glenohumeral joint stability. Clin Orthop. 1993;20-28.

68. Lorne E, Gagey O, Quillard J, Hue E, Gagey N. The fibrous frame of the deltoid muscle. Clin Orthop. 2001;386:222-225.

69. Ludewig P, Borstad J. The Shoulder Complex. In: Levangie PK, Norkin CC, eds. Joint Structure and Function: A Comprehensive Analysis, 5th edition. Philadelphia: F.A. Davis Co.; 2011:231-270.

70. Ludewig P, Phadke V, Braman J, Hassett D, Cieminski C, LaPrade R. Motion of the shoulder complex orientation multiplanar humeral elevation. J Bone Jt Surg. 2009;91A:378-389.

71. Ludewig P, Reynolds J. The association of scapula kinematics and glenohumeral joint pathologies. J Orthop Sports Phys Ther. 2009;39:90-104.

72. Lugo R, Kung P, Ma CB. Shoulder biomechanics. Eur J Radiol. 2008;68:16-24.

73. MacDonald K, J Bridger, Cash C, Parkin I. Transverse humeral ligament: does it exist? Clin Anat. 2007;20:663-667.

74. Maenhout A, Benzoor M, Werin M, Cools A. Scapular muscle activity in a variety of plyometric exercises. J Electromyogr Kinesiol. 2016;27:39-45.

75. Maenhout A, Praet K, Pizza L, Herzeele M, Cools A. Electromyographic analysis of knee push up plus variations: what is the influence of the kinetic chain on scapular muscle activity? Br J Sports Med. 2010;44:1010-1015.

76. Magarey M, Jones M. Dynamic evaluation and early management of altered motor control around the shoulder complex. Man Ther. 2003;8:195-206.

77. Martin C, Bideau B, Bideau N, Nicolas G, Delamarche P, Kulpa R. Energy flow analysis during the tennis serve: comparison between injured and non-injured tennis players. Am J Sports Med. 2014;42:2751-2760.

78. Massimini D, Boyer P, Papannagari R, Gill T, Warner J, Li G. In-vivo glenohumeral translation and ligament elongation during abduction and abduction with internal and external rotation. J Orthop Surg Res. 2012;7:29.

79. McCann P, Wooten M, Kadaba M, Bigliani L. A kinematic and electromyographic study of shoulder rehabilitation exercises. Clin Orthop. 1993;288:179-188.

80. McQuade K, Borstad J, de Oliveira A. Critical and theoretical perspective on scapular stabilisation: What does it really mean, and are we on the right track? Phys Ther. 2016;96:1162-1169.

81. Mirkovic M, Green R, Taylor N, Perrott M. Accuracy of clinical tests to diagnose superior labral anterior and posterior (SLAP) lesions. Phys Ther Rev. 2005;10:5-14.

82. Mochizuki T, Sugaya H, Uomizu M, et al. Humeral insertion of the supraspinatus and infraspinatus. New anatomical findings regarding the footprint of the rotator cuff. J Bone Jt Surg 2008;90A:962-969.

83. Moore KL. Clinically Oriented Anatomy 8th edition. Philadelphia: Wolters Kluwer; 2017.

84. Moseley H, Overgaard B. The anterior capsular mechanism in recurrent anterior dislocation of the shoulder: morphological and clinical studies with special reference to the glenoid labrum and the glenohumeral ligaments. J Bone Jt Surg. 1962;44B:913-927.

85. Nagai K, Tateuchi H, Takashima S, et al. Effects of trunk rotation on scapular kinematics and muscle activity during humeral elevation. J Electromyogr Kinesiol. 2013;23:697-687.

86. Nakamura Y, Tsuruike M, Ellenbecker T. Electromyographic activity of scapular muscle control in free-motion exercise. J Athl Train. 2016;51:195-204.

87. Pagnani M, Deng X, Warren R, Torzilli P, O'Brien S. Role of the long head of the biceps brachii in glenohumeral stability: a biomechanical study in cadavers. J Sh Elbow Surg. 1996;5:255-262.

88. Palastanga N, Field D, Soames R. Anatomy and Human Movement, 5th edition. Oxford: Butterworth-Heinemann; 2006.

89. Payne L, Deng X-H, Craig E, Torzilli P, Warren R. The combined dynamic and static contributions to subacromial impingement: a biomechanical analysis. Am J Sports Med. 1997;25:801-808.

90. Perry J. Normal upper extremity kinesiology. Phys Ther. 1978;58:265-278.

91. Pieper H-G. Humeral torsion in the throwing arm of handball players. Am J Sports Med. 1998;26:247-253.

92. Pontillo M, Spinelle B, Sennett B. Prediction of in-season shoulder injury from preseason testing in division 1 collegiate football players. Sports Health. 2014;6:497-503.

93. Poppen N, Walker P. Forces at the glenohumeral joint in abduction. Clin Orthop. 1978;135:165-170.

94. Poppen N, Walker P. Normal and abnormal motion of the shoulder. J Bone Jt Surg 1976;58A:195-201.

95. Rahu M, Kolts I, Poldoja E, Kask K. Rotator cuff tendon connections with the rotator cable. Knee Surg Sports Traumatol Arthrosc. 2017;25:2047-2050.

96. Rathi S, Taylor NF, Green RA. A comparison of glenohumeral joint translation between young and older asymptomatic adults using ultrasonography: a secondary analysis. Physiother Theory Pract. 2019;1-9.

97. Rathi S, Taylor NF, Green RA. The effect of in vivo rotator cuff muscle contraction on glenohumeral joint translation: an ultrasonographic and electromyographic study. J Biomech. 2016;49:3840-3847.

98. Reagan KM, Meister K, Horodyski MB, Werner DW, Carruthers C, Wilk K. Humeral retroversion and its relationship to glenohumeral rotation in the shoulder of college baseball players. Am J Sports Med. 2002;30:354-360.

99. Reed D, Cathers I, Halaki M, Ginn K. Does supraspinatus initiate shoulder abduction? J Electromyogr Kinesiol. 2013;23:425-429.

100. Reed D, Cathers I, Halaki M, Ginn KA. Does load influence shoulder muscle recruitment patterns during scapular plane abduction? J Sc Med Sport. 2016;19:755-760.

101. Reed D, Halaki M, Cathers I, Ginn K. Does load influence shoulder muscle recruitment patterns during scapular plane abduction? J Sc Med Sport. 2016;19:755-760.

102. Reed D, Halaki M, Ginn K. The rotator cuff muscles are activated at low levels during shoulder adduction: an experimental study. J Physio. 2010;56:259-264.

103. Reinold M, Wilk K, Flesig G, et al. Electromyographic analysis of the rotator cuff and deltoid musculature during common shoulder external rotation exercises. J Orthop Sports Phys Ther. 2004;34:385-394.

104. Richardson E, Lewis J, Gibson J, et al. The role of the kinetic chain in shoulder rehabilitation: does incorporating the trunk and lower limb exercise regimes influence shoulder muscle recruitment patterns? Systematic review of electromyographic studies. BMJ Open Sports Exerc Med. 2020;6 (1):e000683.

105. Robb A, Fleisig G, Wilk K, Macrina L, Bolt B, Pajaczkowski J. Passive ranges of motion of the hips and their relationship with pitching biomechanics and ball velocity in professional baseball pitchers. Am J Sports Med. 2010;38:2487-2493.

106. Saha A. Dynamic stability of the glenohumeral joint. Acta Orthop Scand. 1971;42:491-505.

107. Sahara W, Sugamoto K, Murai M, Tanaka H, Yoshikawa H. The three-dimensional motions of glenohumeral joint under semi-loaded condition during arm abduction using vertically open MRI. Clin Biomech. 2007;22:304-312.

108. Sangwan S, Green RA, Taylor NF. Stabilizing characteristics of rotator cuff muscles: a systematic review. Disabil Rehabil. 2015;37:1033-1043.

109. Scher S, Anderson K, Weber N, Bajorek J, Rand K, Bey M. Associations among hip and shoulder range of motion and shoulder injury in professional baseball players. J Athl Train. 2010;45:191-197.

110. Sciascia A, Cromwell R. Kinetic chain rehabilitation: a theoretical framework. Rehabil Res Pract 2012;1-9.

111. Sharkey NA, Marder RA. The rotator cuff opposes superior translation of the humeral head. J Bone Jt Surg 1995;23A:270-275.

112. Smith J, Dahm D, Kotajarvi B, et al. Electromyographic activity in the immobilised shoulder girdle musculature during ipsilateral kinetic chain exercises. Arch Phys Med Rehabil. 2007;88:1377-1383.

113. Soames R, Palastanga R. Anatomy and Movement: Structure and Function, 7th edition. Elsevier; 2019.

114. Soslowsky LJ, Flatow EL, Bigliani LU, Mow VC. Articular geometry of the glenohumeral joint. Clin Orthop. 1992;285:181-90.

115. Soslowsky LJ, Flatow EL, Bigliani LU, Pawluk RJ, Ateshian GA, Mow VC. Quantitation of in situ contact areas at the glenohumeral joint: a biomechanical study. J Orthop Res. 1992;10:524-534.

116. Standring S. Gray's Anatomy, 40th edition. London: Elsevier; 2008.

117. Steinbeck J, Liljenqvist U, Jerosch J. The anatomy of the glenohumeral ligamentous complex and its contribution to anterior shoulder stability. J Sh Elbow Surg. 1998;7:122-126.

118. Tsuruike M, Ellenbecker T. Serratus anterior and lower trapezius muscle activities during multi-joint isotonic scapular exercises and isometric contractions. J Athl Train. 2015;50:199-210.

119. Uhl T, Muir T, Lawson L. Electromyographic assessment of passive, active assisted and active shoulder rehabilitation exercises. Am J Phys Med Rehabil. 2010;2:132-141.

120. Vahlensieck M, Haack Ka, Schmidt HM. Two portions of the supraspinatus muscle: a new finding about the muscle's macroscopy by dissection and magnetic resonance imaging. Surg Radiol Anat. 1994;16:101-104.

121. van Linge B, Mulder JD. Function of the supraspinatus muscle and its relation to the supraspinatus syndrome: an experimental study in man. J Bone Jt Surg. 1963;45B:750-754.

122. Vangsness C, Ennis M, Taylor J, Atkinson R. Neural anatomy of the glenohumeral ligaments, labrum and subacromial bursa. Arthroscopy. 1995;11:180-184.

123. Warner J, Caborn D, Berger R, Fu F, Seel M. Dynamic capsuloligamentous anatomy of the glenohumeral joint. J Sh Elbow Surg. 1993;2:115-133.

124. Wattanaprakornkul D, Cathers I, Halaki M, Ginn KA. The rotator cuff muscles have a direction specific recruitment pattern during shoulder flexion and extension exercises. J Sc Med Sport. 2011;14:376-382.

125. Wattanaprakornkul D, Halaki M, Boettcher C, Cathers I, Ginn K. A comprehensive

analysis of muscle recruitment patterns during shoulder flexion: an electromyographic study. Clin Anatomy. 2011;24:619-626.

126. Wickham J, Pizzari T, Stansfeld K, Burnside A, Watson L. Quantifying 'normal' shoulder muscle activity during abduction. J Electromyogr Kinesiol. 2010;20:212-222.

127. Wilk K, Arrigo A, Hooks T, Andrews J. Rehabilitation of the overhead athlete: there is more to it than just external/internal rotation strengthening. PM & R. 2016;8:S78-S90.

128. Williamson PM, Hanna P, Momenzadeh K, et al. Effect of rotator cuff muscle activation on glenohumeral kinematics: a cadaveric study. J Biomech. 2020;105:109798.

129. Witherspoon J, Smirnova I, McIff T. Neuroanatomical distribution of mechanoreceptors in the human cadaveric shoulder capsule and labrum. J Anat. 2014;225:337-345.

130. Wright A, Wassinger C, Frank M, Michener L, Hegedus E. Diagnostic accuracy of scapular physical examination tests for shoulder disorders: a systematic review. Br J Sports Med. 2013;47:886-892.

131. Wuelker N, Korell M, Thren K. Dynamic glenohumeral joint stability. J Sh Elbow Surg. 1998;7:43-52.

132. Wuelker N, Plitz W, Roetman B, Wirth CJ. Function of the supraspinatus muscle: abduction of the humerus studied in cadavers. Acta Orthop Scand. 1994;65:442-446.

133. Wuelker N, Wirth CJ, Plitz W, Roetman B. A dynamic shoulder model: reliability testing and muscle force study. J Biomech. 1995;28:489-499.

134. Yamauchi Y, Hasegawa S, Matsumura A, Nakamura M, Ibuki S, Ichihashi N. The effect of trunk rotation during shoulder exercises on activity of the scapula muscles and scapular kinematics. J Sh Elbow Surg. 2015;24:955-964.

5 Lifestyle factors

Graham Burne, Michael Mansfield, Lennard Voogt, Jessica Dukes, Jeremy Lewis

Introduction

Due to associated morbidity and often slow and incomplete resolution of symptoms, shoulder pain presents a substantial challenge for individuals and healthcare providers.[121] Our contemporary understanding of shoulder pain as a personal, complex and heterogeneous experience for a given individual challenges the traditional biomedical approach,[169] and strongly supports embracing a more comprehensive, person-centered, biopsychosocial model of care.[69-71,143] Most nontraumatic diseases or conditions, such as diabetes, hypertension, and depression, as well as idiopathic shoulder pain, appear to evolve as a consequence of multiple, complex and interwoven factors.[195] Therefore offering a single intervention, such as an injection, or an exercise program, or surgery, to treat the person presenting with shoulder pain, arguably would not represent best care.

Lifestyle is a manner of living that involves interests, beliefs, opinions, and behaviors. An individual may have varying amounts of control of their lifestyle, ranging from substantial control to almost none. No one has total control. Lifestyles may be classified as healthy or unhealthy. Determining if a lifestyle is healthy or not is complex, and in part is based upon research evidence, societal and cultural norms, governmental policy, industry, media, environmental, economic, and personal factors, and social determinants of health. Subsequently, ascribing individual blame for a lifestyle choice deemed to be unhealthy is indisputably inappropriate. Due to its complexity in cause and solution, resolving the burden imposed by unhealthy lifestyles is a "super wicked" problem.[120]

Lifestyles deemed to be unhealthy have become increasingly recognized as factors that may cause, contribute to, be associated with, or be a consequence of, musculoskeletal-related health concerns.[158] Therefore addressing unhealthy lifestyles with appropriate behavioral interventions (see Chapter 13) must be considered as part of the management plan for an individual presenting with musculoskeletal shoulder pain.

Smoking, excessive alcohol consumption, poor diet, inadequate sleep, physical inactivity, and obesity, individually, or in combination, are behaviors associated with unhealthy lifestyles. There are myriad ways of defining and describing healthy and unhealthy lifestyles. One term that is being used with increasing frequency is metabolic health. Metabolism involves all the biochemical process that occur within in our bodies to maintain life. As such, defining metabolic health is complicated. Good metabolic health has been described as having natural (i.e., not medicine-controlled) and ideal levels of blood sugar, blood pressure, levels of fat in the blood (triglycerides and cholesterol), and ideal waist measurement (no excess visceral fat). Healthy lifestyles contribute to good metabolic health. Only 12% of adults living in the USA are metabolically healthy, implying 7 in 8 are not.[11]

Unhealthy lifestyles may lead to poor metabolic health, which will increase the risk of being diagnosed with a lifestyle-related metabolic disorder (LRMD). LRMDs include disorders of glucose metabolism, such as diabetes and hyperglycemia, and lipid metabolism, such as hypercholesterolemia and dyslipidemia. The term metabolic syndrome (MetS) is used to describe the combination of diabetes, hypertension and obesity, and being diagnosed with MetS increases the risk of cardiovascular disease and stroke.[64,107] MetS, unhealthy lifestyle behaviors, and poor metabolic health are associated with musculoskeletal disorders, including those involving the shoulder.[33] In this chapter we use the term LRMDs, and we define it as an unhealthy lifestyle with the increased risk of being diagnosed with one or more metabolic disorders.

LRMDs are not only established risk factors for noncommunicable diseases (NCDs) such as type II diabetes mellitus (T2DM), and cardiovascular disease (CVD), but also neurodegenerative diseases and cancer.[184] Research evidence suggests that lifestyle factors such as physical inactivity, obesity, T2DM, poor sleep, poor diet, and smoking, are associated with persistent pain.[47] As such, targeting modifiable lifestyle factors may contribute to improved outcomes for people seeking care for musculoskeletal shoulder conditions, and should form an integral part of management in nonsurgical and surgical management.[117] However, it must be acknowledged that our understanding of LRMDs and shoulder pain is still at an early stage.

Rotator cuff related shoulder pain (RCRSP) was a term proposed by Lewis[121] and involves the rotator cuff muscles, their concomitant tendons, bone interfaces, surrounding bursa, and complex pain neurophysiology. It is an overarching term suggested to replace subacromial impingement syndrome, rotator cuff tendinopathy, and partial and full thickness rotator cuff tears. RCRSP is the most common musculoskeletal condition involving the shoulder (see Chapter 19) and is usually managed with advice, exercise therapy, injections, and surgery. LRMDs may contribute to the onset and perpetuation of RCRSP, and vice versa.[54] As such, potential interactions between LRMDs and musculoskeletal conditions are an important consideration when managing RCRSP.[199] This chapter discusses the potential interdependence of LRMDs and musculoskeletal pain and disability, focusing on RCRSP.

Lifestyle and musculoskeletal conditions involving the shoulder

Lifestyle factors, such as poor diet, cigarette smoking, poor sleep and physical inactivity contribute to metabolic disease,[29] and the resulting LRMDs detrimentally impact on physical and mental well-being, participation in valued activities, and on an individual's quality of life. LRMDs pose escalating harm to the current and future health of all societies and this crisis is now a global health priority.[189] Although LRMDs have an acknowledged pathophysiological link to CVD and T2DM, musculoskeletal complications that potentially result from LRMDs are not as well researched or considered.[47] In the same manner lifestyle education and support for behavioral change is essential in the management of cardiovascular, respiratory, mental health, and neurological conditions, it should also be essential in the management of musculoskeletal conditions, including those involving the shoulder. The potential shared causality of LRMDs and musculoskeletal disease is often given inadequate or no attention in healthcare training, and subsequently it is only given limited consideration in clinical practice.[38,129,138,141] Addressing lifestyle factors in a sensitive manner should become the norm for every clinical encounter with people seeking care for musculoskeletal shoulder problems.[207] This would undoubtedly contribute to improving the health of the individual, and contribute to healthcare sustainability by reducing the financial burden of care.

Research has established a link between RCRSP and LRMDs such as obesity, body mass index (BMI) and central adiposity,[57,67,82,165,166,173,193,197,203] insulin resistance,[46,115,126,147,164,191,197] hypertension,[10,81,123] CVD,[10,197] dyslipidemia,[4,35,112] MetS,[33,165] smoking, [17,26,28,37,53,106,172,197] and alcohol intake.[159] The emerging interpretation is that LRMDs lead to metabolically mediated damage to musculoskeletal tissues through a pathophysiologic non-resolving systemic inflammatory state that influences healing and pain resolution.[21,174,175,209]

Inflammation is integral to the development and perpetuation of LRMDs.[201] Inflammation is a coordinated and complex response to harmful stimuli, and aims to restore body function back to its normal homeostatic baseline. Classic inflammation is described as the principal response of the body invoked to deal with injuries, the hallmarks of which include tumor (swelling), rubor (redness), dolor (pain) and calor (heat).[114] This short-term adaptive response is a crucial component of tissue repair and involves integration of many complex signals in distinct cell regulation.[65] The traditional features commonly associated with inflammation do not apply to LRMDs.[118] Persistent inflammatory states do not benefit from the contribution to healing afforded by acute inflammation, as reported in many LRMDs including MetS, hypertension, T2DM, obesity and dyslipidemia.[59,103,118] They also adversely affect outcomes of people diagnosed with SARS-CoV-2 (COVID-19).[8,157,208]

Furthermore, exogenous exposure to pro-inflammatory cytokines, or endogenous high levels of pro-inflammatory cytokines, is associated with damage across all musculoskeletal tissues.[47] An exposome is the measure of all the exposures of an individual in a lifetime and how those exposures relate to health. An individual's exposure begins before birth and includes exposures from environmental and occupational sources.[206]

What is chronic low-grade inflammation?

Inflammation is involved in the pathogenesis of many LRMDs. The cause of this inflammation is multifactorial with few, if any, of the classic features of inflammation observed. Therefore, it would be useful to set out a distinct form or subclass of inflammation, sometimes referred to as "metainflammation",[59] "low-grade" or "chronic low-grade inflammation" (CLGI). CLGI has key differences to a classic inflammatory response.[140]

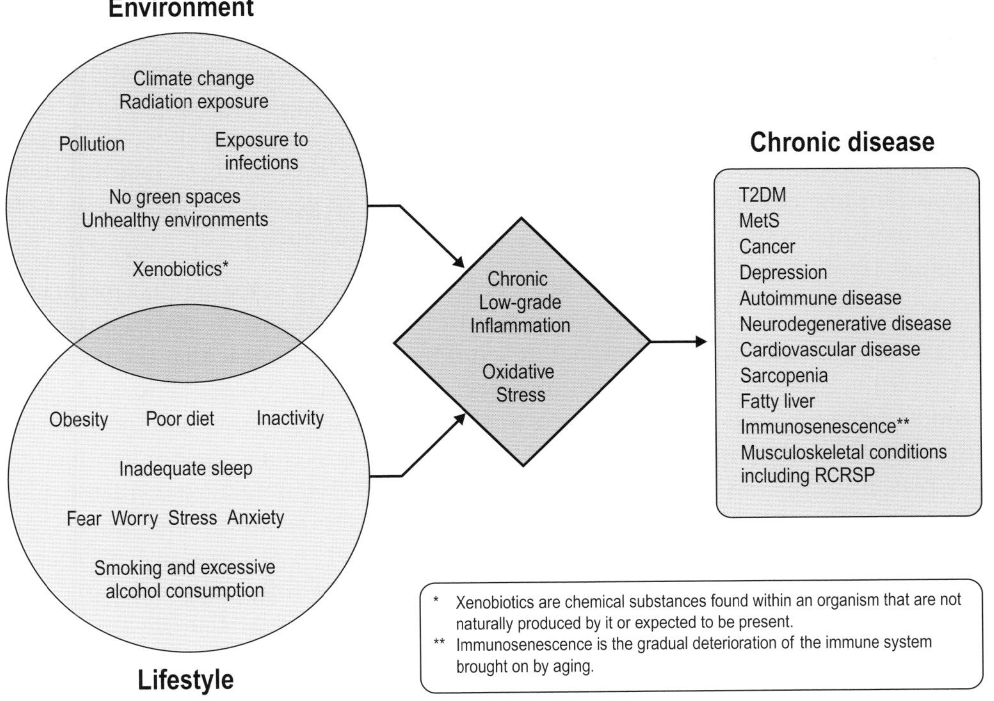

FIGURE 5.1
The potential relationship between an individual's exposome, including unhealthy lifestyle behaviors, leading to chronic low-grade inflammation (CLGI), resulting in persistent disease, including RCRSP.[33]

T2DM, type 2 diabetes mellitus; RCRSP, rotator cuff related shoulder pain.

Figure 5.1 illustrates the potential relationship between an individual's exposome, including unhealthy lifestyle behaviors, leading to CLGI, resulting in persistent disease, including RCRSP. Table 5.1 details the differences between acute inflammation and CLGI.

Low-grade systemic inflammation is characterized by subtly elevated acute-phase proteins, elevated levels of active inflammatory cytokines and oxidative stress,[5,79,103,118,133,156,178] with reduced numbers of neutrophils classically associated with acute inflammation.[39] Systemic metabolic stress such as altered lipid metabolism and insulin sensitivity promotes CLGI, which has been associated with disease risk and/or progression of musculoskeletal conditions such as osteoarthritis, and cervical and low back pain.[96,97,135,136,170,202] Compared to acute inflammation, CLGI: increases inflammatory markers marginally with ensuing chronic, rather than acute, allostasis; exerts effects systemically rather than locally; and, most of its characteristics tend to perpetuate disease.[95,140] Stress and anxiety, reduced sleep, sedentary living, smoking, and high glycemic index foods promote cellular release of inflammatory mediators, most notably the pro-inflammatory cytokines such as interleukin-1β (IL-1),

Table 5.1 Acute inflammation versus chronic low-grade systemic inflammation[66]

	Acute inflammation	Chronic low-grade systemic inflammation
Trigger	Infection, cellular stress, trauma	"Exposome", metabolic dysfunction, tissue damage, environment
Tissue injury	Present	Absent
Duration	Short-term	Persistent, non-resolving
Location	Local	Systemic
Magnitude	High-grade	Low-grade
Outcomes	Healing, tissue repair	Collateral damage, i.e., oxidative stress
Impact on lifestyle	Yes	Yes
Biomarkers	IL-1, IL-6, TNF-α, CRP – accepted biomarkers that predict morbidity or mortality	Silent – no standard biomarker able to predict morbidity or mortality

"Exposome", the measure of all the exposures of an individual in a lifetime and how those exposures relate to health.
CRP, C-reactive protein; IL-1, interleukin-1β, IL-6, interleukin-6; TNF-α, tumor necrosis factor-α.

interleukin-6 (IL-6), tumor necrosis factor-α (TNF-α), adiponectin, and restinin, while depressing anti-inflammatory cytokines (interleukin-4 and interleukin-10).[128] These individually or collectively interact with various biological processes that suppress or enhance inflammation.[3,162,167] In other words, immune cells release the same mediators whether there is overt tissue injury or noxious homeostatic challenges, such as adiposity, diabetes, inadequate sleep, stress and anxiety, smoking and a high glycemic meal.[24,99,113,131,132,154,155,177]

While we readily recognize the effect of inflammation in the acute phase processes, CLGI is not typically considered as a factor that may perpetuate the symptoms in musculoskeletal conditions.[19,170] For those with RCRSP, the ongoing detrimental impact of CLGI may be a reason for the less-than-ideal reduction in symptoms associated with common interventions: exercise, injections, and surgery. Raised circulating proinflammatory cytokines may aggravate shoulder symptoms by maintaining inflammation. Moreover, they play a crucial role in the apoptosis process, particularly in that induced by oxidative stress, leading to tendon degeneration.[203] Addressing CLGI through lifestyle behavioral change (see Chapter 13) may contribute to reducing symptoms and disability, and may contribute to reducing the need for injections and surgery.

Lifestyle-related metabolic disorders and chronic low-grade inflammation in relation to rotator cuff related shoulder pain

While causality has not been established, associations between CLGI biomarkers and RCRSP may exist. The impact by which LRMDs and CLGI may contribute to RCRSP is unclear but potential mechanisms are explored in the following section.

Adiposity, insulin resistance and dyslipidemia

Excess adiposity (fat tissue) is not an inert passive structure but a dynamic, metabolically active organ.[19] It secretes biologically active molecules – adipokines, chemokines, and inflammatory proteinoids – which individually or collectively interact with various biological processes that suppress or enhance inflammation.[3,162,167] Adipokines such as IL-1, IL-6 and TNF-α are classic pro-inflammatory cytokines released from fatty tissue. Increased expression of IL-1 and IL-6 has been observed in the subacromial bursa of people undergoing rotator cuff surgery.[27,198] Associations have also been found between increased expression of TNF-α within the subacromial bursa analyzed after rotator cuff surgery.[50] Concomitantly, reduced levels of interleukin-10 (IL-10) have been detected in people who are obese, have dyslipidemia, and insulin resistance.[13]

IL-10 is an anti-inflammatory cytokine that modulates the immune system by antagonizing the activities of pro-inflammatory cytokines.[182] It is possible that the increased pro-inflammatory adipocytokine expression and anti-inflammatory adipocytokine suppression is a risk factor for developing RCRSP.[166] Hyperglycemia is pro-inflammatory and results in the release of inflammatory mediators and cytokines. Glucose increases the expression of pro-inflammatory cytokines TNF-α and IL-6. In samples of rotator cuff tendon tissues from people with and without diabetes acquired during surgery to repair partial thickness rotator cuff tears, over-expression of IL-6 was demonstrated in people with diabetes when compared with control samples.[43]

Diabetes has been associated with increased risk of persistent rotator cuff tendinopathy.[3,164] In diabetes, advanced glycation end products (AGEs) are precipitated in the tendons of the rotator cuff and may alter the physiological behavior of tendons.[60] This AGE accumulation has been shown to affect collagen crosslinking, reduce proteoglycan content, and activate catabolic cytokines, which lead to tendon thickening and matrix degeneration.[3,34,164] Hence, this cascade may predispose individuals with T2DM to shoulder pain.[3] This deregulation of the tendon matrix is associated with an up-regulation of pro-inflammatory cytokines as the anti-inflammatory actions of insulin are impaired, which may lead to symptoms and functional impairments of the affected tendon.[1] Multifunctional (pro-inflammatory or anti-inflammatory) proteins (leptin, adiponectin, resistin and vistafin) have been identified within the adipocytes. Adipocytes release adipokines such as leptin, adiponectin, vistafin, and resistin as a signaling mechanism, in addition to passively storing energy, which can cause and exacerbate CLGI.[47]

There is an association between leptin and pain related to arthrosis of the shoulder.[68] Leptin is produced by adipocytes, enhancing inflammation by stimulating pro-inflammatory cytokines in pathological conditions such as diabetes.[111] Adiponectin is primarily secreted from white adipose tissue and may have pro- and anti-inflammatory effects. Adiponectin contributes to the prevention of diabetes and CVD. Adiposity may result in relatively low serum levels of adiponectin due to relatively higher serum levels of TNF-α and IL-6 resulting in chronic inflammation.[111] Decreased adiponectin levels may have a central role in conditions such as diabetes and MetS,[109] and may have an association with shoulder pain.[68]

There is uncertainty regarding a relationship between hypercholesterolemia and RCRSP. Longo et al.[127] reported no association between elevated total cholesterol and rotator cuff injury. The mean triglyceride concentration (1.49 mmol/L) was under the threshold of 1.50 mmol/L for 62.5% of subjects to meet the diagnostic criteria required for accumulative LRMDs conditions such as MetS. In contrast, Abboud et al.[4] reported a correlation between rotator cuff tears and increased cholesterol levels, in particular elevated low-density lipoprotein cholesterol (LDL-C) and low high-density lipoprotein cholesterol (HDL-C) levels, in keeping with MetS diagnostic criteria.

The mechanism by which dyslipidemia may be involved with shoulder pain is also unknown. It is hypothesized that due to catabolism of HDL-C, increased LDL-C could initiate and maintain CLGI within the rotator cuff tendon, as shown by in vivo studies on rotator cuff tendon in mice.[2,3] Dyslipidemia is a known precursor to hypertension and CVD.[85] This may contribute to RCRSP, as subsequent endothelial damage caused by hypertension and deregulated lipid metabolism has been associated with tissue damage in tendons.[190] Gumina et al.[81] noted hypertension was associated with a two-fold incidence of large rotator cuff tears, and four-fold incidence of massive rotator cuff tears. The tissue damage in the presence of hypertension has been linked to hypovascularity and hypoxia, ultimately depriving tissues of appropriate nutrient exchange.[139] This deregulation of the tendon matrix may contribute to symptoms and functional impairments associated with RCRSP.[1]

Cigarette smoking

Thousands of chemical compounds are inhaled when smoking a cigarette,[183] including free radicals, metals, tars and other substances that induce inflammatory responses in bodily tissue and increase oxidative stress,[22] most of which exert adverse effects on the cells of the respiratory tract.[186] Apart from contributing to the pathogenesis of chronic respiratory disease,[44] hypertension, CVD and cancer, cigarette smoke is a recognized risk factor for other LRMDs such as atherosclerosis and T2DM.[186]

The pro-inflammatory properties of cigarette smoke are well known.[44,89] Cigarette smoke promotes CLGI by inducing the production of pro-inflammatory cytokines, such a TNF-α, IL-1, IL-6, and IL-8, alongside immunosuppressive properties.[181] Specifically, the effects of cigarette smoke have been related to nicotine, which was shown to decrease anti-inflammatory IL-10 production.[12] The negative effects of cigarette smoke due to nicotine or other substances is not clear.[131] Nicotine and carbon monoxide decrease micro-perfusion and tissue oxygenation, leading to tissue hypoxia,[100,119] and lower cellular oxygen levels are associated with increased tendon degeneration.[20,137,144] This physiological process of dysregulation of cell density could interfere with the assembly and maintenance of a healthy, load-bearing extracellular matrix of rotator cuff tendons.[131]

The imbalance between oxidants and antioxidants resulting from exposure to tobacco smoke leads to oxidative stress, and the increased expression of inflammatory cytokines and decreased expression of anti-inflammatory cytokines may have a negative effect on tendon quality in the rotator cuff. People who smoke are more prone to persistent pain, early-onset rotator cuff tendinopathy (RCRSP), long head of biceps tendinopathy, reduced functional outcome after rotator cuff surgery, and reduced healing ability after surgical repair.[17,22,37,102,110,180]

Depression

Psychological factors such as depression and low pain self-efficacy have been associated with prognostic indicators of poorer outcomes when assessing shoulder pain.[40,73] People with CLGI frequently report poor self-rated health, including depression,[42,98,104,137,145] a known risk factor for persistent pain.[41,171] Pro-inflammatory cytokines influence the production and metabolism of neurotransmitters, such as serotonin and dopamine, which play critical roles in mood regulation.[9] When CLGI has been artificially induced in people through cytokine therapy (interferon, which causes immune cells to release pro-inflammatory cytokines), it can lead to depressed mood, fatigue, lethargy, irritability, social withdrawal, lack of concentration and severe depression, which resolve when cytokine therapy is withdrawn.[98]

The relationship between depression and CLGI appears to be bidirectional: growing evidence posits that CLGI is associated with increased risk of depression,[194] and continued exposure to psychological stressors reciprocally elevate CLGI.[194] A bidirectional relationship between depression and LRMDs also seems to be present, highlighting that there are complex interconnections between CLGI, LRMDs and depression, each having an effect on one another to perpetuate the CLGI state.[36] Depression not only substantially impacts quality of life and elevates CLGI, but it also compromises strategies that may mediate the effects of CLGI. Depression has been shown to impact weight loss, by reducing compliance to treatment or weight management strategies, which may mediate the effects of CLGI when managing RCRSP.[36] Whether CLGI is a driver or result of psychological disorder is unclear.

Clinicians should consider these complex biopsychosocial relationships when caring for a person with shoulder pain, with depression as a co-morbidity.[19] For milder forms of depression, treatment guidelines now recommend addressing lifestyle factors before commencing pharmacotherapy.[134] Clinicians may feel they do not have the competence or support to make appropriate decisions in this area, and formalized signposting or considering behavior change strategies (see Chapter 13) would be well placed within their management of RCRSP. This suggests that taking a true biopsychosocial approach (see Chapter 6), inclusive of the complex multidirectional relationship of lifestyle factors, psychological factors and CLGI, and not just a biomechanical approach to people presenting with shoulder symptoms, including RCRSP, may lead to enhanced outcomes.

Diet

Correlations between poor diet and health problems such as obesity, T2DM and MetS are well known.[58,75] Diets high in red meat, full-fat dairy products, and foods containing highly refined added sugars, starch, and saturated fatty acids may be associated with higher risk of cardiovascular diseases and impaired production of anti-inflammatory cytokines.[58,75,146,179] High-fat meals, those rich in saturated fats, may increase levels of pro-inflammatory cytokines such as IL-18, and may be associated with the increased risk of oxidative stress and inflammation.[75,146] Increased levels of IL-6 as a consequence of suboptimal diet negatively impacts insulin resistance in men, and obese men and women.[58,179]

Encouraging consumptions of fruit, vegetables and fiber can support reducing the risk of cardiovascular disease and CLGI.[142,179] There is no specific or universally accepted diet to treat inflammation.[58] However, evolving research has led to some promising findings in weight management, lower pro-inflammatory cytokine levels, reduced insulin resistance, and total levels of cholesterol and decreased prevalence of MetS when dietary patterns included more whole grains, vegetables, nuts and olive oil.[58,142]

Psychological stress

Psychological stress has a negative impact on cardiovascular disease and CLGI.[149,185] Cytokines respond to mental stress; the production of pro-inflammatory cytokines such as IL-6, TNF-α and IL-1 are associated with poor working environments, academic examinations, and acute trauma in adults.[185] This suggests that CLGI may be involved in the pathways by which psychosocial factors influence cardiovascular disease risk and other pain states. It is important to appreciate that there will be differences in the production and regulation of cytokines associated with CLGI, which may impact on the severity of symptoms. Developing robust strategies to identify and manage psychological stress can be complex and requires a coordinated approach.

Sleep health

Sleep serves to optimize and maintain homeostasis across myriad physiological systems,[61] and is essential for immune, cardiovascular, neurological, and musculoskeletal system function.[176] Reduced sleep is associated with CLGI and increased pain.[84,99,196] Two to seven days of sleep deprivation is associated with variations in IL-6, IL-1, IL-17 (interlueukin-17), CRP and TNF-α levels in adults.[84,196] Long-term sleep restriction may lead to reduction in immune system effectiveness.[84,99,148,149]

Although suboptimal sleep is common in musculoskeletal conditions,[16] its impact on development, perpetuation, recurrence, and persistence of symptoms is yet to be understood.[52] Disturbed sleep is often regarded as the consequence of musculoskeletal conditions, but there is evidence to suggest that poor sleep may be an independent risk factor for musculoskeletal symptoms.[6] Further, a bidirectional relationship has been established between poor sleep and pain; however, sleep disturbances may be a more reliable predictor of pain than pain is for predicting poor sleep.[61] In addition, poor sleep has been found to increase the likelihood of experiencing lower back pain by 52%,[7] and can predict both changes in pain,[108] and the progression of local musculoskeletal symptoms to widespread pain.[205] Mechanisms hypothesized to cause this include down-regulation of endogenous opioid pathways, changes in immune system function,[23] and an increase in pro-inflammatory cytokines.[78,88,160]

Sleep disturbance is experienced by many people diagnosed with RCRSP,[74,130] with one systematic review reporting significant improvements in sleep quality following rotator cuff tendon repairs.[125] Equivocally, two observational studies reported no correlation between sleep quality and rotator cuff full thickness tears or tendinopathy.[105,168] Reyes et al.[168] did report that massive rotator cuff tears (with retraction) were associated with poor sleep. Further investigation is required to determine whether RCRSP leads to poor sleep and/or if poor sleep impacts on the development or prognosis of RCRSP.

Sleeping position has been theorized to be a contributing factor to the development of RCRSP, with possible causative factors being altered blood flow at the anterior humeral circumflex artery[188] and increased subacromial pressures.[204] However, a cross-sectional study failed to find any correlation between sleep position and shoulder pain.[93] Melatonin is a hormone released to promote sleep. There is emerging evidence that melatonin imbalances may play a role in nocturnal pain associated with RCRSP and frozen shoulder.[83] It remains unclear whether rotator cuff tears influence sleep quality.

Whether poor sleep leads to shoulder pain or shoulder pain leads to poor sleep, or if the relationship is bidirectional, or even if a definitive relationship exists, remains uncertain. However, poor sleep, as with poor diet and inadequate physical activity, detrimentally impacts on well-being, and as such, clinicians should consider assessing sleep health as part of routine assessment. If considered to be suboptimal, then strategies to improve sleep should be incorporated in the holistic management of people presenting with shoulder pain. This may require a multidisciplinary team approach and needs to consider: stress and anxiety; physical activity levels; timing, portion size, and type of food intake; alcohol, caffeine, and smoking use and behavior; adiposity; sleep timing and regularity, shift work, travel across time zones, and sleep environment. Many of these factors are modifiable and although additional research is required, they should be considered as targets for management as part of a holistic, individualized, person-centered plan.

Physical inactivity

Physical inactivity and CLGI appear to be associated.[51] A direct link between physical inactivity and accumulation of visceral fat has been established,[200] demonstrating inactive people accumulate visceral fat, without a change in total fat mass.[18,25,76] Visceral fat has a stronger association with increased risk of developing metabolic disorders (hypertension, dyslipidemia, insulin resistance) and CVD.[14] Adults who are physically inactive have elevated CRP and adipokine (IL-6 and leptin) levels. This association is reported in objective measures of activity levels and with people that self-report as inactive. Physical inactivity and abdominal adiposity are also associated with CLGI.[32] This places the body and tissues under metabolically induced stress conditions, and subsequent subtle and sustained up-regulation of CLGI. It is possible that the resultant increased pro-inflammatory adipocytokine expression and anti-inflammatory adipocytokine suppression, as discussed, is a risk factor for developing RCRSP.[166]

The cytokine profile induced by physical activity and exercise is typically anti-inflammatory.[161] Physical inactivity may lead to visceral fat accumulation-induced chronic inflammation and is accompanied by fatigue and muscle wasting.[86,92] The associations between persistent systemic inflammation and reduced physical activity are independent of obesity status and adiposity.[66] This may mean that people who are physically inactive, despite optimal obesity status, are at risk of developing and maintaining persistent inflammation. Physically inactive adults have reduced metabolic resistance, with increased levels of C-reactive protein (CRP) and pro-inflammatory cytokines such as IL-6 and TNF-α.[66,86,92] This leads to an immune response with a reduction in T-regulatory cells that may magnify CLGI, and trigger a cascade of inflammation-related pathophysiologic mechanisms, such as endothelial dysfunction and sarcopenia.[66,86,92]

The interaction between IL-6 and IL-6 receptor (IL-6R) may have an interesting bidirectional relationship. In adults who are physically active, IL-6 levels may be down-regulated during exercise, whereas IL-6R levels are up-regulated in skeletal muscle tissue, suggesting IL-6 resistance.[86] This biological balance suggests that adults who are physically inactive may in fact have poor regulation of IL-6 that in turn may contribute to the maintenance of CLGI. Clinicians should consider the impact of facilitating positive behavior change to reduce the risk of developing CLGI, and reverse the negative consequences of physical inactivity.

Multiple agencies and networks including healthcare systems, society, government, media, education systems, social, familial, and occupational networks, local community groups and public health strategies, all have a role to play in reducing the impact of all LRMDs and CLGI on individuals. Table 5.2 details CLGI guidance for clinicians wishing to communicate these issues to people seeking care for their shoulder symptoms (see Chapter 11).

Although associations have been reported, no inference should be made regarding causation. No study to date has reported biomarkers that might represent potential mediators between LRMDs and RCRSP and this requires further research. Furthermore, the evidence supporting the influence of CLGI biomarkers and their association with symptoms in either the acute or persistent stages of RCRSP is lacking.[77] It is recommended that LRMDs be considered within the wider management of RCRSP, including the understanding of underlying pain mechanisms (see Chapter 7) and interactions between psychosocial and work-related factors.[124] Clinicians should, however, remain cognizant of lifestyle behaviors and cardiometabolic status; in particular, how metabolic stress may precipitate CLGI and its potential negative impact on RCRSP. Developing CLGI may vary in time of onset, expression, and impact between individuals, making specific cause–effect relationships challenging to identify. Nonetheless, it is known that CLGI, while nonspecific in terms of symptoms, is the pathophysiological state found in many LRMDs, and may contribute to RCRSP and its perpetuation.

Table 5.2 Predictors of a chronic low grade inflammation state

Lifestyle and related metabolic disorders (LRMDs)	Abnormal value	Systemic response or interpretation?
Obesity		
Women (waist:hip ratio)	>0.85 = high risk	Associated with CLGI
Men (waist:hip ratio)	>1.0 = high risk	
Insulin resistance		
Fasting blood glucose	>200 mg/dL	Associated with CLGI
Metabolic syndrome		
Fasting blood glucose	>100 mg/dL	3 or more (National Cholesterol Education Programme Adult Treatment Panel III (NCEP ATP III) criteria)[80] Associated with CLGI
Triglycerides	>150 mg/dL	
High density lipoprotein (HDL)	<50 mg/dL for women; <40 mg/dL men	
Blood pressure	>130/85	
Waist circumference	>35 inches in women; >40 inches in men	
Lack of sleep	<6 hours	Associated with CLGI
Stress		Associated with CLGI
Sedentary living		Associated with CLGI
Depression		Associated with CLGI
Smoking		Associated with CLGI
Unhealthy alcohol use		Associated with CLGI

CLGI, chronic low-grade inflammation.

Lifestyle-related metabolic disorders and pain

Pain is a complex phenomenon that is influenced by a multitude of interacting and varying factors.[192] Biological, psychological, sociocultural, and lifestyle factors all color individual pain experiences and give them their specific meaning.[30] Pain is a complex phenomenon and cannot be reduced to a single factor. The complexity of pain should be clearly acknowledged and addressed in musculoskeletal rehabilitation.[30] Therefore, biopsychosocial models of pain and disability are recommended clinical guidelines for musculoskeletal rehabilitation, including shoulder rehabilitation.

The specific roles that biopsychosocial factors play in individual shoulder pain problems may differ between individuals and may also vary over time and, hence, their relative relevance may vary during rehabilitation.[15,48] For instance, shoulder pain experienced at a moment in time may be due to inflammatory processes in shoulder tissues and nociceptive activity, that may be modulated by central neurophysiological processes that amplify or suppress this information to varying degrees. Besides that, psychological processes relating to specific pain beliefs or expectations, attention to pain and/or negative emotions, may influence pain intensity during its time course and may be influenced by avoiding or confronting behavioral responses. All these processes have been described within shoulder rehabilitation.[40,49]

Stress, poor sleep, poor eating habits and limited physical activity and/or highly sedentary behavior have been discussed within the context of musculoskeletal pain and rehabilitation.[56,90,151,163] The biology of prolonged psychological distress (increased activity in the hypothalamic–pituitary axis, and sympathetic arousal),[90] poor sleep (increased glial cell activity),[152] limited physical activity and/or sedentary behavior (associated with low grade neuroinflammatory processes) and poor eating habits (increased glial cell activity)[55] may have a negative effect on the biology of pain by facilitating central sensitization, and impaired top-down nociceptive modulation and/or neuroimmunological processes.

The importance of living well

In a prospective study of 23,000 people (aged 35–65 years old),[62] those adhering to four recommendations: 30 minutes of exercise 5 times per week, maintaining a body mass index of less than 30 kg/m^2, no tobacco use, and eating a healthy diet, had an overall 78% decreased risk of developing a chronic disease condition over an 8-year timeframe. Furthermore, in individuals adhering to these four recommendations, there was a 93% reduced risk of T2DM, an 81% reduced risk of myocardial infarction, a 50% reduction in stroke, and a 36% reduction in the risk of the development of cancer.[62]

Given the potential relationship between LRMDs, CLGI and RCRSP, our approach to managing RCRSP needs to broaden beyond injections, surgery and rehabilitation, in combination or in isolation.[19] Since the experience of pain, physical inactivity, and CLGI appear to be interconnected,[51] examples of how improving lifestyle factors may enhance clinical outcomes, including quality of life and pain, need to be discussed with patients.[116]

Physical activity is associated with very few adverse events,[31,72,101] and plays a pivotal role in maintaining health,[87] whereas inactivity is a strong independent risk factor for many persistent diseases,[32] including persistent musculoskeletal pain.[94] A direct link between physical inactivity and accumulation of visceral fat has been established.[18,25,76,200] Physical inactivity and abdominal adiposity are also associated with CLGI,[32] and it is possible that the resultant increased pro-inflammatory adipocytokine expression and anti-inflammatory adipocytokine suppression is a risk factor for developing RCRSP,[166] with physical activity and lifestyle change being a safe and inexpensive way to counterbalance this.[32]

Translation into practice

Healthy living and lifestyle choices address principles that contribute to health, well-being and joy.[45] Sensitively discussing with patients that they may not achieve the anticipated benefits of a particular management strategy (such as rehabilitation, injection, or surgery) that they are hoping for in the presence of CLGI is important. Healthy living is complex, and influenced by environmental and psychosocial factors often outside the control of the individual, such as work and living conditions, health literacy, relationships and responsibilities, culture, public policy, media, and social influences.[32] We urge caution and sensitivity when discussing this, and no blame should be attributed to the individual.

People diagnosed with RCRSP should derive considerable confidence that exercise therapy is associated with successful outcomes.[121,122] We argue that persistent RCRSP be considered in the same way we consider most persistent health problems – for example, diabetes, depression, and hypertension. None of these conditions can currently be "cured", but with a combination of diet, lifestyle management (smoking cessation, sleep, stress management, and exercise) supported, if required, with medication, the disability associated with these health concerns may be reduced. No one single intervention works in isolation. In the case of diabetes, once blood sugars are brought within a range we consider normal, it will require a lifetime's management to maintain the improvements achieved. We believe that aligning this philosophy in the management of persistent musculoskeletal conditions generally, and RCRSP specifically, will enhance outcomes.[122]

The degree to which LRMDs and CLGI impact RCRSP is unclear; facilitating healthy living behaviors may have the potential to improve local and systemic outcomes for the individual, including life-long health and well-being compared with invasive interventions and their related sequelae and side effects. Evidence suggests that lifestyle factors such as smoking, physical inactivity, sedentary behavior, stress, inadequate sleep and unhealthy diet play a cardinal role in CLGI and persistent pain.[150,153] Current interventions that partly address one or two lifestyle factor(s) in people with persistent pain, at best offer modest effect sizes in reducing pain and related disability.[63,91,150] Given the many lifestyle factors, research is needed to identify characteristics of those individuals with RCRSP who will require one, or multiple interventions.

Conclusion

Lifestyle factors may detrimentally impact on an individual's quality of life, and burden our healthcare systems.[187] Clinicians should remain cognizant that CLGI[19] may cause, contribute to, or perpetuate RCRSP.[33] Clinicians in the future may be able to identify individual lifestyle factors that are relevant for a given individual, and modification of them may reduce the impact of RCRSP. Until then, we believe that there is a strong case for sensitively discussing, as part of a robust clinical reasoning framework, all potential lifestyle factors that need to be considered to enhance surgical and rehabilitation outcomes in the management of RCRSP.

References

1. Abate M, Di Carlo L, Salini V, Schiavone C. Risk factors associated to bilateral rotator cuff tears. Orthopaedics & Traumatology: Surgery & Research. 2017;103:841-845.
2. Abate M, Schiavone C, Salini V. Sonographic evaluation of the shoulder in asymptomatic elderly subjects with diabetes. BMC Musculoskeletal Disorders. 2010;11:278.
3. Abate M, Schiavone C, Salini V, Andia I. Occurrence of tendon pathologies in metabolic disorders. Rheumatology. 2013;52:599-608.
4. Abboud JA, Kim JS. The effect of hypercholesterolemia on rotator cuff disease. Clinical Orthopaedics and Related Research. 2010;468:1493-1497.
5. Abraham TM, Pedley A, Massaro JM, Hoffmann U, Fox CS. Association between visceral and subcutaneous adipose depots and incident cardiovascular disease risk factors. Circulation. 2015;132:1639-1647.
6. Afolalu EF, Ramlee F, Tang NK. Effects of sleep changes on pain-related health outcomes in the general population: a systematic review of longitudinal studies with exploratory meta-analysis. Sleep Medicine Reviews. 2018;39:82-97.
7. Amiri S, Behnezhad S. Sleep disturbances and back pain. Neuropsychiatrie. 2020;34:74-84.
8. An L, Li W, Shi H, et al. Gender difference of symptoms of acute coronary syndrome among Chinese patients: a cross-sectional study. European Journal of Cardiovascular Nursing. 2019;18:179-184.
9. Anisman H, Merali Z, Hayley S. Neurotransmitter, peptide and cytokine processes in relation to depressive disorder: comorbidity between depression and neurodegenerative disorders. Prog Neurobiol. 2008;85:1-74.
10. Applegate KA, Thiese MS, Merryweather AS, et al. Association between cardiovascular disease risk factors and rotator cuff tendinopathy: a cross-sectional study. Journal of Occupational and Environmental Medicine. 2017;59:154-160.
11. Araújo J, Cai J, Stevens J. Prevalence of optimal metabolic health in American adults: National Health and Nutrition Examination Survey 2009–2016. Metabolic Syndrome and Related Disorders. 2018;17:46-52.
12. Arnson Y, Shoenfeld Y, Amital H. Effects of tobacco smoke on immunity, inflammation and autoimmunity. J Autoimmun. 2010;34:J258-265.
13. Aroor AR, McKarns S, DeMarco VG, Guanghong J, Sowers JR. Maladaptive immune and inflammatory pathways lead to cardiovascular insulin resistance. Metabolism: Clinical and Experimental. 2013;62:10.
14. Atkins JL. Effects of sarcopenic obesity on cardiovascular disease and all-cause mortality. In: Walrand S, eds. Nutrition and Skeletal Muscle. Academic Press; 2019:93-103.
15. Bachasson D, Singh A, Shah SB, Lane JG, Ward SR. The role of the peripheral and central nervous systems in rotator cuff disease. J Shoulder Elbow Surg. 2015;24:1322-1335.
16. Batmaz I, Sarıyıdız MA, Göçmez C, Bozkurt M, Yıldız M, Cevik R. Sleep disturbance in lumbar spinal stenosis. Journal of Musculoskeletal Pain. 2014;22:247-250.
17. Baumgarten KM, Gerlach D, Galatz LM, et al. Cigarette smoking increases the risk for rotator cuff tears. Clinical Orthopaedics and Related Research. 2010;468:1534-1541.
18. Belavý DL, Möhlig M, Pfeiffer AF, Felsenberg D, Armbrecht G. Preferential deposition of visceral adipose tissue occurs due to physical inactivity. Int J Obes (Lond). 2014;38:1478-1480.
19. Bennett JM, Reeves G, Billman GE, Sturmberg JP. Inflammation. Nature's way to efficiently respond to all types of challenges: implications for understanding and managing "the epidemic" of chronic diseases. Front Med (Lausanne). 2018;5:316.
20. Benson RT, McDonnell SM, Knowles HJ, Rees JL, Carr AJ, Hulley PA. Tendinopathy and tears of the rotator cuff are associated

with hypoxia and apoptosis. J Bone Joint Surg Br. 2010;92:448-453.

21. Berenbaum F. Osteoarthritis as an inflammatory disease (osteoarthritis is not osteoarthrosis!). Osteoarthritis Cartilage. 2013;21:16-21.

22. Berk M, Williams LJ, Jacka FN, et al. So depression is an inflammatory disease, but where does the inflammation come from? BMC Medicine. 2013;11:200-200.

23. Besedovsky L, Lange T, Born J. Sleep and immune function. Pflügers Archiv-European Journal of Physiology. 2012;463:121-137.

24. Bierhaus A, Humpert PM, Nawroth PP. Linking stress to inflammation. Anesthesiol Clin. 2006;24:325-340.

25. Biolo G, Ciocchi B, Stulle M, et al. Metabolic consequences of physical inactivity. J Ren Nutr. 2005;15:49-53.

26. Bishop JY, Santiago-Torres JE, Rimmke N, Flanigan DC. Smoking predisposes to rotator cuff pathology and shoulder dysfunction: a systematic review. Arthroscopy. 2015;31:1598-1605.

27. Blaine TA, Kim Y-S, Voloshin I, et al. The molecular pathophysiology of subacromial bursitis in rotator cuff disease. Journal of Shoulder and Elbow Surgery. 2005;14:S84-S89.

28. Bodin J, Serazin C, Roquelaure Y, et al. Effects of individual and work-related factors on incidence of shoulder pain in a large working population. Journal of Occupational Health. 2012;54:278-288.

29. Börnhorst C, Russo P, Veidebaum T, et al. The role of lifestyle and non-modifiable risk factors in the development of metabolic disturbances from childhood to adolescence. Int J Obes (Lond). 2020;44:2236-2245.

30. Brodal P. A neurobiologist's attempt to understand persistent pain. Scand J Pain. 2017;15:140-147.

31. Bruce B, Fries JF, Lubeck DP. Aerobic exercise and its impact on musculoskeletal pain in older adults: a 14-year prospective, longitudinal study. Arthritis Res Ther. 2005;7:R1263-1270.

32. Burini RC, Anderson E, Durstine JL, Carson JA. Inflammation, physical activity, and chronic disease: An evolutionary perspective. Sports Medicine and Health Science. 2020;2:1-6.

33. Burne G, Mansfield M, Gaida JE, Lewis JS. Is there an association between metabolic syndrome and rotator cuff-related shoulder pain? A systematic review. BMJ Open Sport & Exercise Medicine. 2019;5:e000544.

34. Burner T, Gohr C, Mitton-Fitzgerald E, Rosenthal AK. Hyperglycemia reduces proteoglycan levels in tendons. Connective Tissue Research. 2012;53:535-541.

35. Cancienne JM, Brockmeier SF, Werner BC, Rodeo SA. Perioperative serum lipid status and statin use affect the revision surgery rate after arthroscopic rotator cuff repair. The American Journal of Sports Medicine. 2017;45:2948-2954.

36. Capuron L, Lasselin J, Castanon N. Role of adiposity-driven inflammation in depressive morbidity. 2017;42(1):115-128.

37. Carbone S, Gumina S, Arceri V, Campagna V, Fagnani C, Postacchini F. The impact of preoperative smoking habit on rotator cuff tear: cigarette smoking influences rotator cuff tear sizes. J Shoulder Elbow Surg. 2012;21:56-60.

38. Chatterjee R, Chapman T, Brannan MGT, Varney J. GPs' knowledge, use, and confidence in national physical activity and health guidelines and tools: a questionnaire-based survey of general practice in England. British Journal of General Practice. 2017;67:e668.

39. Chatzigeorgiou A, Karalis KP, Bornstein SR, Chavakis T. Lymphocytes in obesity-related adipose tissue inflammation. Diabetologia. 2012;55:2583-2592.

40. Chester R, Jerosch-Herold C, Lewis J, Shepstone L. Psychological factors are associated with the outcome of physiotherapy for people with shoulder pain: a multicentre longitudinal cohort study. Br J Sports Med. 2018;52:269-275.

41. Cho C-H, Jung S-W, Park J-Y, Song K-S, Yu K-I. Is shoulder pain for three months or longer correlated with depression, anxiety, and sleep disturbance? Journal of Shoulder and Elbow Surgery. 2013;22:222-228.

42. Christian LM, Glaser R, Porter K, Malarkey WB, Beversdorf D, Kiecolt-Glaser JK. Poorer self-rated health is associated with elevated inflammatory markers among older adults. Psychoneuroendocrinology. 2011;36:1495-1504.

43. Chung SW, Lee YS, Kim JY, Choi BM, Oh KS, Park JY. Altered gene and protein expressions in torn rotator cuff tendon tissues in diabetic patients. Journal of Orthopaedic Research. 2017; 33(3):518-526.e1.

44. Churg A, Zay K, Shay S, et al. Acute cigarette smoke-induced connective tissue breakdown requires both neutrophils and macrophage metalloelastase in mice. Am J Respir Cell Mol Biol. 2002;27:368-374.

45. Cloninger CR, Salloum IM, Mezzich JE. The dynamic origins of positive health and wellbeing. International Journal of Person Centered Medicine. 2012;2:179-187.

46. Cole A, Gill TK, Shanahan EM, Phillips P, Taylor AW, Hill CL. Is diabetes associated with shoulder pain or stiffness? Results from a population based study. Journal of Rheumatology. 2009;36:371-377.

47. Collins KH, Herzog W, MacDonald GZ, et al. Obesity, metabolic syndrome, and musculoskeletal disease: common inflammatory pathways suggest a central role for loss of muscle integrity. Front Physiol. 2018;9:112.

48. Coronado RA, Seitz AL, Pelote E, Archer KR, Jain NB. Are psychosocial factors associated with patient-reported outcome measures in patients with rotator cuff tears? A systematic review. Clin Orthop Relat Res. 2018;476:810-829.

49. De Baets L, Matheve T, Meeus M, Struyf F, Timmermans A. The influence of cognitions, emotions and behavioral factors on treatment outcomes in musculoskeletal shoulder pain: a systematic review. Clin Rehabil. 2019;269215519831056.

50. Dean BJF, Franklin SL, Carr AJ. A systematic review of the histological and molecular changes in rotator cuff disease. Bone & Joint Research. 2012;1:158-166.

51. Dean E, Gormsen Hansen R. Prescribing optimal nutrition and physical activity as "first-line" interventions for best practice management of chronic low-grade inflammation associated with osteoarthritis: evidence synthesis. Arthritis. 2012;2012:560634.

52. Dean E, Soderlund A. What is the role of lifestyle behaviour change associated with non-communicable disease risk in managing musculoskeletal health conditions with special reference to chronic pain? BMC Musculoskelet Disord. 2015;16:87.

53. Djerbi I, Chammas M, Mirous MP, Lazerges C, Coulet B, French Society For Shoulder and Elbow. Impact of

cardiovascular risk factor on the prevalence and severity of symptomatic full-thickness rotator cuff tears. Orthopaedics & Traumatology, Surgery & Research. 2015;101: (6 Suppl):S269-73.

54. Dominick CH, Blyth FM, Nicholas MK. Unpacking the burden: understanding the relationships between chronic pain and comorbidity in the general population. Pain. 2012;153:293-304.

55. Elma O, Yilmaz ST, Deliens T, et al. Do nutritional factors interact with chronic musculoskeletal pain? A systematic review. J Clin Med. 2020;9:10.

56. Elma O, Yilmaz ST, Deliens T, et al. Nutritional factors in chronic musculoskeletal pain: unravelling the underlying mechanisms. Br J Anaesth. 2020;125:e231-e233.

57. Ertan S, Ayhan E, Guven MF, Babacan M, Kesmezacar H, Akgun K. Medium-term natural history of subacromial impingement syndrome. Journal of Shoulder and Elbow Surgery. 2015;24:1512-1518.

58. Esposito K, Giugliano D. Diet and inflammation: a link to metabolic and cardiovascular diseases. European Heart Journal. 2006;27:15-20.

59. Esser N, Legrand-Poels S, Piette J, Scheen AJ, Paquot N. Inflammation as a link between obesity, metabolic syndrome and type 2 diabetes. Diabetes Research and Clinical Practice. 2014;105:141-150.

60. Fessel G, Li Y, Diederich V, et al. Advanced glycation end-products reduce collagen molecular sliding to affect collagen fibril damage mechanisms but not stiffness. PLOS ONE. 2014;9:e110948.

61. Finan PH, Goodin BR, Smith MT. The association of sleep and pain: an update and a path forward. The Journal of Pain. 2013;14:1539-1552.

62. Ford ES, Bergmann MM, Kröger J, Schienkiewitz A, Weikert C, Boeing H. Healthy living is the best revenge: findings from the European Prospective Investigation Into Cancer and Nutrition-Potsdam study. Arch Intern Med. 2009;169:1355-1362.

63. Foster NE. Barriers and progress in the treatment of low back pain. BMC Medicine. 2011;9:108.

64. Freiberg MS, Cabral HJ, Heeren TC, Vasan RS, Curtis Ellison R. Alcohol consumption and the prevalence of the metabolic syndrome in the U.S. Diabetes Care. 2004;27:2954.

65. Freire MO, Van Dyke TE. Natural resolution of inflammation. Periodontology 2000. 2013;63:149-164.

66. Furman D, Campisi J, Verdin E, et al. Chronic inflammation in the etiology of disease across the life span. Nat Med. 2019;25:1822-1832.

67. Gaida JE, Ashe MC, Bass SL, Cook JL. Is adiposity an under-recognized risk factor for tendinopathy? A systematic review. Arthritis Care & Research. 2009;61:840-849.

68. Gandhi R, Perruccio AV, Rizek R, Dessouki O, Evans HMK, Mahomed NN. Obesity-related adipokines predict patient-reported shoulder pain. Obesity Facts. 2013;6:536-541.

69. Gatchel RJ. Comorbidity of chronic pain and mental health disorders: the biopsychosocial perspective. Am Psychol. 2004:59(8):795-805.

70. Gatchel RJ, Peng YB, Peters ML, Fuchs PN, Turk DC. The biopsychosocial approach to chronic pain: scientific advances and future directions. Psychol Bull. 2007;133:581-624.

71. Gatchel RJ, Turk DC. Criticisms of the biopsychosocial model in spine care: creating and then attacking a straw person. Spine (Phila Pa 1976). 2008:2831-2836.

72. Geneen LJ, Moore RA, Clarke C, Martin D, Colvin LA, Smith BH. Physical activity and exercise for chronic pain in adults: an overview of Cochrane Reviews. Cochrane Database Syst Rev. 2017;1:CD011279.

73. Gill TK, Taylor AW, Hill CL, Shanahan EM, Buchbinder R. Shoulder pain in the community: an examination of associative factors using a longitudinal cohort study. Arthritis Care and Research. 2013;65:2000-2007.

74. Gillespie MA, Mącznik A, Wassinger CA, Sole G. Rotator cuff-related pain: Patients' understanding and experiences. Musculoskeletal Science and Practice. 2017;30:64-71.

75. Giugliano D, Esposito K. Mediterranean diet and cardiovascular health. Annals of the New York Academy of Sciences. 2005;1056:253-260.

76. Goedecke JH, Micklesfield LK. The effect of exercise on obesity, body fat distribution and risk for type 2 diabetes. Med Sport Sci. 2014;60:82-93.

77. Gold JE, Hallman DM, Hellström F, et al. Systematic review of biochemical biomarkers for neck and upper-extremity musculoskeletal disorders. Scandinavian Journal of Work, Environment and Health. 2016;42:103-124.

78. Grandner MA, Buxton OM, Jackson N, Sands-Lincoln M, Pandey A, Jean-Louis G. Extreme sleep durations and increased C-reactive protein: effects of sex and ethnoracial group. Sleep. 2013;36:769-779.

79. Grundy SM. Metabolic syndrome pandemic. Arteriosclerosis, Thrombosis, and Vascular Biology. 2008;28:629.

80. Grundy SM, Cleeman JI, Daniels SR, et al. Diagnosis and management of the metabolic syndrome. Circulation. 2005;112:2735.

81. Gumina S, Arceri V, Carbone S, et al. The association between arterial hypertension and rotator cuff tear: the influence on rotator cuff tear sizes. Journal of Shoulder and Elbow Surgery. 2013;22:229-232.

82. Gumina S, Candela V, Passaretti D, et al. The association between body fat and rotator cuff tear: the influence on rotator cuff tear sizes. Journal of Shoulder and Elbow Surgery. 2014;23:1669-1674.

83. Ha E, Lho Y-M, Seo H-J, Cho C-H. Melatonin plays a role as a mediator of nocturnal pain in patients with shoulder disorders. JBJS. 2014;96:e108.

84. Haack M, Sanchez E, Mullington JM. Elevated inflammatory markers in response to prolonged sleep restriction are associated with increased pain experience in healthy volunteers. Sleep. 2007;30:1145-1152.

85. Halperin RO, Sesso HD, Ma J, Buring JE, Stampfer MJ, Michael Gaziano J. Dyslipidemia and the risk of incident hypertension in men. Hypertension. 2006;47:45.

86. Hamer M, Sabia S, Batty GD, et al. Physical activity and inflammatory markers over 10 years: follow-up in men and women from the Whitehall II cohort study. Circulation. 2012;126:928-933.

87. Hawley JA, Holloszy JO. Exercise: it's the real thing! Nutr Rev. 2009;67:172-178.

88. Heffner KL, France CR, Trost Z, Ng HM, Pigeon WR. Chronic low back pain, sleep disturbance, and interleukin-6. The Clinical Journal of Pain. 2011;27:35.

89. Hellermann GR, Nagy SB, Kong X, Lockey RF, Mohapatra SS. Mechanism of cigarette smoke condensate-induced acute

inflammatory response in human bronchial epithelial cells. Respir Res. 2002;3:22.

90. Hendrix J, Nijs J, Ickmans K, Godderis L, Ghosh M, Polli A. The interplay between oxidative stress, exercise, and pain in health and disease: potential role of autonomic regulation and epigenetic mechanisms. Antioxidants (Basel). 2020;9:10.

91. Henschke N, Ostelo RW, van Tulder MW, et al. Behavioural treatment for chronic low-back pain. Cochrane Database Syst Rev. 2010;2010:CD002014.

92. Henson J, Yates T, Edwardson CL, et al. Sedentary time and markers of chronic low-grade inflammation in a high risk population. PloS One. 2013;8:e78350-e78350.

93. Holdaway LA, Hegmann KT, Thiese MS, Kapellusch J. Is sleep position associated with glenohumeral shoulder pain and rotator cuff tendinopathy: a cross-sectional study. BMC Musculoskeletal Disorders. 2018;19:1-8.

94. Holth HS, Werpen HKB, Zwart J-A, Hagen K. Physical inactivity is associated with chronic musculoskeletal complaints 11 years later: results from the Nord-Trøndelag Health Study. BMC Musculoskeletal Disorders. 2008;9:159-159.

95. Hotamisligil GS. Inflammation and metabolic disorders. Nature. 2006;444:860-867.

96. Hoy D, Geere JA, Davatchi F, Meggitt B, Barrero LH. A time for action: opportunities for preventing the growing burden and disability from musculoskeletal conditions in low- and middle-income countries. Best Pract Res Clin Rheumatol. 2014;28:377-393.

97. Hussain SM, Urquhart DM, Wang Y, et al. Fat mass and fat distribution are associated with low back pain intensity and disability: results from a cohort study. Arthritis Res Ther. 2017;19:26.

98. Irwin MR. Inflammation at the intersection of behavior and somatic symptoms. The Psychiatric Clinics of North America. 2011;34:605-620.

99. Irwin MR, Carrillo C, Olmstead R. Sleep loss activates cellular markers of inflammation: sex differences. Brain Behav Immun. 2010;24:54-57.

100. Jensen JA, Goodson WH, Hopf HW, Hunt TK. Cigarette smoking decreases tissue oxygen. Arch Surg. 1991;126:1131-1134.

101. Kaleth AS, Saha CK, Jensen MP, Slaven JE, Ang DC. Effect of moderate to vigorous physical activity on long-term clinical outcomes and pain severity in fibromyalgia. Arthritis Care Res (Hoboken). 2013;65:1211-1218.

102. Kane SM, Dave A, Haque A, Langston K. The incidence of rotator cuff disease in smoking and non-smoking patients: a cadaveric study. Orthopedics. 2006;29:363-366.

103. Kassi E, Pervanidou P, Kaltsas G, Chrousos G. Metabolic syndrome: definitions and controversies. BMC Medicine. 2011;9:48-48.

104. Khairova RA, Machado-Vieira R, Du J, Manji HK. A potential role for pro-inflammatory cytokines in regulating synaptic plasticity in major depressive disorder. Int J Neuropsychopharmacol. 2009;12:561-578.

105. Khazzam MS, Mulligan E, Shirley Z, Brunette M. Sleep quality in patients with rotator cuff disease. Orthopaedic Journal of Sports Medicine. 2015;3:2325967115S2325900001.

106. Kirsch Micheletti J, Bláfoss R, Sundstrup E, Bay H, Pastre CM, Andersen LL. Association between lifestyle and musculoskeletal pain: cross-sectional study among 10,000 adults from the general working population. BMC Musculoskeletal Disorders. 2019;20:609.

107. Klatsky AL. Alcohol-associated hypertension: when one drinks makes a difference. Hypertension. 2004:805-806.

108. Koffel E, Kroenke K, Bair MJ, Leverty D, Polusny MA, Krebs EE. The bidirectional relationship between sleep complaints and pain: analysis of data from a randomized trial. Health Psychology. 2016;35:41.

109. Krysiak R, Handzlik-Orlik G, Okopien B. The role of adipokines in connective tissue diseases. European Journal of Nutrition. 2012;51:513-528.

110. Kukkonen J, Kauko T, Virolainen P, Äärimaa V. Smoking and operative treatment of rotator cuff tear. Scand J Med Sci Sports. 2014;24:400-403.

111. Lago F, Dieguez C, Gómez-Reino J, Gualillo O. The emerging role of adipokines as mediators of inflammation and immune responses. Cytokine & Growth Factor Reviews. 2007;18:313-325.

112. Lai J, Robbins CB, Miller BS, Gagnier JJ. The effect of lipid levels on patient-reported outcomes in patients with rotator cuff tears. JSES Open Access. 2017;1:133-138.

113. Lamon BD, Hajjar DP. Inflammation at the molecular interface of atherogenesis: an anthropological journey. Am J Pathol. 2008;173:1253-1264.

114. Larsen GL, Henson PM. Mediators of inflammation. Annu Rev Immunol. 1983;1:335-359.

115. Laslett LL, Burnet SP, Redmond CL, McNeil JD. Predictors of shoulder pain and shoulder disability after one year in diabetic outpatients. Rheumatology. 2008;47:1583-1586.

116. Lee H, Wiggers J, Kamper SJ, et al. Mechanism evaluation of a lifestyle intervention for patients with musculoskeletal pain who are overweight or obese: protocol for a causal mediation analysis. BMJ Open. 2017;7:e014652.

117. Lee JA, Cha YH, Kim SH, Park HS. Impact of combined lifestyle factors on metabolic syndrome in Korean men. Journal of Public Health. 2017;39:82-89.

118. León-Pedroza JI, González-Tapia LA, del Olmo-Gil E, Castellanos-Rodríguez D, Escobedo G, González-Chávez A. Low-grade systemic inflammation and the development of metabolic diseases: from the molecular evidence to the clinical practice. Cirugía y Cirujanos (English Edition). 2015;83:543-551.

119. Leow YH, Maibach HI. Cigarette smoking, cutaneous vasculature, and tissue oxygen. Clin Dermatol. 1998;16:579-584.

120. Levin K, Cashore B, Bernstein S, Auld G. Overcoming the tragedy of super wicked problems: constraining our future selves to ameliorate global climate change. Policy Sciences. 2012;45:123-145.

121. Lewis J. Rotator cuff related shoulder pain: Assessment, management and uncertainties. Manual Therapy. 2016;23:57-68.

122. Lewis J, O'Sullivan P. Is it time to reframe how we care for people with non-traumatic musculoskeletal pain? British Journal of Sports Medicine. 2018;52:1543.

123. Lin K-T, Lai S-W, Hsu S-D, et al. Shoulder pain and risk of developing hypertension and cardiovascular disease: a nationwide population-based cohort study in Taiwan. Journal of Medical Sciences. 2019;39:127-134.

124. Littlewood C, May S, Walters S. Epidemiology of rotator cuff tendinopathy: a systematic review. Shoulder & Elbow. 2013;5:256-265.

125. Longo UG, Facchinetti G, Marchetti A, et al. Sleep disturbance and rotator cuff tears: a systematic review. Medicina. 2019;55:453.

126. Longo UG, Franceschi F, Ruzzini L, Spiezia F, Maffulli N, Denaro V. Higher fasting plasma glucose levels within the normoglycaemic range and rotator cuff tears. British Journal of Sports Medicine. 2009;43:284-287.

127. Longo UG, Franceschi F, Spiezia F, Forriol F, Maffulli N, Denaro V. Triglycerides and total serum cholesterol in rotator cuff tears: do they matter? British Journal of Sports Medicine. 2010;44:948-951.

128. Longo UG, Petrillo S, Berton A, et al. Role of serum fibrinogen levels in patients with rotator cuff tears. International Journal of Endocrinology. 2014;2014:685820.

129. Lowe A, Littlewood C, McLean S, Kilner K. Physiotherapy and physical activity: a cross-sectional survey exploring physical activity promotion, knowledge of physical activity guidelines and the physical activity habits of UK physiotherapists. BMJ Open Sport & Exercise Medicine. 2017;3:e000290.

130. Lowe CJM, Moser J, Barker K. Living with a symptomatic rotator cuff tear 'bad days, bad nights': a qualitative study. BMC Musculoskeletal Disorders. 2014;15:1-10.

131. Lundgreen K, Lian OB, Scott A, Nassab P, Fearon A, Engebretsen L. Rotator cuff tear degeneration and cell apoptosis in smokers versus nonsmokers. Arthroscopy. 2014;30:936-941.

132. Maes M, Song C, Lin A, et al. The effects of psychological stress on humans: increased production of pro-inflammatory cytokines and a Th1-like response in stress-induced anxiety. Cytokine. 1998;10:313-318.

133. Makki K, Froguel P, Wolowczuk I. Adipose tissue in obesity-related inflammation and insulin resistance: cells, cytokines, and chemokines. ISRN Inflammation. 2013;2013:139239.

134. Malhi GS, Outhred T, Hamilton A, et al. Royal Australian and New Zealand College of Psychiatrists clinical practice guidelines for mood disorders: major depression summary. Med J Aust. 2018;208:175-180.

135. Mäntyselkä P, Kautiainen H, Vanhala M. Prevalence of neck pain in subjects with metabolic syndrome - a cross-sectional population-based study. BMC Musculoskeletal Disorders. 2010;11:171-171.

136. March L, Smith EU, Hoy DG, et al. Burden of disability due to musculoskeletal (MSK) disorders. Best Pract Res Clin Rheumatol. 2014;28:353-366.

137. Matthews TJ, Hand GC, Rees JL, Athanasou NA, Carr AJ. Pathology of the torn rotator cuff tendon. Reduction in potential for repair as tear size increases. J Bone Joint Surg Br. 2006;88:489-495.

138. Mayor S. GPs rarely use interventions for weight management in obese and overweight patients, study finds. BMJ. 2015;350:h142.

139. McMaster WG, Kirabo A, Madhur MS, Harrison DG. Inflammation, Immunity, and hypertensive end-organ damage. Circulation Research. 2015;116:1022-1033.

140. Medzhitov R. Origin and physiological roles of inflammation. Nature. 2008;454:428-435.

141. Meijer E, Verbiest MEA, Chavannes NH, et al. Smokers' identity and quit advice in general practice: general practitioners need to focus more on female smokers. Patient Educ Couns. 2018;101:730-737.

142. Melo HM, Santos LE, Ferreira ST. Diet-derived fatty acids, brain inflammation, and mental health. Frontiers in Neuroscience. 2019;13:265-265.

143. Miaskowski C, Paul SM, Cooper B, et al. Identification of patient subgroups and risk factors for persistent arm/shoulder pain following breast cancer surgery. European Journal of Oncology Nursing. 2014;18:242-253.

144. Millar NL, Reilly JH, Kerr SC, et al. Hypoxia: a critical regulator of early human tendinopathy. Ann Rheum Dis. 2012;71:302-310.

145. Miller AH, Maletic V, Raison CL. Inflammation and its discontents: the role of cytokines in the pathophysiology of major depression. Biological Psychiatry. 2009;65:732-741.

146. Miller WM, Nori Janosz KE, Zalesin KC, McCullough PA. Optimal dietary intake for cardiovascular risk reduction. Current Cardiovascular Risk Reports. 2009;3:95.

147. Miranda H, Punnett L, Viikari-Juntura E, Heliövaara M, Knekt P. Physical work and chronic shoulder disorder. Results of a prospective population-based study. Annals of the Rheumatic Diseases. 2008;67:218-223.

148. Mullington JM, Haack M, Toth M, Serrador JM, Meier-Ewert HK. Cardiovascular, inflammatory, and metabolic consequences of sleep deprivation. Prog Cardiovasc Dis. 2009;51:294-302.

149. Mullington JM, Simpson NS, Meier-Ewert HK, Haack M. Sleep loss and inflammation. Best practice and research. Clinical Endocrinology & Metabolism. 2010;24:775-784.

150. Nijs J, D'Hondt E, Clarys P, et al. Lifestyle and chronic pain across the lifespan: an inconvenient truth? P M & R. 2020;12:410-419.

151. Nijs J, Elma O, Yilmaz ST, et al. Nutritional neurobiology and central nervous system sensitisation: missing link in a comprehensive treatment for chronic pain? Br J Anaesth. 2019;123(5):539-543.

152. Nijs J, Loggia ML, Polli A, et al. Sleep disturbances and severe stress as glial activators: key targets for treating central sensitization in chronic pain patients? Expert Opin Ther Targets. 2017;21:817-826.

153. Norde MM, Fisberg RM, Marchioni DML, Rogero MM. Systemic low-grade inflammation-associated lifestyle, diet, and genetic factors: a population-based cross-sectional study. Nutrition. 2020;70:110596.

154. O'Keefe JH, Bell DS. Postprandial hyperglycemia/hyperlipidemia (postprandial dysmetabolism) is a cardiovascular risk factor. Am J Cardiol. 2007;100:899-904.

155. O'Keefe JH, Gheewala NM, O'Keefe JO. Dietary strategies for improving post-prandial glucose, lipids, inflammation, and cardiovascular health. J Am Coll Cardiol. 2008;51:249-255.

156. Odegaard JI, Chawla A. Pleiotropic actions of insulin resistance and inflammation in metabolic homeostasis. Science. 2013;339:172-177.

157. Palmieri L, Vanacore N, Donfrancesco C, et al. Clinical characteristics of hospitalized individuals dying with COVID-19 by age group in Italy. The Journals of Gerontology. Series A, Biological Sciences and Medical Sciences. 2020;75:1796-1800.

158. Parreira PCS, Maher CG, Ferreira ML, et al. A longitudinal study of the influence of comorbidities and lifestyle factors on low back pain in older men. Pain. 2017;158:1571-1576.

159. Passaretti D, Candela V, Venditto T, Giannicola G, Gumina S. Association between alcohol consumption and rotator cuff tear. Acta Orthopaedica. 2016;87:165-168.

160. Patel SR, Zhu X, Storfer-Isser A, et al. Sleep duration and biomarkers of inflammation. Sleep. 2009;32:200-204.

161. Pedersen BK, Akerström TC, Nielsen AR, Fischer CP. Role of myokines in exercise and metabolism. J Appl Physiol (1985). 2007;103:1093-1098.

162. Pietrzak M. Adhesive capsulitis: an age related symptom of metabolic syndrome and chronic low-grade inflammation? Medical Hypotheses. 2016;88:12-17.

163. Polli A, Ickmans K, Godderis L, Nijs J. When environment meets genetics: a clinical review of the epigenetics of pain, psychological factors, and physical activity. Archives of Physical Medicine and Rehabilitation. 2019;100:1153-1161.

164. Ranger TA, Wong AMY, Cook JL, Gaida JE. Is there an association between tendinopathy and diabetes mellitus? A systematic review with meta-analysis. British Journal of Sports Medicine. 2016;50:982.

165. Rechardt M, Shiri R, Karppinen J, Viikari-Juntura E, Jula A, Heliovaara M. Lifestyle and metabolic factors in relation to shoulder pain and rotator cuff tendinitis: a population-based study. BMC Musculoskeletal Disorders. 2010;11:165.

166. Rechardt M, Shiri R, Lindholm H, Karppinen J, Viikari-Juntura E. Associations of metabolic factors and adipokines with pain in incipient upper extremity soft tissue disorders: a cross-sectional study. BMJ Open. 2013;3:10.

167. Rechardt M, Viikari-Juntura E, Shiri R. Adipokines as predictors of recovery from upper extremity soft tissue disorders. Rheumatology. 2014;53:2238-2242.

168. Reyes BA, Hull BR, Kurth AB, Kukowski NR, Mulligan EP, Khazzam MS. Do magnetic resonance imaging characteristics of full-thickness rotator cuff tears correlate with sleep disturbance? Orthopaedic Journal of Sports Medicine. 2017;5:2325967117735319.

169. Ristori D, Miele S, Rossettini G, Monaldi E, Arceri D, Testa M. Towards an integrated clinical framework for patient with shoulder pain. Archives of Physiotherapy. 2018;8:7.

170. Robinson WH, Lepus CM, Wang Q, et al. Low-grade inflammation as a key mediator of the pathogenesis of osteoarthritis. Nature reviews. Rheumatology. 2016;12:580-592.

171. Rubin DI. Epidemiology and risk factors for spine pain. Neurol Clin. 2007;25:353-371.

172. Safran MR, Graham SM. Distal biceps tendon ruptures: incidence, demographics, and the effect of smoking. Clin Orthop Relat Res. 2002;275-283.

173. Sansone V, Consonni O, Maiorano E, Meroni R, Goddi A. Calcific tendinopathy of the rotator cuff: the correlation between pain and imaging features in symptomatic and asymptomatic female shoulders. Skeletal Radiology. 2016;45:49-55.

174. Seaman DR. Body mass index and musculoskeletal pain: is there a connection? Chiropractic & Manual Therapies. 2013;21:15-15.

175. Shiri R, Karppinen J, Leino-Arjas P, Solovieva S, Viikari-Juntura E. The association between obesity and low back pain: a meta-analysis. Am J Epidemiol. 2010;171:135-154.

176. Siengsukon CF, Al-Dughmi M, Stevens S. Sleep health promotion: practical information for physical therapists. Physical Therapy. 2017;97:826-836.

177. Simpson N, Dinges DF. Sleep and inflammation. Nutr Rev. 2007;65:S244-252.

178. Singh AK, Kari JA. Metabolic syndrome and chronic kidney disease. Current Opinion in Nephrology and Hypertension. 2013;22:198-203.

179. Singh RB, De Meester F, Mechirova V, Pella D, Otsuka K. Fatty acids in the causation and therapy of metabolic syndrome. In: Wild-Type Food in Health Promotion and Disease Prevention. Humana Press; 2008.

180. Smuck M, Schneider BJ, Ehsanian R, Martin E, Kao MJ. Smoking is associated with pain in all body regions, with greatest influence on spinal pain. Pain Med. 2020;21:1759-1768.

181. Sopori M. Effects of cigarette smoke on the immune system. Nat Rev Immunol. 2002;2:372-377.

182. Srikanthan K, Feyh A, Visweshwar H, Shapiro JI, Sodhi K. Systematic review of metabolic syndrome biomarkers: a panel for early detection, management, and risk stratification in the West Virginian population. International Journal of Medical Sciences. 2016;13:25-38.

183. Stedman RL. The chemical composition of tobacco and tobacco smoke. Chem Rev. 1968;68:153-207.

184. Stefan N, Birkenfeld AL, Schulze MB. Global pandemics interconnected: obesity, impaired metabolic health and COVID-19. Nature Reviews Endocrinology. 2021;17:135-149.

185. Steptoe A, Willemsen G, Owen N, Flower L, Mohamed-Ali V. Acute mental stress elicits delayed increase in circulating inflammatory cytokine levels. Clinical Science. 2001;101:185-192.

186. Strzelak A, Ratajczak A, Adamiec A, Feleszko W. Tobacco smoke induces and alters immune responses in the lung triggering inflammation, allergy, asthma and other lung diseases: a mechanistic review. International Journal of Environmental Research and Public Health. 2018;15:1033.

187. Sturmberg J. Health System Redesign. How to Make Health Care Person-Centered, Equitable, and Sustainable. Springer; 2018.

188. Terabayashi N, Watanabe T, Matsumoto K, et al. Increased blood flow in the anterior humeral circumflex artery correlates with night pain in patients with rotator cuff tear. Journal of Orthopaedic Science. 2014;19:744-749.

189. The Lancet. Making more of multimorbidity: an emerging priority. Lancet. 2018;391:1637.

190. Tilley BJ, Cook JL, Docking SI, Gaida JE. Is higher serum cholesterol associated with altered tendon structure or tendon pain? A systematic review. British Journal of Sports Medicine. 2015;49:1504-1509.

191. Titchener AG, White JJE, Tambe AA, Clark DI, Hinchliffe SR, Hubbard RB. Comorbidities in rotator cuff disease: a case-control study. Journal of Shoulder and Elbow Surgery. 2014;23:1282-1288.

192. Tracey I, Mantyh PW. The cerebral signature for pain perception and its modulation. Neuron. 2007;55:377-391.

193. Tülay K, Arslan A, Özdemir F, Acet G. Clinical features of patients diagnosed with degenerative rotator cuff tendon disease: a 6-month prospective-definitive clinical study from turkey. Journal of Physical Therapy Science. 2017;29:1433-1437.

194. Valkanova V, Ebmeier KP, Allan CL. CRP, IL-6 and depression: a systematic review and meta-analysis of longitudinal studies. J Affect Disord. 2013;150:736-744.

195. van Hecke O, Torrance N, Smith BH. Chronic pain epidemiology–where do

lifestyle factors fit in? British Journal of Pain. 2013;7:209-217.

196. van Leeuwen WM, Lehto M, Karisola P, et al. Sleep restriction increases the risk of developing cardiovascular diseases by augmenting proinflammatory responses through IL-17 and CRP. PLoS One. 2009;4:e4589.

197. Viikari-Juntura E, Shiri R, Solovieva S, et al. Risk factors of atherosclerosis and shoulder pain – Is there an association? A systematic review. European Journal of Pain. 2008;12:412-426.

198. Voloshin I, Gelinas J, Maloney MD, O'Keefe RJ, Bigliani LU, Blaine TA. Proinflammatory cytokines and metalloproteases are expressed in the subacromial bursa in patients with rotator cuff disease. Arthroscopy. 2005;21:1076.e1071-1076.e1079.

199. Wearing SC, Hennig EM, Byrne NM, Steele JR, Hills AP. Musculoskeletal disorders associated with obesity: a biomechanical perspective. Obesity Reviews. 2006;7:239-250.

200. Wedell-Neergaard A-S, Eriksen L, Grønbæk M, Pedersen BK, Krogh-Madsen R, Tolstrup J. Low fitness is associated with abdominal adiposity and low-grade inflammation independent of BMI. PloS One. 2018;13:e0190645-e0190645.

201. Wellen KE, Hotamisligil GS. Inflammation, stress, and diabetes. J Clin Invest. 2005;115:1111-1119.

202. Welsh P, Woodward M, Rumley A, Lowe G. Associations of plasma pro-inflammatory cytokines, fibrinogen, viscosity and C-reactive protein with cardiovascular risk factors and social deprivation: the fourth Glasgow MONICA study. British Journal of Haematology. 2008;141:852-861.

203. Wendelboe AM, Gren LH, Alder SC, White Jr GL, Lyon JL, Hegmann KT. Associations between body-mass index and surgery for rotator cuff tendinitis. Journal of Bone and Joint Surgery–Series A. 2004;86:743-747.

204. Werner CM, Ossendorf C, Meyer DC, Blumenthal S, Gerber C. Subacromial pressures vary with simulated sleep positions. Journal of Shoulder and Elbow Surgery. 2010;19:989-993.

205. Wiklund T, Gerdle B, Linton SJ, Dragioti E, Larsson B. Insomnia is a risk factor for spreading of chronic pain: a Swedish longitudinal population study (SwePain). European Journal of Pain. 2020;24:1348-1356.

206. Wild CP. Complementing the genome with an "exposome": the outstanding challenge of environmental exposure measurement in molecular epidemiology. Cancer Epidemiology and Prevention Biomarkers. 2005;14:1847-1850.

207. World Health Organization. ICD-10: International Statistical Classification of Diseases and Related Health Problems: Tenth Revision. Geneva: World Health Organization; 2004.

208. Zhou F, Yu T, Du R, et al. Clinical course and risk factors for mortality of adult inpatients with COVID-19 in Wuhan, China: a retrospective cohort study. The Lancet. 2020;395:1054-1062.

209. Zhuo Q, Yang W, Chen J, Wang Y. Metabolic syndrome meets osteoarthritis. Nat Rev Rheumatol. 2012;8:729-737.

6 Integrating a biopsychosocial approach

Rachel Chester, Kieran O'Sullivan, Liesbet De Baets, Tamar Pincus

Introduction

This chapter focusses on the importance of integrating a biopsychosocial (BPS) approach into clinical practice. It begins with an introduction to the BPS model, and a comparison with the biomedical model. This is followed by a summary of the evidence underpinning the association of biopsychosocial factors with the onset, presentation, and outcome of people seeking care for shoulder pain. Common misunderstandings about the "bio" component of the biopsychosocial model are then presented. This is followed by a section exploring differences between yellow and orange flags, when to treat, and when to refer on to experts in mental health. We discuss some of the common challenges faced by practitioners when implementing a biopsychosocial approach. The final section contains tips for practitioners and three case studies from our own practice as examples of integrating a biopsychosocial approach.

The biopsychosocial approach

The biopsychosocial model is a framework that draws together biomedical, psychological and social perspectives to provide an integrated model of health.[13] Although the primary focus of this book is musculoskeletal shoulder pain, the "bio" or "biomedical" in the biopsychosocial model refers to all body systems. The psychological perspective refers to the mind and how it influences thoughts, emotions, and behavior. The social perspective refers to the role of others, for example, family, friends, work colleagues, or health practitioners. It also refers to the cultural, socioeconomic, medicolegal, and physical environment. Taking a biopsychosocial approach means that the clinician becomes "involved in the full range of difficulties patients (people) bring, not just the biomedical."[44]

The traditional biomedical model focuses on diagnosing a pathoanatomical or pathophysiological source of pain and disability, where treatment is expected to abolish pain, correct disability, and restore health for the individual. However, as with other musculoskeletal conditions, such as low back pain, there is not always an identifiable pathological driver for shoulder complaints. When local tissue damage is present, its severity is not generally associated with the individual's perceived shoulder pain and disability.[38] In addition, the relationship between tissue healing and pain is not linear. Pain and disability can regularly outlast the time that damaged tissue requires to recover.[22] In summary, the biomedical model assumes a linear, unidirectional path of cause and effect. Alone it rarely provides an adequate framework to explain the patient's clinical presentation, and their engagement and response to treatment.

A person's experience of their shoulder condition is unique and will be associated with many factors. These include their beliefs, concerns, emotions, previous experience, expectations, work situation, family, and peer influences. Many biological, psychological, and social factors will influence, and in turn be influenced by, the patient's response to their shoulder condition, their ability to cope, remain at work or leisure, and engage with treatment. Rather than being mere confounding factors within a biomedical model, psychological and social factors are integral to being human.

Instead of viewing biomedical and psychosocial factors as mutually exclusive, the biopsychosocial model considers the broad spectrum of factors from cellular to societal level.[13] Since its inception, there have been several adaptations by various authors to the model. These include for example, the biopsycho-ecological model, which emphasizes the importance of the physical as well as the social environment,[45] and the holistic framework, where communication and the therapeutic alliance provide a scaffold for humanistic individualized care, in which the biopsychosocial approach forms themes rather than distinctive well-defined components.[7]

Evidence that psychosocial factors are important

Psychosocial factors may be risk factors to developing shoulder pain in the future, or precipitating factors that trigger the onset of shoulder pain at a specific time point. They can also be associated with, and may predict the natural course of symptoms or the outcome from treatment. In the latter context, some psychosocial factors will facilitate recovery while others will be barriers to the patient's recovery or ability to self-manage.

People with higher levels of pain-related worry and distress, depressive symptoms, feelings of helplessness, pain-related fear, poor sleep quality, or lower expectation of recovery generally report higher levels of shoulder pain and disability.[20,50] A perceived change in symptoms is not only related to changes in biomechanics and biological factors; psychological and social factors are also associated with the improvement and deterioration of symptoms. Patient expectation of recovery, the individual's belief of the extent to which they will improve with a specific treatment or not, is emerging as one of the most consistent predictors of outcome for both shoulder surgery and physiotherapy.[5,9,20,27,28] People who expect a better outcome have less pain and disability at follow-up than those who expect a poorer outcome. This concurs with research for other musculoskeletal regions,[16] and exploring expectations with patients at the earliest opportunity is important.

Another important factor that may predict treatment outcome is the individual's perceptions about their own ability to control, manage and cope with their pain.[9,16,19] This is known as pain self-efficacy, and is an important predictor of patient-rated pain and disability weeks and months after beginning a course of physical therapy.[5,6] Pain self-efficacy is a self-assessment by the patient of their ability to succeed at a specific task, despite their pain.[1] In this context, high self-efficacy can empower a patient to commit, persist, and explore strategies to enable them to face the challenges of shoulder pain.[1] There is currently insufficient research exploring the role of pain self-efficacy as a predictor of positive or negative outcomes for people undergoing shoulder surgery.

The importance of psychological factors may differ according to the treatment. For people undergoing surgery, high levels of pain-related fear before surgery predicts a poor surgical outcome.[9] However, from the research available, this does not appear to be the case for physical therapy (physiotherapy) interventions.[9] This may be because the active management approach used in physical therapy exposes patients to the activities they may fear, and consciously or unconsciously decreases pain-related fear. We recommend appropriately targeting activities associated with pain and fear before and after surgery.

Social factors commonly associated with persistent symptoms, and assessed for those with musculoskeletal conditions, include demographics, social support by friends and family, the strength of the therapeutic alliance, and occupation. The therapeutic alliance, also known as the therapeutic relationship, refers to the relationship between health provider and patient, which is based on trust and whose focus is the patient's needs. Lower socioeconomic status, such as having a low income or a low level of education, have been linked with poorer outcomes,[12,29] as has being involved in ongoing litigation.[14,37] Interestingly, research demonstrates that detailed consideration of social, demographic and patient-reported information alone can predict sick leave in people with shoulder pain so well that the results of imaging investigations provide no further value in this respect.[31]

"Significant others" such as the patient's spouse, partner, parent, children, or friends may be a help or a hindrance in recovery. For people off work, research has shown that significant others can facilitate return to work by providing emotional, practical and participatory support.[42] In contrast, patients whose family and friends are of the opinion that their condition will deteriorate if they return to work are less likely to return to work.[42] This overprotective behavior may unconsciously increase fear, encouraging dependency and attention-seeking behaviors. It may also explain why, for example, some patients at their initial consultation appear enthusiastic about self-management, but at their follow-up appointment appear to have reservations and have not enacted the agreed actions. We recommend exploring the role of family and friends with the patient. Questions to open up the conversation could include for example, "What do you think your partner would think of our plan?" at the first appointment, or "What did your partner think of our plan?" at the follow up.

The beliefs and attitudes of practitioners are also important and may influence the illness perceptions and health behaviors of their patients. There is evidence that patients' attitudes and beliefs often match those of the practitioner treating them. Practitioners who adopt a biomedical rather than a biopsychosocial approach are more likely to advise patients to limit or avoid return to work and physical activities, and their patients are more likely to have increased certified sick leave.[8,15] However, practitioners who build a strong therapeutic alliance, in which they facilitate a shared discussion about the patients' beliefs and attitudes with respect to the patients' shoulder symptoms may achieve better outcomes.

For patients who may feel stigmatized by a biopsychosocial approach, discussing the relationship between biomedical and psychosocial factors and their effect on symptoms may be a useful starting point.[8] It is important to identify if patients are confused by conflicting diagnoses and advice offered by different clinicians, or information they have seen or heard. Questions to open the conversation might include, "Does this match with the explanation your primary care physician (GP) provided?", or, "Is there anything that appears to contradict what you've been told previously?"

Physical and psychological stressors at work are potential risk factors for developing persistent shoulder pain, the risk increasing as the frequency of these stressors increase.[10] High perceived job demands, poor job control and decision latitude, job insecurity, and poor support from supervisors and colleagues are potential risk factors for shoulder pain.[24,47] Physical, biomechanical, and organizational aspects of work are also important. There is evidence of associations between shoulder pain and physical aspects of the work environment, such as overhead work and shoulder load.[39,47,49] These factors (physical, biomechanical, organizational, social, and psychological) can interact and co-contribute to shoulder pain. This may in part explain why single factors in the workplace do not contribute to pain among all employees equally, and why there is a paucity of convincing evidence for an effective treatment approach.[24,47] Psychological and social processes, such as increased pain self-efficacy and perceived social support, may be additional mechanisms by which physical interventions in this context are effective.

The evidence presented in this chapter is a summary of research evidence demonstrating that psychosocial factors are important. However, it is important to acknowledge that the relative importance of any one psychosocial factor, or combination, will differ for the patient in front of you and their unique set of circumstances and biological make up. Do not "write a patient off" because they are experiencing some of the common barriers cited in the research. Work with those factors that appear important barriers or facilitators to recovery and self-management for the individual patient. Box 6.1 summarizes our top tips for exploring psychosocial factors with patients.

Box 6.1 Top tips for exploring psychosocial factors with patients

Questionnaires are sometimes misused to replace real dialogue.

If you choose to use a questionnaire to explore psychosocial factors, we recommend:

- Using individual item responses as an introduction to a topic rather than focusing on total scores.
- Discussing the patient's strengths as well as barriers to recovery.

We prefer asking patients openly about the things that may predict their response to treatment – there are no fixed questions. Examples of questions we use to introduce some key topics include:

Preferences and expectations

- What are your expectations of this appointment?
- How much do you expect your symptoms to change as a result of treatment?
- What do you hope will be different as a result of surgery?

Self-efficacy

- How confident do you feel in your ability to continue at work, despite your shoulder pain?
- How confident do you feel in your ability to carry out these exercises at home?
- How confident do you feel in your ability to stick to the 3-week post-operative immobilization period?

Concerns, worries and anxieties

- Do you have any worries or concerns about your symptoms?
- Do you have any concerns about your symptoms in the future?
- Do you have any concerns about the treatment?

Questions specific to work or leisure

- Can you perform your job as you want?

(Continued)

- How does your shoulder problem affect your sport or leisure activities?
- Do you feel that our plan fits with your home and work commitments?

The role of friends and family

- What does your partner think you should do?
- What do you think your partner would think of our plan?

Conflicting advice from different clinicians

- Does this tally with the explanation your family doctor/surgeon/therapist provided?

Barriers to recovery

- What do you think could get in the way of progress?
- What do you think might help you in your recovery?

The "bio" in the biopsychosocial model

Several chapters within this text discuss specific "tissue" contributors to shoulder pain, either related to acute trauma (e.g., fracture, tendon rupture), or associated with tissue pathology and/or mechanical loading. Rather than revisit these topics, here we reflect on some common misconceptions of the biopsychosocial model and the wider meaning of the "bio" component beyond "issues in the tissues". Even when there is an obvious tissue-based pathology, such as a traumatic fracture of the neck of the humerus, we cannot provide holistic advice and treatment specific to the individual if the impacts on their home, social, and work circumstances have not been explored.

The patient's concerns and beliefs, such as pain self-efficacy and level of confidence to self-manage, goals, and preferences for treatment, are important and may determine whether they choose to follow advice regarding management. Psychosocial factors are highly likely to positively and negatively impact on the outcome, even when there is identifiable tissue damage, for example post surgery[36] or after significant trauma.[3] A contemporary biopsychosocial approach considers all contributory domains, for all patients, with acute or persistent symptoms. In this way, the risk of mind–body dualism is minimized, and management options are based on the patient's needs.

Biological changes with respect to tissue status are important factors to consider when applying mechanotherapy principles, such as progressive tissue loading.[46] However, among people with persistent pain, a host of other biological changes across the endocrine, immune, and nervous systems are evident.[32,51] There is evidence of systemic inflammation among people with poor sleep,[18] high stress,[43] depression,[35] and with particular dietary choices,[2] and the experience of shoulder pain may be associated with comorbid presentations and lifestyle. While there is an appreciation of how lifestyle factors may alter allostatic load in conditions such as hypertension,[30] there is less awareness of the impact in people with persistent pain.[40] There is evidence that exercise can reduce systemic inflammation,[23] however, the mechanisms by which this occurs are uncertain. For example, there is evidence that the beneficial effects of exercise for tendinopathy may not be due to changes in the macro structure of the tendon.[11] This suggests that the biological benefits of exercise-based rehabilitation may be mediated by systemic responses (e.g., lowered inflammation, better mood, better sleep) as well as local responses (e.g., muscle strength, tissue tolerance to load).

In summary, the presence of significant pathophysiology and/or tissue damage does not reduce the importance of psychosocial factors, which are always important to explore. Clinicians need appreciate that "bio" refers to more than macrostructural changes in tissue status.

Making sense of psychological factors

Clinically, identifying the biological cause of symptoms is generally considered of paramount importance in musculoskeletal healthcare, and responding to patients' psychosocial issues is often viewed as a secondary issue. Providing a structural diagnosis, estimating how long symptoms will remain, and what management to consider, commonly dominate the clinical consultation process. Discussion pertaining to recovery expectations, beliefs about symptoms, mood, concerns, and well-being, can easily become optional add-ons once the biomedical picture has been presented. However, exploring psychosocial factors in parallel to physical symptoms may save time, help develop the therapeutic alliance, increase adherence to management, and may lead to improved outcomes.

People want their symptoms, including pain, to improve so that they may participate in activities that have value to them. As such, talking about pain and symptoms is important. For people with nontraumatic presentations this may involve exploring thoughts of how symptoms arose and how they affect daily activities. It will also involve discussing the person's concerns and expectations of treatment. Some people will welcome the opportunity to discuss the impact of their symptoms on their life, and this may be explored by inviting the patient to respond to questions such as, "What is it like living with this pain/your symptoms?"

At all stages, clinicians should aim to validate the patient's beliefs and experiences. On occasion, the patient's concerns may impede effective management and recovery and need to be addressed by the treating clinician. In this context, they are often referred to as "yellow flags" – defined as "normal but unhelpful psychological reactions."[33] Examples include fear avoidance, low pain self-efficacy, pain-related worrying, and frustration at not knowing what to do to move forwards. There are also people with more severe psychological or psychiatric problems, which are often described as "orange flags."[33] Examples include more severe anxiety or clinical depression that are poorly controlled.

As with any other comorbidity, the presence of psychiatric problems does not exclude the possibility of a biological contribution to shoulder pain, but they may get in the way of treatment and recovery. Some psychiatric problems may be ongoing, and require communication with the existing healthcare team to enable a safe (multidisciplinary) approach that does not exacerbate existing problems. However, some problems may be new or exacerbated by the presence of shoulder pain and require swift referral to the appropriate healthcare provider.

Psychological factors should be considered in two commonly overlapping groups: those associated with distress, and those associated with stress. One way of considering these is to explore factors that stop people metaphorically moving forwards. Those that feel distress are often "stuck" inside their head with ruminating thoughts about loss, accompanied by guilt and sadness, and characterized by a lack of energy. Those that are experiencing high stress are "stuck" in constant processing of the next up-coming threat, accompanied by worry, irritation, and high arousal. Broadly speaking, distress involves a negative self-focus, with low mood, and depression-like symptoms such as lack of energy, crying, and a sense of hopelessness. Stress involves a state of agitation focused outwards towards a threatening world, and it includes excessive worry and inability to concentrate. The result of both is similar, in that patients withdraw from their life/activities into a negative place closely focused around their shoulder pain and symptoms. Often this includes reduced physical activity, withdrawal from normal daily activities, and isolation from family and friends. Developing strategies to enable people to participate in valued activities should therefore be equally important as reducing physical impairments, such as pain.

When to treat and when to refer on

The experience of pain-related distress and stress differs between people. For clinicians, the challenge is differentiating between psychological issues that: 1) have occurred as a result of living with pain; 2) arise from a combination of being in pain and holding certain attitudes, beliefs and coping mechanisms; and 3) are independent of the pain experience. All three categories compromise patients' well-being.

When pain persists, especially if uncertainty about the cause exists and uncertainty regarding the future is a concern, low mood, worry, and helplessness are understandable and normal responses. People need to voice their concerns. Pain interrupts not only what we do, but also how we think and behave.[48] Effective clinicians take the time to listen, acknowledge and validate the thoughts and feelings expressed by patients. Excellent practitioners find ways of helping people evaluate their feelings and thoughts, change their lifestyle when that is indicated, and adjust. Validation that the individual's experiences, concerns and beliefs are respected, combined with shared problem-solving and techniques to promote pain self-efficacy and self-management, are arguably more important than identifying a structural cause for the symptoms when the latter may be unrealistic (see Chapter 15).

Sometimes, people get "stuck" in a place from which they find it difficult to progress, often because they are fearful, mourning the things they used to be able to do, angry at their own body, significant others, healthcare providers, or are just overwhelmed. Healthcare practitioners might perceive this as lack of cooperation, low adherence, and refusal to take responsibility and move on. Good communication between the patient and healthcare practitioner is important because these factors will get in the way of providing effective treatment.

Most people who are seen for shoulder conditions will require support to help cope with their symptoms. Some will have psychological issues or "orange flags" that are independent of their shoulder pain and symptoms.[26,33] In the same way many people live with diabetes, high blood pressure, and asthma, many also live with disorders adversely affecting mental health, the most common being depression, different types of anxiety, schizophrenia, bipolar disorder, obsessive-compulsive disorder, and post-traumatic stress disorder (PTSD) – whether diagnosed or otherwise. Most of the time, with those living with mental health disorders and presenting with shoulder pain, the practitioner may not even be aware of the comorbid mental health problem. However, knowing about the problem is important, as it may be directly connected to the shoulder pain. As with all health concerns that fall outside the remit of the clinician and require specialist care, it is important to suggest the need for, or facilitate, expert help. See Box 6.2 for our top tips relating to yellow and orange flags.

Box 6.2 Top tips relating to yellow and orange flags

Yellow flags are normal but potentially unhelpful psychological reactions when patients struggle to deal with the emotional baggage that comes with pain.

- Explore and gently challenge your patient's beliefs and behaviors.

Orange flags are more severe psychological problems for which liaison with the patient's existing healthcare provider is important.

- As with other comorbidities it doesn't always mean physical rehabilitation to the shoulder is contraindicated.
- When urgent referral is required due to an exacerbation or emerging condition, recognize the boundaries of your scope of practice and refer on quickly.

The clinical challenge

It is tempting to ignore bizarre behaviors exhibited by patients and focus only on the shoulder pain, but this is a mistake, and arguably, a neglect of duty of care. If patients speak quickly, using sentences that have no obvious connection, and demonstrate signs of agitation, routine assessment and management will probably be inappropriate. Patients who are unable to concentrate and understand explanations may also be unable to consent to assessment, participate in shared decision-making, and be adherent with treatment. Ignoring signs of mental confusion and anguish, which some consider outside their remit, equates to ignoring a high-risk clinical presentation. In other words, if the clinician notices that the patient is in a mental crisis, they have a duty of care to gently explore the situation with the patient, and to do their best to get them to the appropriate healthcare provider.

In the first instance this will most likely be their primary care (general) practitioner, unless the patient appears to be a danger to themselves or others, in which case the practitioner must call emergency services. In non-life-threatening situations, rather than ignore, clinicians might embrace the situation, and try to help the patient themselves (Figure 6.1). This is particularly common in cases where the patient discloses a long history of being ignored, dismissed, neglected, and misbelieved, and can be a mistake. However empathic the clinician may be, and no matter how good their relationship is with the patient, recognizing skill limitations is imperative. Always be prepared to refer the individual to a more appropriate healthcare provider.

Clinicians may feel that they have neither the skills nor confidence to address the psychological and social components of a biopsychosocial approach,[17] for example, when trying to help patients deal with the emotional baggage that comes with pain, or perhaps more challenging, help those patients who are failing to deal with their pain. Patients' fear avoidance, low pain self-efficacy, and inability to self-manage can be a normal result of living with pain, or holding certain beliefs, and clinicians can help patients address and often overcome these. However, misunderstanding these can result in practitioners blaming and judging patients. These feelings can get in the way of reflective practice, listening to the patient in a nonjudgmental way, empathizing with, and validating their experience. This will in turn be

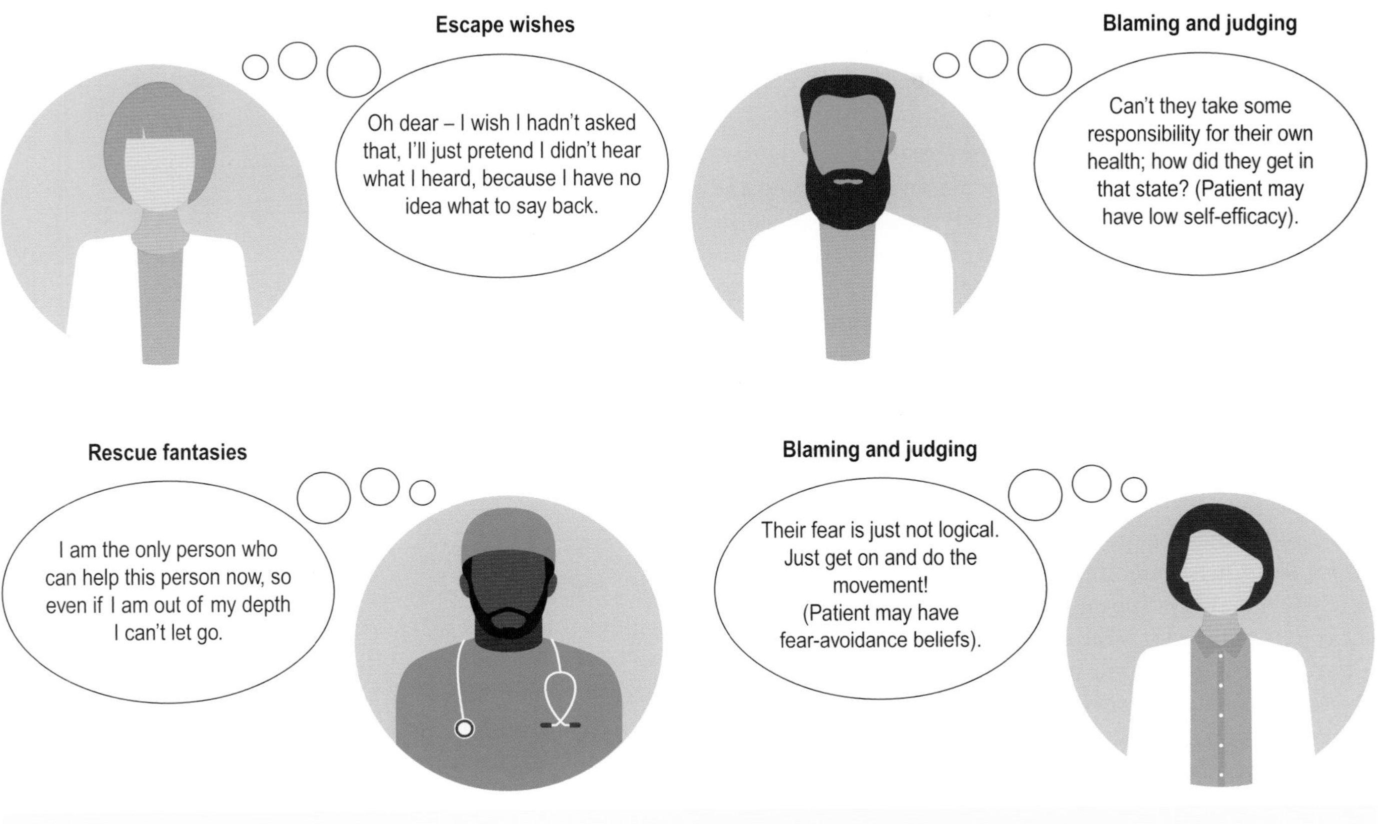

FIGURE 6.1
Clinical responses that lead to suboptimal care.

detrimental to the therapeutic alliance and may become a barrier to the patient's confidence or desire to self-manage.

Clinicians often experience helplessness when information is not forthcoming, and do not know how to interpret the information they do have. In the following section we have provided some additional suggestions for the busy clinician, followed by examples of biopsychosocial approaches from our own practices.

Tips for practitioners

Assessment

A key component of taking a history should be focusing on the patient's *i*deas, *c*oncerns and *e*xpectations (ICE)[41] with respect to their experience of shoulder symptoms. Some clinicians may find it easier to ask their patients to answer these questions in a questionnaire prior to meeting face to face, and use the responses as discussion points. As clinicians we need to hypothesize the biologic and biomechanical basis for the shoulder problem the patient presents with (the bio), and endeavor to contextualize the social context the individual lives in, as well as the impact of living with shoulder symptoms (the illness), together with the patient's expectation of those providing care.

Questionnaires as an adjunct to conversation

Some clinicians use questionnaires as a starting point to explore their patient's beliefs and concerns. Some questionnaires cover a range of psychosocial factors, usually including one question or item to measure each factor. The total scores of these questionnaires gives an indication of psychosocial status but *will not* provide information on the difficulties experienced by individuals. Examples of screening questionnaires are the short form Örebro MSK Pain Screening Questionnaire[25] and the Keele STarT MSK Tool.[4] Typically, these questionnaires were developed to differentiate between those who require minimal or more extensive approaches to care. This concept is known as screening and matching. However, rather than only acting as screening and stratification tools, we suggest also using these questionnaires as tools to highlight which psychosocial factors might benefit from further exploration during the consultation by looking at single item scores, rather than the total of the questionnaire. Factors can thus be identified that could hinder recovery, or on a more positive note, where the patient is coping well.

Questionnaires also have their drawbacks and limitations, and clinicians and researchers can be divided on their usefulness. Questionnaires can be burdensome to complete, and may not always appear that relevant to people who have come to the clinic for treatment of their shoulder symptoms – particularly if they are specific to just one or a few psychological constructs, such anxiety and depression. In addition, questionnaires can sometimes be used as a shortcut, a tool perceived to avoid the necessity of verbally exploring awkward psychosocial issues. However, doing so can often be a barrier to effective communication. Imagine going to your family doctor and the only opportunity to discuss your biggest fears and concerns about your health problem was via a questionnaire. So many psychological phenomena are rich constructs specific to the patient and their individual context, and so cannot be captured using questionnaires. If questionnaires are utilized, they should be used as an adjunct to, and not instead of, effective communication.

Physical examination

The physical examination can sometimes reflect the patient's underlying behavior with respect to their beliefs and concerns. While slow, stiff or guarded movement may occur in response to pain, or biological impairments in mobility or strength, such movement may also be linked to fear, and catastrophizing.[9] These avoidant or protective movement responses can often reflect underlying beliefs that moving the shoulder may cause further harm. Eliminating these avoidance behaviors can become a target for treatment.[9,34] However, rather than forcing the patient to do something that is symptom-provoking, it is first important to establish what the individual is fearful of. A common concern is the fear to move because it will hurt, and hurt means damage. Commonly, patients who have been (mis)informed that their symptoms are caused by acromial impingement on the tendon, may equate the experience of pain to more tendon damage. By understanding this, clinicians may consider some behavioral approaches to help patients make sense of their situation.

One simple example is the use of behavioral experiments during the physical examination to test if the patient's hypotheses, and ours, are accurate. For example, if the patient is moving very cautiously when trying to lift their arm overhead, we can ask them what they think will happen if they move faster. Typically, patients express concern that faster movement will increase pain. By using examples where moving slowly is more difficult (e.g., walking down stairs, or even trying a movement with the opposite shoulder) patients can be encouraged to try faster movement – which can often lead to less pain, tension and effort. Shoulder symptom modification procedures are another example and are discussed in more detail in Chapter 36. See Box 6.3 for our top tips on integrating the psychosocial into a clinical assessment.

Box 6.3 Top tips for integrating the psychosocial into a clinical assessment

- Always ask your patient about their ideas, concerns, and expectations with respect to their shoulder pain.
- Use questionnaires as an adjunct to and not instead of effective communication.
- Use the physical examination to assess and if appropriate challenge avoidant or overly protective movement.

Case studies

The following examples have been selected from our own clinical caseloads to demonstrate integrating a biopsychosocial approach into everyday practice. The clinical details are accurate, but names have been changed to protect anonymity.

These cases illustrate that a biopsychosocial approach can be integrated into everyone's practice and typically, the approach includes common aspects of rehabilitation such as exercise, and lifestyle advice. It requires that we reflect upon the words we use, ensuring we select and tailor education appropriately, and acknowledge that patient beliefs may not be the same as ours, or easy to change.

Rachel's case: the patient who would not exercise

History

Maureen, a 73-year-old retired nurse diagnosed with a degenerative rotator cuff tear, reported that the onset of her symptoms was associated with mild trauma several years ago. Maureen lived alone and prior to her symptoms, played bowls. She wanted surgery, but following an explanation of why it would not help, was referred to a physical therapist (physiotherapist) who "made her" do exercises. Maureen did not attend her follow-up appointment. A year later she attended my clinic, expressing her frustration that we didn't "realize how badly damaged her shoulder was." Despite my attempts to educate her, Maureen "couldn't see the point of exercises."

Stop and think

Are we happier seeing people who already like activity and exercise, and understand how it can help their symptoms improve? Why doesn't Maureen help herself, get on and do the exercises? Is she being lazy? Is she looking for a magic wand? *Or* is she afraid? Are her exercises painful? Does she think her injury means exercise will cause more damage? What do we mean by exercise? To some people, exercise is fun, enjoyable and confidence-building. For Maureen, exercise may be boring and associated with feelings of physical inadequacy. Are people like Maureen, who don't change their beliefs despite our "education", being awkward? *Or* does Maureen, who held many strong opinions including the need for surgery, understandably, just want to take back control?

Reflect and plan

Maureen had a "real" biological tissue injury. However, it was lack confidence in her own ability to be active that limited her progress. By asking Maureen about her ideas, concerns, and preferences, it became clear that she liked "movements" to do at home, whereas "exercises" implied using "boring equipment" like resistance bands. I asked Maureen if she'd like to try exploring coping and self-management strategies together, given her disappointment at not being offered surgery. This allowed Maureen to make her own decision to proceed. Respecting Maureen's expertise in terms of her lived experience of pain and providing an opportunity for shared decision-making empowered Maureen, who very quickly returned to bowls and her previous social activities. See Box 6.4 for Rachel's top tips.

Box 6.4 Top tips from Rachel's case study

- **Some patients do not enjoy exercise but do enjoy physical activity (see Chapter 30).**

Make sure you explore this as not all patients feel comfortable volunteering this information and instead may choose to be non-adherent to "exercises".

- **Don't be afraid to explore ideas with your patient.**

Accept that sometimes the only way to find a solution may be teamwork. Clinicians may need to support patients to self-manage.

Liesbet's case: the patient who was too compliant

History

Maria, a 57-year-old manager, presented with an 8-month history of "frozen shoulder". When first seen, Maria hadn't worked for 2 months due to shoulder pain and had been receiving treatment from a physical therapist (physiotherapist) for 8 months. She did her exercises 6 times per day, including nighttime when she woke with pain. Maria was tired and upset that despite her compliance, her shoulder had not improved.

Stop and think

While we want patients to adhere to our advice, doing exercises 6 times per day, and at night when she should be resting, is clearly unhelpful. Was her work ethic or personality reflected in how she was exercising? Maria had complied with the physical therapist's instructions, without questioning whether the exercises were helping within an expected time frame. Clinicians often focus on the physiological parameters of exercise (repetitions, sets, degree of resistance), and do not explore the context of the exercise, and how they make a person feel in terms of both pain and emotion.

Reflect and plan

I had to be careful with my words – I did not want Maria to feel that all her efforts had been wasted and that she was responsible for her poor recovery. She was clever, and if I had said that she exercised too much, and that insomnia was negatively influencing her recovery, she could have interpreted it that she was responsible for her non-recovery. I felt this would reduce her resilience and engagement with rehabilitation. I asked, "How do the exercises make you feel?", to which she replied, "I do exercises, they hurt, they make me feel I want to cry, they interrupt my rest, they do not make me better, so why am I actually doing them?" Rather than telling her, Maria had found the solution for herself and was motivated to change her behavior.

From that moment on, she found the resilience to restart and reshape her rehabilitation, which began with stopping her shoulder exercises and increasing walking, as this was a valued activity for her. In the following sessions, we talked about the evidence for managing frozen shoulders and the importance of listening to your body to work out what is best for you within your lifestyle. In Maria's case, acknowledging how distressing the pain was and how difficult the rehabilitation process had been were critical initial steps. This was later followed by talking about the importance of good sleep for her shoulder pain, as well as her overall health. See Box 6.5 for Liesbet's top tips.

> **Box 6.5** Top tips from Liesbet's case study
>
> - **Complete adherence can be just as unhealthy as non-adherence.**
>
> Some patients need agency to make amendments according to their lifestyle and the effectiveness of the exercises.
>
> - **Explore the context of the exercises: how do the exercises make your patient feel.**
>
> Do they empower them and help their activity and self-efficacy, or are they disempowering? Asking your patients this can be the opening for change.

Kieran's case: the distressed man who "knew" he was not stressed

History

Michael (48 years old) presented with bilateral shoulder pain. He worked as a manual laborer in construction until 1 year ago when his employment was stopped due to an economic downturn. He had intermittent shoulder pain for many years, without any specific trauma, and it was more troublesome in the previous 9 months. He lived with his wife and 4 children. He reported several markers of poor general health (poor sleep, low energy, 8 kg weight gain) and psychological well-being (e.g., "angry", "fed up", fear about ability to work) in the last year. He had visited his family doctor, multiple physical therapists, and a surgeon in the previous year looking for a solution for his pain. They were all "useless" in his opinion, with one of them suggesting the pain was "all in his head", even though his MRI scan clearly showed his shoulders were "worn down" (mild bilateral degenerative changes on MRI).

Stop and think

Did the practitioners suggest his pain was "all in his head", or is that what Michael inferred? Will he trust any clinician now? Who told him his shoulders were "worn down"? Why is he not working now – is it due to shoulder pain, limited employment being available, or job dissatisfaction? Was his anger related to the economic downturn and his concerns for his family's future? How has his role in the family changed in the last year? How can I evaluate his emotional status, as he might not like me asking about his feelings?

Reflect and plan

Michael discussed at length the burden of the last year, and his anger that despite working for his employer for many years, he only received basic statutory redundancy pay. He was under severe financial strain, seeing limited prospects

Box 6.6 Top tips from Kieran's case study

- **Listen carefully to the words patients use.**

Asking about stress can be provocative for some people, as they associate this with weakness. Being angry, perhaps with the unfairness of a situation, is not the same as being stressed.

- **Don't rush into "education" – help people figure some things out for themselves.**

As clinicians we may have (accurately!) identified poor general health and psychological well-being as significant contributors to ongoing pain, and clear barriers to recovery. However, rushing into educating patients about these factors can backfire, with patients (often inaccurately) thinking it only applies if pain is purely psychosomatic or exaggerated.

for future employment, especially if his pain continued. His wife had to return to work, but he struggled with the increased role he had in the home, including cooking and homework. In Michael's case, I needed to establish a good rapport by listening intently and empathically, and demonstrate to him that I took his problem seriously by evaluating what *he* considered to be important (his scan, and his range of movement). This allowed me to reassure him of the integrity of his shoulder structures, and the safety of being active. We discussed how poor sleep and anger can really increase pain, similarly to how they affect other health complaints such as blood pressure and headaches. Thereafter, discussing the importance of general health and making a specific plan (better sleep, playing cards to relax, restarting physical activity) to address these components was easier. See Box 6.6 for Kieran's top tips.

Summarizing the case studies

While exercise is a common and important aspect of rehabilitation, it is important to be aware of what exercise means to people, and the context within which it takes place. Maureen had low self-efficacy in terms of formal exercise, but had high self-efficacy and motivation for playing bowls, as this was something she had enjoyed for years and was a valued part of her social life. There are times when we must strike a balance between what might be considered an "optimum" exercise program based on strength and conditioning principles (e.g., parameters such as repetitions, sets, load) and factors which are related to people continuing with an activity long-term (e.g., preference, cost, access). In contrast to Maureen, Maria had been over-exercising and her experience, far from enjoyable, was frustrating and painful. Arguably the emphasis she placed on exercise might have been better placed on sleep, especially considering the role of fatigue in ongoing pain.

The case studies also illustrate how traditional biomedical aspects can be incorporated into a biopsychosocial approach. For example, we have reasons to be skeptical about the value of many components of a physical examination, including the so-called shoulder special orthopedic tests. Similarly, imaging findings may be over-valued and may lead to inappropriate concern and harms. However, there is value in a comprehensive physical examination, and we can help patients reframe and make sense of imaging findings.[21] In this manner, we can combine a comprehensive physical examination with the results of imaging tests (where available) to reassure patients of the integrity of their shoulder structures, and the safety of activity. This was important for both Maureen and Michael, who regained confidence to use their shoulders using a valued activity approach, and not formal exercise (Chapter 36), which in turn helped their mental health.

When trying to take a biopsychosocial approach goes wrong

While the focus of this chapter is promoting meaningful discussions with patients about what is going on in their lives, and whether their pain relates to some of these aspects, we can increase psychological distress by handling these discussions poorly. A commonly cited barrier to meaningful engagement with patients is inadequate time.[17] In our view trying to squeeze in a rushed discussion on important but sensitive aspects of a person's life will usually be unhelpful. This might explain reports of a backfire effect where patients such as Michael become angry at the perceived implication that the pain is "all in their head" or exaggerated. In our experience, using the person's own words for their situation can be valuable, as it both demonstrates we are paying attention, but also the language they use (e.g., frustration versus stress) may be less likely to be deemed offensive. It is also important to consider that addressing mild to moderate psychosocial factors may be achieved through simple normalization of a person's situation as the pain resolves, such as resumption of hobbies, work, and perceived role in the home. While a patient's response to pain might reflect some longstanding underlying traits (e.g., anxiety), any discussions around these should not be associated with blaming the patient.

There will clearly be times when a person's situation will require additional support. Family doctors can help facilitate components of care such as imaging, medication, and onward referral for psychological, dietary, and sleep services for example. Family doctors are also likely to have a good insight into the person's long-term health status. There is now increased recognition of the value of social care, and this may include coordinating workplace support when needed and where available, or referral to community support (e.g., group runs, active retirement groups). Despite integrating a biopsychosocial approach, clinicians will still be faced with patients who struggle or choose not to engage. Finally, taking a biopsychosocial approach can be hard work, and clinicians must recognize the importance of looking after their own health as well as that of their patients. Box 6.7 summarizes our top tips for using a biopsychosocial approach.

Box 6.7 Top tips for using a biopsychosocial approach

The biopsychosocial approach:

- Is important for all patients because they are people with ideas, concerns, beliefs, and expectations living in a social context.
- Is about basing your communication and education on sound biomechanical and psychosocial principles to help your patients move towards healthier attitudes and health behaviors. It is not about becoming a psychologist.
- Uses an integrated approach rather than battling between the bio, psycho and social. For example, consider exploring your patient's fear avoidance beliefs and exercise self-efficacy during the clinical examination.
- Taking a biopsychosocial approach gets easier with time, and will enrich your practice and lead to greater patient satisfaction.

References

1. Bandura A. Self-efficacy: toward a unifying theory of behavioral change. Psychological Review. 1977;84:191.
2. Barbaresko J, Koch M, Schulze MB, Nöthlings U. Dietary pattern analysis and biomarkers of low-grade inflammation: a systematic literature review. Nutrition Reviews. 2013;71:511-527.
3. Busse J, Heels-Ansdell D, Makosso-Kallyth S, et al. Patient coping and expectations predict recovery after major orthopaedic trauma. British Journal of Anaesthesia. 2019;122:51-59.
4. Campbell P, Hill JC, Protheroe J, et al. Keele Aches and Pains Study protocol: validity, acceptability, and feasibility of the Keele STarT MSK tool for subgrouping musculoskeletal patients in primary care. Journal of Pain Research. 2016;9:807.
5. Chester R, Jerosch-Herold C, Lewis J, Shepstone L. Psychological factors are associated with the outcome of physiotherapy for people with shoulder pain: a multicentre longitudinal cohort study. British Journal of Sports Medicine. 2018;52:269-275.
6. Chester R, Khondoker M, Shepstone L, Lewis JS, Jerosch-Herold C. Self-efficacy and risk of persistent shoulder pain: results of a Classification and Regression Tree (CART) analysis. British Journal of Sports Medicine. 2019;53:825-834.
7. Daluiso-King G, Hebron C. Is the biopsychosocial model in musculoskeletal physiotherapy adequate? An evolutionary concept analysis. Physiother Theory Pract. 2020;1-17.
8. Darlow B, Fullen BM, Dean S, Hurley DA, Baxter GD, Dowell A. The association between health care professional attitudes and beliefs and the attitudes and beliefs, clinical management, and outcomes of patients with low back pain: a systematic review. European Journal of Pain. 2012;16:3-17.
9. De Baets L, Matheve T, Meeus M, Struyf F, Timmermans A. The influence of cognitions, emotions and behavioral factors on treatment outcomes in musculoskeletal shoulder pain: a systematic review. Clinical Rehabilitation. 2019;33:980-991.
10. Djade CD, Porgo TV, Zomahoun HTV, Perrault-Sullivan G, Dionne CE. Incidence of shoulder pain in 40 years old and over and associated factors: A systematic review. European Journal of Pain. 2020;24:39-50.
11. Docking SI, Cook J. How do tendons adapt? Going beyond tissue responses to understand positive adaptation and pathology development: A narrative review. Journal of Musculoskeletal & Neuronal Interactions. 2019;19:300.
12. Engebretsen KB, Brox JI, Juel NG. Patients with shoulder pain referred to specialist care; treatment, predictors of pain and disability, emotional distress, main symptoms and sick-leave: a cohort study

with a six-months follow-up. Scandinavian Journal of Pain. 2020;20(4):775-783.

13. Engel GL. The need for a new medical model: a challenge for biomedicine. Science. 1977;196:129-136.

14. Fujihara Y, Shauver MJ, Lark ME, Zhong L, Chung KC. The effect of workers' compensation on outcome measurement methods after upper extremity surgery: a systematic review and meta-analysis. Plastic and Reconstructive Surgery. 2017;139:923.

15. Gardner T, Refshauge K, Smith L, McAuley J, Hübscher M, Goodall S. Physiotherapists' beliefs and attitudes influence clinical practice in chronic low back pain: a systematic review of quantitative and qualitative studies. Journal of Physiotherapy. 2017;63:132-143.

16. Hayden JA, Wilson MN, Riley RD, Iles R, Pincus T, Ogilvie R. Individual recovery expectations and prognosis of outcomes in non-specific low back pain: prognostic factor review. Cochrane Database of Systematic Reviews. 2019:CD011284.

17. Holopainen R, Simpson P, Piirainen A, et al. Physiotherapists' perceptions of learning and implementing a biopsychosocial intervention to treat musculoskeletal pain conditions: a systematic review and metasynthesis of qualitative studies. Pain. 2020;161:1150-1168.

18. Irwin MR, Olmstead R, Carroll JE. Sleep disturbance, sleep duration, and inflammation: a systematic review and meta-analysis of cohort studies and experimental sleep deprivation. Biological psychiatry. 2016;80:40-52.

19. Jackson T, Wang Y, Wang Y, Fan H. Self-efficacy and chronic pain outcomes: a meta-analytic review. The Journal of Pain. 2014;15:800-814.

20. Kennedy P, Joshi R, Dhawan A. The effect of psychosocial factors on outcomes in patients with rotator cuff tears: A systematic review. Arthroscopy: The Journal of Arthroscopic & Related Surgery. 2019;35:2698-2706.

21. Lærum E, Indahl A, Sture Skouen J. What is "The Good Back-Consultation"? A combined qualitative and quantitative study of chronic low back pain patients' interaction with and perceptions of consultations with specialists. Journal of Rehabilitation Medicine. 2006;38:255-262.

22. Lewis J. Rotator cuff related shoulder pain: Assessment, management and uncertainties. Man Ther. 2016;23:57-68.

23. Liberman K, Forti LN, Beyer I, Bautmans I. The effects of exercise on muscle strength, body composition, physical functioning and the inflammatory profile of older adults: a systematic review. Current Opinion in Clinical Nutrition and Metabolic Care. 2017;20:30-53.

24. Linaker CH, Walker-Bone K. Shoulder disorders and occupation. Best Practice & Research in Clinical Rheumatology. 2015;29:405-423.

25. Linton SJ, Nicholas M, MacDonald S. Development of a short form of the Örebro Musculoskeletal Pain Screening Questionnaire. Spine. 2011;36:1891-1895.

26. Main CJ, George SZ. Psychologically informed practice for management of low back pain: future directions in practice and research. Physical Therapy. 2011;91:820-824.

27. Martinez-Calderon J, Meeus M, Struyf F, Morales-Asencio JM, Gijon-Nogueron G, Luque-Suarez A. The role of psychological factors in the perpetuation of pain intensity and disability in people with chronic shoulder pain: a systematic review. BMJ open. 2018;8:e020703.

28. Martinez-Calderon J, Struyf F, Meeus M, Luque-Suarez A. The association between pain beliefs and pain intensity and/or disability in people with shoulder pain: a systematic review. Musculoskeletal Science and Practice. 2018;37:29-57.

29. Miedema HS, Feleus A, Bierma-Zeinstra SM, Hoekstra T, Burdorf A, Koes BW. Disability trajectories in patients with complaints of arm, neck, and shoulder (CANS) in primary care: prospective cohort study. Physical Therapy. 2016;96:972-984.

30. Mocayar Maron FJ, Ferder L, Saraví FD, Manucha W. Hypertension linked to allostatic load: from psychosocial stress to inflammation and mitochondrial dysfunction. Stress. 2019;22:169-181.

31. Moll LT, Schmidt AM, Stapelfeldt CM, et al. Prediction of 2-year work participation in sickness absentees with neck or shoulder pain: the contribution of demographic, patient-reported, clinical and imaging information. BMC Musculoskeletal Disorders. 2019;20:1-11.

32. Moseley GL, Butler DS. Fifteen years of explaining pain: the past, present, and future. The Journal of Pain. 2015;16:807-813.

33. Nicholas MK, Linton SJ, Watson PJ, Main CJ, "Decade of the Flags" Working Group. Early identification and management of psychological risk factors ("yellow flags") in patients with low back pain: a reappraisal. Physical Therapy. 2011;91:737-753.

34. O'Sullivan PB, Caneiro J, O'Keeffe M, et al. Cognitive functional therapy: an integrated behavioral approach for the targeted management of disabling low back pain. Physical Therapy. 2018;98:408-423.

35. Osimo EF, Cardinal RN, Jones PB, Khandaker GM. Prevalence and correlates of low-grade systemic inflammation in adult psychiatric inpatients: an electronic health record-based study. Psychoneuroendocrinology. 2018;91:226-234.

36. Ravindra A, Barlow JD, Jones GL, Bishop JY. A prospective evaluation of predictors of pain after arthroscopic rotator cuff repair: psychosocial factors have a stronger association than structural factors. Journal of Shoulder and Elbow Surgery. 2018;27:1824-1829.

37. Rodeghero JR, Cleland JA, Mintken PE, Cook CE. Risk stratification of patients with shoulder pain seen in physical therapy practice. Journal of Evaluation in Clinical Practice. 2017;23:257-263.

38. Sciascia AD, Jacobs CA, Morris BJ, Kibler WB. The degree of tissue injury in the shoulder does not correlate with pain perception. Journal of Shoulder and Elbow Surgery. 2017;26:e151-e152.

39. Seidler A, Romero Starke K, Freiberg A, Hegewald J, Nienhaus A, Bolm-Audorff U. Dose–response relationship between physical workload and specific shoulder diseases: a systematic review with meta-analysis. International Journal of Environmental Research and Public Health. 2020;17:1243.

40. Sibille KT, McBeth J, Smith D, Wilkie R. Allostatic load and pain severity in older adults: results from the English Longitudinal Study of Ageing. Experimental Gerontology. 2017;88:51-58.

41. Silverman J, Kurtz S, Draper J. Skills for communicating with patients. Oxford: Radcliffe Medical Press; 1998.

42. Snippen NC, de Vries HJ, van der Burg-Vermeulen SJ, Hagedoorn M, Brouwer S. Influence of significant others on work participation of individuals with chronic diseases: a systematic review. BMJ Open. 2019;9:e021742.

43. Speer K, Upton D, Semple S, McKune A. Systemic low-grade inflammation in

post-traumatic stress disorder: a systematic review. Journal of Inflammation Research. 2018;11:111.

44. Stewart M, Brown J, Weston W, McWhinney I, McWilliam C, Freeman T. Patient-Centred Medicine: Transforming the Clinical Method. London: Sage; 1995.

45. Stineman MG, Streim JE. The biopsycho-ecological paradigm: a foundational theory for medicine. PM&R. 2010;2:1035-1045.

46. Thompson WR, Scott A, Loghmani MT, Ward SR, Warden SJ. Understanding mechanobiology: physical therapists as a force in mechanotherapy and musculoskeletal regenerative rehabilitation. Physical Therapy. 2016;96:560-569.

47. Van der Molen HF, Foresti C, Daams JG, Frings-Dresen MH, Kuijer PPF. Work-related risk factors for specific shoulder disorders: a systematic review and meta-analysis. Occupational and Environmental Medicine. 2017;74:745-755.

48. Vlaeyen JW, Crombez G. Behavioral conceptualization and treatment of chronic pain. Annual Review of Clinical Psychology. 2020;16:187-212.

49. Wærsted M, Koch M, Veiersted KB. Work above shoulder level and shoulder complaints: a systematic review. International Archives of Occupational and Environmental Health. 2020;1-30.

50. Wong WK, Li MY, Yung PS, Leong HT. The effect of psychological factors on pain, function and quality of life in patients with rotator cuff tendinopathy: a systematic review. Musculoskelet Sci Pract. 2020;47:102173.

51. Zouikr I, Karshikoff B. Lifetime modulation of the pain system via neuroimmune and neuroendocrine interactions. Frontiers in Immunology. 2017;8:276.

Pain neuroscience: where is my shoulder pain coming from?

7

Benjamin JF Dean, Derek Griffin

Introduction

A holistic understanding of pain relies upon a broad base of knowledge in a wide range of areas, ranging from philosophy to neuroscience and immunology. In contemporary healthcare practice, a mixture of factors including specialization, protectionism, and vested interests mean that pain science is not always communicated effectively. The aim of this chapter is to present an overall perspective on pain science, specifically focusing on the shoulder in a way that is clinically relevant and meaningful, building on previous work,[15] that may be useful to read alongside this chapter.

A philosophical perspective on pain

There are numerous definitions of pain available in dictionaries, from specialist societies, and from expert individuals. For example the *Oxford Dictionary* defines pain as: "a highly unpleasant physical sensation caused by illness or injury", while the *Cambridge Dictionary* defines pain as: "a feeling of physical suffering caused by injury or illness". The International Association for the Study of Pain (IASP) has recently presented a revised definition of pain[34]: "An unpleasant sensory and emotional experience associated with, or resembling that associated with, actual or potential tissue damage".

All definitions try to define pain objectively, however pain is inherently a subjective phenomenon and has diverse meanings to different people. Ludwig Wittgenstein (1889–1951) is widely regarded as one of the greatest philosophers of all time, and his "private language argument" has clear relevance to definitions of pain, as Richard Floyd explains[19]:

The first point he makes is that the word "pain" is an expression of the sensation rather than a description of it, as we've seen. It's not a description of pain behaviour either: "the verbal expression of pain replaces crying and does not describe it" (section 244). In section 246 Wittgenstein discusses our knowledge of our sensations. He concludes that it is nonsense to say that "I know I am in pain" as it means nothing more than that "I am in pain." It makes more sense to say that while other people can doubt that I am in pain, I cannot.

"Pain" is therefore a construct of human language, a means of communicating our internal state and is sculpted within our immensely social environments, thus demonstrating that context is key, and highlighting how pain can mean very different things to different people. The conclusion of Wittgenstein's argument is interpreted as:[19]

Wittgenstein's position therefore seems to be that sensations definitely are private, and that sensation words do not have sensations themselves as their meaning, and in fact the exact nature of the sensation has no bearing on the meaning (use) of the word whatsoever. The word merely indicates that a certain kind of sensation is present.

There are many interpretations of Wittgenstein's argument, and it unearths a controversy which dates back to the 17th century, when Descartes proposed his theory that the intensity of pain was directly related to the amount of associated tissue injury, and that pain was processed in one distinct pathway.[6,55] Several early theories of pain relied upon this "dualistic" Descartian philosophy, seeing pain as the consequence of the stimulation of specific peripheral "pain receptors". Over the past 100 years, two opposing theories were developed, namely specificity theory and pattern theory. The specificity theory was based upon the dualistic Descartian model and viewed pain as a distinct modality of sensory input with its own apparatus, while pattern theory described pain resulting from the intense stimulation of nonspecific receptors.[55] In 1965, Melzack and Wall published their seminal work on the gate theory of pain, which produced evidence for a model in which pain perception was influenced by both sensory input and the central nervous system.[51] Advances in neuroscience, immunology, psychology, and molecular medicine have subsequently expanded our overall understanding of the experience of pain.

This philosophical context is important as it helps break down the very essence of pain as an inherently subjective construct of human language. Flaws in definitions become clearer if we accept there is much we do not understand. For example, pain is not always unpleasant, pain does not have to be emotional, and why is pain termed to be a "physical sensation"? Then there are the real-world practical implications that we experience daily in clinical practice.

Is the elderly patient who limps into the clinic with a clearly antalgic gait in pain even though they insist it is not pain, but just a minor discomfort? Does pain disappear when a patient receives education, and their fears are allayed by explaining how certain sensations are not something that necessitates abrupt cessation of all painful activity?

Fundamentally perhaps Wittgenstein described the problem exactly, when remarking that "pain" is an expression of the sensation rather than a description of it, and even more fundamentally once appreciated from this perspective, any attempts to define "pain" are by implication, ill-fated. After all, when thinking about the way people experiencing pain are treated, clinicians do not treat the pain, but try to influence factors leading to the experience of this sensation, reducing the impact it has on the individual. Perhaps this is also why measuring pain itself is problematic from both a practical perspective and a philosophical one; generally measuring the way pain has an impact is far more reliable and potentially useful. Ultimately the presence or absence of pain is defined by the individual, by the patient in a clinical setting, and context is vital in describing the meaning and impact of pain for that person. Pain without context ceases to be of meaning, and although pain can be reduced to a unidimensional variable, such as occurs when using the visual analogue scale for pain, one must be very careful to note the context within which this has been done.

Putting pain in context

Pain is an essential part of an organism's evolutional fight for survival, to reproduce and propagate its genetic material. This is demonstrated by various genetic abnormalities that result in deficiencies in nociceptive processing that may be extremely harmful to the individual.[36,61] Without pain perception, neuropathic damage ensues, illustrating the vital function of pain to protect the individual organism from the very real threat of tissue damage. Pain perception is a complex process, and numerous genes have been implicated and may differ between individuals. Obviously genetic and environmental differences mean that there is significant heterogeneity within a population in the ways individuals will respond to different potentially noxious stimuli, such as acute tissue trauma or persistent age-related degenerative conditions such as osteoarthritis.

There will be advantages and disadvantages to different pain sensitivity profiles or phenotypes; if a particular phenotype results in an increased chance of survival to reproduce, then this phenotype will become more predominant, meaning that over time evolution has sculpted the traits we see in our patient population of today. It is worth considering that there is vast diversity in pain phenotype within a population – some will experience pain without any abnormal pathology, while some will tolerate a substantial amount of abnormal pathology without experiencing symptoms. Certainly, is it possible that different pain phenotypes will have different propensities for survival and reproduction in the modern age, and that this may be influenced to a degree by the way in which pain is treated by modern medicine.

Before explaining the scientific basis underpinning our understanding of peripheral and central sensory processing, it is important to highlight the context within which this understanding has been obtained. This understanding has developed from a multitude of different sources including in vitro research on both animal and human cells, as well as in vivo research on both animal and human subjects. Much research has been done using non-real world acutely painful stimuli, for example using iatrogenic tissue trauma, thermal stimuli, or noxious chemicals. The implication of the detached and artificial basis for much of our knowledge base, combined with the use of overly confusing and complex terminology, has made the task for clinicians of translating the scientific knowledge into something meaningful to support clinical practice almost unsurmountable.

The science of pain with a focus on the shoulder

Peripheral receptors

Sensory receptors are specialized structures that respond to physical stimuli. Classifications may be based on the structure of the receptor (morphology, i.e., free nerve endings versus various types of encapsulated receptors), or on the way which they respond to stimuli (i.e., thermoreceptors, mechanoreceptors). They may also be subclassified based on the presence of chemical markers. All classifications are simplifications of the real world and it is important to appreciate that receptors are sometimes not quite as distinct in type as they appear in classification systems. While the dynamic nature of the way in which they respond to various stimuli is often not captured in classification systems, the threshold for a response and the pattern of a response can change over time, depending on changes that may occur in the receptor and its local environment.

Sensory receptors are supplied by afferent nerves of different sizes, degrees of myelination and conduction velocities. Broadly they can be broken down into three main groups: thick diameter myelinated group II or Aβ fibers, small diameter myelinated group III or Aδ fibers, and unmyelinated group IV or C fibers.[21] Sensory receptors are sometimes simply referred to by the type of nerves which innervate them, for example Aδ nerve endings. In simple terms, receptors respond to stimuli by "firing", sending an electrical message onwards and up the sensory chain (Figure 7.1).

A nociceptor can be defined as a high-threshold sensory receptor that is capable of transducing and encoding noxious stimuli. Nociceptors may respond to thermal, mechanical, and chemical stimuli, and may be subclassified based on four criteria: myelination of nerve supply, types of stimuli that evoke a response, response characteristics, and specific chemical markers. Nociceptors exhibit a high degree of functional and chemical plasticity, which means that their threshold and responsiveness, as well as the dynamics of their synaptic contacts, are regulated in a way that may respond to changes mediated by activity, inflammation, and axonal injury (Figures 7.2 and 7.3).

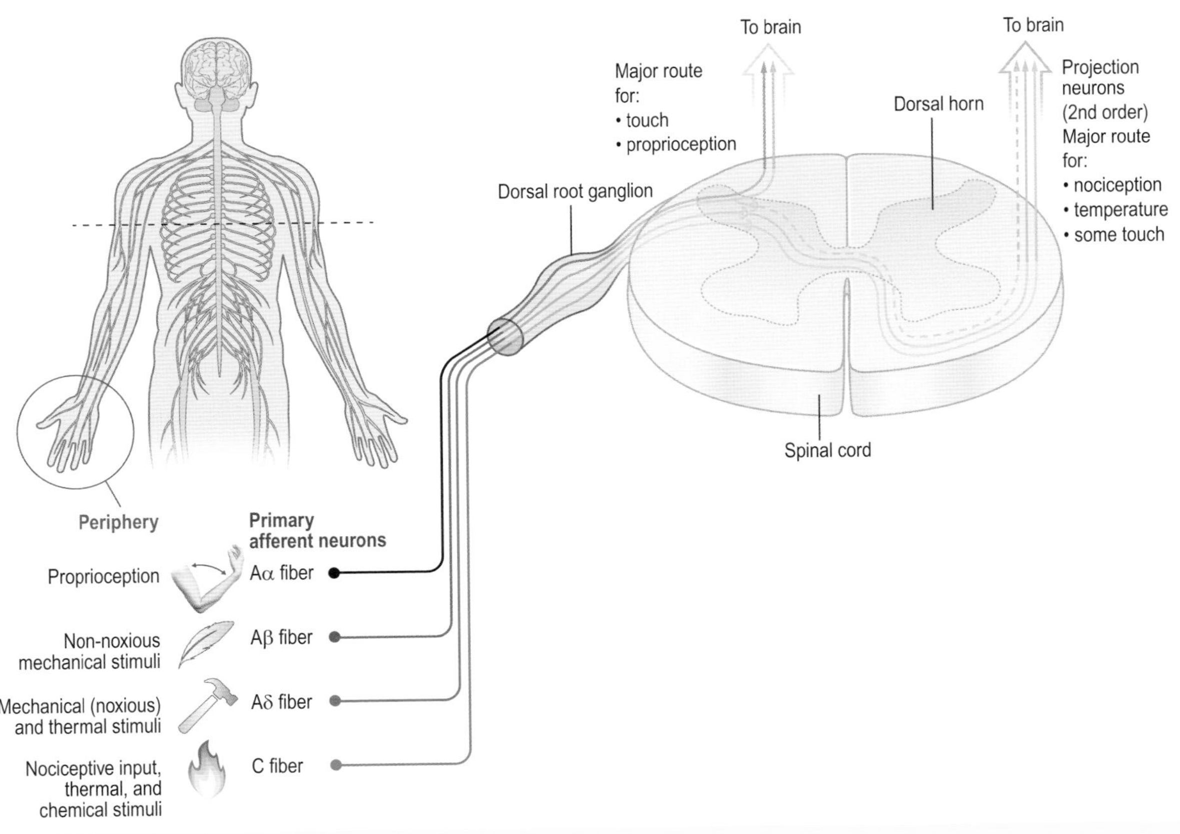

FIGURE 7.1

Primary afferent neurons detect sensations and convert these into electrical signals that travel from the periphery to the central nervous system. They detect different types of input. Aδ and C fibers transmit nociceptive inputs (warning signals), along with other information, e.g., temperature and intense pressure.

(Reproduced with permission from Moloney N, Hartman M. Pain Science – Yoga – Life: Bridging Neuroscience and Yoga for Pain Care. Edinburgh: Handspring Publishing; 2020.)

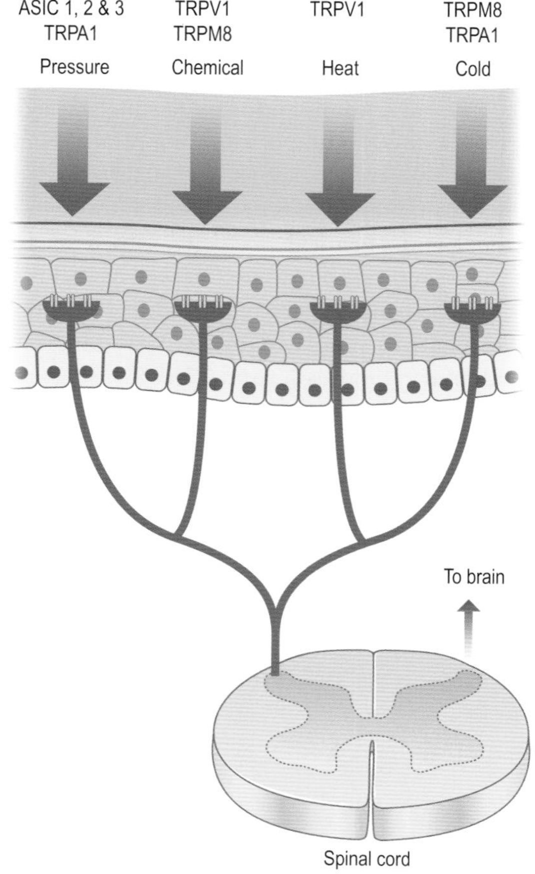

FIGURE 7.2

Nociceptive pain is generated by the activation of nociceptors that respond to thermal, chemical, and mechanical stimuli.

(Reproduced with permission from Austin P. Chronic Pain: A Resource for Effective Manual Therapy. Edinburgh: Handspring Publishing; 2017.)

The mechanoreceptor is a common type of sensory receptor which responds to mechanical stimuli and the most common include Meissner corpuscles, Merkel cell–neurite complexes, Pacinian corpuscles, and free nerve endings. The term proprioceptor is used to describe a type of mechanoreceptor whose role relates to responding to the mechanics associated with muscles and joints. Proprioceptors include muscle spindles, Golgi tendon organs, and Ruffini-type receptors. Importantly, mechanoreceptors can be classified as low-threshold mechanoreceptors (LTMs) or high-threshold mechanoreceptors (HTMs), depending on their threshold for response.

There is a significant crossover between the properties of both nociceptors and mechanoreceptors, and in fact HTMs may also be described as nociceptors. This highlights that creating a neat distinction between mechanoreceptors and nociceptors is rather arbitrary and misleading, particularly given how dynamic a receptor's response threshold may be. This may also explain why the terms nociceptor and nociception are confusing and problematic in practical terms; the plasticity of the nervous system means that static definitions cannot capture the dynamic shifting complexity of the real world. Simplistically, receptors supplied by Aβ nerve endings are LTMs, and those supplied by Aδ nerve endings may be either HTMs or LTMs. HTMs supplied by Aδ nerve endings and most C fiber nerve endings can be called nociceptors. Many LTMs fire in the innocuous range but have a far stronger response in the noxious range, showing how the categorization of receptors as either nociceptors or not can be somewhat problematic.

Shoulder anatomy and receptors

A typical joint is innervated by a nerve that consists of thick diameter myelinated Aβ, small diameter myelinated Aδ, and a high proportion of unmyelinated C fibers. C fibers are further subdivided into an even mixture of either sensory afferents or sympathetic efferents. The nerves that innervate muscle are made up of motor neurons, sensory neurons, and postganglionic sympathetic neurons. In joints, articular Aβ fibers terminate as corpuscular endings of the Ruffini, Golgi and Pacini types in the joint capsule, ligaments, menisci and periosteum.[21] Articular Aδ and C fibers terminate as non-corpuscular or free nerve endings in the capsule, fatty tissue, ligaments, menisci, periosteum, and synovium. In muscle, thick myelinated afferents terminate as organized endings such as muscle spindles and tendon organs, while Aδ and C fibers terminate as free nerve endings.[21]

The neural anatomy of the shoulder has been described in detail,[15,23,71] and the following is a summary. A multitude of nerves contribute to the innervation of the shoulder joint, including the subscapular (C5/6), axillary (C5/6), lateral pectoral (C5/6) and suprascapular (C5/6) nerves. The subscapular nerve supplies a small portion of the anterior joint and the subscapularis muscle. The axillary nerve supplies the anteroinferior and posterior capsule, as well as the teres minor and deltoid muscles. The lateral pectoral nerve

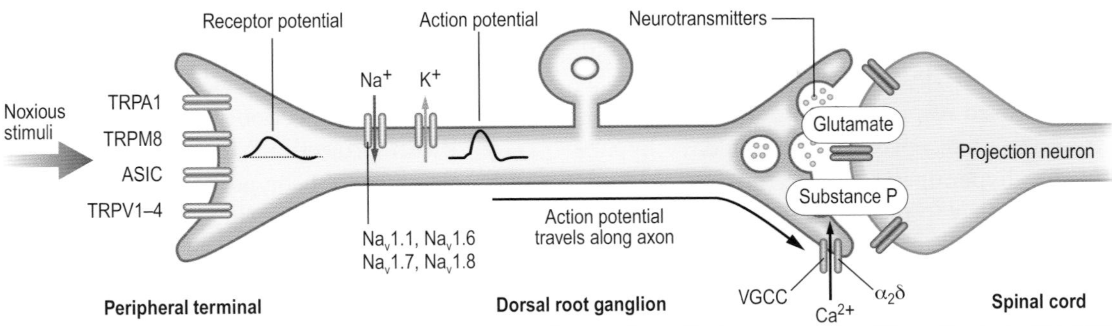

FIGURE 7.3

A schematic diagram of ion channels involved in nociceptive function. Peripheral terminals respond to noxious stimulation (e.g., tissue damage) through receptors and ion channels including TRP and ASIC channels. Once a defined threshold of depolarization is reached, Na_v channels are activated and an action potential is generated. The action potential is transmitted along the axon to the presynaptic terminal where calcium influx through voltage-gated calcium channels (VGCCs) triggers the release of neurotransmitters from the presynaptic terminals.

(Reproduced with permission from Austin P. Chronic Pain: A Resource for Effective Manual Therapy. Edinburgh: Handspring Publishing; 2017.)

supplies some of the anterior capsule, the coracoacromial (C-A) and coracohumeral (C-H) ligaments, the subacromial bursa, the anterior acromioclavicular joint (ACJ), as well as the pectoralis major muscle. The suprascapular nerve supplies the superior capsule, the coracoclavicular ligaments, posterior ACJ, subacromial bursa, posterior and inferior capsule, as well as the supraspinatus and infraspinatus muscles.

Several studies have investigated the neurohistology of the shoulder.[25,35,53,66,70] The rotator cuff is densely innervated with both mechanoreceptors and nociceptors, with these being particularly concentrated at the musculotendinous junction.[2,53] Perhaps this dense innervation is related to the transition that occurs in this highly specialized region between muscle and tendon, where it may be hypothesized that zones of transition are also inherently more at risk of injury and pathology. The capsule is densely innervated with mechanoreceptors, and free nerve endings have been demonstrated in the biceps tendon, capsule and labrum.[2,31,67] The concentration of receptors is more dense in areas of greater mechanical stress.[2] The subacromial bursa is also innervated by both mechanoreceptors and nociceptors.[35]

Sensory pathways

Acute tissue damage results in numerous chemical and cellular changes that may then directly or indirectly lead to the activation of peripheral nociceptors. This involves damage-associated molecular patterns (DAMPs) that are recognized by the receptors of immune cells, as well as other chemicals, cytokines, cell types and signaling pathways.[58] Noxious mechanical, thermal and chemical stimulation may directly activate ion channels on nociceptors or increase the sensitivity of ion channels to other stimuli; essentially anything that results in the activation of enough ion channels can reach the critical threshold for evoking an electrical response or action potential in the nociceptive neuron.[18] This local process resulting in the increased responsiveness of nociceptive neurons and/or the response to normally subthreshold inputs is called peripheral sensitization. There is an abundance of basic science and translational research demonstrating that pro-nociceptive tissue changes occur in common shoulder pathologies, such as tendinopathy and osteoarthritis.[1,11,13,14,16,20,52]

Primary hyperalgesia is simply hypersensitivity at the site of injury and is synonymous with peripheral sensitization. The site of injury is also termed the primary zone, a concept easier to relate to acute injury or experimentally induced pain than persistently painful degenerative conditions. Primary hyperalgesia relates to both heat and mechanical stimuli. Hyperalgesia to light touch is termed allodynia, punctate hyperalgesia is in response to a pinprick or monofilament, while pressure or impact hyperalgesia is in response to pressure to the skin and deeper tissue.

The presence of hyperalgesia is thus part of a completely normal pain response, which may manifest by a lowered threshold to stimulation (less pressure reproducing the same pain), an increased response to suprathreshold stimuli, or the expansion of receptive field. Secondary hyperalgesia is defined as hyperalgesia outside the original zone of injury and relates solely to mechanical stimuli. The activation of nociceptors within the primary zone leads to a so-called flare response, extending outside of this zone through the spreading chemical activation of adjacent nociceptors. Experiments by La Motte et al. have shown that the development of secondary hyperalgesia requires the central nervous system, and it cannot be fully accounted for by the peripheral flare response.[39] The secondary hyperalgesia has been shown to be mediated by the A fiber nociceptors, as it can be obliterated by selective A fiber blockade.[39,74]

Secondary hyperalgesia is therefore a manifestation of central sensitization, which is described as an increased responsiveness of nociceptive neurons in the central nervous system (CNS) to normal or subthreshold afferent input. Punctate and light touch hyperalgesia (allodynia) are the two forms of secondary hyperalgesia that can be observed, and both appear to be mediated by LTMs. The precise mechanisms underlying central sensitization are complex and remain poorly understood. Currently it appears that multiple agents including unmyelinated C fiber nociceptors, LTMs, nociceptive neurons in the dorsal horn of the spinal cord, pre-synaptic interneurons, and descending modulatory pathways are all involved in central sensitization.[15] Central sensitization is hypothesized to occur in numerous clinical situations including the acutely inflamed joint, the arthritic hip and knee, and the painful shoulder.[26]

The spinal dorsal horn receives inputs from many primary afferent nerve fibers including those from nociceptors and mechanoreceptors. Primary afferents are generally excitatory and rely on glutamate as a neurotransmitter (glutaminergic). The primary afferent fibers may synapse with either projection cells which travel in rostral parts of the spinal cord to the higher brain centers, or interneurons which remain in the spinal cord and contribute to local neuronal circuits. Interneurons can be either inhibitory, using GABA/glycine as their neurotransmitter, or excitatory (glutaminergic). The dorsal horn also receives descending input from the brain, and stimulation of these descending inhibitory circuits produces analgesia. These descending systems are also known as the descending pain modulatory system (DPMS). Nociceptive information is transmitted from the spinal cord to the brain via multiple ascending pathways including direct projections to the thalamus (spinothalamic tract), direct projections to homeostatic control regions, and projections to the hypothalamus and ventral forebrain. The periaqueductal gray (PAG) and reticular formation are important parts of the spinobulbar system. The thalamus is of key significance in pain perception and has ascending projections to the primary and secondary somatosensory cortices, the anterior insular cortex, and the cingulate cortex. Central pain perception involves multiple other regions such as the amygdala, prefrontal cortex, cerebellum, and basal ganglia. The key modulatory circuits include the rostral ventromedial medulla (RVM) and PAG, which exert bidirectional control over dorsal horn nociceptive transmission. This network receives numerous inputs from areas which include the amygdala, the anterior cingulate cortex, and the anterior insula – providing a mechanism for the way in which emotion may affect pain perception (Figure 7.4).

Epidemiology of shoulder pain

Broadly, epidemiology is the study of how often a disease occurs in different people and why. Caution is needed when assessing the epidemiological evidence as not all studies are of high quality, studies may overstate their findings as causative without adequate methodology to support such claims, and poor study design can leave results highly subject to bias. There is, however, a reasonable body of evidence relating to shoulder pain which we shall summarize within this section.

Shoulder pain is common, being the third most prevalent musculoskeletal symptom after back and knee pain.[69] The prevalence and incidence vary hugely in the general population depending on the demographic, as well as the way one measures the presence or absence of pain.[44] The prevalence and incidence of shoulder pain which results in a healthcare consultation increases with age, with a plateau reached around 50 to 60 years of age.[43,69] Age (being older than 50 years) is a strong risk factor for both shoulder pain and rotator cuff tendinopathy, while other factors associated with shoulder pain include female sex, ethnicity, obesity, smoking, depression, anxiety, mental stress, and diabetes.[4,8,24,29,40,49,54] Higher pain intensity, higher levels of

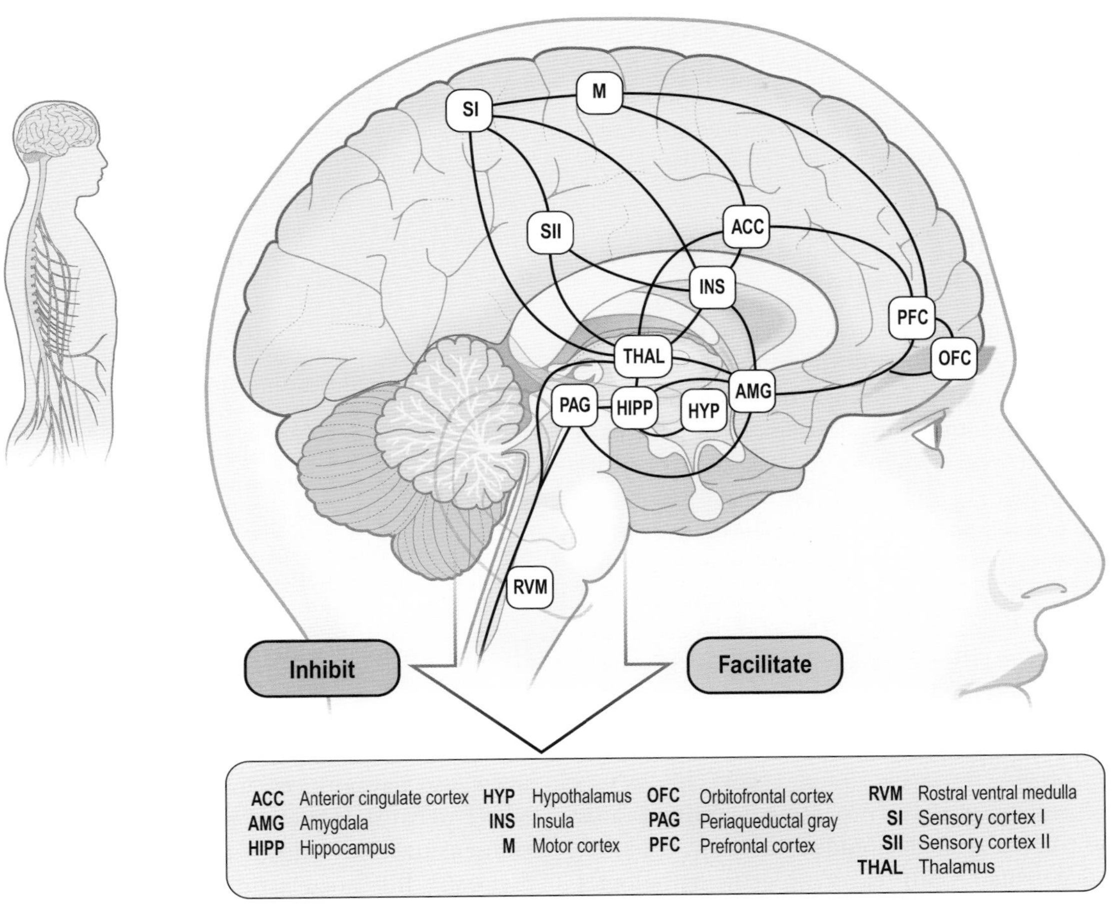

FIGURE 7.4

The nervous system: the "brain pharmacy" and descending modulation of nociception. The PAG/RVM can inhibit or facilitate nociception, turning the dial up or down on nociception. When neurotransmitters that inhibit nociception are released, nociceptive signals are turned down, resulting in less pain. When neurotransmitters that facilitate nociception are released, nociceptive signals are turned up, resulting in more pain.

(Reproduced with permission from Moloney N, Hartman M. Pain Science – Yoga – Life: Bridging Neuroscience and Yoga for Pain Care. Edinburgh: Handspring Publishing; 2020.)

disability, multiple pain sites, the presence of concomitant neck pain, and a longer duration of symptoms are associated with a poorer prognosis.[38,47] Occupational risk factors include a higher physical workload, lower supervisor support, low social support, lower level of job control, repetitiveness of tasks, working at high levels of abduction, and the use of vibrating tools.[4,24,29,40,54,56] High levels of self-efficacy and expectations of recovery are associated with lower levels of pain and disability.[49]

There is a reasonable body of evidence to support a link between structure and pain. A prospective cross-sectional study by Hinsley et al. demonstrated that the chances of shoulder symptoms significantly increase as the degree of rotator cuff structural failure increases, and that the average size of symptomatic rotator cuff tears was significantly greater than that for asymptomatic rotator cuff tears.[33] Yamaguchi et al. have shown that tear size is an important factor in the development of pain, while rotator cuff tears become increasingly common with age.[72] The development of pain in shoulders is associated with an increase in tear size.[37,46] Broadly the epidemiological evidence supports the concept of the biopsychosocial framework given the multiple factors associated with shoulder pain across all domains.

A clinical focus of pain mechanisms involved in shoulder pain

Understanding the mechanisms behind an individual's pain experience may have implications for the choice of therapeutic intervention. A number of potentially confusing and sometimes unhelpful descriptors of pain have emerged in recent years such as 'central neuropathic', 'peripheral neuropathic', 'primary chronic', 'secondary chronic', 'nociceptive', and 'nociplastic'. These descriptors may be more relevant to laboratory experimentation than clinical practice, where patients may not present with one acute and specific clinical problem. The experience of pain is rarely packaged neatly into a silo, and pain may have multiple contributory peripheral and central factors. The art of clinical practice is to acknowledge, appreciate, accept, and manage uncertainty.

The role of peripheral tissue processes is most obvious in the case of trauma-related shoulder pain (e.g., fracture, dislocation, acute rotator cuff tear) or specific pathologies corresponding with the expected clinical signs and symptoms (e.g., frozen shoulder, osteoarthritis). Inflammation leading to peripheral sensitization and altered mechanical loading patterns can result in what is sometimes referred to as the nociceptive pain phenotype. The typical clinical presentation is one of pain that is reasonably well localized, is primarily movement-evoked (intermittent), and with a consistent pattern of aggravating and easing factors.[65] Validated screening questionnaires such as painDETECT provide a relatively simple way of assessing a patient's pain phenotype, with higher scores being associated with a higher pain intensity, depression, and a reduced quality of life, indicative of a more neuropathic or nociplastic phenotype.[22]

However, a high percentage of individuals presenting with shoulder pain in primary care, based on their report of symptoms and clinical examination, may not be recognized to have an identifiable pathological driver of their symptoms, or report a specific traumatic event.[43] Several diagnostic labels have been used in the literature to describe this group including "rotator cuff related shoulder pain", "subacromial impingement or pain syndrome" or simply "nonspecific shoulder pain".[41,62] Identifying a specific structure as a source of symptoms is difficult, given the relatively high prevalence of imaging abnormalities in the absence of symptoms, and the poor sensitivity of clinical special tests to inform a structural diagnosis.[3,32]

Studies examining the somatosensory profile of individuals with unilateral shoulder pain have demonstrated reduced pressure pain thresholds both locally at the site of pain and in remote body regions, as well as impaired conditioned pain modulation.[9,60] These findings point to enhanced pro-nociceptive mechanisms within the central nervous system (central sensitization, impaired descending inhibition) in addition to peripheral nociceptive processes. Where central processes dominate the clinical picture, patients may present with high pain intensity, multiple areas of pain, spontaneous as well as movement-evoked pain (often constant), regional or widespread tenderness on palpation, and pain that may be less responsive to interventions targeted at peripheral tissues.[28] This pattern of signs and symptoms can be referred to as the nociplastic pain phenotype (https://www.iasp-pain.org/resources/terminology/?navItemNumber=576#Pain). However, a key misconception is that central sensitization is always predominantly driven by central factors in this nociplastic picture. Central sensitization is present after acute trauma, and in this situation primarily caused by the peripheral activation of nociceptors, for example after a burn or fracture, and clearly this serves a vital purpose in protecting the injured body part from further damage.[61] Central sensitization is also common in conditions like osteoarthritis, even when the pathology is well localized to a specific structure, thus demonstrating the real world complexity of pain phenotyping.[27,68]

There is emerging evidence that factors other than physical ones, including depression, anxiety, sleep, and lower expectations of recovery are associated with pain and disability among individuals with shoulder pain.[59,73] This is further supported by a recent clinical trial in the primary care setting whereby over 50% of individuals with shoulder pain reported additional health complaints, 70% were overweight or obese, and almost one in four individuals had widespread pain.[64] Psychosocial, lifestyle, and general health factors may negatively impact on the pain experience via neuroimmune modulation of peripheral and central nociceptive processing, or by influencing the individual's coping strategies and behavioral responses (e.g., avoidance behavior), which can also impact on tissue health.[49] These mechanisms are not mutually exclusive, and underlie the complexity of how both peripheral and central processes interact to shape the individual's pain experience. It must also be acknowledged that systemic disease such as hypertension, atherosclerosis, metabolic syndrome, and diabetes are associated with an increased risk of peripheral structural pathologies such as osteoarthritis and tendinopathy.

There is a belief that a peripheral structural intervention is not the best way to address central sensitization. This can be a misconception, as a hip replacement is a highly effective intervention for hip osteoarthritis and reverses central sensitization in this context.[27] This emphasizes the difficulty in diagnosing and treating musculoskeletal pain, as dichotomizing the pain phenotype does not necessarily help guide intervention. The role of surgery remains controversial and highly debated, however, there is clearly a role for structural interventions, particularly for specific acute traumatic injuries, and within specific contexts, for more persistent cases.[30] Certainly, when surgery is undertaken it should be as part of a holistic package of care tailored to the individual's needs. While there is a rationale for being extremely careful when dealing with the more nociplastic pain phenotype, we must also consider the potential for more proximal structural drivers such as cervical radiculopathy, and consider gathering more diagnostic information, such as using targeted local anesthetic injections. Although greater pain radiation and a more neuropathic or nociplastic pain phenotype is associated with poorer clinical outcomes after surgery, this does not mean that patients do not still gain significantly from surgical intervention.[26] Consequently, it is vital to recognize these factors and ensure that the patient is fully aware of the expected outcome, as well as any potential harms of an intervention.

The recent emergence of primary and secondary chronic musculoskeletal pain is controversial, and arguably tries to force a binary choice upon clinicians when many people experiencing pain are within the middle ground, as in the center of a Venn diagram. Primary being chronic pain in the absence of another condition causing the pain, secondary being chronic pain caused by another condition such as tendinopathy or osteoarthritis. In reality, the latter is simply a hypothesis, and the best epidemiological evidence can only describe the structural abnormalities that may increase the risk of pain.

In this categorical system, there is no certainty that the basis for the pain in the secondary classification can be identified. Again, in the real world, patients are complex and heterogeneous; some may have a single structural abnormality that is highly likely to account for their symptoms, some have no structural abnormality and multiple non-structural risk factors for their pain, while the majority are located somewhere in between, and this artificial dichotomization of primary versus secondary chronic (persistent) pain is arguably unhelpful and potentially counterproductive.

Assessment and management of individuals with shoulder pain

There is consensus that the assessment and management of individuals with musculoskeletal disorders should be guided by a biopsychosocial framework (Chapter 6). This will include an initial evaluation to identify individuals with specific pathologies and/or signs and symptoms suggestive of red flags or systemic pathologies requiring further investigations, or referral for medical/surgical management (Chapter 8). A comprehensive assessment will aim to identify all the relevant factors which may be contributing to an individual's clinical presentation. While an understanding of pain mechanisms can guide assessment and management, the clinician should recognize that factors across the biopsychosocial spectrum are interrelated, will vary from individual to individual, and will influence both peripheral and central neuroimmune processes. Therefore, it is essential that the assessment and treatment of individuals with shoulder pain remains person-centered, and avoids unhelpful reductionist approaches targeting "peripheral versus central" processing or "physical versus psychosocial" factors. Supporting the need for a multidimensional assessment, Chester et al., in a longitudinal analysis involving more than 1000 people with shoulder pain, showed that levels of self-efficacy, employment status and expectations of recovery were better predictors of outcome than physical examination findings.[7]

While our understanding of the biopsychosocial model as it relates to pain has been derived primarily from research investigating spinal pain, there is no reason why we should not apply these principles to other regions such as the shoulder.[28] Through a combination of attentive history taking, information gained from standardized questionnaires, as well as clinical examination findings, a biopsychosocial profile of the individual with pain may be established irrespective of the primary location of pain.[50] This approach is applicable across various musculoskeletal pain disorders and may help in formulating an individual-specific treatment plan. Knowledge of the likely pain mechanisms involved will not be as helpful without an understanding of the biopsychosocial variables, both modifiable and non-modifiable, that influence these mechanisms.

Emerging treatment frameworks termed psychologically informed practice emphasize the need to account for and address patients' beliefs, attitudes, expectations, emotional responses, and coping strategies as part of a multidimensional, person-centered approach to assessment and management.[45] Whereas traditional biomedical models of care have emphasized symptom reduction as the primary treatment endpoint, treatment approaches embedded within a biopsychosocial model of care also focus on reducing long-term disability.

Using knowledge of pain to enhance outcomes and minimize harm

Many interventions are proposed for people with shoulder pain. While specific factors related to each intervention are plausible, there are several observations that challenge the assumption that specific factors alone can explain outcome. There is a growing recognition of the role of contextual factors to explain outcomes in people with musculoskeletal pain,[62] such as the therapeutic alliance between the healthcare provider and the patient, patient-specific factors like expectations and previous experiences, as well as factors related to the treatment setting. For example, it is estimated that up to 75% of the total treatment effect across a wide range of therapies (both pharmacological and non-pharmacological) for osteoarthritis is attributable to contextual factors rather than to the specific effects of the treatment.[75] Similarly, de Baets et al. showed that baseline self-efficacy levels and expectations of recovery were predictive of outcomes for individuals with shoulder pain attending physical therapy (physiotherapy)[12] (see Chapter 6).

While a detailed discussion of how these contextual factors impact on outcomes is beyond the scope of this chapter, behavioral responses (e.g., higher levels of self-efficacy leading to more task engagement and greater ability to employ active coping strategies) or neurobiological processes (e.g., placebo analgesia) are implicated. It is also important to remember that a large proportion of this contextual treatment effect is simply related to measurement error and natural improvement over time. Clinicians must be careful in interpreting these findings as it is tricky to unpick association from causality. Frequently, higher self-efficacy and positive expectations are associated with lower levels of disability and pain, as well as better outcomes. However, this relationship is highly complex and the degree to which self-efficacy is truly modifiable is uncertain, as many clinical trials in this area lack an adequate comparator and are highly biased in favor of the self-efficacy based intervention.[48]

Interventions that solely target impairments are therefore inadequate, and clinicians must recognize the important role of contextual factors. Particular attention should be paid to adopting an empathic communication style, validating the patient's symptoms and experiences, listening to and addressing patients' concerns and worries, providing accurate and evidence-based education to optimize treatment expectations, preparing the patient to better deal with adverse effects such as a pain flare up, and engaging in collaborative goal setting.[48] Contextual factors also have the potential to negatively impact on outcomes. In a qualitative study, patients with a diagnosis of "subacromial impingement" viewed their diagnosis through a biomedical lens and relied on imaging to determine this diagnosis.[10] The emphasis on pathology and structure negatively impacted on their beliefs regarding non-surgical interventions such as exercise therapy. Clinicians should therefore be mindful of the terminology they use to describe a patient's symptoms, and should provide an optimistic diagnosis grounded in biopsychosocial reasoning. This parallels work in the low back pain literature showing that individuals who conceptualize pain as a pathoanatomical entity had inferior outcomes.[5] In the absence of trauma, or signs and symptoms suggestive of serious or systemic pathology, care should be taken to avoid unnecessary use of imaging. This may be associated with worse clinical outcomes and higher utilization of more invasive interventions including injections or surgery, which carry additional risk without consistent evidence of achieving superior outcomes.[57] Care should also be taken in framing the results of any investigation, including imaging, in a manner that is specifically designed to reassure and not provoke fear.

Case example

A 45-year-old woman complains of left-sided (nondominant) shoulder pain for the previous 6 months. She has noticed that her pain has worsened in the last 2 months and her sleep is now disturbed. Her shoulder pain is predominantly movement-related especially with reaching overhead, carrying any weight in her left hand and when washing and drying her hair. She uses anti-inflammatories intermittently that give her pain relief. She has noticed that the increase in pain with movement is now lasting longer than before, often into the following day depending on how much she is doing. She recently had an MRI scan of her shoulder which showed a "partial tear" of supraspinatus. She has started to rely on her right shoulder/arm for everyday function as she is unsure how much she should be doing with her left arm, especially if there is a chance of further damaging it.

She has a history of low back and neck pain, and her right knee has been sore in recent months but not as bothersome as her shoulder pain. She says she gets regular "aches and pains" in different body regions but puts this down to "wear and tear" from her busy lifestyle and work. The last year has been challenging as she has lost her job as a chef during the COVID-19 pandemic. She has two children, one of whom is due to start university soon, and she is concerned regarding her financial situation. She previously was an avid runner but has not been exercising in recent months as she finds it difficult to self-motivate to exercise alone.

Commentary

Mechanisms can be inferred from the clinical presentation and examination findings, however, the management approach will depend on the individual's story and the identification of modifiable factors across the biopsychosocial spectrum, known to modulate the pain experience. There are several features in the above case presentation consistent with nociceptive pain. The pain onset was linked to a specific activity, the pain in her shoulder is predominantly movement related, localized to the upper arm and relieved with anti-inflammatory medication. However, the presence of multisite pain and a recent increase in the activity–pain response relationship could suggests components of nociplastic pain (historically this may have been described as central sensitization).

From a clinical standpoint, knowledge of the underlying pain mechanism(s), while useful, cannot guide the treatment approach without knowledge of the modifiable and non-modifiable factors contributing to an individual's pain experience based on the clinical history and examination. This case study highlights several factors that the clinician should consider. This individual's shoulder pain should be considered on the background of a multisite pain phenotype. She also presents with uncertainty relating to the meaning of her movement-related pain as she is concerned that pain may cause "more" damage. Disturbed sleep, recent stress in relation to her job loss and the financial implications, weight gain, the long-term consequences of the COVID-19 pandemic, and low motivation for activity/exercise are of relevance.

There is consensus in the scientific community that movement or exercise-based rehabilitation is usually appropriate for individuals with nontraumatic shoulder pain in the absence of sinister or red flag pathologies.[17,42] Specifically, in relation to the case study, the exercise intervention will be guided based on symptom irritability and specific impairments identified during the examination, but should also target activities that the patient is avoiding or reports difficulty with. This will usually be progressed in a graded manner and the patient should be reassured that it is safe to exercise with a tolerable level of pain.

This individual is concerned that pain with movement is a sign that she could be causing more damage. Counselling the patient that pain does not by default imply damage can be very helpful in encouraging activity engagement, thereby reducing functional disability and enhancing self-efficacy. A more pragmatic approach would be to ensure that any pain experienced is tolerable and returns to pre-activity levels within a reasonable timeframe, usually no more than 24 hours. If an increase in pain is sufficient to negatively impact on this individual's sleep or daily activities, then it is important that the individual is facilitated to modify her daily activities or exercise program.

A flare up of pain, while not uncommon, can be distressing for patients. This individual should be educated at an early point in their care on the meaning of flare ups and how best to cope with them. Understanding that a flare up is common and not usually a sign of further injury or damage may be helpful. Rather than seeing a pain flare up as a set-back, it is often a useful time to reflect on the situation and identify potential triggers. This provides an ideal opportunity for the patient to reflect on the contextual nature of pain, and how factors across the biopsychosocial spectrum might be involved in their individual experiences.

A challenge for the clinician in treating individuals with shoulder pain is to educate the individual in a meaningful way on the role of non-shoulder factors in influencing the pain experience. Patients often report that the pain education they have received has not been relevant to their situation.[63] Reflective questioning is a useful clinical strategy that encourages patients to reflect on their own situation and experiences. This provides the ideal time to discuss and reflect on the multidimensional influences on pain illustrated by examples from the patient's own account of their symptoms. Reflective questioning relevant to the case study may include questions such as, "How does your pain respond to stress?", "Have you noticed any association between your shoulder pain and pain in other parts of your body?", or, "How does not running make you feel, and what might be the benefits of getting back to running?"

It is also important at an early stage to set realistic expectations, as optimal outcomes can take many weeks or even months to achieve. Unrealistic expectations may result in premature disengagement from the treatment plan, as the patient often feels the treatment approach is unsuccessful. This may also have adverse consequences on how the individual views their pain problem or the probability of a successful resolution. This can fuel the cycle of pain and disability.

From the case presentation, this person has reduced her activity levels in recent months. Therefore, general exercise in addition to shoulder-specific exercise should be encouraged and facilitated. The benefits of general exercise on other outcomes like sleep quality, weight management, and mental health are also clearly relevant. If deemed appropriate, referral to other specialties could be considered to comprehensively address the factors contributing to pain and disability. In relation to this case study, if, for example, it appears that the patient is not coping with her recent job loss and the associated stress, then liaising with the general practitioner or local community psychological services may be required.

While this treatment plan is for illustration purposes only, it highlights the complexity facing clinicians daily, and the need to consider a broad range of factors for treatment planning. None of the factors identified from the case study are mutually exclusive; instead, they interact in a non-linear manner which adds to the overall complexity. After a comprehensive evaluation of the patient, the clinician should be able to answer some simple questions: what can I change; what can I change that is meaningful to the patient; what are the barriers to change; and, who or what is required to facilitate the change? A person-specific treatment plan can then be developed.

Conclusions

While many questions remain unanswered as the science continues to evolve, one thing is certain – pain is a highly complex personal experience and cannot be explained solely using a biomedical framework. The reasons and mechanisms underlying the effectiveness of interventions are complex and may often be counterintuitive in terms of the why. It is possible that many treatments with apparently distinct and specific effects actually work through multiple shared mechanisms. For example, engaging with an exercise program may increase levels of self-efficacy or reduce fear avoidance behavior; alternatively, educational, or cognitive behavioral treatments may have similar effects. Further work investigating mediators of change may offer insight into which factors are important and/or necessary to change to enhance clinical outcomes. In the meantime, patient-centered approaches that are grounded in a biopsychosocial framework, promote self-management, and build resilience are to be encouraged.

References

1. Ackermann P, Franklin SL, Dean BJ, Carr AJ, Salo PT, Hart DA. Neuronal pathways in tendon healing and tendinopathy: update. Frontiers in Bioscience. 2014;19:1251-78.
2. Backenköhler U, Strasmann TJ, Halata Z. Topography of mechanoreceptors in the shoulder joint region: a computer-aided 3D reconstruction in the laboratory mouse. The Anatomical Record. 1997;248:433-441.
3. Barreto RPG, Braman JP, Ludewig PM, Ribeiro LP, Camargo PR. Bilateral magnetic resonance imaging findings in individuals with unilateral shoulder pain. Journal of Shoulder and Elbow Surgery. 2019;28:1699-1706.
4. Bodin J, Ha C, Chastang JF, et al. Comparison of risk factors for shoulder pain and rotator cuff syndrome in the working population. American Journal of Industrial Medicine. 2012;55:605-615.
5. Briggs AM, Jordan JE, Buchbinder R, et al. Health literacy and beliefs among a community cohort with and without chronic low back pain. Pain. 2010;150:275-283.
6. Candlish S, Candlish G. Private Language. Available at: https://plato.stanford.edu/entries/private-language/.
7. Chester R, Khondoker M, Shepstone L, Lewis JS, Jerosch-Herold C. Self-efficacy and risk of persistent shoulder pain: results of a Classification and Regression Tree (CART) analysis. British Journal of Sports Medicine. 2019;53:825-834.
8. Cole A, Gill TK, Shanahan EM, Phillips P, Taylor AW, Hill CL. Is diabetes associated with shoulder pain or stiffness? Results from a population based study. The Journal of Rheumatology. 2009;36:371-377.
9. Coronado RA, Simon CB, Valencia C, George SZ. Experimental pain responses support peripheral and central sensitization in patients with unilateral shoulder pain. The Clinical Journal of Pain. 2014;30:143–151.
10. Cuff A, Littlewood C. Subacromial impingement syndrome: what does this mean to and for the patient? A qualitative study. Musculoskeletal Science and Practice. 2018;33:24-28.
11. Dakin SG, Martinez FO, Yapp C, et al. Inflammation activation and resolution in human tendon disease. Science Translational Medicine. 2015;7:311ra173.
12. De Baets L, Matheve T, Meeus M, Struyf F, Timmermans A. The influence of cognitions, emotions and behavioral factors on treatment outcomes in musculoskeletal shoulder pain: a systematic review. Clinical Rehabilitation. 2019;33:980-991.
13. Dean B, Franklin S, Carr A. A systematic review of the histological and molecular changes in rotator cuff disease. Bone & Joint Research. 2012;1:158-166.
14. Dean BJF, Franklin SL, Murphy RJ, Javaid MK, Carr AJ. Glucocorticoids induce specific ion-channel-mediated toxicity in human rotator cuff tendon: a mechanism underpinning the ultimately deleterious effect of steroid injection in tendinopathy? British Journal of Sports Medicine. 2014;48:1620-1626.
15. Dean BJF, Gwilym SE, Carr AJ. Why does my shoulder hurt? A review of the neuroanatomical and biochemical basis of shoulder pain. British Journal of Sports Medicine. 2013;47:1095-1104.
16. Dean BJF, Snelling SJ, Dakin SG, Murphy RJ, Javaid MK, Carr AJ. Differences in glutamate receptors and inflammatory cell numbers are associated with the resolution of pain in human rotator cuff tendinopathy. Arthritis Research & Therapy. 2015;17:1-10.
17. Doiron-Cadrin P, Lafrance S, Saulnier M, et al. Shoulder rotator cuff disorders: a systematic review of clinical practice guidelines and semantic analyses of recommendations. Archives of Physical Medicine and Rehabilitation. 2020;101:1233-1242.
18. Dubin AE, Patapoutian A. Nociceptors: the sensors of the pain pathway. The Journal of Clinical investigation. 2010;120:3760-3772.
19. Floyd R. The Private Language Argument. Available at: https://philosophynow.org/issues/58/The_Private_Language_Argument
20. Franklin SL, Dean BJ, Wheway K, Watkins B, Javaid MK, Carr AJ. Up-regulation of glutamate in painful human supraspinatus tendon tears. The American Journal of Sports Medicine. 2014;42:1955-1962.
21. Freeman M, Wyke B. The innervation of the knee joint. An anatomical and histological study in the cat. Journal of Anatomy. 1967;101:505.
22. Freynhagen R, Baron R, Gockel U, Tölle TR. PainDETECT: a new screening questionnaire to identify neuropathic components in patients with back pain. Current Medical Research and Opinion. 2006;22:1911-1920.
23. Gardner E. The innervation of the shoulder joint. The Anatomical Record. 1948;102:1-18.
24. Gill T, Shanahan EM, Taylor A, Buchbinder R, Hill C. Shoulder pain in the community: an examination of associative factors using a longitudinal cohort study. Arthritis Care & Research. 2013;65:2000-2007.
25. Guanche CA, Noble J, Solomonow M, Wink CS. Periarticular Neural Elements in the Shoulder Joint. Thorofare, NJ: Slack Inc.; 1999.
26. Gwilym S, Oag H, Tracey I, Carr A. Evidence that central sensitisation is present in patients with shoulder impingement syndrome and influences the outcome after surgery. The Journal of Bone and Joint Surgery. 2011;93:498-502.
27. Gwilym SE, Filippini N, Douaud G, Carr AJ, Tracey I. Thalamic atrophy associated with painful osteoarthritis of the hip is reversible after arthroplasty: a longitudinal voxel-based morphometric study. Arthritis & Rheumatism. 2010;62:2930-2940.
28. Hainline B, Turner JA, Caneiro J, Stewart M, Moseley GL. Pain in elite athletes – neurophysiological, biomechanical and psychosocial considerations: a narrative review. British Journal of Sports Medicine. 2017;51:1259-1264.
29. Hanvold TN, Wærsted M, Mengshoel AM, Bjertness E, Twisk J, Veiersted KB. A longitudinal study on risk factors for neck and shoulder pain among young adults in the transition from technical school to working life. Scandinavian Journal of Work, Environment & Health. 2014;597-609.
30. Haque A, Pal Singh H. Does structural integrity following rotator cuff repair affect functional outcomes and pain scores? A meta-analysis. Shoulder & Elbow. 2018;10:163-169.
31. Hashimoto T, Hamada T, Sasaguri Y, Suzuki K. Immunohistochemical approach for the investigation of nerve distribution in the shoulder joint capsule. Clinical Orthopaedics and Related Research. 1994;273-282.
32. Hermans J, Luime JJ, Meuffels DE, Reijman M, Simel DL, Bierma-Zeinstra SM. Does this patient with shoulder pain have rotator cuff disease?: The Rational Clinical Examination systematic review. JAMA. 2013;310:837-847.

33. Hinsley H, Nicholls A, Daines M, Wallace G, Arden N, Carr A. Classification of rotator cuff tendinopathy using high-definition ultrasound. Muscles, Ligaments and Tendons Journal. 2014;4:391.

34. IASP. IASP Announces Revised Definition of Pain. Available at: https://www.iasp-pain.org/PublicationsNews/NewsDetail.aspx?ItemNumber=10475.

35. Ide K, Shirai Y, Ito H, Ito H. Sensory nerve supply in the human subacromial bursa. Journal of Shoulder and Elbow Surgery. 1996;5:371-382.

36. James S. Human pain and genetics: some basics. British Journal of Pain. 2013;7:171-178.

37. Keener JD, Galatz LM, Teefey SA, et al. A prospective evaluation of survivorship of asymptomatic degenerative rotator cuff tears. The Journal of Bone and Joint Surgery. 2015;97:89.

38. Kooijman MK, Barten D-JA, Swinkels IC, et al. Pain intensity, neck pain and longer duration of complaints predict poorer outcome in patients with shoulder pain – a systematic review. BMC Musculoskeletal Disorders. 2015;16:1-9.

39. LaMotte RH, Shain CN, Simone DA, Tsai E. Neurogenic hyperalgesia: psychophysical studies of underlying mechanisms. Journal of Neurophysiology. 1991;66:190-211.

40. Leclerc A, Chastang J, Niedhammer I, Landre M, Roquelaure Y. Incidence of shoulder pain in repetitive work. Occupational and Environmental Medicine. 2004;61:39-44.

41. Lewis J. Rotator cuff related shoulder pain: assessment, management and uncertainties. Manual Therapy. 2016;23:57-68.

42. Lewis J, McCreesh K, Roy J-S, Ginn K. Rotator cuff tendinopathy: navigating the diagnosis-management conundrum. Journal of Orthopaedic & Sports Physical Therapy. 2015;45:923-937.

43. Linsell L, Dawson J, Zondervan K, et al. Prevalence and incidence of adults consulting for shoulder conditions in UK primary care; patterns of diagnosis and referral. Rheumatology. 2006;45:215-221.

44. Luime J, Koes B, Hendriksen I, et al. Prevalence and incidence of shoulder pain in the general population; a systematic review. Scandinavian Journal of Rheumatology. 2004;33:73-81.

45. Main CJ, George SZ. Psychologically informed practice for management of low back pain: future directions in practice and research. Physical Therapy. 2011;91:820-824.

46. Mall NA, Kim HM, Keener JD, et al. Symptomatic progression of asymptomatic rotator cuff tears: a prospective study of clinical and sonographic variables. The Journal of Bone and Joint Surgery. 2010;92:2623.

47. Mallen CD, Peat G, Thomas E, Dunn KM, Croft PR. Prognostic factors for musculoskeletal pain in primary care: a systematic review. British Journal of General Practice. 2007;57:655-661.

48. Marks R. Self-efficacy and arthritis disability: an updated synthesis of the evidence base and its relevance to optimal patient care. Health Psychology Open. 2014;1:2055102914564582.

49. Martinez-Calderon J, Meeus M, Struyf F, Morales-Asencio JM, Gijon-Nogueron G, Luque-Suarez A. The role of psychological factors in the perpetuation of pain intensity and disability in people with chronic shoulder pain: a systematic review. BMJ Open. 2018;8:e020703.

50. Meisingset I, Vasseljen O, Vøllestad NK, et al. Novel approach towards musculoskeletal phenotypes. European Journal of Pain. 2020;24:921-932.

51. Melzack R, Wall PD. Pain mechanisms: a new theory. Science. 1965;150:971-979.

52. Millar NL, Reilly JH, Kerr SC, et al. Hypoxia: a critical regulator of early human tendinopathy. Annals of the Rheumatic Diseases. 2012;71:302-310.

53. Minaki Y, Yamashita T, Takebayashi T, Ishii S. Mechanosensitive afferent units in the shoulder and adjacent tissues. Clinical Orthopaedics and Related Research. 1999;369:349-356.

54. Miranda H, Viikari-Juntura E, Martikainen R, Takala E, Riihimäki H. A prospective study of work-related factors and physical exercise as predictors of shoulder pain. Occupational and Environmental Medicine. 2001;58:528-534.

55. Murat A. Pain. *The Stanford Encyclopedia of Philosophy* (Spring 2019 Edition), Edward N. Zalta (ed.). Available at: https://plato.stanford.edu/archives/spr2019/entries/pain/.

56. Nambiema A, Bertrais S, Bodin J, et al. Proportion of upper extremity musculoskeletal disorders attributable to personal and occupational factors: results from the French Pays de la Loire study. BMC Public Health. 2020;20:1-13.

57. Nazari G, MacDermid JC, Bryant D, Athwal GS. The effectiveness of surgical vs conservative interventions on pain and function in patients with shoulder impingement syndrome. A systematic review and meta-analysis. PloS One. 2019;14:e0216961.

58. Neher MD, Weckbach S, Flierl MA, Huber-Lang MS, Stahel PF. Molecular mechanisms of inflammation and tissue injury after major trauma: is complement the "bad guy"? Journal of Biomedical Science. 2011;18:1-16.

59. Nicholls EE, van der Windt DA, Jordan JL, Dziedzic KS, Thomas E. Factors associated with the severity and progression of self-reported hand pain and functional difficulty in community-dwelling older adults: a systematic review. Musculoskeletal Care. 2012;10:51-62.

60. Noten S, Meeus M, Stassijns G, Van Glabbeek F, Verborgt O, Struyf F. Efficacy of different types of mobilization techniques in patients with primary adhesive capsulitis of the shoulder: a systematic review. Archives of Physical Medicine and Rehabilitation. 2016;97:815-825.

61. Peddareddygari LR, Oberoi K, Grewal RP. Congenital insensitivity to pain: a case report and review of the literature. Case Rep Neurol Med. 2014;2014:141953.

62. Ristori D, Miele S, Rossettini G, Monaldi E, Arceri D, Testa M. Towards an integrated clinical framework for patient with shoulder pain. Archives of Physiotherapy. 2018;8:1-11.

63. Robinson V, King R, Ryan CG, Martin DJ. A qualitative exploration of people's experiences of pain neurophysiological education for chronic pain: the importance of relevance for the individual. Manual Therapy. 2016;22:56-61.

64. Roddy E, Ogollah RO, Oppong R, et al. Optimising outcomes of exercise and corticosteroid injection in patients with subacromial pain (impingement) syndrome: a factorial randomised trial. British Journal of Sports Medicine. 2021;55:262-271.

65. Smart KM, Blake C, Staines A, Thacker M, Doody C. Mechanisms-based classifications of musculoskeletal pain: part 1 of 3: symptoms and signs of central sensitisation

in patients with low back (±leg) pain. Manual Therapy. 2012;17:336-344.

66. Soifer TB, Levy HJ, Soifer FM, Kleinbart F, Vigorita V, Bryk E. Neurohistology of the subacromial space. Arthroscopy: The Journal of Arthroscopic & Related Surgery. 1996;12:182-186.

67. Solomonow M, Guanche C, Wink C, Knatt T, Baratta RV, Lu Y. Mechanoreceptors and reflex arc in the feline shoulder. Journal of Shoulder and Elbow Surgery. 1996;5:139-146.

68. Soni A, Wanigasekera V, Mezue M, et al. Central sensitization in knee osteoarthritis: relating presurgical brainstem neuroimaging and PainDETECT-based patient stratification to arthroplasty outcome. Arthritis & Rheumatology. 2019;71:550-560.

69. Urwin M, Symmons D, Allison T, et al. Estimating the burden of musculoskeletal disorders in the community: the comparative prevalence of symptoms at different anatomical sites, and the relation to social deprivation. Annals of the Rheumatic Diseases. 1998;57:649-655.

70. Vangsness Jr CT, Ennis M, Taylor JG, Atkinson R. Neural anatomy of the glenohumeral ligaments, labrum, and subacromial bursa. Arthroscopy: The Journal of Arthroscopic & Related Surgery. 1995;11:180-184.

71. Wrete M. The innervation of the shoulder-joint in man. Cells Tissues Organs. 1949;7:173-190.

72. Yamaguchi K, Ditsios K, Middleton WD, Hildebolt CF, Galatz LM, Teefey SA. The demographic and morphological features of rotator cuff disease: a comparison of asymptomatic and symptomatic shoulders. JBJS. 2006;88:1699-1704.

73. Zhang Y, Duffy J, de Castillero E. Relationships of musculoskeletal disorders, sleep disturbances, and depression among hospital nurses. Sleep. 2017;40:A410.

74. Ziegler E, Magerl W, Meyer R, Treede R-D. Secondary hyperalgesia to punctate mechanical stimuli: central sensitization to A-fibre nociceptor input. Brain. 1999;122:2245-2257.

75. Zou K, Wong J, Abdullah N, et al. Examination of overall treatment effect and the proportion attributable to contextual effect in osteoarthritis: meta-analysis of randomised controlled trials. Annals of the Rheumatic Diseases. 2016;75:1964-1970.

Red flags, inflammatory conditions, and sinister shoulder pathology

8

Laura Finucane, Christopher Mercer, Alastair Hepburn, Raja Bhaskara Rajasekaran, Thomas Cosker

Introduction

Most musculoskeletal conditions involving the shoulder are benign and respond to a wait and watch approach or appropriate nonsurgical management. However, in a small proportion, symptoms that appear to be musculoskeletal in origin are caused by more serious pathologies or non-musculoskeletal sources. These pathologies may masquerade as musculoskeletal conditions in the early stages of the disease, presenting the clinician with a diagnostic challenge. Missed or delayed diagnosis of serious disease may have devastating consequences for patients. Early diagnosis and intervention are essential as this will lead to better outcomes. The clinician should always consider a broad range of differential diagnoses and aim to exclude serious pathology masquerading as a musculoskeletal condition, with the help of red flags.[28]

Red flags are potential warning signs that may indicate the presence of serious pathology.[26] Clinicians must be aware of potential red flags at all stages during every patient encounter, including face to face and telehealth appointments. In most situations, one new red flag on its own may not be enough to cause immediate concern, but it must be closely monitored. Multiple red flags, or in some cases where there is a significant medical history (e.g., past history of cancer) with concerning presenting features, one red flag, may be enough to consider further investigation depending on the context in which it is present.[20]

Some of the more common pathologies that mimic musculoskeletal conditions are presented in this chapter. It is essential that clinicians are aware of these, as early identification may lead to better outcomes.[20] All the pathologies discussed in this chapter may initially be "diagnosed" as variants of musculoskeletal shoulder pain. The presence of red flags, relevant risk factors and non-mechanical symptoms, should challenge the clinician's diagnosis, if the patient is not responding in the manner and timeline anticipated.

Malignancy

Primary bone and soft tissue tumors

Bone and soft tissue tumors are rare in incidence and account for less than 1% of all diagnosed malignancies.[22] In 2010, there were 531 new cases (around 10 per week) of primary bone tumors in the United Kingdom, in stark contrast to nearly 55,200 new cases of breast cancer reported every year. The rarity of these cases coupled with the heterogeneity in presentation pose a challenge to clinicians in diagnosis, because they commonly present to musculoskeletal services as mechanical conditions.[27] Cases of suspected tumors warrant management by specialists trained in musculoskeletal oncology to achieve optimal outcomes. Early referral is paramount since these tumors often grow rapidly, and outcome is directly related to the size at presentation. The upper extremity is the third most common site of occurrence of these tumors, with wide variation in their histological presentation.[11]

Symptoms and presentation

In the case of bone tumors, the commonest symptom is a constant, dull aching pain around the shoulder joint. Swelling and tenderness with persistent non-mechanical pain around the shoulder joint that increases at night warrants urgent evaluation to rule out a primary tumor.[21] A painful soft tissue mass that is greater than 5 cm (1.97 in), rapidly increasing in size, associated with non-mechanical pain, deep to the fascia, and with recurrence following excision, should be suspected as a tumor and requires urgent investigation and specialist referral.[21,74] Importantly, soft tissue tumors may not always be painful, with up to 71% of people with soft tissue sarcomas only seeking help when the lump increases in size.[21] Clinicians need to be aware that bone and soft tissue tumors have a bimodal age-specific incidence rate, with peaks in incidence seen in teenagers and young adults (around the second and third decades) and elderly patients.[21]

Malignant tumors commonly present with swelling around the shoulder that has been insidious in onset. Infiltration of soft tissues and muscles around the shoulder results in restricted shoulder movements usually associated with pain.[74] In elderly people, metastases to the shoulder are not uncommon and are usually associated with pain and loss of movement. Imaging is important to differentiate tumors from other causes of pain and loss of movement.[12]

Evaluation and investigations

Following clinical examination of the involved shoulder, imaging is important in the diagnosis of a malignant bone tumor involving the shoulder (Table 8.1).

Table 8.1 Summary of the most appropriate investigation for diagnosis and onward management

Modality	Primary tumors	Secondary tumors	Visceral	Rheumatology
Plain radiographs	A radiograph may establish the presence of visible moth-eaten periosteal reaction, characteristic of aggressive tumors.	A radiograph may show bone destruction which is typical of lung cancer, and bone sclerosis, which is typical of prostate cancer; destruction and sclerosis patterns are both common with breast cancer. A radiograph is used to establish risk of pathological fracture. [51]	Conventional radiography has limited diagnostic value in the assessment of most patients with abdominal pain.	Plain radiographs may show erosive change in primary inflammatory arthritides such as RA.
MRI	Used to evaluate the exact extent of the disease and assess the soft tissue involvement extension. STIR in addition to conventional T1 and T2 images help in evaluation of bone tumors and differentiation from infection and edema.[25]	MRI is used as the gold standard in detecting MBD. Where MBD is suspected, consider including the whole spine as MBD is more common in the axial skeleton.[68]	MRI is an emerging technique for the evaluation of abdominal pain that avoids ionizing radiation.[8]	May demonstrate synovitis (particularly if gadolinium contrast is used), effusion and erosion, as well as background rotator cuff pathology and degenerative change. However, in practice MRI is rarely used in the routine management of primary inflammatory arthritis, ultrasound being preferred.
CT	CT to evaluate the lesion involving the shoulder has a limited role, but can be used to define the size of the tumor and determine the presence of peripheral or satellite lesions.[53]	If there are contraindications for MRI, consider CT scan.	CT is the investigation of choice for general acute abdominal pain. CT is the most sensitive technique for depicting free intraperitoneal air and is valuable for determining the cause of any perforation.[67]	CT will demonstrate erosive and degenerative change; rarely used in practice by rheumatologists, more commonly used by orthopedic surgeons for perioperative planning.
Biopsy	Biopsy is mandatory for histological confirmation, operability assessment and therapy planning.[53] Usually a percutaneous needle biopsy under fluoroscopic guidance/ ultrasound guidance through the anterior fibers of the deltoid muscle is recommended.	Biopsy will help determine the primary cancer where there is suspicion of metastasis.		Synovial biopsy of the shoulder may demonstrate chronic inflammation in RA but is seldom used in practice unless co-existing pathology is suspected, such as infection.
Ultrasound			Ultrasonography is the initial imaging test of choice for patients presenting with right upper quadrant pain.	
Blood and urine tests	Blood tests reveal M proteins produced by myeloma cells and also another abnormal protein produced by myeloma cells – beta-2-mirogobulin. Urine samples reveal Bence Jones proteins characteristic of multiple myeloma.	There is no combination of inflammatory markers that can be used as a reliable rule-in or rule-out test strategy. The decision to test must be made in the context of other clinical findings.[75]		Raised inflammatory markers (ESR and CRP) are typical, but not universal in RA and PMR; rheumatoid factor is positive in approximately 85% of patients with RA; anti-CCP antibodies are predictive of erosive disease in RA.

Anti-CCP, anti-cyclic citrullinated peptides; CRP, C-reactive protein; CT, computerized tomography; ESR, erythrocyte sedimentation rate; MBD, metastatic bone disease; MRI, magnetic resonance imaging; PMR, polymyalgia rheumatica; RA, rheumatoid arthritis; STIR, Short TI Inversion Recovery.

Biopsy and histopathology analysis

"When tumor is the rumor, tissue is the issue": this adage remains relevant for suspected musculoskeletal tumors. For lesions in the shoulder, needle biopsy is recommended, followed by histopathological analysis to confirm diagnosis. Outcomes may be enhanced if the biopsy is performed by the treating surgeon, and histological analysis by an experienced pathologist.

Common malignant tumors of the shoulder and management

Multiple myeloma is a malignant tumor of bone marrow. It affects approximately 20 per million people each year. Most cases are seen in people aged 50–70 years old.[48] In the early stages there may be no symptoms or possibly vague symptoms such as fatigue and lethargy. Over time, bone pain, anemia and kidney dysfunction and general malaise ensue. It is an important differential in the work up of any suspected bone malignancy, and while it affects the entire skeleton, the shoulder is a common site. Blood investigations enable clinicians to reach the diagnosis, and with modern chemotherapy regimens, patients have better prognosis.[48]

Osteosarcoma is the second most common bone cancer. Annually it occurs in 2–3 per million people. Most cases occur in teenagers and young adults. Most osteosarcomas occur around the knee, followed by the hip, with the shoulder being the third most common site. Treatment involves neoadjuvant chemotherapy with the aim to shrink the tumor and decrease spread. Following chemotherapy, wide excision surgery is advised with at least a 2 cm (0.8 in) margin from the edges of the tumor.

Ewing's sarcoma most commonly occurs in people aged 5–20 years old. Radiotherapy and chemotherapy need to be considered prior to or after surgery, depending on the disease progression in concurrence with the clinical oncology team. However, clinicians need to be mindful that prosthesis surgery in the upper extremity may be associated with challenges in functional outcomes, and complications including dislocation.[38]

Chondrosarcoma occurs most commonly in people aged 40–70 years old. Unlike osteosarcoma and Ewing's sarcoma, adjuvant therapy has a limited role in chondrosarcoma. Surgical resection of these tumors with adequate margins is the most appropriate management.

Myxofibrosarcoma is one of the most common soft tissue tumors that occurs mainly in people aged 50–70 years old, and is slightly more common in men than women. They are slow growing and painless,[72] and have a high rate of local recurrence and high risk of metastases.[16]

Liposarcoma accounts for up to 18% of all soft tissue sarcomas and can occur most commonly in the trunk, limbs, and abdomen. They are rare in people younger than 30 years old, and may present as a painful mass. These are low-grade neoplasms that rarely metastasize.[13]

Pancoast tumors represent 3–5% of all lung cancers, with a predilection to bony metastases.[15] The major risk factor is smoking, followed by older age, and they affect men more than women. These tumors develop in the apices of the lungs and infiltrate the thoracic inlet, which leads to a constellation of symptoms depending on which structures are invaded and compressed within this area. The tumor may invade muscles, upper ribs, thoracic vertebral bodies, subclavian vessels, the brachial plexus, and the thoracic autonomic chain, specifically the stellate ganglion.[53] Symptoms may include cough, hemoptysis, and dyspnea but are uncommon in the initial stages of the disease due to the tumor's location.[15] In the early stages the most reported symptom is shoulder pain due to the invasion of the pleura, upper ribs and brachial plexus. Symptoms may radiate down the arm in a typical ulnar nerve distribution, with physical signs relating to the invasion and compression of nervous, vascular, and bony structures within the thoracic inlet.[53]

- Tumors located in the anterior compartment of the thoracic inlet will affect the first intercostal nerve and upper ribs, subclavian and jugular veins, presenting with pain in the upper anterior chest wall and venous thrombosis.
- Tumors within the middle compartment will affect the brachial plexus, subclavian artery and phrenic nerves causing neurological symptoms of pain and paresthesia in the upper limb, potential paralysis of the diaphragm and arterial thrombosis.
- Tumors within the posterior compartment will affect the scalene muscles, subclavian and vertebral artery,

stellate ganglion, the sympathetic chain, long thoracic and accessory nerves, and vertebral bodies. Pain is reported within the axilla and medial aspect of the arm, and initial irritation of the sympathetic chain and specifically the stellate ganglion causes flushing and increased sweating ipsilaterally. Further invasion of the sympathetic chain may cause Horner's syndrome in 40% of cases,[43] which is associated with ipsilateral drooping of the eyelid, constricted pupil and lack of sweating (ptosis, miosis, and anhidrosis).[53]

Management

All suspected malignant bone and soft tissue tumors of the shoulder require urgent onward referral and diagnostic work up (Table 8.1). Management and discussion in a sarcoma multidisciplinary team (MDT) ensures better coordination and communication to facilitate the most appropriate management.[53]

Box 8.1 Case study

A 22-year-old student presented to his general practitioner with a 3-month history of persistent pain, weight loss, and swelling in his left shoulder. There was no history of trauma. The swelling was approximately the size of a tennis ball. He did not have a fever, and on palpation no increased temperature was felt in the region of the swelling. Active and passive shoulder movements were limited.

An urgent plain radiograph of the left shoulder demonstrated a lesion in the humerus (Figure 8.1A), which prompted an urgent referral to a specialist unit. Further imaging (Figure 8.1B) confirmed an aggressive expansive lesion breaching the left proximal humeral cortex. Ultrasound-guided needle biopsy through the anterior deltoid muscle confirmed a high-grade osteosarcoma (Figure 8.1C) that was managed with neoadjuvant chemotherapy, followed by extra-articular wide excision surgery and prosthetic replacement (Figure 8.1D).

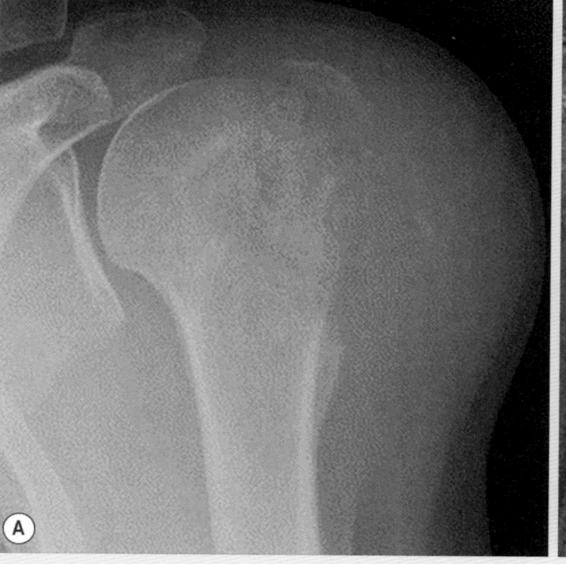

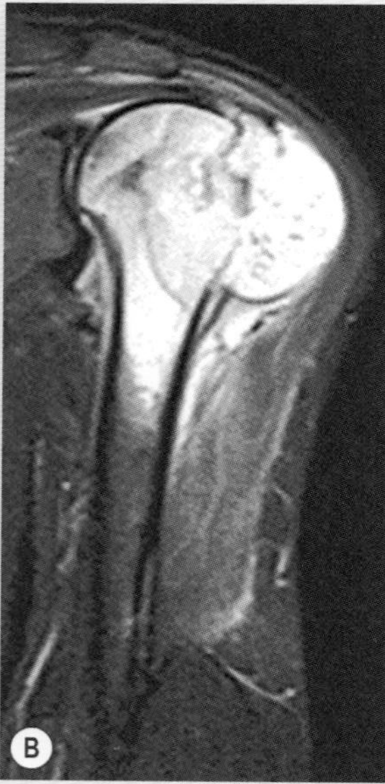

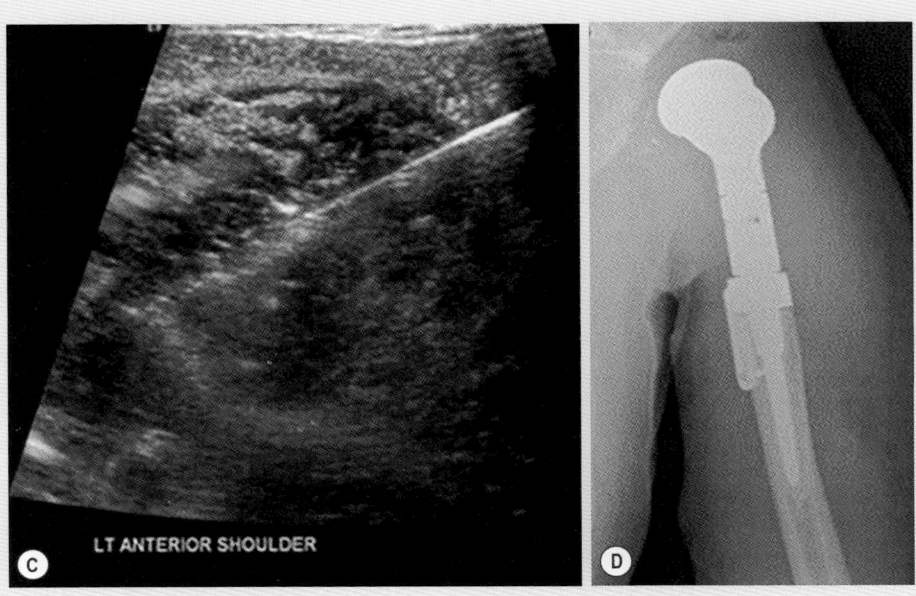

FIGURE 8.1
22-year-old student diagnosed with an osteosarcoma in the left humeral head. (A) Plain radiograph, (B) MRI, (C) ultrasound-guided needle biopsy, (D) wide resection and prosthetic replacement after neo-adjuvant chemotherapy.

Secondary cancers

Metastatic bone disease (MBD) tends to occur more commonly in the spine, but can affect the proximal long bones such as the humerus causing shoulder pain as the first presenting symptom.[51] The five most common cancers to metastasize to bone are of the breast, prostate, lung, kidney and thyroid.[12] MBD of the long bones occurs more commonly in people with breast and lung cancers.[39,55] A past history of cancer is a red flag and has a moderate diagnostic accuracy in relation to the development of MBD,[73] increasing the likelihood of serious pathology by 7% in primary care and 33% in emergency care.[34] A past history of cancer (particularly in cancers with a predilection to bone) should raise the clinician's index of suspicion of serious pathology, but on its own would not be sufficient to act on, as not all primary cancers go on to metastasize. Likewise, the absence of a history of cancer should not reassure the clinician of the lack of serious pathology, as MBD may be the first sign of an undiagnosed primary cancer.[29]

More effective medical treatment of primary cancers has led to longer life expectancies, but places survivors at greater risk of developing MBD.[5] MBD may occur as long as 10–20 years after a diagnosis of primary breast cancer. [45] MBD in the shoulder, particularly in relation to breast and lung cancers, may lead to a misdiagnosis of frozen shoulder, especially as frozen shoulder has a prolonged natural history.[60] Widespread MBD and visceral involvement are the consequences of untreated or late diagnosis and are associated with a poor prognosis.[69]

Clinical presentation

Pain arising from MBD is caused by a combination of ischemic, inflammatory, and neuropathic processes, and is the consequence of destruction or compression of the bone and surrounding tissues.[17] Pain related to MBD may fluctuate, adding to the challenge of early identification, as individuals appear to respond to nonsurgical treatment.[29]

An intermittent localized ache is characteristic of bone pain and may be the first symptom. Pain may also be aggravated by movement.[36] Clearly these descriptors are also present in people with benign conditions.[19] However, in those individuals who have recurrent shoulder problems, an important question to ask is whether the type of pain they are experiencing is similar to previous episodes. In MBD, often the individual will report that this new onset of symptoms is different to the symptoms they have previously experienced, reporting a difference in the quality, location and type of pain.[20]

It is not until the late stages of MBD that pain becomes constant and unremitting, accompanied with significant night pain. Night pain is a common feature in musculoskeletal disorders, and a distinction needs to be made between night pain that is mechanical or caused by MBD. Where the individual describes being woken, with the need to get up and walk to ease the pain during the night, or that they are unable to sleep lying flat and routinely sleep upright in a chair, should raise concern.[19]

Physical examination

Objective findings may mimic rotator cuff pathology or frozen shoulder.[40,55] Tenderness in the greater tuberosity region of the humeral head may be a feature of a pathological fracture.[40] In the late stages, individuals may develop systemic features; a feeling of being unwell, fatigue, fever, or unexplained weight loss. Careful questioning possibly supported by investigations will help establish the relationship between symptoms and serious pathology.[20] If MBD is suspected, urgent referral for further investigation (Table 8.1) and specialist MDT management is essential.[12]

Visceral conditions

Visceral pain is extremely common and is experienced by more than 20% of the population.[31,77] The estimates of prevalence for dyspepsia, constipation and irritable bowel syndrome varies between conditions, and ranges between 1 in 10 to 1 in 2 people.[10,62] Almost all of the visceral organs have the potential to produce symptoms that masquerade as musculoskeletal pain in the thoracic spine, scapular, and shoulder region. Figure 8.2 illustrates the pain referral patterns of the visceral organs.

Visceral pain presentation

Visceral pain is most commonly described as a poorly defined, diffuse and vague,[9,24,61,62] although it may be experienced as sharp, stabbing, colicky pain.[56] Visceral pain generally starts in the midline and then radiates peripherally, and may produce somatic-type symptoms or symptoms in more distal areas.[23,24] A full and thorough clinical examination is required to eliminate the viscera as a potential source of shoulder pain.

Clinical examination

Identifying viscerally referred shoulder pain is a clinical challenge, but clinicians should always consider it as a possible source of the patient's symptoms. Clinicians should ask patients about visceral function, particularly about organs that may refer to the shoulder. This should include a past or current history of cardiac, respiratory, and gastrointestinal symptoms, investigations or concerns, with a clear explanation of the purpose of the questions.

Liver

The liver is the largest organ, responsible for a wide range of tasks, including toxin breakdown, fighting infection, and metabolism of nutrients. Symptoms commonly occur in the later stages of liver disease,[79] and may be experienced as local, right lower thoracic, and right shoulder pain.[54] People with a history of high alcohol intake, obesity, hepatitis, hemochromatosis, or primary biliary cirrhosis may be more likely to develop shoulder symptoms referred from their liver.[2] Clinicians should also be watchful for and question the patient about jaundice, a pruritic rash, yellowing of the eyes, dark circles around the eyes, sweating, fever, strong body odor, bad breath, pale or gray stools, dark urine, fatigue, weight loss, nausea and vomiting, bloating, and testicular swelling.

Gall bladder

Gallstones affect between 5–25% of the population and are more common in women, people who are obese,

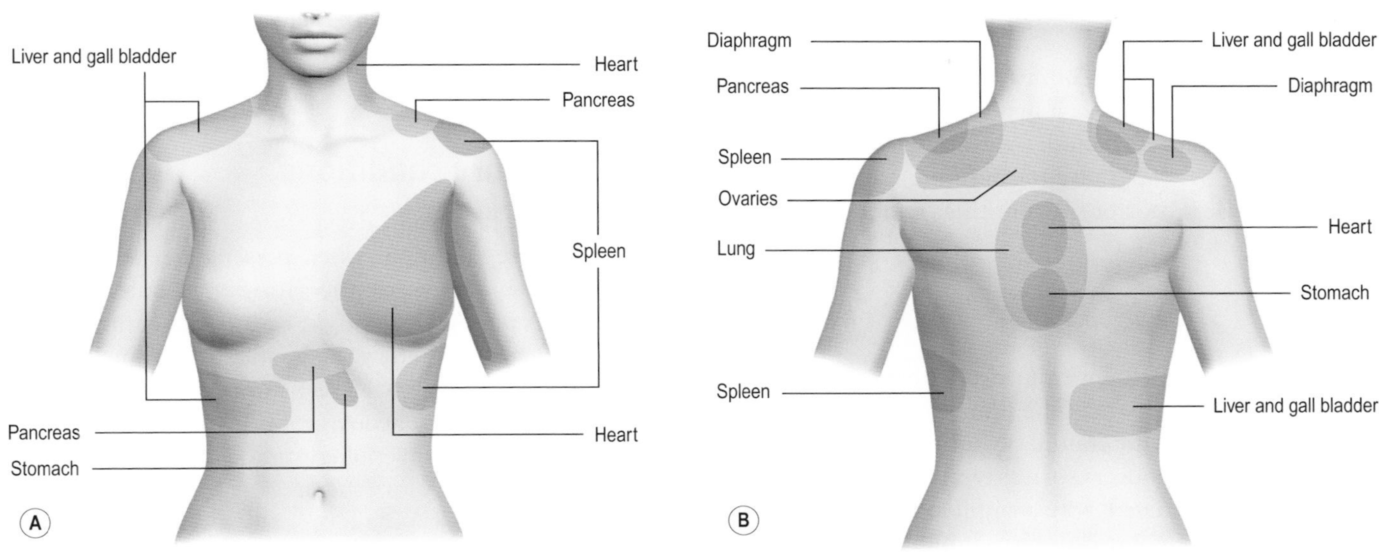

FIGURE 8.2
(A) Anterior and (B) posterior pain referral patterns of visceral organs.
(Based on original drawings by Mr Allan Mercer.)

and older age groups.[32] The gall bladder is positioned below the liver and pain referral occurs in a similar pattern to the liver. Symptoms are commonly caused by calculous cholecystitis (95% of cases), where the cystic duct between the liver and gall bladder becomes blocked and inflamed due to a build-up of biliary sludge/stones.[49] The gall bladder stores bile to help with digestion, so symptoms usually relate to ingestion of fatty, spicy, processed, and high carbohydrate foods. People may initially experience colic-type symptoms, giving severe pain for up to half an hour that then recedes, and may progress to a constant ache.

Pancreas

Pancreatitis is associated with diabetes, high alcohol intake, obesity, and gallstones, though often the cause is unclear. Pancreatic cancer is often hard to detect until the latter stages of the disease and may be associated with general fatigue, weight loss, fever, jaundice, and changes to stools (lighter in color) and urine (darker in color). Pain is predominantly experienced in the epigastric region; the pancreas can also refer to the mid thoracic spine, and there are also documented cases of metastatic disease from the pancreas causing cervical and left or right shoulder pain.[1,46]

Heart

Chest pain and shortness of breath are common symptoms of cardiac disease. Referred pain in the neck, thorax, jaw, throat, and left shoulder and arm may be experienced. Typically, symptoms are activity-related but may occur because of unhealthy stress. Paresthesia, dizziness, nausea and anxiety, or a sense of impending doom are other cardiac-related symptoms.

Lung/pleura

Depending on the area and nature of the pathology, the lungs and pleura may refer to the thorax, or to either shoulder.[44,57,76] Referred pain may be associated with dyspnea, cough or hemoptysis. A smoking history and detailed medical history of any lung disease should be elicited.

Stomach

Stomach pathology most commonly refers to the epigastric region or causes dysphagia; it may refer to the mid to upper thoracic spine and left shoulder. Associated symptoms may include flatus, belching, a feeling of fullness and abdominal bloating, nausea, heartburn, vomiting, reflux, weight loss, and anorexia.

Spleen

The spleen is in the left upper quadrant next to the stomach and is an important part of the immune system. It may be damaged by abscess or traumatic injury.[66,71] Liver disease, anemia, and blood cancers such as lymphoma and leukemia may also be associated with symptoms.[78] If enlarged or infected, the spleen may cause irritation of the diaphragm, and refer pain to the left shoulder via the phrenic nerve (C3, C4, C5).[18] Associated symptoms may be bruising easily and fatigue.

Ovaries

Although unusual, the ovaries may refer pain to the shoulders. Large ovarian cysts may cause pressure on the diaphragm, or ruptured cysts and blood within the peritoneum can also cause irritation of the diaphragm and referral to the shoulder via the phrenic nerve.[50] Shoulder pain will be non-mechanical and may be associated with abdominal pain, nausea and vomiting, and changes to menses.

Physical examination

If there are any suspicions of visceral causes for shoulder symptoms then abdominal inspection, palpation, and auscultation should be performed. If this is not within your scope of practice, appropriate referral is required.

The abdomen should be inspected for: asymmetry, or any obvious lumps and bumps; any signs of injury; bruising (Grey Turner sign that may indicate internal bleeding); skin changes such as spider nevi (present in liver disease); and pulsatile masses that may indicate abdominal aortic aneurysm. Palpation should be performed in a structured and methodical way. The aim is to determine whether there are any painful areas, and whether there are any firm and palpable/pulsatile masses within the abdomen. It may also be possible to reproduce the patient's symptoms with palpation, so it is important to monitor their specific symptoms throughout the process.

Inflammatory conditions

Although soft tissue and degenerative pathology are considerably more common, when presented with a patient with shoulder symptoms the clinician should consider whether this presentation might be the first manifestation of a systemic inflammatory rheumatic disease, such as polymyalgia rheumatica (PMR) or rheumatoid arthritis (RA). These form a heterogeneous group of immune-mediated disorders of unknown etiology that usually require systemic immunomodulatory therapies.

Polymyalgia rheumatica

PMR should be the first inflammatory rheumatic condition to consider when assessing a person with shoulder pain. PMR is a common clinical syndrome of unknown etiology seen in people over the age of 50, characterized by pain and stiffness in the neck, shoulders, pelvic girdle and hips. Symptoms are usually symmetrical but may be assymetrical. The stiffness is particularly severe after rest and may prevent the patient getting out of bed. The onset can be abrupt or more insidious and, along with the related condition giant cell arteritis, may present with a low-grade fever. These conditions therefore both need to be considered in the investigation of a pyrexia of unknown origin. In addition to fever, people with PMR may be systemically unwell, experiencing general malaise, fatigue and weight loss.[14]

As with PMR, the prevalence of rotator cuff related shoulder pain (RCRSP) and symptomatic osteoarthritis (OA) in the glenohumeral and/or acromioclavicular joints also increases with age. This may complicate the clinical picture, and diagnoses of RCRSP and OA based on imaging alone must be avoided. The primary underlying pathology in PMR is a synovitis and subacromial bursitis. Shoulder stiffness in PMR usually affects all directions of movement and needs to be considered with other causes of shoulder stiffness. There is usually minimal tenderness or weakness in PMR, and swelling is rare.

Typically, PMR causes a fairly marked acute phase response, with elevation of the inflammatory markers erythrocyte sedimentation rate (ESR) and C-reactive protein (CRP), which are also used to help guide the response to treatment. Very occasionally inflammatory markers are normal, creating a diagnostic challenge for the clinician. A quick and dramatic response to low doses (15 mg/day) of corticosteroids is a classic feature of PMR. It is not uncommon to require corticosteroids for several years, and to avoid relapse, the dose must be tapered gradually.[65]

Rheumatoid arthritis

Rheumatoid arthritis (RA) is the most common autoimmune chronic inflammatory rheumatic disease, with a population prevalence of 0.5–1%,[63] and is more common in women of childbearing age. The shoulder is involved in 50–60% of cases of RA and, like PMR, symptoms tend to be symmetrical. However, patients are more likely to present with symptoms in other regions first, and RA most commonly presents as a symmetrical polyarthritis affecting the small joints of the hands and feet. The onset may be acute, but is more often subacute or insidious, the latter usually resulting in a poorer prognosis as it is more difficult to control with immunosuppressive drugs. There is also a greater risk of developing erosive joint damage.[33] Patients presenting with an early inflammatory polyarthritis, in whom a firm diagnosis is yet to be established, are more likely to eventually be diagnosed with RA if they have shoulder involvement.[6]

Rheumatologists often observe a history of previous soft tissue disorders, including adhesive capsulitis and rotator cuff tendonitis in patients with newly diagnosed RA. The possibility that a patient may be developing the latter or another systemic inflammatory arthritis should always be considered in patients who appear to have multiple soft lesions of increasing frequency. Indeed, tenosynovitis appears as a common early finding in patients with RA, particularly in those patients who have anti-cyclic citrullinated peptide (anti-CCP) antibodies.[41] In the elderly, a PMR-like presentation of RA is well recognized.

Classic deformities are observed in the hands in people diagnosed with RA, but deformity is rare in the shoulder except in severe or suboptimally treated disease. If the disease remains active with uncontrolled inflammation, irreversible damage, deformity, and instability may occur.[70] Synovitis in the shoulder may lead to effusions, which can extend into the subacromial and subdeltoid spaces, particularly in the presence of rotator cuff damage. As in the hands, secondary muscle wasting is observed. Persistent rheumatoid effusions usually contain thick, inspissated inflammatory fluid, sometimes containing cholesterol crystals in addition to neutrophils, monocytes and synoviocytes. The fluid may become loculated, and therefore difficult to aspirate, and fistulae may form.[4]

In the person with RA involving the shoulder, a loss of external rotation is a common sign although more typically a global restriction of movement is observed, similar to that seen in PMR, particularly with more advance disease.[52] Anterior upper arm pain and tenderness in the bicipital groove is common and may indicate bicipital tendon involvement. There is a risk of bicipital tendon rupture if persistent inflammation is left unchecked.[64]

The management of RA requires a multidisciplinary team, using both pharmacological and non-pharmacological approaches. Suppression of the underlying inflammatory disease using anti-inflammatory and immunosuppressive drug therapy is required.[65] Specific to the shoulder, in addition to arthrocentesis for larger effusions, corticosteroid injections to the glenohumeral joint and subacromial bursa are used to control symptoms. Intramuscular corticosteroid injections are also used, especially during an acute flare of symptoms. These are frequently administered into the deltoid muscle which increases the possibility of subcutaneous fat atrophy. Osteonecrosis of the humeral head may occur in RA or develop secondary to systemic corticosteroid therapy.[47]

Other primary inflammatory arthropathies

Shoulder symptoms are associated in the seronegative inflammatory arthritis group of diseases, although are less common than in RA.[58] Asymmetrical disease is more likely in people with seronegative arthropathies. For example, the disease is asymmetric in approximately 50% of those diagnosed with psoriatic arthritis. Enthesitis tends to be the predominant underlying pathology in this group of diseases, rather than synovitis.[37] Additional involvement of the sternoclavicular joint often points to one of the seronegative arthropathies rather than RA. Synovitis in the sternoclavicular joint causes localized swelling and tenderness, with pain in the joint on arm elevation. Severe symptoms in a less commonly affected joint such as this should raise the

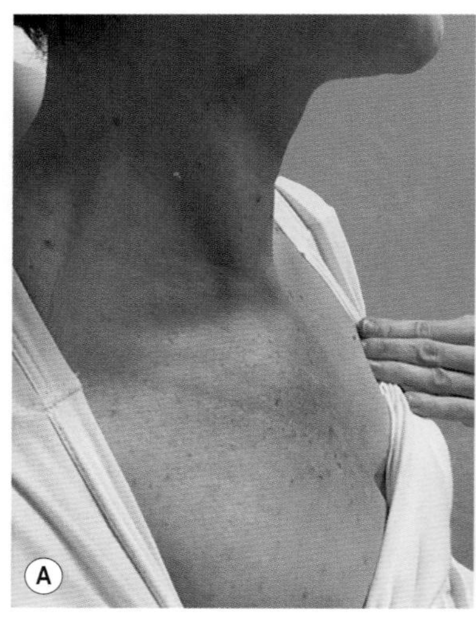

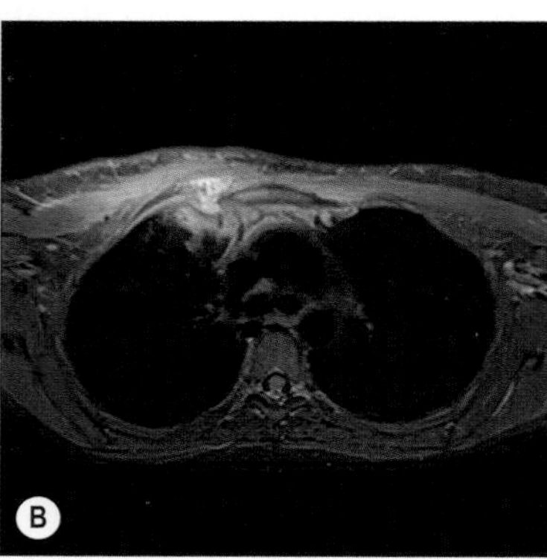

FIGURE 8.3

(A) Infection due to *Staphylococcus aureus* in the right sternoclavicular joint in a 40-year-old woman with psoriatic arthritis treated with sulfasalazine and the TNF-inhibitor adalimumab. (B) Axial MRI at the level of the sternoclavicular joints showing increased signal on T2-weighted images due to soft tissue swelling, bone edema and expansion.

index of suspicion for more serious complications such as infection (Figure 8.3). As in RA, there is a risk of rupture of the long head of biceps in psoriatic arthritis.[7]

Crystal arthropathies

Gout is the most common inflammatory arthritis affecting middle-aged men, and is caused by the deposition of monosodium urate crystals in the joint. This leads to an intense inflammatory response. It most commonly affects lower limb joints, particularly the first metatarsophalangeal joint (podagra); involvement of the shoulder is extremely unusual. However, shoulder involvement in pseudogout (calcium pyrophosphate deposition disease (CPPD)) is common.[59] This is another common form of inflammatory arthritis in the elderly, usually presenting with abrupt-onset severe pain and restricted movement, often accompanied by marked tenderness and erythema. Desquamation over the joint as the acute arthritis settles is a clue to the diagnosis. Chondrocalcinosis is usually seen on radiographs of the affected joint. As with gout, treatment of the acute attack involves NSAIDs, colchicine and corticosteroids (both orally and by injection).

Lupus, inflammatory myositis, and other autoimmune connective tissue disorders

Arthralgia is a very common symptom in systemic lupus erythematosus (SLE), but joint swelling due to synovitis is much less pronounced compared to RA. The inflammatory arthritis seen in SLE is non-erosive. When erosions are found on imaging, this suggests the presence of overlapping RA (formerly termed "rhupus"). Although synovitis in smaller joints is more common, the shoulder may be involved in SLE, as it may in all other multisystem autoimmune connective tissue disorders, such as Sjögren's syndrome and scleroderma (systemic sclerosis). In the latter, dermal fibrosis leads to skin thickening. Although rare, this can affect the shoulder girdle area, with consequent restriction of movement. Subcutaneous and periarticular calcinosis around the shoulder is also described. Fibrosis of ligaments and the joint capsule also contributes to restriction of movement in scleroderma, and fibrosis in the synovium is also observed. Compared to that seen in RA, the synovitis seen in SLE and scleroderma is generally less intense, and erosion is less common.[3]

The primary inflammatory muscle diseases polymyositis and dermatomyositis may present with shoulder pain and stiffness mimicking PMR, but unlike the latter, weakness is a far more pronounced symptom and sign. A proximal myopathy will unusually be apparent on clinical examination, with additional (and usually more severe) lower limb involvement. Dermatomyositis causes typical skin changes such as a heliotrope rash around the eyes, a "shawl" rash on the upper chest, and Gottron's papules on the hands.

Blood tests in patients with polymyositis and dermatomyositis will usually show elevated levels of muscle enzymes such as creatine kinase. Dermatomyositis can be a paraneoplastic phenomenon; testing for myositis-specific antibodies can assist in assessing the patient's risk of an associated malignancy. As in other inflammatory rheumatic conditions such as RA and PMR, corticosteroids are essential in the management of inflammatory myopathies, but additional immunosuppressive drugs are invariably also used for their steroid-sparing and immunomodulatory effects. Patients with autoimmune connective tissue disorders such as SLE, scleroderma, and primary inflammatory myositis have an increased risk of requiring rotator cuff surgery compared to age- and sex-matched controls.[35]

Involvement of the shoulder is also seen in people with the multisystem chronic granulomatous disease sarcoidosis, although is rare relative to other regions such as the ankle and hands.[42] A chronic destructive arthropathy may develop, and synovial biopsy may reveal the presence of typical non-caseating granulomas, although more typically shows nonspecific inflammatory change.

Shoulder pain may be experienced in people with the small vessel vasculitides associated with anti-neutrophil cytoplasmic antibodies (ANCA), such as granulomatosis with polyangiitis, but a true inflammatory arthritis in these diseases is rare.

Conclusion

While most people presenting with shoulder and thoracic pain will not have a serious pathology, the clinician should always consider a range of differential diagnoses as a potential source of symptoms, especially if symptoms are atypical or not responding to treatment. Knowledge of these conditions and their presentation will ensure timely investigation and management and overall better outcomes. In summary, "Things are not always what they seem – be informed and awake."[30]

References

1. Amer S, Manzar HS, Horsley-Silva JL. Shoulder pain as the first sign of pancreatic cancer: 111. American Journal of Gastroenterology. 2015;110:S45-S46.
2. Banks SE, Riley TR, 3rd, Naides SJ. Musculoskeletal complaints and serum autoantibodies associated with chronic hepatitis C and nonalcoholic fatty liver disease. Digestive Diseases and Sciences. 2007;52:1177-1182.
3. Baron M, Lee P, Keystone EC. The articular manifestations of progressive systemic sclerosis (scleroderma). Annals of the Rheumatic Diseases. 1982;41:147-152.
4. Bassett LW, Gold RH, Mirra JM. Rheumatoid bursitis extending into the clavicle and to the skin surface. Annals of the Rheumatic Diseases. 1985;44:336-340.
5. Biermann JS, Holt GE, Lewis VO, Schwartz HS, Yaszemski MJ. Metastatic bone disease: diagnosis, evaluation, and treatment. JBJS. 2009;91:1518-1530.
6. Brinkmann GH, Norli ES, Kvien TK, et al. Disease characteristics and rheumatoid arthritis development in patients with early undifferentiated arthritis: a 2-year follow-up study. J Rheumatol. 2017;44:154-161.
7. Carpenito G, Gutierrez M, Ravagnani V, Raffeiner B, Grassi W. Complete rupture of biceps tendons after corticosteroid injection in psoriatic arthritis "Popeye Sign": role of ultrasound. Journal of Clinical Rheumatology. 2011;17:108.
8. Cartwright SL, Knudson MP. Diagnostic imaging of acute abdominal pain in adults. American Family Physician. 2015;91:452-459.
9. Cervero F. Neurophysiology of gastrointestinal pain. Baillière's Clinical Gastroenterology. 1988;2:183-199.
10. Chang L. Epidemiology and quality of life in functional gastrointestinal disorders. Alimentary Pharmacology & Therapeutics. 2004;20:31-39.
11. Cleeman E, Auerbach JD, Springfield DS. Tumors of the shoulder girdle: a review of 194 cases. Journal of Shoulder and Elbow Surgery. 2005;14:460-465.
12. Coleman R, Holen I. Bone metastases. In: Abeloff's Clinical Oncology, 5th edition. Philadelphia: Elsevier; 2014.
13. Conyers R, Young S, Thomas DM. Liposarcoma: molecular genetics and therapeutics. Sarcoma. 2010;2011: 483154.
14. Dejaco C, Brouwer E, Mason JC, Buttgereit F, Matteson EL, Dasgupta B. Giant cell arteritis and polymyalgia rheumatica: current challenges and opportunities. Nature Reviews Rheumatology. 2017;13:578.
15. Detterbeck FC. Pancoast (superior sulcus) tumors. The Annals of Thoracic Surgery. 1997;63:1810-1818.
16. Dewan V, Darbyshire A, Sumathi V, Jeys L, Grimer R. Prognostic and survival factors in myxofibrosarcomas. Sarcoma. 2012;2012:830879.
17. Falk S, Bannister K, Dickenson AH. Cancer pain physiology. British Journal of Pain. 2014;8:154-162.
18. Fernández-López I, Peña-Otero D, de los Ángeles Atín-Arratibel M, Eguillor-Mutiloa M. Influence of the phrenic nerve in shoulder pain: a systematic review. International Journal of Osteopathic Medicine. 2020;36:36-48.
19. Finucane L, Greenhalgh S, Selfe J. What are the red flags to aid the early detection of metastatic bone disease as a cause of back pain? Physiotherapy Practice and Research. 2017;38:73-77.
20. Finucane LM, Downie A, Mercer C, et al. International Framework for Red Flags for Potential Serious Spinal Pathologies. Journal of Orthopaedic & Sports Physical Therapy. 2020;1-23.
21. George A, Grimer R. Early symptoms of bone and soft tissue sarcomas: could they be diagnosed earlier? The Annals of The Royal College of Surgeons of England. 2012;94:261-266.

22. Gerrand C, Athanasou N, Brennan B, et al. UK guidelines for the management of bone sarcomas. Clin Sarcoma Res. 2016;6:7.

23. Gerwin RD. Myofascial and visceral pain syndromes: visceral-somatic pain representations. Journal of Musculoskeletal Pain. 2002;10:165-175.

24. Giamberardino MA, Affaitati G, Costantini R. Visceral referred pain. Journal of Musculoskeletal Pain. 2010;18:403-410.

25. Golfieri R, Baddeley H, Pringle JS, Souhami R. The role of the STIR sequence in magnetic resonance imaging examination of bone tumours. The British Journal of Radiology. 1990;63:251-256.

26. Goodman CC, Snyder TK. Differential Diagnosis for Physical Therapists. Screening for Referral. St Louis: Elsevier; 2013.

27. Gosling LC, Rushton AB. Identification of adult knee primary bone tumour symptom presentation: a qualitative study. Manual Therapy. 2016;26:54-61.

28. Greenhalgh S, Finucane LM, Mercer C, Selfe J. Safety netting; best practice in the face of uncertainty. Musculoskeletal Science & Practice. 2020;48:102179-102179.

29. Greenhalgh S, Selfe J. Red Flags and Blue Lights. Managing Serious Spinal Pathology, 2nd edition. Edinburgh: Elsevier; 2019.

30. Grieve G. Masqueraders. In: Boyling G, Palastanga N, eds. Grieve's Modern Manual Therapy, 2nd edition. Edinburgh: Churchill Livingston; 1994.

31. Grundy L, Erickson A, Brierley SM. Visceral pain. Annual Review of Physiology. 2019;81:261-284.

32. Gurusamy KS, Davidson BR. Gallstones. BMJ. 2014;348:g2669.

33. Hart FD. Presentation of rheumatoid arthritis and its relation to prognosis. Br Med J. 1977;2:621-624.

34. Hartvigsen J, Hancock MJ, Kongsted A, et al. What low back pain is and why we need to pay attention. The Lancet. 2018;391:2356-2367.

35. Huang LH, Yeung CY, Shyur SD, Lee HC, Huang FY, Wang NL. Diagnosis of Henoch-Schonlein purpura by sonography and radionuclear scanning in a child presenting with bilateral acute scrotum. Journal of Microbiology, Immunology, and Infection. 2004;37:192-195.

36. Jimenez-Andrade J-M, Mantyh PW. Bone cancer pain. International Association for the Study of Pain. 2009;17:2.

37. Kaeley GS, Eder L, Aydin SZ, Gutierrez M, Bakewell C. Enthesitis: a hallmark of psoriatic arthritis. Semin Arthritis Rheum. 2018;48:35-43.

38. Kassab M, Dumaine V, Babinet A, Ouaknine M, Tomeno B, Anract P. Twenty-nine shoulder reconstructions after resection of the proximal humerus for neoplasm with mean 7-year follow-up. Revue de Chirurgie Orthopedique et Reparatrice de L'appareil Moteur. 2005;91:15-23.

39. Kelly M, Lee M, Clarkson P, O'Brien PJ. Metastatic disease of the long bones: a review of the health care burden in a major trauma centre. Canadian Journal of Surgery. 2012;55:95.

40. Kim SY, Jung MW, Kim JM. The shoulder pain due to metastatic breast cancer: a case report. Korean Journal of Pain. 2011;24:119-122.

41. Kleyer A, Krieter M, Oliveira I, et al. High prevalence of tenosynovial inflammation before onset of rheumatoid arthritis and its link to progression to RA-A combined MRI/CT study. Semin Arthritis Rheum. 2016;46:143-150.

42. Kobak S, Sever F, Usluer O, Goksel T, Orman M. The clinical characteristics of sarcoid arthropathy based on a prospective cohort study. Therapeutic Advances in Musculoskeletal Disease. 2016;8:220-224.

43. Komaki R. Preoperative radiation therapy for superior sulcus lesions. Chest Surg Clin North Am. 1991;1:13-35.

44. Kumar A, Mireles-Cabodevila E, Mehta AC, Aboussouan LS. Sudden onset of dyspnea preceded by shoulder and arm pain. Annals of the American Thoracic Society. 2016;13:2261-2265.

45. Lee SJ, Park S, Ahn HK, et al. Implications of bone-only metastases in breast cancer: favorable preference with excellent outcomes of hormone receptor positive breast cancer. Cancer Research and Treatment. 2011;43:89.

46. Lieb JG, Forsmark CE. Review article: pain and chronic pancreatitis. Aliment Pharmacol Ther. 2009;29:706-719.

47. Mont MA, Payman RK, Laporte DM, Petri M, Jones LC, Hungerford DS. Atraumatic osteonecrosis of the humeral head. Journal of Rheumatology. 2000;27:1766-1773.

48. Nau KC, Lewis WD. Multiple myeloma: diagnosis and treatment. American Family Physician. 2008;78:853-859.

49. Njeze GE. Gallstones. Niger J Surg. 2013;19:49-55.

50. Nyhsen C, Mahmood SU. Life-threatening haemoperitoneum secondary to rupture of simple ovarian cyst. Case Reports. 2014;2014:bcr2014205061.

51. Oliver TB, Bhat R, Kellett CF, Adamson DJ. Diagnosis and management of bone metastases. J R Coll Physicians Edinb. 2011;41:330-338.

52. Olofsson Y, Book C, Jacobsson L. Shoulder joint involvement in patients with newly diagnosed rheumatoid arthritis: prevalence and associations. Scandinavian Journal of Rheumatology. 2003;32:25-32.

53. Panagopoulos N, Leivaditis V, Koletsis E, et al. Pancoast tumors: characteristics and preoperative assessment. Journal of Thoracic Disease. 2014;6:S108.

54. Park SH, Lee PB, Seo MS, Lim YH, Oh YS. Referred shoulder pain due to liver abscess: a case report. The Korean Journal of Pain. 2005;18:267-270.

55. Pedersen AB, Horváth-Puhó E, Ehrenstein V, Rørth M, Sørensen HT. Frozen shoulder and risk of cancer: a population-based cohort study. British Journal of Cancer. 2017;117:144-147.

56. Pusceddu MM, Gareau MG. Visceral pain: gut microbiota, a new hope? Journal of Biomedical Science. 2018;25:73.

57. Reamy BV, Williams PM, Odom MR. Pleuritic chest pain: sorting through the differential diagnosis. American Family Physician. 2017;96:306-312.

58. Riente L, Delle Sedie A, Filippucci E, et al. Ultrasound imaging for the rheumatologist XLV. Ultrasound of the shoulder in psoriatic arthritis. Clin Exp Rheumatol. 2013;31(3):329-33.

59. Rosenthal AK, Ryan LM. Calcium pyrophosphate deposition disease. New England Journal of Medicine. 2016;374:2575-2584.

60. Sano H, Hatori M, Mineta M, Hosaka M, Itoi E. Tumors masked as frozen shoulders: a retrospective analysis. Journal of Shoulder and Elbow Surgery. 2010;19:262-266.

61. Sengupta JN. Visceral pain: the neurophysiological mechanism. In: Sensory Nerves. Springer; 2009:31-74.

62. Sikandar S, Dickenson AH. Visceral pain: the ins and outs, the ups and downs. Current Opinion in Supportive and Palliative Care. 2012;6:17.

63. Silman AJ, Pearson JE. Epidemiology and genetics of rheumatoid arthritis. Arthritis Res. 2002;4 Suppl 3:S265-272.

64. Smith AM, Sperling JW, Cofield RH. Rotator cuff repair in patients with rheumatoid arthritis. JBJS. 2005;87:1782-1787.

65. Smolen JS, Landewé RBM, Bijlsma JWJ, et al. EULAR recommendations for the management of rheumatoid arthritis with synthetic and biological disease-modifying antirheumatic drugs: 2019 update. Ann Rheum Dis. 2020;79:685-699.

66. Söyüncü S, Bektaş F, Cete Y. Traditional Kehr's sign: left shoulder pain related to splenic abscess. Turkish Journal of Trauma & Emergency Surgery. 2012;18:87-88.

67. Stoker J, van Randen A, Laméris W, Boermeester MA. Imaging patients with acute abdominal pain. Radiology. 2009;253:31-46.

68. Sutcliffe P, Connock M, Shyangdan D, Court R, Kandala N, Clarke A. A systematic review of evidence on malignant spinal metastases: natural history and technologies for identifying patients at high risk of vertebral fracture and spinal cord compression. Health Technology Assessment. 2013;17:1.

69. Svensson E, Christiansen CF, Ulrichsen SP, Rørth MR, Sørensen HT. Survival after bone metastasis by primary cancer type: a Danish population-based cohort study. BMJ Open. 2017;7:e016022.

70. Taylor P. Update on the diagnosis and management of early rheumatoid arthritis. Clinical Medicine. 2020;20:561-564.

71. Van Manen L, Heidt J. Acute abdominal pain, painful left shoulder and near collapse. Neth J Med. 2014;72:282-286.

72. Vanhoenacker FM, Verstraete KL. Soft tissue tumors about the shoulder. In: Seminars in Musculoskeletal Radiology. Thieme Medical Publishers; 2015:284-299.

73. Verhagen AP, Downie A, Maher CG, Koes BW. Most red flags for malignancy in low back pain guidelines lack empirical support: a systematic review. Pain. 2017;158:1860-1868.

74. Vodanovich DA, Choong PF. Soft-tissue sarcomas. Indian Journal of Orthopaedics. 2018;52:35-44.

75. Watson J, Jones HE, Banks J, Whiting P, Salisbury C, Hamilton W. Use of multiple inflammatory marker tests in primary care: using Clinical Practice Research Datalink to evaluate accuracy. British Journal of General Practice. 2019;69:e462-e469.

76. Welch WC, Erhard R, Clyde B, Jacobs GB. Systemic malignancy presenting as neck and shoulder pain. Archives of Physical Medicine and Rehabilitation. 1994;75:918-920.

77. Wesselmann U, Baranowski AP, Börjesson M, et al. Emerging therapies and novel approaches to visceral pain. Drug Discovery Today: Therapeutic Strategies. 2009;6:89-95.

78. Wu CM, Cheng LC, Lo GH, Lai KH, Cheng CL, Pan WC. Malignant lymphoma of spleen presenting as acute pancreatitis: a case report. World Journal of Gastroenterology. 2007;13:3773-3775.

79. Younossi ZM. Non-alcoholic fatty liver disease: a global public health perspective. Journal of Hepatology. 2019;70:531-544.

The past, present, and future of shoulder surgery

9

Tony Kochhar, Baljinder Singh Dhinsa, Balraj Jagdev, Jeremy Lewis

The past

Hippocrates (c.460–c.370 BCE), Classical Greek physician and frequently referred to as the Father of Medicine, argued that illness had a natural cause at a time when most people attributed sickness to superstition. He has been credited with many accomplishments that may have become conflated, including the Hippocratic Oath, which is attributed to him, but was probably not written by him. Hippocrates first discussed his experience of the dislocated shoulder and reduction maneuvers in his *Corpus*.[1] He is attributed in saying that following relocation, the shoulder muscles must be exercised to avoid future dislocations. Prior to Hippocrates, the ancient Egyptians had developed procedures to reduce dislocated shoulders. Figure 9.1 depicts the oldest known image of a shoulder dislocation and an attempt at reduction.[16]

In the 4th century BCE, several techniques attributed to Hippocrates were described to reduce a shoulder dislocation (Figure 9.2). Hippocrates also suggested that shoulder cauterization should follow reduction in the management of recurrent dislocations. The technique involved the use of red-hot irons to produce deep eschars targeting the axilla and the inferior joint.[1,58] Following the cauterization the arm was bound in shoulder internal rotation. The method is as follows:

It deserves to be known how a shoulder which is subject to frequent dislocations should be treated. The cautery should be applied thus: burn the skin at the front of the humerus, then by all means the arm is to be bound by the side night and day, and even when the ulcers are completely healed, the arm must be bound to the side for a long time, and the wide space into which the humerus used to escape will become contracted.

The aim of the procedure was to develop contracted scar tissue to reduce recurrent dislocations. This appears to be Hippocrates' preferred method, to avoid potential nerve and blood vessel injury that were associated with circumferential cauterization of the shoulder performed by Hippocrates' contemporaries.

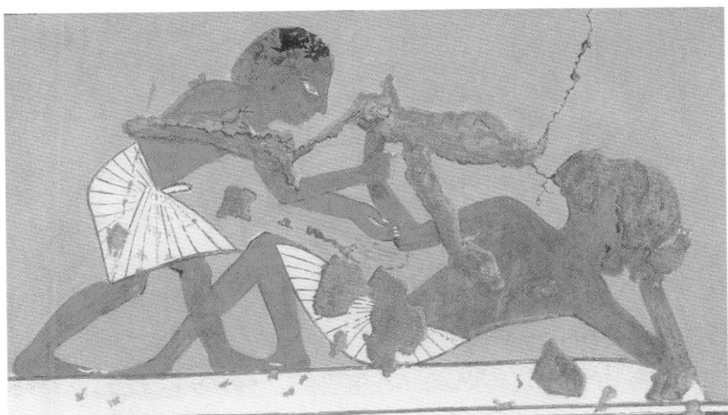

FIGURE 9.1
Detail from *Building a Catafalque, Tomb of Ipuy* (c.1279–1213 BCE), depicting a physician reducing a dislocated shoulder.
(Metropolitan Museum of Art, USA. Creative Commons 1.0 Universal (CC0 1.0)).

Alexander Monro, in 1788, is credited with being the first to define tears of the rotator cuff.[62] Soon after this, the earliest described surgical interventions for the shoulder were procedures for wound management, with the first reported invasive procedure being a disarticulation (surgical separation) of the shoulder joint in 1796.[10] The patient was a soldier with an infected gunshot wound.

In 1822, Adam Hunter (1794–1843) described supraspinatus tears associated with dislocations and hypothesized the role of supraspinatus in initiating shoulder abduction and augmenting the function of the deltoid.[17,30] Sir Astley Cooper (1768–1841) utilized cadaveric studies to demonstrate the resting position of the humeral head in relation to glenoid following dislocations, and mentioned the associated injuries to the joint capsule and rotator cuff muscles. The potential for concomitant brachial plexus injuries associated with dislocations were also described.[17,22]

Kocher's landmark paper in 1870 detailed the closed technique for shoulder reduction, and in the same year, Hüter reported the first repair of the rotator cuff.[56] The technique involved re-attaching the injured supraspinatus tendon to the humeral diaphysis during a humeral head resection for chronic shoulder dislocation. It was ten years later, in

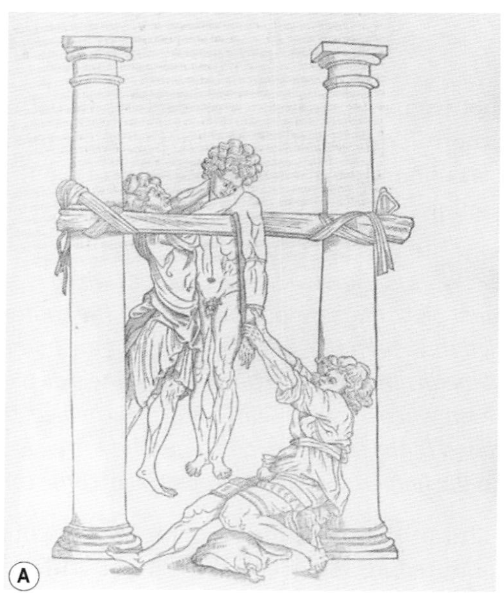
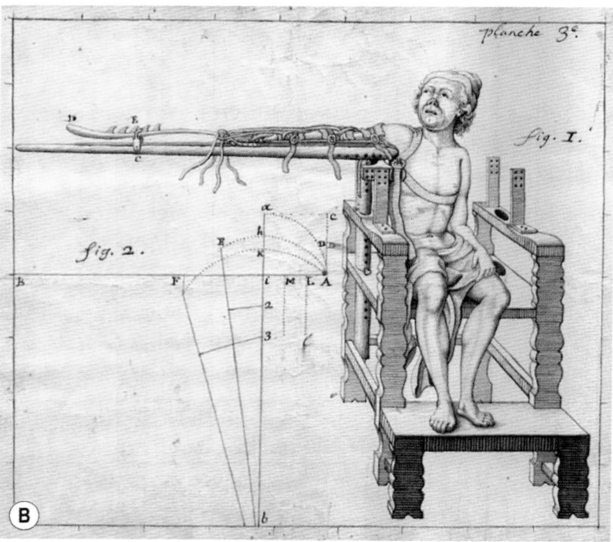

FIGURE 9.2

Methods attributed to Hippocrates to reduce dislocated shoulders.

(A, From *Guidi's Chirurgia* by Guido Guidi (Vidus Vidius) (1544). B, *Ambe of Hippocrates* by Claude-Nicholas Le Cat (1742)).

cadaveric studies, that a posterior impaction injury to the humeral head following dislocation was noted. The suggestion was that this was sustained by direct impact of the humeral head against the anterior margin of the glenoid cavity.[28,59] This was later to be called a Hill-Sachs lesion, named after two radiologists, Harold Hill and Maurice Sachs from San Francisco in 1940.

Shoulder instability continued to dominate clinical literature, with Eduard Albert performing a scapula-humeral fusion for recurrent shoulder instability in 1887.[55] A further injury associated with shoulder dislocation, and possibly a causative factor for recurrent instability, was described by Broca and Hartmann in 1890. This was a combination injury to the anterior glenoid rim, tear of the capsule and antero-inferior labrum. This would be later called a Bankart lesion in 1923, named after British orthopedic surgeon Arthur Bankart (1879–1951).[4]

Towards the end of the 19th century, in 1895, the discovery of X-rays by Wilhelm Röntgen (1845–1923) improved understanding of shoulder pathology. At the same time Jules Péan (1830–1898) is credited with performing the first total shoulder replacement in Paris. Using an anterior approach, he performed a two-stage shoulder arthroplasty on a waiter, using a prosthesis combining platinum and a paraffin-hardened rubber head.[5] Due to infection, the prosthesis had to be removed two years later.

At the beginning of the 20th century, Georg Perthes (1869–1927) performed a repair of the detached glenoid labrum using horseshoe-shaped nails fixated to the glenoid edge.[53] In 1906, Perthes described open repair of the supraspinatus tendon with the use of suture anchors,[53] and in 1911, Ernest Amory Codman (1869–1940) described a procedure using sutures to repair the supraspinatus tendon.[15] Codman described the subacromial space and the effect that shoulder abduction had in narrowing the space.[9] He also described the appearance of inflamed subacromial bursa in operative cases and advocated the use of splints following surgery during the recovery period to avoid abduction.[14]

In 1947, Osmond-Clark described a procedure being performed independently by doctors Putti (from 1923) and Platt (from 1925) as the Putti-Platt procedure. The procedure was used to treat habitual dislocation of the shoulder. When discussing Bankart lesions, Platt, based in Manchester (UK) stated:

I soon found there was no single and constant Bankartian lesion capable of being repaired by a standard procedure. It therefore occurred to me to make sure by stitching the distal end of the divided subscapularis tendon to the cartilaginous remains of the glenoid margin. This provided a primary barrier to redislocation of the head forwards and inwards under the subscapularis. It then appeared logical to stitch the proximal divided end of the subscapularis to the anterior capsule, thus providing an overlap and shortening of the tendon.

Over time it has become apparent that the procedure was associated with limitation of shoulder external rotation, and recurrent dislocation when performed in isolation.[42,52]

Harrison McLaughlin (1906–1970) reported his advancement technique for repair of massive and retracted supraspinatus tears in 1944.[39] With this technique, he attached the stump of the tendon more proximal to its anatomical footprint on the greater tuberosity. For instability due to glenoid injury, the Bristow-Latarjet procedure (transfer of the coracoid process to a deficient anterior glenoid rim) was first described in 1954, to recreate a stable glenoid surface, and using the conjoint tendon as an anterior stabilizer.[27,35]

When Charles Neer (1917–2011) discussed the late management of unimpacted shoulder fracture-dislocations, he hypothesized the benefit of a replacement prosthesis for the excised humeral head to act as a fulcrum and improve range of motion.[48] Initial plastic-based prostheses were abandoned after incidences of implant attrition and fatigue lead to breakage and foreign body reaction.[72] Krueger reported on the first implanted metal shoulder replacement (hemiarthroplasty) in 1952, for a patient with avascular necrosis, and the patient had a pain-free, well-functioning shoulder.[72] Of note, this technique involved preservation of the rotator cuff insertions. Excellent outcomes in pain relief and range of motion were also reported by Neer in a case series of hemiarthroplasties performed for post-traumatic intractable pain following proximal humeral fracture dislocation.[47]

The 1960s brought advancements in surgical and examination techniques, resulting in more lesions being associated as causative for recurrent shoulder instability. McLaughlin[40] noted findings of insufficient middle and inferior glenohumeral ligaments, with subsequent anterior joint laxity and instability. Cadaveric and fetal investigations performed by Moseley and Övergaard (1962) confirmed these findings, and suggested that while Bankart lesions were commonly seen, they were not the only cause for recurrent instability.[43] The role of the subscapularis muscle as a dynamic restraint to dislocations was confirmed by the presence of laxity in the above studies, as well as by DePalma in 1967.[18]

While there were major advancements in shoulder arthroscopy in the 1970s, particularly with the use of fiber-optic technology by Watanabe,[8] most procedures remained open. Lateral or total acromionectomy was routinely performed to reduce subacromial impingement with shoulder abduction.[2,26,36] However, Neer reported that such procedures weaken the deltoid function, and reduce power and range of motion of the shoulder.[51] He went further and suggested that subacromial impingement resulted from the supraspinatus tendon abutting the anterior-inferior edge of the acromion, rather than lateral edge during arm elevation. Subsequently, in 1972 he described an alternative procedure involving open anterior acromioplasty which protected the deltoid muscle and allowed better exposure for subacromial decompression and rotator cuff repair.[44]

Neer expanded his indications for hemiarthroplasty to include glenohumeral arthritis with an intact rotator cuff. His series reported good long-term outcomes in reduction of pain in 1974.[45] In the same year, Neer developed the first functional total shoulder replacement by combining his vitallium hemiarthroplasty with a high-density polyethylene glenoid resurfacing component.[45] The published results demonstrated this joint replacement to be reliable and durable for the management of glenohumeral arthritis.

As the utilization of anatomical shoulder replacements increased in the 1970s, it became apparent that those with poor rotator cuff function demonstrated variable outcomes in strength and range of motion,[47] as well as signs of joint instability with superior humeral head migration.[38] Attempts to manage these difficult cases with a constrained or fixed fulcrum system, led to high rates of failure secondary to prosthetic loosening at the glenoid, fractures, and pain resulting from forces applied across the shoulder.[21] The reverse polarity principle was developed to help those patients with a deficient rotator cuff and joint instability, by reversing the ball and socket of the shoulder. With early generation designs, the center of rotation was recreated at the anatomical center of the shoulder. Reeves designed the first reverse shoulder system, which unfortunately was associated with high rates of loosening of the glenoid component.[57]

In 1980, Neer described the inferior capsular shift technique to treat involuntary inferior and multidirectional instability.[50] The procedure involved reducing the redundant and lax anterior, posterior, and inferior joint capsule and ligaments with a "shift" of a flap of capsule in all three planes. In 1983 he associated rotator cuff tears with attrition secondary to impingement wear rather than direct trauma.[46,49] He also reported a subacromial impingement classification system, which was based on the progressive pathological changes evidenced, from edema and hemorrhagic changes to acromial spur formation and rotator cuff tears.[46] In 1985, Ellman described an arthroscopic technique for subacromial decompression and acromioplasty, as well as treatment of calcific tendonitis.[20] Outcomes were similar to Neer's open acromioplasty, while minimizing complications associated with the open approach and allowing earlier return to function.

Evolution of anatomic total shoulder replacements continued, with second generation systems being modular, allowing options to size the humeral head, neck, and shaft to improve conformity to individual anatomy.[24] Reports showed that the prosthetic head was often oversized and mispositioned in relation to the glenoid, with subsequent abnormal load of the glenoid component.[9,24] Grammont (1985) proposed a new principle for reverse polarity shoulder systems, implementing a distalization of the center of rotation of the shoulder. This change increased the deltoid lever arm, compensated for a deficient supraspinatus muscle, and reduced shear stresses on the glenoid component.[6] In the 1990s, further work was performed to understand the three-dimensional geometry of the proximal humerus,[9] allowing evolution in the design of anatomic and reverse polarity shoulder replacements.[6]

The first arthroscopic Bankart repair series was reported in 1987,[41] with the initial use of trans-glenoid sutures evolving to suture anchors by 1991.[69] During arthroscopic assessment of the shoulder, Wolf confirmed that avulsion of the glenohumeral ligaments at their humeral attachment (HAGL) was another cause of shoulder instability in the absence of a Bankart lesion.[68] These lesions were difficult to diagnose with an open approach, as they can be obscured, and therefore the view afforded by arthroscopy was advantageous. The use of arthroscopy helped identify other anatomical anomalies, such as superior labral anterior and posterior (SLAP) tears in 1990,[63] and the Burford complex in 1994.[67] Levy discussed the use of arthroscopically assisted repair of partial and complete rotator cuff tears through a limited deltoid splitting approach,[37] reporting improvement in pain, function, and strength at one year follow-up.

In the early 2000s, Purchase and Wolf described the arthroscopic remplissage procedure to "fill in" the cavity caused by a Hill-Sachs lesion, by fixing the posterior capsule and infraspinatus tendon to the injured surface with suture anchors.[54] Lafosse reported an arthroscopic variant of the Bristow-Latarjet procedure,[34] which allowed for better exposure of the coracoid process and accurate visualization in the bone block placement at the anterior glenoid, thus reducing the risk of impingement against the humeral head. More recently, there have been advances in restoring the anatomic footprint to improve the healing and mechanical strength of repaired rotator cuff tendons with the use of double row suture techniques to increase tendon–bone contact area. There has also been the introduction of all-suture anchors, to reduce bone loss associated with traditional suture anchors, with encouraging initial results.[19]

Early cell-based therapies have included the use of GRAFTJACKET™ (Wright Medical Technological, Inc., Arlington, TN) Regenerative Tissue matrix as scaffold to augment tendon repairs, or as an interpositional graft. The scaffold becomes revascularized and repopulated with host cells to allow the host tissue to intergrate.[60]

The indications for reverse shoulder arthroplasty have evolved over the past decade to include proximal humerus fractures, irreparable rotator cuff tears, glenohumeral arthritis, and failed rotator cuff repairs. This is principally due to increasing confidence in the prosthesis and technique with good survivorship and functional results.[3]

The present

The history of shoulder surgery has mostly followed a repeating pattern: definition of a clinical problem, a surgical suggestion to address the problem, clinical observations of the benefit of the procedure, research findings, and refinement, followed by evolution, or abandonment of the procedure. The real test of the success for a surgical procedure is that the benefit outweighs the harms and risks of surgery, and if this benefit and post-surgical recovery is an improvement to the natural history of the pathology itself or, indeed, of nonsurgical treatment.

The evolution of shoulder surgery has kept pace with changes in society, such as increased life expectancy and, for many, the unrealistic expectation of a life devoid of any persistent pain, and the need to fix problems immediately. The findings from relatively recent research suggest that a number of procedures may not be able to "fix" problems as originally anticipated.

The Can Shoulder Arthroscopy Work (CSAW) Trial demonstrated little, if any, difference between placebo shoulder arthroscopy and the arthroscopic subacromial decompression procedure, for people diagnosed with subacromial impingement.[7] The imaging study by Girish et al.[25] is one of many that have demonstrated findings reported as pathological change, e.g., acromial spurs, tendinosis and some tendon tears, some labral tears, and changes associated with osteoarthritis, may be as common in people with and without symptoms, and may in fact represent normal morphological differences and/or age-related changes. The implication is clear: not all observed changes described as pathology require surgical intervention.

Yamamoto et al[70] demonstrated that a substantial proportion of the population develops asymptomatic degenerate rotator cuff tears. Therefore, the conviction that all rotator cuff tears require surgery has shifted: when a patient presents with shoulder pain and a tear is identified, they can be either prioritized for surgery followed by rehabilitation, or selected for nonsurgical rehabilitation. The historical assumption of an unquestionable relationship between tear and symptoms is now questionable.

Our current knowledge is far from complete, and as discussed in Chapter 10, many uncertainties remain, including interpretation of study findings. For example, in the placebo arm of the CSAW study, the participants were randomized to a diagnostic arthroscope, which involves visualization and high-pressure irrigation of the bursa. This may have had a therapeutic benefit. The Finnish Subacromial Impingement Arthroscopy Controlled Trial (FIMPACT) compared subacromial decompression (arthroplasty) against arthroscopic visualization, designated as the placebo arm. In this group, the: "bursal tissue was bluntly stretched with a trocar or resected on the tendon side".

The debridement procedure was considered non-therapeutic, however this is not certain. Although ethical consideration and approval would be mandatory, skin incisions, with no arthroscopic insertion, and the same post-operative protocol would arguably have been a more convincing placebo.

Pragmatic trials, such as CSAW and FIMPACT are becoming increasingly popular as they more closely investigate real-life practice situations, however the associated confounding factors may impact on the research findings and certainty in extrapolating the findings. Some may argue that it would be unethical to only cut and thereby damage the skin in a placebo group and not introduce an arthroscope in the shoulder. It may also be unethical to perpetuate many current surgical procedures without knowing how they compare to natural history, and nonsurgical interventions.

Currently, new procedures are being developed and tested. They aim to preserve the fundamental importance of the biomechanics of the shoulder joints and muscles, especially of the rotator cuff. Examples include superior capsular reconstruction, balloon interpositional arthroplasty, tendon transfer surgery, and reverse geometry total shoulder arthroplasty. Each of these procedures aims to reestablish shoulder homeostasis by restoring the normal arthrokinematics and force couples provided by the muscles and tendons acting on the shoulder. There have been several recent advances in arthroplasty that produce better functional outcomes and survivorship data, whether this be anatomic, resurfacing, or reverse polarity arthroplasty. This has been directed by component alignment, modularity, patient-specific kit and prosthesis, as well as bone-preserving arthroplasty and arthroscopic-assisted arthroplasty.[12,29,65]

Scaffolds are currently used for bone healing as well as cartilage regeneration, for example matrix-induced autologous chondrocyte implantation. As with many advances, the drive is to make things smaller and therefore deliverable through less invasive methods, and this is the direction of nano-scaffolds, which may use nanoparticles to deliver the scaffold to specific locations.[11,71]

There has also been a shift to early rehabilitation for soft tissue surgery and day surgery arthroplasty procedures, which has become an increasingly important option when suggesting surgery in 2020 and most of 2021 with respect to the SARs-CoV-2 (COVID-19) pandemic. The use of regional blocks, with or without general anesthetic, has been reported to reduce opioid usage, time in recovery, and stay in hospital. It also permits an earlier start to rehabilitation.

The (near and far) future

With the utilization of platelet-rich plasma (PRP) preparations and mesenchymal stem cells, we are taking the first steps towards understanding the possibilities of biologic enhancements. There remains a high rate of failure reported following rotator cuff repair, and it is hypothesized that growth factors, stem cells, and other types of tissue engineering may help to augment rotator cuff repairs and hopefully improve outcomes.[31,32,66] The next step is to find methods to secure growth factors at targeted sites to help aid healing, translating the use of induced pluripotent stem cells (IPSC) seen in animal laboratory studies to humans.[11,23,61,64,71]

Shoulder surgery is not a single entity. The evolution therefore must be considered in its separate components. Those components include arthroplasty surgery, soft tissue reconstruction, and fracture surgery. With regards to shoulder joint replacement surgery, not only the clinical effectiveness and safety of the procedure, but also the longevity of the implants are key determinants of the effectiveness of the procedure. Computer-assisted surgery may see the evolution to augmented reality (see Chapter 30) for arthroplasty surgery as well as for fracture fixation. It allows the superimposition of computer-generated images onto real-world images, and allows interaction with both at the same time.[13] This technology presents exciting possibilities, with encouraging pre-clinical results, yet consideration for mainstream integration should only be considered when the clinical data and health economic analyses are available.[33]

With regards to soft tissue reconstruction, especially the rotator cuff, as described, surgical practice has focused on restoring normal biomechanics, namely axes of movement and the force couples acting on the shoulder. However, questions remain: current research suggests that people seeking care for rotator cuff-deficient shoulders can improve function and reduce symptoms with nonsurgical interventions and time. The benefits demonstrated so far are incomplete and only short- to mid-term data are available. The relationship between improved clinical symptoms in the presence of aberrant biomechanics requires deeper understanding.

The use of synthetic biology – the alteration of genomes – is another developing biotechnology, not only in soft tissue reconstruction but also in fracture surgery. The work of ribonucleic acid (RNA) interference, which blocks messenger RNA and thus prevents it from producing proteins, effectively inactivates a specific gene. This technology could be used to prevent disease within the shoulder, such as cartilage or tendon degeneration, and to augment healing in combination with other regeneration strategies, such as IPSC. The delivery to the target zone and the control of its actions needs further work, but there are encouraging signs.[11,23,61]

We are a long way from understanding and controlling/optimizing stem cells. Early-stage therapies are controversial, and the results are not proven; however, in the future, appropriate injections of biologics may not simply aid healing along with other treatment modalities, but instead stimulate control and possibly become the main interventions that are offered.

Implant design and materials will improve load sharing and therefore fracture healing as well as implant longevity. In the last 40 years we have seen improvements in material science and locking/fixation mechanisms, for example, titanium alloys superseding stainless steel, and locking plate technology/minimally invasive percutaneous plating (MIPO) techniques.

The future of shoulder surgery has great potential and may take many directions, but with every advancement, the sage and timeless words of Sir William Osler (1849–1919) are to be heeded: "The good physician treats the disease, the great physician treats the patient who has the disease."

References

1. Adams F. On the Articulations. Translation of the Corpus Hippocraticum. Massachusetts Institute of Technology. Available at: http://classics.mit.edu// Hippocrates/artic.html.
2. Armstrong JR. Excision of the acromion in treatment of the supraspinatus syndrome; report of 95 excisions. J Bone Joint Surg Br. 1949;31B(3):436-442.
3. Bacle G, Nove-Josserand L, Garaud P, Walch G. Long-term outcomes of reverse total shoulder arthroplasty. A follow-up of a previous study. The Journal of Bone and Joint Surgery. 2017;99(6):454-461.
4. Bankart ASB. Recurrent or habitual dislocation of the shoulder joint. Br Med J. 1923;2(3285):1132-1133.
5. Bankes MJ, Emery RJ. Pioneers of shoulder replacement: Themistocles Gluck and Jules Emile Péan. J Shoulder Elbow Surg. 1995;4(4):259-62.
6. Baulot E, Sirveaux F, Boileau P. Grammont's idea: the story of Paul Grammont's functional surgery concept and the development of the reverse principle. Clin Orthop Relat Res. 2011;469(9):2425-2431.
7. Beard D, Rees J, Rombach I, Cooper C et al. CSAW Study Group. The CSAW Study (Can Shoulder Arthroscopy Work?)–a placebo-controlled surgical intervention trial assessing the clinical and cost effectiveness of arthroscopic subacromial decompression for shoulder pain: study protocol for a randomised controlled trial. Trials. 2015;16:210.
8. Bigony L. Arthroscopic surgery. Orthopaedic Nursing. 2008;27(6):349-354.
9. Boileau P, Walch G. The three-dimensional geometry of the proximal humerus. JBJS (Br). 1997;79-B(5), 857-865.
10. Burd W, Anderson. History of a case terminating successfully, after amputation was performed at the shoulder-joint. Ann Med (Edinb). 1797;2:282-291.
11. Burkhart SS. Expanding the frontiers of shoulder arthroscopy. J Shoulder Elbow Surg. 2011;20:183-191.
12. Cabarcas BC, Cvetanovich GL, Espinoza-Orias AA, Inoue N, Gowd AK, Bernardoni E, Verma NN. Novel 3-dimensionally printed patient-specific guide improves accuracy compared with standard total shoulder arthroplasty guide: a cadaveric study. JSES Open Access. 2019 15;3(2):83-92.
13. Chytas D, Malahias M-A, Nikolaou VS. Augmented reality in orthopedics: current state and future directions. Front Surg. 2019;6(38): 1-7.
14. Codman EA. On stiff and painful shoulders: the anatomy of the subdeltoid or subacromial bursa and its clinical importance; subdeltoid bursitis. Boston Medical and Surgical Journal. 1906;154:613-620.
15. Codman EA. Complete rupture of the supraspinatus tendon. Operative treatment with report of two successful cases. 1911. Journal of Shoulder and Elbow Surgery. 2011;20(3), 347-349.
16. Colton C. Orthopaedic challenges in Ancient Egypt. Bone & Joint 360. 2013;2(2), 2-7.
17. Cooper A. A treatise on dislocations and on fractures of the joints. Clinical Orthopaedics and Related Research. 2007;458:6-7.
18. DePalma AF, Cooke AJ, Prabhakar M. The role of the subscapularis in recurrent anterior dislocations of the shoulder. Clinical Orthopaedics and Related Research. 1967;54:35-50.
19. Dhinsa BS, Bhamra JS, Aramberri-Gutierrez M, Kochhar T. Mid-term clinical outcome following rotator cuff repair using all-suture anchors. Journal of Clinical Orthopaedics & Trauma. 2019;10(2):241-243.
20. Ellman H. Arthroscopic subacromial decompression: analysis of one- to three-year results. Arthroscopy. 1987;3(3):173-181.
21. Flatow EL, Harrison AK. A history of reverse total shoulder arthroplasty. Clinical Orthopaedics and Related Research. 2011;469(9):2432-2439.
22. Flower WH. On pathologic changes produced in the shoulder joint by traumatic dislocation. Trans Path Soc London. 1861;12:179-200.
23. Fogerty S, Dumont GD, Lafosse L. (iii) Shoulder arthroscopy: the past, present and future directions. Orthopaedics and Trauma. 2014:28(6):378-387.
24. Fukuda H, Mikasa M. Trends in modern shoulder surgery: personal observations. Journal of Orthopaedic Science. 2007;12(1), 4-13.
25. Girish G, Lobo LG, Jacobson JA, Morag Y, et al. Ultrasound of the shoulder: asymptomatic findings in men. AJR Am J Roentgenol. 2011 Oct;197(4):W713-9.
26. Hammond G. Complete acromionectomy in the treatment of chronic tendinitis of the shoulder. J Bone Joint Surg Br.1971; 53(1):173-180
27. Helfet AJ. Coracoid transplantation for recurring dislocation of the shoulder. J Bone Joint Surg Br. 1958;40-B(2):198-202.
28. Hill HA, Sachs MD. The grooved defect of the humeral head. Radiology. 1940;35(6):690-700.
29. Hu H, Liu W, Zeng Q, Wang S, Zhang Z, Liu J, Zhang Y, Shao Z, Wang B. The personalized shoulder reconstruction assisted by 3d printing technology after resection of the proximal humerus tumours. Cancer Management and Research. 2019;11:10665-10673.
30. Hunter A. On dislocation of the hip and shoulder joints. Transactions. Medico-Chirurgical Society of Edinburgh. 1824;1:170-183.
31. Isaac C, Gharaibeh B, Witt M, Wright VJ, Huard J. Biologic approaches to enhance rotator cuff healing after injury. J Shoulder Elbow Surg. 2012;21:181-190.
32. Kim SJ, Yeo SM, Noh SJ, Ha CW, Lee BC, Lee HS, Kim SJ. Effect of platelet-rich plasma on the degenerative rotator cuff tendinopathy according to the compositions. J Orthop Surg Res. 2019;14(1):408.
33. Kriechling P, Roner S, Liebmann F, Casari F, Furnstahl P, Wieser K. Augmented reality for base plate component placement in reverse total shoulder arthroplasty: a feasibility study. Arch Orthop Trauma Surg. 2020. doi: 10.1007/s00402-020-03542-z.
34. Lafosse L, Lejeune E, Bouchard A, Kakuda C, Gobezie R, Kochhar T. The arthroscopic Latarjet procedure for the treatment of anterior shoulder instability. Arthroscopy. 2007;23(11), 1242.e1-1242.e5.
35. Latarjet M. Treatment of recurrent dislocation of the shoulder. Lyon Chir. 1954;49(8):994-997.

36. Leach RE, O'Connor P, Jones R. Acromionectomy for tendinitis of the shoulder in athletes. Phys Sportsmed. 1979;7(4):96-107.

37. Levy HJ, Uribe JW, Delaney LG. Arthroscopic assisted rotator cuff repair: preliminary results. Arthroscopy. 1990;6(1):55-60.

38. Marmor L. Hemiarthroplasty for the rheumatoid shoulder joint. Clin Orthop Relat Res. 1977;122:201-203.

39. McLaughlin HL. Lesions of the musculotendinous cuff of the shoulder. The exposure and treatment of tears with retraction. JBJS. 1944;26(1):31-51.

40. McLaughlin HL. Recurrent anterior dislocation of the shoulder. The American Journal of Surgery. 1960;99(5), 628-632.

41. Morgan CD, Bodenstab AB. Arthroscopic Bankart suture repair: technique and early results. Arthroscopy.1987;3(2):111-122.

42. Morrey BF, Janes JM. Recurrent anterior dislocation of the shoulder. Long-term follow-up of the Putti-Platt and Bankart procedures. JBJS. 1976; 58(2):252-256.

43. Moseley HF, Övergaard B. The anterior capsular mechanism in recurrent anterior dislocation of the shoulder. JBJS (Br). 1962; 44-B(4):913-927.

44. Neer CS. Anterior acromioplasty for the chronic impingement syndrome in the shoulder: a preliminary report. J Bone Joint Surg Am. 1972;54(1):41-50.

45. Neer CS. Replacement arthroplasty for glenohumeral osteoarthritis. JBJS.1974:56;(1):1-13.

46. Neer CS. Impingement lesions. Clin Orthop. 1983;173:70-77.

47. Neer CS. The classic: articular replacement for the humeral head. 1955. Clin Orthop Relat Res. 2011;469(9):2409-2421.

48. Neer CS, Brown TH, McLaughlin HL. Fracture of the neck of the humerus with dislocation of the head fragment. The American Journal of Surgery. 1953;85(3):252-258.

49. Neer CS, Craig EV, Fukuda H. Cuff-tear arthropathy. JBJS. 1983;65-A(9):1232-1244.

50. Neer CS, Foster CR. Inferior capsular shift for involuntary inferior and multidirectional instability of the shoulder. A preliminary report. JBJS. 1980;62:(6):897-908.

51. Neer CS, Marberry TA. On the disadvantages of radical acromionectomy. J Bone Joint Surg Am. 1981;63(3):416-419.

52. Osmond-Clarke, H. Habitual dislocation of the shoulder. JBJS (Br). 1948;30-B(1):19-25.

53. Perthes. Über Operationen bei habitueller Schulterluxation. Deutsche Zeitschrift Für Chirurgie. 1906;85(1):199-227.

54. Purchase RJ, Wolf EM, Hobgood ER, Pollock ME, Smalley CC. Hill–Sachs 'remplissage': an arthroscopic solution for the engaging Hill–Sachs lesion. Arthroscopy. 2008;24:723-726.

55. Randelli P, Cucchi D, Butt U. History of shoulder instability surgery. Knee Surgery, Sports Traumatology, Arthroscopy. 2016;24(2):305-329.

56. Randelli P, Cucchi D, Ragone V, de Girolamo L, Cabitza P, Randelli M. History of rotator cuff surgery. Knee Surgery, Sports Traumatology, Arthroscopy. 2014;23(2): 344-362.

57. Reeves B, Jobbins B, Dowson D, Wright V. A total shoulder endo-prosthesis. Engineering in Medicine. 1972;1(3), 64-67.

58. Regauer M, Polzer H, Mutschler W. Neurovascular complications due to the Hippocrates method for reducing anterior shoulder dislocations. World J Orthop. 2014;5(1):57-61.

59. Rockwood CA, Wirth MA, Fehringer EV, Matsen FA, Sperling JW, Lippitt SB. The Shoulder, 5th edition. Philadelphia: Elsevier; 2018.

60. Sharma N, Refaiy A, Sibly TF. Short-term results of rotator cuff repair using GRAFTJACKET as an interpositional tissue-matched thickness graft. J Orthop. 2018; 15(2):732-735.

61. Singh JA. Stem cells and other innovative intra-articular therapies for osteoarthritis: what does the future hold? BMC Med. 2012;10:44.

62. Smith JG. The classic: pathological appearances of seven cases of injury of the shoulder-joint: with remarks. Clin Orthop Relat Res. 2010;468(6): 1471-1475.

63. Snyder SJ, Karzel RP, Pizzo WD, Ferkel RD, Friedman MJ. SLAP lesions of the shoulder. Arthroscopy. 1990;6(4):274-279.

64. Striano RD, Malanga GA, Bilbool N, Azatullah K. Refractory shoulder pain with osteoarthritis, and rotator cuff tear, treated with micro-fragmented adipose tissue. Orthop Spine Sports Med. 2018;2(1): JOSSM 014.

65. Tashjian RZ, Chalmers PN. Future frontiers in shoulder arthroplasty and the management of shoulder osteoarthritis. Clin Sports Med. 2018;37(4):609-630.

66. Tsekes D, Konstantopoulos G, Khan WS, Rossouw D, Elvey M, Singh J. Use of stem cells and growth factors in rotator cuff tendon repair. European Journal of Orthopaedic Surgery & Traumatology. 2019:29:747-757.

67. Williams MM, Snyder SJ, Buford Jr D. The Buford complex, the "cord-like" middle glenohumeral ligament and absent anterosuperior labrum complex: a normal anatomic capsulolabral variant. Arthroscopy. 1994;10(3):241-247.

68. Wolf EM, Cheng JC, Dickson K. Humeral avulsion of glenohumeral ligaments as a cause of anterior shoulder instability. Arthroscopy. 1995;11(5), 600-607.

69. Wolf EM, Wilk RM, Richmond JC. Arthroscopic Bankart repair using suture anchors. Operative Techniques in Orthopaedics. 1991;1(2), 184-191.

70. Yamamoto A, Takagishi K, Osawa T, Yanagawa T, et al. Prevalence and risk factors of a rotator cuff tear in the general population. J Shoulder Elbow Surg. 2010;19(1):116-20.

71. Zhang B, Huang J, Narayan RJ. Gradient scaffolds for osteochondral tissue engineering and regeneration. Journal of Materials Chemistry B. 2020;8:8149-8170.

72. Zilber S. Shoulder arthroplasty: historical considerations. The Open Orthopaedic Journal. 2017;11(6);1100-1107.

10 Clinical uncertainties: what do and don't we know about the shoulder?

Jeremy Lewis, Chad Cook, Alessandra N Garcia, Kevin Hall, Paul Salamh, Fiona Sandford

Introduction

The human shoulder is an engineering masterpiece. It can move through an arc of 80° in 30 milliseconds – moving at 9000° per second – and working with the kinetic chain, propel baseballs at speeds of up to 170 km per hour (106 mph) with incredible precision (see Chapter 2 and Chapter 38). Elite swimmers may perform more than 6000 stroke cycles per day and more than 2 million stroke cycles per year when training (see Chapter 39). The shoulder demands high and sustained force production, incredible flexibility, and precise motor control to participate in lead and speed climbing, as well as bouldering (Chapter 40). Tai Chi (Chapter 42) and yoga (Chapter 43) require shoulder flexibility, strength, and the ability to maintain sustained positions for extended periods, coupled with unhurried, and breathtakingly fast movements, and meticulous control. Due to the placement of the scapula, orientation of the glenoid fossa and the surrounding muscles and tendons, the shoulder participates in high speed, powerful and accurate actions as well as purposeful placement and stabilization of the upper to perform intricate precision activities, such as threading a needle, or putting the last building block on the top of a wooden tower when playing Jenga™.

Based on the incredible versatility and comprehensive range of functions, shoulder symptoms that most commonly present as pain, stiffness, instability, and weakness, in isolation or combination, result in profound morbidity. Shoulder symptoms adversely affect every aspect of daily life, impacting on the simplest of tasks such as dressing, attending to personal hygiene, and carrying light objects, as well as more demanding requirements – vocational and sporting pursuits, hobbies, playing an instrument, and pushing, pulling, lifting, and carrying heavier items. For many people with shoulder symptoms, the detrimental impact on sleep and resulting fatigue, is voiced as their biggest concern.

Musculoskeletal problems involving the shoulder permeate into every aspect of life. In Chapter 1, people experiencing shoulder symptoms clearly articulate the profound impact that symptoms impose daily, often for protracted periods of time. To provide best care, clinicians not only need to synthesize the available research evidence, but also need to know the knowledge gaps where we do not have evidence to translate into practice, and how should we practice in these circumstances. Addressing these issues is the focus of this chapter.

Clinical practice in an uncertain environment

In 2018, 33,100 peer-reviewed English-language journals and 9,400 non-English-language journals collectively published over 3 million articles. Since the dissemination of scientific information began, the publishing industry has steadily increased its output, on average, by 3–3.5% per year. A quick search of PubMed (PubMed.gov), one of many article indexing sites, indicates that well over 90,000 articles specific to the shoulder have been published to date. As is apparent in this chapter and throughout this book, despite the continued escalation of evidence, not all clinically relevant questions for managing shoulder disorders have been answered.

Editors of reputable journals understandably only want to report high quality randomized clinical trials (RCT), as they help to answer important questions and provide clinicians with the confidence to use or reject specific treatment approaches. However, what should we do when the person in front of us, seeking care for their musculoskeletal shoulder problem, has diabetes, essential hypertension, long-haul (long) covid, and is pregnant? A combination of comorbidities that is unlikely to have ever been investigated in an RCT investigating shoulder pain, and more than likely to be in the list of exclusion criteria.

Making decisions in the absence of evidence is less challenging than it may appear. There is a diverse body of literature that has demonstrated that the incompleteness of knowledge is not simply a void about which nothing can be said or done.[41] It is certainly one of the biggest dilemmas when providing evidence-based care, but it is one that can be overcome by understanding what the absence of evidence means in the current evidence-based environment.

Absence of evidence is not evidence of absence[2]

When we are told that "there is no evidence that a treatment has an effect," we should first ask whether we are dealing with an absence of evidence, i.e., there no information at all to support or refute a particular intervention, or are we dealing with convincible information that an intervention lacks a clinical effect. Since evidence is fluid and new treatments require studies to investigate their effectiveness, it is highly likely we will face future situations of absence of evidence.

From the moment the SARS-CoV-2 (COVID-19) virus was identified, the global community was faced with an absence of evidence that required addressing on an unprecedented scale. We have gained substantial knowledge relating to COVID-19 since the end of 2019, but a vast absence of evidence still exits. Many of the decisions made during the pandemic were made in the absence of irrefutable evidence and was a clear example of the expression: "If you need to be certain you are right before you move, you will probably never move." We observed governments, health authorities, communities and individuals make decisions on the best information they had, and often, especially in the early stages of the pandemic, there was virtually none. Some clearly made much better decisions than others. When a path was erroneous, another was tried and, over time, more robust evidence became available, and the decisions made and directions taken improved. The history of musculoskeletal practice has not been dissimilar. Many researchers and clinicians argue that we should not do anything until evidence exists. Philosophically that makes sense, but probably it would result in never moving. We need to do much better when an absence of evidence is identified and take lessons from the SARS-CoV-2 pandemic, and work much more collaboratively to address the many uncertainties that exist.[47]

Do not discount clinical experience

Clinical expertise includes the general basic skills of clinical practice as well as the experience of the individual practitioner.[28] Clinical expertise, patient preferences and relevant published scientific information, inform decision-making for each individual patient. Whereas population health statistics suggest a pattern of care that is beneficial for the masses, the uniqueness of each patient demands a rational approach by the expert practitioner.

Weak evidence may not be meaningful enough to influence clinical practice

Evidence of absence suggests something is missing or that it does not exist. In some cases, evidence may exist but may be unreliable, lack credibility, or have notable flaws that questions its clinical applicability: the studies may be too small to detect an effect or a difference; the effect or difference may be very small, suggesting little or no clinical significance; there may be too few data or not enough studies; and the evidence may be of very low quality having been derived from poorly designed work (see: https://www.evidentlycochrane.net/teapots-and-unicorns-absence-of-evidence-is-not-evidence-of-absence/). Bias (for multifarious reasons) may have played a part in the design, conduct, interpretation, conclusions, and dissemination of the study findings. With our still very basic level of understanding, no one is currently privileged enough to know how best to assess and manage musculoskeletal problems involving the shoulder.

Systematic reviews and meta-analyses have long been placed at the top of the pyramid of evidence. However, an overemphasis on faulty, poorly designed research has led to some clinicians questioning cumulative review articles.[28] Understanding how strong the present literature is (evidence of absence), as well as whether evidence is missing or does not exist (absence of evidence), improves the likelihood of optimal decision-making.

The human shoulder is a masterpiece, a wonder of form and function, and how to best manage the biopsychosocial challenges imposed by our collective fledgling level of knowledge when an individual seeks care for the shoulder symptoms they are experiencing is a formidable challenge. All masterpieces can be interpreted, and reinterpreted, in countless ways, and for musculoskeletal conditions involving the shoulder, it may remain that way for decades, and even centuries to come.

The purpose of this book is to synthesize current knowledge to support clinicians assisting people seeking care for musculoskeletal conditions involving the shoulder, and the purpose of this chapter is to discuss issues commonly asked by patients or considered by clinicians, and summarize what we currently know and what we still need to know to offer best care. In future editions of this textbook our hope is that what we know becomes a bigger part of the chapter and what we do not yet know, concomitantly reduces in size. We hope that researchers, current and future, pick up on some of the areas highlighted to help close the knowledge gap.

How this chapter is organized

The first section of this chapter presents a narrative style response to the question, "What do we know and what don't we know?" In this section, we discuss questions commonly asked by patients or considered by clinicians, such as, "Should I take any supplements for my shoulder pain?", "Should I include posterior shoulder stretches in my management plan?", "Should I recommend surgery or not?", and finally, "Should I put my faith in clinical guidelines?"

The second section uses a Delphi-style process to build consensus and generate ideas for future research. Colleagues who work as clinicians and/or researchers with expertise in musculoskeletal problems involving the shoulder were asked to contribute, along with people who are currently living with or have experienced shoulder conditions. Participants were invited to provide responses to three questions posed of them: 1) What do we really know?; 2) What do we think we know, but actually don't?; and 3) What we really don't know but need to know? Multiple responses from one or more contributors have been merged under one section. The topics are presented alphabetically and not in order of importance.

What do we know and what don't we know?

Questions commonly asked by patients or considered by clinicians

Should I take any dietary supplements for my shoulder pain?

People experiencing shoulder pain may consider using dietary supplements as a treatment option. Influencing factors may be the Internet, health food shops, supplement industry, experiences of trusted family members and friends, and clinician recommendations. The dietary supplement industry is massive and growing. It is estimated that up to 40% of adults in the UK regularly use supplements, and currently spend approximately £450 million (US$ 586 million) a year.[83] In the USA, the amount spent in 2019 was US$ 32 billion.

Supplements may be considered following a clinical, lay, or (Internet-assisted) self-diagnosis of bursitis, capsulitis, or tendinitis, with the rationale of reducing inflammation and oxidative stress, as both are considered to contribute to the pathophysiological pathways involved in persistent pain,[5,68] including persistent musculoskeletal pain.[19] Inflammatory processes are known to induce oxidative stress (excessive production of free radicals or reactive oxygen species) and reduce cellular antioxidant defense.[40] Radák et al.[63] reported that mature rats fed a restricted diet (resulting in a relative reduction of free radicals) demonstrated significantly less tendon degeneration in comparison to rats fed a normal diet. The Western-style diet has become characterized by the consumption of highly processed and refined foods, with high contents of sugars, salt, and fat and protein from red and processed meat.[6,14] This diet high in saturated fatty acids,[3,50] trans-fatty acids,[4,55] and a high omega-6:omega-3 PUFA (polyunsaturated fatty acids) ratio[22,58] from food is associated with increased levels of inflammatory markers in serum. This results in excessive production of pro-inflammatory mediators and subsequent reduction of anti-inflammatory mediators including antioxidants.

Meta-analyses and systematic reviews suggest that omega-3 fatty acids have a therapeutic role in the reduction of pain associated with rheumatoid arthritis, with doses of 3–6 g/day appearing to have a greater effect.[1,20,42] Sandford et al.[66] investigated the efficacy of omega-3 PUFA supplements compared to a matched placebo alongside an exercise intervention for rotator cuff related shoulder pain (RCRSP). Study results demonstrated statistically and clinically significant improvements in disability and pain in both group's participants at 2, 3, 6, and 12 months. The omega-3 PUFA group demonstrated a more rapid improvement in disability of 64% from baseline at 3 months, compared to 42% in the placebo group, using the Shoulder Pain and Disability Index (SPADI) (95%CI: −15.6 to −0.9, p=0.03), but no discernible difference was noted between the two groups using the Oxford Shoulder Score and pain numerical rating scores. One other randomized controlled trial investigating the efficacy of omega-3 PUFA supplements for the treatment of tendinopathies has also been conducted. The double-blinded study by Mavrogenis et al.[51] reported a significant improvement in pain after 32 days of supplementation with omega-3 PUFA and an antioxidant pill in recreational athletes with tendinopathies. However, methodological limitations included participant selection bias, an absence of intention to treat analysis, and broad inclusion criteria. Poor clarity surrounding confounding factors, including the implications of using therapeutic ultrasound in treatment packages further limited the potential impact of findings.

Dietary supplements containing curcumin (derived from turmeric) have been reported to produce anti-inflammatory effects and provide analgesia for musculoskeletal pain.[13] However, Gaffey et al.[18] concluded in their systematic review that there is insufficient evidence to support the use of curcuminoids in the treatment of musculoskeletal pain. Their use has been investigated in combination with other supplements in the shoulder. Tendisulfur Forte containing methylsulfonylmethane, hydrolyzed swine collagen (Type I and Type II), L-arginine, L-lysine, vitamin C, condroitin sulfate, glucosamine, extract of *Curcuma longa* (curcuminoids), dry *Boswellia serrata* extract (acetyl-11-keto-b-boswellic acid (AKBA)), and myrrh was investigated by Vitali et al.[75] Thirty people with shoulder tendinopathy (diagnosis of which was not clearly defined) were treated with extracorporeal shock wave therapy and 15 also took the Tendisulfur Forte supplement for two months. In the treatment arm there was significant difference in the visual analogue pain scores at 60 days, and nonsteroidal anti-inflammatory medication consumption was significantly reduced at 30 and 60 days. There were clear methodological limitations, including a small sample size and lack of randomization. Previous studies investigating the use of curcuminoids in patients recovering from surgery following rotator cuff repairs did not show any change in long-term pain.[23,54]

As such, there is insufficient evidence to provide support to recommend dietary supplements as a standalone or adjunct treatment in the management of musculoskeletal problems involving the shoulder. Rigorous clinical trials are required to address this, as the industry is large and growing and the natural components of dietary supplements are relatively abundant and inexpensive. Supplements cannot be patented and because of this, there is little incentive to invest in research.[73] Currently, it may be more appropriate to optimize diet than to recommend supplements, except in cases where there is a definitive need and evidence to support their use.

Should I stretch the posterior shoulder capsule?

Posterior shoulder tightness (PST) has been described as an important physical impairment in the management of shoulder pain and disability in both sporting[8,72,77] and non-sporting populations.[46,79] Many authors recommend posterior shoulder intervention within their treatment algorithm for RCRSP[15,49] and as a component of the interventions in RCTs.[33,36] Despite these recommendations, there are many uncertainties relating to the role of PST in shoulder pain and the impact of treatment of PST on shoulder pain and disability.

Although the term "posterior shoulder tightness" is prevalent in the literature, its definition is elusive. Some definitions imply an anatomical source responsible for the deficit in range,[12,65] although this cannot be confirmed either through clinical examination or medical imaging. Other studies have used a deficit of internal rotation,[79,80] horizontal adduction[46] or low flexion[64] to define PST, and have considered a side-to-side difference ranging from 7–20° as an indication that PST is present.[11,64] This lack of clarity over the definition of PST may result in heterogeneity of studied populations.

Defining PST more clearly is important for research and clinical practice. A working definition has been provided by Hall et al.:[27] a side-to-side difference of 10° or more in 2 out of 3 clinical tests, or a difference of 20° or more in a single test. The three clinical tests used to identify PST are glenohumeral joint internal rotation, horizontal adduction, and low flexion. Several authors have described the prevalence of PST in samples of people with shoulder pain.[46,56,71] However, due to the lack of clarity in how the samples were selected, the various methods used to define PST, and the small sample sizes of the study populations, the available results should be interpreted with caution. If a correlation were established between PST and shoulder pain, several possibilities might explain the observed relationship:

1. PST is a cause of shoulder pain.
2. Shoulder pain is a cause of PST.
3. There is no causal connection between PST and shoulder pain.
4. PST and shoulder pain have no causal connection but may have a common cause.
5. PST causes shoulder pain, and shoulder pain causes PST.

These possibilities are under-represented in the literature relating to PST. It is widely acknowledged that PST might be a cause of shoulder pain, but the possibility that shoulder pain causes PST is rarely discussed.[26]

Most of the mechanistic research on PST assumes that the observed deficit in range is caused by contracture of the posterior capsule. This contracture is believed to alter glenohumeral joint kinematics, resulting in shoulder pain. There are, however, several inconsistencies with this theory. Firstly, there is no convincing evidence that the capsule is responsible for PST. Imaging studies have demonstrated increased thickness of the posterior capsule in the throwing arm of baseball pitchers,[70] but there is no evidence that these hyperplastic changes result in tissue shortening. In addition, cadaveric studies investigating the effect of experimentally shortening the posterior capsule on glenohumeral joint kinematics often shorten it by 20–40% of its total length. This extreme shortening is unlikely to represent natural change and challenges the validity of the findings.

Several studies have reported reductions in PST following joint mobilization.[11,71] The manual forces used clinically were between 3–14 kg,[78] while the posterior glenohumeral joint capsule has a modulus of elasticity of 683 kg/cm^2.[34] It is therefore unlikely that even the most carefully applied, capsule-specific mobilizations would reach the elastic limit of the tissue in question. The increase in range following treatment is therefore unlikely to result from structural changes in the posterior capsule; perhaps the original deficit was also unrelated to the structure of the posterior capsule? The current evidence suggests that only weak recommendations can be made from low quality studies to support the use of manual therapy treatments in sporting and non-sporting symptomatic populations.[11,79] Other possible causes of PST include humeral retroversion, glenoid retroversion, muscular stiffness due to reflex afferent discharge from mechanoreceptors,[21] or muscular guarding in response to pain.[32]

Further research is required to establish if PST is due to posterior capsular tightness in isolation or additional causes, such as active muscle guarding. Establishing pathophysiology may lead to better management. If the loss of internal rotation range is due to glenoid retroversion, no amount of stretching or strengthening will change this. Research needs to establish if there is a causal relationship between PST and shoulder pain. A well-designed randomized controlled trial would address the uncertainty relating to the additional benefit posterior shoulder treatment adds to a multimodal exercise and education program.

To operate, or not to operate? – that is the question

Arguably the most debated surgical procedure performed on the shoulder has been subacromial decompression (SAD) for what is often referred to as subacromial impingement syndrome (SIS). This procedure was originally described by Neer[57] based on the theory that the acromion was responsible for the impingement of various shoulder structures, more specifically the supraspinatus tendon, ultimately leading to pain and dysfunction. Removing a portion of the acromion, in theory, would eliminate the impingement. However, this theory had never properly been tested until recently despite the popularity of this procedure. Significant evidence through randomized controlled trials has shown that there are no differences in outcomes between exercise and SAD surgery among those with SIS at 1, 2, 4, 5, and 10-year follow-ups.[24,25,37–39] Furthermore, evidence through randomized controlled placebo trials among those with SIS have demonstrated no difference among those having had the SAD procedure performed, compared to those having only diagnostic arthroscopy performed. These trials along with other evidence, including systematic reviews on the topic, have led to changes in clinical practice guidelines and a Rapid Recommendation by the *British Medical Journal* providing a strong recommendation against SAD surgery for people with SIS.[35,45,74]

The evidence regarding surgical and nonsurgical treatment among those with degenerative full thickness rotator cuff tears is somewhat less clear when compared to those with SIS. Evidence has historically supported the use of nonsurgical treatment for rotator cuff tears as the first line of treatment followed by surgical repair for those not reaching their desired goals.[67] Emerging evidence has begun to investigate the comparison of surgical versus nonsurgical treatment among those with rotator cuff tears.

Kuhn et al.[43] performed a prospective multicenter cohort study investigating the effectiveness of physical therapy on treating nontraumatic full thickness rotator cuff tears with a two-year follow-up. The authors demonstrated that physical therapy significantly reduced the need for surgery among 75% of the patients at two years. Carr et al.[9] performed a randomized controlled trial looking at the effectiveness of open versus arthroscopic repair for those with rotator cuff tears. An interesting finding from this study was the relatively high retear rate among both procedures. However, among those with a retorn rotator cuff following their repair, there was no significant difference in their Oxford Shoulder Score compared to those with an intact repair, which may challenge the structural importance of the repair on patient outcomes.

However, there are those who argue that if the rotator cuff tear is not repaired, the patient is simply delaying the inevitable, as the tear will progressively become worse and ultimately lead to surgery anyhow. Evidence to the contrary can be found in the work of Boorman et al.[7] who examined those with chronic full thickness rotator cuff tears. All individuals participated in a three-month home exercise program. After three months, those who were asymptomatic did not undergo surgery and those that remained symptomatic underwent rotator cuff repair. Follow-up was performed at 5 years with no significant difference between groups.

Finally, a recent systematic review looking at operative versus non-operative treatment for full thickness rotator cuff tears was performed to help provide consensus from the current available evidence.[60] Surprisingly, the review resulted in only three articles being retained for analysis. The results from the limited evidence revealed a statistically significant difference between both Constant and visual analogue pain scores favoring the surgical group; however, these differences were small and did not meet the minimal difference to be considered clinically important. Perhaps the most surprising finding from this study is the lack of high-level evidence investigating surgical versus nonsurgical care among those with rotator cuff tears currently.

Standardized management recommendations

When considering standardized management recommendations for shoulder conditions, it is common to turn to clinical practice guidelines. For example, studies investigating physical therapy treatment choices for shoulder pain by surveys completed by clinicians revealed that most of the delivered treatments were aligned with guideline recommendations (93%). However, the percentage of treatments not recommended in guidelines and inconclusive treatments (e.g., acupuncture, electrical stimulation, ice, ultrasound,[44] massage and TENS for nonspecific shoulder pain),[53, 81] or that had not yet been investigated was also high (90% and 79%).[81]

When the guidelines are current, valid, and of high quality, they support shared decision-making and clinical confidence.[62] Unfortunately, this is not the case for the majority of current clinical practice guidelines pertaining to musculoskeletal shoulder conditions. A recent review of musculoskeletal clinical practice guidelines revealed that, of the clinical practice guidelines retained, only one related to the management of rotator cuff syndrome in the workplace was of high quality.[48] When translating the conclusion of clinical practice guidelines into practice, clinicians must remain circumspect as to the value of the evidence that was available to generate the guidelines.

Modified Delphi technique responses

Acute traumatic rotator cuff tears

1. **What we really do know:**
    - Delayed diagnosis of acute rotator cuff tears may result in impairment of shoulder function, even if patients undergo surgery.[29]
2. **What we think we know but actually don't:**
    - Surgery is commonly presented as the best treatment for traumatic rotator cuff tendon tears, but we don't actually know why.
3. **What we really don't know and need to know:**
    - What is the most effective treatment for acute tears?
    - Why with atraumatic cuff tears are we comfortable not pointing to the tear as the source of pain, but in traumatic tears we lean towards the tear being the source of pain? Maybe something to do with the chemical makeup in synovial fluid following the acute tear?
    - Clinical utility of orthopedic physical examination tests on acute tears.

Adjunct treatments

1. **What we really do know:**
    - In some individuals, taping and bracing may be effective in relieving pain, as well as improving

range of motion, provided these techniques are used in conjunction with an evidence-based physical therapy (physiotherapy) program.

- Manual therapy is effective for some individuals with shoulder pain when embedded in an exercise program and used sparingly and early in management. The recommendation for its inclusion is "strong", but "strong" does not mean a large treatment effect.[59]

2. **What we think we know but actually don't:**

   The following are commonly considered factual but may not be correct:

   - Shoulder symptoms will improve if we improve posture, and address abnormal muscle timing and abnormal movement patterns.
   - Including manual therapy in management will benefit most people (≥80%) with shoulder conditions.
   - The more you practice manual therapy and the more techniques and skills you acquire, the more clinical outcomes will concomitantly improve.

3. **What we really don't know and need to know:**

   - Do taping and bracing when added to another treatment, such as exercise, enhance the treatment response (i.e., result in faster, and better outcomes)?
   - If taping and bracing do enhance outcomes, then we need to know why.
   - Are there specific clinical parameters or conditions where taping and bracing is more (or less) likely to help?
   - What additional (adjunct) treatments, such as manual therapy, taping, bracing, and modalities, improve outcome when used independently or incorporated into other interventions, such as exercise, and by how much and for how long, and what is the associated cost?
   - Are manual therapy procedures (such as mobilization with movement, mobilization, Mechanical Diagnosis and Therapy®), valid screening tools to identify cervicothoracic referred shoulder pain?
   - Are all hands-on interventions (e.g., trigger point therapy, acupressure, joint mobilization techniques) identical physiologically with the only difference being the philosophy behind why the "touch" is being applied?

Assessment

1. **What we really do know:**

   - Pain can be referred from the spine to the shoulder region.

2. **What we think we know but actually don't:**

   - We think we know how to rule out the spine during a routine orthopedic assessment for patients presenting with shoulder pain, but there is no gold standard.

3. **What we really don't know and need to know:**

   - What are the most important components of assessment for people seeking care experiencing shoulder pain?
   - Can we/should we develop assessment approaches to provide individualized treatment plans?
   - We don't know how to rule out the spine for patients presenting with shoulder pain but need to know.
   - We don't know what impairments are relevant in individual patients' presentations. We need to know this (through reasoned analysis) to avoid assuming a given factor is necessarily always relevant and must be addressed or, conversely, is never relevant and can be ignored.

Calcific tendinopathy

1. **What we really do know:**

   - Some people with calcific deposits in the rotator cuff tendons experience debilitating symptoms, while others remain asymptomatic.

2. **What we think we know but actually don't:**
   - We think that calcific deposits of the rotator cuff are associated with pain and shoulder dysfunction, but we actually do not know that at all. They may be part of the normal healing process and may in fact be protective against rotator cuff tears, irrespective of the pain that some people experience.
3. **What we really don't know and need to know:**
   - We do not know why calcific deposits occur in the rotator cuff tendons, or what causes some people to experience shoulder pain while others experience no pain or dysfunction at all. We need to know this to provide better education and management.

Communication

1. **What we really do know:**
   - Acknowledgment and validation are important in healthcare communication.
   - The words we use when talking about shoulder pain can have either a beneficial or detrimental impact on people's lives.
   - Different labels used by doctors for rotator cuff disease may influence people to say yes to surgery when there are other options.[82]
2. **What we think we know but actually don't:**
   - How to hear, how to acknowledge, and how to validate a patient's stories and experiences; we think that we do it, yet patients continue to say they feel unheard, disbelieved or dismissed, and invalidated.
   - We assume that obtaining a qualification as a healthcare professional automatically leads to effective patient education skills. Education is a crucial component of modern-day healthcare, yet less than 1% of undergraduate healthcare training is devoted to developing the necessary knowledge and skills needed to guide and facilitate people living with shoulder pain.
3. **What we really don't know and need to know:**
   - How best to acknowledge and validate an individual's beliefs and lived experiences.
   - How best to provide education for a given individual.
   - How best to promote behavioral change in clinical practice and how to tailor it to a given individual.
   - How best to develop meaningful, solution-focused approaches to shoulder rehabilitation.
   - How people with shoulder pain who *don't* seek care find solutions to overcome their symptoms. We need to ask, "What are these individuals doing and how are they doing it?" to achieve effective and independent self-management.
   - How many people are living with persistent shoulder symptoms who never seek care, and why not.
   - What is the best way to present the shared decision-making model to patients with shoulder pain?
   - How do we build relationships/communication with other care providers so that there is some agreement on the best value-based care to present to the patient?

Exercise and rehabilitation

1. **What we really do know:**
   - The long head of biceps tendon may be involved in shoulder pain and dysfunction.
   - Exercise is (to a degree) effective for the treatment of soft tissue/rotator cuff related shoulder pain.
   - Self-management and confidence are important for long-term benefit.
   - Strengthening and motor control exercises are effective in decreasing pain and improving function. Motor control exercises appear to have a quicker response than strengthening programs.

2. **What we think we know but actually don't:**
   - The function of the long head of the biceps tendon at the shoulder. Our current understanding of its role relies heavily on (outdated) kinematic studies performed on cadavers, usually on an isolated tendon removed from the surrounding anatomy, which does not accurately represent the forces or functional anatomy of this tendon in vivo.
   - People with shoulder pain get better because they improve their shoulder muscle strength and that getting stronger is the reason rehabilitation is successful for most shoulder conditions.
   - We believe that specific exercises are better than general exercises for most shoulder conditions, but we don't actually know.
   - How to support patient self-management and adherence.
   - Whether we need to reduce impairments (decreased strength/reduced range of motion/abnormal movement patterns) to improve clinical outcomes for a person experiencing shoulder pain.
   - We think we know which shoulder exercises rehabilitate specific shoulder muscles and the best way to progress these exercises. But this "understanding" does not have consensus and is most often based on a simplistic mechanistic understanding of the action of a muscle. This does not adequately address the complex motor control aspect of normal shoulder muscle function.
3. **What we really don't know and need to know:**
   - Are whole body exercise programs such as Tai Chi and yoga and the incorporated breathing and relaxation techniques more effective on impairment and disability than local exercise treatments?
   - How can we best assess the long head of biceps tendon clinically? What do responses to clinical tests and imaging findings actually mean?
   - How can we treat long head of biceps tendinopathy when we still don't understand its exact role in the shoulder? What is the best treatment?
   - We don't know if immersive virtual reality (VR) as an intervention will reduce shoulder impairment and disability and improve motor control in people experiencing shoulder symptoms.
   - We don't know if VR is of any additive value to usual care. We don't know if there are any individual characteristics that suggest VR will bring about better outcomes than no, or usual, intervention.
   - If immersive VR helps to decrease impairment and increase function, then we need to know why.
   - Will patients be more compliant with their rehabilitation program when using VR in the clinic, and/or at home, than they are with current rehabilitation programs?
   - What is the best rehabilitation approach for the management of rotator cuff related shoulder pain?
   - What are the parameters of exercise that are related to outcomes?
   - How to support self-management and adherence.
   - Studies show that people are not stronger following strengthening exercises and don't really move better following motor control exercises (when looking at mean group changes). So why are these exercises effective?
   - How treatments work. For example, if exercise helps, what is the mechanism of recovery? Does it help through reducing systemic inflammation, reducing fear, restoring confidence, placebo, improving load tolerance, restoring biochemical homeostasis in the shoulder tissues, promoting muscle hypertrophy and tendon stiffness, or combinations of potential effects?

Frozen shoulder

1. **What we really do know:**
   - It is not self-limiting for everyone.
   - Intra-articular corticosteroid injections may offer clinically important improvements in pain in the short term.
   - Currently, it is a condition based on a diagnosis of exclusion.

2. **What we think we know but actually don't:**
   - We think we understand the pathophysiology, but we don't.
   - Corticosteroid injections target inflammatory processes in frozen shoulder, but there is no certainty.
   - That it passes through defined stages in defined timelines, and it always gets better.
3. **What we really don't know and need to know:**
   - Is there a central sensitization/nociplastic component to the pain?
   - The best management for this condition.
   - How best to diagnose the condition in its early stages.
   - Does calling the condition "frozen shoulder" cause harm for people diagnosed with a frozen shoulder?
   - Do corticosteroid injections target inflammation, myofibroblasts, both, something else?
   - What do people with frozen shoulders think and feel about their treatment, particularly with reference to injection therapy?
   - Do hydrodistension (arthro-distention) procedures really help in the management of frozen shoulder?
   - What is the best combination of pharmaceutical agents to inject when performing hydrodistension?
   - During hydrodistension, is there a need for the capsule to rupture or not?
   - Is muscle guarding the basis for the "frozen" shoulder in some individuals (and not a capsular contraction), and what are those individuals' characteristics?

Injection therapy

1. **What we really do know:**
   - Although not without harms, it is likely to help reduce pain in the early (pain > stiffness) stage of a frozen shoulder.
   - For rotator cuff related shoulder pain, the benefit of injection therapy is highly variable and short lived.
2. **What we think we know but actually don't:**
   - That ultrasound guidance for injections contributes to better safety and/or effectiveness when performing injections for shoulder conditions.
   - We think nonsurgical treatments such as injections improve pain and function in people diagnosed with shoulder osteoarthritis, but the evidence is limited.
3. **What we really don't know and need to know:**
   - What is the efficacy of injection therapy in shoulder osteoarthritis, and the most effective injectate?
   - Does saline perform as well as corticosteroid in people with rotator cuff related shoulder pain?
   - What are the long-term tissue effects of corticosteroids on shoulder tissues?

Lifestyle

1. **What we really do know:**
   - A high-fat diet negatively affects tendon quality, increasing the risk of rupture and tendinopathy.[16]
2. **What we think we know but actually don't:**
   - The secretion of adipokines is strictly related to fat ingestion and body composition and can potentially act on tendon physiology and injury.
3. **What we really don't know and need to know:**
   - Central obesity, insulin resistance, adipokines, chronic low-grade inflammation, and fat intake play a role in disrupting tendon healing and contribute to tendinopathy. Research is needed to define the molecular pathways involved and identifiable biomarkers that correlate with/predict pathogenesis.

Pain

1. **What we really do know:**
   - Many factors contribute to the experience of pain.
   - Pain severity and disability are not consistent with findings from medical imaging or the

clinical examination. In other words: pain is often disproportionate and unpredictable.

- Shoulder pain can be referred from the cervical region.
- Immersive virtual reality (VR) technology can provide effective short-term pain relief for various clinical pain conditions. Studies using functional magnetic resonance imaging have reported a reduction in activity in five areas of the brain related to pain processing when using VR.[30,31]

2. **What we think we know but actually don't:**
   - The actual meaning(s) of pain to people experiencing shoulder pain.
   - That shoulder pain causes secondary changes in the cervical musculature.
   - In some people with persistent shoulder pain, nociplastic pain is the cause. As such, phenotyping patients is crucial to steer treatment.
   - That the treatments for pure nociceptive pain versus nociplastic pain are different.
3. **What we really don't know and need to know:**
   - How can we improve pain-related outcomes? Which factors to modify in which individuals?
   - We do not know if the changes in the cervical region identified clinically are primary, secondary, or coincidental findings, but understanding this phenomenon more precisely through basic research may improve management.
   - The clinical classification of a shoulder pain patient where pain is driven by peripheral factors or in the phenotype where altered central pain processing is the underlying driver.
   - How best to assess the complex mechanisms underlying shoulder pain and dysfunction and how they interact, e.g., biomechanical, neurophysiological, psychological, social, lifestyle, and cultural determinants.
   - Can virtual reality interventions be used to effectively manage pain and support rehabilitation for people with musculoskeletal shoulder pain? If it is beneficial, are their conditions and/or individuals where it is more (or less) beneficial? Do software design and preference impact outcome? Does a "reward" system enhance outcome?

Pathology and symptoms

1. **What we really do know:**
   - Shoulder pain is rarely related to "pathology" seen on imaging.
2. **What we think we know but actually don't:**
   - Shoulder special tests enable us to make a structural diagnosis, but this is not correct.
3. **What we really don't know and need to know:**
   - We don't understand why some people experience pain and others don't – it is clearly broader than pathoanatomical findings. How do we determine the contribution of factors for any given individual?
   - How do psychosocial factors and social determinants of health impact pain, and how can we best assess and manage these factors?
   - Does treatment influence pathology, even at a biochemical level?

Pediatric shoulder problems

1. **What we really do know:**
   - That a growing child has a musculoskeletal system that differs from adults.
2. **What we think we know but actually don't:**
   - The natural course of atraumatic shoulder instability.
3. **What we really don't know and need to know:**
   - The lived experience of children and adolescents experiencing shoulder problems. What do they understand, what is the impact on their life and what outcomes of treatment matter most to them?

Psychosocial factors

1. **What we really do know:**
    - Psychosocial factors are associated with recovery from and prognosis of shoulder pain.
    - Persistent shoulder pain is closely associated with depression and anxiety.[10]
2. **What we think we know but actually don't:**
    - We think psychosocial interventions benefit people with shoulder pain, but we don't really know.
    - We think that patients don't like discussing psychosocial factors, but there isn't evidence for this.
3. **What we really don't know and need to know:**
    - Do psychosocial interventions reduce the progression from acute to persistent shoulder pain?
    - Do psychosocial interventions improve outcomes in the presence of persistent shoulder pain?

Suprascapular nerve blocks

1. **What we really do know:**
    - Suprascapular nerve blocks (SSNB) are not routinely used in the management of shoulder pain.
2. **What we think we know but actually don't:**
    - We think SSNBs are effective in the short term, but we don't know.
3. **What we really don't know and need to know:**
    - Are SSNBs effective and safe, for which patient groups, at what stage, and for how long do they benefit? What are the definitive harms?

Surgery versus nonsurgical interventions

1. **What we really do know:**
    - Subacromial decompression surgery for individuals with shoulder impingement syndrome has no greater benefit than nonsurgical treatment.
    - Nonsurgical treatment for many individuals with atraumatic rotator cuff tears, even full thickness, can produce comparable clinical outcomes to surgery.
2. **What we think we know but actually don't:**
    - That all elective surgical procedures, exercise, manual therapy, or injection techniques have efficacy beyond their contextual effects.
3. **What we really don't know and need to know:**
    - In the management of Grade III acromioclavicular joint injuries, are there any early prognostic factors to direct treatment to a surgical or nonsurgical path?
    - How should we tailor treatments (surgical or nonsurgical) for individual patients? What are the relevant determinants in individual situations?
    - How specific should our treatments be?
    - We don't know the precise mechanism(s) by which therapeutic interventions effect change. We have moved from a predominately biomedical explanation regarding altered biomechanics and tissue stiffness to a predominately neuroprocessing explanation of neuromodulation. Neither should be fully accepted or dismissed as we need to know more about the contribution and interplay of these different mechanisms.

Swimmer's shoulder

1. **What we really do know:**
    - Shoulder pain in swimmers is a significant problem.[52,69]
    - Swimmers with shoulder external rotation range outside 93–100° are at risk of developing shoulder pain.[76]
    - Tendinopathic change in supraspinatus, subscapularis, and long head of biceps is the predominant pathological process observed in the shoulders of swimmers.[61,69]
    - There is an acute swim training response in supraspinatus tendon (which is greater in sprint training than distance), and evidence of rotator cuff tendon changes on magnetic resonance imaging in swimmers with or without shoulder pain.[61]

2. **What we think we know but actually don't:**
   - Swimmer's shoulder pain commonly occurs when rotator cuff tendons fail to adapt to the training load over time.
   - Subscapularis tendon has the same acute response to training as supraspinatus.
   - Shoulder muscle strength may be protective for swimmers' shoulders.
   - Change in load is a risk factor for shoulder pain, but is an acute to chronic workload model useful and what is the optimal ratio?[17]
3. **What we really don't know and need to know:**
   - What is the optimal amount of swim training load for different ages/level?
   - The cumulative effect of swim training on rotator cuff tendon thickness and how long it takes to return to baseline thickness.
   - Is monitoring tendon thickness with ultrasound useful in a prediction model?
   - Muscle performance, including parameters such as rate of force development, endurance, and force production in relation to training load and shoulder pain in swimmers, needs further investigation.
   - Can we develop an effective shoulder pain prevention program for swimmers, and what does it look like?

Conclusion

We know that a graduated exercise-based approach has the most compelling level of evidence (albeit it is no silver bullet) for the management of most musculoskeletal problems involving the shoulder. We know that psychological variables are hugely influential and are likely as prevalent as in other body regions (although the directionality of the contribution of these areas needs further study). There is controversy regarding the pathogenesis of selected tissues as pain generators for patients with shoulder pain. Lastly, we know most clinical so-called special tests used in clinical practice have notable overlap and do not function as "stand alone" measures for diagnosis. There are still a great number of health providers who follow a pathogenesis-based diagnostic process. Based on clinical testing or imagery, many diagnosticians will label a shoulder disorder and design a treatment regimen that is based on this label. We do not know the true extent to which a 'pathology' contributes to the patient's pain experience, nor do we know if this defined treatment regimen is why patients improve. We are also unable to define a logical pattern associated with risk factors for shoulder pain, and we do not understand the role of a psychologically informed treatment approach on individuals with shoulder pain. Research priority should be given to: 1) understanding the prognosis for shoulder pain, as this has the potential to improve management and reduce unnecessary care, and 2) phenotyping may improve our ability to refine management options.

The information provided by this chapter helped us to identify knowledge gaps that researchers may consider as priorities to address to facilitate improved care, as we broaden and deepen our understanding of shoulder-related conditions. The responses also provide an opportunity for clinicians to reflect and consider where a paucity of knowledge relating to musculoskeletal problems involving the shoulder challenges our practice, and how we should use that information in our clinical decision-making and management planning.

Acknowledgements

We would like to wholeheartedly thank the following people for their contribution to this chapter: Amee Seitz, Angela Spontelli Gisselman, Beate Dejaco, Ben Dean, Bill Vicenzino, César Fernández-de-las-Peñas, Christopher Mercer, Chris Worsfold, Christine Bilsborough Smith, Craig Boettcher, Craig Wassinger, Danielle Hollis, Derek Griffin, Emma Salt, Eric Hegedus, Gajan Rajeswaren, Gwendolen Jull, Helen Walker, Hubert van Griensven, Ian Horsley, Jean-Sébastian Roy, Jenny McConnell, Jillian McDowell, Joel Bialosky, Joletta Belton, Karen Ginn, Karen McCreesh, Kieran O'Sullivan, Lennard Voogt, Liesbet de Baets, Lorenzo Masci, Mark Jones, Mike Stewart, Mike Cummings, Mira Meeus, Niamh Brady, Panos Barlas, Rachel Chester, Rod Whiteley, and Sally McLaine.

References

1. Abdulrazaq M, Innes JK, Calder PC. Effect of ω-3 polyunsaturated fatty acids on arthritic pain: a systematic review. Nutrition. 2017;39:57-66.

2. Altman DG, Bland JM. Absence of evidence is not evidence of absence. BMJ. 1995;311:485.

3. Arya S, Isharwal S, Misra A, et al. C-reactive protein and dietary nutrients in urban Asian Indian adolescents and young adults. Nutrition. 2006;22:865-871.

4. Ascherio A, Katan MB, Zock PL, Stampfer MJ, Willett WC. Trans fatty acids and coronary heart disease. New England Journal of Medicine. 1999;340:1994-1998.

5. Birklein F, Schmelz M. Neuropeptides, neurogenic inflammation and complex regional pain syndrome (CRPS). Neuroscience Letters. 2008;437:199-202.

6. Bjørklund G, Aaseth J, Doşa MD, et al. Does diet play a role in reducing nociception related to inflammation and chronic pain? Nutrition. 2019;66:153-165.

7. Boorman RS, More KD, Hollinshead RM, et al. What happens to patients when we do not repair their cuff tears? Five-year rotator cuff quality-of-life index outcomes following nonoperative treatment of patients with full-thickness rotator cuff tears. J Shoulder Elbow Surg. 2018;27:444-448.

8. Burkhart SS, Morgan CD, Kibler WB. The disabled throwing shoulder: spectrum of pathology Part I: pathoanatomy and biomechanics. Arthroscopy. 2003;19:404-420.

9. Carr A, Cooper C, Campbell MK, et al. Effectiveness of open and arthroscopic rotator cuff repair (UKUFF): a randomised controlled trial. The Bone & Joint Journal. 2017;99-b:107-115.

10. Cho CH, Jung SW, Park JY, Song KS, Yu KI. Is shoulder pain for three months or longer correlated with depression, anxiety, and sleep disturbance? J Shoulder Elbow Surg. 2013;22:222-228.

11. Cools AM, Johansson FR, Cagnie B, Cambier DC, Witvrouw EE. Stretching the posterior shoulder structures in subjects with internal rotation deficit: comparison of two stretching techniques. Shoulder & Elbow. 2012;4:56-63.

12. Dashottar A, Costantini O, Borstad J. A comparison of range of motion change across four posterior shoulder tightness measurements after external rotator fatigue. International Journal of Sports Physical Therapy. 2014;9:498-508.

13. Di Pierro F, Zacconi P, Bertuccioli A, et al. A naturally-inspired, curcumin-based lecithin formulation (Meriva formulated as the finished product Algocur) alleviates the osteo-muscular pain conditions in rugby players. Eur Rev Med Pharm Sci. 2017;21:4935-4940.

14. Dragan S, Şerban M-C, Damian G, Buleu F, Valcovici M, Christodorescu R. Dietary patterns and interventions to alleviate chronic pain. Nutrients. 2020;12:2510.

15. Ellenbecker TS, Cools A. Rehabilitation of shoulder impingement syndrome and rotator cuff injuries: an evidence-based review. Br J Sports Med. 2010;44:319-327.

16. Elli S, Schiaffini G, Macchi M, Spezia M, Chisari E, Maffulli N. High-fat diet, adipokines and low-grade inflammation are associated with disrupted tendon healing: a systematic review of preclinical studies. British Medical Bulletin. 2021;10.1093/bmb/ldab007.

17. Feijen S ST, Kuppens K, Tate A, Struyf F. Prediction of shoulder pain in youth competitive swimmers: the development and internal validation of a prognostic prediction model. The American Journal of Sports Medicine. 2020;19:1-8.

18. Gaffey A, Slater H, Porritt K, Campbell JM. The effects of curcuminoids on musculoskeletal pain: a systematic review. JBI Evidence Synthesis. 2017;15:486-516.

19. Gallo J, Raska M, Kriegova E, Goodman SB. Inflammation and its resolution and the musculoskeletal system. Journal of Orthopaedic Translation. 2017;10:52-67.

20. Gioxari A, Kaliora AC, Marantidou F, Panagiotakos DP. Intake of ω-3 polyunsaturated fatty acids in patients with rheumatoid arthritis: a systematic review and meta-analysis. Nutrition. 2018;45:114-124.e114.

21. Guanche C, Knatt T, Solomonow M, Lu Y, Baratta R. The synergistic action of the capsule and the shoulder muscles. Am J Sports Med. 1995;23:301-306.

22. Guebre-Egziabher F, Rabasa-Lhoret R, Bonnet F, et al. Nutritional intervention to reduce the n− 6/n− 3 fatty acid ratio increases adiponectin concentration and fatty acid oxidation in healthy subjects. European Journal of Clinical Nutrition. 2008;62:1287-1293.

23. Gumina S, Passaretti D, Gurzì M, Candela V. Arginine L-alpha-ketoglutarate, methylsulfonylmethane, hydrolyzed type I collagen and bromelain in rotator cuff tear repair: a prospective randomized study. Current Medical Research and Opinion. 2012;28:1767-1774.

24. Haahr JP, Andersen JH. Exercises may be as efficient as subacromial decompression in patients with subacromial stage II impingement: 4-8-years' follow-up in a prospective, randomized study. Scand J Rheumatol. 2006;35:224-228.

25. Haahr JP, Ostergaard S, Dalsgaard J, et al. Exercises versus arthroscopic decompression in patients with subacromial impingement: a randomised, controlled study in 90 cases with a one year follow up. Ann Rheum Dis. 2005;64:760-764.

26. Hall K, Borstad JD. Posterior shoulder tightness: to treat or not to treat? J Orthop Sports Phys Ther. 2018;48:133-136.

27. Hall K, Lewis J, Moore A, Ridehalgh C. Posterior shoulder tightness: an intersession reliability study of 3 clinical tests. Archives of Physiotherapy. 2020;10:14-14.

28. Haynes RB, Devereaux PJ, Guyatt GH. Clinical expertise in the era of evidence-based medicine and patient choice. BMJ Evidence-Based Medicine. 2002;7:36-38.

29. Hegedus EJ, Goode AP, Cook CE, et al. Which physical examination tests provide clinicians with the most value when examining the shoulder? Update of a systematic review with meta-analysis of individual tests. British Journal of Sports Medicine. 2012;46:964-978.

30. Hoffman HG, Richards TL, Bills AR, et al. Using FMRI to study the neural correlates of virtual reality analgesia. CNS Spectrums. 2006;11:45-51.

31. Hoffman HG, Richards TL, Van Oostrom T, et al. The analgesic effects of opioids and immersive virtual reality distraction: evidence from subjective and functional brain imaging assessments. Anesthesia and Analgesia. 2007;105:1776-1783.

32. Hollmann L, Halaki M, Kamper SJ, Haber M, Ginn KA. Does muscle guarding play a role in range of motion loss in patients with frozen shoulder? Musculoskelet Sci Pract. 2018;37:64-68.

33. Holmgren T, Bjornsson Hallgren H, Oberg B, Adolfsson L, Johansson K. Effect

of specific exercise strategy on need for surgery in patients with subacromial impingement syndrome: randomised controlled study. BMJ. 2012;344:e787.

34. Itoi E, Grabowski JJ, Morrey BF, An KN. Capsular properties of the shoulder. Tohoku J Exp Med. 1993;171:203-210.

35. Karjalainen TV, Jain NB, Page CM, et al. Subacromial decompression surgery for rotator cuff disease. Cochrane Database Syst Rev. 2019;1:CD005619.

36. Keene DJ, Soutakbar H, Hopewell S, et al. Development and implementation of the physiotherapy-led exercise interventions for the treatment of rotator cuff disorders for the 'Getting it Right: Addressing Shoulder Pain' (GRASP) trial. Physiotherapy. 2020;107:252-266.

37. Ketola S, Lehtinen J, Arnala I, et al. Does arthroscopic acromioplasty provide any additional value in the treatment of shoulder impingement syndrome?: a two-year randomised controlled trial. J Bone Joint Surg Br. 2009;91:1326-1334.

38. Ketola S, Lehtinen J, Rousi T, et al. No evidence of long-term benefits of arthroscopicacromioplasty in the treatment of shoulder impingement syndrome: five-year results of a randomised controlled trial. Bone & Joint Research. 2013;2:132-139.

39. Ketola S, Lehtinen JT, Arnala I. Arthroscopic decompression not recommended in the treatment of rotator cuff tendinopathy: a final review of a randomised controlled trial at a minimum follow-up of ten years. Bone Joint J. 2017;99-B:799-805.

40. Khansari N, Shakiba Y, Mahmoudi M. Chronic inflammation and oxidative stress as a major cause of age-related diseases and cancer. Recent Patents on Inflammation & Allergy Drug Discovery. 2009;3:73-80.

41. Knaapen L. Being 'evidence-based' in the absence of evidence: the management of non-evidence in guideline development. Social Studies of Science. 2013;43:681-706.

42. Kostoglou-Athanassiou I, Athanassiou L, Athanassiou P. The effect of omega-3 fatty acids on rheumatoid arthritis. Mediterranean Journal of Rheumatology. 2020;31:190.

43. Kuhn JE, Dunn WR, Sanders R, et al. Effectiveness of physical therapy in treating atraumatic full-thickness rotator cuff tears: a multicenter prospective cohort study. J Shoulder Elbow Surg. 2013;22:1371-1379.

44. Kulkarni R, Gibson J, Brownson P, et al. BESS/BOA patient care pathways: subacromial shoulder pain. Shoulder Elb. 2015;7:135-143.

45. Lähdeoja T, Karjalainen T, Jokihaara J, et al. Subacromial decompression surgery for adults with shoulder pain: a systematic review with meta-analysis. Br J Sports Med. 2020;54:665-673.

46. Land H, Gordon S, Watt K. Clinical assessment of subacromial shoulder impingement – which factors differ from the asymptomatic population? Musculoskeletal Science and Practice. 2017;27:49-56.

47. Lewis J, Mc Auliffe S, O'Sullivan K, O'Sullivan P, Whiteley R. Musculoskeletal physical therapy after COVID-19: time for a new "normal". JOSPT. 2021;51:5-7.

48. Lin I, Wiles LK, Waller R, et al. Poor overall quality of clinical practice guidelines for musculoskeletal pain: a systematic review. Br J Sports Med. 2018;52:337-343.

49. Ludewig PM, Braman JP. Shoulder impingement: biomechanical considerations in rehabilitation. Manual Therapy. 2011;16:33-39.

50. Margioris AN. Fatty acids and postprandial inflammation. Current Opinion in Clinical Nutrition & Metabolic Care. 2009;12:129-137.

51. Mavrogenis S, Johannessen E, Jensen P, Sindberg C. The effect of essential fatty acids and antioxidants combined with physiotherapy treatment in recreational athletes with chronic tendon disorders: a randomised, double-blind, placebo-controlled study. Physical Therapy in Sport. 2004;5:194-199.

52. McMaster WC, Troup J. A survey of interfering shoulder pain in United States competitive swimmers. Am J Sports Med. 1993;21:67-70.

53. Members PP, Experts CS, Albright J, et al. Philadelphia Panel evidence-based clinical practice guidelines on selected rehabilitation interventions for shoulder pain. Physical Therapy. 2001;81:1719-1730.

54. Merolla G, Dellabiancia F, Ingardia A, Paladini P, Porcellini G. Co-analgesic therapy for arthroscopic supraspinatus tendon repair pain using a dietary supplement containing Boswellia serrata and Curcuma longa: a prospective randomized placebo-controlled study. Musculoskeletal Surgery. 2015;99:43-52.

55. Mozaffarian D, Aro A, Willett WC. Health effects of trans-fatty acids: experimental and observational evidence. European Journal of Clinical Nutrition. 2009;63:S5-S21.

56. Myers JB, Laudner KG, Pasquale MR, Bradley JP, Lephart SM. Glenohumeral range of motion deficits and posterior shoulder tightness in throwers with pathologic internal impingement. Am J Sports Med. 2006;34:385-391.

57. Neer CS, 2nd. Anterior acromioplasty for the chronic impingement syndrome in the shoulder: a preliminary report. J Bone Joint Surg Am. 1972;54:41-50.

58. Olsen KS, Fenton C, Frøyland L, Waaseth M, Paulssen RH, Lund E. Plasma fatty acid ratios affect blood gene expression profiles: a cross-sectional study of the Norwegian women and cancer post-genome cohort. PLoS One. 2013;8:e67270.

59. Pieters L, Lewis J, Kuppens K, et al. An update of systematic reviews examining the effectiveness of conservative physical therapy interventions for subacromial shoulder pain. Journal of Orthopaedic & Sports Physical Therapy. 2020;50:131-141.

60. Piper CC, Hughes AJ, Ma Y, Wang H, Neviaser AS. Operative versus nonoperative treatment for the management of full-thickness rotator cuff tears: a systematic review and meta-analysis. J Shoulder Elbow Surg. 2018;27:572-576.

61. Porter KN, Talpey S, Pascoe D, Blanch PD, Walker HM, Shield AJ. The effect of swimming volume and intensity on changes in supraspinatus tendon thickness. Physical Therapy in Sport. 2020;47:173-177.

62. Qaseem A, Forland F, Macbeth F, Ollenschläger G, Phillips S, van der Wees P. Guidelines International Network: toward international standards for clinical practice guidelines. Ann Intern Med. 2012;156:525-531.

63. Radák Z, Naito H, Kaneko T, et al. Exercise training decreases DNA damage and increases DNA repair and resistance against oxidative stress of proteins in aged rat skeletal muscle. Pflügers Archiv. 2002;445:273-278.

64. Rosa DP, Camargo PR, Borstad JD. Effect of posterior capsule tightness and humeral retroversion on 5 glenohumeral joint range of motion measurements: a cadaveric study.

The American Journal of Sports Medicine. 2019;47:1434-1440.

65. Salamh PA, Liu X, Hanney WJ, Sprague PA, Kolber MJ. The efficacy and fidelity of clinical interventions used to reduce posterior shoulder tightness: a systematic review with meta-analysis. Journal of Shoulder and Elbow Surgery. 2019;28:1204-1213.

66. Sandford FM, Sanders TA, Wilson H, Lewis JS. A randomised controlled trial of long-chain omega-3 polyunsaturated fatty acids in the management of rotator cuff related shoulder pain. BMJ Open Sport & Exercise Medicine. 2018;4:e000414.

67. Schmidt CC, Jarrett CD, Brown BT. Management of rotator cuff tears. The Journal of Hand surgery. 2015;40:399-408.

68. Seaman DR. The diet-induced proinflammatory state: a cause of chronic pain and other degenerative diseases? Journal of Manipulative and Physiological Therapeutics. 2002;25:168-179.

69. Sein ML, Walton J, Linklater J, et al. Shoulder pain in elite swimmers: primarily due to swim-volume-induced supraspinatus tendinopathy. Br J Sports Med. 2010;44:105-113.

70. Takagishi K, Makino K, Takahira N, Ikeda T, Tsuruno K, Itoman M. Ultrasonography for diagnosis of rotator cuff tear. Skeletal Radiol. 1996;25:221-224.

71. Tyler TF, Nicholas SJ, Roy T, Gleim GW. Quantification of posterior capsule tightness and motion loss in patients with shoulder impingement. Am J Sports Med. 2000;28:668-673.

72. Tyler TF, Roy T, Nicholas SJ, Gleim GW. Reliability and validity of a new method of measuring posterior shoulder tightness. J Orthop Sports Phys Ther. 1999;29:262-269; discussion 270-264.

73. Umhau JC, Garg K, Woodward AM. Dietary supplements and their future in health care: commentary on draft guidelines proposed by the Food and Drug Administration. Antioxid Redox Signal. 2012;16:461-2.

74. Vandvik PO, Lähdeoja T, Ardern C, et al. Subacromial decompression surgery for adults with shoulder pain: a clinical practice guideline. BMJ. 2019;364:l294.

75. Vitali M, Naim Rodriguez N, Pironti P, et al. ESWT and nutraceutical supplementation (Tendisulfur Forte) vs ESWT-only in the treatment of lateral epicondylitis, Achilles tendinopathy, and rotator cuff tendinopathy: a comparative study. Journal of Drug Assessment. 2019;8:77-86.

76. Walker H, Gabbe B, Wajswelner H, Blanch P, Bennell K. Shoulder pain in swimmers: a 12-month prospective cohort study of incidence and risk factors. Phys Ther Sport. 2012;13:243-249.

77. Wilk KE, Macrina LC, Fleisig GS, et al. Correlation of glenohumeral internal rotation deficit and total rotational motion to shoulder injuries in professional baseball pitchers. The American Journal of Sports Medicine. 2011;39:329-335.

78. Witt DW, Talbott NR. In-vivo measurements of force and humeral movement during inferior glenohumeral mobilizations. Man Ther. 2016;21:198-203.

79. Yang J-l, Chen S-y, Hsieh C-L, Lin J-j. Effects and predictors of shoulder muscle massage for patients with posterior shoulder tightness. BMC Musculoskeletal Disorders. 2012;13:1-8.

80. Yang JL, Jan MH, Chang CW, Lin JJ. Effectiveness of the end-range mobilization and scapular mobilization approach in a subgroup of subjects with frozen shoulder syndrome: a randomized control trial. Man Ther. 2012;17:47-52.

81. Zadro J, O'Keeffe M, Maher C. Do physical therapists follow evidence-based guidelines when managing musculoskeletal conditions? Systematic review. BMJ Open. 2019;9:e032329.

82. Zadro JR, O'Keeffe M, Ferreira GE, et al. Diagnostic labels for rotator cuff disease can increase people's perceived need for shoulder surgery: an online randomized controlled experiment. J Orthop Sports Phys Ther. 2021;1-45.

83. Euromonitor International. Vitamins in the United Kingdom. Oct 2020. Available at: https://www.euromonitor.com/vitamins-in-the-united-kingdom/report.

Part 2
Assessment and management

11 Communicating with people experiencing shoulder pain

Mike Stewart, Joletta Belton, Stephen Loftus, Tamar Pincus, Peter O'Sullivan, Jeremy Lewis

Introduction: Joletta's experience

In *Experiencing Chronic Pain in Society*, Lous Heshusius writes that she always yearns for a doctor to really listen.[23] Those words resonated deeply with my own yearning, and leant insight into my experiences of seeking care for pain. I never really felt listened to. I rarely felt heard or seen, believed, or validated. Rather, I had to continually prove that I was in pain, that it was real, that I was suffering. And in having to prove my pain, having to prove my worth, my humanity, my value. To prove that, yes, I was deserving of care. It was exhausting and demoralizing.

At the same time, the clinicians I saw for my pain were very kind and caring. I knew they wanted to help me and wanted me to get better, and I did not want to let them down. I desperately wanted their treatments to work, not just for myself, but also for them. So where did things go so wrong? If I knew they cared and wanted me to get better, why did I also feel so unheard and invalidated?

When we talk about communication in healthcare, it is usually related to how to *tell* information to a patient, such as what information to give and how to give it. I was told a great many things during my care. I was told that my pain was everything from weakness, instability, poor posture, and misalignments, to various forms of dysfunctions and disorders, to tears, impingements, and the joint being "bone-on-bone". I was told what should be done, when it was to be done, and that, in the end, I would be "fixed".

When I was asked about my experience, I was expected to tell a very specific and narrowly focused story about the presenting complaint. So, I listed symptoms, when they started, how long they had lasted, how intense my pain was on scales that were meaningless to me, what "quality" the pain had within a defined set of options, what treatments I'd undergone, what treatments *I'd* failed...and that became the story of my pain. But it was not *my* story. It was a clinical story of a painful joint that did not respond to treatment; I hardly seemed relevant at all.[36] My knowledge and expertise, my life and experiences, my worries and fears, values and goals, hopes and dreams, were not there. The *me* in my story was missing altogether.

Yet pain is about so much more than symptoms, pain scores, and diagnoses. It was incredibly distressing to have pain I could not make sense of, and that didn't respond to treatment as expected. And I lost so much: my career, my financial security, my friends, family, and future. I lost my ability to sit, drive, go out socially, or do everyday things that made me feel like myself. So, I was not myself. I was isolated, withdrawn, alone. My life was upended, the world as I knew it turned upside down. It was not my tissues that were threatened by pain, it was my identity, my *self – my very existence* – that was threatened by pain. Yet my losses, my distress, were rarely acknowledged; the story of *my* pain never heard.

In not being heard, I did not feel *known*.[3] If *I* was not known, how could *my* pain be understood? If my pain was not understood, how could I ever find a way forward? So, I kept hoping that someone would truly listen. That someone would hear my suffering, acknowledge my difficulties, and address my concerns. I desperately needed to make sense of things. Arthur Frank writes of how we need to tell stories to work through the situation we find ourselves in. If the story continues to be told, the work of that situation continues to need doing.[17]

The most important aspect of communication is often not what is *told*, but what is *heard*. When I was finally asked to tell *my story*, and was truly listened to, I was able to gain critical distance from the tale and begin to reflect on what was being told. Only then could I start to make sense of things and work through the situation I found myself in. While I understand why many clinicians want to just move on and get to the "important stuff", I couldn't move on until my story was heard, acknowledged, and validated. That *was* the important stuff. Once that burden was lifted, I had more capacity for taking on new information and was better able to find possible paths forward.

The stories we create together during the clinical encounter have to make both biological and biographical sense. The story must apply to *me*. When it doesn't, it's just a story about pain, or a diagnosis, or a shoulder. A story of a problem, the person lost altogether.[3] This is important, because the story told in my medical record, filled with language of damage, disorders, deviations, and dysfunctions, became part of the story I told myself: I was broken, weak, unstable, dysfunctional, unable, incapable, unworthy...

I am not alone in this – many people seeking care feel invalidated, made to feel that our pain isn't real, isn't legitimate, or is somehow exaggerated or "all in our head". We despair when we are abandoned and are told "nothing more can be done".[54] Yet we are empowered when we are heard, acknowledged, and known. When we are understood, we can begin to make sense of our experience and find our path forward.

Changing how we communicate offers the opportunity to dramatically improve healthcare and treatment outcomes. Conversations and dialogue can invite the change that clinicians and patients alike are so often seeking.[30,36] Communication that includes listening, respect, and validation can foster trust and promote the cocreation of new, more therapeutic narratives that facilitate change, promote healing, and alleviate suffering.

Thank you for listening.

Communicating effectively

Communication is arguably the principal component of shoulder rehabilitation. It does not matter what we know if we cannot communicate it in a meaningful, respectful, sensitive, and effective manner.[19] Joletta's healthcare experience highlights the need for clinicians to listen to personal narratives so that we may tailor our communication to individual needs. Communication permeates every aspect of healthcare practice and is about building relationships, trust, and a strong therapeutic alliance. Gaining the trust of a person seeking care without effective communication is unachievable, and places the provision of support, reassurance, validation, hope, empowerment, resilience, and self-efficacy at risk.[18]

It would be naive to suggest that all forms of communication are helpful. Unfortunately, some of the most persuasive messages received by people living with shoulder pain may either knowingly or unwittingly contain toxic messages that cause anxiety, escalate vulnerability, diminish self-efficacy and disempower (see Chapter 1).[12] As with all human interaction, the most charismatic and gifted communicators are also capable of causing the most harm.[42] In a speech to the Royal College of Surgeons in London (UK) in 1923, the author Rudyard Kipling stated, "Words are, of course, the most powerful drug used by mankind." The words we choose in our clinical practice have the capacity both to support and to cause lasting harm.[2] Words have the ability to both positively and negatively affect the way another person thinks, feels and acts,[52] and can either make or break a positive clinical outcome.[10]

It is our aim throughout this chapter to provide practical support, guidance and clinical companionship so that you may feel less alone in dealing with these everyday challenges, while hopefully enabling you to feel better equipped to help more people and, in turn, to feel more fulfilled in your role as a healthcare professional. There is no such thing as perfect communication, and there is not simply one method of communication to learn. We all make mistakes, and we can all try to do better. We all have strengths, and we all have areas that may require development. This is as true for us as authors and experienced clinicians as it is for everybody.

We can define communication as "the exchange of information, thoughts and feelings among people using speech and other means."[28] Effective communication requires a collaborative, two-way understanding between equals. Communication is both a comprehensively researched science and a much-contemplated art. Effective communicators understand when to lead or walk ahead of patients, when to walk beside them, and when to follow. The development of effective communication skills for people living with shoulder pain begins with an acknowledgement of two key concepts:

1. The answers to other people's problems often lie in their words and thoughts, not ours.
2. To empower others, we must first be prepared to lose some of our own power.

Although building relationships through communication might sound simple, and many clinicians feel that they are already equipped with the necessary skills, the reality is frequently different. Meaningful and effective rapport building is often challenging to achieve in practice, as communication is nuanced, context dependent, and idiosyncratic.[7] As Bullington reminds us, "To encounter another human is to encounter another world."[4] In the "other world", customs, culture, language, communication, beliefs, and behaviors may be very different from the world inhabited by the clinician. In the same way that you would feel privileged when travelling to an unfamiliar country, and you would be careful to respect the cultural practices and customs, you need to do the same when "travelling" to the "other world" inhabited by the patient in front of you.

Most people presenting with a shoulder problem describe pain as their primary concern. Eccleston and Crombez[12] referred to pain as "an ideal habitat for worry to flourish." When travelling to the world inhabited by the patient we need be sensitive, as something said in a short sentence has the ability to harm for months, years and even a lifetime, such as: "The X-ray of your shoulder shows substantial degeneration, and the bone-on-bone appearance is more typical of someone 30 years older than you. A joint replacement is the only thing that will help you, but you are too young for the procedure. The pain will only get worse. You will need to learn to live with it and adapt." Clearly, words communicated in this manner will, for some, only increase worry and concern, and words like toothpaste: once out, are impossible to put back in.

Building rapport and developing collaborative relationships with people who have shoulder pain

The goals of patients and clinicians might seem simple. Both want to find out what went wrong, and 'fix' the problem, or, in the absence of a cure, to manage it. The reality of the situation is more complex. As outlined in Joletta's narrative, the list of symptoms, treatments tried, and hypothesized diagnoses failed to capture her story. She felt distressed, and as her distress was ignored, she felt unheard. Some patients talk about their distress as "the cry that is never heard". To respond to this cry, we need to learn to listen out for it, and when we hear it, we need to make sure people know we have heard it.

For clinicians, shoulder pain presents a high level of uncertainty about prognosis, which can be influenced by many factors, including psychological and social (see Chapter 6). Many clinicians focus their efforts on trying to form and then confirm a biomechanical hypothesis to explain the presenting symptoms. The result of this is an almost subconscious switch away from information that is not congruent with this focus. For example:

Clinician: *What brought you here today?*

Patient: *It's my shoulder. The pain is awful. I feel that it is taking over my life ... There are so many things I can't do. I tried to wait for it to go away by itself, but it's been three months now, and I am at my wits' end.*

Clinician: *OK, you said three months; did it come on suddenly, did you do something to injure it?*

The patient's narrative weaves a story around suffering, but the clinician immediately moves on to establish facts. Often, in these circumstances, patients start repeating themselves, re-emphasizing and even augmenting their testimony of suffering. Alternatively, they might become monosyllabic, drop eye contact, and appear to disengage. These are all indications of someone who is communicating something very important, who feels unheard. Sometimes, patients get frustrated and show signs of agitation, or even anger. Substantial evidence has demonstrated that people living with pain feel both unbelieved and unaccepted, especially in the context of diagnostic uncertainty.[49] The clinician's failure to acknowledge suffering in the narrative may be perceived as another brick added to the wall of rejection, feeling dismissed and being left unvalidated. One of the fastest and most immediate ways to reduce patients' agitation and enhance disclosure and therapeutic alliance is through validation. As Edmond and Keefe[14] have eloquently stated:

Validation, then, involves expressing that another person's disclosure is understandable and legitimate, and conveys acceptance of that disclosure, whether or not the person communicating validation agrees with the content of that disclosure. By understandable and legitimate, we mean both that the listener hears and comprehends the content of the disclosure, and that the listener conveys that, given the circumstances, the content of that disclosure is reasonable and valid.

Marsha Linehan, a key validation theorist,[32] suggests that validation is a process in which a listener communicates that a person's thoughts and feelings are understandable and legitimate. This empathic form of communication is absent from most consultations for people presenting with shoulder problems. It is puzzling to observe clinicians who are extremely competent at showing empathy and responding to pain and need in their family and friends forget, or stop themselves, from showing a similar natural response towards their patients. In part at least it is because of the widely held belief that showing empathy to expressions of suffering will result in increased complaining and illness-behaviors.

This belief, based on an operant conditioning model, regards empathic responses (including validation of pain and suffering) as a social reinforcement that acts to maintain the behavior immediately preceding the response.[14]

However, in an excellent review of validation in the context of pain, Edmond and Keefe[14] present an alternative model, which hypothesizes that once validation has happened, patients trust the clinician more, they feel better about their problem and, importantly, both their report of pain and their pain behaviors decrease. A review of evidence, though scarce, suggests that these ideas are correct. In a study observing communications between people living with pain and their romantic partners, validation was associated with lower perceived support entitlement, and was not associated with reports of pain and mood.[5] Students undergoing a pain tolerance task who received validation expressed less worry than those who didn't.[34] Finally, a group of pain patients who perceived themselves to have received very low validation were found to have significantly more pain interference and low mood after rehabilitation treatment.[13]

In direct contrast to validation, which aims to acknowledge individual suffering, is generic reassurance. Generic reassurance consists of giving patients optimistic messages that there is no need to worry, the clinician is experienced and has seen it all before, everything will be alright – without any specific information that relates to the individual. This type of reassuring communication might make patients feel worse, especially in complex cases where pain has gone on for some time. Studies in primary care indicate that such reassurance is associated with worse outcomes, even when immediate satisfaction is high,[45] and in patients with back pain, such statements have been associated with increased depression three months later in patients who were prone to depression during the consultation.[24]

What all the studies show is that patients want and need clear explanations about their pain, and a pain management plan that they understand.

Listening to people

The history-taking was so structured, so searching, so thorough, that I felt that, for the first time, my pain was being listened to. The consultation was, in itself, therapeutic.

Hilary Mantel[39]

When we stop and reflect upon patient experiences such as those expressed by the esteemed writer, Hilary Mantel, we may begin to recall our own similar experiences from clinical practice. Perhaps that time when your communication skills alone, without the use of additional interventions, resulted in therapeutic gain. When they occur, these satisfyingly simple experiences may leave us all confused, trying to comprehend what just happened. While the person living with shoulder pain may offer reflective feedback, "I feel much better now that we have talked, but we haven't really done any treatment yet have we?", the clinician may also wonder about the foundational nature of treatment and therapy. What was it that made Mantel's experience so positive? Why and how did she perceive the consultation to be therapeutic? Some of the possible answers to these questions involve listening.

Linton[33] argues that there are three steps to good communication: listen, listen, and listen. Listening begins with an active acknowledgement that the other person needs to be heard. When we reflect upon the considerable number of factors that impact on our time, it is little wonder that we can find it hard to listen. Lawn et al.[31] explored the barriers to a narrative approach within healthcare consultations. They found a lack of training, poor interdisciplinary communication, and a variety of time constraints to be key factors. Padfield et al.[43] also found that time constraints within practice settings posed a logistical obstacle for many participants when attempting to explore patient narratives.

Following several years of interviewing clinicians, researchers, and people in pain, the healthcare journalist Judy Foreman concluded that, "There is an appalling mismatch between what people in pain need and what healthcare professionals know."[15] The following statement highlights just one typical example of how this gap may manifest itself within clinical practice:

She told me that the high point of her life was playing the organ for her church choir. She lived for the twice-a-week practices and Sunday performances. Now, with pain immobilizing her elbow, she could no longer manage the keyboard. Her days held nothing that she looked forward to. The constant aching had robbed her of any hope. Life seemed empty of everything except pain. When I asked her if she had explained this to the staff in the clinic, she replied that they had not asked. Her medical history, as one might expect, read exactly like the history of an elbow.[41]

During illness, it is not just the body that is threatened, but also the person's whole identity.[36] As a clinician, it is therefore essential to ensure a collaborative, narrative approach that is intrinsically linked to individual values.[44,48] Padfield et al.[43] suggest an inherent dilemma exists in many clinical consultations, with clinicians and patients searching for separate goals with separate meanings. Frankel and Levinson[18] reviewed audio recordings of 125 doctors, and found correlations between communication style and malpractice claims. Interestingly, no difference was found between the amount and quality of information provided by the clinicians. The difference found was closely linked to the clinicians' ability to relate to the patient's narrative.[18] This highlights the necessity for clinicians to actively listen and respond to the person's idiosyncratic story. These crucial skills have been found to be both undervalued and lacking in clinical practice.[8,11,26,51] Figure 11.1 demonstrates the types of communication that are common within healthcare settings.

At its best, a consultation represents the coming together of two people with each person openly and honestly sharing their knowledge and experience with the other. Coulter and Collins[9] argue that while the clinician may have knowledge regarding diagnosis, disease etiology, prognosis, treatment options and outcome probabilities, the process of healthcare is left somewhat incomplete if we fail to recognize the patient's knowledge and expertise regarding their values, preferences, attitudes to risk, social circumstances and experience of illness. A core principle of healthcare communication is that if we, as clinicians, are talking more than our patients, there is something wrong. See Reflective exercise 11.1.

Reflective exercise 11.1

Read and reflect on the following statements. What are your thoughts? Do you recognize these rationales when caring for people with shoulder pain? Have you overheard similar ideas within clinics? What do you notice about the words that are used within the statements?

1. *"I have to say I don't particularly ask the patient what they want. I think giving them so much choice, they can often get confused. It is almost too much for them."* Clinician
2. *"I must admit for every patient I have coming in through my door, I pretty much will always give them exercise. I don't think about it too hard, it's just part and parcel of the package that I like to give."* Physical therapist
3. *"Overall, the physical assessment plays a very large role in the choice of exercises. I tend to work out what I think is best."* Physical therapist

Adapted from Stenner et al.[51]

To empower others, we, as clinicians, must first be prepared to lose some of our power. Much of this power is held within the words we use and the knowledge we have gained. This incredible knowledge comes with a curse.[46] The more comfortable we become with what we know, the more we lose sight of the fact that other people may not know what we know. To highlight this problem, and to show some potential solutions for use in practice, the following case study (Figure 11.2) shows excerpts of dialogue from a consultation. Unspoken thoughts, beliefs and actions are shown within bold parentheses.

Figure 11.2 depicts how easily our cognitive biases may, unwittingly, distort reality. We construct a subjective social reality that is based upon our perception of sensory input.[16] In Figure 11.2, the clinician recognizes the patient's misinterpretation of "degenerative changes" as

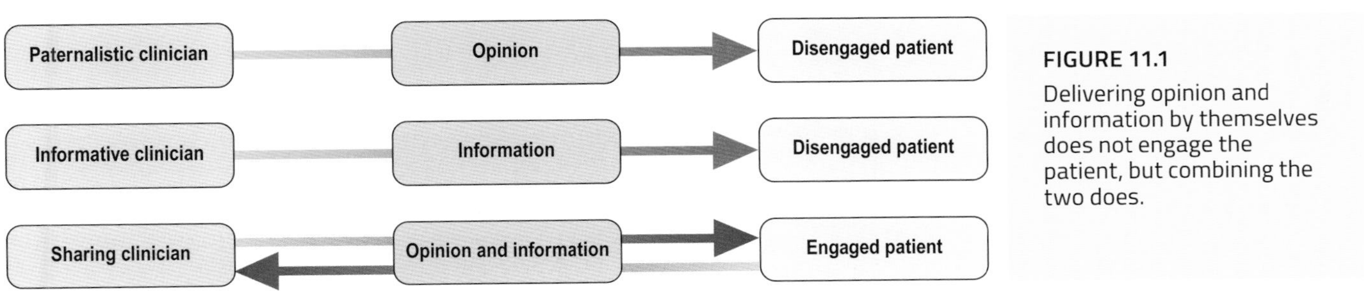

FIGURE 11.1
Delivering opinion and information by themselves does not engage the patient, but combining the two does.

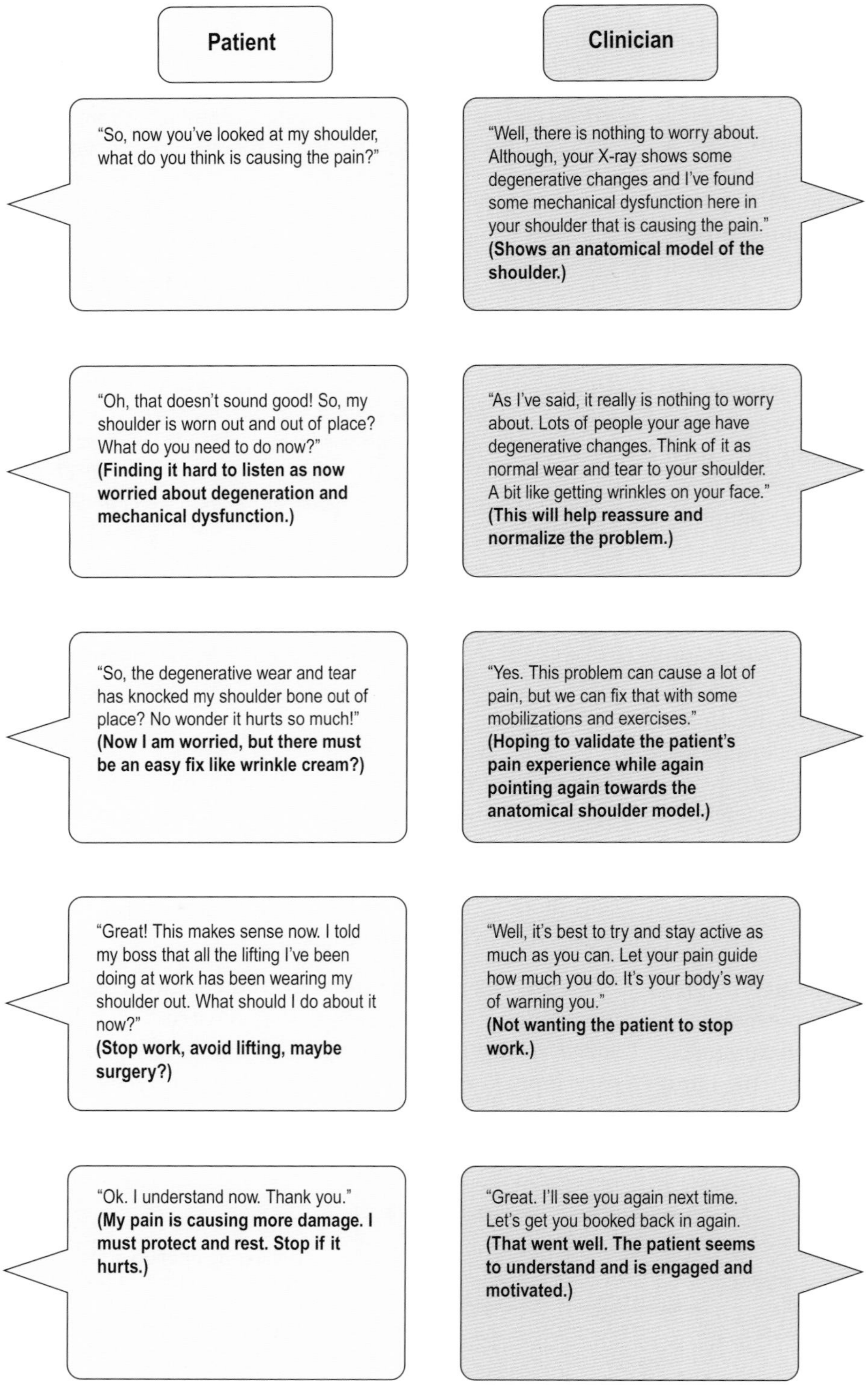

FIGURE 11.2
Patients can interpret different meanings to those intended by the clinician.

Reflective exercise 11.2

1. List any potential communication barriers and/or facilitators which may improve communication that you have noticed within Figure 11.2.
2. Now consider how you might rewrite the dialogue in Figure 11.2 to better share opinions and information between the clinician and patient, and therefore improve communication.

"worn out" and attempts to minimize the harm through saying "wear and tear." However, without realizing the hidden impact, the clinician has unwittingly confirmed the patient's belief that lifting at work has led to a "worn out" shoulder. This, in turn, reinforces the patient's pain behavior. Barker et al.[1] reported that patients often misinterpret medical terminology, with "wear and tear" being perceived as "something is rotting away." This finding was supported by Padfield et al.[43] who asked participants to display their perceptions of pain by creating photographic images to represent their beliefs. "Wear and tear" was depicted as a piece of rotten, unhealthy fruit. See Reflective exercise 11.2.

Following careful consideration of the evidence and with an awareness of the issues raised, let us now contemplate how the dialogue in Figure 11.2 might be handled differently (Figure 11.3).

Table 11.1 details a solution-focused approach to some common communication challenges that are encountered in clinical practice settings. Please take some time either on your own or with colleagues to reflect upon these issues. Can you think of any other problems you might add to this table or any additional solutions you could try using in clinic?

The role of narrative

Human beings are narrative creatures. We live and breathe stories from an early age. We live out life stories that gives those same lives meaning. When patients present to us with problems, such as shoulder pain, it is because that shoulder pain is interfering, in some way, with the life story they want and had anticipated to live out. When patients must contend with pain, especially on a long-term basis, then the pain can become a central part of the life story that may then become an illness narrative.[17] It is important for patients to share these stories with clinicians, and it is even more important for patients to know that we, the clinicians, have not only heard but accepted, and validated, those stories.

It is surprising how often patients do not feel that their clinicians have done this. This chapter begins with one example, Joletta's experience, but there are many reports of patients who feel their stories have not been heard, and the result can be a mixture of anger, disillusionment, and frustration. However, if patients do feel they have been heard and understood, then that fact alone can be therapeutic.[35] Knowing that their story matters, and has been validated by those with clinical knowledge, is an important first step in therapy. Narrative plays a key role throughout communication in clinical practice, not only in assessment but all the way through to completion of therapy.

Mattingly[40] describes the important role of narrative in her description of a clinician who is introducing a new patient to a rehabilitation center. The center focuses on the rehabilitation of young men who have become permanently impaired following traffic accidents, and who need to learn to live out new lives with disability. Mattingly is essentially outlining what is a new narrative trajectory into the future. Mattingly calls this "therapeutic emplotment".[40] Without this narrative trajectory towards a new and meaningful life story, the various rehabilitation activities and therapies would be essentially meaningless for the patient. The new narrative trajectory is an important part of the therapy, and it has a key role in evidence-based therapy.

When Sackett et al.[47] promoted an evidence-based approach to clinical practice, they emphasized three aspects. These were, firstly, the best available evidence, secondly, the expertise and experience of the clinician and, thirdly, the values and desires of the patient. The narrative trajectory needs to integrate all these aspects. However, it is particularly in the values and desires of the patient that narrative plays a key role. Careful attention to the patient's

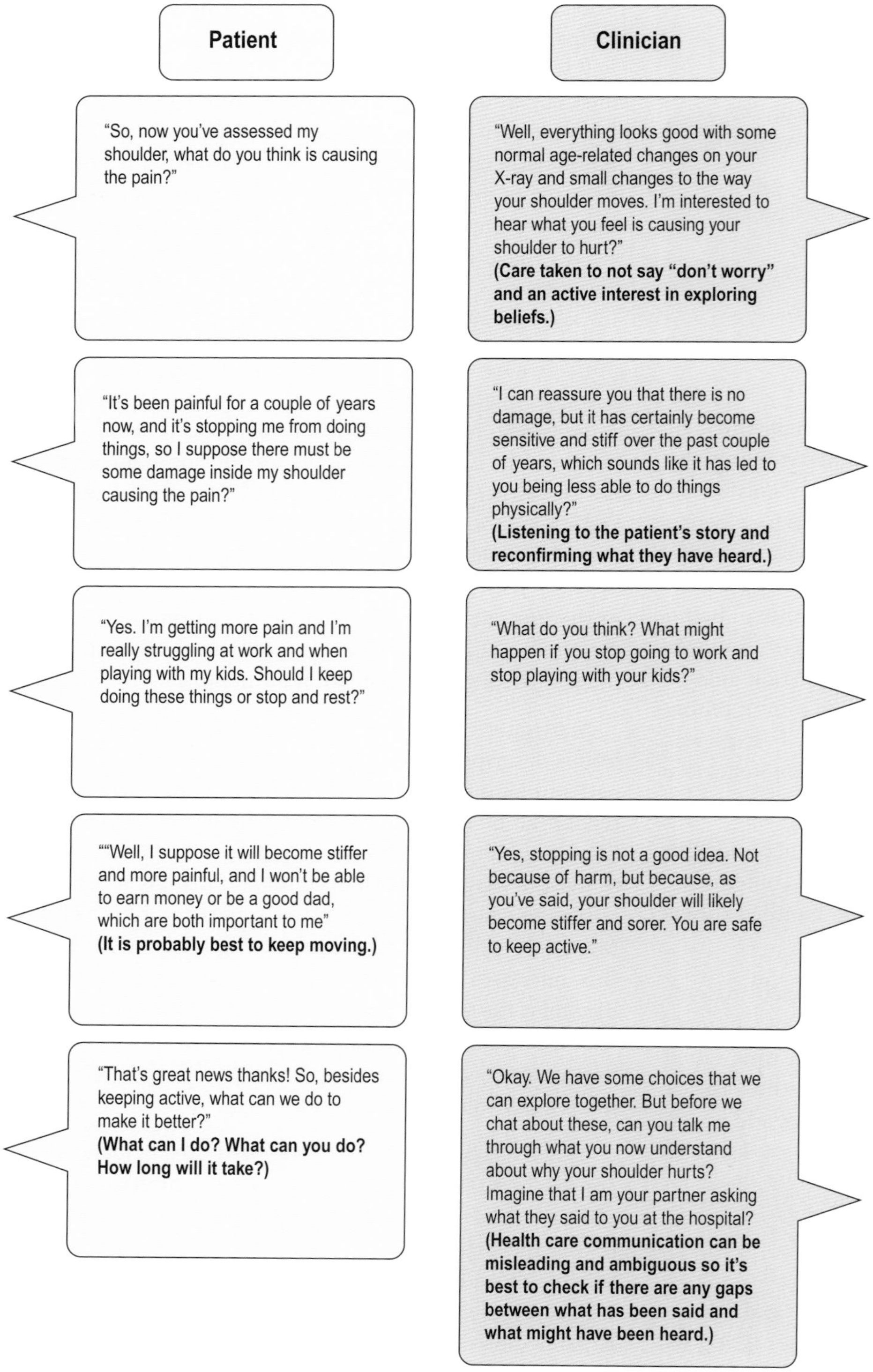

Patient

"So, now you've assessed my shoulder, what do you think is causing the pain?"

Clinician

"Well, everything looks good with some normal age-related changes on your X-ray and small changes to the way your shoulder moves. I'm interested to hear what you feel is causing your shoulder to hurt?"
(Care taken to not say "don't worry" and an active interest in exploring beliefs.)

Patient

"It's been painful for a couple of years now, and it's stopping me from doing things, so I suppose there must be some damage inside my shoulder causing the pain?"

Clinician

"I can reassure you that there is no damage, but it has certainly become sensitive and stiff over the past couple of years, which sounds like it has led to you being less able to do things physically?"
(Listening to the patient's story and reconfirming what they have heard.)

Patient

"Yes. I'm getting more pain and I'm really struggling at work and when playing with my kids. Should I keep doing these things or stop and rest?"

Clinician

"What do you think? What might happen if you stop going to work and stop playing with your kids?"

Patient

""Well, I suppose it will become stiffer and more painful, and I won't be able to earn money or be a good dad, which are both important to me"
(It is probably best to keep moving.)

Clinician

"Yes, stopping is not a good idea. Not because of harm, but because, as you've said, your shoulder will likely become stiffer and sorer. You are safe to keep active."

Patient

"That's great news thanks! So, besides keeping active, what can we do to make it better?"
(What can I do? What can you do? How long will it take?)

Clinician

"Okay. We have some choices that we can explore together. But before we chat about these, can you talk me through what you now understand about why your shoulder hurts? Imagine that I am your partner asking what they said to you at the hospital?
(Health care communication can be misleading and ambiguous so it's best to check if there are any gaps between what has been said and what might have been heard.)

FIGURE 11.3

Reducing communication gaps and misunderstandings requires a collaborative approach.

Table 11.1 A solution-focused approach to clinical communication challenges

Problems	Solutions
I find it difficult to pay attention to what the patient is saying.	• Take the time to listen. • Remove distractions (phones, computer, paperwork). • Make eye contact. • Nod to show you understand. • Confirmation and "playback", e.g., "So, let me check I've heard you correctly. It sounds like…"
I find it hard to get people to talk about how their shoulder pain affects their life.	• Connect with the patient from the very beginning of the session by going off topic. • Use prompts to facilitate conversations about wider issues e.g., "It is often hard to live with pain. Can you talk to me about how it impacts on your life?" • Get creative! Encourage expression through written narratives, art and metaphors.
I worry that I don't have time to fully listen and connect with patients.	• Make the most of the time of you have by allowing the patient to talk uninterrupted for the first two minutes. • Acknowledge time constraints, e.g., "We have 30 minutes together so how can we make best use of this time?" • Make use of blended learning and "homework", e.g., "Can you make a list of things we need to talk about so that we can discuss them next time?"
I find my need to fix the patient's problem and to share my knowledge with them prevents me from listening to what they need.	• Focus on shifting from a "fix it" mindset to a "sit with it mindset". • Do not assume that you are on the same page. Check, clarify and confirm meanings. • Follow the 3 rules of facilitation: listen, find out what they need, then tailor how you guide them.

story can reveal just what someone's values and desires are. If we ignore the patient's values and desires (or appear to), then assessment and therapy are likely to fail, even if technically correct.

Beyond this, the reality is that clinical practice can be complex, and there is often insufficient evidence to provide complete certainty. A narrative approach to practice accommodates this:

Narrative allows for conflict, uncertainty, different levels of meaning and differing opinions, where factual knowledge alone is insufficient. Narrative can give us sufficient understanding to negotiate between conflicting options and make decisions under conditions of uncertainty. [37]

This need to cope with complexity and uncertainty can be thought of in terms of interpretive gaps. No story can ever say everything that can be said. What is said contrasts with what is not said. This means that every story has interpretive gaps, that may be opened up to allow for further development and complexity as someone's story develops. As we saw from Joletta's experience, if patients feel ignored then there will be disillusionment, disengagement, and little inclination for compliance with healthcare, no matter how sound the evidence for that care may be. This means that the patient's story needs to be woven into the management plan in a way that each patient can see that their narrative trajectory includes their values and desires. All this means that when patients present, we need to pay careful attention to how we communicate, and let them tell their stories.

Every health profession has protocols for listening to stories and gathering the information needed.[38] Beginners must learn these by heart and practice using them so that they become second nature. With experience, clinicians learn to modify these protocols according to the needs of the patient. A narrative approach to assessment emphasizes the questions, who, what, where, when, how, and above all, why. How do patients tell us their stories? Can we also hear the music, the tone of voice? What can we observe from the body language? What might the patient avoid saying and why?

Reflective exercise 11.3

At the start of the assessment, ask this question from Charon[6] who opens her interviews with: "Tell me what you think I should know about your situation". Charon also notes that she will consciously sit on her hands when she asks this question to stop herself from picking up a pen and starting to make notes. Patients, even if quite verbose, will rarely talk for longer than three minutes if we do not interrupt them.

The story that the patient tells is only part of the picture. Greenhalgh[22] describes three texts that need to be integrated to come up with a full story: the experiential text – what the patient says; the physical text – information gained from the physical examination; and the instrumental text – information from investigations, such as radiographs and blood tests. The clinician needs to integrate all these texts to come up with a clinical version of the patient story that promises a narrative trajectory into the future. See Reflective exercise 11.3.

Enabling people to talk about their experience of living with shoulder pain

Living with pain can be a hugely distressing experience. Pain is a simple four-letter word that belies myriad subjective human beliefs and emotions. Far from the uncomplicated, cathartic expression of "Ouch!" that is commonly associated with an experience of pain, the distress that frequently accompanies persistent shoulder pain is characteristically wrapped within feelings of depression, anxiety, isolation, uncertainty and chaos.[4,33] From this chaotic blend of emotions comes a desire to seek meaning.[4] Mantel[39] states that, "Pain cannot easily be divided from the emotions surrounding it. Apprehension sharpens it, hopelessness intensifies it, loneliness protracts it by making hours seem like days. The worst pain is unexplained pain."

Although they remain frequently implicit, metaphors influence how we facilitate others, and how others attempt to reach out to make sense of their experiences. We turn to metaphors when conveying human experiences that are most resistant to expression.[20] Pain is one such experience. Metaphors contain the ability to provide a bridge between subjective experience and clinical descriptions.[36] With this in mind, we must appreciate the extent to which people living with shoulder pain use metaphors to express their experiences. We must also develop communication skills that create a path towards therapeutic gains. For those who find their experience of shoulder pain difficult to communicate, it's important to consider how we might elicit their own patient-generated metaphors so as to develop a shared understanding and foster empathetic connections.

In their qualitative study entitled, "I feel so stupid because I can't give a proper answer..." Clarke et al.[7] found that older adults who live with pain used metaphors and similes to convey their distress. When asked to explain a feeling of embarrassment when being unable to explain his pain to healthcare professionals, one participant stated, "I don't have the vocabulary and I haven't got the medical vocabulary. I don't have the jargon to explain what I'm feeling." However, when given enough space and time during the interview, the same participant drew upon his experience of working within the dairy industry to metaphorically describe his experience of pain as a "sort of bubbling" sound like you might hear within a refrigeration pipe. By recognizing the importance of linking meaningful lived experiences to bodily sensations, and thus by using a narrative approach to clinical encounters, metaphors may enable us to link the abstract to what is already known.

Shinebourne and Smith[50] argued that patient-generated metaphors act as a linguistic "safe bridge" through which people can express emotions that are too distressing to communicate literally. With a limited ability to detect when people are attempting to cross this bridge through metaphoric expression, healthcare professionals risk squandering opportunities for a meaningful reconceptualization of shoulder pain and ultimately, a safe and confident return to physical activities. As clinicians, we must strive to identify our patients' own metaphors to explore meaning, and to foster empathetic and therapeutic connections. Gray et al.[21] argued that for health psychology to remain relevant to the lives of people in pain, clinicians must seek a narrative approach that focuses on preserving the context in which stories and metaphors are told. See Reflective exercise 11.4.

Metaphors, particularly visual representations of metaphoric expressions such as the circles seen below, permit a means of shared communication that move beyond words.

Reflective exercise 11.4

Making use of patient-generated metaphors

Patient: "It's so frustrating. I just feel like I'm going round in circles without any answers."

Clinician: "Living with shoulder pain can be very frustrating. I'm interested in something you've just said. Do you mind if we try something?"

Patient: "Yes ok."

Clinician: "You just said that you feel like you're going round in circles with your shoulder pain. If I were to draw what that looks like, would it look like this?"

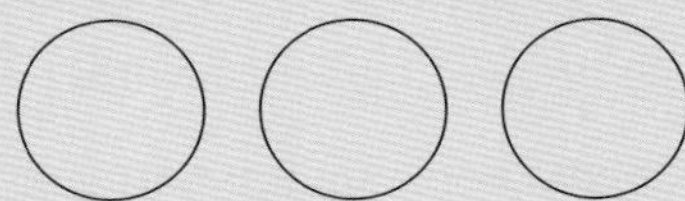

Patient: "Yes. I suppose so. I feel as if I am trapped in an endless loop."

Clinician: "If a friend of yours said that they were going around in circles, what would your advice be? What things might you suggest that they could do to change the situation?"

Patient: "I would advise them to pause and think about how they might break the cycle. Maybe they could create an opening and find another way out. They could also reverse the cycle or find a lever that might slow it down and eventually stop the spinning. You know, like slowing down a waltzer ride at the fairground?"

Clinician: "That sounds like a good plan. Without a good understanding, pain can be confusing and chaotic like a waltzer ride. Shall we explore some ways to help you take back control?"

Patient: "Yes. That sounds like a great idea!"

Images extend the boundaries of our linguistic constraints by providing a window through which we may explore otherwise hard to reach beliefs and emotions about shoulder pain. They can also enable a sense of connection from within an otherwise isolating and chaotic internal pain experience. Words are limiting, but art elicits an emotional response.[27] Padfield et al. [43] reported that metaphoric images which had been created by people living with pain offer, "a narrative space for people to step into, the possibility of some kind of identification and empathy with the other... some kind of slippery surface for further narrative."

Metaphors pervade all aspects of everyday life including our language, thoughts and actions.[29] They enable us to link the abstract to what is already known. Metaphors provide us all with shared expressive phrases for dialogue that can lead to emotional relief and behavioral change, but they can also accelerate the process towards disease, disability and depression, and hinder meaningful reconceptualization of pain.[53] Hurwitz[25] argues that, "pain not only hurts and demands relief, it also scares, baffles, enrages, isolates, resists medical treatment and demands interpretation." As clinicians, we have a professional and moral duty to guide people in pain towards a meaningful, scientifically informed understanding so that we might empower them towards recovery. Our metaphoric expressions, particularly those created by people living with shoulder pain, can assist us all when attempting to seek order amidst the chaos of an uncertain pain experience.

No one cares how much you know until they know how much you care

It is not uncommon for a person with a health concern to experience anxiety and fear when they decide to see a health professional. There are myriad reasons, such as:

Will the doctor take me seriously? Will the physical therapist give me a chance to explain all my concerns? Will I receive substandard care because my ethnicity, race, religion, skin color, body shape, lifestyle choice, sex or gender identification is different from the health provider? I am scared I may need to undress to show the clinician my shoulder. Will I be respected? I have seen so many healthcare providers for my problem, they have all given me different explanations for my problem, promised me the treatment they are offering will work (it never has) – will this person be the same? Will this clinician suggest my problem is in my head like the last one?

I am so scared of what the doctor will find. I am so scared I will need an injection. I am so scared I will need surgery. I am so scared I'll be told that this will never resolve.

The doctor didn't introduce themself last time but called me by my first name, I felt so disrespected and powerless. Why did the clinician keep referring to my pain, I clearly said it was an ache? I didn't understand a word the clinician told me last time; will it be the same this time? Does the health professional know how hard it is for me to travel to/make time to come to the clinic? I've got to get back to work, how long will I have to wait this time? Will I be rushed in and out like last time?

What were all those weird tests I underwent last time? I have no idea what they were for. Why didn't the clinician want to know what it is like living with this problem? Why didn't the doctor discuss with me the different treatment approaches for my problem? The physical therapist said it's my posture, the doctor said it's a tear, why aren't they saying the same thing? Will the doctor focus on me, or take phone calls like last time? Will I be asked personal details again in the waiting room…?

The list is disturbing long, and worryingly, these and additional concerns have been voiced by those seeking help for their shoulder symptoms. We are sure you can add many more examples.

The aim of this section is to provide some simple suggestions to demonstrate, to the person seeking care, that you care, and acknowledge that the most important person in the consultation isn't the health professional, but unquestionably, is the individual that has made the decision, and often the considerable effort, to seek care.

Before the patient sees or speaks to you

Imagine these two scenarios. You are the patient and you have been given the telephone number of the clinic to call and book an appointment. In scenario one, a member of the administration team answers your call, is clearly rushed, doesn't seem to care that you can't take time off work or your studies, are caring for an elderly parent/disabled child, can't make 8:00 am as you have to take a bus and it will take over an hour in peak traffic to arrive, and seemingly can't get you off the phone quickly enough. You leave the conversation feeling underwhelmed at the lack of personal care you have received, and are concerned that this may reflect the care you will receive when you see the clinician.

In scenario two, a member of the administration team answers your call, introduces themselves, warmly thanks you for calling, apologizes for any delay explaining why, asks how they may help you, asks the time that would be most convenient for you and tries to accommodate, asks for your contact information, for example an email, and informs you that you will be sent the time of your appointment, clinic contact information should you need to make a change or if you have any follow up questions, and information pertaining to what you should bring and wear for the first visit. The conversation comes to an end with the person on the other end of the phone saying, "We're looking forward to meeting you and will do our utmost to help you in the best way possible". The caring professional interaction impresses you and you are confident you have made the right decision regarding your health.

Whether patients book an appointment by calling your clinic, a hospital department, or a remote call center, you must ensure the process is simple, accountable, not rushed, responsive, reassuring, professional, and caring. Try calling your own clinic to make an appointment to understand the process the patient will experience. Equally, make time to be the person who answers the calls, to appreciate the process from the administration team's perspective, and effect changes to ensure the first contact is provided at the highest standard possible. If providing optimal healthcare is important to you, then so should be the system that patients will use to access the care you will offer. Patients, whenever possible, should be offered the opportunity to attend with a chaperone, either one that is provided by your facility or a valued person the patient wishes to attend with. Of course, people may prefer to attend alone but, if they choose a chaperone, this person may support the patient, reminding them of questions they wanted to ask, provide comfort in a potentially distressing environment, and discuss the outcome of the clinical visit after it has concluded.

The waiting area

The great amounts of space given over to healthcare waiting areas need to function as more than just places to wait. As much as possible, they should be designed to respect patients' privacy, reflect your professional values, be a reassuring space, and an environment that provides information and education. They may also be used to collect valuable clinical information to reduce the burden on both patients and clinicians: patients often do not understand why the clinician's focus during a consultation is on completing questionnaires, when their main aim is to discuss their concerns and receive treatment.

It does not matter if your waiting area is small or large, maximize its use. Inform patients that they will need to complete information prior to seeing you and, if needed, this can be done with an official interpreter or trusted chaperone. Using paper-based or electronic systems, the waiting area can be used to collect valuable data. You can ask patients to complete appropriate psychosocial questions, generic and specific disability questionnaires, and complete their own body charts or symptom diagrams. They can detail comorbidities, medications, and past surgical and medical history. Lifestyle questions such as sleeping, smoking, nutrition and current and past exercise and activity participation can also be completed. Red flag screening can also be undertaken in the waiting area, and all information can be reviewed in the clinic with the clinician asking pertinent follow-up questions. By doing this, essential information is collected, and better use can be made of the clinician's time with the patient. It avoids the frustration experienced by patients who would prefer to interact with clinicians and not use the time filling in forms.

Those few patients who prefer not to do this in the waiting area may, of course, complete these forms in the consultation room. However, collecting information in the waiting room or before the patient attends the clinic does not negate the need for effective communication that is underpinned by listening, empathizing and validation in the clinical area.

You may also use your waiting areas as a place to communicate health information. One suggestion is to set up a television screen or monitor and run short and carefully selected healthcare videos. Examples could include videos that present the value of physical activity and exercise, the importance of sleep, stress reduction, smoking cessation, and balancing nutrition to optimize health. Such resources may be provided by professional bodies, healthcare funders and charities, social media websites, or be made specifically for your clinic.

The very first meeting

You might first meet the patient in the waiting area, the clinic room, or via a telephone or video consultation. The suggestions are the same. Introduce yourself, using your full name (not your title and surname), your profession and grade, and consider inviting the patient to call you by your first name. Ask the patient how they would like to be addressed and use this consistently. If you are walking back to your clinic room with the patient, do not walk in front of the patient, walk by their side. If you are meeting the patient in your clinic room, make sure when they come in, you are focused on them, and not attending to paperwork or your phone.

The first question

After you have invited the patient to sit down and have established how you will refer to each other and you have thanked the patient for coming to see you, you may like to consider asking a question not at all related to the reason the patient has come to see you. Nothing complicated, political, or controversial, such as "Was it easy for you to get here?", "Did you get caught in the rain?" By doing this you have demonstrated you are interested in the individual, and you care more about the individual than just their shoulder.

Setting the scene

The patient may be nervous and uncertain as to what will happen during the clinical visit. You can alleviate their concerns by setting the scene. Inform the patient of the time you have available and what will happen during that time, for example: "We have 30 minutes and during this time I would like to discuss with you how your problem started and how it has been affecting you. Once we have had a chance to talk, I will ask your permission to examine your shoulder, and I will explain what I am going to do at each stage. Once the assessment is complete, I would like to sit down again with you and discuss what I have learnt. You will have the opportunity to ask any questions you have relating to what I have found. After that I would like to discuss with you the different ways we can manage your shoulder symptoms, presenting the benefits and any risks (harms), expected outcomes, time frames, and what you will need to do for the different options, and together we can decide how best to move forward."

The second question

Once you have set the scene, invite the patient to share the reason why they have come to see you. You may currently be using invitations such as, "Please tell me about your shoulder problem, when it started and how it's been affecting you." Although this will get the patient talking, it is very shoulder symptom-centered and the patient will probably focus on their shoulder problem. We suggest using a less structured opening statement, such as "Please tell me your story," as it is more person-centered and may provide the opportunity for you to listen to what is most important to the person in front of you.

Most people will focus on their shoulder concern, but here are examples of actual responses, each given by a different person when invited to tell their story:

My aunt had bone cancer – I'm worried I may have cancer too.

I told my family doctor I fell, which is true, but I didn't say it was because I drank too much. I'm so worried I am drinking too much – I think that's my biggest problem.

I've told everyone I fell, it's not true. My shoulder is not my main problem, it was just a way for me to get here – I am in an abusive relationship and have been physically abused by my partner.

I'm so depressed.

I usually tell people I fell, but actually I was tortured, and I was chained by one arm to a wall for three days. When I was allowed to sleep, the weight of my body caused my shoulder to dislocate.

Maybe by walking next to the person from the waiting area, asking the patient how they want to be addressed, asking a question to demonstrate your interest in the person in front of you, setting the scene, and then saying, "please tell me your story," on this occasion the person will feel that they will be listened to. When the individual starts to reply, never ask for points of clarification, and allow the patient to complete their first sentence without interruption. Most people will complete their opening sentence in a few minutes. By not interrupting, they will feel more valued, and that their concerns are important to you. Once they have completed their first sentence, thank the patient for sharing their concerns and then follow up with other relevant questions and points of clarification, following the suggestions made earlier in this chapter.

The physical examination

Clinicians with more experience typically spend more time listening and communicating with patients and less time physically examining. The opposite is true for more recently graduated clinicians. Try and limit the physical examination to procedures that have relevance to the patient, are supported by the available evidence, and provide meaningful information. Inform the patient of the next stage in the physical examination and why you think it is relevant:

- "I would like to see how your shoulder moves and how much it moves because..."
- "The way we will assess your movement is..."
- "What I would like you to do is..."
- "Is this OK?"
- "I would like to assess the strength of your shoulder muscles because..."
- "The way we will assess your strength is..."

Shared decision-making

Shared decision making aims to address the asymmetrical relationship between clinician and patient. When the physical examination is complete, invite the patient to sit down. Thank them for providing all the information that they have, and for allowing you to examine their shoulder. You have a duty of care to provide the patient with information about the available treatment options in an unbiased manner, outlining the intended benefits, potential harms (risks), time frames, effort required and realistic outcomes. This opens the process known as shared decision-making and is outlined in detail in Chapter 13. The patient may ask you what you would do: answer them honestly. Pretend the person in front of you is your mother, father, child, very best friend, any loved one: what would you tell them? Tell the person in front of you the same.

Has the patient understood?

Kieran O'Sullivan PhD is a professor at Limerick University in Ireland. He has suggested a method of determining if a patient has understood the information you have discussed. Start by asking the patient who they will tell the information to. This helps you to further understand the patient's social network, and whether there is a person that they trust to discuss their condition with, and how it will be managed. The second question is simply, "What will you tell them?" The patient's answer to this is important, as it will demonstrate to the clinician whether the information that was discussed has been received and interpreted in the way it was intended. If it has not, then it is incumbent on the clinician to present the information in an alternative manner.

Education

Clinicians frequently report that they don't have the time to communicate educational information satisfactorily. Where possible, emailing patients healthcare information, together with links to carefully selected videos that communicate important healthcare information will also facilitate patient understanding and education. The clinician may consider suggesting that the patient watch one video every few days or once a week, and watch it with a family member or valued friend. At the end of the video, the clinician may encourage the patient to discuss the relevance of the video to their experience.

Another way to facilitate a deeper level of education, beyond just watching or reading, is to ask the patient to write the title of the video they watched, or the infographic or article they read, and to answer two questions: 1) What did you consider to be the most valuable message in the video or article?; and 2) What didn't make sense? When the patient attends your clinic for follow-up consultations, the clinician may ask the patient what video they watched, what they thought of it, what was the most important message, and ask what was difficult or confusing to understand. When the patient volunteers what was difficult to understand, the clinician can focus on education about this topic, discussing and providing additional resources as required, facilitating patient-centered education.

Conclusion

In summary, communication is a crucial foundation for effective healthcare for people living with shoulder pain. Joletta's experience highlights a distressing personal account of feeling unheard and invalidated. While the evidence shows that such experiences are not uncommon within clinical practice, it is our hope that this chapter has enabled you to reflect upon the importance of communication, and has helped to provide you with practical methods to develop your communication skills.

References

1. Barker KL, Reid M, Lowe CJM. Divided by a lack of common language? A qualitative study exploring the use of language by health professionals treating back pain. BMC Musculoskeletal Disorders. 2009;10:1-10.
2. Biro D. The Language of Pain. New York: W.W. Norton & Company; 2010.
3. Brody H. "My story is broken; can you help me fix it?" Medical ethics and the joint construction of narrative. Literature and Medicine. 1994;13:79-92.
4. Bullington J, Nordemar R, Nordemar K, Sjöström-Flanagan C. Meaning out of chaos: a way to understand chronic pain. Scandinavian Journal of Caring Sciences. 2003;17:325-331.
5. Cano A, Leong L, Heller JB, Lutz JR. Perceived entitlement to pain-related support and pain catastrophizing: associations with perceived and observed support. Pain. 2009;147:249-254.
6. Charon R. Narrative Medicine: Honoring the Stories of Illness. Oxford University Press; 2008.
7. Clarke A, Anthony G, Gray D, et al. "I feel so stupid because I can't give a proper answer..." How older adults describe chronic pain: a qualitative study. BMC Geriatrics. 2012;12:1-8.
8. Cooper K, Smith BH, Hancock E. Patient-centredness in physiotherapy from the perspective of the chronic low back pain patient. Physiotherapy. 2008;94:244-252.
9. Coulter A, Collins A. Making Shared Decision-Making a Reality. London: King's Fund; 2011.
10. Darlow B, Dowell A, Baxter GD, Mathieson F, Perry M, Dean S. The enduring impact of what clinicians say to people with low back pain. The Annals of Family Medicine. 2013;11:527-534.
11. Dierckx K, Deveugele M, Roosen P, Devisch I. Implementation of shared decision making in physical therapy: observed level of involvement and patient preference. Physical Therapy. 2013;93:1321-1330.
12. Eccleston C, Crombez G. Worry and chronic pain: a misdirected problem-solving model. Pain. 2007;132:233-236.
13. Edlund SM, Wurm M, Holländare F, Linton SJ, Fruzzetti AE, Tillfors M. Pain patients' experiences of validation and invalidation from physicians before and after multimodal pain rehabilitation: associations with pain, negative affectivity, and treatment outcome. Scandinavian Journal of Pain. 2017;17:77-86.
14. Edmond SN, Keefe FJ. Validating pain communication: current state of the science. Pain. 2015;156:215.
15. Foreman J. A Nation in Pain: Healing our Biggest Health Problem. Oxford University Press; 2014.
16. Fox E. Rainy Brain, Sunny Brain: The New Science of Fear and Optimism. Harper Collins; 2012.
17. Frank AW. The Wounded Storyteller: Body, Illness, and Ethics. University of Chicago Press; 2013.
18. Frankel RM, Levinson W. Back to the future: can conversation analysis be used to judge physicians' malpractice history? Communication & Medicine. 2014;11:27.
19. Gardner H, Winner E. First intimations of artistry. In: Strauss S, ed. U-Shaped

Development. New York: Academic Press; 1982. pp.147-168.

20. Geary J. I is An Other: The Secret Life of Metaphor and How it Shapes the Way We See the World. New York: HarperCollins; 2011.

21. Gray RE, Fergus KD, Fitch MI. Two Black men with prostate cancer: a narrative approach. British Journal of Health Psychology. 2005;10:71-84.

22. Greenhalgh T. Narrative based medicine in an evidence-based world. BMJ. 1999;318:323-325.

23. Heshusius L. Experiencing Chronic Pain in Society. Arroyo Grande: CreateSpace Independent Publishing Platform; 2017.

24. Holt N, Mansell G, Hill JC, Pincus T. Testing a model of consultation-based reassurance and back pain outcomes with psychological risk as moderator: a prospective cohort study. The Clinical Journal of Pain. 2018;34:339.

25. Hurwitz B. In: Padfield D, ed. Perceptions of Pain, first edition. Stockport: Dewi Lewis Publishing; 2003. p.10.

26. Jones L, Roberts L, Little P, Mullee M, Cleland J, Cooper C. Shared decision-making in back pain consultations: an illusion or reality? European Spine Journal. 2014;23:13-19.

27. Kenny DT. Constructions of chronic pain in doctor–patient relationships: bridging the communication chasm. Patient Education and Counseling. 2004;52:297-305.

28. Kourkouta L, Papathanasiou IV. Communication in nursing practice. Materia Socio-Medica. 2014;26:65.

29. Lakoff G, Johnson M. Metaphors We Live By. University of Chicago Press; 2008.

30. Launer J. Narrative-based practice in health and social care: conversations inviting change. Routledge; 2018.

31. Lawn S, Delany T, Sweet L, Battersby M, Skinner T. Barriers and enablers to good communication and information-sharing practices in care planning for chronic condition management. Australian Journal of Primary Health. 2015;21:84-89.

32. Linehan MM. Validation and psychotherapy. In: Bohart AC, Greenberg LS, eds. Empathy Reconsidered: New Directions in Psychotherapy. American Psychological Association; 1997;353-392.

33. Linton SJ. Understanding Pain for Better Clinical Practice: A Psychological Perspective. Elsevier; 2005.

34. Linton SJ, Boersma K, Vangronsveld K, Fruzzetti A. Painfully reassuring? The effects of validation on emotions and adherence in a pain test. European Journal of Pain. 2012;16:592-599.

35. Loftus S. Embodiment in the practice and education of health professionals. In: Green B, Hopwood N, eds. The Body in Professional Practice, Learning and Education. Springer; 2015;139-156.

36. Loftus S. Pain and its metaphors: a dialogical approach. Journal of Medical Humanities. 2011;32:213-230.

37. Loftus S, Greenhalgh T. Towards a narrative mode of practice. In: Education for Future Practice. Sense Publishers; 2010;85-96.

38. Loftus S, Mackey S. Interviewing patients and clients. Communicating in the Health Sciences. 2012;187-194.

39. Mantel H. Giving up the Ghost: A memoir. Macmillan; 2003.

40. Mattingly C. The concept of therapeutic 'emplotment'. Social Science & Medicine. 1994;38:811-822.

41. Morris DB. The Culture of Pain. University of California Press; 1991.

42. Moynihan R, Cassels A. Selling sickness: How the world's biggest pharmaceutical companies are turning us all into patients. Greystone Books; 2008.

43. Padfield D, Janmohamed F, Zakrzewska JM, Pither C, Hurwitz B. A slippery surface… can photographic images of pain improve communication in pain consultations? International Journal of Surgery. 2010;8:144-150.

44. Parsons S, Harding G, Breen A, et al. Will shared decision making between patients with chronic musculoskeletal pain and physiotherapists, osteopaths and chiropractors improve patient care? Family Practice. 2012;29:203-212.

45. Pincus T, Holt N, Vogel S, et al. Cognitive and affective reassurance and patient outcomes in primary care: a systematic review. Pain. 2013;154:2407-2416.

46. Pinker S. The Sense of Style: The Thinking Person's Guide to Writing in the 21st Century. Penguin Books; 2015.

47. Sackett D, Straus S, Richardson W, Rosenberg W, Haynes R. Evidence-based medicine: How to teach and practice EBM, second edition. Edinburgh: Churchill Livingstone; 2000.

48. Schoeb V, Staffoni L, Parry R, Pilnick A. "What do you expect from physiotherapy?": a detailed analysis of goal setting in physiotherapy. Disability and Rehabilitation. 2014;36:1679-1686.

49. Serbic D, Pincus T. Chasing the ghosts: the impact of diagnostic labelling on self-management and pain-related guilt in chronic low back pain patients. Journal of Pain Management. 2013;6:25-35.

50. Shinebourne P, Smith JA. The communicative power of metaphors: an analysis and interpretation of metaphors in accounts of the experience of addiction. Psychol Psychother. 2010;83:59-73.

51. Stenner R, Swinkels A, Mitchell T, Palmer S. Exercise prescription for non-specific chronic low back pain (NSCLBP): a qualitative study of patients' experiences of involvement in decision making. Physiotherapy. 2016;102:339-344.

52. Stewart M, Loftus S. Sticks and stones: the impact of language in musculoskeletal rehabilitation. Journal of Orthopaedic & Sports Physical Therapy. 2018;48:519-522.

53. Stewart M, Ryan S-J. Do metaphors have therapeutic value for people in pain? A systematic review. Pain and Rehabilitation. 2019;2020:10-23.

54. Toye F, Seers K, Hannink E, Barker K. A mega-ethnography of eleven qualitative evidence syntheses exploring the experience of living with chronic non-malignant pain. BMC Medical Research Methodology. 2017;17:1-11.

What shoulder outcomes to assess and how to measure them 12

Joy MacDermid, Rochelle Furtado, Jean-Sébastien Roy

Considering the "why" and "what" of outcome measures

Measurement is critical to all parts of clinical practice and research. What we choose to measure and how well we measure those constructs influences our quality of care because we treat what we measure, and because ongoing adjustments to our management are informed by valid assessments of previous treatment response. Measurement supports patient self-efficacy and adherence, since sharing meaningful data pertaining to prognosis or recovery motivates patients and thus indirectly influences outcomes. Therefore, the initial step in selecting a measurement strategy is defining what we want to measure, why we want to measure it, and how the measures will be used.

In clinical practice, we typically call measurements outcome measures (OMs). Although technically diagnostic measures such as imaging and blood tests are a specific subgroup of OMs, they are considered separately in Chapter 14. Given the many ways we use OMs, it is important to select them based on content and measurement properties. As an example, global rating of change scores (GRC) are sometimes used as a quick measure of change, but by design are subject to recall bias.[96]

Understanding what construct or trait to measure is a critical step in an evaluation strategy. Finding measures that assess the appropriate components and scope of that trait is fundamental to the validity of our measurements (content validity). For example, shoulder instability and shoulder arthritis have very different clinical profiles, and the items that are relevant to these clinical populations will differ. OMs include objective measures like nerve conduction, self/patient-reported OMs (PROMs), clinician-based OMs (CBOMs), and performance-based OMs (PBOMs). Some shoulder function PROMs sample a specific list of tasks (e.g., the Shoulder Pain and Disability Index (SPADI)), others present a unique list of tasks to each patient through computer adaptive testing (CAT), and others require patients to make their own list of tasks (Patient-Specific Functional Scale (PSFS)).

PROMs can assess different perspectives of a construct such as disability by rating the ability/difficulty doing a task, satisfaction in how a task is done (e.g., Canadian Occupational Performance Measure), or frequency a task is performed.[171] Positive/negative framing of items, e.g., ability/disability, may also influence responses.[171] Some measures focus on the affected shoulder (e.g., SPADI), and others consider disability at the person level (e.g., Disability Arm Shoulder Hand (DASH)). Some use visual analogue scales (VAS) where a continuous line is rated, others use numeric rating scales of 0 to 10 with descriptive anchors, or Likert scales where discrete categories are individually described. In addition to content, these structural differences influence measurement properties, relevance to patients, and how different OMs relate to each other.

Using The International Classification of Functioning, Disability and Health (ICF) as a model[193] (Figure 12.1), we can assess impairments in body structure, e.g., imaging, body functioning, shoulder strength, and disability which encompasses activity limitations and participation restrictions. Most PROMs have items that cross multiple aspects of ICF, and ICF linkage has been increasingly used to describe OM content.[8,38,53,117,127,169] Objective and performance-based impairment tests are critical to understanding the mechanisms that underlie pathology/disability and whether interventions modify their intended targets. PROMs are needed to understand the patient experience and how a shoulder condition affects overall functioning and quality of life.

OMs taken at a specific timepoint describe current status. These scores may be used to make comparisons between a patient and clinical or normative data to quantify the severity of an impairment/disability. More commonly, we use OMs at multiple timepoints to measure change related to treatment, aging, disease, or natural course of recovery. To do this successfully, we select OMs that can detect change (i.e., are responsive), that inform clinical decision-making, and where the quantity of change has a true meaning across the scale (interval level scaling). Responsiveness studies, particularly those with head-to-head comparisons between OMs, can guide selection of an OM that is optimal for measuring clinical change over time and provide useable benchmarks such as clinically important difference/change

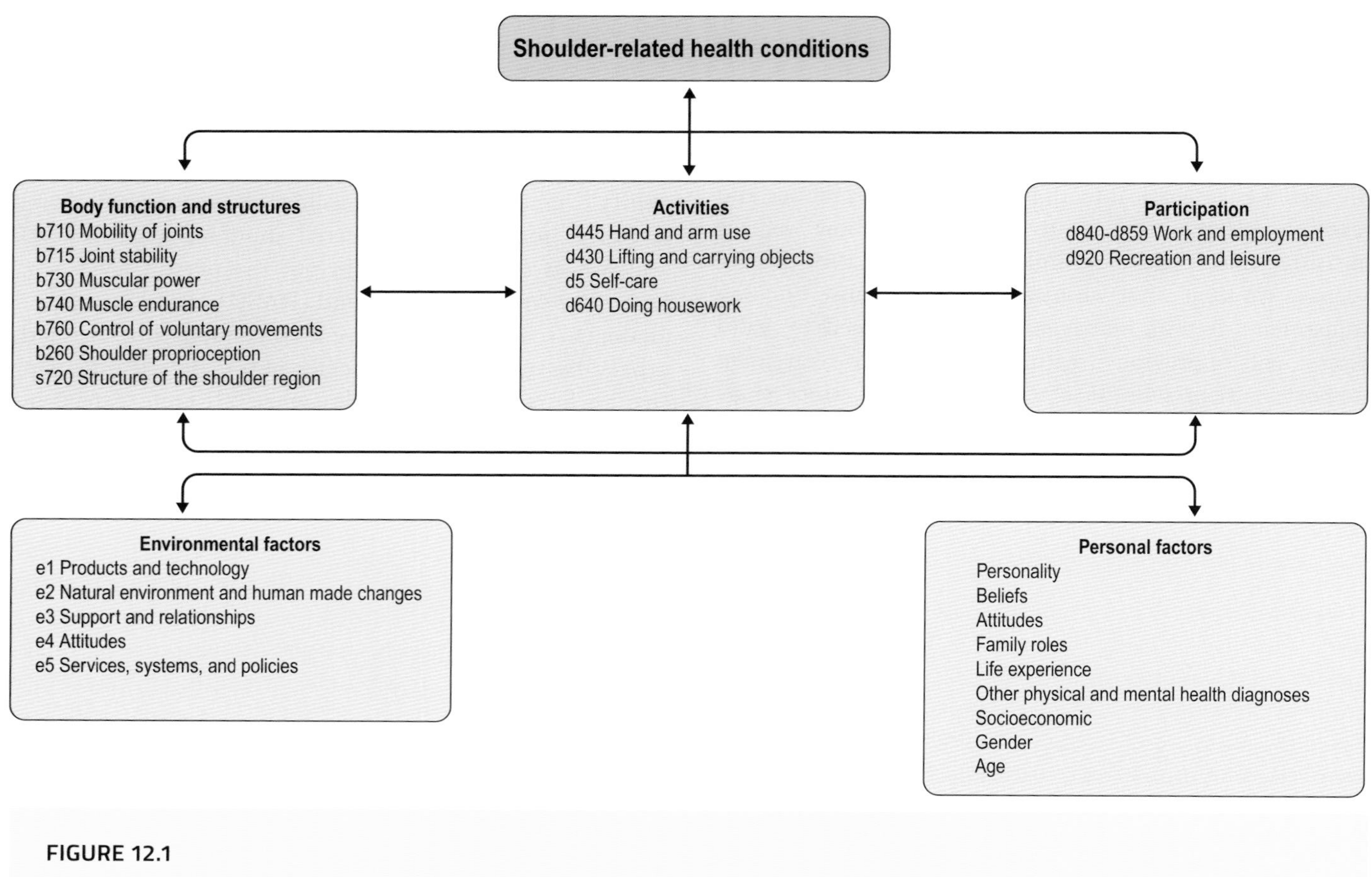

FIGURE 12.1
The ICF conceptual model as it relates to shoulder conditions.

(CID/CIC). Responsiveness varies by context, patient population and intervention.

Sometimes we are interested in discriminating between different individuals or subgroups at a specific point in time to make a diagnosis, or determine membership in a specific subclass with clinical meaning, e.g., readiness for return to sport/work, or clinical subgroups that might need different treatment approaches. For example, work disability scales are often used to discriminate those who are capable of performing their work roles versus those who are not.[178] Neuropathic pain scales indicate those needing different pain management. The characteristics that make a good discriminative test are different to those that make an OM responsive. For example, discriminative/diagnostic tools might function well with yes/no response options, whereas Likert or 0–10 scales are used to optimize responsiveness.

Some OMs are intended to predict a future outcome such as a complication/adverse event or return to work/sport. Prediction OMs, like prediction rules, should assess the items/factors that are most associated with a specific future outcome. In some cases, measures may serve multiple purposes, but it is important to understand the measurement strengths and limitations of any OM when using it for different types of clinical decisions. Systematic reviews that synthesize the evidence on shoulder OMs[172,175,178,179,182] are valuable for clinicians to understand the overall measurement capabilities of different tools (Table 12.1).

Table 12.1 Summary of shoulder outcome measures

Construct assessed	Measure	Burden: Number of items, time to complete	Score range	Minimal detectable change	Clinically important difference
Generic health status	EQ-5D-5L	5 items, <5 minutes Low burden	0–1	Not reported	0.03–0.52
Generic health status	SF-36	36 items, 10–60 minutes High burden	0–100	Not reported	Not reported
Generic health status	PROMIS-UE	29 items, 10 minutes Low burden	0–10	Not reported	4.2
Pain and function	ASES	11 items, <5 minutes Low burden	0–100	10.5 (90% CI)	6.4 points
Disability and function	DASH	30 items, <30 minutes Low burden	0–100	10.7	10.2 points
Pain, disability, and function	SPADI	13 items, 5–10 minutes Low burden	0–130	18.1 (90% CI)	13.2 points
Pain and function	OSS	12 items, 10 minutes Low burden	0–60	11.4 (90% CI)	12 points
Function	SST	12 items, 2–3 minutes Low burden	0–100	32.3 (95%CI)	2.4–9.7 points
Pain, function, and satisfaction	PSS	20 items, 10–15 minutes Low burden	0–100	Not reported	Not reported
Shoulder instability	MISS	22 items, 10–15 minutes Low burden	0–100	5.5 points	Not reported
Quality of life with RCDs	RC-QOL	34 items, 15–20 minutes Low burden	0–100	n/a	11 points
Quality of life with RCDs	WORC	21 items, <10 minutes Low burden	0–1400	16.7	34
Shoulder instability	WOSI	21 items, <10 minutes Low burden	0–2100	339.3	10% change
Pain	NPRS	1 item, <1 minute Low burden	0–10	2 points	1 point or 15% change
Pain	MPQ	78 items, 30 minutes High burden	0–78	Not reported	Not reported
Pain	BPI	10 Items, 10 minutes Low burden	0–10	Not reported	2.2 points
At-work disability and productivity loss	WLQ	25 items, 5–10 minutes Low burden	0–100	0.77–0.97	13 points
Work instability	WIS	23 items, 5–10 minutes Low burden	0–23	0.86–0.93	Not reported
Ability to concentrate on work despite disability	SPS	6-items, 5–10 minutes Low burden	0–100	0.71–0.80	Not reported

(Continued)

Table 12.1 *(Continued)*					
Construct assessed	**Measure**	**Burden: Number of items, time to complete**	**Score range**	**Minimal detectable change**	**Clinically important difference**
Global rate of change	SANE	1 item, < 1 minute Low burden	0–100	7–9%	15%
Function	PSFS	1 item, 1–5 minutes Low burden	0–10	2 points	1.2 points

Legend: ASES, American Shoulder and Elbow Surgeons Standardized Assessment; BPI, Brief Pain Inventory; DASH, Disabilities of the Arm, Shoulder and Hand questionnaire; EQ-5D-5L, EuroQol-5 Dimensions-5 Levels; MISS, Melbourne Instability Shoulder Scale; MPQ, McGill Pain Questionnaire; NRPS, Numerical Pain Rating Scale; OSS, Oxford Shoulder Score; PROMIS-UE, Patient-Reported Outcomes Measurement Information System Upper Extremities; PSFS, Patient Specific Functional Score; PSS, University of Pennsylvania Shoulder Score; RCDs, rotator cuff disorders; RC-QOL, Rotator Cuff Quality of Life; SANE, Single Assessment Numeric Evaluation; SF-36, Short Form-36; SPADI, Shoulder Pain and Disability Index; SPS, Stanford Presentism Scale; SST, Simple Shoulder Test; WIS, Work Instability Scale; WLQ, Work Limitations Questionnaire; WORC, Western Ontario Rotator Cuff Index; WOSI, Western Ontario Shoulder Instability Index.

Integrate outcome measures into clinical decision-making

OMs can be useful when integrated into clinical decision-making, but do not replace clinical interviews or physical examination.[153] To reduce reporting errors, clinicians should consider literacy and check forms for errors.[25]

Clinical experience using OMs develops therapist skills in judging whether a score is appropriate for a patient given the type of health condition, intervention and stage of recovery. This is enhanced by comparing scores to benchmarks obtained from clinic-specific databases or published literature on similar patients. Acute shoulder conditions typically have a 3–6 month period of rapid improvement followed by a slower period of recovery which can extend for years.[63,133] Methods like growth curves are increasingly being used to describe recovery trajectories, and the factors that modify them,[150] which can be useful to map patient progress.

All OMs are associated with measurement error, which must be considered when making clinical decisions. We can use a reliability ratio, e.g., Intraclass Correlation Coefficients (ICCs), to relate measurement error to the variability in a population. Then we choose an OM that achieves an appropriate reliability ratio benchmark (ICCs >0.75 for group decisions and 0.90 for individual patient decisions). We use absolute error indices to quantify measurement error in specific units, e.g., minimal detectable change (MDC), or limits of agreement (LoA). We can use these numbers to adjust our point-estimate OM score into intervals around which we have more confidence. The sample standard deviation (SD) and intraclass correlation coefficient (ICC) help us to calculate the standard error of measurement (SEM; $SEM = (SD \times \sqrt{1\text{-}ICC})$), which conveys how much a score is likely to vary with repeated measurements of the same patient (without true change). We use SEM to calculate MDC_{90} ($1.64 * SEM * \sqrt{2}$), the interval within which there is a 90% chance that a patient's true score falls.

For example, a patient with rotator cuff pathology might score 44/100 (where 0 is no disability) on the DASH, but with a SEM of 4.4, the MDC_{90} provides 90% confidence that the true score is likely to fall between 39.5 and 48.5.[136] MDC assumes that measurement error is symmetrical and unbiased. The Bland and Altman approach evaluates whether there is a systematic mean difference (bias) between two raters/OM or assessment intervals (where no true change has occurred), and provides an interval of 2SD around that difference (limits of agreement, LoA). This can be important to evaluate whether factors like instrument limitations, patient fatigue or learning have affected scores.

PROMs are subject to recalibration or response shift over time, e.g., rethinking priorities or changing usual activities.[187] Response shift, where people recalibrate how they score, can be challenging to detect. Measurement error should be random unless a systematic bias occurs. When setting short-term goals, we want to ensure that we are exceeding expected measurement error and can use MDC_{90} as an appropriate target in goal setting.

When setting longer-term patient goals or targets in clinical studies, we consider what change is clinically important. Values used include the minimally or clinically important change (MIC/CIC) also called the minimally or clinically important difference (MID/CID). MIC/MID is the smallest change in score that is perceived as important by patients, clinicians, researchers, or funding bodies.[209] We often apply CID as a single number benchmark, although it is possible to calculate the associated confidence interval around the CID, or the accuracy of CID in distinguishing meaningful change using the area under the curve, sensitivity, and specificity.[207]

A few caveats that must be remembered when using MDC or MIC as benchmarks: numbers vary across different populations, different treatment approaches and timepoints, and there are dangers in applying simplistic rules to CID.[78] Further, Rasch analysis of shoulder questionnaires has illustrated that most of the measures we use do not provide interval level scaling as originally constructed. This means changes in one part of the scale may not be the same at other points in the range. In some cases, interval level scoring can be achieved through Rasch analysis and rescoring algorithms.[20,37,91] Unfortunately, such solutions are not always stable. For example, Rasch analyses of the SPADI in different samples has provided different solutions.[20,37,91] For all these reasons, MDC and MIC are useful but imperfect benchmarks that should be used to inform, but not dictate, decisions about whether changes in OM scores are meaningful. Patient Acceptable Symptom State (PASS) is rarely reported but a useful target benchmark, since it represents the score on an OM that patients consider acceptable to remain in.

When using OMs to predict a future outcome, we can use relative risk or odds ratios to describe how likely a person is to have a specific outcome based on their current score/status, or mathematical equations that consider multiple factors to estimate a future score/outcome. When OMs are used for discriminative or predictive purposes, we should be aware of, and transparent about, the accuracy of the decision-making rules/cut-offs. This is important given the potential downsides to misclassification error that results in patients acquiring labels that can be detrimental to their care and outcomes.

Progress on development of core sets

In the past decade there has been a trend for OM developers, experts, users, and consumers to collaborate on the development of core OM sets. Advantages to this consistency include ease of data pooling for meta-analysis, comparability of constructs/measures over different studies, leveraging of clinical data, and ease of conducting multisite research. Challenges to achieving agreement on core OMs include that the OMs with the most evidence are not necessarily the best, and flawed measures in common use may be retained due to limited evidence on better alternatives. There may be multiple acceptable OMs, and individual teams or researchers may be reluctant to give up ones that are working well for them, which can hamper implementation of core sets. Finally, different consensus groups often come to different conclusions.

The core domains recommended by a consensus panel for shoulder conditions include an inner core of physical function/activity, global perceived effect, and adverse events.[27,69] The middle core consists of sleep, participation, and emotional well-being (originally called psychological functioning). A content analysis of shoulder measures indicated that most shoulder PROMs represent these core domains.[169] However, a core set of measures has not been published. A review of measures used in shoulder clinical research indicates wide diversity in OM use,[160] so agreement on future OM use may be difficult to achieve. Fortunately, PROMs that measure the same construct are often highly correlated, suggesting that we would come to similar results with any of the validated measures.

Shoulder impairment outcomes

https://apps.who.int/classifications/icfbrowser/

The physical examination of the shoulder usually includes the assessment of outcomes that in ICF language include impairments in body structure of the shoulder region (ICF-s720), e.g., imaging or humeral head positioning;[111]

or body functions such as mobility of joints (b710), joint stability (b715), muscular power (b730), muscle endurance (b740), proprioception (b260), or control of voluntary movement (b760).[160] This chapter will focus on routine shoulder impairment outcomes, e.g., range of motion (ROM) and muscle performance testing, and other important shoulder impairment outcomes such as scapular control. These outcomes should be initially examined on both shoulders so that any side-to-side differences can be identified.[85]

Joint mobility (ICF-b710)

The primary role of the shoulder is to position the hand in space to perform functional activities.[85,122] In the ICF, mobility of joint function (b710) is defined as "the range and ease of movement of a joint". Assessment of shoulder range of movement (ROM) is an integral part of the routine physical examination of the shoulder[160] and assists with diagnosis, identifies movement restriction treatment targets, and determines patient progress relative to the initial deficits.[152] ROM should be evaluated in a series of movements: flexion, extension, abduction, cross-body adduction, external rotation, internal rotation, and hand-behind-back. These measures can be taken actively and passively with the patient sitting, lying, or standing, and studies show that reliable ROM measures can be achieved with different types of active or passive movement.[9,42,77,128,132,152,183,212,222] Passive ROM can be further qualified using the magnitude of the resistance or pain with movement (such as characterized with a movement diagram) which demonstrates moderate to high intra- and interrater reliability.[34] To optimize the validity of the ROM examination, it is important to limit trunk (i.e., trunk extension during forward flexion) and scapula (i.e., scapular protraction during internal rotation at 90° of abduction) compensations.[42]

Universal goniometers and inclinometers (including those integrated in smartphones) can be used to assess shoulder ROM. Goniometry demonstrates excellent intrarater reliability and moderate to excellent interrater reliability in individuals with or without shoulder pain.[42,77,109,110,152,183,212] The MDC values do not appear to favor one instrument over the other, and vary between 5° and 23° for active and between 3° and 21° for passive shoulder ROM.[42,77,109,110,152,183,212]

Muscle strength (ICF-b730)

The shoulder is inherently unstable.[4] Scapulothoracic and scapulohumeral muscles are essential to maintain shoulder stability and mobility, and their strength and endurance should be assessed.[174] The muscle groups usually targeted are the humeral flexors, extensors, abductors, external rotators and lateral rotators, as well as the scapular elevators, depressors, protractors and retractors. In some populations, such as manual workers and athletes, it may be important to also assess muscle groups at the trunk or lower limb as weakness in these areas may lead to an overutilization of the shoulder.[103]

In clinical settings, shoulder muscle strength can be roughly estimated using manual muscle testing (MMT). However, it is preferable to quantify performance using either a small hand-held dynamometer (HHD), which measures maximal voluntary strength during an isometric contraction, or a large stationary dynamometer which measures maximal voluntary isometric, isotonic or isokinetic (concentric and eccentric) strength. Using standardized positioning and appropriate stabilization to minimize substitution and extraneous movements is essential to obtaining reliable scores.[56,174] Comparing scores over time, or to clinical/normative data should be done across similar test procedures, and must be disaggregated by age and sex differences given the marked impact these have on muscle performance.[176]

For humeral flexors, extensors, abductors, and internal and external rotators, the intra- and interrater reliability of both HHD and stationary dynamometer varies from good to excellent.[173] MDC has been reported as 29 to 40 Newtons (N) using HHD, and 21 to 57 N using a stationary dynamometer for maximal isometric strength, 21% to 43% for humeral internal/external rotators, and abductors/adductors maximal isokinetic strength.[142] Responsiveness to change has been reported as moderate using HHD for humeral abductors, flexors and external rotators.[141,205] Additional studies are needed as these indices have been rarely characterized and often include small samples.

For scapular elevators, depressors, protractors and retractors, the reliability of strength measures have been rarely assessed, and the studies that have investigated them suggest a lack of precision, as they report poor to excellent intrarater reliability for HHD[18,30,76,119,196,202] with high MDC

(MDC of 127 N for protractors).[205] Finally, clinicians using MMT should bear in mind that its validity has been questioned, as only 20% of maximal strength is needed to obtain a score of 4 (out of 5).[54] Good to excellent intrarater reliability and moderate to good interrater reliability has been obtained for MMT of humeral muscles,[76] while only poor interrater reliability has been achieved for scapular muscles.[60] Given validity concerns and the need for interval level scaling, dynamometers are preferable.

Muscle endurance (ICF-b740)

The ICF defines this as "sustaining muscle contraction for the required period of time", and has rarely been studied as an isolated construct as it is often embedded in a performance-based functional test (see below). An endurance protocol for shoulder rotators performing isotonic contractions was proposed which used resistance set at 50% of each subject's peak torque, and evaluated the reduction in force over 60 continuous repetitions, which demonstrated excellent test-retest reliability (ICC >0.84).[174] Others have used isokinetic contractions to study shoulder endurance/fatigue, although evidence on the reliability of these protocols is limited.[12,32,208] This area requires further research, considering the role of the shoulder muscles in sustained stabilization of the upper extremity in many aspects of functioning.

Shoulder proprioception (ICF-b260)

Proprioception is defined in the ICF as "sensory functions of sensing the relative position of body parts", i.e., the control of movement and maintaining of positions. It is affected in shoulder disorders[3,19] and changed with rehabilitation[2] or surgical intervention.[211] Measures of proprioception include kinesthesia, joint position sense, and ability to detect vibrations, force production or changes in limb velocity.[4] The most used proprioceptive tests assess kinesthesia as the threshold to detect passive motion or joint position. Measures[3,4,19] include a variety of test protocols that differ on whether active or passive movement is used, instructions, and what is used as a criterion measure. A systematic review concluded that a passive protocol with an isokinetic dynamometer for internal rotation at 90° of shoulder abduction was the most reliable,[4] although other protocols with simple equipment such as goniometers, inclinometers, laser pointers or accelerometers/inertial sensors have adequate reliability.[4] Joint position sense has moderate to good test-retest reliability (MDC varying from 2° to 6°).[4]

Scapular position (ICF-s720) and control (ICF-b760)

Proper scapular mobility and control are essential since approximately 35% of shoulder mobility in elevation depends on the scapulothoracic joint, and the scapula provides a stable base for the rotator cuff muscles. The presence of scapular dyskinesis (aberrant scapular posture and movement) has been suggested as a factor contributing to the persistence of shoulder pain.[28,81,104] Two categories of scapular position and mobility have been proposed: linear and angular measures of scapular position, and qualitative observation of scapular movement.[44,116,123,139,156,157,191,192]

Linear measures are used to assess the scapular position relative to a fixed point on the spinal column. The Lateral Scapular Slide Test (LSST) evaluates scapular position (distance between scapular inferior angle and thoracic spinous process on same horizontal plane) with the arms in three positions: arms in resting position, hands on the hips, and arms at 90° of abduction.[44,103,123] Other examples include linear measures developed to evaluate protraction (distance between posterior angle of acromion or base of scapular spine, and the spinous process)[44,123,156] or depression (vertical distance between posterior angle of acromion and C7)[28] of the scapula in the resting position.

Angular measures evaluate angular position of the scapula in upward rotation. Different methods have been proposed, either using mathematical formulas based on the distances between bony landmarks, or using an inclinometer positioned along the scapular spine.[70,92,123,186,190,219] Lewis and Valentine[123] proposed a measure of scapular tilting using an inclinometer placed between the root of the scapular spine and the inferior angle of the scapula. Most studies suggest good to excellent reliability for linear and angular measures of scapular position.

Scapular control can also be qualitatively evaluated by observing scapular movement during arm elevation. For example, Kibler et al.[105,204] described three abnormal movement patterns (prominence of the inferomedial angle, medial border or superior scapular border) that are used to characterize an altered scapular control during arm elevation (low to moderate intra- and interrater reliability). In the Scapular Dyskinesis Test (SDT), the patient elevates his or her arm with a dumbbell in their hand and the clinician rates the movement as being normal, slightly abnormal, or abnormal (moderate interrater agreement).[139,201]

Current evidence indicates limited discriminative validity which suggests that these measures should be limited to characterizing scapular position and movement.[46,113] Systematic reviews[45,46] found insufficient evidence to recommend any scapular measures.

Performance-based functional tests

Instruments such as the Simple Shoulder Endurance Test (SSET)[88] and Functional Impairment Test-Head, Neck/Shoulder/Arm (Fit-HaNSA)[74,75,115,134,176] are composite tests that reflect integration or "weak links" in impairments like pain, muscle endurance, weakness, mobility, sensory integration, and motor control. In the ICF, they are measures of capability to perform such activities as: "Carrying, moving, and handling objects (d430-d449)." In the SSET, patients must screw and unscrew bolts with their arm at 45° of elevation. At 2, 4, and 6 minutes after the start of the test, a weight of 0.45 kg is added to the patient's wrist. The test ends when the patient can no longer perform the task. The SSET showed moderate test-retest reliability (r = 0.59 to 0.60).[88] The FIT-HaNSA consists of 3 subtasks: repetitive placing of a weighted object at waist height and then eye level, followed by sustained manipulation/assembly in an overhead position, that are performed sequentially with each task lasting up to 5 minutes. The test is terminated when the patient has too much discomfort or is unable to complete the task, and is scored on 3 subtest times combined to a total score. The test requires purchase or assembly[64] of a shelving type unit for tasks to be performed. Excellent reliability and construct validity has been reported for the FIT-HaNSA in individuals with or without a shoulder disorder,[74,115,134,176] or with Grade 2 whiplash with neck/arm pain.[162]

Composite clinician-based outcome measures (CBOMs)

Some clinicians and researchers like to have a summary measure that is considered a global indicator. These scores can be constructed by pooled weighting of different outcome measures in a clinical trial or by creation of a pooled index.

Constant

https://www.orthopaedicscore.com/scorepages/constant_shoulder_score.html

The Constant was designed to provide "an overall clinical functional assessment".[40] Items on subjective function are rated 0–5 for 35 points, and physical assessment of active ROM and strength are responsible for the remaining 65 points.[40] Variations include whether the examiner asks items or they are self-reported, and how ROM and strength are measured. Composite CBOMs like the Constant have been widely criticized by measurement experts since weighting is arbitrary and different constructs are added together, which is against the principle of specificity of measurement; systematic reviews criticize the quality of the psychometric evidence and lack of standardized procedures.[179] Despite these major flaws, it is a popular measure in outcome studies. If used for research, there should be substantial efforts made to standardize procedures (devices, examiner procedures, positioning) to improve reliability.[82,179] Clinical usefulness is minimal as therapists need to track specific constructs.

Patient-reported pain and disability measures

No single PROM has established itself as the "gold" standard. Clinicians can select from an array of different PROMs with different measurement structures, content and measurement abilities.[130,136] Below we describe the most frequently used, assessed, and cited PROMs for shoulder disorders.

PROMs for generic health status, utility and QoL measures in shoulder conditions

Generic PROMs are designed to consider overall health, well-being, or quality of life (QoL) which includes physical, psychological, and social health. Advantages include a global perspective and the ability to compare across different health conditions. Generic OMs may be used to determine burden of illness, describe the cumulative effects of multiple health problems,[221] or consider how mental and physical might interact.[133] Utility measures (e.g., EQ-5D) have the additional benefit of supporting economic analyses. However, health status (e.g., SF-36) and utility OMs are typically less responsive when compared to condition or joint-specific OMs[133] and therefore, less than ideal as primary OMs for measuring response to treatment in individual patients or in clinical trials.

1) EuroQol 5L-5D (EQ-5D-5L)

https://euroqol.org/eq-5d-instruments/

The EQ-5D-5L is a utility measure that assesses across 5 levels of severity in 5 different dimensions of health[80,164] and has a single global item. A systematic review of its use in upper extremity orthopedic conditions concluded that it has good reliability and validity, as well as moderate responsiveness.[71] Advantages include its ease of application, that it is translated into more than 200 languages, that it is free for unfunded studies or clinical use, and that there is a wide pool of comparative data.[224] Registration is required. Older versions exists, and comparability across the 5L and 3L can be computed.[87] The MCID for EQ-5D index ranged from 0.03 to 0.52 and the MID is 0.08.

2) 36-Item Short Form Health Survey (SF-36)

https://www.rand.org/health-care/surveys_tools/mos/36-item-short-form/survey-instrument.html

The SF-36 is a health status measure with 8 subscales: physical functioning, physical role, bodily pain, general health, vitality, social functioning, emotional role, and mental health.[217,218] It should be reported by 8 subscale scores (/100) and/or 2 norm-references summary scores representing physical and mental health.[216] The summary scores can also be measured with the shorter SF-12.[216] Although the SF-36 was not designed as a single summary score, a scoping review revealed it has been used that way.[124] The SF-12/36 are less responsive than shoulder or rotator cuff specific measures, and MCIDs and MDCs have yet to be assessed in shoulder populations.[133] Advantages include its widespread use, comprehensive nature, large pool of comparative norms or clinical data, mapping to utility through the SF-6D,[184] and validation in musculoskeletal disorders. Disadvantages include scoring complexity and potential challenges in free access to the tool.

3) Patient-Reported Outcomes Measurement Information System-Upper Extremities (PROMIS-UE)

https://www.healthmeasures.net/explore-measurement-systems/promis

http://www.healthmeasures.net/explore-measurement-systems/nih-toolbox

PROMIS and the NIH toolbox provide an array of recently developed OMs that have an emerging pool of psychometric evidence. Registration is required. Although PROMIS developed CAT, it has also developed new standard items scales. Item banks regarding upper extremity function have been constructed and validated across several upper extremity populations.[89,98,99] The PROMIS-UE can be administered as a CAT or a 7-item standardized item short-form. Some studies have used the PROMIS physical function scale rather than the UE OMs. PROMIS OMs have undergone extensive testing in shoulder populations.[7,16,17,52,58,151,155,161,180] Strengths include brevity and the focus on function separate from symptoms. It has been suggested that PROMIS CAT performs as well or better than standardized shoulder scales,[16,161,180] but some found poor correlation to standardized shoulder OMs.[161] CAT does require computer-based administration which can be an implementation barrier for some contexts or patient populations, or an advantage in others. CAT can lower responder burden, but clinicians cannot review changes on the same items over time, and the time saved compared to standard item shoulder OMs is minimal.[147] The MCID for PROMIS UE CAT has been reported between 3 and 5 in shoulder arthroplasty or rotator cuff disorders.[59,73]

Single item global PROMs

1) Single Assessment Numeric Evaluation (SANE)

https://orthop.washington.edu/sites/default/files/files/POOS-12_SANE.pdf

The Single Assessment Numeric Evaluation is a single-item, global PROM that is considered a measure of function. The response to a question of: "On a scale from 0% to 100%, how would you rate your (e.g., shoulder) today, with 100% being normal?",[225] is completed by writing in a number. Strengths include the low burden, use across multiple musculoskeletal problems, and that when administered on two occasions, it is a more valid method for assessment of global change (limits recall bias). Weaknesses include that patient interpretation of "normal" may vary, and that the construct being measured is unclear. The SANE has shown to be a reliable, valid and responsive tool to be used for shoulder pathologies.[154] The MDC is reported to be 7–9 % and the MCID is 15%.

2) Single Item Measures of Change

Global rating of change (GRC) or global perceived effect (GPE) are single item PROMs administered at follow-up where the patient rates their change or treatment effectiveness, ranging from worse, to no change, to better. These are typically used to create subgroups in validation of OMs and are reliable.[21] They can have different numbers of intervals and anchors and are inherently subject to recall bias.[21,96]

Standard-item region/joint-specific PROMs for the shoulder

Standard-item region/joint-specific PROMs using a standardized set of items for assessment of the shoulder are outlined below.

1) American Shoulder and Elbow Surgeons Standardized Assessment (ASES)

https://www.orthopaedicscore.com/scorepages/patient_completed_score.html

The ASES measures functional limitations and shoulder pain.[166] The ASES has two subscales including a single item pain (0–10) and 10 functional (4-point Likert) items. Pain and function are weighted equally and the total score ranges from 0 to 100 points, where 0 = worst and 100 = best. A systematic review reported that the ASES is a reliable and valid tool, but further work is needed to estimate its longitudinal responsiveness properties in different contexts.[178] It has been reported to be reliable in paper or mobile versions,[86] although one study suggested inadequate test-retest reliability of the pain dimension, and that the "do usual sports" item has a high rate of missing data, especially for older people.[210] The MDC is 10.5 (90% CI) and MCID is 15.5 (15% total difference).[93] Patients treated with a shoulder arthroplasty consider an ASES score of 76 to be a Patient Acceptable Symptom State (PASS).[31]

2) Disabilities of the Arm, Shoulder and Hand questionnaire (DASH)

https://dash.iwh.on.ca/about-dash

The full 30-item DASH was developed to measure disability in people with upper extremity conditions, although it also includes items that measure symptoms.[14] The score ranges from 0–100 (100 the worst) and can be compared to normative scores[1] as well as extensive data from clinical populations. A systematic review reported that the DASH is reliable and valid.[178] In 2005, the DASH was reduced to the 11-item QuickDASH.[15] It has similar measurement properties as the full DASH, and reduces response burden.[135] Advantages of the DASH include use across multiple upper extremity conditions, a large pool of comparative data, and that many translations are available on the DASH website. The MDC is 10.7 (90% CI) and MCID is 10.2 points.

3) Shoulder Pain and Disability Index (SPADI)

https://orthotoolkit.com/spadi/

The SPADI measures both shoulder pain and function[167] in separate subscales. There are 5 items in the pain subscale and

8 items in the disability subscale, each scored from 0 (best) to 10 (worst) either as a VAS or more commonly as an NRS. Multiple studies and systematic reviews have demonstrated its reliability, validity, and responsiveness.[24,170,178] An advantage is the separation of the constructs of pain and disability which are often combined in other PROMs, although a total score which rates each at 50% is also commonly used. The MDC is 18.1 (90% CI)[178] and MCID is 14–21/100.[47]

4) Oxford Shoulder Score (OSS)

http://www.orthopaedicscore.com/scorepages/oxford_shoulder_score.html

The Oxford Shoulder Score (OSS) is a 12-item PROM developed to evaluate the outcome of many types of shoulder surgery, excluding instability.[48] The OSS contains two subscales, pain (20 points) and activities of daily living (40 points). Scores range from 0 to 60, with a higher score being associated with increased disability. Based on a systematic review, the OSS has shown to be reliable, valid (only construct validity is reported) and sensitive to change (effect sizes reported). Responsiveness indices/studies and translation studies are still limited[185] compared to other PROMs. The MCID is 6 (13% total difference).[93]

5) Simple Shoulder Test (SST)

https://orthotoolkit.com/simple-shoulder/

The SST measures functional limitations of an affected shoulder in people with shoulder dysfunction.[125] It consists of 12 items with dichotomous response options (yes/no), and the scaling increases by progressive item difficultly (Guttman scaling). The score is the number of the items that the patient indicates they can do. A systematic review reported the SST as a reliable and valid tool, but further data on its longitudinal responsiveness properties are required.[178] Strengths are its low patient and clinician burden, and widespread use. Few translations are published. The MDC is 32.3 (95% CI) and MCID is 2.4 to 9.7 points.

6) University of Pennsylvania Shoulder Score (PSS)

https://orthotoolkit.com/penn-shoulder-score/

The PSS is a 100-point scale that consists of 3 subscales of pain, function and satisfaction.[118] The pain and satisfaction items use a 10-point NRS to determine how much pain or how satisfied the respondent reports with their level of function. The function subsection is based on a sum of 20 items, each with a 4-point Likert scale. A small number of studies suggest that PSS is reliable, valid and responsive.[118] Limitations include limited comparative data, and the combination of different constructs into a global score.

Condition-specific PROMs

Condition/disease-specific OMs are those that assess the impact of a single symptom, health state, or diagnosis.

1) Western Ontario Rotator Cuff Index (WORC) and Short-WORC

https://journals.lww.com/jorthotrauma/fulltext/2006/09001/western_ontario_rotator_cuff_index__worc_.48.aspx

The Western Ontario Rotator Cuff Index[106,107] is a disease-specific QoL PROM focusing on rotator cuff disease. The WORC originally consisted of 21 visual analog scale (VAS) items, organized in 5 subscales: physical symptoms, sports/recreation, work, lifestyle, and emotions. Scoring differences appear in the literature (/2100 vs percentage), although the developer suggested summation (/2100). Normative values have been established.[101] The WORC was recently abbreviated from 21 to 7 VAS items (/700) by retaining items from the work and lifestyle subscales. The Short-WORC was subsequently validated in a numeric (0–10) version[49,50] which is scored as a percentage (0–100%). One systematic review reported that it is valid, reliable, and responsive with an MDC_{90} of 16.7/100 and MIC of 34/100, and another reported an MCID of 276 (13% total difference).[93] Some studies suggest it more responsive than shoulder joint-specific OMs.[49]

2) Rotator Cuff Quality of Life (RC-QoL)

https://pubmed.ncbi.nlm.nih.gov/11075319/

The RC-QoL is a disease-specific quality of life measure for people with rotator cuff pathology.[23,84] The 34 items in the RC-QoL were derived through a clinimetric process that was built on previous literature, expert opinions, and patient interviews. A small pool of evidence supports its reliability,[57] validity,[23] and responsiveness; MDC is 3, MCID ranges from 7 to 14 points.[57]

3) Melbourne Instability Shoulder Scale (MISS)

https://pubmed.ncbi.nlm.nih.gov/15723010/

The MISS[220] is a 22-item OM for shoulder instability with 4 domains: pain (4 items), instability (5 items), function (8 items), and occupation and sports (5 items), with scores on a 5-point Likert scale. A limited number of studies indicate the MISS is reliable, valid and responsive (MDC = 5.5 points).[171,223] More psychometric evidence is needed.

4) Western Ontario Shoulder Instability Index (WOSI)

https://orthotoolkit.com/wosi/

The WOSI[180] has 4 domains: physical symptoms (10 items), sports/recreation/work (4 items), lifestyle (4 items), and emotions (3 items), and scored using a VAS (scored/2100). The WOSI is shown to be reliable, valid, and responsive,[223] and was found to have the most support evidence for an instability-specific OM.[223] The MCID is 10% and MDC is 339.3/2100.

Symptom-specific PROMs

Symptom-specific PROMs measure the severity and/or impact of symptoms like fatigue, pain intensity or pain interference. The National Institutes of Health (NIH) Toolbox suggests measurement of pain intensity (NRS) and pain interference,[41] and provides a website for a variety of OMs.

https://www.healthmeasures.net/explore-measurement-systems/nih-toolbox

1) Numerical Pain Rating Scale (NPRS)

https://www.orthopaedicscore.com/scorepages/VAS_score.html

The NPRS is single numeric item PROM with anchors from 0–10. Unlike a VAS, it can be administered verbally or in text. The question framing, time frame and anchors vary across studies. The NIH toolbox recommends asking "In the past 7 days, how would you rate your pain on average?" with anchors of "no pain" to "extreme pain".[160] Advantages of the NPRS are its ease of application in text or verbal formats, simplicity for scoring, generic use, and extensive evidence that it is reliable, valid and responsive in many conditions[35,83] including those with shoulder pain.[149] The MDC is 2 points and MCID is 1 point.

2) McGill Pain Questionnaire (MPQ)

https://eprovide.mapi-trust.org/instruments/short-form-mcgill-pain-questionnaire

The McGill Pain Questionnaire was one of the first PROMs to focus on pain qualities.[143] It has been used in many different diagnoses, including shoulder pathology.[95] The original version was based solely on words (78 words in 20 different pain quality items), but shortened versions[55] have reduced the number of words and introduced numeric scales to quantify both quality and intensity of pain. The most recent version of the 22-item SF-MPQ-V2 (items rated 0–10) has less burden, retains a focus on pain typology, and contains items that differentiate neuropathic pain.[159] A downside compared to other pain scales is response burden and fewer psychometric studies.[94,126]

3) Brief Pain Inventory (BPI)

https://www.mdanderson.org/research/departments-labs-institutes/departments-divisions/symptom-research/symptom-assessment-tools/brief-pain-inventory.html

The Brief Pain Inventory measures the intensity of pain (sensory dimension) and interference of pain in the patient's life (reactive dimension).[39] It has a long form for research and short for form for clinical practice (7 and 10 item versions exist).[163] It has been used with cancer and non-cancer pain,[6,100] including MSK disorders[131] and shoulder disorders.[226] Some studies support 2 subscales,[131] while one large study suggested that it should be interpreted as two separate subscales (Affective Interference, Physical Interference) with the sleep item removed or interpreted separately for optimal fit to the Rasch model (interval level scaling).[213] The BPI has been translated into many languages. It is reliable, valid, and responsive (MCID = 2.2 points in MSK disorders). The BPI was shortened to 9 items (BPI-SF).[140]

Disability- (activity/participation) specific OMs

Some OMs are designed to assess a specific activity limitation or participation restriction e.g., return to sports or work.

1) Work Limitations Questionnaire (WLQ)

https://www.tuftsmedicalcenter.org/research-clinical-trials/institutes-centers-labs/center-for-health-solutions/available-questionnaires

The Work Limitations Questionnaire[120,121] is used to evaluate at-work disability and productivity loss.[5,8,175] It is available in multiple versions with different numbers of items (e.g., 8, 25, 26), subscales or scoring formats. Therefore, care must be used when selecting a WLQ version.[175,200] The WLQ-25 has four subscales: time demands, physical demands, mental/interpersonal demands, and output demands.[197] In a systematic review, the WLQ-25 demonstrated good reliability, validity and responsiveness properties (MCID =13 points, MDC=0.77–0.97).[175]

2) Work Instability Scale (WIS)

https://eprovide.mapi-trust.org/instruments/rheumatoid-arthritis-work-instability-scale

The Work Instability Scale is a 23-item PROM developed using Rasch analysis to measure work instability in people with rheumatoid arthritis,[68] defined as a mismatch between an individual's functional ability and their work tasks that places the individual at risk for work disability. While the WIS was originally developed for arthritis patients, it has been validated for many upper limb musculoskeletal disorders. The MDC is reported as 0.86–0.93.[165,198,199]

3) Stanford Presenteeism Scale (SPS)

https://pubmed.ncbi.nlm.nih.gov/11802460/

The 6-item SPS measures the impact of a worker's perceived ability to concentrate on work tasks despite the distractions of health impairments and pain.[112] The SPS contains 6 items on a 5-item Likert scale. In a systematic review, the SPS was shown to have good reliability and validity properties, but limited responsiveness (MDC = 0.71–0.80).[175]

Person-specific PROMs

Person-specific OMs have items chosen by the patient. Typically, patient-specific PROMs will be more responsive than standard-item scales since the person picks the items most salient to their condition.

1) Patient Specific Functional Scale (PSFS)

https://www.sralab.org/rehabilitation-measures/patient-specific-functional-scale

The PSFS[189] asks patients to identify 3–5 important activities that they are unable to perform or are having difficulty with as a result of their problem, and then rate the difficulty. The PSFS has shown to be a reliable, valid, and responsive tool to be used for shoulder, and many other musculoskeletal pathologies.[114] Strengths include patient-centeredness, relation to functional goals, and high responsiveness. A weakness is that the scores cannot be compared across individuals or norms, since the items are not standard. In upper extremity disorders, the MCID is reported as 1.2 points and the MDC is 2 points.[79,108]

2) The Canadian Occupational Performance Measure (COPM)

https://www.thecopm.ca/

The COPM requires the patient to pick aspects of occupational performance and rate them on difficulty and satisfaction. The COPM requires specific training and is integrated into treatment planning, which account for much longer administration time.

Patient-reported psychological measures

Psychological PROMs are often used to predict whether patients will likely have a positive recovery trajectory/outcome, or are at risk of a poor recovery/outcome.[10,65] They are increasingly used with a focus on biopsychosocial shoulder rehabilitation. Psychosocial health is complex, with many overlapping constructs which complicate assessment (Figure 12.2). Psychological PROMs are useful to identify modifiable predictors at a stage when the outcome trajectory can be improved.[66] However, there are potential risks in identifying people as being depressed, pain catastrophizers, helpless or overly anxious, if these labels are used to explain suboptimal outcomes rather than improve them. Labelling patients may result in inferior care if clinicians or patients see their situation as more hopeless. Psychological PROMs measure perceived states that can be realistic, or not. Negative realistic assessments that reflect severe injury or impairment are not the same as exaggerated psychological responses. For example, patients with an amputation and neuropathic pain will answer a "pain catastrophizing" or self-efficacy PROM differently than patients with a minor injury.

The goal of using psychological OMs is not to make a diagnosis, but to identify beliefs and symptoms that may be barriers to recovery which can preferably become treatment targets. Psychological features of illness are tempered with clinical experience/judgement that differentiate appropriate negative statements of status from negative thinking by considering multiple factors, including responses on OMs, injury/disease severity, progress, behaviors, context, culture and attitudes. We know that prior life experiences and trauma affect how patients present and communicate,[209] and we must practice trauma-informed care.[11,158] Every health condition involves physical, psychological, and social responses that can improve in parallel with the health condition, so we can monitor this with OMs. Biopsychosocial treatment is effective in managing shoulder conditions.[72,97] Despite increasing interest in the psychosocial aspects of managing shoulder conditions, evidence on prognosis and treatment targeting is limited and equivocal,[10,138] so we do not know which OM constructs or cut-offs will best triage patients into different treatment pathways.

Symptom/construct-defined psychological measures

1) The Patient Health Questionnaire (PHQ)

https://strokengine.ca/en/assessments/patient-health-questionnaire-phq-9/

The PHQ exists in multiple versions including a PHQ-9 and PHQ-2,[137,203] and is one of the more commonly used prognostic OMs. It measures depressive symptoms and has been used as a screening tool for people with shoulder conditions, where it predicts greater disability.[144,215] Since one item refers to suicidal ideation, hospital and research users

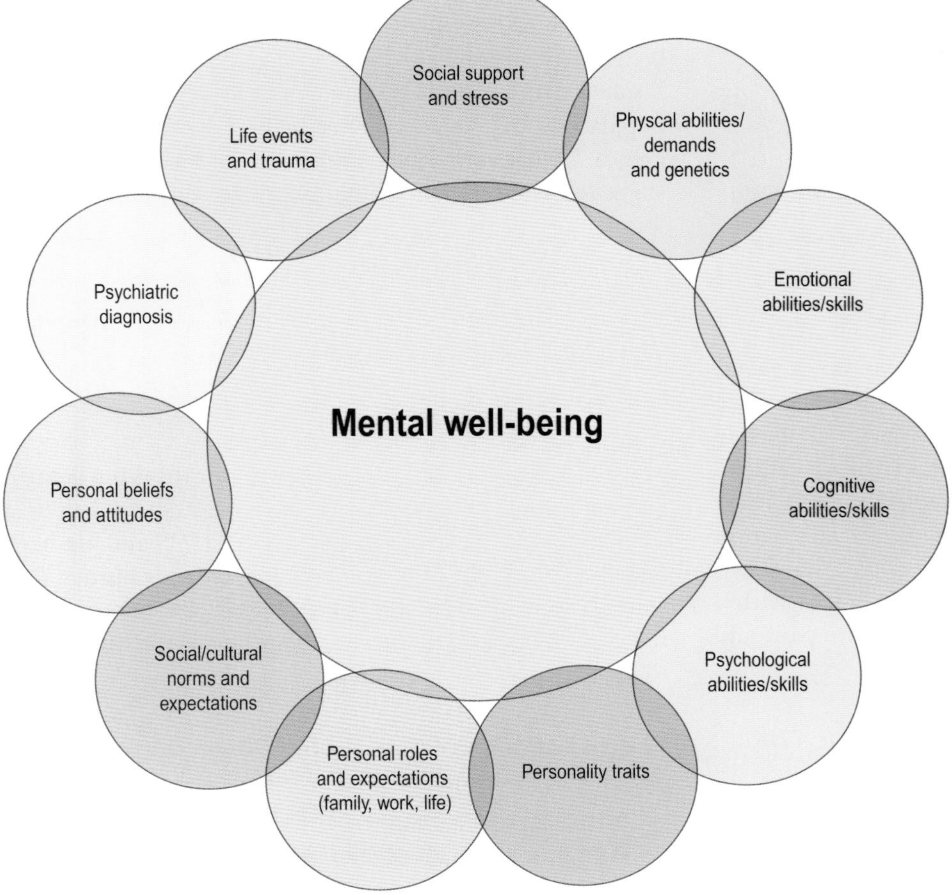

FIGURE 12.2
Constructs that affect mental health and well-being that contribute to psychological PROM scores.

may need to have a plan in place for people who endorse this item.

2) The Hospital Anxiety and Depression Scale (HADS)

https://strokengine.ca/en/assessments/hospital-anxiety-and-depression-scale-hads/

The HADS has one subscale of 7 items (rated 0–3) that assesses depression, with 5 items on an inability to experience pleasure, and 2 about appearance and feelings of slowing down. Seven items form the anxiety subscale, from which 2 assess autonomic anxiety (panic and butterflies in the stomach), and 5 assess tension and restlessness. A higher score indicates higher distress. HADS has been used to differentiate subgroups of patients with shoulder conditions.[36,51,226]

3) The General Health Questionnaire-28 (GHQ-28)

https://www.gl-assessment.co.uk/products/general-health-questionnaire-ghq/

The GHQ-28 measures psychological well-being in 28 items designed to identify whether an individual's current mental state differs from his/her typical state. Factor analysis established 4 subscales: somatic symptoms, anxiety/insomnia, social dysfunction and severe depression.[188] It has been used for screening or prognosis in MSK conditions. A downside is that it must be purchased.

4) Fear-Avoidance Beliefs Questionnaire (FABQ)

https://www.sralab.org/rehabilitation-measures/fear-avoidance-beliefs-questionnaire

The FABQ focuses on how a patient's fear-avoidance beliefs about physical activity and work may affect their MSK pain and disability, including shoulder disorders.[148] It has 16 items scored 0–6 on which a patient rates their agreement, from 0 = completely disagree, to 6 = completely agree. There is a maximum score of 96. There are two subscales within the FABQ: the work subscale (FABQw) with 7 questions (/42) and the physical activity subscale (FABQpa) with 4 questions (/24). It has been used to differentiate pain and disability outcomes in shoulder conditions.[148]

5) Tampa Scale of Kinesiophobia (TSK-11 or 17)

https://orthotoolkit.com/tampa-scale/

The TSK assesses self-reported fear of movement[146] based on the model of fear-avoidance (fear of work-related activities, fear of movement, and fear of reinjury). It consists of two subscales: Activity Avoidance due to perceived risk of pain or injury, and Somatic Focus that reflects beliefs of having a serious condition. The TSK has 17 questions rated 1–4, with some items having reverse scoring. The total score ranges from 17–68, where 17 means no kinesiophobia, 37 means it is present, and 68 means it is severe. The shorter TSK-11 score ranges from 11–44 and is prognostic in shoulder disorders.[148]

6) Pain Self Efficacy Questionnaire (PSEQ)

https://orthotoolkit.com/pseq/

PSEQ measures confidence to perform certain tasks despite pain. It is a 10-item questionnaire where items are rated from 0 (not at all confident) to 6 points (completely confident). Limited data supports psychometric properties in shoulder populations[144,145] as a predictor of pain and disability outcomes.[33] A 2-item version correlates to DASH scores, and was suggested as a screening OM in upper extremity populations.[26]

7) Pain Catastrophizing Scale (PCS)

https://www.physio-pedia.com/Pain_Catastrophizing_Scale

The PCS assesses the extent of catastrophic thinking defined as rumination, magnification, and helplessness.[195] It is a 13-item scale, with a total range of 0 to 52,[43,144] and has been widely translated.[90] A 4-item version reduces burden and shows strong measurement properties.[214] The name may be misused to label or blame patients, whereas the intention is to identify modifiable risk factors.

8) Injustice Experience Questionnaire (IEQ)

https://eprovide.mapi-trust.org/instruments/injustice-experience-questionnaire

The IEQ is a 12-item PROM where patients report the frequency with which they experience different thoughts about unfairness in relation to their injury.[194] It has 2 two correlated factors: severity/irreparability of loss, and blame/unfairness. Perceived injustice has been reported as being a distinct construct,[194] and a systematic review found strong evidence that it is associated with pain intensity, disability-related variables, and mental health outcomes in MSK conditions.[29] The IEQ is now licensed and distributed by Mapi Research Trust on behalf of Dr Michael Sullivan. It has been validated in injured workers[102] and fibromyalgia.[168]

9) Life Orientation Test-Revised (LOT-R)

https://osf.io/atgm9/

LOT-R[181] is a 10-item scale with negative and positive items, where 3 items measure optimism, 3 items measure pessimism, and 4 items serve as fillers. Respondents rate each item on a 4-point scale where 0 = strongly disagree, 1 = disagree, 2 = neutral, 3 = agree, and 4 = strongly agree. Optimism has been shown to moderate the influence of pain catastrophizing on shoulder pain.[43]

Multi-construct prognostic measures

In contrast to PROMs that focus on specific constructs, some psychological PROMs assess an array of prognostic items with a focus on overall prediction.

Örebro Musculoskeletal Pain Screening Questionnaire (OMPSQ)

https://orthotoolkit.com/ompsq-sf/

ÖMPSQ was designed to identify psychosocial factors associated with future disability called "yellow flags". It has been shown to complement clinician perceptions.[13] Ten, 12, and 21-item versions exist. It has been most used in low back pain. The ÖMSQ-12 content-retention version was recommended for broad musculoskeletal caseloads.[62]

Process of care/patient satisfaction

Measures of process of care, including satisfaction with care, focus on the delivery of care. A review highlighted that patient satisfaction PROMs have little standardization, low reliability and uncertain validity.[67] We found that satisfaction was poorly related to PROMs, impairments, or expert case review in patients following shoulder arthroplasty.[177] Despite these limitations it is often considered an important administrative measure to evaluate health service delivery, and can be mandated by some organizations or included in core sets.

Adherence is an important process measure since it can inform adjustments to treatment programs to modify outcomes. However, it can be challenging to measure. A review of 61 options found no conclusive winner.[22] Adherence PROMs are often context-specific.[61] A 5-item measure for upper extremity patients considers exercise, activity modifications, use of devices/aids, home program, and overall engagement.[129] It has versions for patient and clinician to complete to capture both perspectives.

Limitations

All OMs have strengths and limitations. PROMs may have measurement flaws such as inadequate targeting to the health condition or treatment being evaluated, lack of interval scaling, floor/ceiling effects, inadequate responsiveness, inappropriately high health literacy demands, high burden, lack of adequate cross-cultural translation and other flaws. Impairment measures, even when taken with instrumented tools, can lack precision across the full scale, have instrument-related floor or ceiling effects, be subject to calibration errors, lack reliability between examiners, and have limited association to important clinical outcomes. Both self-report and performance-based measures are subject to purposeful or involuntary lack of sincere/true effort or response. The possibility that important aspects of symptoms or disability were missed, or that patients were mislabelled or misclassified should be considered as a potential harm. Clinicians mitigate potential adverse effects of inappropriate OMs by selecting the best possible measures, cross-referencing different types of evaluation, repeating evaluations over time, and considering health literacy and the effects of social context.

Conclusion

The process of outcome evaluation requires purposeful selection of measures for tracking impacts on mechanisms or impairments that are treatment targets, prognostic measures, and measures of important health outcomes that reflect patient priorities including activity and participation. Clinical measurement science has greatly improved the scope of measures that have been validated to assess status, change and prognosis in people with shoulder conditions, although gaps remain.

References

1. Aasheim T, Finsen V. The DASH and the QuickDASH instruments. Normative values in the general population in Norway. J Hand Surg Eur Vol. 2014. doi:10.1177/1753193413481302.

2. Ager AL, Borms D, Bernaert M, et al. Can a conservative rehabilitation strategy improve shoulder proprioception? A systematic review. J Sport Rehabil. 2021. doi:10.1123/jsr.2019-0400.

3. Ager AL, Borms D, Deschepper L, et al. Proprioception: how is it affected by shoulder pain? A systematic review. J Hand Ther. 2020. doi:10.1016/j.jht.2019.06.002.

4. Ager AL, Roy JS, Roos M, Belley AF, Cools A, Hébert LJ. Shoulder proprioception: how is it measured and is it reliable? A systematic review. J Hand Ther. 2017. doi:10.1016/j.jht.2017.05.003

5. Amick BC, Lerner D, Rogers WH, Rooney T, Katz JN. A review of health-related work outcome measures and their uses, and recommended measures. Spine (Phila Pa 1976). 2000;25(24):3152-3160. doi:10.1097/00007632-200012150-00010

6. de Andrés Ares J, Cruces Prado LM, Canos Verdecho MA, et al. Validation of the Short Form of the Brief Pain Inventory (BPI-SF) in Spanish patients with non-cancer-related pain. Pain Pract. 2015. doi:10.1111/papr.12219

7. Anthony CA, Glass NA, Hancock K, Bollier M, Wolf BR, Hettrich CM. Performance of PROMIS Instruments in Patients with Shoulder Instability. Am J Sports Med. 2017. doi:10.1177/0363546516668304

8. Arumugam V, Macdermid JC, Grewal R. Content analysis of work limitation, stanford presenteeism, and work instability questionnaires using international classification of functioning, disability, and health and item perspective framework. Rehabil Res Pract. 2013. doi:10.1155/2013/614825

9. Awan R, Smith J, Boon AJ. Measuring shoulder internal rotation range of motion: a comparison of 3 techniques. Arch Phys Med Rehabil. 2002. doi:10.1053/apmr.2002.34815

10. De Baets L, Matheve T, Meeus M, Struyf F, Timmermans A. The influence of cognitions, emotions and behavioral factors on treatment outcomes in musculoskeletal shoulder pain: a systematic review. Clin Rehabil. 2019. doi:10.1177/0269215519831056

11. Bath H. The three pillars of trauma-informed care. Reclaiming Children and Youth. 2008. Available at: https://www.hope.ms.gov/sites/mccj/files/Hope%20training%20January%202021/read_3%20Pillars%20of%20TIC.pdf

12. Beach ML, Whitney SL, Dickoff-Hoffman SA. Relationship of shoulder flexibility, strength, and endurance to shoulder pain in competitive swimmers. J Orthop Sports Phys Ther. 1992. doi:10.2519/jospt.1992.16.6.262

13. Beales D, Kendell M, Chang RP, et al. Association between the 10 item Örebro Musculoskeletal Pain Screening Questionnaire and physiotherapists' perception of the contribution of biopsychosocial factors in patients with musculoskeletal pain. Man Ther. 2016. doi:10.1016/j.math.2016.03.010

14. Beaton DE, Katz JN, Fossel AH, Wright JG, Tarasuk V, Bombardier C. Measuring the whole or the parts? Validity, reliability and responsiveness of the Disabilities of the Arm, Shoulder and Hand outcome measure in different regions of the upper extremity. J Hand Ther. 2001. doi:10.1016/S0894-1130(01)80043-0

15. Beaton DE, Wright JG, Katz JN, et al. Development of the QuickDASH: comparison of three item-reduction approaches. J Bone Jt Surg - Ser A. 2005. doi:10.2106/JBJS.D.02060

16. Beckmann JT, Hung M, Bounsanga J, Wylie JD, Granger EK, Tashjian RZ. Psychometric evaluation of the PROMIS Physical Function Computerized Adaptive Test in comparison to the American Shoulder and Elbow Surgeons score and Simple Shoulder Test in patients with rotator cuff disease. J Shoulder Elb Surg. 2015. doi:10.1016/j.jse.2015.06.025

17. Beleckas CM, Padovano A, Guattery J, Chamberlain AM, Keener JD, Calfee RP. Performance of Patient-Reported Outcomes Measurement Information System (PROMIS) Upper Extremity (UE) versus physical function (PF) computer adaptive tests (CATs) in upper extremity clinics. J Hand Surg Am. 2017. doi:10.1016/j.jhsa.2017.06.012

18. Beshay N, Lam PH, Murrell GAC. Assessing the reliability of shoulder strength measurement: hand-held versus fixed dynamometry. Shoulder Elb. 2011. doi:10.1111/j.1758-5740.2011.00137.x

19. Blasier RB, Carpenter JE, Huston LJ. Shoulder proprioception: effect of joint laxity, joint position, and direction of motion. Orthop Rev. 1994;23(1):45-50.

20. Boake BR, Childs TK, Soules TD, Zervos DL, Vincent JI, MacDermid JC. Rasch analysis of the Shoulder Pain and Disability Index (SPADI) in a postrepair rotator cuff sample. J Hand Ther. 2020. doi:10.1016/j.jht.2020.09.001

21. Bobos P, Ziebart C, Furtado R, Lu Z, MacDermid JC. Psychometric properties of the global rating of change scales in patients with low back pain, upper and lower extremity disorders. A systematic review with meta-analysis. J Orthop. 2020. doi:10.1016/j.jor.2020.01.047

22. Bollen JC, Dean SG, Siegert RJ, Howe TE, Goodwin VA. A systematic review of measures of self-reported adherence to unsupervised home-based rehabilitation exercise programmes, and their psychometric properties. BMJ Open. 2014. doi:10.1136/bmjopen-2014-005044

23. Boorman RS, More KD, Hollinshead RM, et al. The Rotator Cuff Quality-of-Life Index predicts the outcome of nonoperative treatment of patients with a chronic rotator cuff tear. J Bone Jt Surgery-American Vol. 2014. doi:10.2106/JBJS.M.01457

24. Bot SDM, Terwee CB, Van Der Windt DAWM, Bouter LM, Dekker J, De Vet HCW. Clinimetric evaluation of shoulder disability questionnaires: a systematic review of the literature. Ann Rheum Dis. 2004. doi:10.1136/ard.2003.007724

25. Bourget-Murray J, Frederick A, Murphy L, French J, Barwood S, LeBlanc J. Establishing user error on the patient-reported component of the American Shoulder and Elbow Surgeons Shoulder Score. Orthop J Sport Med. 2020. doi:10.1177/2325967120910094

26. Briet JP, Bot AGJ, Hageman MGJS, Menendez ME, Mudgal CS, Ring DC. The Pain Self-Efficacy Questionnaire: validation of an abbreviated two-item questionnaire. Psychosomatics. 2014. doi:10.1016/j.psym.2014.02.011

27. Buchbinder R, Page MJ, Huang H, et al. A preliminary core domain set for clinical trials of shoulder disorders: a report from

the OMERACT 2016 shoulder core outcome set special interest group. J Rheumatol. 2017. doi:10.3899/jrheum.161123

28. Burn MB, McCulloch PC, Lintner DM, Liberman SR, Harris JD. Prevalence of scapular dyskinesis in overhead and nonoverhead athletes: a systematic review. Orthop J Sport Med. 2016. doi:10.1177/2325967115627608

29. Carriere JS, Donayre Pimentel S, Yakobov E, Edwards RR. A systematic review of the association between perceived injustice and pain-related outcomes in individuals with musculoskeletal pain. Pain Med. 2020. doi:10.1093/pm/pnaa088

30. Celik D, Dirican A, Baltaci G. Intrarater reliability of assessing strength of the shoulder and scapular muscles. J Sport Rehabil. 2017. doi:10.1123/jsr.2012-0007

31. Chamberlain AM, Hung M, Chen W, et al. Determining the patient acceptable symptomatic state for the ASES, SST, and VAS pain after total shoulder arthroplasty. J Shoulder Elb Arthroplast. doi:10.1177/2471549217720042

32. Chandler TJ, Kibler WB, Stracener EC, Ziegler AK, Pace B. Shoulder strength, power, and endurance in college tennis players. Am J Sports Med. 1992. doi:10.1177/036354659202000416

33. Chester R, Khondoker M, Shepstone L, Lewis JS, Jerosch-Herold C. Self-efficacy and risk of persistent shoulder pain: results of a Classification and Regression Tree (CART) analysis. Br J Sports Med. 2019. doi:10.1136/bjsports-2018-099450

34. Chesworth BM, MacDermid JC, Roth JH, Patterson SD. Movement diagram and "end-feel" reliability when measuring passive lateral rotation of the shoulder in patients with shoulder pathology. Phys Ther. 1998;78(6):593-601.

35. Chiarotto A, Maxwell LJ, Ostelo RW, Boers M, Tugwell P, Terwee CB. Measurement properties of visual analogue scale, numeric rating scale, and pain severity subscale of the Brief Pain Inventory in patients with low back pain: a systematic review. J Pain. 2019. doi:10.1016/j.jpain.2018.07.009

36. Cho CH, Jung SW, Park JY, Song KS, Yu KI. Is shoulder pain for three months or longer correlated with depression, anxiety, and sleep disturbance? J Shoulder Elb Surg. doi:10.1016/j.jse.2012.04.001

37. Christensen KB, Thorborg K, Hölmich P, Clausen MB. Rasch validation of the Danish version of the Shoulder Pain and Disability Index (SPADI) in patients with rotator cuff-related disorders. Qual Life Res. 2019. doi:10.1007/s11136-018-2052-8

38. Cieza A, Stucki G. Content comparison of Health-Related Quality of Life (HRQOL) instruments based on the International Classification of Functioning, Disability and Health (ICF). Qual Life Res. doi:10.1007/s11136-004-4773-0

39. Cleeland CS, Ryan KM. Pain assessment: global use of the Brief Pain Inventory. Annals Acad Med Singapore. 1994;23(2):129–138.

40. Constant CR, Murley AH. A clinical method of functional assessment of the shoulder. Clin Orthop Relat Res. 1987. doi:10.1097/00003086-198701000-00023

41. Cook KF, Dunn W, Griffith JW, et al. Pain assessment using the NIH Toolbox. Neurology. 2013. doi:10.1212/WNL.0b013e3182872e80

42. Cools AM, De Wilde L, Van Tongel A, Ceyssens C, Ryckewaert R, Cambier DC. Measuring shoulder external and internal rotation strength and range of motion: comprehensive intra-rater and inter-rater reliability study of several testing protocols. J Shoulder Elb Surg. 2014. doi: 10.1016/j.jse.2014.01.006.

43. Coronado RA, Simon CB, Lentz TA, Gay CW, Mackie LN, George SZ. Optimism moderates the influence of pain catastrophizing on shoulder pain outcome: a longitudinal analysis. J Orthop Sports Phys Ther. 2017. doi:10.2519/jospt.2017.7068

44. da Costa BR, Armijo-Olivo S, Gadotti I, Warren S, Reid DC, Magee DJ. Reliability of scapular positioning measurement procedure using the Palpation Meter (PALM). Physiotherapy. 2010. doi:10.1016/j.physio.2009.06.007

45. D'hondt NE, Kiers H, Pool JJM, Hacquebord ST, Terwee CB, Veeger DHEJ. Reliability of performance-based clinical measurements to assess shoulder girdle kinematics and positioning: systematic review. Phys Ther. 2017. doi:10.2522/ptj.20160088

46. D'hondt Ne, Pool JJM, Kiers H, Terwee CB, Veeger HEJ. Validity of clinical measurement instruments assessing scapular function: Insufficient evidence to recommend any instrument for assessing scapular posture, movement, and dysfunction: a systematic review. J Orthop Sports Phys Ther. 2020. doi:10.2519/jospt.2020.9265

47. Dabija DI, Jain NB. Minimal clinically important difference of shoulder outcome measures and diagnoses: a systematic review. Am J Phys Med Rehabil. 2019. doi:10.1097/PHM.0000000000001169

48. Dawson J, Rogers K, Fitzpatrick R, Carr A. The Oxford Shoulder Score revisited. Arch Orthop Trauma Surg. 2009. doi:10.1007/s00402-007-0549-7

49. Dewan N, Macdermid JC, Macintyre N. Validity and responsiveness of the short version of the Western Ontario Rotator Cuff Index (Short-WORC) in patients with rotator cuff repair. J Orthop Sports Phys Ther. 2018. doi:10.2519/jospt.2018.7928

50. Dewan N, MacDermid JC, MacIntyre NJ, Grewal R. Reproducibility: reliability and agreement of short version of Western Ontario Rotator Cuff Index (Short-WORC) in patients with rotator cuff disorders. J Hand Ther. 2016. doi:10.1016/j.jht.2015.11.007

51. Ding H, Tang Y, Xue Y, et al. A report on the prevalence of depression and anxiety in patients with frozen shoulder and their relations to disease status. Psychol Heal Med. 2014. doi:10.1080/13548506.2013.873814

52. Dowdle SB, Glass N, Anthony CA, Hettrich CM. Use of PROMIS for patients undergoing primary total shoulder arthroplasty. Orthop J Sport Med. 2017. doi:10.1177/2325967117726044

53. Drummond AS, Sampaio RF, Mancini MC, Kirkwood RN, Stamm TA. Linking the Disabilities of Arm, Shoulder, and Hand to the International Classification of Functioning, Disability, and Health. J Hand Ther. 2007. doi:10.1197/j.jht.2007.07.008

54. Dvir Z. Grade 4 in manual muscle testing: the problem with submaximal strength assessment. Clin Rehabil. 1997. doi:10.1177/026921559701100106

55. Dworkin RH, Turk DC, Trudeau JJ, et al. Validation of the short-form McGill Pain Questionnaire-2 (SF-MPQ-2) in acute low back pain. J Pain. 2015. doi:10.1016/j.jpain.2015.01.012

56. Edouard P, Samozino P, Julia M, et al. Reliability of isokinetic assessment of shoulder-rotator strength: a systematic review of the effect of position. J Sport Rehabil. 2011. doi:10.1123/jsr.20.3.367

57. Eubank BH, Mohtadi NG, Lafave MR, Wiley JP, Emery JCH. Further validation and reliability testing of the Rotator Cuff Quality of Life Index (RC-QOL) according to the Consensus-Based Standards for the Selection of Health Measurement Instruments (COSMIN) guidelines. J Shoulder Elb Surg. 2017. doi:10.1016/j.jse.2016.07.030

58. Fisk F, Franovic S, Tramer JS, et al. PROMIS CAT forms demonstrate responsiveness in patients following arthroscopic rotator cuff repair across numerous health domains. J Shoulder Elb Surg. Published 2019. doi:10.1016/j.jse.2019.04.055

59. Franovic S, Kuhlmann N, Schlosser C, Pietroski A, Buchta AG, Muh SJ. Role of preoperative PROMIS scores in predicting postoperative outcomes and likelihood of achieving MCID following reverse shoulder arthroplasty. Semin Arthroplasty. 2020. doi:10.1053/j.sart.2020.05.008

60. Frese E, Brown M, Norton BJ. Clinical reliability of manual muscle testing. Middle trapezius and gluteus medius muscles. Phys Ther. 1987. doi:10.1093/ptj/67.7.1072

61. Frost R, Levati S, McClurg D, Brady M, Williams B. What adherence measures should be used in trials of home-based rehabilitation interventions? A Systematic review of the validity, reliability, and acceptability of measures. Arch Phys Med Rehabil. 2017. doi:10.1016/j.apmr.2016.08.482

62. Gabel CP, Burkett B, Melloh M. The shortened Örebro musculoskeletal screening questionnaire: evaluation in a work-injured population. Man Ther. 2013. doi:10.1016/j.math.2013.01.002

63. Galatz LM, Griggs S, Cameron B, Iannotti JP. Prospective longitudinal analysis of postoperative shoulder function. J Bone Jt Surg. 2001;83(7):1052-1056.

64. Galea V, Pierrynowski M, MacDermid J, Gross A. Upper limb neuromuscular strategies are altered in patients with mechanical neck disorders compared with asymptomatic volunteers. Crit Rev Phys Rehabil Med. 2012;24(1-2):69-84.

65. George SZ, Parr JJ, Wallace MR, et al. Biopsychosocial influence on exercise-induced injury: genetic and psychological combinations are predictive of shoulder pain phenotypes. J Pain. 2014. doi:10.1016/j.jpain.2013.09.012

66. Gibson E, Sabo MT. Can pain catastrophizing be changed in surgical patients? A scoping review. Can J Surg. 2018. doi:10.1503/cjs.015417

67. Gill L, White L. A critical review of patient satisfaction. Leadersh Heal Serv. 2009. doi:10.1108/17511870910927994

68. Gilworth G, Chamberlain MA, Harvey A, et al. Development of a work instability scale for rheumatoid arthritis. Arthritis Care Res. 2003. doi:10.1002/art.11114

69. Goldhahn J, Beaton D, Ladd A, Macdermid J, Hoang-Kim A. Recommendation for measuring clinical outcome in distal radius fractures. Osteoporos Int. 2012;23:S341.

70. Greenfield B, Catlin PA, Coats PW, Green E, McDonald JJ, North C. Posture in patients with shoulder overuse injuries and healthy individuals. J Orthop Sports Phys Ther. 1995. doi:10.2519/jospt.1995.21.5.287

71. Grobet C, Marks M, Tecklenburg L, Audigé L. Application and measurement properties of EQ-5D to measure quality of life in patients with upper extremity orthopaedic disorders: a systematic literature review. Arch Orthop Trauma Surg. 2018. doi:10.1007/s00402-018-2933-x

72. Guerrero AVS, Maujean A, Campbell L, Sterling M. A systematic review and meta-analysis of the effectiveness of psychological interventions delivered by physiotherapists on pain, disability and psychological outcomes in musculoskeletal pain conditions. Clin J Pain. 2018. doi:10.1097/AJP.0000000000000601

73. Haunschild ED, Gilat R, Fu MC, et al. Establishing the minimal clinically important difference, patient acceptable symptomatic state, and substantial clinical benefit of the PROMIS Upper Extremity questionnaire after rotator cuff repair. Am J Sports Med. 2020. doi:10.1177/0363546520964957

74. Hawkes DH, Alizadehkhaiyat O, Fisher AC, Kemp GJ, Roebuck MM, Frostick SP. Normal shoulder muscular activation and co-ordination during a shoulder elevation task based on activities of daily living: an electromyographic study. J Orthop Res. 2012. doi:10.1002/jor.21482

75. Hawkes DH, Alizadehkhaiyat O, Kemp GJ, Fisher AC, Roebuck MM, Frostick SP. Shoulder muscle activation and coordination in patients with a massive rotator cuff tear: an electromyographic study. J Orthop Res. 2012. doi:10.1002/jor.22051

76. Hayes K, Walton JR, Szomor ZL, Murrell GAC. Reliability of 3 methods for assessing shoulder strength. J Shoulder Elb Surg. doi:10.1067/mse.2002.119852

77. Hayes K, Walton JR, Szomor ZL, Murrell GAC. Reliability of five methods for assessing shoulder range of motion. Aust J Physiother. 2001. doi:S0004-9514(14)60274-9

78. Hays RD, Woolley JM. The concept of clinically meaningful difference in health-related quality-of-life research: how meaningful is it? Pharmacoeconomics. 2000. doi:10.2165/00019053-200018050-00001

79. Hefford C, Abbott JH, Arnold R, Baxter GD. The Patient-Specific Functional Scale: validity, reliability, and responsiveness in patients with upper extremity musculoskeletal problems. J Orthop Sport Phys Ther. 2012. doi:10.2519/jospt.2012.3953

80. Herdman M, Gudex C, Lloyd A, et al. Development and preliminary testing of the new five-level version of EQ-5D (EQ-5D-5L). Qual Life Res. 2011. doi:10.1007/s11136-011-9903-x

81. Hickey D, Solvig V, Cavalheri V, Harrold M, Mckenna L. Scapular dyskinesis increases the risk of future shoulder pain by 43% in asymptomatic athletes: a systematic review and meta-analysis. British Journal of Sports Medicine. 2018. doi:10.1136/bjsports-2017-097559

82. Hirschmann MT, Wind B, Amsler F, Gross T. Reliability of shoulder abduction strength measure for the Constant-Murley score. Clin Orthop Relat Res. 2010. doi:10.1007/s11999-009-1007-3

83. Hjermstad MJ, Fayers PM, Haugen DF, et al. Studies comparing numerical rating scales, verbal rating scales, and visual analogue scales for assessment of pain intensity in adults: a systematic literature review. J Pain Symptom Manage. 2011. doi:10.1016/j.jpainsymman.2010.08.016

84. Hollinshead RM, Mohtadi NGH, Vande Guchte RA, Wadey VMR. Two 6-year follow-up studies of large and massive rotator cuff tears: comparison of outcome measures. J Shoulder Elb Surg. 2000. doi:10.1067/mse.2000.108389

85. Holmes RE, Barfield WR, Woolf SK. Clinical evaluation of nonarthritic shoulder pain: diagnosis and treatment. Phys Sportsmed. 2015. doi:10.1080/00913847.2015.1005542

86. Hou J, Li Q, Yu M, et al. Validation of a mobile version of the American Shoulder and Elbow Surgeons Standardized Shoulder Assessment Form: an observational randomized crossover trial. JMIR Mhealth Uhealth. 2020. doi:10.2196/16758

87. Van Hout B, Janssen MF, Feng YS, et al. Interim scoring for the EQ-5D-5L: mapping the EQ-5D-5L to EQ-5D-3L value sets. Value Heal. 2012. doi:10.1016/j.jval.2012.02.008

88. Hughes RE, Johnson ME, Skow A, An KN, O'Driscoll SW. Reliability of a simple shoulder endurance test. J Musculoskelet Res. 1999. doi:10.1142/S0218957799000208

89. Hung M, Voss MW, Bounsanga J, Crum AB, Tyser AR. Examination of the PROMIS upper extremity item bank. J Hand Ther. 2017. doi:10.1016/j.jht.2016.10.008

90. Ikemoto T, Hayashi K, Shiro Y, et al. A systematic review of cross-cultural validation of the pain catastrophizing scale. Eur J Pain (UK). 2020. doi:10.1002/ejp.1587

91. Jerosch-Herold C, Chester R, Shepstone L, Vincent JI, MacDermid JC. An evaluation of the structural validity of the shoulder pain and disability index (SPADI) using the Rasch model. Qual Life Res. 2018. doi:10.1007/s11136-017-1746-7

92. Johnson MP, McClure PW, Karduna AR. New method to assess scapular upward rotation in subjects with shoulder pathology. J Orthop Sports Phys Ther. 2001. doi:10.2519/jospt.2001.31.2.81

93. Jones IA, Togashi R, Heckmann N, Vangsness CT. Minimal clinically important difference (MCID) for patient-reported shoulder outcomes. J Shoulder Elb Surg. 2020;29(7):1484-1492. doi:10.1016/j.jse.2019.12.033

94. Jumbo SU, MacDermid JC, Kalu ME, Packham TL, Athwal GS, Faber KJ. Measurement properties of the Brief Pain Inventory-Short Form (BPI-SF) and the revised short Mcgill Pain Questionnaire-version-2 (SF-MPQ-2) in pain-related musculoskeletal conditions: a systematic review protocol. Arch Bone Jt Surg. 2020. doi:10.22038/abjs.2020.36779.1973

95. Jumbo SU, MacDermid JC, Packham TL, Athwal GS, Faber KJ. Reproducibility: reliability and agreement parameters of the Revised Short McGill Pain Questionnaire Version-2 for use in patients with musculoskeletal shoulder pain. Health Qual Life Outcomes. 2020. doi:10.1186/s12955-020-01617-4

96. Kamper SJ, Maher CG, Mackay G. Global rating of change scales: a review of strengths and weaknesses and considerations for design. J Man Manip Ther. 2009. doi:10.1179/jmt.2009.17.3.163

97. Karjalainen KA, Malmivaara A, van Tulder MW, et al. Multidisciplinary biopsychosocial rehabilitation for neck and shoulder pain among working age adults. Cochrane Database Syst Rev. 2003. doi:10.1002/14651858.cd002194

98. Kazmers NH, Hung M, Bounsanga J, Voss MW, Howenstein A, Tyser AR. Minimal clinically important difference after carpal tunnel release using the PROMIS Platform. J Hand Surg Am. doi:10.1016/j.jhsa.2019.03.006

99. Kazmers NH, Qiu Y, Yoo M, Stephens AR, Tyser AR, Zhang Y. The minimal clinically important difference of the PROMIS and QuickDASH instruments in a nonshoulder hand and upper extremity patient population. J Hand Surg Am. 2020. doi:10.1016/j.jhsa.2019.12.002

100. Keller S, Bann CM, Dodd SL, Schein J, Mendoza TR, Cleeland CS. Validity of the Brief Pain Inventory for use in documenting the outcomes of patients with noncancer pain. Clin J Pain. 2004;20(5):309-318.

101. Kemp SE, Urband CE, Haase LR, Obermeier MC, Sikka RS, Tompkins M. Normative values of the Western Ontario Rotator Cuff (WORC) Index for the general population in the USA. J ISAKOS. 2020. doi:10.1136/jisakos-2019-000418

102. Kennedy L, Dunstan DA. Confirmatory factor analysis of the injustice experience questionnaire in an Australian compensable population. J Occup Rehabil. 2014. doi:10.1007/s10926-013-9462-9

103. Kibler WB. The role of the scapula in athletic shoulder function. Am J Sports Med. 1998. doi:10.1177/03635465980260022801

104. Kibler WB, Ludewig PM, McClure PW, Michener LA, Bak K, Sciascia AD. Clinical implications of scapular dyskinesis in shoulder injury: the 2013 consensus statement from the "scapular summit." Br J Sports Med. 2013. doi:10.1136/bjsports-2013-092425

105. Kibler WB, Uhl TL, Maddux JWQ, Brooks P V, Zeller B, McMullen J. Qualitative clinical evaluation of scapular dysfunction: a reliability study. J Shoulder Elb Surg. 2002. doi:10.1067/mse.2002.126766

106. Kirkley A, Alvarez C, Griffin S. The development and evaluation of a disease-specific quality-of-life questionnaire for disorders of the rotator cuff: the Western Ontario Rotator Cuff index. Clin J Sport Med. 2003. doi:10.1097/00042752-200303000-00004

107. Kirkley A, Griffin S, Dainty K. Scoring systems for the functional assessment of the shoulder. J Arthrosc Relat Surg. 2003. doi:10.1016/j.arthro.2003.10.030

108. Koehorst MLS, Van Trijffel E, Lindeboom R. Evaluative measurement properties of the patient-specific functional scale for primary shoulder complaints in physical therapy practice. J Orthop Sports Phys Ther. 2014. doi:10.2519/jospt.2014.5133

109. Kolber MJ, Hanney WJ. The reliability and concurrent validity of shoulder mobility measurements using a digital inclinometer and goniometer: a technical report. Int J Sports Phys Ther. 2012; 7(3):306-13.

110. Kolber MJ, Vega F, Widmayer K, Cheng MSS. The reliability and minimal detectable change of shoulder mobility measurements using a digital inclinometer. Physiother Theory Pract. 2011. doi:10.3109/09593985.2010.481011

111. Konieczka C, Gibson C, Russett L, et al. What is the reliability of clinical measurement tests for humeral head position? A systematic review. J Hand Ther. 2017. doi:10.1016/j.jht.2017.06.010

112. Koopman C, Pelletier KR, Murray JF, et al. Stanford Presenteeism Scale: health status and employee productivity. J Occup Environ Med. 2002. doi:10.1097/00043764-200201000-00004

113. Koslow PA, Prosser LA, Strony GA, Suchecki SL, Mattingly GE. Specificity of the lateral scapular slide test in asymptomatic competitive athletes. J Orthop Sports Phys Ther. 2003. doi:10.2519/jospt.2003.33.6.331

114. Kowalchuk-Horn K, Jennings S, Richardson G, VanVliet D, Hefford C, Abbott JH. The Patient-Specific Functional Scale: psychometrics, clinimetrics, and application as a clinical outcome measure. J Orthop Sports Phys Ther. 2011. doi:10.2519/jospt.2012.3727

115. Kumta P, MacDermid JC, Mehta SP, Stratford PW. The FIT-HaNSA

demonstrates reliability and convergent validity of functional performance in patients with shoulder disorders. J Orthop Sports Phys Ther. 2012. doi:10.2519/jospt.2012.3796

116. Larsen CM, Juul-Kristensen B, Lund H, Søgaard K. Measurement properties of existing clinical assessment methods evaluating scapular positioning and function. A systematic review. Physiother Theory Pract. 2014. doi:10.3109/09593985.2014.899414

117. Lee HJ, Song JM. Linking of items in two function-related questionnaires to the International Classification of Functioning, Disability and Health: Shoulder Pain. J Korean Phys Ther. 2018. doi:10.18857/jkpt.2018.30.6.239

118. Leggin BG, Michener LA, Shaffer MA, Brenneman SK, Iannotti JP, Williams GR. The Penn shoulder score: reliability and validity. J Orthop Sports Phys Ther. 2006;36(3):138-151.

119. Leggin BG, Neuman RM, Iannotti JP, Williams GR, Thompson EC. Intrarater and interrater reliability of three isometric dynamometers in assessing shoulder strength. J Shoulder Elbow Surg. 1967. doi:10.1016/S1058-2746(96)80026-7

120. Lerner D, Amick BC, Lee JC, et al. Relationship of employee-reported work limitations to work productivity. Med Care. 2003. doi:10.1097/01.MLR.0000062551.76504.A9

121. Lerner D, Reed JI, Massarotti E, et al. The Work Limitations Questionnaire's validity and reliability among patients with osteoarthritis. J Clin Epidemiol. 2002. doi:10.1016/S0895-4356(01)00424-3

122. Lewis JS. Subacromial impingement syndrome: a musculoskeletal condition or a clinical illusion? Phys Ther Rev. 2011. doi:10.1179/1743288X11Y.0000000027

123. Lewis JS, Valentine RE. Intraobserver reliability of angular and linear measurements of scapular position in subjects with and without symptoms. Arch Phys Med Rehabil. 2008. doi:10.1016/j.apmr.2008.01.028

124. Lins L, Carvalho FM. SF-36 total score as a single measure of health-related quality of life: scoping review. SAGE Open Med. 2016. doi:10.1177/2050312116671725

125. Lippitt SB, Harryman DT, Matsen FA. Practical tool for evaluation of function: the Simple Shoulder Test. In: The Shoulder: A Balance of Mobility and Stability. American Academy of Orthopedic Surgery; 1993. pp. 501-518.

126. Lovejoy TI, Turk DC, Morasco BJ. Evaluation of the psychometric properties of the revised short-form McGill pain questionnaire. J Pain. 2012. doi:10.1016/j.jpain.2012.09.011

127. Lu Z, MacDermid JC, Rosenbaum P. A narrative review and content analysis of functional and quality of life measures used to evaluate the outcome after TSA: an ICF linking application. BMC Musculoskelet Disord. 2020. doi:10.1186/s12891-020-03238-w

128. Lunden JB, Muffenbier M, Giveans MR, Cieminski CJ. Reliability of shoulder internal rotation passive range of motion measurements in the supine versus sidelying position. J Orthop Sports Phys Ther. 2010. doi:10.2519/jospt.2010.3197

129. MacDermid J. Health literacy, adherence and fidelity. In: Skirven T et al. (eds). Rehabilitation of The Hand, 6th edition. Elsevier Inc.; 2018.

130. MacDermid J. A primer on outcome measures for surgical interventions. In: Thoma A, Sprague S, Voineskos SH, Goldsmith CH (eds). Evidence-Based Surgery. Springer; 2019. doi:10.1007/978-3-030-05120-4_7

131. MacDermid J, Jumbo S, Kalu M, Packham T, Athwal G, Faber K. Measurement properties of the Brief Pain Inventory-Short Form (BPI-SF) and the revised Short-Form McGill Pain Questionnaire-Version-2 (SF-MPQ-2) in pain-related musculoskeletal conditions: a systematic review. Ann Rheum Dis. 2019. doi:10.1136/annrheumdis-2019-eular.3525

132. MacDermid JC, Chesworth BM, Patterson S, Roth JH. Intratester and intertester reliability of goniometric measurement of passive lateral shoulder rotation. J Hand Ther. 1999. doi:10.1016/S0894-1130(99)80045-3

133. MacDermid JC, Drosdowech D, Faber K. Responsiveness of self-report scales in patients recovering from rotator cuff surgery. J Shoulder Elb Surg. 2006. doi:10.1016/j.jse.2005.09.005

134. MacDermid JC, Ghobrial M, Badra Quirion K, et al. Validation of a new test that assesses functional performance of the upper extremity and neck (FIT-HaNSA) in patients with shoulder pathology. BMC Musculoskelet Disord. 2007. doi:10.1186/1471-2474-8-42

135. MacDermid JC, Khadilkar L, Birmingham TB, Athwal GS. Validity of the QuickDASH in patients with shoulder-related disorders undergoing surgery. J Orthop Sports Phys Ther. 2015. doi:10.2519/jospt.2015.5033

136. MacDermid JC, Stratford P. Applying evidence on outcome measures to hand therapy practice. J Hand Ther. 2004. doi:10.1197/j.jht.2004.02.005

137. Manea L, Gilbody S, McMillan D. A diagnostic meta-analysis of the Patient Health Questionnaire-9 (PHQ-9) algorithm scoring method as a screen for depression. Gen Hosp Psychiatry. 2015. doi:10.1016/j.genhosppsych.2014.09.009

138. Martinez-Calderon J, Struyf F, Meeus M, Luque-Suarez A. The association between pain beliefs and pain intensity and/or disability in people with shoulder pain: a systematic review. Musculoskelet Sci Pract. 2018. doi:10.1016/j.msksp.2018.06.010

139. McClure P, Tate AR, Kareha S, Irwin D, Zlupko E. A clinical method for identifying scapular dyskinesis, part 1: Reliability. J Athl Train. 2009. doi:10.4085/1062-6050-44.2.160

140. Mease PJ, Spaeth M, Clauw DJ, et al. Estimation of minimum clinically important difference for pain in fibromyalgia. Arthritis Care Res. 2011. doi:10.1002/acr.20449

141. van Meeteren J, Roebroeck ME, Selles RW, Stam HJ. Responsiveness of isokinetic dynamometry parameters, pain and activity level scores to evaluate changes in patients with capsulitis of the shoulder. Clin Rehabil. 2006. doi:10.1191/0269215506cr983oa

142. van Meeteren J, Roebroeck ME, Stam HJ. Test-retest reliability in isokinetic muscle strength measurements of the shoulder. J Rehabil Med. 2002. doi:10.1080/165019702753557890

143. Melzack R. The short-form McGill pain questionnaire. Pain. 1987. doi:10.1016/0304-3959(87)91074-8

144. Menendez ME, Baker DK, Oladeji LO, et al. Psychological distress is associated with greater perceived disability and pain in patients presenting to a shoulder clinic. J Bone Joint Surg Am. 2015. doi: 10.2106/JBJS.O.00387.

145. Miles CL, Pincus T, Carnes D, Taylor SJC, Underwood M. Measuring pain self-

efficacy. Clin J Pain. 2011. doi:10.1097/AJP.0b013e318208c8a2

146. Miller R, Kori S, Todd D. The Tampa Scale: a measure of kinesiophobia. Clin J Pain. 1991. doi:10.1097/00002508-199103000-00053

147. Minoughan CE, Schumaier AP, Fritch JL, Grawe BM. Correlation of PROMIS Physical Function Upper Extremity Computer Adaptive Test with American Shoulder and Elbow Surgeons shoulder assessment form and Simple Shoulder Test in patients with shoulder arthritis. J Shoulder Elb Surg. 2018. doi:10.1016/j.jse.2017.10.036

148. Mintken PE, Cleland JA, Whitman JM, George SZ. Psychometric properties of the Fear-Avoidance Beliefs Questionnaire and Tampa Scale of Kinesiophobia in patients with shoulder pain. Arch Phys Med Rehabil. 2010. doi:10.1016/j.apmr.2010.04.009

149. Mintken PE, Glynn P, Cleland JA. Psychometric properties of the shortened Disabilities of the Arm, Shoulder, and Hand Questionnaire (QuickDASH) and numeric pain rating scale in patients with shoulder pain. J Shoulder Elb Surg. 2009. doi:10.1016/j.jse.2008.12.015

150. Modarresi S, Suh N, Walton DM, MacDermid JC. Depression affects the recovery trajectories of patients with distal radius fractures: a latent growth curve analysis. Musculoskelet Sci Pract. 2019. doi:10.1016/j.msksp.2019.07.012

151. Morgan JH, Kallen MA, Okike K, Lee OC, Vrahas MS. PROMIS physical function computer adaptive test compared with other upper extremity outcome measures in the evaluation of proximal humerus fractures in patients older than 60 years. Journal of Orthopaedic Trauma. 2015. doi:10.1097/BOT.0000000000000280

152. Mullaney MJ, McHugh MP, Johnson CP, Tyler TF. Reliability of shoulder range of motion comparing a goniometer to a digital level. Physiother Theory Pract. 2010. doi:10.3109/09593980903094230

153. Nabhan D, Taylor D, Hedges A, Bahr R. The value of the patient history in the periodic health evaluation: patient interviews capture 4 times more injuries than electronic questionnaires. J Orthop Sport Phys Ther. 2021. doi:10.2519/jospt.2021.9821

154. Nazari G, MacDermid JC, Bobos P, Furtado R. Psychometric properties of the Single Assessment Numeric Evaluation (SANE) in patients with shoulder conditions. A systematic review. Physiother (UK). 2020. doi:10.1016/j.physio.2020.02.008

155. Nicholson AD, Kassam HF, Pan SD, Berman JE, Blaine TA, Kovacevic D. Performance of PROMIS Global-10 compared with legacy instruments for rotator cuff disease. Am J Sports Med. 2019. doi:10.1177/0363546518810508

156. Nijs J, Roussel N, Vermeulen K, Souvereyns G. Scapular positioning in patients with shoulder pain: a study examining the reliability and clinical importance of 3 clinical tests. Arch Phys Med Rehabil. 2005. doi:10.1016/j.apmr.2005.03.021

157. Odom CJ, Taylor AB, Hurd CE, Denegar CR. Measurement of scapular asymmetry and assessment of shoulder dysfunction using the Lateral Scapular Slide Test: a reliability and validity study. Phys Ther. 2001. doi:10.1093/ptj/81.2.799

158. Oral R, Ramirez M, Coohey C, et al. Adverse childhood experiences and trauma informed care: the future of health care. Pediatr Res. 2016. doi:10.1038/pr.2015.197

159. Packham TL, Bean D, Johnson MH, et al. Measurement properties of the SF-MPQ-2 neuropathic qualities subscale in persons with CRPs: validity, responsiveness, and Rasch analysis. Pain Med (US). 2019. doi:10.1093/pm/pny202

160. Page MJ, Huang H, Verhagen AP, Gagnier JJ, Buchbinder R. Outcome reporting in randomized trials for shoulder disorders: literature review to inform the development of a core outcome set. Arthritis Care Res. 2018. doi:10.1002/acr.23254

161. Patterson BM, Orvets ND, Aleem AW, et al. Correlation of Patient-Reported Outcomes Measurement Information System (PROMIS) scores with legacy patient-reported outcome scores in patients undergoing rotator cuff repair. J Shoulder Elb Surg. 2018. doi:10.1016/j.jse.2018.03.023

162. Pierrynowski M, McPhee C, Mehta SP, MacDermid JC, Gross A. Intra and inter-rater reliability and convergent validity of FIT-HaNSA in individuals with Grade II whiplash associated disorder. Open Orthop J. 2016. doi:10.2174/1874325001610010179

163. Raman J, MacDermid JC, Walton D, Athwal GS. Rasch analysis indicates that the Simple Shoulder Test is robust, but minor item modifications and attention to gender differences should be considered. J Hand Ther. 2017. doi:10.1016/j.jht.2017.01.005

164. van Reenen M, Oppe M. EQ-5D-3L user guide: basic information on how to use the EQ-5D-3L instrument. EuroQol Res Found. 2015. Available at: https://nanopdf.com/queue/eq-5d-3l-user-guide_pdf?queue_id=-1&x=1625695349&z=MmEwMDoyM2M0OjgyNGE6ZGUwMDplNDZmOmZmOGQ6YjdlNTpiNTEy

165. Revicki D, Ganguli A, Kimel M, et al. Reliability and validity of the Work Instability Scale for Rheumatoid Arthritis. Value Heal. 2015. doi:10.1016/j.jval.2015.09.2941

166. Richards RR, An KN, Bigliani LU, et al. A standardized method for the assessment of shoulder function. J Shoulder Elb Surg. 1994. doi:10.1016/s1058-2746(09)80019-0

167. Roach KE, Budiman-Mak E, Songsiridej N, Lertratanakul Y. Development of a shoulder pain and disability index. Arthritis Care Res. 1991. doi:10.1002/art.1790040403

168. Rodero B, Luciano J V., Montero-Marín J, et al. Perceived injustice in fibromyalgia: psychometric characteristics of the Injustice Experience Questionnaire and relationship with pain catastrophising and pain acceptance. J Psychosom Res. 2012. doi:10.1016/j.jpsychores.2012.05.011

169. Røe Y, Buchbinder R, Grotle M, et al. What do the OMERACT shoulder core set candidate instruments measure? An analysis using the refined international classification of functioning, disability, and health linking rules. J Rheumatol. 2020. doi:10.3899/jrheum.190832

170. Røe Y, Soberg HL, Bautz-holter E, Ostensjo S. A systematic review of measures of shoulder pain and functioning using the International Classification of Functioning, Disability and health (ICF). BMC Musculoskelet Disord. 2013. doi:10.1186/1471-2474-14-73

171. Rosa D, MacDermid J, Klubowicz D. A comparative performance analysis of the International Classification of Functioning, Disability and Health and the Item-Perspective Classification framework for classifying the content of patient-reported outcome measures. Health Qual Life Outcomes. 2021. doi: 10.1186/s12955-021-01774-0.

172. Rouleau DM, Faber K, MacDermid JC. Systematic review of patient-administered shoulder functional scores on instability. J Shoulder Elb Surg. 2010. doi:10.1016/j.jse.2010.07.003

173. Roy J-S, Fremont P, Dionne C, MacDermid JC. Treatment and return to work of workers suffering from rotator cuff disorders: a knowledge review. 2017. DOI:10.13140/RG.2.2.15416.75520

174. Roy J-S, Ma B, MacDermid JC, Woodhouse LJ. Shoulder muscle endurance: the development of a standardized and reliable protocol. Sport Med Arthrosc Rehabil Ther Technol. 2011. doi:10.1186/1758-2555-3-1

175. Roy J-S, MacDermid JC, Amick BC, 3rd, et al. Validity and responsiveness of presenteeism scales in chronic work-related upper-extremity disorders. Phys Ther. 2011. doi:10.2522/ptj.20090274

176. Roy J-S, MacDermid JC, Boyd KU, Faber KJ, Drosdowech D, Athwal GS. Rotational strength, range of motion, and function in people with unaffected shoulders from various stages of life. Sports Med Arthrosc Rehabil Ther Technol. 2009. doi:10.1186/1758-2555-1-4

177. Roy J-S, MacDermid JC, Goel D, Faber KJ, Athwal GS, Drosdowech DS. What is a successful outcome following reverse total shoulder arthroplasty? Open Orthop J. 2010. doi:10.2174/1874325001004010157

178. Roy J-S, MacDermid JC, Woodhouse LJ. Measuring shoulder function: a systematic review of four questionnaires. Arthritis Care Res. 2009. doi:10.1002/art.24396

179. Roy J-S, MacDermid JC, Woodhouse LJ. A systematic review of the psychometric properties of the Constant-Murley score. J Shoulder Elb Surg. 2010. doi:10.1016/j.jse.2009.04.008

180. Saad MA, Kassam HF, Suriani RJ, Pan SD, Blaine TA, Kovacevic D. Performance of PROMIS Global-10 compared with legacy instruments in patients with shoulder arthritis. J Shoulder Elb Surg. 2018. doi:10.1016/j.jse.2018.06.006

181. Scheier MF, Carver CS, Bridges MW. Distinguishing optimism from neuroticism (and trait anxiety, self-mastery, and self-esteem): a reevaluation of the Life Orientation Test. J Pers Soc Psychol. 1994. doi:10.1037/0022-3514.67.6.1063

182. Schmidt S, Ferrer M, González M, et al. Evaluation of shoulder-specific patient-reported outcome measures: a systematic and standardized comparison of available evidence. J Shoulder Elb Surg. 2014. doi:10.1016/j.jse.2013.09.029

183. Shin SH, Ro DH, Lee OS, Oh JH, Kim SH. Within-day reliability of shoulder range of motion measurement with a smartphone. Man Ther. 2012. doi:10.1016/j.math.2012.02.010

184. Slobogean GP, Noonan VK, O'Brien PJ. The reliability and validity of the Disabilities of Arm, Shoulder, and Hand, EuroQol-5D, Health Utilities Index, and Short Form-6D outcome instruments in patients with proximal humeral fractures. J Shoulder Elb Surg. 2010. doi:10.1016/j.jse.2009.10.021

185. Slobogean GP, Slobogean BL. Measuring shoulder injury function: common scales and checklists. Injury. 2011. doi:10.1016/j.injury.2010.11.046

186. Sobush DC, Simoneau GG, Dietz KE, Levene JA, Grossman RE, Smith WB. The Lennie test for measuring scapular position in healthy young adult females: a reliability and validity study. J Orthop Sports Phys Ther. 1996. doi:10.2519/jospt.1996.23.1.39

187. Sprangers MAG, Schwartz CE. Integrating response shift into health-related quality of life research: a theoretical model. In: Social Science and Medicine. 1999. doi:10.1016/S0277-9536(99)00045-3

188. Sterling M. General Health Questionnaire - 28 (GHQ-28). J Physiother. 2011. doi:10.1016/S1836-9553(11)70060-1

189. Stratford P. Assessing disability and change on individual patients: a report of a patient specific measure. Physiother Canada. 1995. doi:10.3138/ptc.47.4.258

190. Struyf F, Nijs J, Baeyens JP, Mottram S, Meeusen R. Scapular positioning and movement in unimpaired shoulders, shoulder impingement syndrome, and glenohumeral instability. Scand J Med Sci Sport. 2011. doi:10.1111/j.1600-0838.2010.01274.x

191. Struyf F, Nijs J, De Coninck K, Giunta M, Mottram S, Meeusen R. Clinical assessment of scapular positioning in musicians: an intertester reliability study. J Athl Train. 2009. doi:10.4085/1062-6050-44.5.519

192. Struyf F, Nijs J, Mottram S, Roussel NA, Cools AMJ, Meeusen R. Clinical assessment of the scapula: a review of the literature. Br J Sports Med. 2014. doi:10.1136/bjsports-2012-091059

193. Stucki G, Kostanjsek N, Üstün B, Cieza A. ICF-based classification and measurement of functioning. Eur J Phys Rehabil Med. 2008. doi:R33Y2008N03A0315

194. Sullivan MJL, Adams H, Horan S, Maher D, Boland D, Gross R. The role of perceived injustice in the experience of chronic pain and disability: scale development and validation. J Occup Rehabil. doi:10.1007/s10926-008-9140-5

195. Sullivan MJL, Bishop SR, Pivik J. The Pain Catastrophizing Scale: development and validation. Psychol Assess. 1995. doi:10.1037/1040-3590.7.4.524

196. Sullivan SJ, Chesley A, Hebert G, McFaull S, Scullion D. The validity and reliability of hand-held dynamometry in assessing isometric external rotator performance. J Orthop Sports Phys Ther. 1988. doi:10.2519/jospt.1988.10.6.213

197. Tang K, Beaton DE, Amick BC, Hogg-Johnson S, Côté P, Loisel P. Confirmatory factor analysis of the Work Limitations Questionnaire (WLQ-25) in workers' compensation claimants with chronic upper-limb disorders. J Occup Rehabil. 2013. doi:10.1007/s10926-012-9397-6

198. Tang K, Beaton DE, Boonen A, Gignac MAM, Bombardier C. Measures of work disability and productivity: Rheumatoid Arthritis Specific Work Productivity Survey (WPS-RA), Workplace Activity Limitations Scale (WALS), Work Instability Scale for Rheumatoid Arthritis (RA-WIS), Work Limitations Questionnaire (WLQ), and Work Productivity and Activity Impairment Questionnaire (WPAI). Arthritis Care Res. 2011. doi:10.1002/acr.20633

199. Tang K, Beaton DE, Lacaille D, et al. The Work Instability Scale for Rheumatoid Arthritis (RA-WIS): does it work in osteoarthritis? Qual Life Res. 2010. doi:10.1007/s11136-010-9656-y

200. Tang K, Pitts S, Solway S, Beaton D. Comparison of the psychometric properties of four at-work disability measures in workers with shoulder or elbow disorders. J Occup Rehabil. 2009. doi:10.1007/s10926-009-9171-6

201. Tate AR, McClure P, Kareha S, Irwin D, Barbe MF. A clinical method for identifying scapular dyskinesis, part 2: validity. J Athl Train. 2009. doi:10.4085/1062-6050-44.2.165

202. Taylor JD, Bandy WD. Intrarater reliability of 1 repetition maximum estimation in determining shoulder internal rotation muscle strength performance. J Strength Cond Res. 2005. doi:10.1519/1533-4287(2005)19<163:IRORME>2.0.CO;2

203. Thombs BD, Benedetti A, Kloda LA, et al. The diagnostic accuracy of the Patient Health Questionnaire-2 (PHQ-2), Patient Health Questionnaire-8 (PHQ-8), and Patient Health Questionnaire-9 (PHQ-9) for detecting major depression: protocol for a systematic review and individual patient data meta-analysis. Syst Rev. 2014. doi:10.1186/2046-4053-3-124

204. Uhl TL, Kibler W Ben, Gecewich B, Tripp BL. Evaluation of clinical assessment methods for scapular dyskinesis. J Arthrosc Relat Surg. 2009. doi:10.1016/j.arthro.2009.06.007

205. Vermeulen HM, de Bock GH, van Houwelingen HC, et al. A comparison of two portable dynamometers in the assessment of shoulder and elbow strength. Physiotherapy. 2005. doi:10.1016/j.physio.2004.08.005

206. de Vet HC, Terwee CB, Ostelo RW, Beckerman H, Knol DL, Bouter LM. Minimal changes in health status questionnaires: distinction between minimally detectable change and minimally important change. Health Qual Life Outcomes. 2006. doi:10.1186/1477-7525-4-54

207. de Vet HCW, Terluin B, Knol DL, et al. Three ways to quantify uncertainty in individually applied "minimally important change" values. J Clin Epidemiol. 2010. doi:10.1016/j.jclinepi.2009.03.011

208. Voight ML, Allen Hardin J, Blackburn TA, Tippett S, Canner GC. The effects of muscle fatigue on and the relationship of arm dominance to shoulder proprioception. J Orthop Sports Phys Ther. 1996. doi:10.2519/jospt.1996.23.6.348

209. Vranceanu AM, Elbon M, Ring D. The emotive impact of orthopedic words. J Hand Ther. 2011. doi:10.1016/j.jht.2010.10.010

210. Vrotsou K, Cuéllar R, Silió F, Garay D, Busto G, Escobar A. Test-retest reliability of the ASES-p shoulder scale. Musculoskelet Sci Pract. 2019. doi:10.1016/j.msksp.2019.02.004

211. Walecka J, Lubiatowski P, Consigliere P, Atoun E, Levy O. Shoulder proprioception following reverse total shoulder arthroplasty. Int Orthop. 2020. doi:10.1007/s00264-020-04756-x

212. Walker H, Pizzari T, Wajswelner H, et al. The reliability of shoulder range of motion measures in competitive swimmers. Phys Ther Sport. 2016. doi:10.1016/j.ptsp.2016.03.002

213. Walton DM, Beattie T, Putos J, Macdermid JC. A Rasch analysis of the Brief Pain Inventory Interference subscale reveals three dimensions and an age bias. J Clin Epidemiol. 2016. doi:10.1016/j.jclinepi.2015.10.022

214. Walton DM, Mehta S, Seo W, MacDermid JC. Creation and validation of the 4-item Brief PCS-chronic through methodological triangulation. Health Qual Life Outcomes. 2020. doi:10.1186/s12955-020-01346-8

215. Wang JC, Chan RC, Tsai YA, et al. The influence of shoulder pain on functional limitation, perceived health, and depressive mood in patients with traumatic paraplegia. J Spinal Cord Med. 2015. doi:10.1179/2045772314Y.0000000271

216. Ware J, Kosinski M, Keller SD. A 12-Item Short-Form Health Survey: construction of scales and preliminary tests of reliability and validity. Med Care. 1996. doi:10.2307/3766749

217. Ware JE. SF-36 Health Survey update. Spine (Phila Pa 1976). 2000. doi:10.1097/00007632-200012150-00008

218. Ware JE, Snow KK, Kosinski M, Gandek B. SF-36 Health Survey Manual and Interpretation Guide. Lincoln, RI: Quality Metric, Inc; 1993.

219. Watson L, Balster SM, Finch C, Dalziel R. Measurement of scapula upward rotation: a reliable clinical procedure. Br J Sports Med. 2005. doi:10.1136/bjsm.2004.013243

220. Watson L, Story I, Dalziel R, Hoy G, Shimmin A, Woods D. A new clinical outcome measure of glenohumeral joint instability: the MISS questionnaire. J Shoulder Elb Surg. 2005. doi:10.1016/j.jse.2004.05.002

221. Wells GA, Russell AS, Haraoui B, Bissonnette R, Ware CF. Validity of quality of life measurement tools - from generic to disease-specific. J Rheumatol. 2011. doi:10.3899/jrheum.110906

222. Werner BC, Holzgrefe RE, Griffin JW, et al. Validation of an innovative method of shoulder range-of-motion measurement using a smartphone clinometer application. J Shoulder Elb Surg. 2014. doi:10.1016/j.jse.2014.02.030

223. Whittle JH, Peters SE, Manzanero S, Duke PF. A systematic review of patient-reported outcome measures used in shoulder instability research. J Shoulder Elb Surg. 2020. doi:10.1016/j.jse.2019.07.001

224. Van Wilder L, Rammant E, Clays E, Devleesschauwer B, Pauwels N, De Smedt D. A comprehensive catalogue of EQ-5D scores in chronic disease: results of a systematic review. Qual Life Res. 2019. doi:10.1007/s11136-019-02300-y

225. Williams GN, Gangel TJ, Arciero R a, Uhorchak JM, Taylor DC. Comparison of the Single Assessment Numeric Evaluation method and two shoulder rating scales. Outcomes measures after shoulder surgery. Am J Sports Med. 1999. doi:10102104

226. Wolfensberger A, Vuistiner P, Konzelmann M, Plomb-Holmes C, Léger B, Luthi F. Clinician and patient-reported outcomes are associated with psychological factors in patients with chronic shoulder pain. Clin Orthop Relat Res. 2016. doi:10.1007/s11999-016-4894-0

Clinical reasoning, behavioral change, and shared decision-making

13

Mark Jones, Kevin Hall, Jeremy Lewis

Introduction

This chapter addresses two inter-related concepts: clinical reasoning and shared decision-making. Clinical reasoning may be defined as, "a reflective process of inquiry and analysis carried out by a health professional in collaboration with the patient with the aim of understanding the patient, their context and their clinical problem(s) in order to guide evidence-based practice."[27,p.379] We provide an overview of what clinical reasoning involves and associated benefits. We take a new perspective by identifying elements common to all analytical thinking and relate each element to examples of what that entails for clinical reasoning in musculoskeletal practice. We then share intellectual standards of critical thinking that can be used to judge the quality of thinking and clinical reasoning.

Shared decision-making (SDM) is the process of developing a therapeutic alliance and facilitating patients' participation in their healthcare. SDM is also identified in professional standards as essential, but it is commonly only superficially understood and often poorly implemented in practice.[15,31,33,55] While there are aspects of SDM applicable to all professions and contexts, we focus on musculoskeletal practice, discussing the application of SDM through the entire clinical interaction and providing examples of where it should occur and what it can achieve.

Clinical reasoning

What does clinical reasoning involve?

Clinical reasoning involves collecting and analyzing patient information. The information gained elicits hypotheses regarding the patient's problem(s) and choices relating to management. It is iterative as information obtained through the interview, physical examination, and during reassessment is constantly reappraised and, if indicated, hypotheses revised. Clinical reasoning is often described as involving nonanalytical and analytical processes.[11,13,34,36,41] Nonanalytical processes include tacit or intuitive knowing (i.e., recognizing problems and solutions without conscious awareness) are ineffective by themselves. In contrast, conscious pattern recognition of problems, causes, and solutions learned through theoretical knowledge (e.g., clinical features of common clinical problems) and reinforced through clinical experience, is a characteristic of expert clinical practice when engaged with familiar presentations.[5,32,37,52] Clinicians should strive to identify common clinical patterns as presented in this book but be cautious of relying on them, because it then becomes difficult to recognize new patterns. We recommend a balance between pattern recognition and the slower analytical hypothesis-oriented process with emphasis on identifying physical, psychosocial, and environmental factors in a patient's presentation. In this chapter we focus on the analytical process of clinical reasoning.

Why is clinical reasoning important?

Clinical reasoning is important for several reasons. Firstly, musculoskeletal problems such as shoulder pain and disability can vary from minor strains that naturally resolve or respond to appropriate advice regarding acute care management, to complex multifactorial presentations that defy the technical rationality of simply applying a "proven" protocol of management. Health professionals must be able to perform comprehensive assessment and analysis across the full scope of factors known to influence health problems, including biological and genetic factors, physical impairments in function and structure, activity and participation restrictions and capabilities, psychosocial and environmental factors.[59] Our current knowledge is incomplete and even where clinical practice guidelines are available, they are not intended to be used prescriptively, and judgment regarding application to patients' individual presentations and circumstances is always required.

Clinical reasoning is analytical thinking in a clinical context, and is important to safeguard against the natural biases in judgment. Over 30 different types of cognitive error associated with clinical judgment have been identified,[12] many of which can be attributed to quick first impressions and decisions based on insufficient information and lack of further deliberation.[34,36] Improving clinical reasoning proficiency not only benefits decisions made in current practice, it also enhances learning and the development of expertise for the benefit of future patients.[7,8,17,32] Expertise in clinical practice arises from excellence in research translation, analytical thinking, and clinical experience.

Elements of analytical thinking applied to clinical reasoning

Like all analytical thinking, clinical reasoning is a hypothesis-oriented, iterative process comprised of key elements.[20] The elements of thinking may be used to examine your own and others' reasoning. Hawkins and colleagues[28] have summarized elements of all analytical thinking relevant to clinical reasoning as follows:

> *Whenever we think, we think for a purpose within a point of view based on assumptions leading to implications and consequences. We use concepts, ideas, and theories to interpret data, facts, and experiences in order to answer questions, solve problems, and resolve issues.*
>
> Hawkins et al.[28,p.5]

Table 13.1 presents elements of analytical thinking[20] with applications of each element to clinical reasoning. It provides a structured and inclusive way to reflect on and critique clinical reasoning. The examples proposed are not exhaustive. Rather than simply teaching and learning a prescribed patient examination and what reasoning should occur, take a step back and consider the "purpose" of your clinical practice. Identify the "questions" you set out to answer to achieve that purpose. Reflect on the "information" you believe important to answering those questions. Consider the "inferences", or categories of clinical judgment you need to formulate and what information specifically informs each category. Review and critique your "theory and conceptual" knowledge underpinning your examination, analysis, and evidence-based management.

Table 13.1 Elements of analytical thinking applied to clinical reasoning in musculoskeletal practice

Elements of analytical thinking	Elements of analytical thinking applied to clinical reasoning to enhance clinical practice
Has purpose(s): Critically reflecting on the "Purpose" of your clinical practice enables you to examine the focus you take and whether anything is lacking.	• Do I understand the patient as a person, their health problem(s), concerns, goals, and their experiences living with their condition(s)? • Have I taken a biopsychosocial approach and analyzed the problem to a level that enables me to offer the most appropriate management for this individual?
Incorporates questions linked to categories of clinical judgment: Examining the "Questions" you set out to answer through your examination and the rationale for each part of the interview and physical assessment ensures you are not simply following someone else's routine, and helps you to relate each section of your examination to the inferences or categories of clinical judgment they inform.	Categories of questions to be answered to understand the patient's health problem(s) and their experiences living with their health problem(s) may include: • Diagnostic categorization: – Symptomatic pathology? – Pathophysiological process (e.g., overload "strain" or tissue reactive process, degenerative, inflammatory, biochemical, ischemic)? – Pain type(s)/mechanism(s)? – Clinical syndrome? – Nonspecific but apparent musculoskeletal pain? – Hypothesized source of symptoms? – Physical impairments? • How is the individual affected? – Activity and participation capabilities and restrictions at work, sport, and socially? – Psychosocial factors? • What factors potentially contribute to the development and ongoing nature of the problem (physical, psychological, socioenvironmental, genetic)? • Are there any safety concerns requiring caution in the physical examination and treatment, specific safety testing or the need for referral for further investigations or to other specialties? • What are the best management options once I have synthesized available research, experienced-based evidence, and patient preferences? • What are the positive and negative factors affecting speed and extent of recovery (i.e., prognosis)?

(Continued)

Table 13.1 *(Continued)*

Elements of analytical thinking	Elements of analytical thinking applied to clinical reasoning to enhance clinical practice
Information used to answer questions: Considering the specific information needed to answer the questions asked facilitates understanding of the purpose and value of each section of your examination and the clinical judgments made.	Multiple sources of information (and knowledge) are utilized. Specific categories of information from the clinician's examination that might inform the questions listed above include: • The main problem(s). • Description, area, behavior, relationship, and history of the problem(s). • Concomitant co-morbidities. • Red flag screening. • The social, cultural, economic, environmental, work, and living circumstances. • Past and present lifestyle factors and exercise participation. • Beliefs. • The individual's understanding of their problem including meaning it has to them (e.g., expectations for recovery, goals, preferences for management). • The presence of any distress (e.g., anxiety, frustration, anger, fear, depression) and its relationship to their problem, and their coping strategies. • The presence of physical impairments in function and structure of the musculoskeletal, neurological, cardiovascular, respiratory, and other systems (as required). • Relationships between symptoms, activity and participation restrictions, and physical impairments.
Identify assumptions: Awareness of common unjustified assumptions in assessment and analysis encourages greater depth of assessment and accuracy of analysis.	Assumptions are taken-for-granted beliefs that may lead to errors of reasoning if based on inappropriate generalizations and insufficient information, for example: • Assuming the information the patient has volunteered (e.g., problem(s), symptoms, activity, and participation) is all that is needed without further screening. • Assuming that you can interpret the meaning in the patient's answers without clarification (e.g., what their understanding means to them with respect to their perception of threat, expectations for recovery, expectations for management and expectations for participation. What specifically is it about an aggravating factor that is a problem?). • Assuming you understand the relevance of a patient's reported distress without clarification. • Assuming you know what the pathology is or isn't, or the source of the individual's symptoms. • Assuming patients who do not do their exercise are unmotivated. • Assuming X is the best way to treat Y because that is what you have always done.
Has implications to other judgments and actions: Individually tailored management, as opposed to simply following a pre-determined protocol, requires understanding the implications of clinical judgments on other judgments and actions.	Clinical judgments have implications for other judgments and actions, for example: • Judgments regarding severity, irritability, inflammation, neuropathy, vascular features, instability, etc., have implications on specific assessments included in the physical examination (e.g., neurological, vascular assessment) and require caution in the extent and strength of assessments performed. • Analysis of mechanism of onset, area, and behavior of symptoms have implications for the diagnostic categorizations, identifying the underlying cause and factors contributing to the problem, and judging what body areas need to be examined. • Judgment regarding dominant pain type has implications to physical examination analysis, management, and prognosis. • Physical and psychosocial examination analyses have implications to management and prognosis.
Embodies a point of view: Recognizing the perspective or point of view you are taking when examining and analyzing a patient's problem enables you to reflect whether other perspectives should also be considered.	All analytical thinking occurs from a point of view, for example: • Biomedical versus biopsychosocial. • Clinician-centered versus patient-centered. • Specific "approaches" to be used in examination, analysis, and management (e.g., injections, surgery, exercise, dry needling, cognitive behavioral therapy, manual therapy disciplines).

Identify "assumptions" inherent in your assessment and management approach and adopt strategies to minimize unjustified assumptions. Check that your reasoning is truly hypothesis-oriented and iterative, in that inferences made have "implications to other judgments and actions". Lastly, reflect on the breadth of your reasoning by recognizing the "point of view" you are taking and ponder whether other perspectives should also be considered.

Intellectual standards for judging the quality of analytical thinking and reasoning

Table 13.2 provides an overview of intellectual standards for judging the quality of analytical thinking.[20] The table can be used to understand the different aspects of quality in thinking and reasoning and to reflect on your own practice and what you consider important to quality examination and reasoning.

Table 13.2 Intellectual standards for judging the quality of analytical thinking[20]

Intellectual standards for judging the quality of analytical thinking	Explanation of the standard	Examples when applied to the clinical examination and clinical reasoning
Depth and breadth	Is the depth and breadth of assessment (e.g., interview and physical examination) sufficient for a thorough, holistic analysis?	• Screening for other symptoms initially not reported by the patient: – Articular associated symptoms (e.g., crepitus, locking joint sensations) – Neural associated symptoms (e.g., numbness, hyperesthesia, paresthesia) – Muscle/soft tissue associated symptoms (e.g., tension, cramp, tenderness) – Vascular associated symptoms (e.g., swelling, changes in color or temperature) • Screening for additional activity restrictions and aggravating factors not volunteered: – Effect of other movements, postures/positions of the affected body part or other body parts capable of referring symptoms to the affected area – Effect of load on the symptoms (e.g., lifting, pushing, pulling) – Effect of compression on the symptoms (e.g., lying on affected side) – Effect of functional activities of daily living (home, work, fitness, sport, leisure) on the symptoms – Relationship to non-musculoskeletal system function (e.g., gastrointestinal, cardiorespiratory) • Screening for psychological factors not spontaneously volunteered: – Patient understanding/beliefs (e.g., regarding the problem, potential for recovery, self-management, self-efficacy) – Patient threat perception (e.g., seriousness of problem, perceived effect on all aspects of life, perceived possibility of recovery) – Presence of distress (e.g., anxiety, anger, fear, depression) and its relationship to the symptoms – Patient coping (e.g., acceptance to catastrophizing continuum) – Coping strategies (pacing and using alternative physical activity to excessive avoidance continuum, use of medication, alcohol/drugs) • Screening for socioenvironmental factors not spontaneously volunteered: – Social and living circumstances – Education and health literacy – Perceived support from home, work, friends – Financial issues • Screening for physical environmental factors not spontaneously volunteered: – Work and home environments – Exercise, training, sport load

(Continued)

Table 13.2 *(Continued)*

Intellectual standards for judging the quality of analytical thinking	Explanation of the standard	Examples when applied to the clinical examination and clinical reasoning
		• Screening for features in the clinical presentation that signal the need for precaution in the physical examination and treatment and need for further medical investigation: – Red flags – Severity of symptoms – Irritability of symptoms – Progression of problem (e.g., rapidly worsening condition) – Distress (e.g., anxiety associated with past clinical experiences) – Co-morbidities
Relevance and significance	Is the relevance and significance attributed to assessment findings justified?	• Relevance and significance attributed to physical impairment findings in physical examination (e.g., posture, active and passive movement, motor control, strength, sensorimotor function, muscle length, soft tissue, neurodynamics, neurological, fitness) can be guided by the following considerations: – Is the physical impairment symptomatic? – Is the physical impairment logically related to the activity and participation restrictions? – What is the extent of the physical impairment (e.g., compared to normal or the asymptomatic side)? – What is the effect of impairment modification or treatment? • Relevance and significance of psychological and social factors can be guided by the following considerations: – Relationship between patient's understanding of their problem and the meaning their understanding has to them with respect to their threat perception, expectations for recovery, expectations for management and their coping strategies. Each must then be judged regarding its relevance and significance (e.g., reasonable, adaptive perspective that may be contributing to the patient's resilience providing protection to maladaptive sensitization and persistence of symptoms versus an unhelpful perspective creating vulnerability and risk for maladaptive sensitization and persistent symptoms – see Edwards et al.[19]) – Relationship of any distress (e.g., anxiety, anger, fear, depression) to the patient's symptoms (historically and behaviorally) – Effect of patient's coping strategies on the symptoms, disability, and recovery – Effect of patient's perceived support on their symptoms, disability, and self-efficacy

Clarity, accuracy, and precision	Is the patient information obtained clear, accurate and precise?
	Is the clinician's analysis and reporting clear, accurate, and precise?
		• Clarity, accuracy, and precision of information obtained influences the quality of clinical reasoning analysis:
		– Recognizing the need to clarify patient answers for precision to ensure accuracy of information analyzed, for example:
		  – Area of symptoms
		  – Clarifying the aggravating activity for precision (e.g., what is it about the movement, activity, posture, that is the problem?)
		  – Clarity and precision regarding irritability of the symptom (e.g., how much it takes to aggravate, severity once aggravated, and time it takes to settle?)
		  – Clarity regarding the relationship of the symptom with other symptoms behaviorally and historically
		  – Clarity regarding explicit coping strategies used and their effectiveness

(Continued)

Table 13.2 *(Continued)*

Intellectual standards for judging the quality of analytical thinking	Explanation of the standard	Examples when applied to the clinical examination and clinical reasoning
		• Clarity, accuracy, and precision of clinician's analysis: – Is the diagnostic classification at an appropriate level of specificity? – Diagnostic specificity is greater for some peripheral contractile (e.g., hamstring), tendon (e.g., Achilles) and ligamentous (e.g., ACL) injuries, but poorer for body regions with anatomical complexity that prevents clinical tissue/structural diagnostic differentiation (e.g., shoulder, spine, hip) – Even when precise tissue source of symptoms cannot be clinically differentiated as in the shoulder, it is important to broadly differentiate between local somatic nociception, spinal somatic referral, visceral referral, neuropathic and vascular, and to rule out potential serious pathologies (fracture, dislocation, infection, malignancy)

Shared decision-making

While clinicians have specialized knowledge about different health problems, diagnostic and impairment tests and evidence-based management strategies, patients have specialized knowledge about their problem(s), personal circumstances, goals, and healthcare preferences. Shared decision-making (SDM), also called collaborative reasoning,[18] is a healthcare collaboration between the clinician and patient (and sometimes trusted family member, close friend or representative) in making choices about care based on provision of the clinician's analysis, evidence-based information about management, outcomes and uncertainties, and the patient's preferences.[10]

SDM draws from both sets of knowledge to assist the patient to make informed healthcare choices. It is particularly important in situations of uncertainty such as when no single option is clearly superior, when patient preferences are strong and when risk of harm exists.[9,29,30] It reflects a patient-centered philosophy of practice that promotes self-efficacy, motivation for change, and active patient participation rather than passive compliance.[16,22] SDM is also an ethical imperative regarding the rights of patients to participate in healthcare decisions promoted by national health policies, the World Health Organization, and international regulatory bodies.

Benefits

The importance of SDM is underscored by theory and evidence that patients who have been given an opportunity to share in healthcare decision-making are empowered to take greater responsibility for their own management, thereby creating greater autonomy and self-efficacy.[18,23,42,51] They are also likely to be more satisfied with their healthcare and achieve better, more meaningful outcomes.[2,23,25,42,56,57] Opportunity to participate will make some patients feel more valued and may facilitate greater motivation for change. Unfortunately, SDM is often poorly implemented in clinical practice[15,33,55] often limited to agreement on a specified plan of management or informed consent for a procedure.[9,18]

What does shared decision-making require?

SDM requires, or at least is benefited by, understanding of behavior change theory that can help clinicians understand patients' readiness and motivation for change and for collaborating and participating in therapy.

Behavior change theory

Behavior change is the modification or transformation of behavior. Behavior change science assumes that: 1) morbidity and mortality are due in part to certain behaviors, and 2) these behaviors are modifiable. There is now a great deal of evidence describing the negative impact of lifestyle factors such as smoking, lack of physical exercise, excessive alcohol intake, and poor diet on medical and musculoskeletal health.[39] Guidelines are available regarding the use of physical activity to promote health: "If physical activity were a drug, we would refer to it as a miracle cure, due to the great many illnesses it can prevent and help treat."[49]

Musculoskeletal clinicians are well placed to promote general health behavior in every contact, but also to use behavior change interventions to promote specific behaviors to help with the management of musculoskeletal conditions. There is a large and growing body of evidence, for example, to support the use of physiotherapist-led exercise in the management of rotator cuff-related shoulder pain. Adherence to home exercise regimes has been shown to be an important predictor of treatment outcome.[3] Despite this, adherence to home exercise is problematic, with 50–70% of people not adhering to their program.[1,48] It is possible that implementing strategies to improve adherence could lead to improved clinical outcomes.

Choosing a theory

There are many theoretical models that have been used to predict or change health behaviors, so choosing the right model is challenging. Following a comprehensive review of behavior change theories, 83 behavior theories were identified containing over 1600 constructs.[44] Capability, opportunity, and motivation have been identified in several models as the primary drivers of behavior change that are essential to address.[44]

Defining what needs to change

Once a target behavior (e.g., walk 10,000 steps/day) has been identified, the next step is to understand why that behavior might be difficult to adopt. Behaviors occur in the context of an individual's other behaviors and the behaviors of those around them. Understanding this complexity is important when developing behavior change interventions, and psychosocial, physical, and cultural factors need to be considered.[43]

Defining how to change it

Once the target behavior has been understood and the behavioral analysis has identified what needs to change, the behavior change wheel[46] (Figure 13.1) can help identify how to change it. This might be through enablement, training, education, modelling, and environmental restructuring. This allows the clinician or researcher to select the right behavior change technique, which is an intervention designed to alter or regulate behavior.[45] Behavior Change Technique Taxonomy (v1) describes 93 consensually agreed and distinct techniques, in 16 categories, that may be used to facilitate behavior change (Table 13.3). These techniques can be used alone or in conjunction with others. However, it is important to appreciate that, when combined, the effects might be interfering (negative), additive, or emergent. When selecting behavior change techniques it is important to ensure that the overall intervention remains practical, affordable, effective, acceptable, and safe.[43]

Well-described and defined behavior change interventions, developed using a theoretical framework, facilitate the accumulation of knowledge about behavior change and enable researchers and clinicians to replicate effective interventions in order to promote healthy behaviors and improve clinical outcomes.

If an individual receiving care is keen to lose weight but is unsure where to begin, the behavior change wheel can be used to develop an individualized behavior change intervention. Weight loss itself is not a behavior; however, several behaviors might be relevant to achieve this target, such as reducing the intake of high calorie foods and/or increasing physical activity. By exploring these behaviors with the person receiving care it may be possible to identify which behavior will yield the greatest return. Activity or food diaries can help provide deeper insight into these behaviors if initially unclear. Trying to change too many variables initially can be overwhelming and it is often more successful to introduce change gradually by targeting one behavior and building on small achievements.[43] If, for example, reducing intake of high calorie snacks is identified as the target behavior, a behavioral analysis using the COM-B model at the center of the behavior wheel will help identify exactly what needs to change.

The "capability" analysis may reveal a lack of understanding of the weekly calorific intake relating to regular snacking on high calorie foods. The "opportunity" analysis may identify social prompts that trigger snacking behavior. The behavioral intervention can then be designed using the relevant intervention functions such as education or environmental restructuring, and behavior change techniques can be selected from the taxonomy.[45] Providing "information about health consequences" and "restructuring the social environment" may be particularly appropriate to this scenario as well as techniques contained within the categories "goals and planning", "monitoring", and "social support".[45]

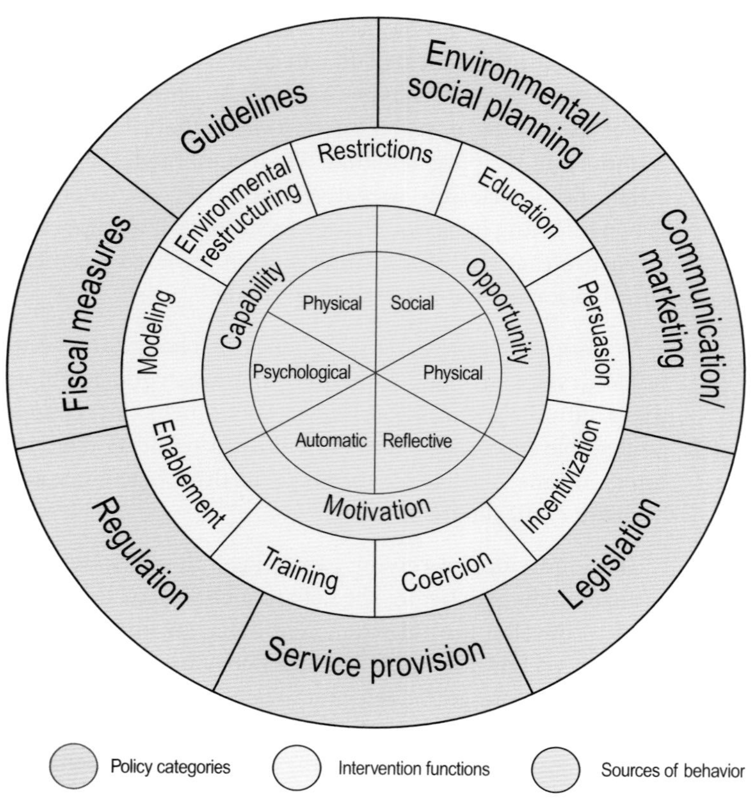

FIGURE 13.1

The Behavior Change Wheel, a framework for characterizing and designing behavior change interventions.

(Reproduced with permission from Michie et al. 2011.[46])

Table 13.3 An example of the categories of behavior change (BC) techniques with an example and descriptor for the category

Category of BC techniques	Example of BC technique within this group	Description of the BC technique
1. Goals and planning	1.2 Problem solving	Analyze, or prompt the person to analyze, factors influencing the behavior, and generate or select strategies that include overcoming barriers and/or increasing facilitators.
2. Feedback and monitoring	2.3 Self-monitoring of behavior	Establish a method for the person to monitor and record their behavior(s) as part of the behavior change strategy.
3. Social support	3.2 Social support (practical)	Advise on, arrange, or provide practical help for the performance of the behavior.
4. Shaping knowledge	4.1 Instruction on how to perform the behavior	Advise or agree on how to perform the behavior (includes skills training).

For a full summary of all 16 categories and 93 BC techniques see Michie et al 2013.[45]

Biopsychosocial practice

Implicit in shared decision-making is:

1) A biopsychosocial philosophy that accepts health problems are influenced by interwoven biological, psychological, social, and physical environmental factors (Figure 13.2) requiring assessment that explicitly evaluates each;[34,59] and
2) Management that promotes patient understanding, self-efficacy and participation.[16,34]

Better understanding of the person seeking care requires understanding of their personal life circumstances and their

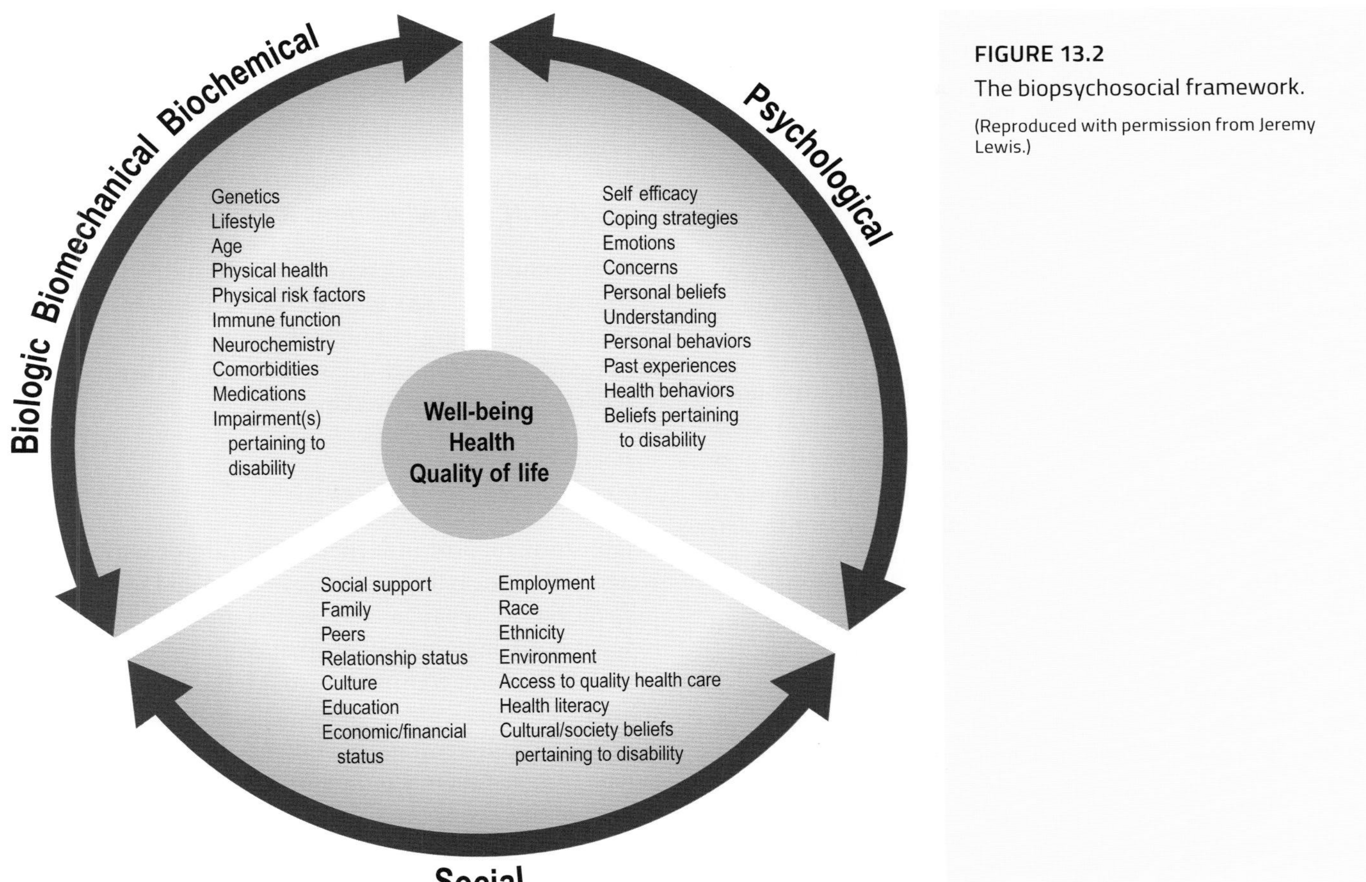

FIGURE 13.2
The biopsychosocial framework.
(Reproduced with permission from Jeremy Lewis.)

experiences living with their problem(s). Understanding patients' perspectives on their experiences includes exploring their understanding of their problem(s) and the meaning their understanding has to them with respect to their expectations for recovery, for management and for their participation and self-efficacy.[4] Analysis needs to consider any perceived threats (e.g., worsening of their condition) and the basis for those perceptions (e.g., past experiences, previous health problem explanations). Understanding the person also includes assessment of any distress they may be experiencing, the source(s) of the distress, the relationship between any distress and their problem(s)/symptom(s), and their coping strategies (e.g., medication, avoidance/load management, exercise). Factors such as high levels of distress, trauma, fear, excessive avoidance, catastrophizing, and perception of low self-worth increase a person's vulnerability, while social support, active coping strategies, acceptance and good self-efficacy promote resilience.[19,50]

Elements of shared decision-making

The elements of SDM include the following:[9,31,56]

- The problem is analyzed.
- Explanation that there is not always one simple method of management, as each patient's problem and personal circumstances are different necessitating an individualized approach.
- The patient is invited to collaborate in the decision-making process.
- Providing the patient with an initial explanation of your analysis of the problem, including factors you believe have contributed to the onset and maintenance of the problem.

- Explaining the treatment options including the process of natural recovery, and that one option is advice on self-management for a specified time (watch and wait) to judge whether additional therapeutic interventions are necessary.
- Elaborating on the benefits and potential harms of the different options with discussion, including opportunity to ask questions, regarding best practice (based on research and your experience) in the context of their preferences, values, and circumstances.

Communication skills are taught in all healthcare undergraduate courses, yet patients' dissatisfaction and complaints are often related to misunderstanding linked to poor communication.[56] It is beyond the scope of this chapter to cover all that comprises good communication and readers are referred to the following online resource for a succinct overview: https://cptbc.org/wp-content/uploads/2020/02/CPTBC-making-a-connection-2019.pdf. However, to provide a framework to illustrate opportunities and strategies to facilitate SDM through the full patient encounter (i.e., as opposed to only when considering treatment options) we summarize a strategy called the "Four Habits Approach to effective clinical communication"[23,54,40,42] (Table 13.4).

Table 13.4 The Four Habits Approach to effective communication for shared decision-making

Habit	Communication behaviors important to shared decision-making
1. Invest in the beginning	• Establishing rapport • Setting the scene • Eliciting full spectrum of patient concerns
2. Elicit the patient's perspective	• Exploring impact of problem(s) on the patient's life • Assessing psychosocial factors • Validating the patient's experiences and beliefs
3. Demonstrate empathy	• Being aware of and responding to the patient's emotions with empathy
4. Invest in the end	• Explanation of analysis • Shared decision-making • Discuss the options • Summarize agreed actions and plans

Adapted from Frankel and Stein[23,p.81] and Matthias, Salyers, and Frankel.[42,p.177]

Further detail relating to these communication behaviors important for SDM are presented in Chapter 11, which provides an in-depth discussion on communication.

Shared decision-making doesn't just happen: when does it start and what does it look like?

The communication behaviors outlined in the Four Habits Approach (Table 13.4) identify key aspects of clinicians' thinking and acting through the entire clinical encounter important to shared decision-making. There are areas where the Four Habits overlap.

Habit 1: establishing rapport

Establishing rapport influences patient information volunteered, willingness to participate in SDM and management, motivation for change and satisfaction.[21,25,38,42] Building rapport is an ongoing process that commences with initial introductions and continues through the examination and subsequent management. There are numerous ways rapport is enhanced but central are demonstrating interest in the person (not just their shoulder problem), empathy, and validation of their concerns.

Habit 1: setting the scene – an informed patient

Inform the patient of the anticipated duration of the consultation and what is planned. For example, you may consider saying, "First I would like to discuss your shoulder problem, how it started and how it's been affecting you; after that with your permission I would like to examine your shoulder. I will explain what I am doing at each stage. Following the assessment, I would like to sit down with you, present what I have learned and discuss with you the available management options and together we can decide the best way to move forwards."

Habit 1: eliciting the full spectrum of patient concerns

Once the patient's main problem(s) are established, clarify additional concerns, including screening other body areas and other symptoms. Clarification of relationships between problems assists in formulating priorities of assessment that can be discussed with the patient.

Habit 2: exploring impact of problem(s) on the patient's life

Valuable questions to consider include, "What is it like living with this problem?" and, "What would life look like (what would you be doing) if you didn't have this problem?" Understanding the impact on function and life participation provides a greater appreciation of the problem than only asking about aggravating and easing factors. It may also provide patient-specific outcome measures for planning short- and long-term goals.

Habit 2: assessing psychosocial factors

Understanding the person behind the problem requires a biopsychosocial approach that explicitly explores the patient's personal social/life circumstances and their perspectives on their problem/pain experiences.[4,26] Patient perspectives on their experiences and social influences (i.e., psychosocial status) incorporates:

- **Patients' understanding/beliefs:** it is important to explore what the symptoms (and diagnosis) mean to the patient regarding recovery, management, outcomes and participation during treatment, especially as patient beliefs and preferences may be based on incorrect or incomplete information.
- **Patients' evaluation of their problem(s):** this includes perception of seriousness, impact on daily life and the future, timescale, and ability to self-manage.
- **Patients' distress:** for example, anxiety, frustration, fear, anger, helplessness, and depression. Assessing the relationship of any distress to the patient's symptoms, both behaviorally and historically, helps determine whether the distress is contributing to the symptoms and disability or perhaps simply coexisting.
- **Patients' resilience resources:** for example, their disposition toward acceptance, problem-solving skills, active coping strategies and good self-efficacy.
- **Patients' coping behaviors and strategies:** for example, passive coping strategies such as excessive avoidance, rest, and medication, and passive treatments versus active coping strategies such as positive thinking, distracting one's attention from pain, pacing, and using physical pain-reducing techniques such as relaxation, exercises and stretching. Key to the clinician's analysis, and later patient explanation, is whether the coping strategies are adaptive (i.e., appropriate for the current stage of the problem) or maladaptive (i.e., unhelpful to the recovery).
- **Patients' goals:** explicit assessment of a patient's goals provides further insight to their expectations for recovery and what is important to them to address and achieve. Assessing goals also provides an opportunity for SDM and participation. Patients can be asked to rank different functional goals by importance and to help break broader goals down into smaller sub-goals. The well-known acronym SMART (or SMARTER) goals is important to ensure the patient is actively involved in decisions made:
  - Specific
  - Measurable
  - Achievable
  - Relevant
  - Time bound
  - Evaluated
  - Reviewed
- **Patients' willingness and ability to change:** patients vary considerably in their motivation for change. Principles of motivational interviewing can be employed to evaluate the importance of change to the patient and their self-efficacy to positively contribute to change.[47]

Habit 2: validating synthesized understanding

Brief summaries of information synthesized (e.g., "Let me see if I have this right" or "I want to make sure I understand", give the patient the opportunity to validate your understanding while also demonstrating empathy.[24]

Habit 3: being aware and responding to patients' emotions with empathy

In a clinical context, empathy refers to clinicians' cognitive abilities to understand what their patients are experiencing and imaginatively project themselves into their patients' situations.[6] When applied in practice, patients are more likely to feel they have been given a voice, heard and believed, thus strengthening the therapeutic alliance important to SDM.[42] Empathic responses, be they expressions (e.g., "that must be difficult") or appropriate touch, provide affirmation and support of the patient's concerns and emotions. Matthias, Salyers and Frankel[42] highlight research demonstrating positive effects of empathy including: "...therapeutic alliance, improved coping, increased trust, improved relationship and satisfaction, reduced pain and even a positive impact on physiological processes".

Habit 4: explanation of analysis

Patients need a clear understanding of their problem(s) including the likely cause or contributing factors. Information may be presented verbally, textually, and/or audio-visually, depending of the individual's preference(s). Key physical impairments should be explained and environmental and psychosocial factors that may be contributing to the presentation should be discussed. Explanations must be free of jargon, meaningfully linked to the patient's presentation and circumstances, and re-assessed for understanding.

Habit 4: interest in shared decision-making

SDM is a continuum with respect to the extent of patient participation.[31] Some patients, possibly based on previous paternalistic healthcare encounters, may not be aware of SDM, or, due to a number of reasons may choose not to participate in the process. While this may change following thorough assessment, explanation, and invitation to participate, autonomy includes exercising the right to relinquish some autonomy and be "directed".[18] The key is ensuring the patient is fully informed of the required assessments and management options and given opportunity to ask questions and discuss their preferences and concerns. Once given this information the patient can relinquish decision-making, although active participation in management should still be encouraged to optimize outcomes and minimize recurrence. For example, management of shoulder pain and minimization of recurrence is improved when the patient can problem-solve regarding load management in their activities of daily living, especially in unusual or unfamiliar activities where there is greater risk the load on the shoulder may exceed their load capacity (strength). Equipped with this knowledge, the patient is better able to either pace a high-risk activity or alter the activity itself (e.g., using a ladder for sustained overhead tasks).

Habit 4: discuss the options

Discussion of management options should include reference to research, best practice guidelines, and personal experience with appropriate explanation that all guidelines need to be tailored to patients' individual clinical presentations and personal circumstances.[35] Likely benefits, uncertainties, and potential harms of options should be discussed, including the concept of recovery through natural history and the option to continue with guided self-management alone.[31]

Discussion regarding exercise dosage should include what is realistic with respect to the patient's lifestyle and any barriers it may present. Explicitly asking about potential barriers upfront (e.g., "What might prevent you from carrying out this plan?") not only facilitates SDM but also promotes problem solving (an important active coping strategy) around strategies to address barriers.

Decision support aids, like clinical guidelines, are based on research evidence, but are developed to inform and assist patients in forming their management preference.[10,29,53,58] These are typically presented visually and have been produced for people with partial rotator cuff tears.[14]

Habit 4: summarize agreed actions and plans

While time is an issue in clinical practice, "investing in the end", like investing in the beginning, will reinforce the therapeutic alliance established through the encounter and further promote SDM. At a minimum, a summary of agreed actions and plans should be reviewed, ideally with a written summary of any agreed and practiced self-management and advice.

Bringing it all together

Box 13.1 The behavioral analysis – adopting a home exercise program for RCRSP

Emily, a 38-year-old woman with a 9-month history of increasingly severe right-sided rotator cuff related shoulder pain presented for physiotherapy. Her functional limitations included significant sleep disturbance and inability to play with her children (aged 5 and 7). She recently left her job as a caregiver due to her pain as well as conflict with her unsupportive employer. She has experienced an increase in anxiety and depression (on a background of chronic depression) since the onset of her shoulder pain. She described financial challenges due to the inability to work and felt trapped by her circumstances.

A thorough examination explored the full spectrum of Emily's concerns and the impact these had on her family, work, and social life followed by a comprehensive physical examination. The thoroughness and empathetic manner combined with the clinician's validation of their understanding of Emily's experiences created an excellent rapport giving her confidence and motivation to proceed with the agreed management plan and goals.

1. **Capability:** Emily describes herself as a non-exerciser. Thinking about doing exercises with her painful shoulder makes her "worried that I'll do it wrong or look stupid". She understands why it is important and recognizes that the weakness in her shoulder is an issue and that it needs to be stronger to do her physical job, but she is very fearful of making the pain worse. She is "not sure how I'll manage if it gets any worse". The behavioral intervention needs to address physical skill and overcoming mental obstacles to perform the behavior.
2. **Motivation:** Emily understands that physiotherapy can help due to her positive experience in the past. She also sees clients at work responding to physiotherapy (positive social norm). She believes it will work but has great difficulty motivating herself due to her depression. The behavioral intervention needs to address behavioral planning and habit formation.
3. **Opportunity:** she is not working now and has the opportunity (time, space, supportive husband) to perform the behavior. She believes the exercises will be helpful. Opportunity will be addressed by providing access to equipment and the use of triggers and reminders.

Intervention functions

Physical and physiological capability will be addressed through training, education, and enablement. Automatic motivation will be addressed through training and environmental restructuring and opportunity will be addressed through restructuring the environment and enablement.

Behavior change techniques

An empathic encouraging ("Social support (unspecified) (behavior change technique 3.1"[45]) collaborative approach to "Goal setting (behavior) (1.1)"[45] incorporating the patient's preferences was adopted. Emily described a preference for a more prescriptive exercise dose ("Action planning 1.4")[45] as she felt making less decisions regarding the sets and repetitions at each exercise session would remove a mental obstacle. Three exercises were identified that related to Emily's functional restrictions and these were demonstrated and rehearsed with feedback in the clinic ("Behavioral practice/rehearsal 8.1")[45] to increase confidence and physical skill.

The meaning of pain or discomfort during exercise was reframed ("Framing/Reframing 13.2")[45] as a sensitive protective response, not indicating injury or damage. Clear guidance and reassurance ("Social support (unspecified) 3.1")[45] was provided regarding the expected sensations using the pain-monitoring model to build confidence. Through discussion with Emily, it was decided that "instruction on how to perform the behavior 4.1"[45] be provided in the form of a video of Emily performing the exercises with voiceover from the physiotherapist providing

(Continued)

guidance, reassurance and encouragement ("Social support (unspecified) 3.1").[45] Watching video of herself performing the exercises in the clinic under supervision may help Emily to overcome mental obstacles and reinforce expected sensory experience.

At the second consultation, home exercise concordance was discussed and the "discrepancy between current behavior and goal (1.6)"[45] was discussed in an empathic manner. Emily did not feel that the use of an exercise diary ("self-monitoring of the behavior 2.3")[45] would be helpful: "I know if I've done them, I don't need a diary for that." Emily was able to provide a clear account of why she fell short of her planned exercise dose and explained that some days her depression saps all motivation. In addition, she found the evenings difficult due to fatigue, and although her husband was around to help with the children and to provide support, she felt that earlier in the day would be easier ("problem solving 1.2").[45] Through collaborative "review [of the] behavior goal(s)(1.5)"[45] a new goal of daily exercise was set. Emily decided to perform the exercises at lunchtime to facilitate "Habit formation (8.3)" by prompting rehearsal and repetition in the same context so that the context starts to elicit the behavior. She "restructured the environment 12.2"[45] by attaching the resistance bands in the kitchen and leaving them in place and set up phone reminders to trigger the behavior ("prompts/cues 7.1").[45]

Behavior change interventions describe the content but not the mode of delivery. Behavior change interventions were tailored to the individual and delivered in a person-centered manner within a framework of positive empathic communication.

Conclusion

Clinical reasoning and shared decision-making are essential competencies in clinical practice. Like all analytical thinking, clinical reasoning is driven by a guiding purpose (e.g., understand the patient's health problems and their experiences to inform health education and best management). Pattern recognition is a recognized feature of expert practice but also a cause of reasoning error when the clinician's analysis is reduced to a few common patterns, highlighting the importance of combining pattern recognition with more deliberative hypothesis testing. Clinical reasoning is underpinned by key biopsychosocial and musculoskeletal theory and concepts essential to accurate judgments. All humans are subject to bias; awareness of common assumptions in clinical practice and in your own reasoning can enhance the accuracy and precision of information obtained and judgments made. Similarly, awareness and critique of your point of view or practice perspective (e.g., biomedical versus biopsychosocial, preferred clinical approach) are elements of skilled analytical thinking that facilitate change and growth in practice.

Using the COM-B model can help clinicians understand an individual's capability, opportunity, and motivation for change. This understanding can help facilitate behavior change through a collaborative process using a tailored behavior change intervention composed of individual techniques that are appropriate and meaningful for that individual, enhancing their desire for change.

Shared decision-making (SDM) is a collaboration between the patient and clinician that occurs throughout the patient encounter. SDM is enhanced through the development of rapport, thorough assessment of patients' concerns, explanations of the clinical process, attending to the patient's perspective, empathy and clear explanation of the clinician's analysis and management options. Successful SDM may empower patients to take greater responsibility in their management, creating greater autonomy and self-efficacy with better, more meaningful outcomes.

References

1. Alexandre NMC, Nordin M, Hiebert R, Campello M. Predictors of compliance with short-term treatment among patients with back pain. Rev Panam Salud Publica. 2002;12:86-94.
2. Arnetz JE, Almin I, Bergström K, Franzén Y, Nilsson H. Active patient involvement in the establishment of physical therapy goals: Effects on treatment outcome and quality of care. Advances in Physiotherapy. 2004;6:50-69.
3. Beinart NA, Goodchild CE, Weinman JA, Ayis S, Godfrey EL. Individual and intervention-related factors associated with adherence to home exercise in chronic low back pain: a systematic review. Spine J. 2013;13:1940-1950.
4. Beneciuk JM, George SZ, Jones MA. Assessment, reasoning and management of psychological factors in musculoskeletal practice. In: Jones MA, Rivett DA (eds). Clinical Reasoning in Musculoskeletal Practice, 4th edition. Edinburgh: Elsevier; 2019:71-88.
5. Boshuizen HPA, Schmidt HG. The development of clinical reasoning expertise. In: Higgs J, Jensen G, Loftus S, Christensen N (eds). Clinical Reasoning in the Health Professions, 4th edition. Edinburgh: Elsevier; 2019.
6. Braude HD. Conciliating cognition and consciousness: the perceptual foundations of clinical reasoning. Journal of Evaluation in Clinical Practice. 2012;18:945-950.
7. Christensen N, Jensen GM. Developing clinical reasoning capability. In: Higgs J, Jensen G, Loftus S, Christensen N (eds). Clinical Reasoning in the Health Professions, 4th edition. Edinburgh: Elsevier; 2019:435-443.
8. Christensen N, Jones MA, Rivett DA. Strategies to facilitate clinical reasoning development. In: Jones MA, Rivett DA (eds). Clinical Reasoning in Musculoskeletal Practice, 4th edition. Edinburgh: Elsevier; 2019:562-282.
9. Costanzo C, Doll J, Jensen GM. Shared decision making in practice. In: Higgs J, Jensen G, Loftus S, Christensen N, eds. Clinical Reasoning in the Health Professions, 4th edition. Edinburgh: Elsevier; 2019:181-190.
10. Coulter A, Collins A. Making shared decision-making a reality. No decision about me, without me. Available at: https://www.kingsfund.org.uk/sites/default/files/Making-shared-decision-making-a-reality-paper-Angela-Coulter-Alf-Collins-July-2011_0.pdf.
11. Croskerry P. Clinical cognition and diagnostic error: applications of a dual process model of reasoning. Adv Health Sci Educ Theory Pract. 2009;14 Suppl 1:27-35.
12. Croskerry P. The importance of cognitive errors in diagnosis and strategies to minimize them. Acad Med. 2003;78:775-780.
13. Croskerry P. A universal model of diagnostic reasoning. Acad Med. 2009;84:1022-1028.
14. Deville G, Gibson J, Lewis J, Guémann M. A patient decision aid to facilitate shared decision-making for patients with shoulder pain associated with a non-traumatic rotator cuff tear. Kinésithérapie. 2020;20:9-21.
15. Dierckx K, Deveugele M, Roosen P, Devisch I. Implementation of shared decision making in physical therapy: observed level of involvement and patient preference. Phys Ther. 2013;93:1321-1330.
16. Dukhu S, Purcell C, Bulley C. Person-centred care in the physiotherapeutic management of long-term conditions: a critical review of components, barriers and facilitators. International Practice Development Journal. 2018;8:1-27.
17. Edwards I, Jones M. Clinical reasoning and expert practice. In: Jensen G, Gwyer J, Hack L, Shepard K, (eds). Expertise in Physical Therapy Practice, 2nd edition. St. Louis: Saunders Elsevier; 2007:192-213.
18. Edwards I, Jones M, Higgs J, Trede F, Jensen G. What is collaborative reasoning? Advances in Physiotherapy. 2004;6:70-83.
19. Edwards RR, Dworkin RH, Sullivan MD, Turk DC, Wasan AD. The role of psychosocial processes in the development and maintenance of chronic pain. The Journal of Pain. 2016;17:T70-T92.
20. Elder L, Paul R. The Thinker's Guide to Analytic Thinking. Tomales, California: Foundation for Critical Thinking Press; 2016.
21. Ferreira PH, Ferreira ML, Maher CG, Refshauge KM, Latimer J, Adams RD. The therapeutic alliance between clinicians and patients predicts outcome in chronic low back pain. Phys Ther. 2013;93:470-478.
22. Fish D, De Cossart L. Clinical thinking, client expectations and patient-centred care. In: Higgs J, Jensen G, Loftus S, Christensen N (eds). Clinical Reasoning in the Health Professions, 4th edition. Edinburgh: Elsevier; 2019:97-107.
23. Frankel RM, Stein T. Getting the most out of the clinical encounter: The four habits model. The Permanente Journal. 1999;3:79-88.
24. Garber MB, Boissonnault WG. The patient interview: The science behind the art of skillful communication. In: Boissonnault WG, VanWye WR (eds). Primary Care for the Physical Therapist: Examination and Triage. St Louis: Elsevier; 2021:39-48.
25. Hall AM, Ferreira PH, Maher CG, Latimer J, Ferreira ML. The influence of the therapist-patient relationship on treatment outcome in physical rehabilitation: a systematic review. Phys Ther. 2010;90:1099-1110.
26. Hammerich AS, Scherer SA, Jones MA. Influence of stress, coping and social factors on pain and disability in musculoskeletal practice. In: Jones MA, Rivett DA (eds). Clinical Reasoning in Musculoskeletal Practice, 2nd edition. Edinburgh: Elsevier; 2019:47-70.
27. Harris P, Nagy S, Vardaxis N. Mosby's Dictionary of Medicine, Nursing and Health Professions, 3rd edition. Edinburgh: Elsevier; 2014.
28. Hawkins D, Elder L, Paul R. The Thinker's Guide to Clinical Reasoning. Tomales, California: Foundation for Critical Thinking Press; 2010.
29. Hoffmann TC, Del Mar CB. Patient expectations of the benefits and harms of treatments, screening, and tests: a systematic review. JAMA Intern Med. 2015;175(2):274-286.
30. Hoffmann TC, Legare F, Simmons MB, et al. Shared decision making: what do clinicians need to know and why should they bother? Med J Aust. 2014;201:35-39.
31. Hoffmann TC, Lewis J, Maher CG. Shared decision making should be an integral part of physiotherapy practice. Physiotherapy. 2020;107:43-49.
32. Jensen GM, Resnick L, Haddad A. Expertise and clinical reasoning. In: Higgs J, Jensen G, Loftus S, Christensen N, eds. Clinical Reasoning in the Health Professions, 4th edition. Edinburgh: Elsevier; 2019:67-76.
33. Jones LE, Roberts LC, Little PS, Mullee MA, Cleland JA, Cooper C. Shared decision-

making in back pain consultations: an illusion or reality? Eur Spine J. 2014;23 Suppl 1:S13-19.

34. Jones MA. Clinical reasoning: Fast and slow thinking in musculoskeletal practice. In: Jones MA, Rivett DA (eds). Clinical Reasoning in Musculoskeletal Practice, 2nd edition. Edinburgh: Elsevier; 2019.

35. Jones MA, Grimmer K, Edwards I, Higgs J, Trede F. Challenges in applying best evidence to physiotherapy. Internet Journal of Allied Health Science Practice. 2006;4:1-8.

36. Kahneman D. Thinking, Fast and Slow. London: Allen Lane; 2011.

37. Kaufmann DR, Yoskowitz NA, Patel VL. Clinical reasoning and biomedical knowledge: Implications for teaching. In: Higgs J, Jensen G, Loftus S, Christensen N (eds). Clinical Reasoning in the Health Professions, 4th edition. Edinburgh: Elsevier; 2019.

38. Klaber Moffett JA, Richardson PH. The influence of the physiotherapist–patient relationship on pain and disability. Physiotherapy Theory and Practice. 1997;13:89-96.

39. Loef M, Walach H. The combined effects of healthy lifestyle behaviors on all cause mortality: a systematic review and meta-analysis. Prev Med. 2012;55:163-170.

40. Lundeby T, Gulbrandsen P, Finset A. The expanded four habits model: a teachable consultation model for encounters with patients in emotional distress. Patient Education and Counseling. 2015;98:598-603.

41. Marcum JA. An integrated model of clinical reasoning: dual-process theory of cognition and metacognition. Journal of Evaluation in Clinical Practice. 2012;18:954-961.

42. Matthias MS, Salyers MP, Frankel RM. Re-thinking shared decision-making: context matters. Patient Education and Counseling 2013;91:176-179.

43. Michie S, Atkins L, West RT. The Behaviour Change Wheel: A Guide to Designing Interventions. London: Silverback Publishing; 2014.

44. Michie S, Campbell R, Brown J, West R, Gainforth H. ABC of Theories of Behavior Change. London: Silverback Publishing; 2014.

45. Michie S, Richardson M, Johnston M, et al. The behavior change technique taxonomy (v1) of 93 hierarchically clustered techniques: building an international consensus for the reporting of behavior change interventions. Ann Behav Med. 2013;46:81-95.

46. Michie S, van Stralen MM, West R. The behaviour change wheel: A new method for characterising and designing behaviour change interventions. Implementation Science. 2011;6:42.

47. Miller WR, Rollnick S. Motivational Interviewing: Helping People Change, 3rd edition. New York: Guilford Publications; 2012.

48. Nelson BW, O'Reilly E, Miller M, Hogan M, Wegner JA, Kelly C. The clinical effects of intensive, specific exercise on chronic low back pain: a controlled study of 895 consecutive patients with 1-year follow up. Orthopedics. 1995;18:971-981.

49. Department of Health and Social Care. UK Chief Medical Officers' Physical Activity Guidelines. Available at: https://assets.publishing.service.gov.uk/government/uploads/system/uploads/attachment_data/file/832868/uk-chief-medical-officers-physical-activity-guidelines.pdf.

50. Pincus T, McCracken LM. Psychological factors and treatment opportunities in low back pain. Best Pract Res Clin Rheumatol. 2013;27:625-635.

51. Sandman L, Munthe C. Shared decision-making and patient autonomy. Theor Med Bioeth. 2009;30:289-310.

52. Schwartz A, Kostopoulou O. Clinical reasoning in medicine. In: Higgs J, Jensen G, Loftus S, Christensen N (eds). Clinical Reasoning in the Health Professions, 4th edition. Edinburgh: Elsevier; 2019.

53. Stacey D, Légaré F, Lewis K, et al. Decision aids for people facing health treatment or screening decisions. Cochrane Database Syst Rev. 2017;4:CD001431.

54. Stein T, Krupat E, Frankel R. Talking with patients: using the four habits model. The Permanente Medical Group. 2011.

55. Stenner R, Swinkels A, Mitchell T, Palmer S. Exercise prescription for patients with non-specific chronic low back pain: a qualitative exploration of decision making in physiotherapy practice. Physiotherapy. 2016;102:332-338.

56. Trede F, Higgs J. Collaborative decision making in liquid times. In: Higgs J, Jensen G, Loftus S, Christensen N (eds). Clinical Reasoning in the Health Professions, 4th edition. Edinburgh: Elsevier; 2019:159-168.

57. Trede F, Higgs J. Collaborative decision making. In: Higgs J, Jones MA, Loftus S, Christensen N (eds). Clinical Reasoning in the Health Professions, 3rd edition. Amsterdam: Butterworth Heinemann Elsevier; 2008:31-41.

58. Trevena L, McCaffrey K. Using decision aids to involve clients in clinical decision making. In: Higgs J, Jensen G, Loftus S, Christensen N (eds). Clinical Reasoning in the Health Professions, 4th edition. Edinburgh: Elsevier; 2019:191-200.

59. World Health Organization. International Classification of Functioning, Disability and Health. Geneva: World Health Organization; 2001.

The role of imaging, blood tests, EMG, and nerve conduction 14

Caroline Alexander, Gajan Rajeswaran, Sanjay Vijayanathan, Dana Lewis, Ann Cools

Introduction

The appropriate use of imaging, blood tests, and electromyographic recordings of muscle activity supports the clinical examination and management of musculoskeletal conditions involving the shoulder. This chapter describes these investigative techniques, using case studies to contextualize their use.

Imaging of the shoulder

Imaging of the shoulder allows assessment and diagnosis of pathology not visible on clinical examination to aid management. Techniques include plain radiograph, ultrasound, computed tomography (CT) and magnetic resonance imaging (MRI), each with advantages and disadvantages dependent on the patient demography, history, and local infrastructure.

Radiograph and CT images are generated by passing X-rays from a source, through the shoulder and onto a digital detector. X-rays are a part of the electromagnetic spectrum (which includes visible light) and are a form of ionizing radiation. The average annual human exposure to natural background radiation from the sun and earth is about 2.4 millisievert (mSv) per year, which is equivalent to 125 chest X-rays.[35] High radiation doses can increase the risk of cancer, but given that the lifetime risk of cancer in the UK is now 1 in 2 people, most medical ionizing radiation exposures will not significantly affect this risk.[41] This is particularly true of a shoulder radiograph (radiation dose of only 0.01 mSv), but the use of shoulder CT (radiation dose of 2.4 to 2.8 mSv) should be undertaken with more caution, particularly in patients who are more susceptible to ionizing radiation.[4,18] For comparison, a return flight to New York, USA from London, UK is equivalent to 0.6 mSv.

Ionizing radiation medical exposure regulations (IRMER) are in place to ensure that radiographs are performed only when needed and using the lowest radiation dose possible. Ultrasound and MRI are imaging tests that do not involve ionizing radiation and are therefore not subject to these regulations and considerations. Some patients will become claustrophobic while having an imaging test, most commonly with MRI. For people known to be claustrophobic, open scanners are available which permit the patient to sit, but produce images of lower quality than conventional MRI.

There are contraindications to imaging that need to be considered. MRI involves placing the patient in a strong magnetic field, so metallic objects within or on the patient might move or heat up during the scan with potentially devastating consequences. It is the responsibility of the referrer to mention these at referral and the patient should be screened again for these prior to entering the scanner. Many newer surgical prostheses such as joint arthroplasties are now MRI compatible, so the details of the device are needed to determine if a scan may be undertaken. Their biggest drawback is the causation of artefact obscuring the area being scanned. Pacemakers may also be MRI compatible and, in some institutions, patients with pacemakers may undergo an MRI scan with appropriate cardiac monitoring.

Incidental findings or "incidentalomas" are findings discovered on an imaging test unrelated to the clinical presentation responsible for the test, and for which the patient is asymptomatic at the time.[31] These may cause significant anxiety for the patient, with an indeterminate diagnosis potentially leading to further/follow-up imaging, biopsy or surgery, each with potential harms and uncertainties.[34] Incidental findings occur with sufficient frequency that it is good practice for clinicians referring for imaging to discuss the possibility of incidental findings with the patient,[46] and include a statement on the imaging report relating to findings observed in people without symptoms.

Imaging costs vary widely. For the purpose of comparison, in a local London, UK National Health Service (NHS) hospital, the tariffs for imaging tests are currently: radiograph – £35 (US $48); diagnostic ultrasound – £71 (US $97); ultrasound-guided injection – £103 (US $140); CT – £169 (US $230); MRI – £268 (US $365).[43] When deciding which imaging test is most appropriate and to ensure healthcare sustainability,[26] the variations in cost should be considered. We will discuss the criteria to consider when choosing a test and illustrate this using clinical scenarios.

Cases

Subacromial pain syndrome

A 53-year-old woman with left-sided shoulder pain presents with what appears to be subacromial pain syndrome. This only requires imaging if nonsurgical management does not achieve the desired goals in an acceptable timeframe. The purpose of imaging in this case is to exclude differential diagnoses and to assess severity of any pathology in order to support treatment plans.[24]

Given its low cost, ready availability and relatively low radiation dose, a shoulder radiograph can be useful as a first-line imaging test, particularly to demonstrate differential diagnoses of glenohumeral osteoarthritis or calcific tendinopathy. Ultrasound imaging may demonstrate a range of findings that suggest subacromial bursitis, tendinosis, partial and full thickness tears, calcification, spur formation, degenerative changes in the acromioclavicular (AC) joint and humeral head (Figure 14.1). Ultrasound provides excellent spatial resolution of the soft tissue structures and given its relatively low cost and no radiation, is probably the best first-line test. If required, a guided injection may be administered concomitantly (see Chapter 23).

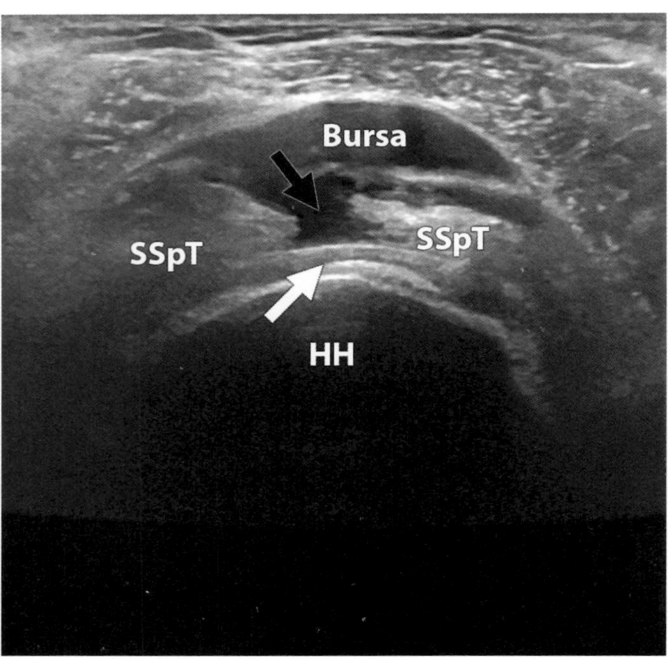

FIGURE 14.1
53-year-old female with left-sided shoulder pain. Transverse section ultrasound image demonstrating severe bursitis with fluid distension of the subacromial-subdeltoid bursa (Bursa) and extension of the fluid into a full thickness supraspinatus tendon (SSpT) tear (black arrow) with the fluid outlining the articular cartilage (white arrow) of the humeral head (HH).

MRI is also an excellent imaging test for subacromial pain syndrome, demonstrating the same pathology as ultrasound though not dynamically. It is much better than ultrasound for assessing the articular, osseous, and muscular pathology (Figure 14.2).

Although calcific tendinopathy is observable in radiographs (Figure 14.3), it is arguable that ultrasound is the best imaging modality to evaluate for the presence and progression of calcification. It shows the intratendinous calcification at its earliest stage and can be used to guide treatment such as barbotage, aspiration and bursal injection (see Chapter 27). It is not particularly effective in assessing for adhesive periarthritis and intraosseous loculation.

CT has no real role in calcific tendinopathy, offering little diagnostic advantage over a radiograph but considerably more radiation dose and cost. It will effectively demonstrate extrusion of the calcification into the bone (intraosseous loculation) and should be considered only for those patients where the presence of intraosseous loculation would affect management and which has not been demonstrated by other imaging tests.

MRI can demonstrate intratendinous calcification but is not as sensitive as ultrasound, and given its much higher cost and reduced availability should only be considered in patients who have not responded to nonsurgical management or in whom the diagnosis of frozen shoulder and intraosseous or dumbbell loculation (where the coracoacromial ligament compresses semisolid sub-bursal calcifications producing a dumbbell configuration) would affect clinical management.

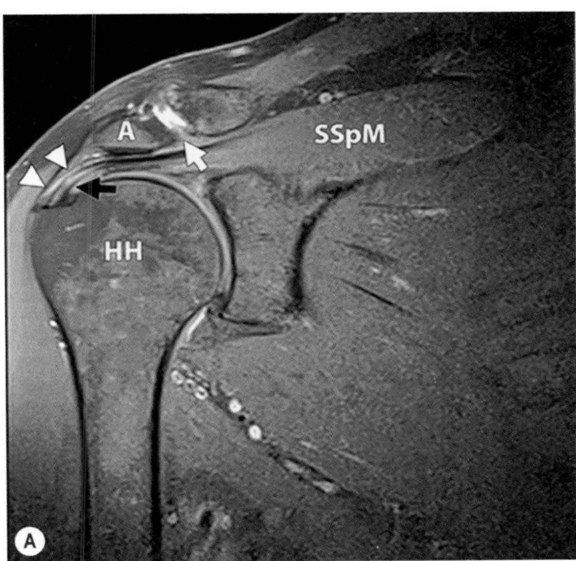

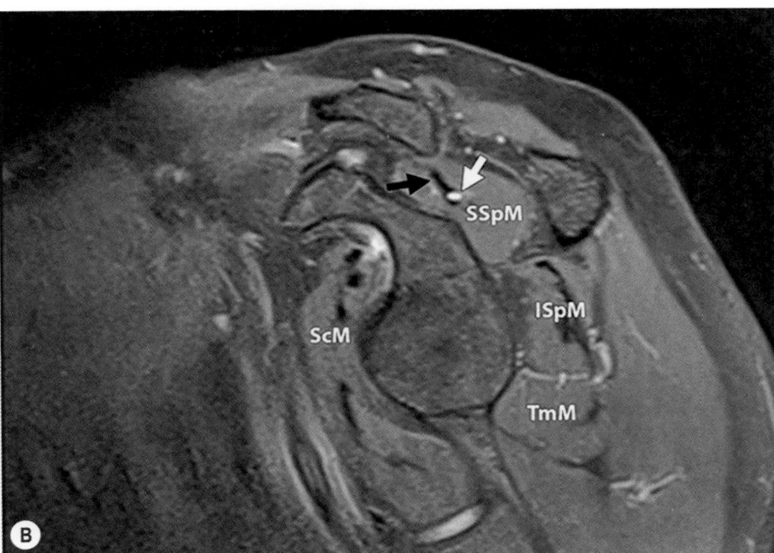

FIGURE 14.2
46-year-old male with right shoulder pain. (A) Coronal fat saturated proton density MRI demonstrating subacromial-subdeltoid bursitis (white arrowheads), AC joint degenerative change and capsulitis (white arrow) as well as supraspinatus tendinopathy and a partial thickness intrasubstance delamination tear (black arrow). (B) Sagittal fat saturated proton density image at the level of the rotator cuff muscles (medial to A) demonstrating that the supraspinatus tendon intrasubstance delamination tear extends to involve the musculotendinous junction of the muscle with a tubular T2 high signal cyst (white arrow) adjacent to the intramuscular tendon (black arrow). This would be difficult to assess with ultrasound. HH, humeral head; ISpM, infraspinatus muscle; ScM, subscapularis muscle; SSpM, supraspinatus muscle; TmM, teres minor muscle.

Adhesive capsulitis (frozen shoulder)

A 56-year-old male presents with left nondominant side shoulder pain and restricted range of motion, particularly in active and passive external rotation. Frozen shoulder is suspected clinically. Here, MRI is the best imaging test to support the clinical hypothesis, usually demonstrating a glenohumeral joint effusion, axillary recess inflammatory change and soft tissue thickening in the rotator interval (Figure 14.4). However, given its high cost, it is usually only used in recalcitrant cases.

The role of ultrasound in frozen shoulder is primarily to guide injections into the glenohumeral joint and the subacromial bursa, as well as guided hydrodilatation procedures rather than to support diagnosis. Typically, nothing abnormal is detected in radiographs of people with frozen shoulders and they are often used to exclude glenohumeral joint osteoarthritis, which is a differential diagnosis. The classical features of the radiograph for osteoarthritis are joint space loss (due to articular cartilage damage), marginal osteophyte formation, subchondral sclerosis and subchondral cystic change.[23] The joint changes are predominantly posterior and the marginal osteophytes are proportionate to the degree of joint space loss (Figure 14.5).[19] These findings are different when compared to an inflammatory arthritis, such as rheumatoid arthritis. Here the joint changes would be concentric rather than predominantly posterior, and marginal osteophytes are small in proportion to the degree of joint space loss with periarticular osteopenia.[23]

Septic arthritis

A 56-year-old male presents with left shoulder pain, swelling, fever and malaise. Although relatively uncommon in the shoulder, septic arthritis is suspected. The best first-line

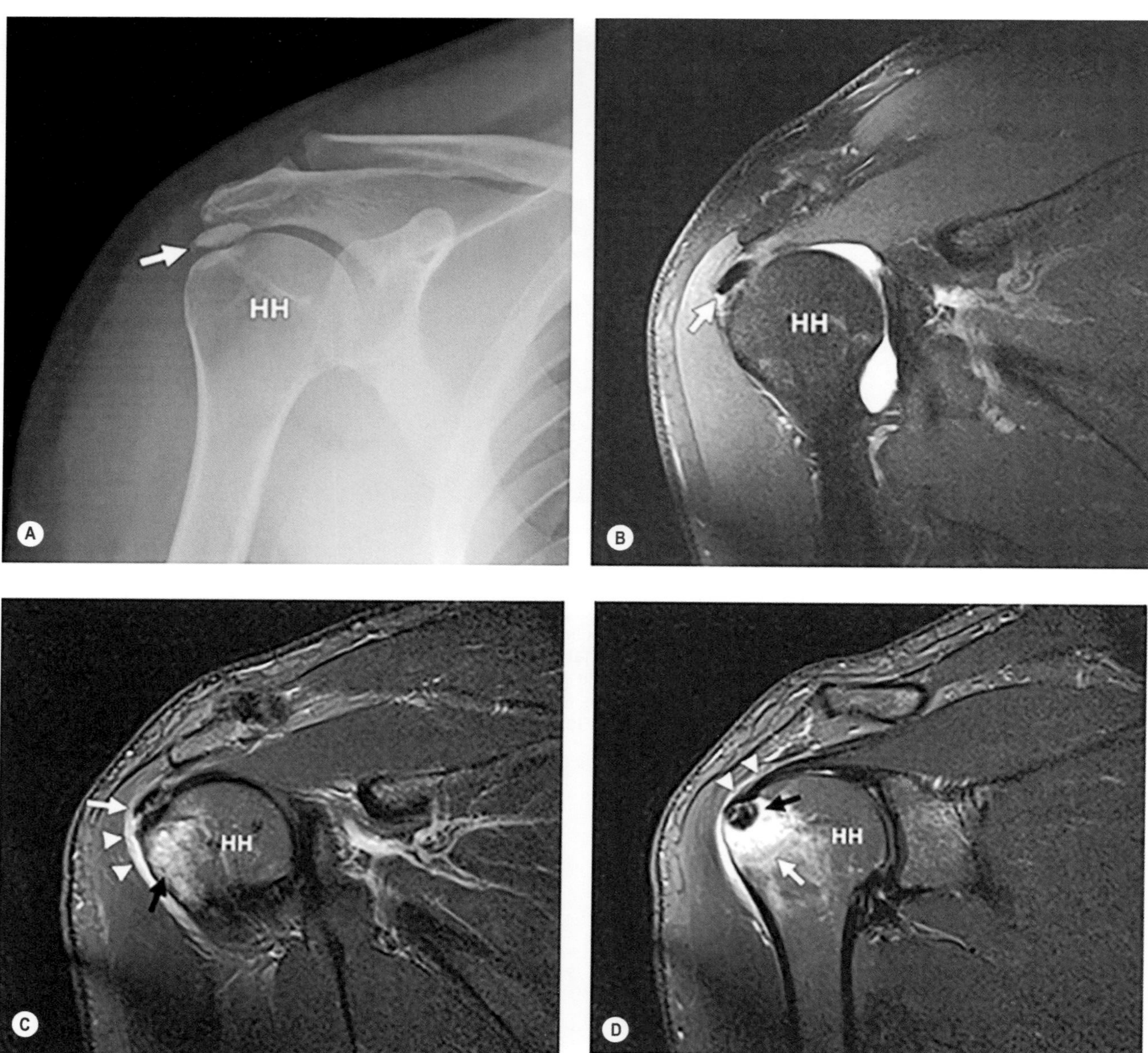

FIGURE 14.3

51-year-old female with acute right shoulder pain. (A) Anterior-posterior radiograph demonstrating an oval shaped focus of soft tissue calcification in the expected position of the supraspinatus tendon, consistent with calcific tendinopathy (arrow). (B) Coronal fat saturated proton density MRI confirming that the soft tissue calcification on the radiograph is within the supraspinatus tendon (arrow). (C) Coronal short tau inversion recovery (STIR) MRI image performed 17 months after recurrence of acute right shoulder pain demonstrating persistent supraspinatus calcific tendinopathy (white arrow), marked subacromial-subdeltoid bursitis (white arrowheads) and new humeral head (HH) bone marrow edema near the tendon insertion (black arrow). (D) Coronal STIR MRI slightly posterior to (C) confirming the presence of adhesive periarthritis secondary to the calcific tendinitis with florid bone marrow edema (white arrow) within the humeral head (HH) as well as intraosseous loculation of calcification (black arrow) adjacent to the supraspinatus tendon (white arrowheads) insertion. These findings would be difficult to assess with ultrasound.

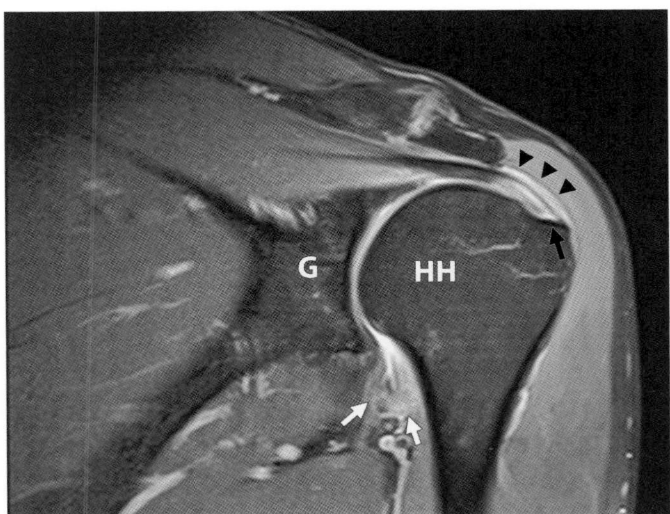

FIGURE 14.4

56-year-old male presenting with left shoulder pain and restricted range of motion, particularly in external rotation. Coronal fat saturated proton density MRI demonstrating a small glenohumeral joint effusion as well as thickening and edema of the inferior axillary recess (white arrows) consistent with adhesive capsulitis. Note is also made of a partial thickness articular surface tear of the supraspinatus tendon with intrasubstance delamination (black arrow) as well as subacromial-subdeltoid bursitis (black arrowheads).

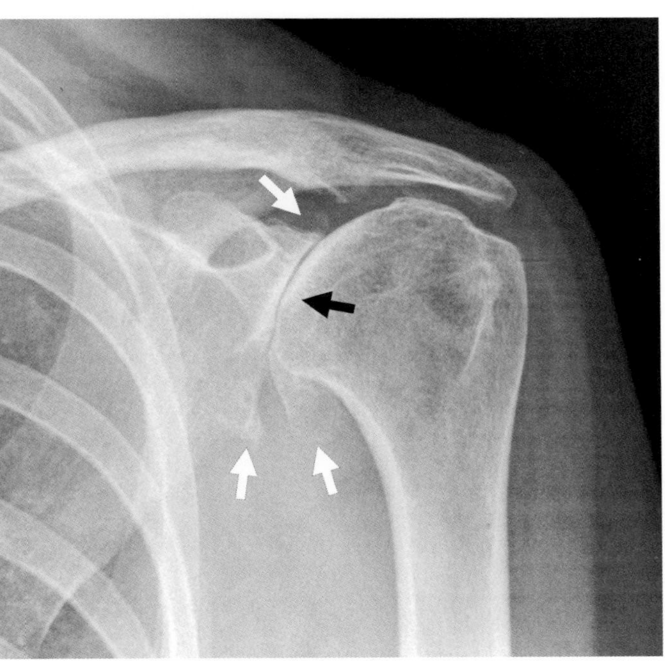

FIGURE 14.5

76-year-old female with left shoulder pain and restricted range of motion. AP radiograph demonstrating significant joint space loss at the glenohumeral joint, with a "bone-on-bone" appearance (black arrow) as well as significant marginal osteophyte formation (white arrows), subchondral sclerosis and subchondral cyst formation in keeping with severe osteoarthritis.

imaging test is a radiograph, due to its excellent ability to confirm the diagnosis and its severity, its low cost, and its ready availability. The joint is best demonstrated on axial and AP views (Figure 14.6).

CT may be used in patients who have relatively severe osteoarthritis who are being considered for surgical management. In this context, CT is often useful for evaluation as it is better at assessing bone stock (the amount of residual glenoid bone volume), glenoid morphology and glenoid version (the angle between the glenoid articular surface and the longitudinal axis of the scapular spine) measurements which are essential for pre-operative planning.

MRI is useful when trying to differentiate between primary osteoarthritis and other causes of arthritis allowing for assessment of synovitis, rotator cuff pathology, bone marrow oedema, and intraosseous fluid collections in the context of infection (see Figure 14.6).

Trauma

A 53-year-old female with right-sided shoulder pain presents following a fall with a direct blow to the shoulder. Humeral, clavicular, and scapular fractures are best assessed initially with a radiograph to support a diagnosis and assess displacement, comminution, and angulation, and can be used for follow-up. At least two views perpendicular to each other are essential to avoid missing a fracture. CT is often used to further assess fractures that may require surgical management, in any plane, allowing better understanding of the fracture morphology. Fractures of the greater tuberosity of the humerus can be missed on radiographs as they are often minimally displaced. The initial radiograph for this patient was normal. If a radiograph is normal and there is a high index of clinical suspicion, MRI is useful as it can confirm the presence of a greater tuberosity fracture and assess for associated rotator cuff tears (Figure 14.7).

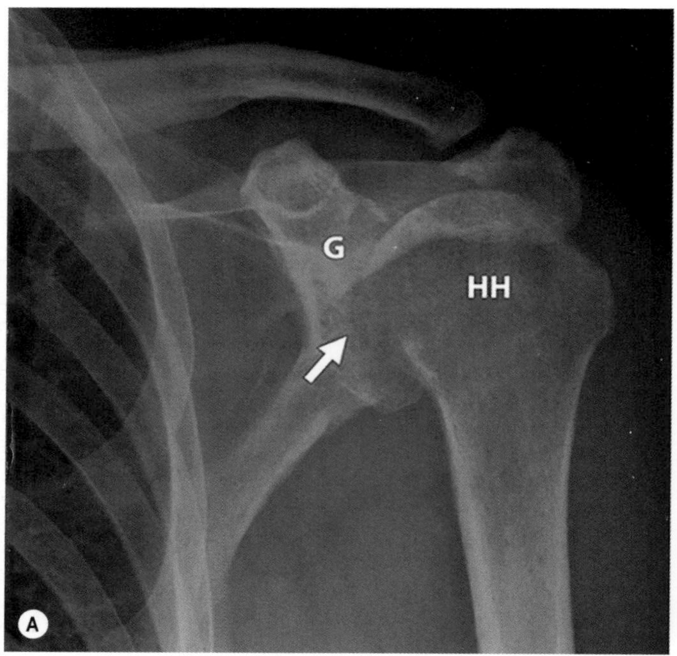

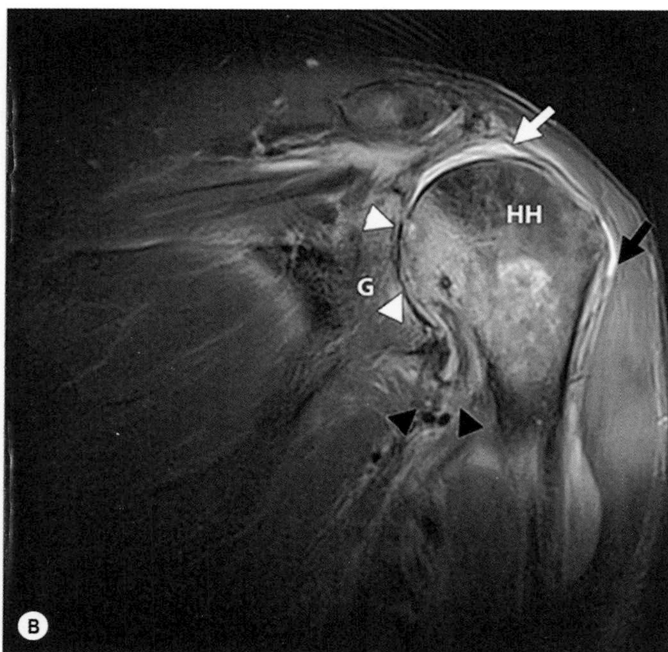

FIGURE 14.6
56-year-old male presenting with left shoulder pain, swelling, fever and malaise. (A) AP radiograph demonstrating glenohumeral joint (G) space loss and subchondral lucency (arrow) suggestive of an erosive arthropathy. (B) Coronal fat saturated proton density MRI demonstrating severe full thickness glenohumeral articular cartilage (G) damage, erosive change and small subarticular fluid collections (white arrowheads), a joint effusion (white arrow) and capsulitis (black arrowheads), and extension of joint fluid into the bursa and lateral margin of the humerus (black arrow) through a full thickness supraspinatus tendon tear (not shown). The appearances are consistent with septic arthritis. This was confirmed by microscopy and culture following arthroscopic joint washout. HH, humeral head.

A 49-year-old male presents with right shoulder pain and swelling following a traumatic fall. The acromioclavicular (AC) area is painful and looks displaced. AC joint separation injuries are assessed with a radiograph in the first instance, to assess for joint subluxation/dislocation and an increase in the AC joint and coracoclavicular distances (Figure 14.8). If surgical management is considered, MRI is useful to assess the AC joint and coracoclavicular ligaments as well as the trapezius and deltoid muscles, which cannot be assessed with a radiograph (Figure 14.8).[1]

A 32-year-old male presents with shoulder pain following trauma, and a glenohumeral joint (GHJ) dislocation is suspected. GHJ dislocation is best assessed with a radiograph in the acute presentation. It may be used to differentiate anterior from posterior dislocation and inform the technique for reduction. The ideal views are anteroposterior in internal and external rotation, scapular "Y", and axillary views, dependent on whether the patient can tolerate them. As the patient has presented with a previous shoulder instability episode, a humeral Hill Sachs lesion or glenoid bony Bankart fracture (both bony impaction injuries due to the posterosuperior humeral head hitting the glenoid during dislocation) is suspected. Therefore, Stryker notch and West Point views can be obtained respectively.[20] For patients with recurrent instability, MRI is useful to evaluate the glenoid labrum and articular cartilage for tears (Figure 14.9).

An MRI arthrogram (performed after a contrast agent is injected into the glenohumeral joint) may be useful to

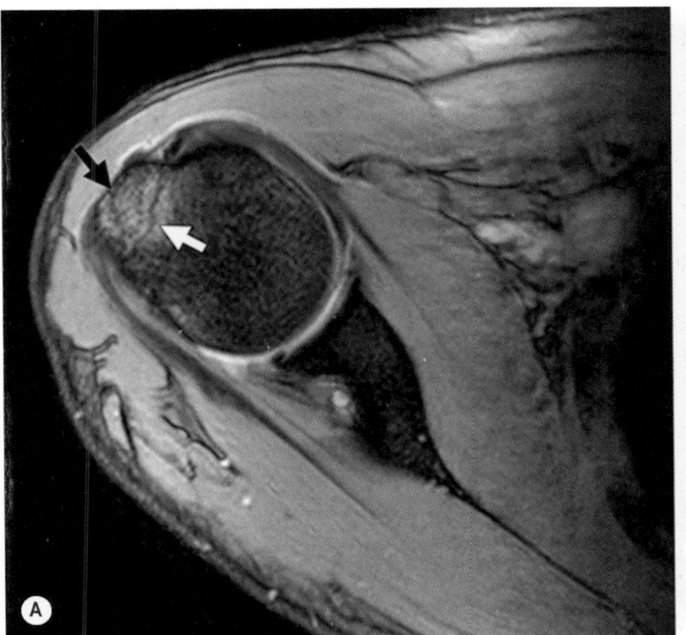

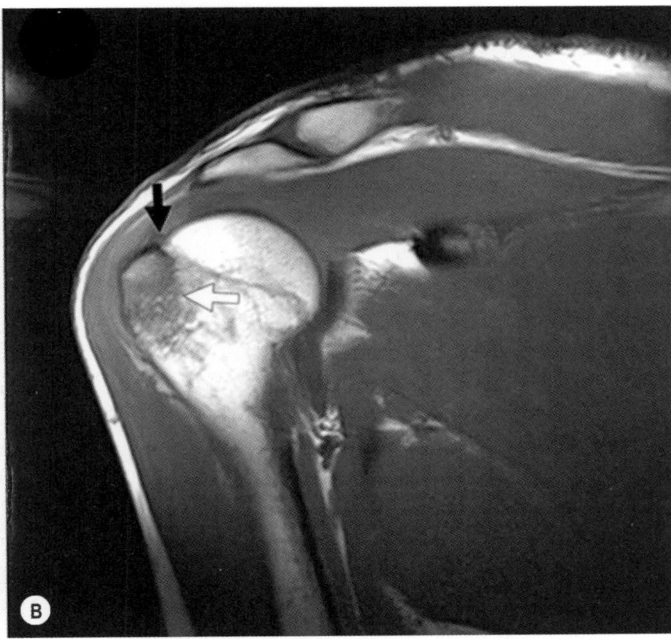

FIGURE 14.7
53-year-old female with right-sided shoulder pain following a fall with a direct blow to the shoulder. The initial radiograph was normal. (A) Axial T2*-weighted gradient echo multiple echo data image combination (MEDIC) MRI showing florid bone marrow oedema in the greater tuberosity of the humerus (black arrow) with a jagged fracture line (white arrow) in keeping with an undisplaced fracture. (B) Coronal T1-weighted MRI showing bone marrow edema in the same place as well as cortical disruption in keeping with a fracture.

further characterize suspected labral tears as intra-articular contrast will highlight any tear present (Figure 14.10). CT is often useful for patients in whom surgical stabilization is considered to assess any Hill Sachs lesion or bony Bankart fracture in more detail.[2]

Bone lesions

A 26-year-old male presents with right shoulder/arm pain without a traumatic incident. One differential diagnosis was a bone lesion (a region within the bone which is damaged). Bone lesions are relatively uncommon and usually unsuspected findings on radiographs or MRI performed to investigate shoulder pain. Imaging plays a vital role in helping to differentiate benign from malignant lesions. The most important radiographic feature of a benign bone lesion is a well marginated border (narrow zone of transition between its border and normal bone; Figure 14.11). If the border is poorly marginated, aggressive causes such as infection and malignancy must be considered. Other signs of an aggressive bone lesion include a periosteal reaction, cortical destruction and an intra- or extra-osseous soft tissue mass.

The most common benign lesion in the shoulder is a simple bone cyst in the humerus, the majority occurring in people under 20 years of age.[32] This is well demonstrated with a radiograph and usually asymptomatic unless complicated by a pathological fracture. Malignant lesions are relatively uncommon in the shoulder and include secondary bone metastases, multiple myeloma, and less commonly primary malignant tumors such as osteosarcoma. A radiograph is usually performed initially and if there are suspicious features, further imaging with MRI or CT (or both) should be performed (see Figure 14.11).

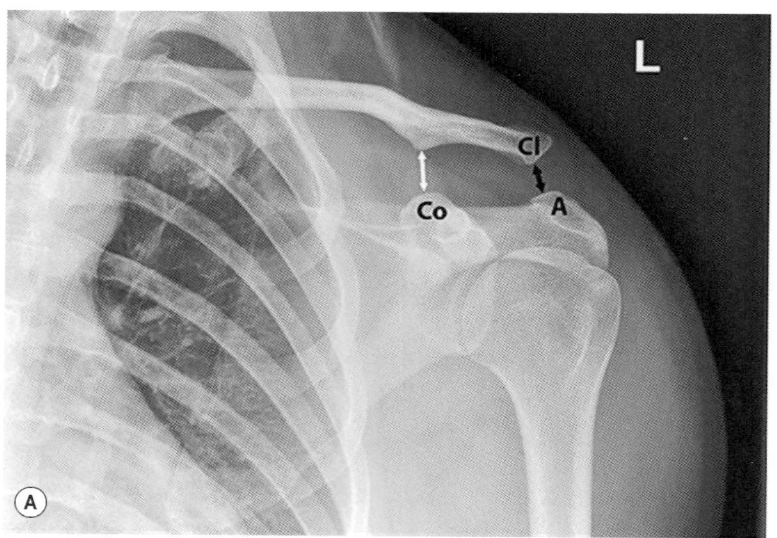

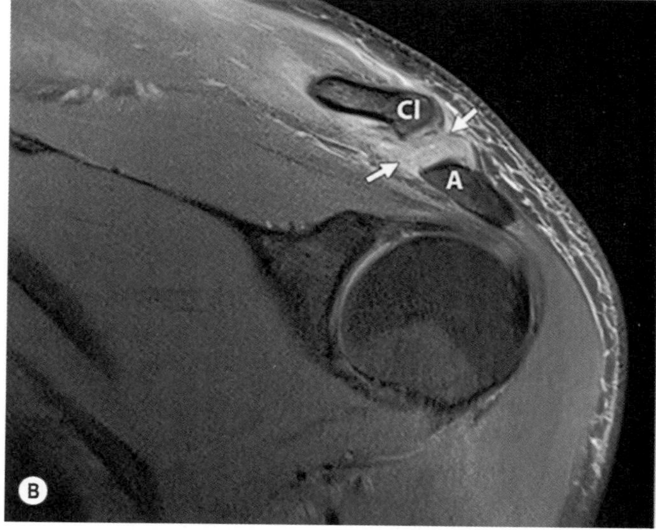

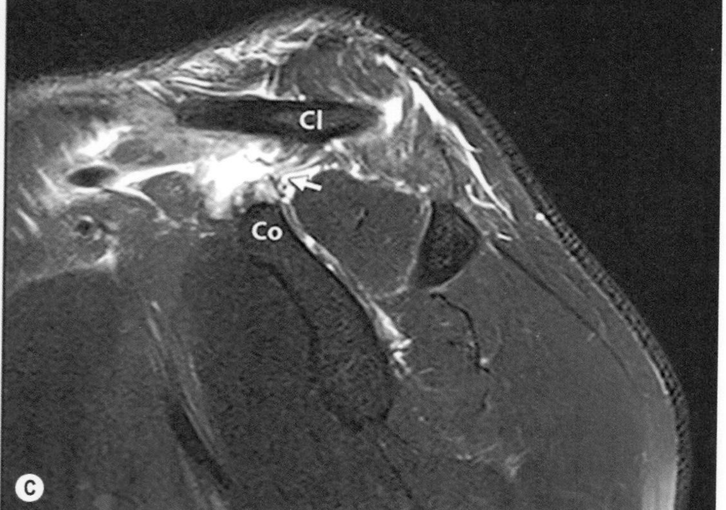

FIGURE 14.8

49-year-old male presenting with right shoulder pain and swelling following a traumatic injury. (A) AP radiograph showing superior displacement of the lateral clavicle (Cl) relative to the acromion (A) with widening of the AC joint space (black arrow) and widening of the coracoclavicular distance (white arrow) consistent with AC joint dislocation. (B) Coronal fat saturated proton density MRI confirming the AC joint dislocation and demonstrating widening of the AC joint and full thickness rupture of the AC joint ligaments (arrows). (C) Sagittal fat saturated proton density MRI showing widening of the coracoclavicular distance with full thickness rupture of the coracoclavicular ligament (arrow). Co, coracoid.

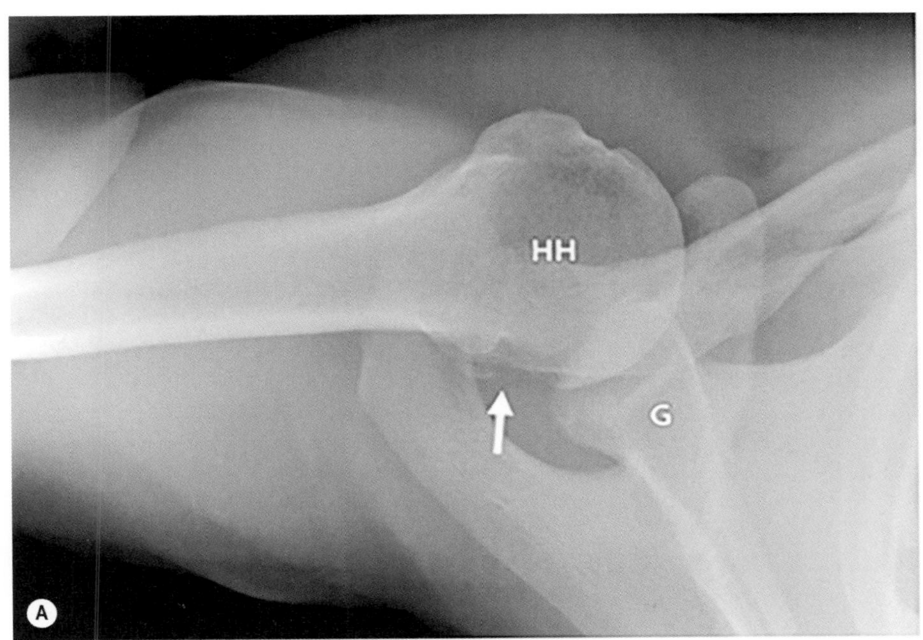

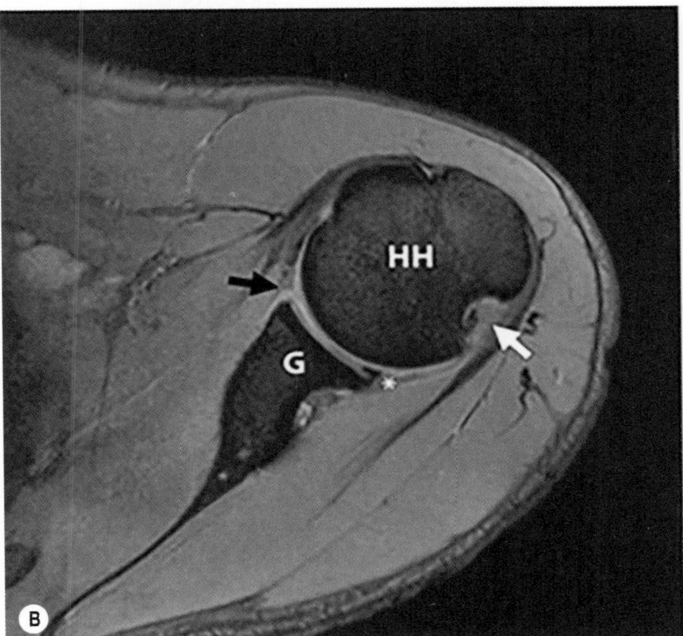

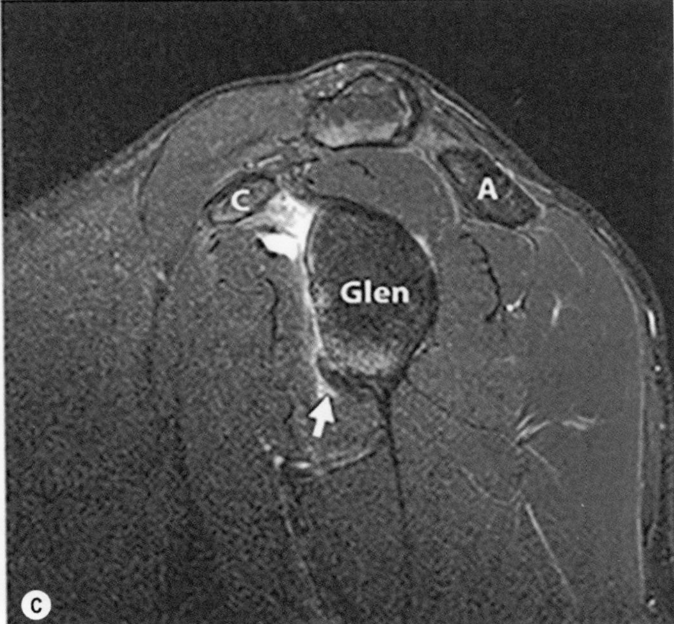

FIGURE 14.9

32-year-old male presenting with shoulder pain and discomfort after a previous shoulder instability episode. (A) Axial radiograph demonstrating normal alignment at the glenohumeral joint (G) but a large concavity (arrow) of the posterior superior humeral head (HH) confirming previous anterior shoulder dislocation. (B) Axial T2*-weighted gradient echo multiple echo data image combination (MEDIC) MRI confirming the presence of the Hill Sachs lesion (white arrow) in the humeral head (HH) with absence of the normal low signal triangular anterior labrum (black arrow) in keeping with a labral tear (compare with the normal posterior labrum (*)). (C) Sagittal short tau inversion recovery (STIR) MRI showing the displaced anterior inferior labral tear (arrow). A, acromion; C, coracoid; Glen, glenoid.

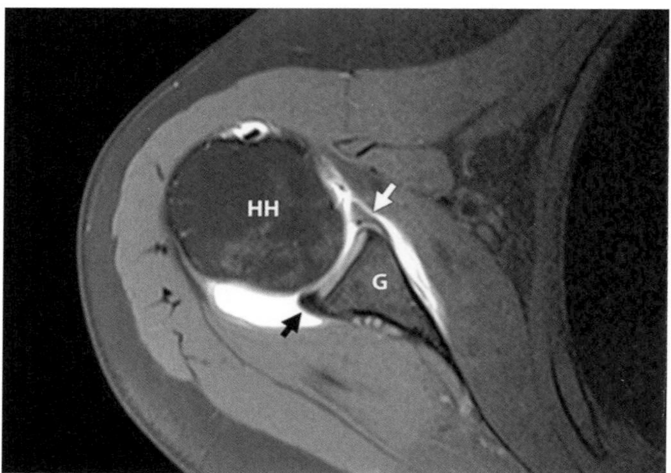

FIGURE 14.10

44-year-old male with right shoulder pain and a history of previous shoulder dislocation episodes. Axial fat saturated T1-weighted MRI arthrogram obtained after contrast injection into the glenohumeral joint. There is medial detachment of the anterior inferior labrum which remains attached to the glenoid by a thin strip of periosteum (white arrow) outlined by contrast. Compare with the normal posterior labrum (black arrow). G, glenoid; HH, humeral head.

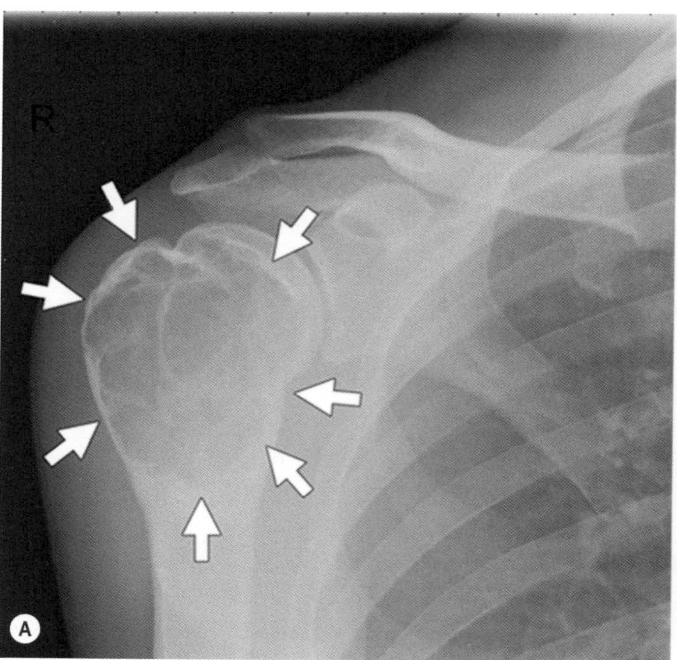

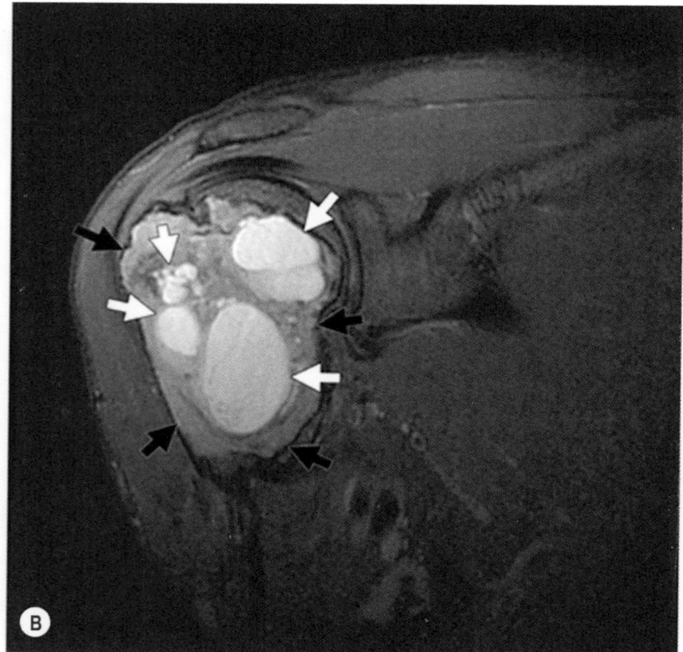

FIGURE 14.11

26-year-old male with right shoulder/arm pain. (A) AP radiograph demonstrating an expansile, subarticular lucent lesion in the proximal humerus with a non-sclerotic margin and no cortical destruction or periosteal reaction (arrows), suggesting a non-aggressive primary bone lesion. (B) Coronal fat saturated proton density MRI which demonstrates both cystic (white arrows) and solid (black arrows) components within the humeral lesion and confirms no cortical destruction or periosteal reaction. There are no demonstrable fluid-fluid levels. The lesion was suspected to represent a giant cell tumor and was referred to a bone tumor center where the patient underwent image-guided biopsy, confirming the suspicion.

Blood tests

From the middle ages to the 18th century, bedside medicine was prevalent; then between 1794 and 1848 came hospital medicine; and from that time forward, laboratory medicine has served as medicine's lodestar.[3]

As a symptom rather than a condition, shoulder pain may be rooted in intrinsic pathological processes, generated from local or referred from distant anatomical structures, or exist as a manifestation of systemic illness. Although laboratory tests do not offer diagnostic certainty when considering the underlying etiological cause, they play a role in the diagnostic work up to either support or refute a potentially long list of differential diagnoses. Diagnostic ambiguity often results from casting the net wide due to the significant phenotypic overlap in how different categories of disease may present.

Thorough assessment of the shoulder will involve taking a careful history and performing a tailored clinical assessment, as well as supportive radiological imaging. In most cases of shoulder joint disease, a full blood count (FBC) and tests for inflammatory markers (CRP/ESR) are sufficient first-line hematological and biochemical tests. More specialist blood tests may be warranted in specific situations (see Table 14.1). To explore the utility of blood tests in the context of shoulder-related symptoms, a case study is presented illustrating the complexity and sometimes formidable challenge of categorizing shoulder-related symptoms.

Case

A 59-year-old female presents with a 3-week history of acute onset, atraumatic, largely symmetrical, dull shoulder and pelvic pain associated with stiffness. She denies radiation or focal neurological deficit. Her symptoms were preceded by a flu-like prodrome and are typically worse in the morning, and she informs that it takes her approximately one hour to get moving. She struggles to brush her hair and open cupboards, and has noted that getting out of her car is getting increasingly more difficult. Her symptoms ease with the use of nonsteroidal anti-inflammatory agents (NSAIDs). She remains systemically well and denies recent history of focal infective symptoms, weight loss, or fevers. She further denies a history of headaches or visual changes.

Her past medical history is significant for diet-controlled diabetes mellitus and hypothyroidism for which she takes daily levothyroxine (100 mcg). She has no known drug allergies. Family history is significant for debilitating maternal rheumatoid arthritis and hypertension. She does not smoke and has one glass of wine on most nights. She works as an accountant and is normally independent in activities of daily living. She lives with her husband and two children and, when well, is moderately physically active during an average week.

On initial examination, there is no joint deformity or focal tenderness. There is perceived weakness of proximal muscles, however, with encouragement and on re-testing power, strength appears normal in all muscle groups bilaterally in both the upper and lower limbs. There is no demonstrable painful arc on shoulder abduction and range of movement is satisfactory with preserved joint stability. Neurologically, tone, reflexes, coordination, and sensory examinations are unremarkable. Her gait is normal; however, she does struggle to get out of the chair without the use of her arms for support. She is understandably concerned and frustrated.

Case reflection

Although suspecting polymyalgia rheumatica (PMR) would be understandable, it would always be a mistake to jump to a conclusion without considering potential differential diagnoses. Supportive blood tests will include an FBC (normochromic normocytic anemia) as well as CRP/ESR (expected to be raised). It is important to consider other subtle elements in the history that may suggest alternative differential diagnoses or even dual pathologies. The individual has known diabetes and although her condition is diet-controlled, which often reassures the healthcare provider that it is well regulated, one must seek biochemical evidence of this (HbA1c – glycated hemoglobin). Diabetes mellitus may be associated with increased risk of infection as well as frozen shoulder, and bilateral presentations have been reported. Although rare, a potential differential diagnosis which requires consideration is a septic GHJ.[25]

This person also has clinical hypothyroidism, which may present with muscle stiffness, while hyperthyroidism (possibly through overtreatment of her hypothyroid state) can feature proximal muscle weakness. Assessment of her

Table 14.1 A summary of conditions that may present with shoulder pain/stiffness and supportive blood work

Disease process	Condition	Common presentation	Blood tests
Inflammatory			
	Rheumatoid arthritis	Symmetrical and deforming polyarthropathy (typically small joints of hands). May involve larger joints such as shoulder, knee and elbow. Morning pain and stiffness is common. Extra-articular manifestations may be present (e.g., compression neuropathies).	FBC (anemia), RF (↑/↔), Anti-CCP (↑/↔), CRP/ ESR (↑)
	Seronegative spondyloarthropathies (e.g., ankylosing spondylitis)	Inflammatory back pain and stiffness associated with peripheral enthesopathy and asymmetrical large joint arthropathy (i.e., shoulder girdle involvement). Extra-articular manifestations may be present (e.g., ocular, cardiovascular, pulmonary, renal, and metabolic).	FBC (anemia), CRP/ESR (↑/↔)
	Systemic lupus erythematosus	Arthralgia (may involve any joint). Multisystem disease with potential of hematological, renal, neuropsychiatric, dermal, mucosal, and serosal involvement.	FBC (pancytopenia), LFTs (impaired), renal function (impaired), ESR (↑), CRP (↔, though ↑ in drug-induced lupus), C3/C4 (↓), ANA/anti-dsDNA/ anti-phospholipid antibody positivity
Metabolic			
	Diabetes (adhesive capsulitis)	Pain, stiffness and restricted movement. Typically asymmetrical.	HbA1c
	Pseudogout. (Gout does not typically involve the shoulder joint)	Mono-/oligo-articular arthropathy with a red, swollen and painful joint associated with reduced mobility.	FBC (elevated WBC may be seen), joint aspiration for culture and polarized light microscopy*
Infective			
	Septic arthritis (uncommon)	Red, hot, swollen joint associated with pain on mobilization. Predisposing risk factors: immunosuppression, IVDU, underlying joint disease, intra-articular instrumentation.	FBC, CRP, blood cultures, joint aspiration for culture*
Neoplastic			
	Primary or metastatic	Weight loss, night sweats, fevers, pathological fracture, known history of malignancy.	FBC (anemia), CRP/ESR (↑), Bone profile (elevated calcium), myeloma screen and tumor markers, imaging +/– histology*
Other: degenerative, traumatic, idiopathic			

*Clinically urgent.
ANA, anti-nuclear antigen; anti-CCP, anti-cyclic citrullinated peptide; anti-dsDNA, anti-double stranded DNA; C3/C4, complement protein-3/-4; CRP, c-reactive protein; CK, creatine kinase; ESR, erythrocyte sedimentation rate; FBC, full blood count; HbA1c, glycated hemoglobin; IVDU, intravenous-drug user; LFTs, liver function tests; RF, rheumatoid factor; WBC, white blood count.

thyroid status is justified here. Moreover, there is a family history of severe rheumatoid arthritis (RA) with polymyalgic onset RA[27] being a recognized phenomenon, which should also be considered as part of the diagnostic work-up. Reassuringly, she did not exhibit features suggestive of a possible paraneoplastic syndrome, a primary muscle disorder (e.g., polymyositis/dermatomyositis) or an immune-mediated process (e.g., systemic lupus erythematosus). Management is largely glucocorticoid based and therefore a routine baseline biochemical profile will be recommended prior to treatment initiation (renal, liver, and bone).

Clearly there is substantial overlap of conditions that need to be considered when an individual presents with a painful shoulder. Diagnostic uncertainty warrants a multidisciplinary team approach coupled with targeted, multimodal investigations. Though not exhaustive, Table 14.1 summarizes a list of conditions which may present with shoulder pain/stiffness, and associated blood tests.

Electromyographic activity and nerve conduction

Electromyography (EMG), or the measurement of the electrical activity in muscles, should be considered as an extension of the clinical examination. It allows the detection of abnormalities in nerve conduction, and can provide objective evidence of peripheral neuropathy.[11] It may also be used to assess and measure muscle recruitment patterns during analytical or functional movements.[15,16] It should be remembered that EMG is not a measure of muscle force.

In the clinical setting, needle or fine wire as well as surface EMG can be performed.[22,28] The choice will depend upon the muscle to be measured (superficial or deeper layers of muscles) and the amount of movement the person will undertake.[10] Needle and fine wire electrodes record potentials from single motor units, that is, from muscle fibers supplied by a single motor neuron. In contrast, surface electrodes pick up from multiple motor units that would encompass more of the electrical activity of the surrounding muscle fibers.[28] A basic assumption in surface EMG is that the recorded potentials originate from the muscle directly under the electrodes. However, potentials from muscles further away may also reach the recording site through volume conduction, thus contributing to the EMG signal. This phenomenon is referred to as "crosstalk".[10,28] Although some limitations need to be acknowledged regarding surface EMG, such as crosstalk, this method is widely used in clinical practice to record superficial muscles.[39]

When analyzing EMG signals, several approaches are available. We can calculate the mean or peak voluntary activity over time.[28] This will inform us about the amount of EMG generated. However, one can't compare the amplitude of raw EMG – that is, one can't compare between one person and another or between one person across different points in time, or compare the amount of raw EMG your patient can generate against the raw amplitude reported in research papers.[7] To make comparisons, the amplitude of the EMG needs to be scaled in a standardized way, which is called normalization. This is commonly achieved by measuring the mean activity as a percentage of the activity during a maximal voluntary isometric contraction (MVIC). This can be problematic when a person is in pain and is unable to produce an MVIC. Different methods may be employed but require some compromise.

Other methods of analysis not requiring normalization of the amount of activity are: determining the onset/offset timing of muscle activity (in msec) in relation to movement or another muscle,[9] or performing a frequency analysis (the number of times the raw signal crosses the zero-line), which contributes to the assessment of fatigue and/or endurance.[28] A novel method for EMG signal analysis is statistical parametric mapping (SPM), which allows comparison between subjects, exercises, and movements, not only in certain predetermined positions as in traditional EMG analysis, but on any given point during the movement.[36] In SPM, the total curves of the EMG signals are statistically compared. An example is given in Figure 14.12.

An example of statistical parametric mapping analysis of the levator scapulae (LS) during elevation in the frontal (black) and sagittal (red) plane (left). The dark pink area denotes an overlap of the standard deviation (SD) of the activity between planes of movement. The right figure illustrates in which part of the movement (dark area above the dotted line) there are significant differences in muscle activity between both planes. The x-axis denotes the time of motion as a percentage of the whole time.

Besides the mean or peak activity, muscle balance ratios may be of interest, comparing activity in one muscle with respect to another.[29] This allows an assessment of the balance of activity between muscles, known to be necessary for dynamic functional joint stability and movement. Regarding the latter, analysis of muscle recruitment during rehabilitation exercises may assist the clinician to guide the patient through an exercise program with specific focus on restoring normal muscle activity and intermuscular balance.

EMG can also be used to assess for neurological injury or disease. Neurological tests may be used to assess altered patterns of activity (e.g., spontaneous firing) that could be observed in some neurological disease, such as chronic radiculopathies, peripheral neuropathies or motor neuron disease.[17] In contrast to recording ongoing activity, EMG can also record responses from artificially stimulating the central or peripheral nervous system.[33,38] These investigative techniques are not used for rehabilitation but can guide

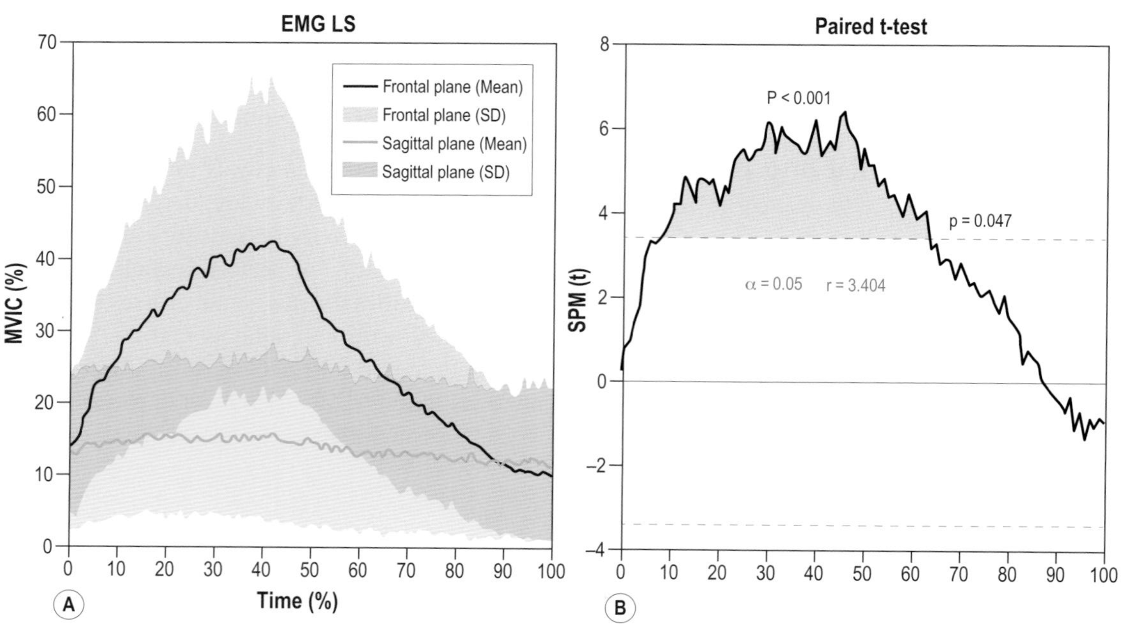

FIGURE 14.12

(A) An example of statistical parametric mapping analysis of the levator scapulae (LS) during elevation in the frontal (black) and sagittal (orange) plane. The dark orange area denotes an overlap of the standard deviation (SD) of the activity between planes of movement. (B) Illustration of part of the movement (dark area above the dotted line) in which there are significant differences in muscle activity between both planes. The x-axis denotes the time of motion as a percentage of the whole time.

prognosis, and assist in diagnosis and defining treatment pathways, as well as support an understanding of the control of the shoulder. Here the response recorded by EMG is evoked rather than voluntarily recruited, and the amplitude, timing and/or change of the response is measured and compared to normal values.

Case

A 29-year-old male presents after a blunt, direct trauma to the lateral chest wall. He is a construction worker, currently unable to perform his job. He feels no pain at rest, however, he cannot elevate his arm above 90°. During this movement, a clear scapular dyskinesis is noticeable, characterized by insufficient upward rotation.

Due to the trauma experienced by the patient, and the subsequent loss of shoulder function, he underwent nerve conduction tests including that of the long thoracic nerve, the nerve supplying serratus anterior. The nerve was supra-maximally stimulated at Erb's point (posterior border of the sternocleidomastoid muscle) to recruit all of the available motor units.[40] The latency and amplitude of the response were slow and small respectively, suggesting a loss of peripheral nerve conduction beyond Erb's point. It should be noted that supra-maximal stimulation of a mixed nerve evokes responses in both the motor and sensory fibers of a mixed nerve. It is challenging to identify sensory loss because the faster latency motor response that is seen earlier in the EMG recording, evokes a response that can superimpose upon the slightly later, slower sensory responses. This mixed pattern of EMG originating from both sensory and motor fibers can be difficult to untangle. Small fiber loss such as that of sensory fibers, would be better investigated using quantitative sensory testing rather than using EMG.[44]

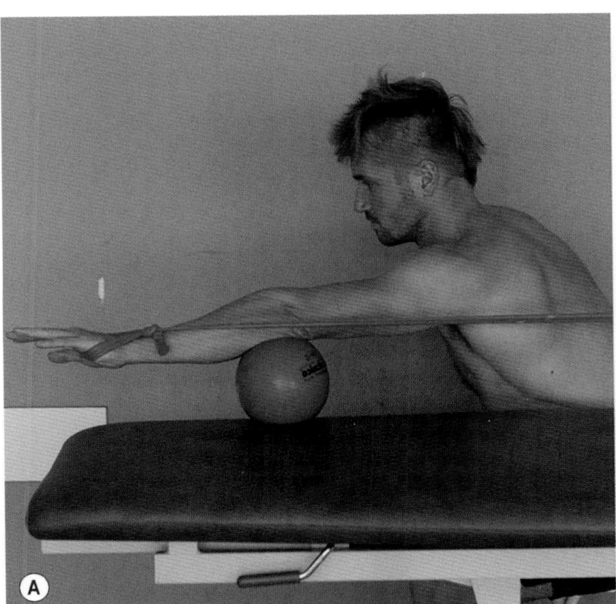

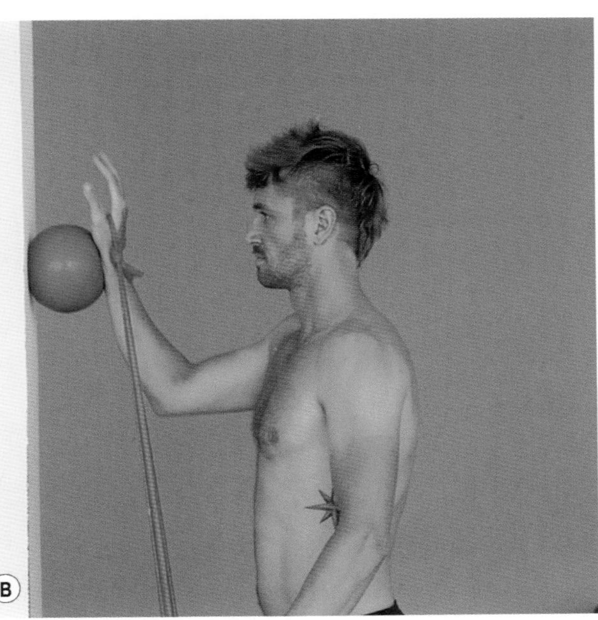

FIGURE 14.13
Closed chain exercises with low load of body weight on the shoulders against resistance: a bench slide (A) and a wall slide (B).

Having confirmed denervation of the serratus anterior (SA), the patient was seen two weeks later. Initial therapeutic strategy focused on elevation exercises with minimal demands for SA, such as bench slides (Figure 14.13A) and wall slides (Figure 14.13B), to maintain mobility into elevation, while waiting for recovery of nerve conduction.[14] The exercises were built into a daily home program and limited to 3 exercises to maximize adherence to the program, with a strength program set at 3 sets of 10 repetitions, loaded such that the last repetition was difficult to complete due to fatigue.

After 4 months, a substantial increase in active elevation was observed, and the patient reported return to professional activity, however, not yet with full functional capacity. Then, more demanding SA exercises were implemented, such as elevation in the scapular plane in open chain, against resistance. In order to maximally activate all scapular muscles, external rotation (ER) components were added to the exercises, such as the ER wall slide (Figure 14.14A), and elevation with ER (Figure 14.14B).[8] After 6 months, the patient was discharged from rehabilitation.

In addition to advice and identifying patient-related goals, exercise prescription is often based on the expected muscle recruitment of the targeted muscles during the specific movements. These muscle recruitment patterns can be defined by EMG activity during the exercises to ensure appropriate recruitment during the task. For that purpose, many studies have been performed investigating specific muscle patterning of the glenohumeral and scapulothoracic muscles during a variety of exercises. With respect to shoulder rehabilitation, the data presented in Box 14.1 is a synthesis of published research and may be considered to aid clinical reasoning when prescribing exercises.

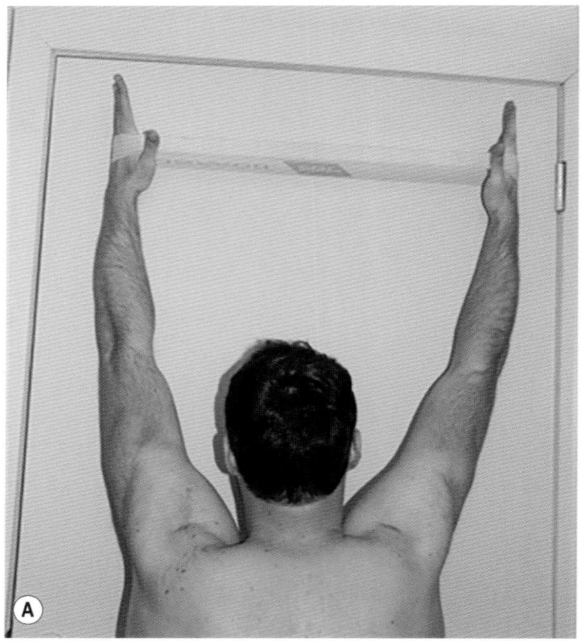

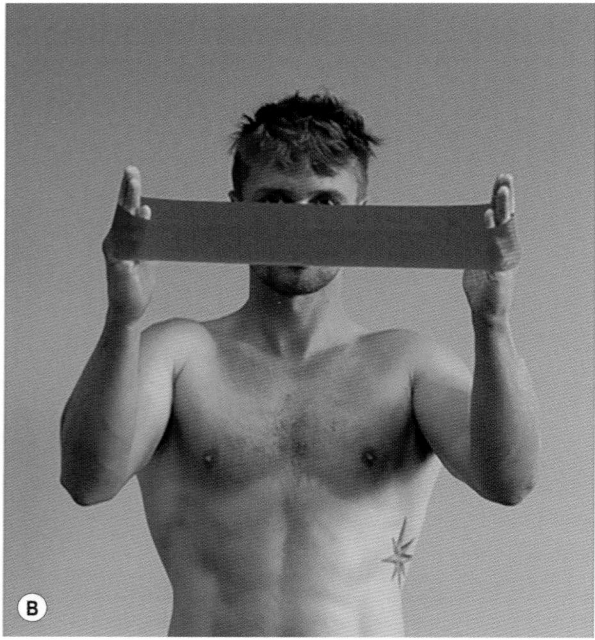

FIGURE 14.14
Exercises into elevation: to maximally activate all scapular muscles, an external rotation wall slide (A), and elevation with external rotation (B).

Box 14.1

- Lower and middle trapezius are mainly activated by adding an external rotation (ER) component to the exercise.[8,13]
- Pectoralis minor may be inhibited by performing ER, by preference in an open kinetic chain.[8]
- Serratus anterior activation is increased during elevation exercises compared to isolated protraction exercises[12] and stepping forwards.[37]
- Rotator cuff (RC) activity is low during low-load closed chain exercises such as bench or wall slides.[14,21]
- Deltoid activity during supine elevation exercises may be increased by increasing trunk inclination.[14]
- Both infra- and supraspinatus activity are high during ER exercises.[21]
- Subscapularis activity may be increased by performing flexion-extension exercises at low elevation angles (below 90°).[30,45]
- Biceps activity is high during plyometric elevation exercises in supination.[5]
- Exercises with an open hand increase middle and lower trapezius activity, whereas making a fist may increase RC activity.[6,42]

References

1. Alyas F, Curtis M, Speed C, Saifuddin A, Connell D. MR imaging appearances of acromioclavicular joint dislocation. Radiographics. 2008;28:463-479; quiz 619.
2. Bencardino JT, Gyftopoulos S, Palmer WE. Imaging in anterior glenohumeral instability. Radiology. 2013;269:323-337.
3. Berger D. A brief history of medical diagnosis and the birth of the clinical laboratory. Part 1: Ancient times through the 19th century. MLO Med Lab Obs. 1999;31:28-30, 32, 34-40.
4. Binkert CA, Verdun FR, Zanetti M, Pfirrmann CW, Hodler J. CT arthrography of the glenohumeral joint: CT fluoroscopy versus conventional CT and fluoroscopy – comparison of image-guidance techniques. Radiology. 2003;229:153-158.
5. Borms D, Ackerman I, Smets P, Van den Berge G, Cools AM. Biceps disorder rehabilitation for the athlete: a continuum of moderate- to high-load exercises. Am J Sports Med. 2017;45:642-650.
6. Borms D, Maenhout A, Cools AM. Incorporation of the kinetic chain into shoulder-elevation exercises: does it affect scapular muscle activity? J Athl Train. 2020;55:343-349.
7. Burden A, Bartlett R. Normalisation of EMG amplitude: an evaluation and comparison of old and new methods. Med Eng Phys. 1999;21:247-257.
8. Castelein B, Cagnie B, Parlevliet T, Cools A. Superficial and deep scapulothoracic muscle electromyographic activity during elevation exercises in the scapular plane. J Orthop Sports Phys Ther. 2016;46:184-193.
9. Cavallari P, Bolzoni F, Bruttini C, Esposti R. The Organization and control of intra-limb anticipatory postural adjustments and their role in movement performance. Front Hum Neurosci. 2016;10:525.
10. Chowdhury RH, Reaz MB, Ali MA, Bakar AA, Chellappan K, Chang TG. Surface electromyography signal processing and classification techniques. Sensors (Basel). 2013;13:12431-12466.
11. Chung T, Prasad K, Lloyd TE. Peripheral neuropathy: clinical and electrophysiological considerations. Neuroimaging Clin N Am. 2014;24:49-65.
12. Cools AM, Borms D, Cottens S, Himpe M, Meersdom S, Cagnie B. Rehabilitation exercises for athletes with biceps disorders and SLAP Lesions: a continuum of exercises with increasing loads on the biceps. Am J Sports Med. 2014;42:1315-1322.
13. Cools AM, Struyf F, De Mey K, Maenhout A, Castelein B, Cagnie B. Rehabilitation of scapular dyskinesis: from the office worker to the elite overhead athlete. Br J Sports Med. 2014;48:692-697.
14. Cools AM, Tongel AV, Berckmans K, et al. Electromyographic analysis of selected shoulder muscles during a series of exercises commonly used in patients with symptomatic degenerative rotator cuff tears. J Shoulder Elbow Surg. 2020;29:e361-e373.
15. Cools AM, Witvrouw EE, Declercq GA, Danneels LA, Cambier DC. Scapular muscle recruitment patterns: trapezius muscle latency with and without impingement symptoms. American Journal of Sports Medicine. 2003;31:542-549.
16. Dark A, Ginn KA, Halaki M. Shoulder muscle recruitment patterns during commonly used rotator cuff exercises: an electromyographic study. Phys Ther. 2007;87:1039-1046.
17. Davalos L, Kushlaf H. Abnormal spontaneous electromyographic activity. StatPearls (online). Treasure Island (FL): StatPearls Publishing; 2021.Available at: https://www.ncbi.nlm.nih.gov/books/NBK482461/
18. De Filippo M, Bertellini A, Sverzellati N, et al. Multidetector computed tomography arthrography of the shoulder: diagnostic accuracy and indications. Acta Radiol. 2008;49:540-549.
19. Dines DM, Laurencin CT, Williams GR (eds). Arthritis and Arthroplasty: The Shoulder. Philadelphia: Saunders Elsevier; 2009.
20. Dumont GD, Russell RD, Robertson WJ. Anterior shoulder instability: a review of pathoanatomy, diagnosis and treatment. Curr Rev Musculoskelet Med. 2011;4:200-207.
21. Edwards PK, Ebert JR, Littlewood C, Ackland T, Wang A. A systematic review of electromyography studies in normal shoulders to inform postoperative rehabilitation following rotator cuff repair. J Orthop Sports Phys Ther. 2017;47:931-944.
22. Farina D, Negro F. Accessing the neural drive to muscle and translation to neurorehabilitation technologies. IEEE Rev Biomed Eng. 2012;5:3-14.
23. Jacobson JA, Girish G, Jiang Y, Resnick D. Radiographic evaluation of arthritis: inflammatory conditions. Radiology. 2008;248:378-389.
24. Kassarjian A, Bencardino JT, Palmer WE. MR imaging of the rotator cuff. Magn Reson Imaging Clin N Am. 2004;12:39-60, vi.
25. Klinger HM, Baums MH, Freche S, Nusselt T, Spahn G, Steckel H. Septic arthritis of the shoulder joint: an analysis of management and outcome. Acta Orthopaedica Belgica. 2010;76:598-603.
26. Lewis JS, Cook CE, Hoffmann TC, O'Sullivan P. The elephant in the room: too much medicine in musculoskeletal practice. J Orthop Sports Phys Ther. 2020;50:1-4.
27. Lopez-Hoyos M, Ruiz de Alegria C, Blanco R, et al. Clinical utility of anti-CCP antibodies in the differential diagnosis of elderly-onset rheumatoid arthritis and polymyalgia rheumatica. Rheumatology (Oxford). 2004;43:655-657.
28. McManus L, De Vito G, Lowery MM. Analysis and biophysics of surface EMG for physiotherapists and kinesiologists: toward a common language with rehabilitation engineers. Front Neurol. 2020;11:576729.
29. Moeller CR, Bliven KC, Valier AR. Scapular muscle-activation ratios in patients with shoulder injuries during functional shoulder exercises. J Athl Train. 2014;49:345-355.
30. Myers JB, Pasquale MR, Laudner KG, Sell TC, Bradley JP, Lephart SM. On-the-field resistance-tubing exercises for throwers: an electromyographic analysis. J Athl Train. 2005;40:15-22.
31. O'Sullivan JW, Muntinga T, Grigg S, Ioannidis JPA. Prevalence and outcomes of incidental imaging findings: umbrella review. BMJ. 2018;361:k2387.
32. Parman LM, Murphey MD. Alphabet soup: cystic lesions of bone. Semin Musculoskelet Radiol. 2000;4:89-101.
33. Pascual-Leone A, Davey N, Rothwell J, Wasserman E, Puri BK. Handbook of Transcranial Magnetic Stimulation 1. London: CRC Press; 2002.
34. Powell DK. Patient explanation guidelines for incidentalomas: helping patients not to fear the delayed surveillance. AJR Am J Roentgenol. 2014;202:W602.

35. **United Nations Scientific Committee on the Effects of Atomic Radiation.** Sources and Effects of Ionizing Radiation. New York: United Nations; 2008.

36. Ribeiro DC, Day A, Dickerson CR. Grade-IV inferior glenohumeral mobilization does not immediately alter shoulder and scapular muscle activity: a repeated-measures study in asymptomatic individuals. J Man Manip Ther. 2017;25:260-269.

37. Richardson E, Lewis JS, Gibson J, et al. Role of the kinetic chain in shoulder rehabilitation: does incorporating the trunk and lower limb into shoulder exercise regimes influence shoulder muscle recruitment patterns? Systematic review of electromyography studies. BMJ Open Sport Exerc Med. 2020;6:e000683.

38. Daube JR, Rubin DI. Clinical Neurophysiology (3rd edition). Oxford: Oxford University Press; 2013.

39. SENIAM. Surface ElectroMyoGraphy for the Non-Invasive Assessment of Muscles. Available at: www.seniam.org.

40. Seror P. The long thoracic nerve conduction study revisited in 2006. Clin Neurophysiol. 2006;117:2446-2450.

41. Smittenaar CR, Petersen KA, Stewart K, Moitt N. Cancer incidence and mortality projections in the UK until 2035. Br J Cancer. 2016;115:1147-1155.

42. Sporrong H, Palmerud G, Herberts P. Hand grip increases shoulder muscle activity: an EMG analysis with static hand contractions in 9 subjects. Acta Orthopaedica Scandinavica. 1996;67:485-490.

43. University College London Hospitals NHS Foundation Trust. Provider to Provider Services 2019-2020 Tariff. Available at: https://www.uclh.nhs.uk/application/files/8416/0490/8552/UCLH_Provider_to_Provider_Tariff_2019-20.pdf.

44. Waldman SD, Waldman HJ, Waldman KA. Evaluation and treatment of peripheral neuropathies. In: Waldman SD, Bloch JI (eds). Pain Management. WB Saunders; 2007:268-278.

45. Wattanaprakornkul D, Cathers I, Halaki M, Ginn KA. The rotator cuff muscles have a direction specific recruitment pattern during shoulder flexion and extension exercises. J Sci Med.Sport. 2011;14:376-82.

46. Weiner C. Anticipate and communicate: ethical management of incidental and secondary findings in the clinical, research, and direct-to-consumer contexts (December 2013 report of the Presidential Commission for the Study of Bioethical Issues). Am J Epidemiol. 2014;180:562-564.

Assessing and classifying musculoskeletal shoulder conditions 15

Angela Cadogan, Jeremy Lewis, Danielle Hollis

Introduction

Globally, musculoskeletal conditions have been a leading cause of disability for the past three decades[70] with shoulder pain being the third most common musculoskeletal complaint.[58] Shoulder pain affects all age groups and is associated with significant disability, reduced health-related quality of life, depression, increased risk of chronic health conditions and loss of functional independence.[15,45,65,70] Traditional methods of assessment adopted by clinicians have attempted to identify the structure (anatomy) and cause (pathology) of symptoms, followed by treatment directed at the pathoanatomic reason for symptoms. The pathoanatomic approach to diagnosis has become a routine and accepted aspect of shoulder assessment with the intended benefits of guiding treatment decisions, informing prognosis, and enhancing healthcare communication.

While the pathoanatomic approach remains an important component of assessment in the context of traumatic injury such as fractures, dislocations, and acute soft tissue ruptures, as well as for other specific conditions such as osteosarcomas, clinical tests lack specificity for most shoulder conditions. In many clinical settings, most people present with nontraumatic shoulder symptoms for which a pathoanatomic diagnosis may not inform best management decisions. In both traumatic and nontraumatic presentations concomitant psychosocial, lifestyle, environmental, contextual, and experiential factors will influence and impact on treatment outcomes. The implication being that an isolated pathoanatomic approach to assessment is insufficient to guide treatment decisions for the majority of people seeking care. As such, there is a need to reframe the classification of shoulder disability and align it with a contemporary understanding of musculoskeletal symptoms.

The limitations and uncertainties surrounding the traditional approach to pathoanatomic diagnosis, designed to identify a causative structure, mean this must now be integrated within an interpretive framework that places the person and their narrative at the center of care. In addition to pathoanatomic factors, this framework requires clinicians to assess the range of health determinants and contextual effects to ensure the provision of a more holistic understanding of the individual and their needs. This chapter aims to: 1) review the validity of typical diagnostic assessment of shoulder pain presentations and discuss the role of pathoanatomic diagnosis, 2) discuss new and emerging evidence for other factors known to influence treatment outcomes, and 3) consider a new model of assessment that may be used to classify shoulder disorders to improve outcomes for a larger proportion of people seeking care.

Traditional approach to shoulder diagnosis

Definition of diagnosis

The term diagnosis originates from Greek "dia" (apart) and "gignōskein" (recognize, know).[46] The meaning of the Greek word "diagignōskein" was therefore "discern or distinguish" and later became "diagnosis" in modern Latin around the 17th century.[46] The word "diagnosis" may be defined as the determination of an individual's clinical presentation by evaluation of the signs, symptoms, and tests.[1,39]

In musculoskeletal shoulder practice, the term "diagnosis" has become synonymous with "pathoanatomic diagnosis". Clinicians have typically performed shoulder assessments in attempts to identify a specific anatomic structure and associated pathology that is assumed to be the cause of the person's symptoms. Some examples of pathoanatomic diagnoses include humeral fracture, subscapularis tear, labral tear, and supraspinatus calcific tendinopathy. While there are other forms of diagnosis, the pathoanatomic diagnostic model has typically formed the basis of musculoskeletal assessment over the last several decades.

Pathoanatomic diagnosis

The pathoanatomic approach to diagnosis can be helpful in guiding the selection of treatments that target a structural lesion or pathology in circumstances where this will positively influence recovery, e.g., surgical fixation of a fracture, surgical repair of a traumatic rotator cuff tear in a young person or surgical replacement of an arthritic glenohumeral joint associated with severe symptoms and morbidity. A pathoanatomic diagnosis may also guide the protection of specific tissues from excessive load during periods of healing, such as in bone, ligament, tendon, and muscle injuries.

Where a pathoanatomic diagnosis is possible it can help those with shoulder conditions to understand their condition and its prognosis, inform their expectations and decisions relating to the available treatment options, and provide a means of communication between health professionals to facilitate access to agreed care pathways for specific conditions.

Limitations of pathoanatomic diagnosis in nontraumatic shoulder pain

The pathoanatomic approach to diagnosis and treatment is predicated upon two assumptions: that we can determine the anatomical source of a patient's symptoms with reasonable consistency, and that doing so will better inform treatment options and improve patient outcomes. While this may hold true in traumatic tissue rupture and for some nontraumatic conditions such as advanced osteoarthritis where surgical treatment has shown clinical benefit, there is increasing evidence that challenges these foundational beliefs in people with nontraumatic shoulder conditions. Concerns with the pathoanatomic approach relating to the validity of the clinical examination to identify the source of pain, the interpretation of the symptomatic relevance of imaging findings, and the outcomes of surgical treatments that target pathoanatomic structures has questioned the widespread applicability of the pathoanatomic model to many nontraumatic shoulder presentations.

Validity of clinical examination tests

Shoulder orthopedic special tests have been widely incorporated into the clinical examination to identify structural pathology or to help rule-in a condition such as rotator cuff tendinopathy or labral tear. They rely on the assumption that a specific structure can be isolated, and that a positive test finding, such as pain, originates from the structure being tested.[49] The ability to isolate shoulder structures during the examination is unquestionably challenged by the complex anatomic connections between the rotator cuff muscles and tendons, the glenohumeral joint capsule, capsular ligaments, and bursal tissue.[13] Therefore the ability of these tests to selectively isolate specific shoulder structures is doubtful, with mounting evidence showing poor specificity of many of these tests for specific shoulder pathologies.[20,22,23,26,27]

Evidence for the accuracy of these tests for identifying specific pathology consistently demonstrates the orthopedic tests to be of limited diagnostic value when compared with imaging or surgical reference standards.[22,26,27] The authors of a recent systematic review and meta-analysis concluded that they could not unequivocally recommend the use of any single test for informing a pathoanatomic diagnosis.[27] Even when these tests were combined, diagnostic utility was limited.[25]

Symptomatic relevance of imaging findings

Radiologic imaging or surgical visualization were the reference standard tests used to identify structural pathology in most of these diagnostic accuracy studies, based upon the assumption that the visualized pathology is the source of pain. The same assumptions are often made in clinical practice when interpreting pathologic findings on diagnostic imaging investigations. There is a high prevalence of imaged pathology in asymptomatic populations. For example, rotator cuff tendinosis, partial and full thickness rotator cuff tears, labral tears, and thickening of the subacromial bursa are evident in many people without symptoms, and with normal function.[31,38,40,50,51,55] The prevalence of these findings increases with advancing age.[38,40,55] This suggests that in some people, degenerative changes in the shoulder may simply be a normal sign of aging (such as gray hair and wrinkles that we cannot feel and only "hurt" when you see them in the mirror!) and therefore, caution should be exercised when interpreting imaging findings, as is the case with nonspecific low back pain.

The results of diagnostic accuracy studies that have used imaging or surgical visualization of pathology such as bursal, labral, and degenerative tendon changes as the reference standard test to estimate diagnostic accuracy of clinical tests must therefore be re-evaluated. The same holds true in clinical practice, where imaging findings must be interpreted in the context of clinical findings and correlated with presenting symptoms and signs to avoid overdiagnosis and inappropriate treatment of asymptomatic pathology. Researchers have used diagnostic injection of local anesthetic as the reference test to compare clinical tests aiming to identify subacromial[6,8] or acromioclavicular joint pain.[7,12,64] Although some tests were helpful for ruling out the pain source, few individual tests demonstrated a clinically meaningful change in the ability to positively identify pain arising from the subacromial region or acromioclavicular joint.

We know that pain is a complex phenomenon with nociceptive, and non-nociceptive causes (see Chapter 7) and there is increasing awareness and appreciation of the myriad factors that can influence the perception of pain. That is to say, the traditional view of musculoskeletal pain as an accurate and infallible indicator of underlying tissue pathology should be reframed in the context of an evolving understanding of pain.

Traumatic and nontraumatic shoulder conditions

Traumatic shoulder conditions

Making a rapid diagnosis of traumatic injuries such as fractures, complex glenohumeral instability, neurovascular injury, and soft tissue ruptures is important to facilitate orthopedic review as surgery may be required. Missing a surgical window of opportunity for these traumatic injuries may result in suboptimal outcomes due to deterioration in muscle quality over time that can negatively affect repairability and result in functional disability.[24] The severity of trauma required to produce significant structural injury may also reduce with age, and with poor tissue health (e.g., osteoporosis), and these factors should be considered when assessing the probability of traumatic structural injury in specific populations.

Nontraumatic shoulder conditions

The assumption that surgical treatment of the pathoanatomic lesion leads to superior outcomes has also been challenged in people with nontraumatic shoulder pain. In people with impingement symptoms, and in those with small, nontraumatic, isolated supraspinatus tears, surgical treatment including subacromial decompression and rotator cuff repair did not result in significantly improved outcomes compared with nonsurgical treatment.[41,42] While surgical procedures may have a place in the continuum of care in the context of people whose symptoms fail to improve with appropriate periods of time and following a course of nonsurgical treatment, there is mounting evidence to suggest that these surgical procedures may not be appropriate first-line treatments for nontraumatic shoulder conditions.

For the majority of those with nontraumatic shoulder symptoms the process of searching for a specific pathoanatomic diagnosis generally does little to inform treatment selection and does not confer significant clinical benefit especially in the early stages of management. Pursuit of a pathoanatomic source of symptoms may lead to overdiagnosis and overtreatment of asymptomatic pathology and has the potential to create fear and anxiety that may lead to maladaptive pain-related beliefs and behaviors in some people, thereby negatively affecting outcomes.

A pathoanatomic diagnosis is not often needed for nontraumatic shoulder conditions early in the clinical pathway. However, it becomes increasingly important to gain further diagnostic clarity when clinical progress is inadequate to help exclude or identify specific conditions to inform treatment selection, provide prognostic information and facilitate continuity of care through the health system according to agreed clinical pathways for specific conditions.

Conditions such as glenohumeral and acromioclavicular osteoarthritis have natural histories characterized by progressive deterioration. When nonsurgical treatments no longer adequately control symptoms, many people experience relief from surgical treatment.[5,9,19] Despite its often-favorable natural history, some people experience persistent symptoms from calcific tendinopathy (see Chapter 27) that do not settle adequately over time. Targeted treatments including injection therapy and surgical treatment have been shown to be beneficial in the treatment of ongoing and functionally limiting symptoms for some nontraumatic shoulder conditions such as frozen shoulder and calcific tendinopathy.[3,17] Table 15.1 categorizes traumatic and nontraumatic conditions that may benefit from targeted treatment if there is insufficient clinical progress.

Table 15.1 Categories of pathoanatomic diagnoses for which specific treatment may be required

Category	Traumatic conditions Orthopaedic review may be required	Nontraumatic conditions Targeted treatments may be required if there is insufficient clinical progress
Unstable shoulder History of instability	Bony Bankart fracture Glenoid labrum tear (large or complex) Humeral avulsion glenohumeral ligaments (HAGL) lesion	
Stiff shoulder Loss of passive movement, especially external rotation	Locked posterior dislocation Humeral fracture	Glenohumeral osteoarthritis Frozen shoulder
Rotator cuff Full passive movement, pain, and weakness with rotator cuff tests	Acute, large, or multi-tendon rotator cuff tear Complete subscapularis tear	Calcific tendinopathy (resorptive)
Acromioclavicular (AC) joint Exclusion of other conditions, observation, palpation and pain on movements that stress the AC joint	Clavicle or scapular fracture High grade dislocation	Acromioclavicular joint arthropathy Clavicular osteolysis
Other conditions	Fractures Acute soft tissue ruptures	Sternoclavicular joint arthropathy

Health

Health is defined as a state of complete physical, mental and social well-being and not merely the absence of disease or infirmity.[68] There is an increasing recognition of a range of contextual and experiential factors as well as other psychosocial factors that influence a person's health status and can moderate treatment outcomes. These factors work in combinations, and interact with each other to influence a person's experience of pain, their level of disability and their response to treatment.[43] In acute, traumatic presentations, restoration of pathoanatomy may be the immediate priority.[44] Later during rehabilitation, and for those with many nontraumatic presentations, these factors are more likely to play a role in the persistence of symptoms and associated disability.

Psychosocial factors

Cognitive and psychosocial factors such as patient expectations of a good treatment outcome and higher levels of pain self-efficacy have been consistently shown to predict better treatment outcomes for pain and function following both surgical[14,59] and nonsurgical (physiotherapy) treatment.[10,16] Baseline measures of shoulder pain and function,[11] distress, anxiety, catastrophizing, and kinesiophobia[37,52,61,67] have also been recognized as mediators of pain and disability in those with shoulder symptoms (see Chapter 6).

Lifestyle factors

Lifestyle factors are modifiable entities relating to a person's choice about social, nutritional, smoking, drug and alcohol intake, recreational and physical activity habits (see Chapter 5). Musculoskeletal conditions, including shoulder conditions share similar lifestyle risk factors to other noncommunicable diseases, such as cardiovascular disease, diabetes, dementia and cancer.[70]

Environmental factors

Environmental factors are external to the individual and beyond their direct control. These factors influence not only individual but also population health. In the context of health, they include policy, access to healthcare, the availability of healthcare services, physical accessibility for those with disabilities, housing and social infrastructure, and cultural factors. The degree to which each of these factors combine and interact with each other to influence outcomes will vary among individuals, even for those with similar clinical presentations. Treatment priorities will depend upon identification of the most influential factors for the individual. For some, biomedical factors specific to the shoulder condition may take priority for management, such as treatment targeting the pathoanatomic lesion (e.g., bony Bankart lesion (glenoid fracture), traumatic rotator cuff tear, or displaced humerus fracture). For others, various psychosocial, lifestyle, or environmental modifiers may present a significant barrier to recovery and may take priority over biomedical factors for management.

Careful and thorough assessment of each of these factors is essential in helping to select interventions that are most likely to have the largest beneficial impact upon outcome for people with shoulder symptoms. Importantly, these factors are rarely managed in isolation, rather they become integrated and prioritized within the wider management program to support concurrent components of treatment.

Contextual factors

In addition to biopsychosocial factors and other health determinants, contextual effects and the lived experience are being increasingly recognized as influencers of health, disability, and response to treatment. For people who present with causal complexity, a "whole person-centered" approach has been suggested that uses the patient narrative (see Chapters 1 and 11) as a starting point for further enquiry rather than beginning with an assessment of individual elements.[21,47]

Contextual effects including characteristics of the treatment provider, the person with symptoms, the relationship between them and features of the treatment itself can all influence clinical outcomes.[56] Recent evidence suggests that diagnostic terminology may create fear, corrupt thoughts, generate negative emotions and prompt actions and behavioral changes that may negatively influence outcome in some people.[53] However, many people still have an expectation of a discussion relating to the cause of their symptoms,[62] and in a cohort of adults attending private clinics, 83% rated diagnosis as being important.[36] People with shoulder pain have also expressed a desire to understand why "it hurts so much" and held well-established biomechanical notions of pain, that appeared to influence their expectations relating to diagnosis and treatment.[35]

Navigating this dilemma represents the art to the science of clinical practice requiring careful communication, explanation and contextualization when conveying information to people with shoulder symptoms, and other musculoskeletal conditions.

Shoulder assessment

The assessment of shoulder symptoms aims to provide the means for helping the clinician make decisions about the most appropriate management for the individual. Contemporary methods of shoulder assessment must therefore be expanded beyond the traditional pathoanatomic approach. The integration of clinical examination findings within an interpretative framework using clinical methods that help to evaluate the contribution of other biopsychosocial, contextual, and experiential factors is required.

Assessment starts with observation of the individual as they enter your clinic and includes verbal and nonverbal communication. It continues during the patient interview and physical assessment where information is gathered, and hypotheses are tested to help screen for indicators of serious medical conditions (see Chapters 8, 13, and 14), identify specific shoulder conditions that may require specific treatment, and further define other symptoms to help guide treatment. Purposeful communication (see Chapters 6, 11, and 36) is central to this process and is supported by the application of meaningful outcome measures (see Chapter 12) and clinical reasoning (see Chapter 13).

Interpretive assessment

Interpretative assessment is central to the integration of further information gained from the clinical examination and results of further investigations. The use of narrative-based clinical tools enables the person with symptoms to be seen as an individual rather than a set of clinical symptoms and signs. Enabling the individual to tell their story enhances person-centered care, improves communication and provides a model of empathy, trust and collaboration to guide treatment decisions.[48] Questioning the individual about their interpretation of health information, understanding of their condition and beliefs, concerns and fears about their symptoms and treatment can help gain an understanding about the possible influence of some contextual effects that may influence treatment response.

Information pertaining to general health, cognitive, psychological, lifestyle, and social factors can be obtained using questionnaires and through careful questioning during the initial and subsequent clinical encounters. Results can help guide decisions regarding the need for further assessment, onward referral, or specific management.

Managing diagnostic uncertainty

Due to uncertainties in diagnosis in those with nontraumatic presentations, in the majority of cases when discussing the findings of the assessment with patients, clinicians (at best) should say: "Based on our discussion and from the physical assessment, supported by the imaging and laboratory tests, it is *likely* that you have [*insert condition*]." This should then be followed by shared decision-making (see Chapter 13). This chapter focuses on supporting clinicians arriving at the point of likely diagnosis. For example, when faced with a combination of shoulder pain and restricted movement, the clinician might categorize this presentation as a stiff and painful shoulder. There are myriad reasons for the clinical presentation of shoulder pain and stiffness including osteoarthritis, avascular necrosis, osteosarcoma, and locked posterior dislocation, and each requires a separate management pathway.

We suggest subclassification is not only possible, but is also desirable, for research purposes and for more appropriately targeted clinical intervention. For example, in an otherwise fit and healthy 50-year-old who is experiencing nondominant-side shoulder pain associated with a 50% loss of active and passive external rotation when compared to the contralateral side, and with nothing abnormal detected on radiograph, it would enable the clinician to subcategorize the presenting pain and stiffness as a primary idiopathic frozen shoulder. The clinician can then inform the patient that they are *likely* to have a frozen shoulder. This would be followed by a discussion about the condition, followed by an unbiased presentation of the different management options, which would include their expected benefits, harms, and timeframes. The option of "watch and wait" should also be considered and discussed.

Clinical examination

Interview

During the interview, important information is gathered about the mechanism of onset of symptoms (traumatic versus nontraumatic), symptom location, severity, nature and behavior, associated symptoms, health history, response to previous treatments and comorbidities. Together, this information is added to demographic data and, later, physical examination findings to help refine the clinical hypotheses (see Chapters 12 and 13).

Physical examination

The aim of the physical examination is to systematically assess the shoulder to identify observable concerns, such as substantial atrophy, structural abnormalities that might suggest a fracture or dislocation, and screening for other concerns, such as melanomas. Palpation is important to detect changes in temperature, identify unexpected lumps, bumps, structural abnormalities, and swelling. There is no evidence that palpation is reliable for the definitive identification of structures.

The physical examination includes screening procedures to implicate or exclude, as best as possible, non-shoulder causes of symptoms, such as referred, cervical, thoracic, and abdominal region pain. The results of basic physical shoulder examination tests such as active and passive movement and muscle performance can provide valuable differential diagnostic information to help identify or exclude local shoulder symptoms. Associated symptoms, commonly pain, stiffness and feelings of instability are recorded during the tests and can help determine whether the primary shoulder problem is related to stiffness, instability, pain, or weakness. Functional movement testing is also important, and joint laxity testing and a comprehensive neurological examination may also be indicated. Table 15.2 details recommendations for the physical examination of a person presenting with shoulder symptoms.

Interpretation of clinical examination findings

Many people present with a variety of symptoms that include pain, stiffness, weakness, and instability. In many cases these symptoms overlap, however, usually there will be a predominant clinical feature. It is possible to formulate clinical hypotheses based on key clinical features gained during the examination: unstable shoulder (interview); stiff shoulder (passive range of motion tests); painful shoulder (active and passive movement, and muscle performance testing); weak shoulder (active and passive movement tests, and muscle performance testing). There are several specific conditions within these categories, and further differential diagnosis may be required if clinically indicated.

Table 15.2 Recommended components of the physical examination of the shoulder

Examination	Purpose
Observation	Identification of: • Substantial atrophy • Bruising, discoloration • Dislocation, fracture • Severe fixed postural abnormality • Potential melanoma or other masses/lumps
Palpation	Identification of: • Temperature changes • Lumps and bumps • Soft tissue swelling and bony abnormalities
Cervical, thoracic, abdominal region assessment	Identification of • Referred pain (see Chapter 16)
Active and passive ranges of physiological movement. May be conducted in standing, sitting, side-lying, supine, prone and when relevant using long (elbow extended) and short (elbow flexed) lever arms to assess symptom reproduction and range of motion.	Bilateral assessment of shoulder: • Flexion • Extension • Abduction (scapular +/– anatomical plane) • External rotation • Internal rotation/hand behind back • Cross body flexion (adduction)/ extension (abduction)
Muscle performance testing. May be conducted in standing, sitting, side-lying, supine, and prone.	Assessment during: • Abduction • Flexion • Extension • External rotation • Internal rotation • Lag signs (for rupture of specific rotator cuff components) May include: • Maximal isometric strength (break test) • Isometric strength (make test) • Repetitions to pain • Repetitions to fatigue • Repetitions to symptoms
Procedures as appropriate	May include: • Neurological tests • Neuromeningeal tests (see Chapter 21) • Hemodynamic tests (see Chapter 22) • Other relevant physiological tests (e.g., respiratory function, hip–waist ratios) • Kinetic chain assessment

(Continued)

Table 15.2 *(Continued)*

Examination	Purpose
Functional assessment	Patient-identified movements or postures that provoke or alleviate symptoms: • Active movements • Functional activities • Postures (see Chapter 20)

Imaging

Due to the lack of specificity of clinical examination tests for specific shoulder conditions, appropriate imaging is often required to confirm or exclude a specific pathoanatomic diagnosis where specific treatment targeting the condition is required, such as surgery or injections. When traumatic conditions are suspected, or in those with non-traumatic conditions that are not responding to treatment, appropriate imaging may be utilized to further clarify the clinical differential diagnosis to help guide management. Patient safety, cost, diagnostic value, and the risk of overdiagnosis and overtreatment also need to be considered when requesting shoulder imaging, and careful correlation of any imaged pathology with the clinical presentation is essential.

Where no guidelines are available, the following may serve as a guide during the diagnostic process for people with shoulder symptoms. Imaging indication guidelines (Box 15.1) support clinical decisions but should not replace clinical judgement. The role of imaging in the assessment and management of shoulder conditions is discussed in more detail in Chapter 14.

Radiographs are the recommended starting point for shoulder imaging and are recommended prior to other imaging investigations for most people with shoulder symptoms.[57,60,66] Other imaging modalities are utilized according to the clinical question. Diagnostic ultrasound visualizes soft tissues and is used as a method of guidance for interventional procedures.[66] Magnetic resonance imaging provides high resolution images used for the visualization of occult fractures, and detailed soft tissue imaging of the quality and integrity of the rotator cuff, bursa, biceps tendon, acromion, acromioclavicular joint, and surrounding bone marrow.[66] Computerized tomography is used to image complex fractures, and for surgical planning, such as prior to arthroplasty.[66] More detail is presented in Chapter 14.

Box 15.1 Indications for imaging

- Red flags.
- Significant trauma.
- First-time and subsequent traumatic shoulder dislocation.
- Suspected acute, traumatic rotator cuff or shoulder muscle-tear.
- Severe pain without identifiable cause.
- To differentiate between conditions where this will alter management.
- Prior to an invasive procedure such as an intra-articular glenohumeral injection for frozen shoulder.
- Unanticipated deterioration in a condition.
- Failure to progress with treatment.

New shoulder classification model

We propose a new model of classifying shoulder symptoms that integrates appropriate use of the traditional approach to diagnosis within an interpretive assessment framework that incorporates other influencing factors to help identify treatment priorities for people with shoulder symptoms. The purpose of classifying is to support clinicians to achieve a working hypothesis to explain the combination of symptoms, communicate this to the patient, and suggest the best possible management. Classification systems will inevitably evolve and change with new knowledge and technological advances, and are intended to be used as a guideline, allowing scope for variation supported by sound clinical reasoning processes to enable the provision of optimal management based upon individual needs.

The following classification system may be used at all levels of healthcare to help guide assessment, diagnostic tests, and treatment decision-making. The model groups individuals according to their predominant presenting clinical feature from which clinical hypotheses can be further refined within each category. The model acknowledges that symptoms and signs often overlap and change over time. Classification models that do not account for overlapping presentations may not reflect clinical reality. This model also allows for movement between categories while still allowing treatment priorities to change according to evolving clinical presentations.

The classification system also acknowledges the interaction between clinical features and other biopsychosocial, pathoanatomic, lifestyle, and environmental factors in determining health and treatment outcomes. These factors surround the clinical categories representing their importance in the assessment and management of people with shoulder conditions. Central to the model is an understanding of the importance of contextual factors and the narrative of the person with shoulder symptoms in both assessment and treatment. The model and explanatory legend are presented in Figure 15.1.

Clinical classification of shoulder disability

Nearly all people who present with musculoskeletal shoulder problems will describe varying combinations of pain, weakness, stiffness and, less commonly, instability. Categorization in this model is intended to be based upon the most significant clinical presentation for the individual. The categories are grouped sequentially to reflect diagnostic reasoning processes, where there is an increase in probability of the person falling into one category if previous categories have been excluded. These categories are not intended to represent strict diagnostic criteria – rather they represent a start point from which further diagnostic reasoning and decisions about further investigations and management can occur.

The clinical examination should be supported by a robust clinical reasoning process. Within each category there are several possible causes for the presenting symptoms including red flag or serious medical conditions, specific traumatic and nontraumatic pathoanatomic shoulder conditions, other clinical syndromes (e.g., impingement, scapular dyskinesis, mechanosensitivity) or persistent pain presentations. The overall clinical reasoning process is informed by the information gathered during the interview and physical examination that is then used to formulate a list of possible hypotheses that are refined with the addition of new information.

A list of possible causes of symptoms in each category are listed under the diagram. These are not exhaustive but provide an indication of some of the more common causes considered to explain the presenting symptoms. Imaging may be required to confirm, exclude, or differentiate between specific conditions to aid in the differential diagnosis process as covered earlier in this chapter.

Not the shoulder

Clinicians need be alert for indicators of serious medical pathology as the cause of the symptoms, even if there has been previous medical assessment. Medical conditions that may present with shoulder girdle and upper limb symptoms include infections, cancer (primary and secondary bone, lung and other cancers), and cardiovascular compromise, all of which are commonly missed in primary care settings.[69] Other conditions that may cause symptoms in the shoulder region include pulmonary or neurologic disease (upper or lower motor neuron), and systemic inflammatory diseases such as rheumatoid arthritis and seronegative spondyloarthropathies.

The assessment of health risk factors, atypical symptoms and signs, involvement of other body systems and assessment of the response to previous treatment may help identify red flag indicators of serious pathology that require medical follow-up.[4] Red flags may also develop between medical consultations, and the clinician should remain vigilant for the development of red flags between sessions. Timeliness of referral for medical assessment is critical in avoiding error-related harm relating to delayed or missed diagnosis.[18] Red flags, inflammatory conditions, and sinister pathology are covered in detail in Chapter 8.

Shoulder symptoms may also arise due to pain referred from somatic (e.g., cervicothoracic region) or visceral structures (e.g., heart, gall bladder). Conducting an appropriate examination for somatic referred pain and being alert for symptoms or signs of visceral body system involvement are important in the screening process for people with shoulder symptoms. This is discussed in Chapter 16.

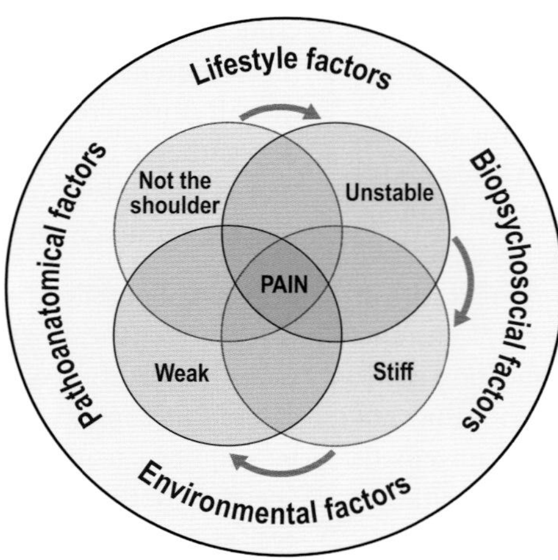

Lifestyle	Biopsychosocial	Environmental	Pathoanatomical
Physical activity **Nutrition** **Sleep** **Smoking** **Stress** **Alcohol** **Recreational drug use**	**Biomechanical/biologic** Variation of movement and/or posture produced by one or multiple variables that results in a physiological (e.g., edema) and/ or functional abnormality (e.g., movement restriction or control) Genetic factors Metabolic factors Hormonal factors Medical comorbidities Musculoskeletal comorbidities Medication Neurophysiologic processes **Psychological** Cognitive, behavioral and emotional factors, mental health, mood, anxiety, and fear that can detrimentally impact on the individual and cause distress **Social** Socioeconomic, family circumstances, personal relationships, occupational, cultural, and religious factors that influence the individual and their health	**Policy** **Healthcare inequalities** **Healthcare access – including availability and use of healthcare services, physical accessibility** **Eligibility for healthcare funding** **Compensation** **Housing and social infrastructure** **Culture**	**Inflammation** **Biochemical imbalance** **Infection** **Neuropathy** **Degeneration** **Soft tissue pathology** **Fracture** **Loose body** **Vascular pathology** **Arthropathy**

FIGURE 15.1
Shoulder classification model.

Unstable shoulder

The key clinical diagnostic feature of the unstable shoulder is a history of instability (subluxation or dislocation). The mechanism and circumstances behind the instability (traumatic versus atraumatic), as well as the frequency, direction, and severity of instability are also key elements of the patient history that help subclassify shoulder instability to help determine whether further investigations are required, as well as guiding the best management for different types of instability. More detail is presented in Chapters 17 and 37.

Traumatic instability

Traumatic instability events may result in structural injury to bone, capsuloligamentous, labral, soft tissue and neurovascular structures. Imaging is generally recommended for all those who suffer a first-time shoulder dislocation around the shoulder to identify or exclude structural pathology. Undiagnosed structural pathology may result in recurrent instability and poor outcomes and there is a higher prevalence of fractures and rotator cuff tears in those over 40 years of age with a first-time traumatic dislocation.[2] The anterior apprehension and relocation tests have shown high levels of accuracy for structural instability lesions, when apprehension is used as the positive test criteria.[25–27] Physical examination tests for labral pathology have shown variable accuracy and should be interpreted with caution.[26,27]

In some cases, surgery may be required for structural injury following shared decision-making. In many cases a trial of nonsurgical treatment and rehabilitation may be offered focusing on respecting the pathoanatomy of any healing tissue, followed by progressive restoration of range of motion, strength and proprioception.

Atraumatic instability

This can be a complex subgroup of the instability population, with younger people primarily affected. Patients with atraumatic instability rarely have structural lesions on imaging, however in some cases, a structural cause of ongoing instability may need to be excluded. For most people, a pathoanatomic diagnostic approach is unhelpful and the mainstay of treatment is physiotherapy, with a focus on neuromuscular rehabilitation that includes assessment and management of important psychosocial, lifestyle, and environmental modifiers of outcome.

Stiff shoulder

The definition of a "stiff shoulder" is a loss of passive range of motion for any reason,[29] and common causes include frozen shoulder and glenohumeral osteoarthritis. However, a range of other traumatic, neoplastic, and neurologic conditions can also cause a loss of passive movement, including a locked posterior glenohumeral dislocation, proximal humerus fracture, osteosarcoma of the proximal humerus, high tone in upper motor neuron conditions, and muscle guarding.[28,30,63] Treatment and prognosis are dependent on the most likely explanation for the presentation and are discussed throughout this book.

Painful shoulder

To be classified in the "painful shoulder" group, pain must be the predominant feature. An important feature of diagnosis for both subacromial and acromioclavicular joint pain conditions is the exclusion of shoulder instability and stiff shoulder conditions as a cause of the pain. In other words, no history of instability, and full or almost full passive range of motion are important clinical features in this category.

Most people present with complaints of pain around the shoulder for which there are many causes. The structures that most commonly cause pain (not already covered in the unstable and stiff shoulder conditions) include subacromial structures (subacromial bursa, rotator cuff tendons and the long head of biceps) and the acromioclavicular joint (ligaments, bone and capsule). Pain will commonly be associated with a degree of weakness identified in muscle performance testing, which may be due to pain inhibition, structural pathology, or disuse atrophy.

Subacromial pain

Several important pathoanatomic hypotheses influence management and prognosis in this group including acute traumatic rotator cuff tears, especially complete subscapularis tears that may require surgical repair. Pain attributed to biceps tendinopathy (see Chapter 26) and calcific tendinopathy (see Chapter 27) may require nuanced intervention. The majority of other painful subacromial conditions are of limited pathoanatomic significance as treatment is primarily impairment- and symptom-based.[32,33] However, conditions that fail to respond to an appropriate period of nonsurgical management may also require additional pain relief interventions, or orthopedic review, hence imaging may play a role in refining the diagnosis later in the clinical course for those who fail to progress.

Clavicular pain

The exclusion of shoulder instability, shoulder stiffness and subacromial pain are important clinical diagnostic features of both acromioclavicular, and the less-often discussed sternoclavicular joint. Full passive range of motion (except for pain and associated mild loss of end range), and minimal pain or weakness with resisted rotator cuff tests, combined with tenderness around the acromioclavicular (or sternoclavicular) joint, and pain provocation in positions that place stress across these joints (end ranges of elevation, cross body movement and, often, hand behind back) are the primary features of pain arising from these joints. Scapular movements may also provoke pain in some people with symptomatic clavicular joints. There are a wide range of pathologies that can affect these joints, and differentiation of specific pathologies may inform management and prognosis if symptoms fail to settle.

Weak shoulder

This category includes people for whom weakness or loss of strength or power in the shoulder is the primary feature, that may occur in the presence of variable amounts of pain, the absence of instability, and full passive motion.

Ruptures

Acute muscle or tendon ruptures, sufficient to cause loss of power in the arm, will commonly require surgical repair, and obtaining an early pathoanatomic diagnosis with imaging confirmation is important in avoiding adverse outcomes from delayed surgical repair. The loss of power may also be associated with pain in acute injury; however, the loss of strength is the predominant feature of concern.

Neuropathies

While some neuropathies present with pain in the early stages, after several weeks, specific muscle weakness and associated atrophy often becomes evident. The differential diagnosis of the pain in the early stages, before the onset of significant weakness, can be difficult; however, once weakness becomes apparent, the differential diagnosis becomes clearer, especially as it is often followed by specific innervation patterns of muscle atrophy. There can be many causes of peripheral neuropathy ranging from trauma to compressive lesions such as tumors or paralabral cysts, to post-viral onset of symptoms.[34,54] A careful history is required, often supported by medical referral, to investigate possible causes and to monitor recovery of nerve function. The prognosis depends upon the etiology and duration of denervation with recovery generally being slow, taking months or years.

Conclusion

Our framework broadly categorizes musculoskeletal shoulder disorders under the chief presenting problem: referred pain, instability or hypermobility, stiffness, or weakness. Pain is common to all of them, but in some cases may not be present. A movement-based diagnosis need not completely dismiss a pathoanatomic one – they can coexist without contradiction.

Incorporation of the traditional pathoanatomic diagnostic model within a broader assessment framework may improve alignment with treatment strategies and better acknowledge the role of lifestyle factors, comorbidities, psychosocial and contextual factors in the experience of shoulder conditions. Making a diagnosis of traumatic structural lesions and other conditions, such as an osteosarcoma, is important and immediate referral is essential; however, for many people who seek care for nontraumatic shoulder symptoms, the utility of a pathoanatomic diagnostic approach is limited. A movement-based classification system that de-emphasizes but incorporates pathoanatomic hypotheses may strike the right balance and is more likely to serve a wider proportion of those who seek care for shoulder symptoms.

References

1. Aggarwal R, Ringold S, Khanna D, et al. Distinctions between diagnostic and classification criteria? Arthritis Care Res. 2015;67:891-897.
2. Atef A, El-Tantawy A, Gad H, Hefeda M. Prevalence of associated injuries after anterior shoulder dislocation: a prospective study. Int Orthop. 2016;40:519-524.
3. Barber FA, Cowden CH, 3rd. Arthroscopic treatment of calcific tendonitis. Arthrosc Tech. 2014;3:e237-e240.
4. Boissonnault WG. Primary Care for the Physical Therapist. Elsevier Inc.; 2005.
5. Cadet E, Ahmad CS, Levine WN. The management of acromioclavicular joint osteoarthrosis: débride, resect, or leave it alone. Instr. Course Lect. 2006;55:75-83.
6. Cadogan A, McNair P, Laslett M, Hing W. Diagnostic accuracy of clinical examination and imaging findings for identifying subacromial pain. PLoS ONE. 2016;11:e0167738.
7. Cadogan A, McNair P, Laslett M, Hing W. Shoulder pain in primary care: diagnostic accuracy of clinical examination tests for non-traumatic acromioclavicular joint pain. BMC Musculoskelet Disord. 2013;14:156.
8. Calis M, Akgun K, Birtane M, Karacan I, Calis H, Tuzun F. Diagnostic values of clinical diagnostic tests in subacromial impingement syndrome. Ann. Rheum. Dis. 2000;59:44-47.
9. Carter MJ, Mikuls TR, Nayak S, Fehringer EV, Michaud K. Impact of total shoulder arthroplasty on generic and shoulder-specific health-related quality-of-life measures: a systematic literature review and meta-analysis. J Bone Joint Surg Am. 2012;94:e127.121-e127.129.
10. Chester R, Jerosch-Herold C, Lewis J, Shepstone L. Psychological factors are associated with the outcome of physiotherapy for people with shoulder pain: a multicentre longitudinal cohort study. British Journal of Sports Medicine. 2018;52:269-275.
11. Chester R, Shepstone L, Daniell H, Sweeting D, Lewis J, Jerosch-Herold C. Predicting response to physiotherapy treatment for musculoskeletal shoulder pain: a systematic review. BMC Musculoskelet Disord. 2013;14:203.
12. Chronopoulos E, Kim TK, Park HB, Ashenbrenner D, McFarland EG. Diagnostic value of physical tests for isolated chronic acromioclavicular lesions. American Journal of Sports Medicine. 2004;32:655-661.
13. Clark JM, Harryman II DT. Tendons, ligaments, and capsule of the rotator cuff. Gross and microscopic anatomy. J. Bone Joint Surg Am. 1992;74:713-725.
14. Coronado RA, Seitz AL, Pelote E, Archer KR, Jain NB. Are psychosocial factors associated with patient-reported outcome measures in patients with rotator cuff tears? A Systematic review. Clinical Orthopaedics and Related Research. 2018;476:810-829.
15. Croft PR, Pope DP, Silman AJ. The clinical course of shoulder pain: prospective cohort study in primary care. BMJ. 1996;313:601-602.
16. De Baets L, Matheve T, Meeus M, Struyf F, Timmermans A. The influence of cognitions, emotions and behavioral factors on treatment outcomes in musculoskeletal shoulder pain: a systematic review. Clin Rehabil. 2019;33:980-991.
17. ElShewy MT. Calcific tendinitis of the rotator cuff. World J Orthop. 2016;7:55-60.
18. Finucane LM, Downie A, Mercer C, et al. International framework for red flags for potential serious spinal pathologies. J Orthop. Sports Phys Ther. 2020;50:350-372.
19. Gancarczyk SM, Ahmad CS. Acromioclavicular arthritis and osteolysis. Operative Techniques in Sports Medicine. 2014;22:214-220.
20. Gismervik SØ, Drogset JO, Granviken F, Rø M, Leivseth G. Physical examination tests of the shoulder: a systematic review and meta-analysis of diagnostic test performance. BMC Musculoskelet Disord. 2017;18:41.
21. Greenhalgh T. Narrative based medicine: narrative based medicine in an evidence based world. BMJ (Clinical research ed.). 1999;318:323-325.
22. Hanchard NCA, Handoll HHG. Physical tests for shoulder impingements and local lesions of bursa, tendon or labrum that may accompany impingement. Cochrane Database Syst Rev. 2008;CD007427.
23. Hanchard NCA, Lenza M, Handoll HHG, Takwoingi Y. Physical tests for shoulder impingements and local lesions of bursa, tendon or labrum that may accompany impingement. Cochrane Database Syst Rev. 2013;CD007427.
24. Hantes ME, Karidakis GK, Vlychou M, Varitimidis S, Dailiana Z, Malizos KN. A comparison of early versus delayed repair of traumatic rotator cuff tears. Knee Surg Sports Traumatol Arthrosc. 2011;19:1766-1770.
25. Hegedus EJ, Cook C, Lewis J, Wright A, Park JY. Combining orthopedic special tests to improve diagnosis of shoulder pathology. Phys Ther Sport. 2015;16:87-92.
26. Hegedus EJ, Goode A, Campbell S, et al. Physical examination tests of the shoulder: a systematic review with meta-analysis of individual tests. British Journal of Sports Medicine. 2008;42:80-92.
27. Hegedus EJ, Goode AP, Cook CE, et al. Which physical examination tests provide clinicians with the most value when examining the shoulder? Update of a systematic review with meta-analysis of individual tests. British Journal of Sports Medicine. 2012;46:964-978.
28. Hollmann L, Halaki M, Kamper SJ, Haber M, Ginn KA. Does muscle guarding play a role in range of motion loss in patients with frozen shoulder? Musculoskelet Sci Pract. 2018;37:64-68.
29. ISAKOS Upper Extremity Committee. ISAKOS Upper Extremity Committee Consensus Statement: Shoulder Stiffness. Berlin: Springer-Verlag; 2014.
30. Itoi E, Arce G, Bain GI, et al. Shoulder Stiffness: Current Concepts and Concerns. Springer; 2015.
31. Lee CS, Goldhaber NH, Davis SM, et al. Shoulder MRI in asymptomatic elite volleyball athletes shows extensive pathology. Journal of ISAKOS: Joint Disorders & Orthopaedic Sports Medicine 2020;5:10-14.
32. Lewis J. Rotator cuff related shoulder pain: assessment, management and uncertainties. Man Ther. 2016;23:57-68.
33. Lewis JS. Rotator cuff tendinopathy: a model for the continuum of pathology and related management. British Journal of Sports Medicine. 2010;44:918-923.
34. Madani A, Creteur V. Nerves around the shoulder: what the radiologist should know. J Belg Soc Radiol. 2017;101:9.
35. Maxwell C, Robinson K, McCreesh K. Understanding shoulder pain: a qualitative evidence synthesis exploring the patient experience. Physical Therapy. 2021;101:pzaa229.

36. McRae M, Hancock MJ. Adults attending private physiotherapy practices seek diagnosis, pain relief, improved function, education and prevention: a survey. J Physiother. 2017;63:250-256.

37. Menendez ME, Baker DK, Oladeji LO, Fryberger CT, McGwin G, Ponce BA. Psychological distress is associated with greater perceived disability and pain in patients presenting to a shoulder clinic. J Bone Joint Surg Am. 2015;97:1999-2003.

38. Milgrom C, Schaffler M, Gilbert S, van Holsbeeck M. Rotator-cuff changes in asymptomatic adults. The effect of age, hand dominance and gender. J Bone Joint Surg Br. 1995;77:296-298.

39. Miller-Keane Encyclopedia and Dictionary of Medicine, Nursing and Allied Health, 7th edition. Diagnosis. Saunders; 2003.

40. Minagawa H, Yamamoto N, Abe H, et al. Prevalence of symptomatic and asymptomatic rotator cuff tears in the general population: from mass-screening in one village. Journal of Orthopaedics. 2013;10:8-12.

41. Moosmayer S, Lund G, Seljom US, et al. Tendon repair compared with physiotherapy in the treatment of rotator cuff tears: a randomized controlled study in 103 cases with a five-year follow-up. J Bone Joint Surg Am. 2014;96:1504-1514.

42. Nazari G, MacDermid JC, Bryant D, Athwal GS. The effectiveness of surgical vs conservative interventions on pain and function in patients with shoulder impingement syndrome. A systematic review and meta-analysis. PloS One. 2019;14:e0216961-e0216961.

43. Office of Disease Prevention and Health Promotion. Determinants of Health. Available at: https://www.healthypeople.gov/2020/about/foundation-health-measures/Determinants-of-Health.

44. Olds M, Coulter C, Marant D, Uhl T. Reliability of a shoulder arm return to sport test battery. Phys Ther Sport. 2019;39:16-22.

45. Ostor AJK, Richards CA, Prevost AT, Speed CA, Hazleman BL. Diagnosis and relation to general health of shoulder disorders presenting to primary care. Rheumatology. 2005;44:800-805.

46. Oxford Online Dictionary. Diagnosis. Available at: https://en.oxforddictionaries.com/definition/diagnosis.

47. Rocca E, Anjum RL. Complexity, reductionism and the biomedical model. In: Anjum RL, Copeland S, Rocca E (eds). Rethinking Causality, Complexity and Evidence for the Unique Patient: A CauseHealth Resource for Healthcare Professionals and the Clinical Encounter. Springer International Publishing; 2020:75-94.

48. Rosti G. Role of narrative-based medicine in proper patient assessment. Supportive Care in Cancer 2017;25:3-6.

49. Salamh P, Lewis J. It is time to put special tests for rotator cuff–related shoulder pain out to pasture. J Orthop Sports Phys Ther. 2020;50:222-225.

50. Sher JS, Iannotti JP, Williams GR, et al. The effect of shoulder magnetic resonance imaging on clinical decision making. Journal of Shoulder and Elbow Surgery. 1998;7:205-209.

51. Shubin Stein BE, Wiater JM, Pfaff HC, Bigliani LU, Levine WN. Detection of acromioclavicular joint pathology in asymptomatic shoulders with magnetic resonance imaging. Journal of Shoulder and Elbow Surgery. 2001;10:204-208.

52. Smedbråten K, Øiestad BE, Røe Y. Emotional distress was associated with persistent shoulder pain after physiotherapy: a prospective cohort study. BMC Musculoskelet Disord. 2018;19:304.

53. Stewart M, Loftus S. Sticks and stones: the impact of language in musculoskeletal rehabilitation. J Orthop Sports Phys Ther. 2018;48:519-522.

54. Sumner AJ. Idiopathic brachial neuritis. Neurosurgery. 2009;65:A150-A152.

55. Tempelhof S, Rupp S, Seil R. Age-related prevalence of rotator cuff tears in asymptomatic shoulders. Journal of Shoulder and Elbow Surgery. 1999;8:296-299.

56. Testa M, Rossettini G. Enhance placebo, avoid nocebo: how contextual factors affect physiotherapy outcomes. Man Ther. 2016;24:65-74.

57. Tuite MJ, Small KM. Imaging evaluation of nonacute shoulder pain. American Journal of Roentgenology. 2017;209:525-533.

58. Urwin M, Symmons D, Allison T, et al. Estimating the burden of musculoskeletal disorders in the community: the comparative prevalence of symptoms at different anatomical sites, and the relation to social deprivation. Ann Rheum Dis. 1998;57:649-655.

59. Vajapey SP, Cvetanovich GL, Bishop JY, Neviaser AS. Psychosocial factors affecting outcomes after shoulder arthroplasty: a systematic review. Journal of Shoulder and Elbow Surgery. 2020;29:e175-e184.

60. Vakil C. Radiation and medical procedures: how do we do no harm? Canadian Family Physician. 2017;63:774-775.

61. Van Der Windt DAWM, Kuijpers T, Jellema P, Van Der Heijden GJMG, Bouter LM. Do psychological factors predict outcome in both low-back pain and shoulder pain? Ann Rheum Dis. 2007;66:313-319.

62. Verbeek J, Sengers MJ, Riemens L, Haafkens J. Patient expectations of treatment for back pain: a systematic review of qualitative and quantitative studies. Spine. 2004;29:2309-2318.

63. Walmsley S, Osmotherly PG, Rivett DA. Movement and pain patterns in early stage primary/idiopathic adhesive capsulitis: a factor analysis. Physiotherapy. 2014;100:336-343.

64. Walton J, Mahajan S, Paxinos A, et al. Diagnostic values of tests for acromioclavicular joint pain. J Bone Joint Surg Am. 2004;86:807-812.

65. Williams A, Kamper SJ, Wiggers JH, et al. Musculoskeletal conditions may increase the risk of chronic disease: a systematic review and meta-analysis of cohort studies. BMC Med. 2018;16:167.

66. Wise JN, Daffner RH, Weissman BN, et al. ACR Appropriateness Criteria® on acute shoulder pain. J Am Coll Radiol. 2011;8:602-609.

67. Wolfensberger A, Vuistiner P, Konzelmann M, Plomb-Holmes C, Léger B, Luthi F. Clinician and patient-reported outcomes are associated with psychological factors in patients with chronic shoulder pain. Clinical Orthopaedics and Related Research. 2016;474:2030-2039.

68. World Health Organisation. Constitution. Available at: https://www.who.int/about/who-we-are/.

69. World Health Organisation. Diagnostic Errors: Technical Series on Safer Primary Care. Geneva: World Health Organisation; 2016.

70. World Health Organisation. Musculoskeletal Conditions. Available at: https://www.who.int/news-room/fact-sheets/detail/musculoskeletal-conditions.

16 Not a shoulder

Chris Worsfold, Jeremy Lewis, Mira Meeus, Gwendolen Jull, Shaun O'Leary, Greg Lynch, Richard Rosedale, Grant Watson, Jillian McDowell, Bill Vicenzino, Brian Mulligan

Introduction

Shoulder pain most commonly arises from local shoulder problems. It may also arise from altered central pain processing, serious pathologies, visceral pathologies, and disorders of the cervicothoracic region. Differentiating a specific pathology that gives rise to pain experienced in the shoulder region is challenging. Clinical practice is akin to being the best (clinical) detective and best crime scene investigator possible, where hypotheses are generated, tested, accepted, or refuted. When refuted, alternative hypotheses should be considered. Clinicians should never unreservedly accept the diagnosis written on the referral or seek symptoms of their favorite diagnosis. Clinicians must remain cognizant to the uncertainty of diagnosis and also consider non-musculoskeletal causes of shoulder pain. The focus of this chapter is to discuss conditions that may present as shoulder pain, whose origins are not from local shoulder structures. This chapter should be read in conjunction with Chapter 8, which discusses red flags, inflammatory conditions and sinister shoulder pathology.

Pain referred to the shoulder region from the cervicothoracic spine

For a person experiencing pain in the shoulder region, regional interdependence refers to the possibility that another region may be responsible for causing or contributing to the presenting local pain and impairment. Referred pain is perceived in areas innervated by different nerves from those that supply the site of real transduction: the nerves supplying the region of referred pain are not engaged nor do they convey any input. As a rule, somatic referred pain is perceived in regions that share the same segmental innervation as the source. For example, shoulder pain, restricted shoulder movement and local muscle inhibition may have a cervical or cervicothoracic source. Full range of shoulder movement is dependent on a mobile cervicothoracic and thoracic spine, hence hypomobility in this region can contribute to a perceived lack of arm elevation.[66] Although definitive statistics are not available, up to 40% of people presenting with shoulder pain may have regional interdependence with the cervicothoracic region.[45]

Although several approaches have been suggested, we do not know the best method of assessing shoulder pain from cervicothoracic structures. In this chapter we will consider three that have gained international acceptance: the Maitland Approach, the McKenzie Method, and the Mulligan Concept. There are clear differences but also notable similarities across these approaches. Research has not been conducted to determine if any of these approaches is more reliable, valid, or effective than another. Since their introduction, research has shaped our understanding of these models of assessment and management, with the original biomechanical hypotheses for these methods now being replaced with the biopsychosocial model, underpinned with clinical reasoning.

An important starting point in the physical examination of the cervicothoracic spine's influence on the shoulder region is the careful assessment of active physiological movements and combinations of these movements, such as combining cervical rotation with side-flexion and then adding cervical flexion and extension if no contraindications exist. When safe and appropriate to do so, clinicians can add gentle pressure in the direction of the physiological cervicothoracic movements if the active movements alone do not reproduce symptoms. The threshold for determining a relationship between the cervicothoracic regions and the shoulder varies between clinical models of assessment. There is also the possibility that persistent shoulder pain (>6 months' duration) may be associated with cervical muscle weakness.[1] Ongoing research is required to establish if a definitive relationship exists, and in which patient populations. The implication may be that neck muscle performance testing and rehabilitation may also be relevant in the assessment and management of shoulder pain. The following sections describe the Maitland, McKenzie, and Mulligan approaches to cervicothoracic assessment and management.

The Maitland Approach

The Maitland Approach to assessment and management of musculoskeletal disorders is grounded in a clinical reasoning process in which hypotheses are proposed, tested, and modified as management progresses. Differential diagnosis of the nature and origin of the disorder is established collaboratively between clinician and patient through the patient interview, physical examination, and judicious monitoring of response to interventions. Cervical musculoskeletal disorders (particularly of cervical segments C4–7 origin) may refer pain to the shoulder and upper arm.[9] There is also a biomechanical interdependence between the cervical spine and shoulder such as shared muscular attachments to the scapula, and dependence on cervicothoracic mobility for elevated shoulder function.[49,60] Therefore, a cervical disorder may lead to shoulder pain, and it may coexist with a shoulder disorder, or it may develop secondarily to a shoulder disorder.

The examination

The Maitland Approach is a layered examination that commences with active listening to the patient's story, with supplementary questioning to gain purposeful information. The clinician listens to gain an understanding of the historical features and current movement, work, or leisure activities or postures that are aggravating pain. First, the clinician listens for a familiar mechanical pattern, because shoulder pain may present from nonmusculoskeletal sources such as the viscera. Secondly, the information from the history is analyzed to determine if the features of postures or activities implicate more the cervical or shoulder region, or both. No decision can be made at this point on the origin of pain but several hypotheses on possible causes and contributors are generated which then direct a focused, patient-centered approach to the physical examination.

The physical examination begins with analysis of the patient's nominated activity that aggravates pain and progresses to movement tests of the cervical and shoulder regions, and finally to precise testing to target specific structures. Again, no one test will provide the answer in differential diagnosis; rather, information is synthesized from each level of testing and hypotheses are tested and modified to reach a provisional differential diagnosis. Integral to that process are evaluations of relevant examination/trial treatment techniques to determine their effect on the shoulder pain in the differential diagnostic process.

The patient's nominated aggravating or functionally limited activity is analyzed, and aberrant postures or movement patterns of the shoulder or neck are modified. Any impact on symptoms and signs adds information about the possible regional and structural source. Answers are not always definitive. For example, modifying the position of the scapula may improve shoulder pain or movement, but this may occur for several reasons (see Chapter 36), one of which may be as a result of altering adverse strains on either neck or shoulder structures.

More definitive information may be acquired in other circumstances. Reaching the arm out sideways as the main aggravating movement could indicate a subacromial nociceptive source or an indication of nerve tissue mechanosensitivity. Nerve tissue mechanosensitivity is suspected if pain responses change when repeating the movement with the addition of a neural sensitizing maneuver, i.e., placing the neck in contralateral lateral flexion, or the wrist in extension. While such observations may not rule out a subacromial source, they add weight to a provisional hypothesis of neural mechanosensitivity and potential dysfunction at a cervical interface. For more information see Chapter 21.

When shoulder pain is thought to arise from the cervical region, it is important to have recorded baseline shoulder information for both the differential examination process and for the assessment of trial treatment effects. Examination includes an analysis of all active and passive shoulder and axioscapular movements assessing for movement quality, range, and symptom provocation. Findings may lead to a more detailed examination of joint (glenohumeral, acromio- and sterno-clavicular joints) and muscle function (axioscapular, glenohumeral muscles). Suspicions that a local shoulder condition may not underlie the clinical presentation might be considered in the absence of relevant deficiencies in the quality or range of shoulder motion, or the absence of symptoms with testing. This would be particularly the case if apparent local shoulder findings were diminished in response to any subsequent intervention to the cervical spine.

The cervical and thoracic region is evaluated. A cervical source of shoulder/arm pain cannot be discarded when cervical movements or combined movements do not reproduce shoulder symptoms. Muscle spasm might modify a spinal segment's contribution to an active cervical movement, nullifying the pain response. A skilled manual examination of the cervical and thoracic regions is required. Pain and abnormal motion principally at the lower cervical segments C4–7 would be signs that may explain shoulder pain.

Similarly, a loss of thoracic segmental mobility may be relevant given the need for thoracic extension as the shoulder is raised into elevation.

A trial treatment of manual therapy to the indicted segment(s) is conducted as part of the hypothesis testing. It is important that the dose of manual therapy during this trial of treatment is sufficient to make a change (e.g., 2–3 minutes as tolerated). Any relevant local shoulder findings are re-evaluated to determine their relationship with the cervical findings. There are three basic outcomes: 1) there is no difference, 2) there is a slight improvement, 3) there is marked improvement. If no difference, a primary cervicothoracic source is unlikely and the clinician in this case should focus on the relevant shoulder findings. If a slight difference, another trial of manual therapy should be undertaken and effect re-evaluated. If marked improvement, there may be a cervicothoracic source of pain.

Notably, marked improvement immediately post treatment does not guarantee a cervical source of symptoms. In some cases, manual therapy may have had a modulatory effect on pain without specifically addressing the cause. Before there can be any confidence that the shoulder pain is of cervicothoracic origin, the improvement (or most of it), must be maintained between treatments. If the patient returns and improvement is lost, either the neck is not the primary source of symptoms, or there are accompanying cervical muscle impairments that need to be addressed and an examination of cervical muscle function[48] is justified, given the physical strain muscles such as levator scapulae and upper trapezius impose to the head/neck complex during shoulder activities.

In summary, the Maitland approach to differential examination for the source of shoulder pain involves a clinical reasoning process informed by a comprehensive layered examination. Reliance is never on one test outcome, but a pattern is sought from historical and physical features and from a diligent evaluation of trial treatment responses.

The McKenzie Method

The McKenzie Method of Mechanical Diagnosis and Therapy (MDT) is a musculoskeletal classification system developed by Robin McKenzie that continues to evolve as guided by ongoing research and evidence. It is an assessment and problem-solving paradigm that enables clinicians to work with patients to formulate appropriate management strategies for their complaint. The clinician conducts a thorough history, investigating how this problem has impacted the patient's life, as well as the effects of specific activities of daily living on the patient's symptoms and movements. During the history, the clinician begins to formulate differential diagnoses, which are then explored further in the physical examination. Utilizing structured testing and a series of loading strategies, the clinician is then able to confirm or refute the postulated classifications, consider the influences on the patient's pain experience, and establish a management strategy.

One challenge for any musculoskeletal clinician is when a patient presents with "shoulder pain" and there is a need to determine whether the complaint is originating from the shoulder region or if it is referred from elsewhere, such as the cervical spine. There are situations, e.g., cervical radiculopathy, where the relationship is usually clearer, however, there are scenarios where the relationship is not so obvious and therefore it is crucial that the assessment is able to effectively rule the cervical spine in or out as the origin of the patient's symptoms. Despite recommendations for the assessment of the neck in patients presenting with shoulder pain[36] and further discussed by Walker et al.,[67] clear guidance for neck assessments supported by higher levels of evidence is not available.[55,62]

The consequences of not undertaking a thorough examination of the neck as a possible cause of a presenting shoulder complaint could lead to suboptimal outcomes for patients if treatment is misdirected.[67] Rosedale et al.[54] published a cohort study assessing the prevalence of spinal origin in patients presenting with isolated extremity pain. In this study of 369 patients, 84 people were referred with shoulder pain and 47.6% (40/84) were found to have symptoms that were originating from the cervical spine following an MDT assessment by trained clinicians, demonstrating the importance of assessing the cervical spine in patients presenting with shoulder pain.

During the MDT assessment, there are certain aspects of the history that are proposed to indicate potential spinal origin. These include location of symptoms (e.g., scapular pain, distal pain below the shoulder), neurological symptoms such as paresthesia, history of neck pain, poor response to previous treatment of the shoulder, or if the patient described their symptoms were worse with sitting, and cervical flexion or rotation. Specific findings from the physical examination can also indicate a potential spinal source of symptoms. These include a change of symptoms with altering the person's posture, e.g., sitting slumped or erect. With respect to range of motion, an important finding of Rosedale et al.'s[54] study was that only 50% of the patients who were classified as "spinal" had any observable loss of spinal mobility. This would question the wisdom of ruling out the spine solely based on reductions in range of motion.

The MDT physical examination first involves the clinician evaluating if a change in spinal posture impacts any shoulder baseline symptoms. The clinician then establishes more comprehensive shoulder baselines; symptom location and intensity, active and passive range of movement and a patient-specific movement that produces the familiar pain. Next, the clinician assesses the spinal range of movement for movement loss to determine if the shoulder pain is reproduced with the neck movement. Finally, the clinician will explore repeated movements of the cervical spine to determine its effect on the shoulder baselines (e.g., pain, range of shoulder movement, quality of shoulder motion).

The assessment would start in the sagittal plane; for example, the patient would perform sets of repeated end range retraction or extension movements of their neck, reporting their symptomatic response. The shoulder baselines are then re-assessed to ascertain if any change has occurred. If the sagittal plane does not cause any lasting change, then the clinician may further explore the sagittal plane in a lying position and/or move on to the frontal plane with repeated movements of cervical lateral flexion or rotation. Once completed, the shoulder baselines will be reassessed. If during any component of this process there is any change in the patient's shoulder symptoms, then a greater suspicion of a cervical region involvement would be considered.

If there appears to be a positive change in the shoulder baselines from assessing the cervical region, the patient will be educated on the response to the neck repeated movements and advised to trial this regime for several days to evaluate if the treatment effect is sustained. Figure 16.1 presents the MDT spinal extremity differentiation algorithm. Figure 16.2 depicts pre and post shoulder range following cervical region repeated movements.

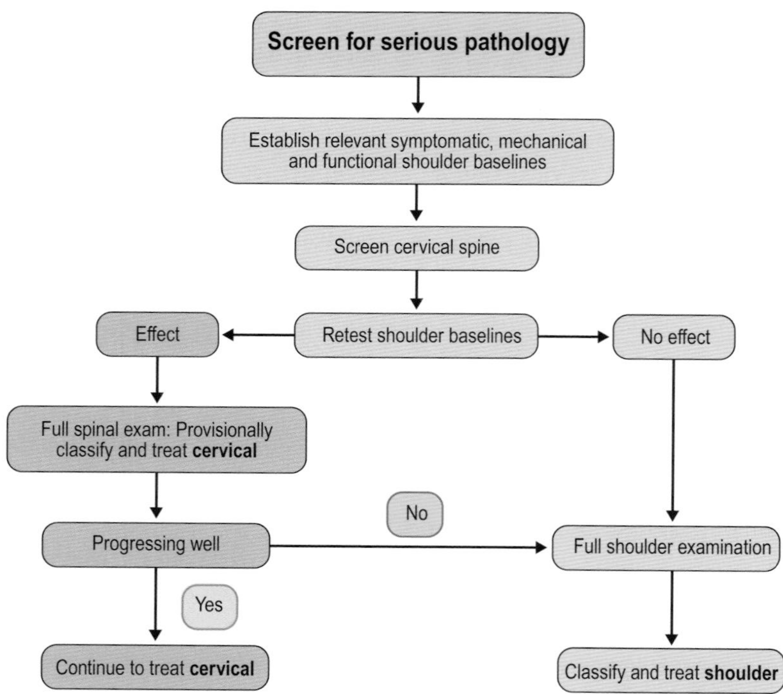

FIGURE 16.1
Spinal extremity differentiation algorithm.

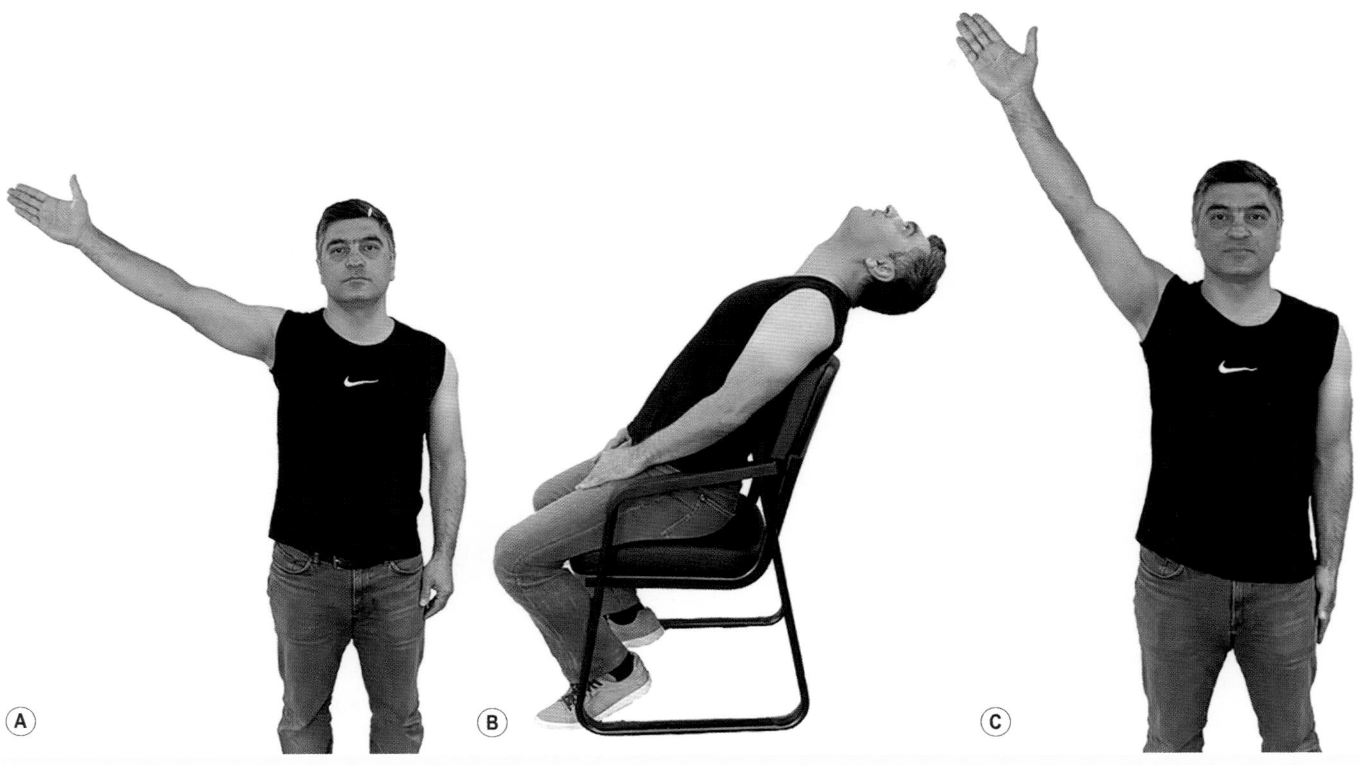

FIGURE 16.2
Pre and post shoulder range following cervical region repeated movements.

In those patients where the spinal source was excluded, a comprehensive assessment of the shoulder would be undertaken and involve a series of repeated shoulder movements including, but not limited to, active movement, passive movement, or resisted tests. The response to the repeated movement testing on the patient's shoulder baselines (symptomatic, mechanical, and functional) would then allow the clinician to classify the patient into a specific subgroup that would dictate the management.

The most common classification would be based on establishing a "Directional Preference" movement (37% in a study by Heidar Abady et al.).[24] The patient would show an immediate change in baselines in response to one specific direction of end range repeated movements. Another common classification would be Contractile Dysfunction (akin to tendinopathy) and would require a graduated loading regime to restore the tissue capacity and the patient's function. If the patient's presentation did not fit the criteria for these classifications, then other MDT classifications would be considered, including post-surgery, structurally compromised (e.g., labral tear), serious pathology (e.g., fracture), and managed appropriately utilizing MDT principles within evidence-based practice.

The Mulligan Concept

The Mulligan Concept is a unique manual therapy approach combining mobilization with an active movement or functional task.[26,46] Although considered treatments, Mobilization with Movements (MWMs) are also examination procedures. The fundamental principle of MWMs, in assessment and treatment, is that any pain occurring on movement must be eliminated when appropriate manual (or treatment belt) forces are applied. The Mulligan

Concept's approach to deciding that the treatment target is *not the shoulder* relies on patient-centered clinical reasoning (see Chapter 13) from information collected during the clinical interview and physical examination.

Clinical interview

Two key components gathered at interview are the patient's aggravating factors and the patient's pain chart. Aggravating factors are the activities that the patient reports exacerbate the chief complaint for which they are seeking treatment. They may be a movement, muscle contraction or functional task. Reported cervical movements or postures which alter or aggravate shoulder pain would lead the clinician to consider targeting management to the cervical spine. The body pain and symptom chart may also implicate a spinal origin if wider, vaguer areas of pain in dermatomal or myotomal patterns over the shoulder girdle were reported. Combined with somatic and nociceptive pain descriptors, this group of symptoms may indicate the cervical spine needs to be included in the physical examination. Pattern recognition is a skill that is thought to increase with practitioner experience (see Chapter 13).

Physical examination

From the aggravating factors and physical examination, a specific movement (task) which reliably reproduces the patient's familiar symptoms may be chosen to test with an MWM. This is termed the Client Specific Impairment Measure (CSIM). MWMs used as examination procedures follow the primary Mulligan Concept clinical reasoning guideline called the PILL response: *p*ain free, *i*nstant and have *l*ong *l*asting effects. That is, the MWM must render the patient's CSIM as PILL after the completion of the MWM and over time between treatments.

The key MWM test utilized by Mulligan Concept practitioners as a screening tool to implicate the cervical spine in upper limb pain is the Spinal Mobilization with Arm Movement (SMWAM).[26] Specifically, Brian Mulligan[47] recommends SMWAMs are considered for patients who report the following pain patterns:

1. Rhomboid region pain felt by a patient during horizontal adduction of the arm.
2. Pain radiating from the neck to the upper arm when the arm is abducted above the horizontal.
3. Pain radiating to the hand with arm movement in more than one direction.

The Mulligan Concept recommends that the cervical spine is routinely screened in all upper limb presentations. Mulligan practitioners use standard orthopedic tests to establish the patient's baseline and to identify their CSIM before applying SMWAM tests to clear the cervical spine. A neurological examination is performed to screen for neurological involvement with reflexes, power, and sensation of the upper limbs tested and recorded. Active range of motion, response to repeated movement, Spurling's test, and Spring tests are also integral to the decision-making process in the physical examination and may guide the selection of the correct CSIM and SMWAM test for the patient.

The benefits of utilizing an SMWAM as a test within a clinical examination is the speed and ease of application and the instant feedback in real time resulting in modification of the patient's CSIM. As a general clinical guideline, the dermatome within which the patient's pain lies is identified, and the corresponding spinal process above the nerve is translated laterally as the upper limb movement is repeated. In the case of the shoulder, it is typically between C3–5.[13]

Clinical example

The patient presents with a painful arc through elevation in the scapular plane (i.e., scaption) of the right shoulder. Pain is experienced locally between the acromion and the deltoid insertion, within the C4 dermatome.[13] C3 would be the target spinous process. The patient's readily reproducible pain on abduction becomes their CSIM, to use during the SMWAM test as the active movement during the mobilization. The patient sits, with the therapist standing behind. The clinician places the medial border of their left thumb against the right lateral aspect of the C3 spinous process (via the soft tissue of the paravertebral muscles). Using their right index and middle finger they perform a transverse glide via the left thumb to the right side of the spinous process of C3, imparting a rotational force onto the segment directed away from the side of pain (Figure 16.3). The translation is sustained as the patient repeats their right arm scaption.

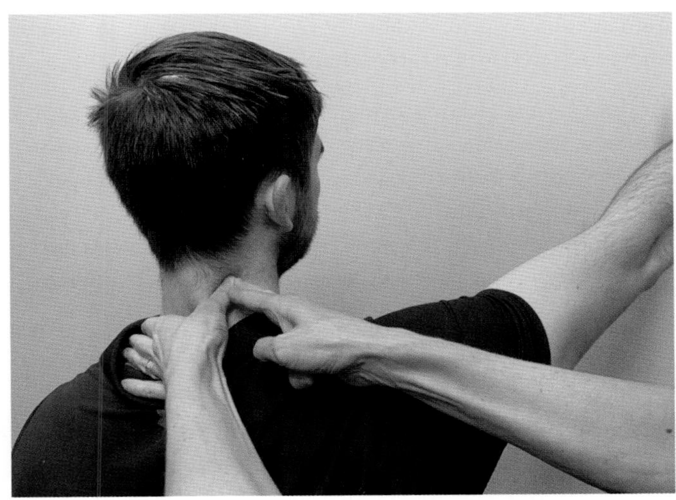

FIGURE 16.3
Single level SMWAM. The spinous process of C3 is translated laterally as the patient moves their right shoulder through scaption.

If successful in abolishing the painful arc, the clinician would interpret this as a successful SMWAM test and hypothesize the pain was of cervical spine origin, or at least treatment of the cervical spine is more likely to lead to successful relief of pain. They would then utilize the SMWAM as a treatment, performing subsequent repetitions relative to the stage of irritability (see Box 16.1 for the "Rule of three").

Box 16.1 Mulligan Concept "Rule of three" for treatment repetitions

- In the Mulligan Concept, a patient would initially receive *three* repetitions of the mobilization with movement technique on the first day before reassessment.
- As irritability reduces, repetitions would then increase to 2–3 sets of 6 with overpressure, and finally 3–5 sets of 10 with overpressure.
- Home exercises would be prescribed to increase the efficacy and long-lasting effect of the MWM.

If the pain on scaption was reduced during the SMWAM but not completely abolished, then subtle changes in the direction and amount of the applied force should be trialed. If still unsuccessful the thumbs would be repositioned to apply force to two segments simultaneously: C3 from the right and C4 from the left, imparting a stronger rotational force moving C3 further to the right relative to C4.

If still no change was experienced in the patient's CSIM, the clinician would trial other segments above and below. Failure to gain a PILL response on the SMWAM test would guide the clinician to considering treatment targeted at the shoulder to manage symptoms. The symptomatic shoulder movements would be assessed next with shoulder MWMs. If shoulder stiffness into end range scaption was the primary comparable sign, the SMWAM would also be trialed at the cervicothoracic junction, from levels C7 to thoracic level T4, as the mobility of this area contributes to successful end range shoulder elevation.

While the SMWAM relies on a positive PILL response, a negative PILL response from MWM targeting the shoulder articulations may inform clinical reasoning and be of clinical importance. For example, the likelihood of shoulder region involvement may be reduced if there was no immediate pain relief when an MWM test was applied to the glenohumeral, scapulothoracic, acromioclavicular or sternoclavicular joints. Furthermore, the clinician should reconsider using MWMs if there was no long-lasting relief from the use of MWMs applied to the shoulder – that is, the CSIM has not improved at the 4th pre-treatment assessment, despite modulating the applied force, increasing total volume of treatment, and fine-tuning of the direction of the applied manual force.

It should be noted in the initial presentation, no more than three MWM test movements may be tolerated by the patient before irritability may increase. The practitioner should proceed with caution in the presence of radicular pain, if neurological signs are stable, and a PILL response is achieved without any exacerbation of neural signs. Clinical experience would suggest that the SMWAM works more effectively for somatic nociceptive pain and stiffness of the shoulder.

In the example that a PILL response was achieved with a SMWAM, the cervical spine becomes the treatment target and not the shoulder. That the treatment was directed at the cervical spine is not in itself diagnostic of the source of shoulder pain. While a mechanical explanation of "gapping the segment" has been proposed by Brian Mulligan,[46] further research is needed to elaborate fully the biomechanical influences of a SMWAM and validate it as a screening tool.

Recommendations

We advocate considering cervicothoracic involvement and management when:

1. assessment of active physiological cervicothoracic movement in isolation or combination reveal
   - cervicothoracic stiffness and/or pain *without* referred shoulder pain
   - cervicothoracic stiffness and/or pain *with* referred shoulder pain
   - no local cervicothoracic stiffness and/or pain *with* referred shoulder pain; and
2. reduction in shoulder symptoms occur in response to
   - repeated neck movement[54]
   - and/or spinal mobilization with arm movement[26]
   - and/or cervicothoracic region mobilization.[39]

Cervical radiculopathy

Cervical radiculopathy occurs when one or more nerves are affected at the level of the nerve root resulting in objective signs of nerve conduction deficit including sensory loss, motor loss, or impaired reflexes. The cause can be disk herniation, spondylosis, or osteophytosis, and prevalence is greatest in the fifth decade.[4] In the context of objective signs of nerve conduction deficit, a combination of a positive Spurling's test, reduction of symptoms with cervical axial traction, and a positive arm squeeze test increases the likelihood of a diagnosis of cervical radiculopathy.[62]

Spurling's neck compression test is performed by extending, laterally flexing, and rotating the neck to the same side and then applying downward axial pressure through the head. The test is considered positive if radicular symptoms radiate into the limb ipsilateral to the side to which the head is laterally flexed and rotated.[40] The test appears to have high specificity and sensitivity (95% and 92% respectively) and good to fair interrater reliability.[40]

The cervical axial traction test is performed in a supine position, with the examiner applying an axial traction force corresponding to 10–15 kg (15–33 lb) to the patient's neck. A decrease in symptoms with traction and an increase or return of symptoms with the release of traction (distraction) is considered a positive outcome suggestive of cervical radiculopathy.[65]

The arm squeeze test is performed by squeezing the patient's middle third of the upper arm with the thumb posteriorly on the triceps muscle and the fingers anteriorly on the biceps muscle. The test is considered positive when the score is 3 points or higher (out of 10) compared to two other areas (acromioclavicular joint and subacromial area).[21]

There appears to be a favorable natural history with substantial improvement in 4–6 months, but time to complete recovery can be between 24–36 months. A small proportion of sufferers have residual pain and disability with a full neurological recovery in most cases, with no myelopathy.[68] In a prospective randomized study[16] of 5- to 8-year outcomes of anterior cervical decompression and fusion (ACDF) combined with a structured physiotherapy program compared to physiotherapy alone in patients with cervical radiculopathy, no significant difference was found between the two patient groups as regards arm pain and health outcome. The combined care group, however, reported a greater reduction in neck disability and pain compared to physiotherapy alone. Self-rating by patients as regards treatment outcome was also superior in the combined care group.

Visceral referred shoulder pain

Shoulder pain referred from the diaphragm via the phrenic nerve (C3,4,5) is common following surgical procedures of the thoracic viscera with incidence ranging from 40% of women who underwent cesarean section[69] to 60% following general thoracic surgery.[50] Danelli et al.[10] have explained the mechanism as one of *irritation* of the diaphragm, pericardium, or mediastinal pleural surfaces. This is supported by evidence that intraperitoneal anesthetic irrigation during surgery appears to reduce the incidence of post-operative shoulder pain (for a review see Fernández-López et al.[17]).

Traumatic diaphragmatic rupture (TDR) is a rare cause of shoulder pain but a common consequence of motor vehicle collisions.[30] While most patients present with symptoms of respiratory distress including dyspnea, shortness of breath, abdominal pain, nausea, and vomiting, King et al.[30] describe a case of a 22-year delay in diagnosing a TDR with the only symptom being shoulder pain. Ten years following unsuccessful physiotherapy and cortisone injections, the patient developed abdominal pain and nausea. Further investigations revealed diaphragmatic hernia on plain radiograph. The natural history as described by King et al.[30] is compelling: the diaphragm is not known to spontaneously heal, and defects may enlarge over time because the abdominal-thoracic pressure gradient of 9–12 mmHg draws abdominal contents through the defect into the pleural cavity.

Pathologies such as splenic abscess, a condition with a high mortality rate, usually characterized by the clinical triad of fever, abdominal pain, and leukocytosis, may present as shoulder pain as the only symptom.[58] The esophagus (innervated by thoracic nerves T4–T6) also refers pain to the shoulder through contact with the central portion of the diaphragm, and increased shoulder pain during or following meals can be a symptom of esophageal pathologies such as cancer.[3] Disorders of the gallbladder (innervated by thoracic nerves T7–T9) such as cholecystitis and cholelithiasis are characterized by fever, weight loss and jaundice, and may also refer pain to the *right* shoulder: a vague cramping, gnawing pain in the posterior aspect of the right shoulder may be one of the first symptoms of gallbladder pathology.[33]

Shoulder pain related to endometriosis and ectopic pregnancy

Endometriosis is experienced in approximately 10% of women during child-bearing years,[64] and may occur in multiple regions of the body.[29] Cyclical right shoulder pain linked with menstrual cycle may be associated with endometriosis[61] and should be considered as a differential diagnosis. Risk factors for endometriosis that may support clinical reasoning include never giving birth, menarche at early age, short (<27 days) menstrual cycles, heavy menstrual periods lasting longer than 7 days, low body mass index, close relatives (mother, aunt, sister) with endometriosis, high concentrations of estrogen, and reproductive tract abnormalities. Endometriosis most commonly occurs in the pelvic peritoneum but it has been reported in the upper abdominal cavity, diaphragm, liver and elsewhere.[29,61]

There are several recognized risk factors associated with ectopic (or extrauterine) pregnancy that include smoking, history of ectopic pregnancy, sexually transmitted infections, and in vitro fertilization (IVF) treatment. Ectopic pregnancies occur in one in 80–90 pregnancies and may be asymptomatic, but if symptoms occur (vaginal bleeding, brown watery discharge, missed period, cramping or pain on one side of the abdomen, gastroenteritis-like symptoms, pain during bowel movements) urgent medical attention is required. Symptoms commonly occur in the first trimester of pregnancy between 4 and 12 weeks of pregnancy (sometimes later). Although commonly associated with other symptoms of ectopic pregnancy, shoulder pain may be a symptom, possibly due to intrabdominal bleeding irritating the diaphragm.[25,63]

In cases of unresolving shoulder pain where diagnosis is unclear, enquiring with respect to recent abdominal surgery (cesarean/thoracotomy), past trauma (blunt force/motor vehicle collision) and recent health changes (e.g. weight loss, fever, and jaundice) may lead to consideration of visceral pathology and referral for further investigations through regionally appropriate clinical pathways. Consideration should be given to the possibility of referred shoulder pain related to endometriosis and extrauterine pregnancy. (See Kinjo[31] for further information.)

Central sensitization

More than half of all people experiencing shoulder pain recover completely within one year, but a substantial proportion report persistent shoulder pain[34,35] and several systematic reviews have suggested central sensitization (CS) may play a role.[48,56] Central sensitization may be defined as an increased responsiveness of nociceptive neurons in the central nervous system to their normal or subthreshold afferent input. This may include increased responsiveness due to dysfunction of endogenous pain control systems.[28] Noten et al.[48] reported moderate evidence for the presence of CS in people with musculoskeletal (MSK) shoulder pain. They concluded that the presence of generalized mechanical hyperalgesia (both locally and distally, e.g., the forearm and hand) and allodynia may indicate the involvement of the central nervous system in a subgroup of those with shoulder pain. Noten et al.[48] concluded that although progress has been made towards a better understanding of neurophysiological pain mechanisms in patients with shoulder pain, the results for endogenous pain modulation are not clear-cut in this respect.[48] Altered endogenous pain modulation may represent an imbalance between excitatory and inhibitory sensory inputs indicating that central sensitization drives their pain experience. The efficacy of top-down pain inhibitory capacity in interaction with increased excitatory input remains questionable in this population; up to now studies evaluating endogenous pain inhibition remain inconclusive.

Research in other MSK populations, such as spinal pain and knee osteoarthritis (OA), have made progress in studying patients along the continuum of nociplastic pain. Central sensitization is a specific neurophysiological phenomenon that may partially account for nociplastic pain. Nociplastic pain is defined as "pain arising from altered nociception despite no clear evidence of actual or threatened tissue damage causing the activation of peripheral nociceptors or evidence for disease or lesion of the somatosensory system causing the pain".[28]

When we consider the continuum of nociplastic pain in other MSK conditions,[11,18] it becomes apparent that subgrouping patients is critical and that a symptom-based (medical diagnosis) classification is not sufficient. Phenotyping patients with a pain mechanism-based approach to pain management, beyond the diagnosis, includes and builds on the biopsychosocial model by defining specific pathobiology in pain processing and pain-relevant psychological factors.[8] As a result, all predisposing, provoking, and perpetuating factors are taken into account, resulting in different phenotypes, such as already elaborated in OA.[53] In line with research in other MSK conditions,[12] some characteristics such as pain sensitization, psychological distress, structural impairments, metabolic factors, and inflammation may possibly be associated with different clinical phenotypes in people with shoulder pain.

Features that are by far the most studied in patients with persistent shoulder pain are the anatomical structures and the biomechanics of the shoulder. Nevertheless, the relation between clinical representation and biomechanical and structural factors is inconsistent[19,20] suggesting that these cannot be the only explanations for persistent shoulder pain. Researchers have investigated *psychosocial factors* that might play a role. Negative emotional and behavioral aspects, such as distress, depression, anxiety, catastrophizing, kinesiophobia, fear-avoidance beliefs or low self-efficacy, affect endogenous pain modulation and can contribute to persistent shoulder complaints.[6,7,38,41–43] Conversely, greater self-efficacy and expectations of recovery are associated with lower levels of pain and disability.[42]

Somatosensory aspects are important biological features. The somatosensory cortex is heavily involved in the perception of sensory features of pain, but pain and somatosensory processing are accomplished in overlapping cortical structures, raising the question whether pain states are associated with alteration of somatosensory function itself. Impaired endogenous pain modulation and altered perception of somatosensory information in the cerebral cortex have been associated with chronicity of rotator cuff-related shoulder pain (RCRSP).[22] In frozen shoulder it is hypothesized that the ongoing inflammation may lead to central sensitization, as inflammatory mediators may play a direct role in the process of central sensitization.[32] People with acute and persistent RCRSP demonstrated lower levels of endogenous pain modulation, but the presence of central sensitization was only found in a minority of individuals with *acute* RCRSP, while most of those with persistent RCRSP (almost 80%) showed reduced pain inhibitory capacity.[22] There are many reasons for ongoing increased pain sensitivity, including failure to modify activity, provocative movements, and load, as well as the nervous system being unable to normalize sensitivity in the acute phase. Ongoing peripheral nociception may lead to neuroplastic changes that contribute to the development of central sensitization and result in persistent pain.[37]

Autonomic nervous system (ANS) *dysfunctions* are rarely studied in shoulder pain research. From the few studies available, changes in autonomic nervous system regulation appear to play a part in the pathogenesis of persistent neck–shoulder pain. Heart rate variability (HRV) is the variation in time between successive heart beats. Measuring HRV is a non-invasive way to identify ANS imbalances. Put simply, the healthier the ANS, the greater the variability between beats, and people with high HRV may have greater cardiovascular fitness and be more resilient to stress. Low HRV is associated with increased risk of cardiovascular disease and death (see Chapter 36). Elevated heart rate and reduced heart rate variability were reported in workers with persistent neck–shoulder pain compared to healthy controls and interestingly it could partly be explained by reduced physical activity in the neck–shoulder pain group.[23] In frozen shoulder, a role for autonomic dysregulation has been suggested as well,[59] analogous to the evidence on altered autonomic function in other persistent pain populations, and more specifically in rheumatic and inflammatory conditions, such as rheumatoid arthritis.[44] Additionally, ongoing nociceptive stimuli arriving at the central nervous system may lead to an increased activity of the sympathetic nervous system, parallel to long-lasting central sensitization.[32,57]

When a person presents with shoulder pain, we are obliged to think beyond local shoulder structures, and the approach should not solely rely on biomechanical diagnosis. Both phenotyping and genotyping people may lead to patient-centered treatment for those with (persistent) shoulder pain and improve their outcomes. Unfortunately, assessing and unravelling the dominance of altered central pain processing in individual patients remains an enigma in clinical practice. In studies, indices of altered nociception/pain sensitivity can be studied at the group level, but interpreting clinical findings in individual patients still relies heavily on the clinical reasoning (see Chapter 13).

Lifestyle factors and shoulder pain

There is a growing body of evidence linking shoulder pain with metabolic risk factors, such as obesity.[5,14,52] There is an increased prevalence of tendinopathies in people with diabetes.[51] Systemic metabolic stress leads to chronic low-grade inflammation, altered lipid metabolism and altered tendon matrix and may be related to shoulder pain. People with metabolic syndrome have a higher risk of rotator cuff tears and more severe rotator cuff tears.[5] Also, the high incidence of frozen shoulder in diabetes mellitus is striking and hypothesized to be due to a faster rate of collagen glycosylation and cross-linking in the shoulder capsule, restricting joint mobility.[27] Dietary behavior may be associated with chronic low-level systemic inflammation,[2] and therefore with persistent pain and pain intensity. Plant-based dietary patterns such as vegetarian and vegan diets might have pain-relieving effects on persistent musculoskeletal pain.[15] Chapter 5 focuses on lifestyle factors and shoulder pain.

Conclusion

Serious non-musculoskeletal visceral pathology may masquerade as musculoskeletal pathology. As clinicians we have an obligation and duty of care to maintain a wide and continuous gaze with any clinical shoulder presentation. We need to be the best clinical detective possible to consider every possible source of symptoms. Recent work on central sensitization implores us not only to consider local shoulder structures and regional interdependence but also to consider a neuroplastic paradigm when assessing a person seeking care for shoulder pain. Lastly, there are striking and reassuring parallels between the three main exponents of manual therapies – Maitland, McKenzie, and Mulligan – in their approach to discriminating between cervical and shoulder disorders. Put simply: the effect of neck movements on shoulder symptoms, whether accessory and passive or physiological and active (or a blended approach) should be examined in all people with shoulder pain, and subsequently targeted with appropriate rehabilitation strategies if found impaired.

References

1. Asker M, Ravnanger J, Bjørnstad T, Skillgate E. Correlation between neck motor control impairment and shoulder pain in elite male handball players. Journal of Science and Medicine in Sport. 2014;18:e76.
2. Barbaresko J, Koch M, Schulze MB, Nöthlings U. Dietary pattern analysis and biomarkers of low-grade inflammation: a systematic literature review. Nutrition Reviews. 2013;71:511-527.
3. Boissonnault WG, Bass C. Pathological origins of trunk and neck pain: part III—diseases of the musculoskeletal system. Journal of Orthopaedic & Sports Physical Therapy. 1990;12:216-221.
4. Boyd EA, Goudreau L, O'Riain MD, Grinnell DM, Torrance GM, Gaylard A. A radiological measure of shoulder subluxation in hemiplegia: its reliability and validity. Arch Phys Med Rehabil. 1993;74:188-193.
5. Burne G, Mansfield M, Gaida JE, Lewis JS. Is there an association between metabolic syndrome and rotator cuff-related shoulder pain? A systematic review. BMJ Open Sport & Exercise Medicine. 2019;5:e000544.
6. Chester R, Jerosch-Herold C, Lewis J, Shepstone L. Psychological factors are associated with the outcome of physiotherapy for people with shoulder pain: a multicentre longitudinal cohort study. British Journal of Sports Medicine. 2018;52:269-275.
7. Chester R, Khondoker M, Shepstone L, Lewis JS, Jerosch-Herold C. Self-efficacy and risk of persistent shoulder pain: results of a Classification and Regression Tree

(CART) analysis. British Journal of Sports Medicine. 2019;53:825-834.

8. Chimenti RL, Frey-Law LA, Sluka KA. A mechanism-based approach to physical therapist management of pain. Physical Therapy. 2018;98:302-314.

9. Cooper G, Bailey B, Bogduk N. Cervical zygapophysial joint pain maps. Pain Med. 2007;8:344-353.

10. Danelli G, Berti M, Casati A, et al. Ipsilateral shoulder pain after thoracotomy surgery: a prospective, randomized, double-blind, placebo-controlled evaluation of the efficacy of infiltrating the phrenic nerve with 0.2% wt/vol ropivacaine. European Journal of Anaesthesiology| EJA. 2007;24:596-601.

11. Davis F, Gostine M, Roberts B, Risko R, Cappelleri JC, Sadosky A. Characterizing classes of fibromyalgia within the continuum of central sensitization syndrome. Journal of Pain Research. 2018;11:2551.

12. Deveza LA, Melo L, Yamato T, Mills K, Ravi V, Hunter D. Knee osteoarthritis phenotypes and their relevance for outcomes: a systematic review. Osteoarthritis and Cartilage. 2017;25:1926-1941.

13. Devinsky O, Feldham E. Examination fo the Cranial and Peripheral Nerves. New York: Churchill Livingstone; 1988.

14. Dominick CH, Blyth FM, Nicholas MK. Unpacking the burden: understanding the relationships between chronic pain and comorbidity in the general population. Pain. 2012;153:293-304.

15. Elma Ö, Yilmaz ST, Deliens T, et al. Do nutritional factors interact with chronic musculoskeletal pain? A systematic review. Journal of Clinical Medicine. 2020;9:702.

16. Engquist M, Löfgren H, Öberg B, et al. A 5-to 8-year randomized study on the treatment of cervical radiculopathy: anterior cervical decompression and fusion plus physiotherapy versus physiotherapy alone. Journal of Neurosurgery: Spine. 2017;26:19-27.

17. Fernández-López I, Peña-Otero D, de los Ángeles Atín-Arratibel M, Eguillor-Mutiloa M. Influence of the phrenic nerve in shoulder pain: a systematic review. International Journal of Osteopathic Medicine. 2020;36:36-48.

18. Ferro Moura Franco K, Lenoir D, Dos Santos Franco YR, Jandre Reis FJ, Nunes Cabral CM, Meeus M. Prescription of exercises for the treatment of chronic pain along the continuum of nociplastic pain: a systematic review with meta-analysis. Eur J Pain. 2021;25:51-70.

19. Frost P, Andersen JH, Lundorf E. Is supraspinatus pathology as defined by magnetic resonance imaging associated with clinical sign of shoulder impingement? J Shoulder Elbow Surg. 1999;8:565-568.

20. Girish G, Lobo LG, Jacobson JA, Morag Y, Miller B, Jamadar DA. Ultrasound of the shoulder: asymptomatic findings in men. AJR Am J Roentgenol. 2011;197:W713-719.

21. Gumina S, Carbone S, Albino P, Gurzi M, Postacchini F. Arm Squeeze Test: a new clinical test to distinguish neck from shoulder pain. European Spine Journal. 2013;22:1558-1563.

22. Haik MN, Alburquerque-Sendín F, Fernandes RAS, et al. Biopsychosocial aspects in individuals with acute and chronic rotator cuff related shoulder pain: classification based on a decision tree analysis. Diagnostics (Basel). 2020;10:928.

23. Hallman DM, Ekman AH, Lyskov E. Changes in physical activity and heart rate variability in chronic neck-shoulder pain: monitoring during work and leisure time. Int Arch Occup Environ Health. 2014;87:735-744.

24. Heidar Abady A, Rosedale R, Chesworth BM, Rotondi MA, Overend TJ. Application of the McKenzie system of Mechanical Diagnosis and Therapy (MDT) in patients with shoulder pain; a prospective longitudinal study. Journal of Manual & Manipulative Therapy. 2017;25:235-243.

25. Hendriks E, Rosenberg R, Prine L. Ectopic pregnancy: diagnosis and management. American Family Physician. 2020;101:599-606.

26. Hing W, Hall T, Rivett DA, Vicenzino B. The Mulligan Concept of Manual Therapy: Textbook of Techniques, 2nd edition. Sydney: Churchill Livingstone; 2019.

27. Hsu JE, Anakwenze OA, Warrender WJ, Abboud JA. Current review of adhesive capsulitis. Journal of Shoulder and Elbow Surgery. 2011;20:502-514.

28. IASP. IASP Terminology. Available at: https://www.iasp-pain.org/Education/Content.aspx?ItemNumber=1698.

29. Kaveh M, Tahermanesh K, Kashi AM, Tajbakhsh B, Mansouri G, Sadegi K. Endometriosis of diaphragm: a case report. International Journal of Fertility & Sterility. 2018;12:263.

30. King BW, Skedros JG, Glasgow RE, Morrell DG. Resolution of chronic shoulder pain after repair of a posttraumatic diaphragmatic hernia: a 22-year delay in diagnosis and treatment. Case reports in orthopedics. 2020;2020:7984936.

31. Kinjo M. Shoulder Pain. Springer; 2018.

32. Konttinen YT, Kemppinen P, Segerberg M, et al. Peripheral and spinal neural mechanisms in arthritis, with particular reference to treatment of inflammation and pain. Arthritis & Rheumatism. 1994;37:965-982.

33. Koopmeiners MB. Screening for gastrointestinal system disease. In: Boissonnault WG (ed). Examination in Physical Therapy Practice: Screening for Medical Disease, 2nd edition. New York: Churchill Livingstone; 1995:

34. Kuijpers T, van der Windt DA, Boeke AJ, et al. Clinical prediction rules for the prognosis of shoulder pain in general practice. Pain. 2006;120:276-285.

35. Kuijpers T, van Tulder MW, van der Heijden GJ, Bouter LM, van der Windt DA. Costs of shoulder pain in primary care consulters: a prospective cohort study in The Netherlands. BMC Musculoskeletal Disorders. 2006;7:1-8.

36. Kulkarni R, Gibson J, Brownson P, et al. Subacromial shoulder pain. Shoulder Elbow. 2015;7:135-143.

37. Kwon M, Altin M, Duenas H, Alev L. The role of descending inhibitory pathways on chronic pain modulation and clinical implications. Pain Practice. 2014;14:656-667.

38. Luque-Suarez A, Martinez-Calderon J, Navarro-Ledesma S, Morales-Asencio JM, Meeus M, Struyf F. Kinesiophobia is associated with pain intensity and disability in chronic shoulder pain: a cross-sectional study. Journal of Manipulative and Physiological Therapeutics. 2020;43:791-798.

39. Maitland GD, Hengeveld E, Banks K, English K. Maitland's Vertebral Manipulation, 7th edition. Edinburgh: Butterworth-Heinemann; 2005.

40. Malanga GA, Landes P, Nadler SF. Provocative tests in cervical spine

examination: historical basis and scientific analyses. Pain Physician. 2003;6:199-206.

41. Martinez-Calderon J, Meeus M, Struyf F, et al. Psychological factors are associated with local and generalized pressure pain hypersensitivity, pain intensity, and function in people with chronic shoulder pain: a cross-sectional study. Musculoskeletal Science and Practice. 2019;44:102064.

42. Martinez-Calderon J, Meeus M, Struyf F, Morales-Asencio JM, Gijon-Nogueron G, Luque-Suarez A. The role of psychological factors in the perpetuation of pain intensity and disability in people with chronic shoulder pain: a systematic review. BMJ Open. 2018;8:e020703.

43. Martinez-Calderon J, Struyf F, Meeus M, Luque-Suarez A. The association between pain beliefs and pain intensity and/or disability in people with shoulder pain: a systematic review. Musculoskeletal Science and Practice. 2018;37:29-57.

44. Meeus M, Vervisch S, De Clerck LS, Moorkens G, Hans G, Nijs J. Central sensitization in patients with rheumatoid arthritis: a systematic literature review. Semin Arthritis Rheum. 2012;41:556-567.

45. Mintken P. Shoulder pain and regional interdependence: contributions of the cervicothoracic spine. Journal of Yoga & Physical Therapy. 2015;5:1.

46. Mulligan BR. Manual Therapy: "NAGS", "SNAGS", "MWMS" etc., 7th edition. Wellington: APN Print Ltd; 2018.

47. Mulligan BR. Spinal mobilisations with arm movement (further mobilisations with movement). Journal of Manual & Manipulative Therapy. 1994;2:75-77.

48. Noten S, Struyf F, Lluch E, D'Hoore M, Van Looveren E, Meeus M. Central pain processing in patients with shoulder pain: a review of the literature. Pain Practice. 2017;17:267-280.

49. Osborn W, Jull G. Patients with non-specific neck disorders commonly report upper limb disability. Manual Therapy. 2013;18:492-497.

50. Pennefather S, Akrofi M, Kendall J, Russell G, Scawn N. Double-blind comparison of intrapleural saline and 0.25% bupivacaine for ipsilateral shoulder pain after thoracotomy in patients receiving thoracic epidural analgesia. British Journal of Anaesthesia. 2005;94:234-238.

51. Ranger TA, Wong AM, Cook JL, Gaida JE. Is there an association between tendinopathy and diabetes mellitus? A systematic review with meta-analysis. British Journal of Sports Medicine. 2016;50:982-989.

52. Rechardt M, Shiri R, Karppinen J, Jula A, Heliovaara M, Viikari-Juntura E. Lifestyle and metabolic factors in relation to shoulder pain and rotator cuff tendinitis: a population-based study. BMC Musculoskelet Disord. 2010;11:165.

53. Roman-Blas JA, Mendoza-Torres LA, Largo R, Herrero-Beaumont G. Setting up distinctive outcome measures for each osteoarthritis phenotype. Therapeutic Advances in Musculoskeletal Disease. 2020;12:1759720X20937966.

54. Rosedale R, Rastogi R, Kidd J, Lynch G, Supp G, Robbins SM. A study exploring the prevalence of Extremity Pain of Spinal Source (EXPOSS). Journal of Manual & Manipulative Therapy. 2020;28:222-230.

55. Rubinstein SM, Pool JJ, Van Tulder MW, Riphagen II, De Vet HC. A systematic review of the diagnostic accuracy of provocative tests of the neck for diagnosing cervical radiculopathy. European Spine Journal. 2007;16:307-319.

56. Sanchis MN, Lluch E, Nijs J, Struyf F, Kangasperko M. The role of central sensitization in shoulder pain: a systematic literature review. In: eds. Seminars in arthritis and rheumatism. 2015;44:710-716.

57. Schaible H-G, Grubb BD. Afferent and spinal mechanisms of joint pain. Pain. 1993;55:5-54.

58. Söyüncü S, Bektaş F, Cete Y. Traditional Kehr's sign: left shoulder pain related to splenic abscess. Turkish Journal of Trauma & Emergency Surgery. 2012;18:87-88.

59. Struyf F, Meeus M. Current evidence on physical therapy in patients with adhesive capsulitis: what are we missing? Clinical Rheumatology. 2014;33:593-600.

60. Theodoridis D, Ruston S. The effect of shoulder movements on thoracic spine 3D motion. Clinical Biomechanics. 2002;17:418-421.

61. Theodosopoulos T, Yiallourou AI, Hatzipappas J, Koutoulidis V, Dadnios N, Contis J. Right-shoulder pain: an unusual sign of hepatic endometriosis. Journal of Gynecologic Surgery. 2014;30:383-385.

62. Thoomes EJ, van Geest S, van der Windt DA, et al. Value of physical tests in diagnosing cervical radiculopathy: a systematic review. Spine J. 2018;18:179-189.

63. van de Ven J, Geomini P. A pregnant woman with acute shoulder pain. Nederlands Tijdschrift voor Geneeskunde. 2017;161:D1136-D1136.

64. Viganò P, Parazzini F, Somigliana E, Vercellini P. Endometriosis: epidemiology and aetiological factors. Best practice and research. Clinical Obstetrics & Gynaecology. 2004;18:177-200.

65. Viikari-Juntura E, Porras M, Laasonen E. Validity of clinical tests in the diagnosis of root compression in cervical disc disease. Spine. 1989;14:253-257.

66. Wainner RS, Whitman JM, Cleland JA, Flynn TW. Regional interdependence: a musculoskeletal examination model whose time has come. J Orthop Sports Phys Ther. 2007;37:658-660.

67. Walker T, Cuff A, Salt E, Lynch G, Littlewood C. Examination of the neck when a patient complains of shoulder pain: a global survey of current practice (2019). Musculoskeletal Care. 2020;18:256-264.

68. Wong JJ, Côté P, Quesnele JJ, Stern PJ, Mior SA. The course and prognostic factors of symptomatic cervical disc herniation with radiculopathy: a systematic review of the literature. The Spine Journal. 2014;14:1781-1789.

69. Zirak N, Soltani G, Hafizi L, Mashayekhi Z, Kashani I. Shoulder pain after caesarean section: comparison between general and spinal anaesthesia. Journal of Obstetrics and Gynaecology. 2012;32:347-349.

The unstable shoulder: assessment and management

17

Jo Gibson, Anju Jaggi, Amee L Seitz, Margie Olds, Lennard Funk

Defining instability

The capsule, labrum, ligaments, bones, and surrounding muscles that make up the shoulder provide a balance of force to maintain stability. Disruption of any of these in isolation or combination may give rise to instability. Instability refers to the inability to maintain the humeral head in the glenoid fossa and may be diagnosed as transient subluxation, partial displacement, and dislocation.[13,60] Instability is associated with symptoms that may include pain, neurovascular compromise, feeling that the shoulder is loose and may give way, and kinesiophobia. In contrast, shoulder laxity is the presence of excessive motion (physiological and accessory) but without symptoms.

Ninety-six percent of shoulder dislocations presenting to accident and emergency departments are anterior shoulder dislocations resulting from a traumatic event, and as such are the most common type.[13] Instability occurs due to a significant force to the shoulder such as a fall or collision. As a result, there may be damage to the structures of the shoulder, which can predispose to recurring symptoms. Up to 97% of individuals sustain a Bankart lesion following a traumatic anterior dislocation;[112] however, this structural lesion is less common in older individuals.[107,112] Atraumatic instability is less common, and prevalence is not fully known, with estimates from 2% to 30%.[81] Instability without a clear mechanism of trauma commonly occurs as a result of repetitive overhead movements or congenital abnormalities often related to hyperlaxity and inadequate muscle control.

Numerous classification systems have been suggested to define instability and direct management. These are predominantly categorized into etiology (traumatic versus atraumatic), frequency, direction, and severity.[122] Most dislocations occur unidirectionally, of which anterior is the most common; some occur in two directions often with an inferior component, termed bidirectional or multidirectional.[79] The term multidirectional has been interpreted and applied differently by many authors due to a reliance on the presence of multidirectional laxity being diagnostic rather than associated with symptoms.[72] Neer and Foster's seminal paper informed the most consistently cited definition of multidirectional instability as excessive joint translations in at least two directions with activity-related pain.[79] Given the significant variations in the definition and classification of this condition, the extrapolation of results from intervention studies is challenging and it is likely that prevalence is over-reported.[60,72,122]

The Stanmore Classification (Figure 17.1) as described by Lewis et al. defines three polar types of instability:[65] Polar I instability is directly related to trauma with evidence of structural deficit within the glenohumeral joint; Polar II atraumatic shoulder instability is also associated with a structural deficit primarily to the soft tissue structures (dysfunctional capsule), but with no bony injury; and Polar III is associated with no structural defect but with abnormal shoulder muscle control sometimes referred to as muscle patterning. The classification is unique in that it recognizes there is a continuum between the groups and that structural integrity and muscles play a role in all types but to a varying degree.[122]

The lack of consensus regarding classification of shoulder instability has led to ongoing confusion and has made comparison of interventions and treatment choices difficult. Only

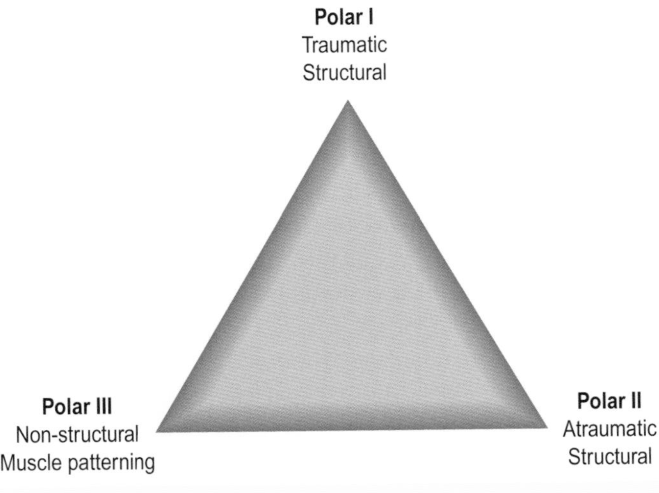

FIGURE 17.1
The Stanmore Classification of Shoulder Instability.

the frequency, etiology, direction, severity (FEDS) classification system has been tested for reliability and content validity.[60] This system categorizes shoulder instability according to patient-perceived FEDS of their symptoms and identifies a primary direction of instability. However, it is of note that the FEDS system eliminates the concept of multidirectional instability and fails to acknowledge that pain could be a secondary sign of subtle instability in some patients.

To date all classification systems have been based on a predominantly biomechanical framework. Surgical and nonsurgical decisions for shoulder instability are, however, also influenced by factors such as age, level of sport, function, and motivation, rather than simply the biological impairment itself.[13,81] Therefore, a biopsychosocial model should be considered in shoulder instability management in line with all musculoskeletal conditions. Although more research is required, pre-screening tools to predict recurrence and/or success of interventions have been explored in traumatic instability to guide clinician decision-making.[85,116]

Epidemiology

Glenohumeral joint instability

Overall incidence rates of shoulder dislocation have been shown to vary between 23.1[64] and 23.9[131] per 100,000 person-years, with a higher incidence in younger men under the age of 20 (98.3 per 100,000 person-years[64]). Cross-sectional epidemiological studies have reported that 72% of all dislocations are in males and that injury rates in young men under 20 are 6.7 times higher than in similarly aged females.[64] Almost 50% of traumatic shoulder dislocations occur in people between the ages of 15 and 29 years, with a second peak in incidence observed in elderly women over the age of 70.[13] Dislocations most commonly occur from a fall (58.8%) and happen at home (47.7%) or at a location of sport or recreation (34.5%). Overall, 48.3% of dislocations occur during sports or recreation activities,[131] with young contact and collision athletes experiencing the highest rate of instability.[24,120] Studies that have evaluated factors that may predispose individuals to traumatic shoulder dislocation have failed to demonstrate any predictive value of shoulder range of movement, scapula dyskinesia, strength deficits, or Beighton scores.[87,92]

Traumatic anterior glenohumeral dislocations are between 15.5 and 21.7 times more common than posterior dislocations.[95,127] The prevalence of traumatic posterior dislocation is reported as 1.1 per 100,000 people per year, with peaks in male patients between the ages of 14 and 19 years (9.21 per 100,000 person-years), males aged 20 to 49 years (2.26 per 100,000 person-years), and in elderly patients over 70 years old.[95,127] Up to 67% of traumatic posterior dislocations result from an acute traumatic event, with most of the remainder (31%) resulting from seizures. Increased glenoid retroversion has been shown to increase the risk of a first-time posterior dislocation.[88]

The true prevalence of atraumatic shoulder instability is difficult to extrapolate from the literature due to the lack of a universally accepted classification system, however, authors report incidence rates of between 4–10%.[81] Most people will have underlying laxity with loss of muscle control. Repetitive microtrauma may give rise to pathological laxity within the capsule restraints when moving the arm at extremes, such as in throwing sports. Nonstructural causes can be congenital, developmental, or psychological.[81]

Risk of recurrence

Almost 90% of recurrent dislocations occur within two years of first-time traumatic anterior shoulder dislocation (FTASD),[93] with recurrence rates inversely related to age. People between the ages of 14 and 25 years are at increased risk of recurrent anterior shoulder instability,[83,84,86] although exact figures are difficult to determine from the literature due to varied study designs, patient demographics, sporting activities and levels. Some studies have reported an increased rate of recurrent shoulder instability in males,[84,123] while others have not.[86,113] Similarly, there is a lack of agreement in the literature with regards to bony Bankart lesions, with some papers showing increased risk of re-dislocation after a bony Bankart lesion,[86] and some authors reporting decreased risk of recurrence.[101] The weight of evidence would support that Hill-Sachs lesions are not a significant univariate risk factor for recurrent instability.[84,123] However, one recent paper[26] has advocated that Hill-Sachs lesions on the humeral head that extend into the path of contact with the glenoid (off-track lesions) significantly increase the risk of recurrent shoulder instability. In other pathological lesions, people with a greater tuberosity fracture were seven times less likely to have recurrent anterior shoulder instability, while those with a nerve palsy were 2.5 times less likely to have recurrent shoulder instability.[84]

Despite many authors reporting sports participation and type of sport as risk factors for recurrence, systematic reviews do not demonstrate a significant difference in the rate of recurrence in athletic and non athletic populations.[67,123] People who work with their arm above shoulder height have a greater risk of recurrence ($p=0.05$) but not when this is adjusted for age, pain rating >8 (on a 10-point pain scale where 10 represents worst pain) and participation in contact sport ($p=0.07$).[99] Those performing hard physical work have also been shown to be at increased risk of recurrent instability when compared to more sedentary workers.[119] People with a positive apprehension test six weeks after a dislocation have been shown to be at increased risk of recurrent instability.[73,100] Kinesiophobia and self-reported pain and disability following FTASD have also been shown to increase the risk of further instability events at 12-month follow-up.[86]

In a recent study, many of these risk factors (age, bony Bankart lesion, hand dominance, immobilization after initial FTASD, kinesiophobia, perceived pain and disability) have been combined in a predictive tool to Predict Recurrent Instability of the Shoulder (PRIS).[85] An online tool (www.margieolds.com/pris) may help identify people who are less likely to have recurrent shoulder instability in the year following a FTASD and facilitate shared decision-making regarding best management.

Recurrence rates following a first time traumatic posterior dislocation are reported as being between 17% and 40%[95,127] with the majority occurring in the first year after initial injury. The four main factors associated a with an increased risk of recurrence are: 1) age under 40 years, 2) dislocation sustained during a seizure, 3) presence of a large reverse Hill-Sachs lesion, and 4) glenoid retroversion.[11]

Acromioclavicular and sternoclavicular joint instability

Acromioclavicular joint (ACJ) instability injuries have a reported incidence of 3–4 cases per 100,000 people per year in the general population.[69] A recent prospective cohort study reported that ACJ injuries accounted for 11% of all shoulder injuries presenting to accident and emergency departments, with 68% of injuries diagnosed as sprains and 32% as dislocations.[109] These injuries are more common in men under the age of 30, and highly associated with sporting activity – particularly high-energy contact sport.[69,109] Atraumatic ACJ instability is extremely rare, with only five case reports being reported in the literature.[4]

Injury to the sternoclavicular joint (SCJ) is uncommon and generally results from a high-energy traumatic impact, with dislocation of the SCJ representing 3% of all dislocations in the shoulder region. Anterior dislocation has been reported to be up to nine times more common than posterior dislocation.[103] Atraumatic dislocation and instability of the SCJ are less frequent and have a high association with hypermobility syndromes.[34]

The individual's perspective

An individual with an unstable shoulder will commonly experience reduced ability to function physically, socially, and emotionally, often associated with fear of movement.[102] Gartsmann et al. reported that the decrease of life quality ranks in severity with other major medical diseases such as hypertension, congestive cardiac failure, acute myocardial infarction, diabetes mellitus and clinical depression.[35] The impact of psychosocial factors and patient expectations on outcome of treatment and self-reported pain and function are well reported in populations with musculoskeletal conditions.[17,71] These cohorts express that clinicians do not appreciate the impact their problem has on their life.[54,74]

The British Prime Minister, army officer, and writer, Sir Winston Churchill, experienced a traumatic anterior shoulder dislocation. When describing his experience, he wrote:

> *Quite an exceptional strain is required to tear the capsule which holds the shoulder joint together, but once the deed is done, a terrible liability remains. I had sustained an injury which was to last me my life, which was to cripple me at polo, to prevent me from ever playing tennis, and to be a grave embarrassment in moments of peril, violence, and effort. It is one of the most unfortunate things ... I try to be philosophic, but it is very hard. Of course, it is better to have bad luck in the minor pleasures of life than in one's bigger undertakings. But I am very low and unhappy about it.*[121]

Functional magnetic resonance imaging (fMRI) studies evaluating people with persistent apprehension following FTASD have demonstrated specific reorganization in functional connectivity of brain regions involved in the cognitive control of motor behavior.[43,105,132] Howard et al. found increased brain activity within specific regions including the primary motor cortex, premotor cortex, and middle frontal gyrus in patients with atraumatic instability (that had proved resistance to traditional rehabilitation approaches) compared to controls.[47] Patients exhibit neural activity similar to that observed in early learning of a motor sequence, which indicates that patients are in some sense working harder or differently to maintain shoulder stability. These studies illustrate the potential impact of emotional and cognitive functions on motor strategies and the perpetuation of feelings of apprehension and instability.[61]

Studies have also shown that both extrinsic and intrinsic factors such as competing interests, kinesiophobia, and internal stressors and motivators can have a major effect on a patient's decision to return to sport following shoulder dislocation and subsequent surgery.[115] This highlights the importance of understanding the patient perspective, and exploring patients' beliefs and expectations regarding their shoulder instability and treatment as underpinning principles of the subjective examination.

Assessment

Patient interview

A clinical diagnosis of shoulder instability is predominantly based on the patient interview and physical examination (see Chapters 11 and 15). It is essential to gain a thorough history to help establish subgroups and to inform management. The instability diagnosis is typically used for those with complaints of subluxations, apprehension, or a feeling that their shoulder is unstable, particularly at end ranges of motion. However, adolescent athletes with instability relating to sporting activity may present with anterior shoulder pain in the region of the long head of biceps. Similarly, people with atraumatic instability may report diffuse glenohumeral pain and fatigue in relation to activity in association with subjective feelings of instability. Many people with posterior instability commonly report pain as their predominant symptom.[7]

Key questions relating to mechanism of onset, age, frequency and direction of instability, provoking movements/activities, impact on function/quality of life, and presence of hypermobility help classify the type of shoulder instability, inform management and prognosis.

Mechanism of onset

Glenohumeral joint instability

Establishing a significant traumatic event resulting in dislocation or onset of instability symptoms is helpful in identifying the likelihood of structural pathology.[81] Berhardson et al. reported the primary mechanism of injury in an anterior instability cohort was a dislocation event, affecting 82.5% patients, of whom 46% required reduction by a medical provider.[7] This contrasted with 78% of those presenting with symptoms consistent with posterior instability who were unable to identify a specific injury. Weightlifting and shoulder pressing (11%) and football "blocking" (10%) were the most common activities in those able to identify a single event.[127]

Individuals participating in overhead sports may have acquired laxity due to the repeated microtrauma of fast or powerful movements at the extremes of range.[127] Patients may have a history of repetitive movement into the symptom-provoking position. Those patients with a background of hyperlaxity or hypermobility may relate symptoms to a change in activity.[81] It is important to explore whether there is a history of subluxation (either voluntary or involuntarily dislocations) during childhood, and whether there are symptoms in any other joints to suggest the potential presence of generalized joint laxity.

Superior labral anterior posterior lesions

Several injury mechanisms have been proposed for the pathogenesis of superior labral anterior posterior (SLAP) tears. Traumatic lesions may result from direct compression loads, such as a fall onto an outstretched arm or onto the point of the shoulder, from direct traction injuries to the shoulder, or as a consequence of bracing in anticipation of a motor vehicle collision.[31]

SLAP lesions can also occur as a result of repetitive overhead activity in individuals participating in overhead sport or with occupations involving repeated overhead loading. In these scenarios, SLAP tears often present with insidious onset and progressive deep shoulder pain, particularly with the arm in abduction and external rotation position. Patients may also report a loss of power and performance during the late-cocking phase of throwing.[12]

Acromioclavicular and sternoclavicular joint instability

Acromioclavicular joint (ACJ) instability is usually traumatic and ranges from subtle instability with pain alone to complete dislocations of varying degrees (see Chapter 24). The two most common mechanisms that account for traumatic ACJ injury are direct and indirect trauma. Direct impact injuries have the highest incidence and occur when a person falls onto the ACJ with their arm at their side in an adducted position.[108,129] An indirect injury to the ACJ may also occur as the result of a fall on an outstretched hand where the humeral head is driven superiorly into the acromion.[108,129]

Traumatic sternoclavicular joint (SCJ) dislocation occurs after high-energy injuries including road traffic accidents, sporting injuries, and falls from height. A direct blow to the anteromedial aspect of the clavicle or a compressive force to the shoulder applied laterally with the arm flexed at the shoulder can cause posterior dislocation of the SCJ. A compressive force applied to the lateral aspect of the shoulder girdle, as when struck from the side, can cause anterior dislocation of the SCJ.[70,94] Studies have shown that the force required to dislocate the SCJ posteriorly is 50% greater than the force needed to dislocate it anteriorly.[103]

Provoking movements and activities

Patients are not always able to specify a direction of instability, however, questioning about those movements that provoke symptoms can help clarify this.[60] In those with anterior instability, provocation of symptoms is common when the shoulder is placed at 90° of abduction and end range external rotation.[7] Those with posterior instability often report provocation with activities at 90° of shoulder flexion and horizontal adduction, and posteriorly directed force or load through the glenohumeral joint.[7]

People with multidirectional instability often report recurrent subluxation events rather than frank dislocation, and may report instability with simple reaching movements below shoulder height. In addition, they may report waking at night with the shoulder subluxated or dislocated.

Impact on function/quality of life

Exploring the individual's experience of instability, the impact on their life, their beliefs, concerns, and expectations of treatment are paramount in highlighting psychosocial factors that may impact management options and outcomes.[17,115] Olds et al. demonstrated an association between fear of injury and self-reported pain and function near the time of injury with recurrent shoulder instability following FTASD at 12-month follow-up.[86] In patients with atraumatic instability, Noorani et al. highlighted that missing school more than 20% of the time, absence from work for more than 3 months, persistent subluxation or dislocation of the glenohumeral joint, and frequent attendance at accident and emergency, may warrant early referral to a specialist multidisciplinary team with psychological support.[81]

Hyperlaxity and hypermobility spectrum disorders

Hyperlaxity can predispose people to symptoms of instability. Hyperlaxity may be either congenital ("born loose") or acquired ("become loose"), and is not always associated with hypermobility spectrum disorders (HSDs) or hereditary connective tissue disorders such as Ehlers Danlos syndrome or Marfan disease.[16] (HSDs are a group of clinically relevant conditions related to joint hypermobility, which are distinguishable from hereditary connective tissues disorders, as the phenotypic domains of HSDs are usually limited to the musculoskeletal system.)

Between 4% and 13% of the population have joint hypermobility that is not associated with systemic disease. Unlike people with traumatic shoulder instability, those with hyperlaxity and instability are more likely to experience episodes of recurrent subluxation than they are to have recurrent dislocation.[53] In those with acquired hyperlaxity, symptoms are commonly unilateral in the dominant shoulder; swimmers, weightlifters, rowers, gymnasts, and those playing racquet, overhead, or throwing sports are the most commonly affected.[53]

It is key to ascertain the mechanism of onset, although people with joint hyperlaxity may require less trauma to sustain a structural lesion than those without.[81] In addition, it is important to question patients about other joints that may be affected, and other symptoms associated with hypermobility spectrum disorder in those with congenital hyperlaxity. The five-point hypermobility questionnaire (Table 17.1) described by Hakim and Grahame is a valid and reliable tool and a useful adjunct to clinical examination in identifying individuals with hypermobility spectrum disorder.[38]

Table 17.1 The five-point hypermobility questionnaire[38]

The 5-point hypermobility questionnaire	
1	Can you now (or could you ever) place your hands flat on the floor without bending your knees?
2	Can you now (or could you ever) bend your thumb to touch your forearm?
3	As a child, did you amuse your friends by contorting your body into strange shapes or could you do the splits?
4	As a child or a teenager, did your kneecap or shoulder dislocate on more than one occasion?
5	Do you consider yourself double-jointed?

Answering yes to 2 or more of these questions indicates hypermobility (sensitivity 85%, specificity 90%).[38]

Physical examination

Special tests

In addition to the factors discussed in the interview and medical history, there are certain clinical tests that have a greater ability to rule in glenohumeral instability and potentially define the direction. Tests for determining the presence of anterior glenohumeral instability include the anterior apprehension test,[98] relocation test,[51] and surprise test.[40] These are symptom reproduction tests, with a test considered positive if it reproduces an apprehension response. These tests are described in Table 17.2. The use of pain as a positive test significantly reduces the diagnostic accuracy of the tests.[32,66] The combination of the apprehension test, relocation and surprise test have the greatest likelihood to rule in anterior instability.[66]

The anterior and posterior drawer tests,[36] load and shift test,[106] and sulcus sign[79] evaluate relative laxity of the joint and do not determine instability unless reproducing instability symptoms. Furthermore, grading of translation and quantification of laxity has poor intertester reliability, with

Table 17.2 Diagnostic accuracy of anterior instability tests using either pain or apprehension as a positive result

Test	Description	Performance	Result	Sensitivity(%)	Specificity (%)
Apprehension[98,32]	Determination if patient is apprehensive or fears glenohumeral joint will go out of place at the extremes of passive motion	With the patient in a supine position and the arm in 90° abduction, the examiner passively moves the arm into external rotation	• Pain • Apprehension	50 72	56 96
Relocation[51,32]	Determination if apprehension or fear elicited via the anterior apprehension test is reduced or eliminated with added manual stability to the glenohumeral joint	With the patient in a supine position and the arm in 90° abduction, the examiner places a hand over the anterior shoulder to apply a posterior directed force. The arm is then passively moved into external rotation.	• Pain • Apprehension	30 81	90 92
Anterior release[40,66] **(surprise test)**	Determination if apprehension or fear that glenohumeral joint will go out of place at the extremes of passive motion occurs when manual stability provided by examiner is unexpectedly removed	With the patient in a supine position and the arm in 90° abduction, the examiner places a hand over the anterior shoulder to apply a posterior directed force. The arm is then passively moved into external rotation. The examiner then removes the hand applying the posterior force.	Pain or apprehension	64	99

risk of false negatives due to patients' inability to relax during testing.[29] Recommendations have been made that physiological measures of hyperlaxity such as external rotation in neutral are more reliable for assessing anterior hyperlaxity, especially if measured in supine.[75,97]

The posterior apprehension test[90] is recommended for the diagnosis of posterior instability with a post-test probability positive likelihood ratio (+LR) of +LR 19 when the test is positive.[50] However, while apprehension increases reliability of anterior instability tests, only a 1/3 of patients with posterior instability with confirmed posterior structural lesions have apprehension or feelings of instability. Most people with posterior instability report positional-specific pain,[23,127] and consequently, pain and apprehension should be considered as positive findings when applying the posterior apprehension test. There is a lack of evidence to support the use of the jerk test, Kim test, posterior impingement sign, and O'Brien test as standalone clinical tests for identifying posterior instability. However, Kim et al. reported that patients who presented with a painful jerk test had a higher failure rate following nonoperative care.[57] While clustering may help support the clinical picture, clinicians must rely on history and recognition of risk factors to support clinical diagnosis.[23]

The hyperabduction test was originally described as an assessment of inferior instability.[33] Although the posterior apprehension test was validated in one study and the hyperabduction test has only been validated as a test for anterior instability, a positive finding of apprehension on any two of these three tests will enable a diagnosis of multidirectional instability. Multidirectional instability has a greater likelihood with the presence of overall generalized laxity, frequently defined using the Beighton Index.[46] The Beighton Index consists of nine dichotomous tests of mobility at the metacarpophalangeal joints of the thumb and fifth finger, knee, elbows, and low back/hamstrings.[6] Authors suggest a score of 5/9 as a cut-off for adolescents and adults (with a relevant history) and 6/9 for prepubescent groups.[55] However, in those that score one point below the threshold, a score of 2 or more on the 5-point hypermobility questionnaire confirms generalized joint hypermobility.[16,55] In the presence of other factors such as features of skin and fascia, and a family history of hypermobility, referral to further rule out genetic connective tissue disorders such as Ehlers-Danlos, Loeys-Dietz, or Marfan syndromes should be considered.[16]

Superior labral lesions

The clinical diagnosis of SLAP lesions remains challenging as they commonly occur in conjunction with other shoulder pathologies and the diagnostic accuracy of reported examination tests is generally poor.[31] In a meta-analysis of pooled diagnostic accuracy values, the physical examination tests that were recommended with caution to confirm the diagnosis of type II to type IV SLAP lesions are the anterior slide, Yergason, and compression rotation test.[45] However, based on this meta-analysis, no test is recommended for ruling out a SLAP lesion. More recent research suggests that any combination of three out of the biceps load I, biceps load II, Speed's, passive compression, and O'Brien's tests would be sufficient to diagnose a SLAP lesion without an MRI or MRA for confirmation due to the excellent sensitivity and specificity of this cluster of tests.[19] However, clustering tests is not without its limitations and in reality, the history of onset and functional limitations are fundamental in informing diagnosis of these lesions.[19,31]

Acromioclavicular joint

In type I and II ACJ injuries, pain provocation tests such as the Paxinos, cross adduction/scarf, O'Brien's active compression, and ACJ resisted extension tests are advocated to confirm the presence of an ACJ injury.[20] However, these tests have limited clinical utility in the absence of a relevant traumatic history and relevant signs and symptoms.[14,59]

In injuries where the clavicle is prominent, it is important to note that this prominence represents depression of the scapula and not true elevation of the clavicle. In patients with clear deformity, researchers have described using the reducibility of the ACJ to help define the lesion, and also assessing anterior-posterior mobility/horizontal stability of the lateral end of clavicle in comparison to the opposite shoulder. Morris et al. highlight the relevance of scapular dyskinesis in combination with perceived laxity on manual assessment as indicating higher grade injuries.[76] There is a lack of research assessing the intertester reliability of these assessment approaches and their utility in informing management.

More recently the shrug test has been described to differentiate a type III injury from a type V injury. The patient is asked to shrug their shoulders, and if the AC joint reduces, this suggests that the deltotrapezial fascia is intact and a type V injury can be ruled out.[20,130]

Sternoclavicular joint

There is a lack of research to support the utility of specific tests when assessing instability in the sternoclavicular joint. Van Tongel et al.[118] describe the protraction test in combination with local palpation as reliable in diagnosing degenerative pathology affecting the SCJ but this has not been investigated in patients with instability. In patients with atraumatic SCJ instability, case series reports advocate the use of symptom modification approaches that assess postural change to influence symptoms.[2,3]

Assessing muscle function

Studies evaluating patients with multidirectional instability provide evidence for altered muscle activity and altered humeral and scapular kinematics in patients compared to controls.[110] Clinical observations supported by fine wire electromyography analysis in patients with atraumatic instability have shown aberrant muscle recruitment patterns associated with the displacement of the humerus on the glenoid/glenohumeral joint.[49] In cohorts with anterior instability, authors report specific strength deficits in both the glenohumeral internal and external rotators, and scapular protractors and retractors.[1,27]

Improved understanding of shoulder muscle function helps guide specific approaches to assessment of the shoulder muscles. Muscles of the shoulder girdle work in a pattern of recruitment to allow for movement and maintain stability at the glenohumeral joint that is dependent on the plane and direction of movement.[8,125] Function at the shoulder girdle relies on muscles that directly influence the scapula (trapezius, serratus anterior, rhomboids, pectoralis minor) and muscles that directly influence the humeral head position (infraspinatus and supraspinatus, subscapularis, deltoid, pectoralis major, and latissimus dorsi). It is important to consider the lines of action of these muscles and the need to work as balanced force couples to maintain stability and function. Additionally, these muscles have dual roles acting to both move the limb as well as to stabilize. As a starting point, it is important to assess muscle performance as this will inform management.

Rotator cuff strength

Testing the rotator cuff (RC) in supine lying in varying degrees of abduction has been shown to be more specific than with the patient in standing positions.[8,21,37] The patient should lie supine with the elbow flexed to 90°, between 45–90° of abduction. A small, rolled towel placed under the arm supports arm weight, and prevents extension of the glenohumeral joint. Active external rotation to the point of apprehension should be performed, followed by resisted external rotation at the limit of the movement to test isometric strength, with the posterior RC in its shortened (inner range) position (Figure 17.2A), and then resisted internal rotation in the same position to test the anterior RC in its lengthened (outer range) position (Figure 17.2B). The arm is then actively moved to maximum internal rotation, ensuring that the scapula does not lift off the from the couch, and resisted external rotation tests the posterior RC in its lengthened position, and resisted internal rotation in this position tests the anterior RC in its shortened position. Use of a handheld dynamometer has been shown to be a reliable method to gain more objective shoulder strength measurements[52] and has been shown to identify weakness of up to 28% in the shoulder in those rated as "normal" with manual muscle testing.[117]

Scapular muscles

Isolated scapular control may be observed by asking the patient to elevate, depress, retract and protract the scapula. Further assessment of the scapulothoracic muscles, such as trapezius and serratus anterior function should be performed. Testing of the trapezius is best performed in prone positions with the patient holding the load of limb in varying degrees of elevation (Figure 17.3A). Serratus anterior should be tested where the strength of isolated protraction can be performed, such as in supine lying or sitting, noting any increased winging when resistance is applied (Figure 17.3B). A loss of scapular upward rotation during elevation of the arm is one of the most consistent kinematic findings in patients with atraumatic instability.[110] The utilization of symptom modification approaches such as the scapular assistance test, or maneuvers that facilitate the scapula during provocative movements (e.g., upward rotation) can help inform rehabilitation strategies to normalize strength and motor control.[124]

Symptom modification

Symptom modification approaches (Figure 17.4) are more fully explored in Chapter 36. The mechanism of effect of

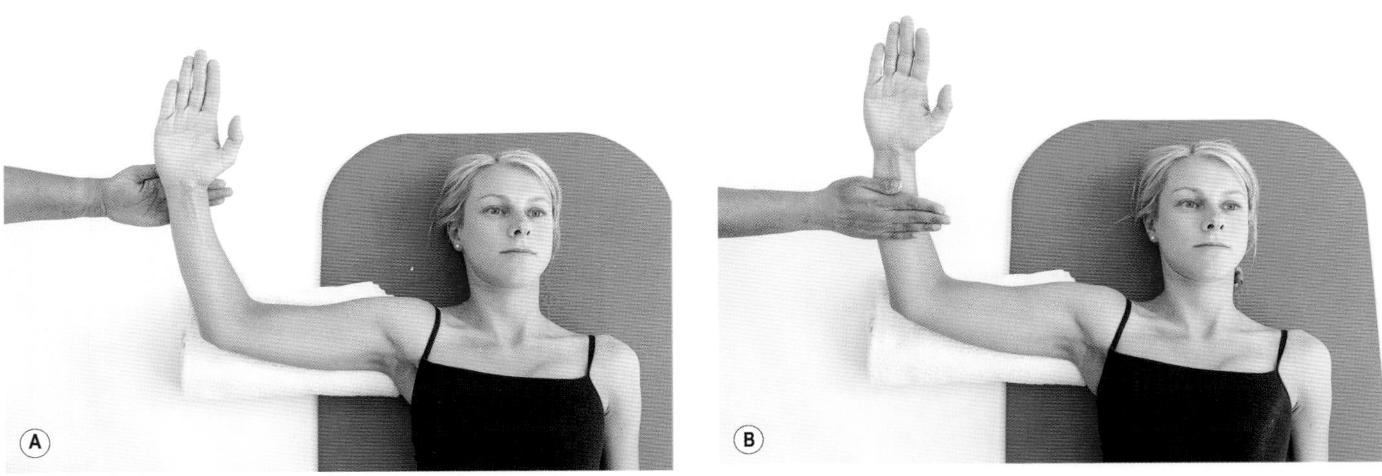

FIGURE 17.2 A&B
Assessment of the rotator cuff in supine.

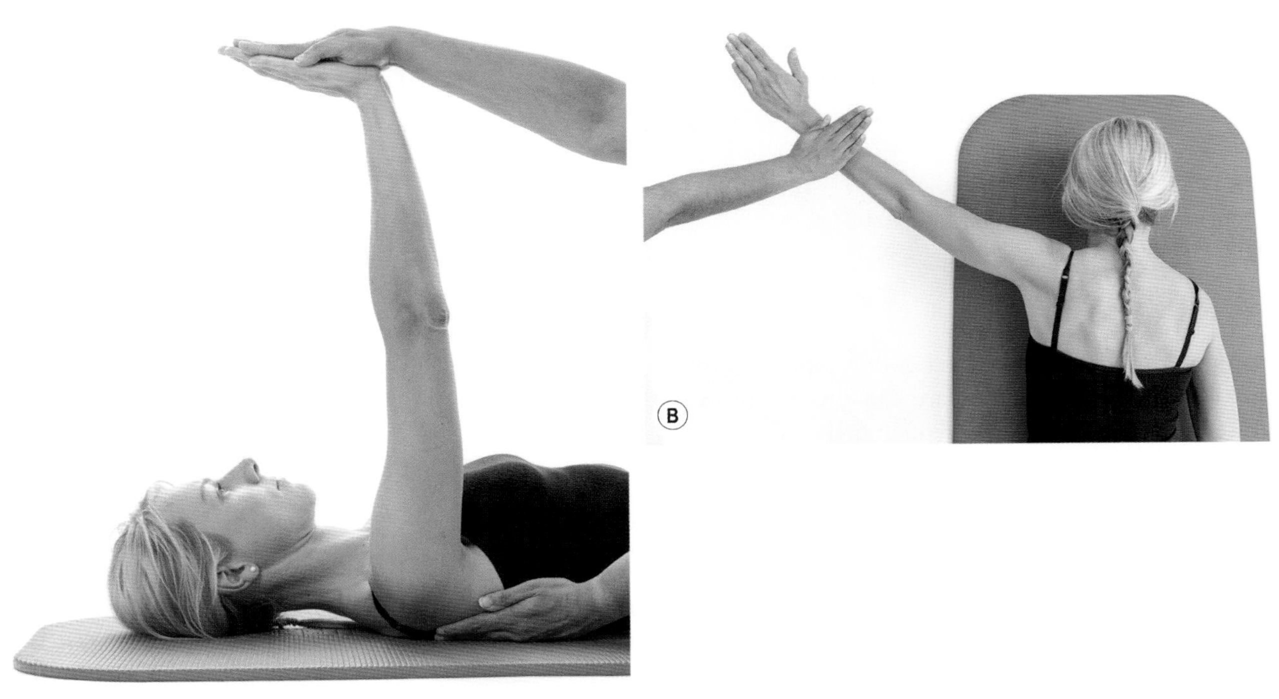

FIGURE 17.3 A&B
Assessment of the scapulothoracic muscles.

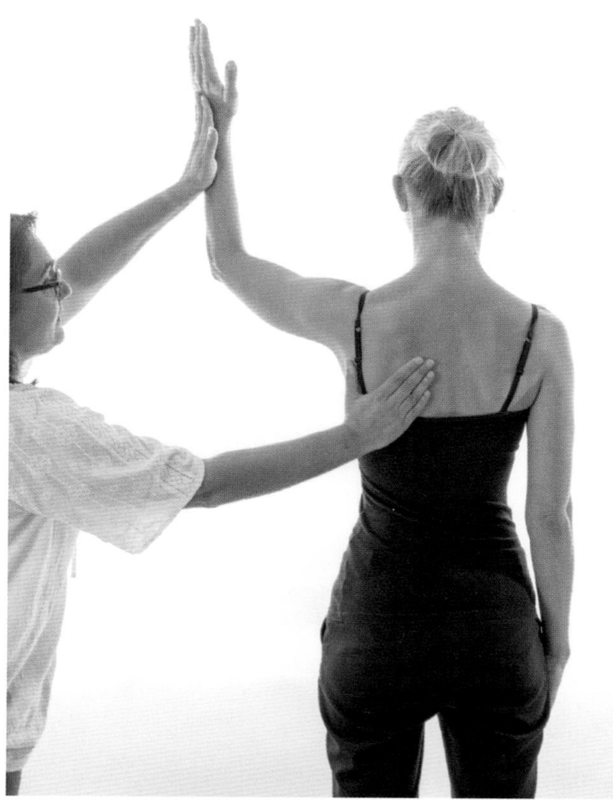

FIGURE 17.4
Symptom modification approaches: facilitation of the posterior rotator cuff and scapula.

these procedures is not clearly understood.[63] Improving the experience of instability by manipulating load and or movement strategy may contribute to reducing the impact of negative influences, such as protective and safety behaviors and kinesiophobia. Specific sensorimotor deficits are well reported in patients with both traumatic and atraumatic shoulder instability.[28,62,78] Tactile input and applied resistance during symptom modification have been shown to influence muscle recruitment and may help normalize body schema.[63,111] There has been increasing interest in the role of the kinetic chain in shoulder pathology and its potential role in rehabilitation; however, to date, evidence is conflicting.[9,91] With respect to informing symptom modification approaches, evidence demonstrates that initiating shoulder exercises with the lower quadrant in the form of step or weight transfer increases local recruitment of the scapular muscles.[91] In those patients who have significant kinesiophobia, this may provide an additional tool to influence instability and challenge negative beliefs and expectations.

Approaches to the objective assessment are informed by the subjective history and aim to confirm the presentation of instability, identify strength deficits in the rotator cuff and scapula muscles and improve a patient's confidence to move and function. This provides targets for rehabilitation and acknowledges the multifactorial nature of an individual's presentation.

Imaging

Plain radiographs are the first-line investigation following traumatic shoulder instability. In the case of glenohumeral joint dislocation they can be used to assess for bony defects of the glenoid (bony Bankart lesions) and humeral head (Hill-Sachs lesion).[13] In the event that such lesions are identified, CT scans with 3D reformatted images can be used to further assess the extent of bony injuries and can help inform surgical approaches when this is indicated. In patients with atraumatic glenohumeral joint instability, particularly for those cases where conservative measures have failed, plain film radiography is useful to exclude an inherent structural abnormality such as glenoid dysplasia.[5]

Magnetic resonance imaging enhanced with intra-articular gadolinium (MR arthrogram) is the gold standard modality for assessing the spectrum of intra-articular soft tissue injuries that are associated with shoulder instability. It has been demonstrated that positioning the arm in the apprehension position (abduction and external rotation) during imaging can increase sensitivity for identifying anterior and superior labral pathology.[128]

Other considerations

Nerve involvement

Potential factors complicating management of traumatic dislocations include concomitant nerve injuries. Risk factors for nerve injury following a FTASD include older patient age, higher energy of the initial trauma, and a longer period from dislocation to its reduction.[41] Nerve injuries following FTASD are predominantly neurapraxia or axonotmesis, with complete nerve disruption seen in less than 3% of patients.[42] The axillary nerve is most commonly involved, both in isolation and in combination with other nerves following FTASD.[96] The risk is greater in older adults over the age of 60 years and particularly in those with an associated rotator cuff tear or greater tuberosity fracture.[96]

A recent systematic review[42] suggested that multi-nerve involvement was more common than isolated nerve injuries following FTASD, which conflicts with previous research.[96] However, there is a consensus that those patients most likely to have multiple nerve involvement are elderly females following a fall and young men after high-energy trauma. Multi-nerve injury patterns include the musculocutaneous nerve, radial nerve and potentially the suprascapular nerve.

This highlights the importance of evaluating the integrity of the axillary nerve and other relevant peripheral nerves following FTASD with sensation and myotome testing. Suspected lesions should be referred for electromyographic studies and nerve conduction testing. However, to minimize the risk of false negatives and gain the most diagnostic information from a single study, testing should be done 3–4 weeks post-injury.[15] Rehabilitation considerations for patients with concomitant nerve involvement include delayed recovery of strength and muscular stability. Thus, delayed return to high-risk positions of combined external rotation and abduction range of motion and strengthening are expected with a course of recovery that may extend over a year.

Rotator cuff tear

Radiologically proven full-thickness rotator cuff tears are common following FTASD in adults over 40 years of age, with incidence increasing in line with age.[104,107] In view of the prevalence of asymptomatic rotator cuff tears in this age group, it can be challenging to distinguish acute tears from normal age-related change.[114] Authors advocate that weakness and loss of function are better indicators for surgery than pain.[25]

Management options

Controversies in management

Management of FTASD is controversial, with many advocating a trial of rehabilitation in all patients. A systematic review of interventions to reduce recurrent instability after FTASD showed that 47% of patients did not experience recurrence of shoulder instability or re-dislocation following nonsurgical management.[56] However, others suggest surgical stabilization as the primary treatment in younger active patients. A Cochrane review[44] with a meta-analysis of four trials compared nonoperative to operative management for patients with FTASD. The review concluded there is limited evidence supporting primary treatment of a stabilization surgery compared to rehabilitation alone in young males engaged in high demand activities. A more recent systematic review and meta-analysis concluded that arthroscopic Bankart repair resulted in a 7-fold lower recurrence rate and a higher rate of return to play following FTASD than nonsurgical management.[48] However, critical review of these data may suggest otherwise. Of the four trials included in Cochrane review, only two were published randomized trials on primary surgery versus rehabilitation.[10,58] Cohorts in both meta-analyses consisted primarily of males (90%) with a mean age of 22 years. In the Cochrane review, participants who were managed with rehabilitation were treated with a post-surgical protocol.

Therefore, we caution in using these results to support primary surgery in patients following FTASD given the rehabilitation program that was provided. First, the rehabilitation programs included 3–4 weeks sling immobilization. Second, formal strengthening in these randomized trials was only initiated 8 weeks after, in lieu of active and active-assisted motion exercises. Lastly, the rehabilitation program did not include key components of rehabilitation shown to be effective following a FTASD including proprioception, coordination, and core dynamic functional exercises.[30]

Contemporary rehabilitation for FTASD should recognize that immobilization for more than one week does not reduce the risk of recurrence.[89] Patients should be encouraged to wean off their sling after one week or as comfort permits. Limiting lengthy immobilization avoids the negative consequences of decreased strength and motor control. Patients should initiate early activation of rotator cuff and scapular positioning musculature in the first week and include activities to address proprioception, motor control[30] and kinesiophobia. More representative, prospective research is needed to compare primary surgical intervention with appropriate contemporaneous rehabilitation strategies.

Atraumatic glenohumeral joint instability

A good clinical history with appropriate imaging, when indicated, helps to determine appropriate management. The literature advocates a structured rehabilitation program for the majority of cases, reporting between 50% and 80% effective outcome; however, this is based on poor quality studies with variable diagnostic criteria and outcomes, and to date there are no good quality trials comparing surgery with rehabilitation. Surgery is intended to reduce the excess capsular volume, thereby reducing laxity, and possibly improving proprioception (see Chapter 41). Initially this was via the open capsular shift procedure, but this has been superseded by arthroscopic approaches.[68] For the right indications, along with appropriate rehabilitation, the outcomes are very good with success rates of over 70%.[126]

Superior labrum anterior to posterior (SLAP) lesions

In patients with an acute mechanism of injury resulting in a SLAP lesion, early arthroscopic intervention may be indicated. Decision-making is based on several factors including the type and extent of SLAP tear, the age of the patient, functional demands, level of sporting activity and surgeon preference.[31] Arthroscopic treatment of symptomatic SLAP lesions following trauma in young athletes leads to good clinical results.[12]

In patients who have a SLAP tear as a result of repeated overhead activity such as in throwing sports, initial treatment should be conservative for a period of 3–6 months. In the event that nonsurgical management is unsuccessful, surgery in the form of either a SLAP repair or biceps tenodesis may be appropriate. However, in overhead throwing athletes the reported results are less successful, with a significant amount of patients failing to return to their pre-injury activity level.[12,31]

Acromioclavicular joint instability

Traditional management for treating traumatic ACJ injuries is based on the Rockwood classification which represents a continuum of increasingly severe soft tissue injury: types 1 and 2 represent injury to the acromioclavicular ligaments (ACL) with preservation of the coracoclavicular ligaments (CCL); type 3 represents disruption to the ACL and some of the CCL ligaments; types 4 and 5 represent disruption of both the ACL and CCL with increasing displacement (posteriorly or inferiorly) and soft tissue involvement. The consensus in the literature is that of nonoperative management of types 1 and 2, and operative treatment of types 4 and 5, with type 3 remaining controversial.[129] However, classifying an injury is imprecise, with poor inter- and intra-observer agreement when classifying according to radiographs, MRI or CT scans.[18,39,80] Increasingly, experts advocate for more emphasis on clinical presentation, patient factors, pain, and functional deficits in informing the role of surgery, than a reliance on imaging.

Generally, most acute injuries can be managed nonoperatively initially, as most patients can functionally compensate for the injury, with little difference between operative and nonoperative management overall.[77] However, some studies suggest certain groups do better with surgical reconstruction, and these include overhead athletes and overhead manual workers.[22] Surgery involves reduction of the ACJ and reconstruction of the CCL and ACL. Most recent studies show that anatomical reconstruction of the ligaments gives better biomechanical outcomes, as the reconstruction mimics the normal three-dimensional properties of the CCL complex.[82] However, there are numerous different techniques, depending on surgeon preference.

Sternoclavicular joint instability

Traumatic subluxation or dislocation of the SCJ usually requires significant force and one should be mindful of associated injuries. Damage or compromise to the posterior mediastinal structures is a risk with a posterior dislocation and should be considered as a potential medical emergency. Rarely the SCJ disc can be damaged, leading to symptoms of clicking and pain in overhead sports; this is sometimes the result of a shearing injury in a normal disc but more commonly due to a tear in a degenerate disc. Most anterior dislocations and posterior subluxations can be managed nonoperatively, while an acute posterior dislocation, particularly in the presence of mediastinal compromise, may require an open reduction and stabilization.[34]

Summary

Shoulder stability is dependent on the capsuloligamentous structures, bony congruency and a balanced net reaction force from the surrounding shoulder musculature.

Shoulder instability encompasses a spectrum of presentations involving the compromise or disruption of any of these factors. The continued lack of consensus with respect to classification systems limits comparison and the understanding of effective treatments for subgroups of instability. However, similarities in classification systems highlight the importance of mechanism of onset (i.e., traumatic or not), together with the presence or lack of structural pathology to inform treatment approaches.

A detailed patient history is essential to extrapolate relevant information regarding the mechanism of onset, frequency of instability and severity of symptoms. Detailed examination of specific strength deficits in comparison to the unaffected shoulder establishes baseline values and directs clinicians to targeted, focused rehabilitation. In addition, increased understanding of the interplay between prognostic factors allows clinicians to engage in shared decision-making regarding treatment options for people with shoulder instability. The influence of psychosocial factors in predicting recurrent instability highlights the importance of understanding the individual's beliefs, expectations, and concerns from the outset.

References

1. Ansanello Netto W, Zanca GG, Saccol MF, Zatiti SCA, Mattiello SM. Scapular muscles weakness in subjects with traumatic anterior glenohumeral instability. Phys Ther Sport. 2018;33:76-81.
2. Armstrong A. Disorders of the Sternoclavicular Joint. Orthopaedics and Trauma. 2018;32:186-199.
3. Athanatos L, Pal Singh H, Armstrong A. The management of sternoclavicular instability. Journal of Arthroscopy and Joint Surgery. 2018;5:126-132.
4. Barchick SR, Otte RS, Garrigues GE. Voluntary acromioclavicular joint dislocation: a case report and literature review. J Shoulder Elbow Surg. 2019;28:e238-e244.
5. Bateman M, Jaiswal A, Tambe A. Diagnosis and management of atraumatic shoulder instability. Journal of Arthroscopy and Joint Surgery. 2018;2018:79-85.
6. Beighton P, Solomon L, Soskolne CL. Articular mobility in an African population. Ann Rheum Dis. 1973;32:413-418.
7. Bernhardson AS, Murphy CP, Aman ZS, LaPrade RF, Provencher MT. A prospective analysis of patients with anterior versus posterior shoulder instability: a matched cohort examination and surgical outcome analysis of 200 patients. Am J Sports Med. 2019;47:682-687.
8. Boettcher CE, Cathers I, Ginn KA. The role of shoulder muscles is task specific. J Sci Med Sport. 2010;13:651-656.
9. Borms D, Maenhout A, Cools AM. Incorporation of the kinetic chain into shoulder-elevation exercises: does it affect scapular muscle activity? J Athl Train. 2020;55:343-349.
10. Bottoni CR, Wilckens JH, DeBerardino TM, et al. A prospective, randomized evaluation of arthroscopic stabilization versus nonoperative treatment in patients with acute, traumatic, first-time shoulder dislocations. Am J Sports Med. 2002;30:576-580.
11. Brelin A, Dickens JF. Posterior shoulder instability. Sports Med Arthrosc Rev. 2017;25:136-143.
12. Brockmeyer M, Tompkins M, Kohn DM, Lorbach O. SLAP lesions: a treatment algorithm. Knee Surg Sports Traumatol Arthrosc. 2016;24:447-455.
13. Brownson P, Donaldson O, Fox M, et al. BESS/BOA patient care pathways: traumatic anterior shoulder instability. Shoulder Elbow. 2015;7:214-226.
14. Cadogan A, McNair P, Laslett M, Hing W. Shoulder pain in primary care: diagnostic accuracy of clinical examination tests for non-traumatic acromioclavicular joint pain. BMC Musculoskelet Disord. 2013;14:156.
15. Campbell WW. Evaluation and management of peripheral nerve injury. Clin Neurophysiol. 2008;119:1951-1965.
16. Castori M, Tinkle B, Levy H, Grahame R, Malfait F, Hakim A. A framework for the classification of joint hypermobility and related conditions. Am J Med Genet C Semin Med Genet. 2017;175:148-157.
17. Chester R, Jerosch-Herold C, Lewis J, Shepstone L. Psychological factors are associated with the outcome of physiotherapy for people with shoulder pain: a multicentre longitudinal cohort study. Br J Sports Med. 2018;52:269-275.
18. Cho CH, Hwang I, Seo JS, et al. Reliability of the classification and treatment of dislocations of the acromioclavicular joint. J Shoulder Elbow Surg. 2014;23:665-670.
19. Clark RC, Chandler CC, Fuqua AC, Glymph KN, Lambert GC, Rigney KJ. Use of clinical test clusters versus advanced imaging studies in the management of patients with a suspected SLAP tear. Int J Sports Phys Ther. 2019;14:345-352.
20. Cook JB, Krul KP. Challenges in treating acromioclavicular separations: current concepts. J Am Acad Orthop Surg. 2018;26:669-677.
21. Dark A, Ginn KA, Halaki M. Shoulder muscle recruitment patterns during commonly used rotator cuff exercises: an electromyographic study. Phys Ther. 2007;87:1039-1046.
22. Deans CF, Gentile JM, Tao MA. Acromioclavicular joint injuries in overhead athletes: a concise review of injury mechanisms, treatment options, and outcomes. Curr Rev Musculoskelet Med. 2019;12:80-86.
23. Dhir J, Willis M, Watson L, Somerville L, Sadi J. Evidence-based review of clinical diagnostic tests and predictive clinical tests that evaluate response to conservative rehabilitation for posterior glenohumeral instability: a systematic review. Sports Health. 2018;10:141-145.
24. Dickens JF, Rue JP, Cameron KL, et al. Successful return to sport after arthroscopic shoulder stabilization versus nonoperative management in contact athletes with anterior shoulder instability: a prospective multicenter study. Am J Sports Med. 2017;45:2540-2546.

25. Dunn WR, Kuhn JE, Sanders R, et al. Symptoms of pain do not correlate with rotator cuff tear severity: a cross-sectional study of 393 patients with a symptomatic atraumatic full-thickness rotator cuff tear. J Bone Joint Surg Am. 2014;96:793-800.

26. Dyrna FGE, Ludwig M, Imhoff AB, Martetschlager F. Off-track Hill-Sachs lesions predispose to recurrence after nonoperative management of first-time anterior shoulder dislocations. Knee Surg Sports Traumatol Arthrosc. 2021;29:2289-2296.

27. Edouard P, Degache F, Beguin L, et al. Rotator cuff strength in recurrent anterior shoulder instability. J Bone Joint Surg Am. 2011;93:759-765.

28. Edouard P, Gasq D, Calmels P, Degache F. Sensorimotor control deficiency in recurrent anterior shoulder instability assessed with a stabilometric force platform. J Shoulder Elbow Surg. 2014;23:355-360.

29. Eshoj H, Ingwersen KG, Larsen CM, Kjaer BH, Juul-Kristensen B. Intertester reliability of clinical shoulder instability and laxity tests in subjects with and without self-reported shoulder problems. BMJ Open. 2018;8:e018472.

30. Eshoj HR, Rasmussen S, Frich LH, et al. Neuromuscular exercises improve shoulder function more than standard care exercises in patients with a traumatic anterior shoulder dislocation: a randomized controlled trial. Orthop J Sports Med. 2020;8:2325967119896102.

31. Familiari F, Huri G, Simonetta R, McFarland EG. SLAP lesions: current controversies. EFORT Open Rev. 2019;4:25-32.

32. Farber AJ, Castillo R, Clough M, Bahk M, McFarland EG. Clinical assessment of three common tests for traumatic anterior shoulder instability. J Bone Joint Surg Am. 2006;88:1467-1474.

33. Gagey OJ, Gagey N. The hyperabduction test. J Bone Joint Surg Br. 2001;83:69-74.

34. Garcia JA, Arguello AM, Momaya AM, Ponce BA. Sternoclavicular joint instability: symptoms, diagnosis and management. Orthop Res Rev. 2020;12:75-87.

35. Gartsman GM, Brinker MR, Khan M, Karahan M. Self-assessment of general health status in patients with five common shoulder conditions. J Shoulder Elbow Surg. 1998;7:228-237.

36. Gerber C, Ganz R. Clinical assessment of instability of the shoulder. With special reference to anterior and posterior drawer tests. J Bone Joint Surg Br. 1984;66:551-556.

37. Ginn KA, Cohen ML. Conservative treatment for shoulder pain: prognostic indicators of outcome. Arch Phys Med Rehabil. 2004;85:1231-1235.

38. Grahame R, Hakim AJ. Hypermobility. Curr Opin Rheumatol. 2008;20:106-110.

39. Granville-Chapman J, Torrance E, Rashid A, Funk L. The Rockwood classification in acute acromioclavicular joint injury does not correlate with symptoms. J Orthop Surg (Hong Kong). 2018;26:2309499018777886.

40. Gross ML, Distefano MC. Anterior release test. A new test for occult shoulder instability. Clin Orthop Relat Res. 1997;105-108.

41. Gutkowska O, Martynkiewicz J, Stepniewski M, Gosk J. Analysis of patient-dependent and trauma-dependent risk factors for persistent brachial plexus injury after shoulder dislocation. Biomed Res Int. 2018;2018:4512137.

42. Gutkowska O, Martynkiewicz J, Urban M, Gosk J. Brachial plexus injury after shoulder dislocation: a literature review. Neurosurg Rev. 2020;43:407-423.

43. Haller S, Cunningham G, Laedermann A, et al. Shoulder apprehension impacts large-scale functional brain networks. AJNR Am J Neuroradiol. 2014;35:691-697.

44. Handoll HH, Almaiyah MA, Rangan A. Surgical versus non-surgical treatment for acute anterior shoulder dislocation. Cochrane Database Syst Rev. 2004;CD004325.

45. Hegedus EJ, Goode AP, Cook CE, et al. Which physical examination tests provide clinicians with the most value when examining the shoulder? Update of a systematic review with meta-analysis of individual tests. Br J Sports Med. 2012;46:964-978.

46. Hegedus EJ, Michener LA, Seitz AL. Three key findings when diagnosing shoulder multidirectional instability: patient report of instability, hypermobility, and specific shoulder tests. J Orthop Sports Phys Ther. 2020;50:52-54.

47. Howard A, Powell JL, Gibson J, Hawkes D, Kemp GJ, Frostick SP. A functional magnetic resonance imaging study of patients with Polar Type II/III complex shoulder instability. Sci Rep. 2019;9:6271.

48. Hurley ET, Manjunath AK, Bloom DA, et al. Arthroscopic Bankart repair versus conservative management for first-time traumatic anterior shoulder instability: a systematic review and meta-analysis. Arthroscopy. 2020;36:2526-2532.

49. Jaggi A, Noorani A, Malone A, Cowan J, Lambert S, Bayley I. Muscle activation patterns in patients with recurrent shoulder instability. Int J Shoulder Surg. 2012;6:101-107.

50. Jia X, Ji JH, Petersen SA, Freehill MT, McFarland EG. An analysis of shoulder laxity in patients undergoing shoulder surgery. J Bone Joint Surg Am. 2009;91:2144-2150.

51. Jobe FW, Kvitne RS, Giangarra CE. Shoulder pain in the overhand or throwing athlete. The relationship of anterior instability and rotator cuff impingement. Orthop Rev. 1989;18:963-975.

52. Johansson FR, Skillgate E, Lapauw ML, et al. Measuring eccentric strength of the shoulder external rotators using a handheld dynamometer: reliability and validity. J Athl Train. 2015;50:719-725.

53. Johnson SM, Robinson CM. Shoulder instability in patients with joint hyperlaxity. J Bone Joint Surg Am. 2010;92:1545-1557.

54. Jones S, Hanchard N, Hamilton S, Rangan A. A qualitative study of patients' perceptions and priorities when living with primary frozen shoulder. BMJ Open. 2013;3:e003452.

55. Juul-Kristensen B, Schmedling K, Rombaut L, Lund H, Engelbert RH. Measurement properties of clinical assessment methods for classifying generalized joint hypermobility: a systematic review. Am J Med Genet C Semin Med Genet. 2017;175:116-147.

56. Kavaja L, Lahdeoja T, Malmivaara A, Paavola M. Treatment after traumatic shoulder dislocation: a systematic review with a network meta-analysis. Br J Sports Med. 2018;52:1498-1506.

57. Kim SH, Park JC, Park JS, Oh I. Painful jerk test: a predictor of success in nonoperative treatment of posteroinferior instability of the shoulder. Am J Sports Med. 2004;32:1849-1855.

58. Kirkley A, Griffin S, Richards C, Miniaci A, Mohtadi N. Prospective randomized clinical trial comparing the effectiveness of immediate arthroscopic stabilization versus immobilization and rehabilitation in

first traumatic anterior dislocations of the shoulder. Arthroscopy. 1999;15:507-514.

59. Krill MK, Rosas S, Kwon K, Dakkak A, Nwachukwu BU, McCormick F. A concise evidence-based physical examination for diagnosis of acromioclavicular joint pathology: a systematic review. Phys Sportsmed. 2018;46:98-104.

60. Kuhn JE. A new classification system for shoulder instability. Br J Sports Med. 2010;44:341-346.

61. Ladermann A, Tirefort J, Zanchi D, et al. Shoulder apprehension: a multifactorial approach. EFORT Open Rev. 2018;3:550-557.

62. Lee JH, Park JS, Hwang HJ, Jeong WK. Time to peak torque and acceleration time are altered in male patients following traumatic shoulder instability. J Shoulder Elbow Surg. 2018;27:1505-1511.

63. Lehman GJ. The role and value of symptom-modification approaches in musculoskeletal practice. J Orthop Sports Phys Ther. 2018;48:430-435.

64. Leroux T, Wasserstein D, Veillette C, et al. Epidemiology of primary anterior shoulder dislocation requiring closed reduction in Ontario, Canada. Am J Sports Med. 2014;42:442-450.

65. Lewis A, Kitamura T, Bayley JIL. (ii) The classification of shoulder instability: new light through old windows! Current Orthopaedics. 2004;18:97-108.

66. Lo IK, Nonweiler B, Woolfrey M, Litchfield R, Kirkley A. An evaluation of the apprehension, relocation, and surprise tests for anterior shoulder instability. Am J Sports Med. 2004;32:301-307.

67. Longo UG, Loppini M, Rizzello G, Ciuffreda M, Maffulli N, Denaro V. Management of primary acute anterior shoulder dislocation: systematic review and quantitative synthesis of the literature. Arthroscopy. 2014;30:506-522.

68. Longo UG, Rizzello G, Loppini M, et al. Multidirectional instability of the shoulder: a systematic review. Arthroscopy. 2015;31:2431-2443.

69. Martetschlager F, Kraus N, Scheibel M, Streich J, Venjakob A, Maier D. The diagnosis and treatment of acute dislocation of the acromioclavicular joint. Dtsch Arztebl Int. 2019;116:89-95.

70. Martetschlager F, Warth RJ, Millett PJ. Instability and degenerative arthritis of the sternoclavicular joint: a current concepts review. Am J Sports Med. 2014;42:999-1007.

71. Martinez-Calderon J, Struyf F, Meeus M, Luque-Suarez A. The association between pain beliefs and pain intensity and/or disability in people with shoulder pain: A systematic review. Musculoskelet Sci Pract. 2018;37:29-57.

72. McFarland EG, Kim TK, Park HB, Neira CA, Gutierrez MI. The effect of variation in definition on the diagnosis of multidirectional instability of the shoulder. J Bone Joint Surg Am. 2003;85:2138-2144.

73. Milgrom C, Milgrom Y, Radeva-Petrova D, Jaber S, Beyth S, Finestone AS. The supine apprehension test helps predict the risk of recurrent instability after a first-time anterior shoulder dislocation. J Shoulder Elbow Surg. 2014;23:1838-1842.

74. Minns Lowe CJ, Moser J, Barker K. Living with a symptomatic rotator cuff tear 'bad days, bad nights': a qualitative study. BMC Musculoskelet Disord. 2014;15:228.

75. Morita W, Tasaki A. Intra- and inter-observer reproducibility of shoulder laxity tests: comparison of the drawer, modified drawer and load and shift tests. J Orthop Sci. 2018;23:57-63.

76. Morris B, Dome D, Sciascia A, Kibler WB. The Scapula and Acromioclavicular Separation and Arthritis. Switzerland: Springer International Publishing; 2017.

77. Murray IR, Robinson PG, Goudie EB, Duckworth AD, Clark K, Robinson CM. Open reduction and tunneled suspensory device fixation compared with nonoperative treatment for type-III and type-IV acromioclavicular joint dislocations: the ACORN prospective, randomized controlled trial. J Bone Joint Surg Am. 2018;100:1912-1918.

78. Myers JB, Wassinger CA, Lephart SM. Sensorimotor contribution to shoulder stability: effect of injury and rehabilitation. Man Ther. 2006;11:197-201.

79. Neer CS, 2nd, Foster CR. Inferior capsular shift for involuntary inferior and multidirectional instability of the shoulder. A preliminary report. J Bone Joint Surg Am. 1980;62:897-908.

80. Ng CY, Smith EK, Funk L. Reliability of the traditional classification systems for acromioclavicular joint injuries by radiography. 2012;4:266-269.

81. Noorani A, Goldring M, Jaggi A, et al. BESS/BOA patient care pathways: atraumatic shoulder instability. Shoulder Elbow. 2019;11:60-70.

82. North AS, Wilkinson T. Surgical reconstruction of the acromioclavicular joint: can we identify the optimal approach? Strategies Trauma Limb Reconstr. 2018;13:69-74.

83. Olds M, Donaldson K, Ellis R, Kersten P. In children 18 years and under, what promotes recurrent shoulder instability after traumatic anterior shoulder dislocation? A systematic review and meta-analysis of risk factors. Br J Sports Med. 2016;50:1135-1141.

84. Olds M, Ellis R, Donaldson K, Parmar P, Kersten P. Risk factors which predispose first-time traumatic anterior shoulder dislocations to recurrent instability in adults: a systematic review and meta-analysis. Br J Sports Med. 2015;49:913-922.

85. Olds M, Ellis R, Kersten P. Predicting Recurrent Instability of the Shoulder (PRIS): a valid tool to predict which patients will not have repeat shoulder instability after first-time traumatic anterior dislocation. J Orthop Sports Phys Ther. 2020;50:431-437.

86. Olds MK, Ellis R, Parmar P, Kersten P. Who will redislocate his/her shoulder? Predicting recurrent instability following a first traumatic anterior shoulder dislocation. BMJ Open Sport Exerc Med. 2019;5:e000447.

87. Owens BD, Campbell SE, Cameron KL. Risk factors for anterior glenohumeral instability. Am J Sports Med. 2014;42:2591-2596.

88. Owens BD, Campbell SE, Cameron KL. Risk factors for posterior shoulder instability in young athletes. Am J Sports Med. 2013;41:2645-2649.

89. Paterson WH, Throckmorton TW, Koester M, Azar FM, Kuhn JE. Position and duration of immobilization after primary anterior shoulder dislocation: a systematic review and meta-analysis of the literature. J Bone Joint Surg Am. 2010;92:2924-2933.

90. Pollock RG, Bigliani LU. Recurrent posterior shoulder instability. Diagnosis and treatment. Clin Orthop Relat Res. 1993;85-96.

91. Richardson E, Lewis JS, Gibson J, et al. Role of the kinetic chain in shoulder rehabilitation: does incorporating the trunk and lower limb into shoulder exercise regimes influence shoulder muscle recruitment patterns? Systematic review of

electromyography studies. BMJ Open Sport Exerc Med. 2020;6:e000683.

92. Roach CJ, Cameron KL, Westrick RB, Posner MA, Owens BD. Rotator cuff weakness is not a risk factor for first-time anterior glenohumeral instability. Orthop J Sports Med. 2013;1:2325967113489097.

93. Robinson CM, Howes J, Murdoch H, Will E, Graham C. Functional outcome and risk of recurrent instability after primary traumatic anterior shoulder dislocation in young patients. J Bone Joint Surg Am. 2006;88:2326-2336.

94. Robinson CM, Jenkins PJ, Markham PE, Beggs I. Disorders of the sternoclavicular joint. J Bone Joint Surg Br. 2008;90:685-696. 1

95. Robinson CM, Seah M, Akhtar MA. The epidemiology, risk of recurrence, and functional outcome after an acute traumatic posterior dislocation of the shoulder. J Bone Joint Surg Am. 2011;93:1605-1613.

96. Robinson CM, Shur N, Sharpe T, Ray A, Murray IR. Injuries associated with traumatic anterior glenohumeral dislocations. J Bone Joint Surg Am. 2012;94:18-26.

97. Ropars M, Fournier A, Campillo B, et al. Clinical assessment of external rotation for the diagnosis of anterior shoulder hyperlaxity. Orthop Traumatol Surg Res. 2010;96:S84-87.

98. Rowe CR, Zarins B. Recurrent transient subluxation of the shoulder. J Bone Joint Surg Am. 1981;63:863-872.

99. Sachs RA, Stone ML, Paxton E, Kuney M, Lin D. Can the need for future surgery for acute traumatic anterior shoulder dislocation be predicted? 2007;89:1665-1674.

100. Safran O, Milgrom C, Radeva-Petrova DR, Jaber S, Finestone A. Accuracy of the anterior apprehension test as a predictor of risk for redislocation after a first traumatic shoulder dislocation. Am J Sports Med. 2010;38:972-975.

101. Salomonsson B, von Heine A, Dahlborn M, et al. Bony Bankart is a positive predictive factor after primary shoulder dislocation. Knee Surg Sports Traumatol Arthrosc. 2010;18:1425-1431.

102. Scott M, Sachinis NP, Gooding B. The role of structured physiotherapy in treating patients with atraumatic shoulder instability: medium term results from a case series. Shoulder Elbow. 2020;12:63-70.

103. Sewell MD, Al-Hadithy N, Le Leu A, Lambert SM. Instability of the sternoclavicular joint: current concepts in classification, treatment and outcomes. Bone Joint J. 2013;95-B:721-731.

104. Shin SJ, Yun YH, Kim DJ, Yoo JD. Treatment of traumatic anterior shoulder dislocation in patients older than 60 years. Am J Sports Med. 2012;40:822-827.

105. Shitara H, Shimoyama D, Sasaki T, et al. The neural correlates of shoulder apprehension: a functional MRI study. PLoS One. 2015;10:e0137387.

106. Silliman JF, Hawkins RJ. Classification and physical diagnosis of instability of the shoulder. Clin Orthop Relat Res. 1993;7-19.

107. Simank HG, Dauer G, Schneider S, Loew M. Incidence of rotator cuff tears in shoulder dislocations and results of therapy in older patients. Arch Orthop Trauma Surg. 2006;126:235-240.

108. Sirin E, Aydin N, Mert Topkar O. Acromioclavicular joint injuries: diagnosis, classification and ligamentoplasty procedures. EFORT Open Rev. 2018;3:426-433.

109. Skjaker SA, Enger M, Engebretsen L, Brox JI, Boe B. Young men in sports are at highest risk of acromioclavicular joint injuries: a prospective cohort study. Knee Surg Sports Traumatol Arthrosc. 2021;29:2039–2045.

110. Spanhove V, Van Daele M, Van den Abeele A, et al. Muscle activity and scapular kinematics in individuals with multidirectional shoulder instability: a systematic review. Ann Phys Rehabil Med. 2021;64:101457.

111. Staker JL, Evans AJ, Jacobs LE, et al. The effect of tactile and verbal guidance during scapulothoracic exercises: an EMG and kinematic investigation. J Electromyogr Kinesiol. 2019;102334.

112. Taylor DC, Arciero RA. Pathologic changes associated with shoulder dislocations. Arthroscopic and physical examination findings in first-time, traumatic anterior dislocations. Am J Sports Med. 1997;25:306-311.

113. te Slaa RL, Brand R, Marti RK. A prospective arthroscopic study of acute first-time anterior shoulder dislocation in the young: a five-year follow-up study. J Shoulder Elbow Surg. 2003;12:529-534.

114. Teunis T, Lubberts B, Reilly BT, Ring D. A systematic review and pooled analysis of the prevalence of rotator cuff disease with increasing age. J Shoulder Elbow Surg. 2014;23:1913-1921.

115. Tjong VK, Devitt BM, Murnaghan ML, Ogilvie-Harris DJ, Theodoropoulos JS. A qualitative investigation of return to sport after arthroscopic Bankart repair: beyond stability. Am J Sports Med. 2015;43:2005-2011.

116. Tokish JM, Thigpen CA, Kissenberth MJ, et al. The Nonoperative Instability Severity Index Score (NISIS): a simple tool to guide operative versus nonoperative treatment of the unstable shoulder. Sports Health. 2020;12:598-602.

117. Tyler TF, Nahow RC, Nicholas SJ, McHugh MP. Quantifying shoulder rotation weakness in patients with shoulder impingement. J Shoulder Elbow Surg. 2005;14:570-574.

118. Van Tongel A, Karelse A, Berghs B, Van Isacker T, De Wilde L. Diagnostic value of active protraction and retraction for sternoclavicular joint pain. BMC Musculoskelet Disord. 2014;15:421.

119. Vermeiren J, Handelberg F, Casteleyn PP, Opdecam P. The rate of recurrence of traumatic anterior dislocation of the shoulder. A study of 154 cases and a review of the literature. Int Orthop. 1993;17:337-341.

120. Wagstrom E, Raynor B, Jani S, et al. Epidemiology of glenohumeral instability related to sporting activities using the FEDS (Frequency, Etiology, Direction, and Severity) classification system: a multicenter analysis. Orthop J Sports Med. 2019;7:2325967119861038.

121. Wallace AL. Faithful but unfortunate: Churchill and his shoulder. Shoulder Elbow. 2019;11:4-8.

122. Warby SA, Watson L, Ford JJ, Hahne AJ, Pizzari T. Multidirectional instability of the glenohumeral joint: etiology, classification, assessment, and management. J Hand Ther. 2017;30:175-181.

123. Wasserstein DN, Sheth U, Colbenson K, et al. The true recurrence rate and factors predicting recurrent instability after nonsurgical management of traumatic primary anterior shoulder dislocation:

a systematic review. Arthroscopy. 2016;32:2616-2625.

124. Watson L, Warby S, Balster S, Lenssen R, Pizzari T. The treatment of multidirectional instability of the shoulder with a rehabilitation program: Part 1. Shoulder Elbow. 2016;8:271-278. 6

125. Wattanaprakornkul D, Cathers I, Halaki M, Ginn KA. The rotator cuff muscles have a direction specific recruitment pattern during shoulder flexion and extension exercises. J Sci Med Sport. 2011;14:376-382.

126. Witney-Lagen C, Hassan A, Doodson A, Venkateswaran B. Arthroscopic plication for multidirectional instability: 50 patients with a minimum of 2 years of follow-up. J Shoulder Elbow Surg. 2017;26:e29-e36.

127. Woodmass JM, Lee J, Wu IT, et al. Incidence of posterior shoulder instability and trends in surgical reconstruction: a 22-year population-based study. J Shoulder Elbow Surg. 2019;28:611-616.

128. Wright A, Monga P. Diagnosing shoulder instability. Journal of Arthroscopy and Joint Surgery. 2018;5:67-70.

129. Yewlett A, Dearden PMC, Ferran NA, Evans RO, Kulkani R. Acromioclavicular joint dislocation: diagnosis and management. 2012;4:81-86.

130. Yoo Y-S. Acromial clavicular joint. In: Bain GI, Di Giacomo G, Itoi E, Sugaya H (eds). Normal and Pathological Anatomy of the Shoulder. Berlin: Springer; 2015.

131. Zacchilli MA, Owens BD. Epidemiology of shoulder dislocations presenting to emergency departments in the United States. J Bone Joint Surg Am. 2010;92:542-549.

132. Zanchi D, Cunningham G, Ladermann A, Ozturk M, Hoffmeyer P, Haller S. Structural white matter and functional connectivity alterations in patients with shoulder apprehension. Sci Rep. 2017;7:42327.

The stiff shoulder 18

Jeremy Lewis, Sarah Boyd, William King, Paul Salamh

Introduction

Concluding that the person in front of you has a less than expected shoulder range of motion, commonly referred to as a stiff shoulder, is not complicated. Methods to arrive at this conclusion come from the patient interview and are confirmed with assessment of active and passive physiological shoulder movements using visual inspection, goniometry, inclinometer measurements, tape measures, movement capturing software and functional tests. The more difficult question to address is *why* the shoulder is stiff.

Attempting to determine what biopsychosocial factors contribute to the presentation of shoulder stiffness for any given individual carries a unique set of challenges and warrants careful consideration. As suggested in Chapter 15 and depicted in Figure 15.1 most people presenting with symptoms occurring from a musculoskeletal condition involving the shoulder will describe pain, loss of movement, weakness, and myriad other symptoms. It is the role of the clinician, working as a clinical detective to integrate the information gathered during the patient interview (Chapter 11), together with clinical reasoning (Chapter 13), and when required, the findings of further investigations (Chapter 14), to hypothesize what the specific combination of pain, stiffness and other symptoms may mean, at this point in time, for the person in front of you, and to you, the clinician.

During the assessment process, the individual will have completed appropriate patient-reported outcome measures (PROMs) as discussed in Chapter 12. These PROMs provide valuable information pertaining to shoulder function, the experience of pain, psychosocial and lifestyle factors, fear avoidance behavior, pain catastrophizing, and depression. Although no outcome measure is perfect for all people, as with other shoulder conditions, the contributing factors relating to shoulder stiffness are likely to be multifarious and all may need to be addressed to reduce the disability caused by the stiffness.

During the interview, the individual may describe difficulty performing routine daily tasks such as dressing, attending to personal hygiene, participating in sports, hobbies, occupation, and other valued daily activities. Through the interview, the clinician will typically learn if the onset was slow or fast, traumatic, nontraumatic, idiopathic, iatrogenic, related to other symptoms, conditions, or comorbidities, and possibly familial.[84,114,165] The clinician will also start to synthesize important information about symptom behavior, and start to appreciate the patient's concerns, fears, expectations, desires, and aims of the clinical relationship. At all stages, the clinician will pay careful attention to the patient's story (see Chapters 1 and 11) and validate their beliefs, concerns, and experiences, aiming to build the strongest therapeutic alliance possible, underpinned by mutual trust and respect.

The heart of the clinical examination is screening for serious (red flag) pathology (see Chapters 8, 13, 14, 15, 24, and 25), such as osteosarcomas and other bone tumors, infections, locked dislocations, or avascular necrosis.[50,84,126] We are fortunate to be amongst the first generations of humans who can see inside the body of people who are alive, and imaging (see Chapter 14), when used appropriately, plays an important role in hypothesis testing, clinical reasoning, and diagnosis for people presenting with shoulder stiffness.

Assessing the active and passive shoulder ranges of physiological motion, as well as assessing movement during relevant functional activities and comparing them (when possible) to the contralateral side along with normative data is essential. When stiffness is the primary limiter of shoulder function, movement may be limited equally when assessing passive and active ranges of motion.[18,165] Additionally, what the patient reports, and what the clinician perceives when testing passive range of motion may support clinical reasoning. For example, a patient may be limited to 15° of external rotation at the glenohumeral joint both actively and passively and report pain, and at this end of available range the clinician may feel substantial movement restriction (stiffness). Pattern recognition, a contemporary understanding of pain science, knowledge of different shoulder conditions and their presentations, and interpretation of imaging investigations, will all support the clinician's understanding of the clinical findings.

Information gained during the patient interview, together with clinical examination, supported by imaging as appropriate, may help explain the presenting combinations of shoulder stiffness, pain, and weakness. Diagnoses such as a locked dislocation, severe osteoarthritis, rotator cuff arthropathy, osteosarcoma, or avascular necrosis, may explain the reasons for the shoulder stiffness and any concomitant symptoms. In other situations where imaging findings, blood tests and other investigations cannot confirm a diagnosis, such as in the case of a frozen shoulder, a clinical hypothesis may be formed, but might never be confirmed. In these situations, the clinician will need to sensitively inform the patient, "...based on our conversation, the clinical assessment, and imaging findings, *it is likely* that you have a frozen shoulder, and this is the reason you are experiencing shoulder pain and restricted movement."

The next stage is to engage in a shared decision-making conversation with the patient outlining the harms, benefits, and requirements of various treatment options (Chapter 13). Although this may appear to be a bridge between the assessment and management of the stiff shoulder, it is also a very important part of the assessment, as we continue to learn more about the patient, their values, beliefs, and expectations surrounding their stiff shoulder, as well as gaining an understanding of the individuals who may support and influence their management decision.[58]

The following sections in this chapter explore the assessment and management for different conditions that are associated with shoulder stiffness. It is not exhaustive, and we have selected examples of common and less common presentations.

Frozen shoulder

History

Frozen shoulder (FS) is a condition that typically involves substantial shoulder pain, movement restriction, and considerable morbidity. Although function improves and disability reduces over time, pain and shoulder stiffness may not resolve for everyone with FS. Despite substantial research, FS remains a complex and poorly understood musculoskeletal condition.[1,27,78,84] One hundred and fifty years ago, Duplay[38, 39] described the disabling combination of shoulder pain and restricted movement as "péri-arthrite scapulo-humérale", attributing the condition to inflammation of the subacromial bursa. With the advent of radiographs, calcific deposits were observed, and for a period of time, the pain and stiffness were attributed by some to this newly observed phenomenon.[7]

Codman[32] initially considered the condition to be an "adherent subacromial bursitis", but after 15 years of clinical observation he rejected this in favor of the term frozen shoulder. He believed the condition involved a non-calcifying tendinitis of the rotator cuff, arguing that calcification represented a different pathology. During a one-year period (c. 1933), Codman treated four people suffering from frozen shoulder, and described the symptoms to consistently involve: slow onset (typically insidious, although trauma or strain may predispose), pain near the insertion of deltoid, inability to sleep on the affected side, painful and incomplete shoulder elevation and external rotation, and, apart from possible bone atrophy, normal shoulder radiographs. He added that although the etiology remained uncertain, and the condition difficult to treat, the disorder would almost certainly resolve. To treat frozen shoulder, Codman advocated hospitalization, with the arm constrained in elevation for one to two weeks. Patients were permitted to get out of bed once a day to perform pendular exercises. Lippmann[88] supported many of Codman's observations, but argued that periarthritis or frozen shoulder resulted from inflammation of the long head of biceps tendon that eventuated in firm adhesions of the tendon to the bicipital sheath and bicipital groove. Based on intraoperative findings in 12 people, Lippmann argued the condition should be called bicipital tenosynovitis and clinically should be regarded as being similar to de Quervain's disease. Soon after this and based on a case series of 10 patients and observations of inflammation, fibrosis, and contraction of the shoulder capsule, and with the axillary fold becoming "adherent" to the humeral head, Neviaser[100] suggested the term adhesive capsulitis better described the pathology – the adhesion being similar to that of an adhesive plaster applied to the skin. Rotation and manipulation of the humerus was advocated to separate the adherent capsule from the humeral head. Later evidence suggested that thickening and contracture of the glenohumeral joint capsule and the coracohumeral ligament and rotator interval was associated with frozen shoulder, without adhesions to the humerus,[16,17,19,141,152] which has led to confusion and fueled the debate as to the best terminology to use to describe this condition.

Terminology

Two terms, frozen shoulder and adhesive capsulitis, are today commonly used interchangeably to describe the condition. Historically, Codman[32] who introduced the term frozen shoulder and Neviaser[100] who introduced adhesive capsulitis were describing different pathologies with seemingly similar clinical presentations. Based on the small number of participants in both original publications and relatively limited subsequent research, it remains uncertain if the original terminology represents the same or separate conditions, separate conditions with some overlap, or a continuum of pathology. In the past decades the two terms have merged and whether capsule contraction, inflammation, or adhesions occur in the same manner in everyone with this condition remains unresolved.[16,89] In summary, it is possible that FS and adhesive capsulitis represent similar clinical presentations with different pathoetiology, or are the same condition, with a range of mechanisms and pathologies leading to the pain and stiffness. As the evidence for adhesions and inflammation remains equivocal,[16,57,89] we favor the term frozen shoulder as it resembles what the patient experiences – a shoulder that freezes, is frozen, then thaws. Whether the term frozen shoulder is the best term, or will stand the test of time, is by no means certain. We suggest that it is the best term currently available.

The uncertainty in terminology has resulted in some clinicians and researchers arguing that both names should be rejected, and that we should simply call the clinical presentation a stiff shoulder. We argue that the term stiff shoulder is too broad, as it is an overarching term for multifarious clinical presentations that involve restricted shoulder motion (as will be discussed in this chapter), that frequently require very different management. For example, frozen shoulders and avascular necrosis may have similar clinical presentations and both sit under the overarching term, stiff shoulder. We suggest that "diagnosing" all those presenting with restricted shoulder range as having a stiff shoulder does not permit for clinical discourse and is unhelpful when formulating inclusion and exclusion criteria for research.

Following this, using the term frozen shoulder, with agreed clinical features, as a subcategory of conditions associated with shoulder stiffness, enables clinicians and researchers to communicate with each other. Diagnosing a suspected frozen shoulder, as a "stiff shoulder" without qualification, as one of many conditions that present as a stiff shoulder, would not facilitate discussion, and would only amplify our current confusion, as well as the confusion faced for those seeking care.

The terms, "primary" and "secondary" frozen shoulder have been introduced into the literature.[89] Primary FS is also known as idiopathic frozen shoulder where onset is not related to trauma, surgery or an associated comorbidity. Secondary FS occurs in the presence of an underlying comorbidity or following surgery or trauma. The secondary form has been further classified into intrinsic, intrinsic iatrogenic, extrinsic, and systemic subcategories. Intrinsic involves other conditions intrinsic to the shoulder (such as rotator cuff pathology), extrinsic involves conditions more remote to the immediate shoulder (such as cervical radiculopathy), and secondary systemic involves associated systemic health conditions such as diabetes mellitus (DM) or a thyroid condition. Intrinsic iatrogenic refers to the development of a frozen shoulder after surgery. Figure 18.1 details the nomenclature commonly used to subclassify frozen shoulder.

Pathophysiology and time course

The complexities of defining and classifying FS mirror attempts to confirm the pathophysiology and course of the condition. Neviaser[100] described an inflammatory process of the shoulder capsule, which informed the terminology of "adhesive capsulitis". This feature was combined with clinical observations and the original "frozen shoulder" terminology leading to the course of the condition being classified in three phases. Phase one "freezing" (inflammatory), phase two "frozen"' (fibrosis), and phase three "thawing" to natural resolution via resolving fibrosis.[99] Inflammation and neovascularity observed in the early phases of the condition and accompanying the most severe pain experience associated with the condition led to a color classification roughly matching the phases using red, pink, and white terminology.[101] These authors added a fourth, "pre-inflammatory" phase, when pain is beginning but there is no stiffness.[101]

Lewis[84] suggested the use of two distinct clinical phases – pain and stiffness. This two-phase description focuses on which of these states is more prevalent, pain > stiffness (first phase) or stiffness > pain (second phase).[84] Regardless of the classification, the speed at which the condition progresses

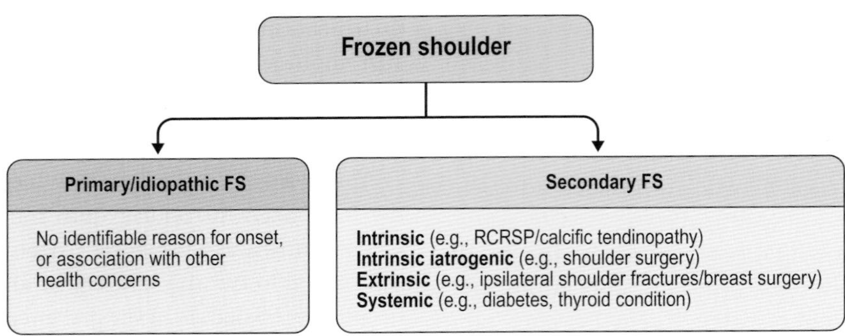

FIGURE 18.1
The nomenclature commonly used to subclassify frozen shoulder. FS, frozen shoulder; RCRSP, rotator cuff related shoulder pain.

appears to be variable, lasting between one and four or more years, with studies reporting the symptoms of FS well beyond this time frame, which challenges the belief that FS is a self-resolving condition.[54,153] There is no certainty why the duration of living with a FS for some people is much longer than others, and why the symptoms apparently resolve in some people whereas others demonstrate ongoing impairments (pain and loss of motion).

Attempts have been made to understand and match the pathophysiology of FS to the various descriptions of phases. Growth factors, cytokines and immune cells have been associated with the proposed inflammation and neovascularity at the start of the condition. However, inflammatory involvement remains equivocal.[16,89] The feature of fibrosis and thickening in various areas of the shoulder capsule and ligaments has been associated with the presence of contractile and tissue matrix proteins, which seems more accepted.[80] The presence of greater myofibroblast staining in an adhesive capsulitis population has also been implicated in the pathophysiology of capsular contracture.[57] A recent review of the biology identified variability in the suggested pathophysiology amongst many studies, perhaps reflecting the variability in the classification systems. However, authors have concluded that inflammation and fibrosis are involved, but not definitively understood, in FS. These features are in some way related to processes involving cytokines, growth factors, matrix metalloproteinases and immune cells.[28,57,119]

Currently the restriction (stiffness) associated with FS is principally considered to be due to contraction of the glenohumeral joint capsule, and when capsular contraction is confirmed the diagnostic term "frozen shoulder contracture syndrome" has been suggested.[84] However, capsular contraction may not be present in everybody presenting with the clinical manifestations of FS. In a small case series, Hollmann et al.[59,60] reported that the stiffness may in fact not be attributable to capsular contraction, and may be due to active muscle guarding. The ongoing uncertainty suggests that many people experiencing stiff shoulders are classified as having a frozen shoulder, but the cause of the stiffness may be variable, and in some people may be a combination of capsular contraction and active muscle guarding.

Epidemiology and associations

In China and Japan, frozen shoulder is colloquially known as the "50-year-old shoulder", which represents the mean age (men 52 years, women 55 years) of onset for most people. The epidemiology of FS is somewhat clearer than the classification and course, however substantial gaps in our knowledge persist. In terms of the general population, the incidence has been estimated at 2.4 per 1000 people and the primary form of FS in up to 5.3% of the population.[70,144] A prevalence of FS has been estimated at a female to male ratio of 7:3, and in a working age population the ratio has been reported as 5:4 (women to men).[132,148] It appears that there is an increased risk of developing FS in people who have diabetes.[81,164] Diabetes has links with obesity, which has also been associated with FS[77]; diabetes and obesity are also features of metabolic syndrome.[20] Proinflammatory lipoproteinemia in metabolic syndrome has been suggested as a causal factor for FS, however, these features require further investigation to understand their influence on the condition,[108] as well as the links of FS to coronary heart disease (CHD).

CHD has been identified as another health condition associated with FS, but given the causative nature of metabolic syndrome on CHD it is unclear whether some or all these associations are of more importance than others for FS.[164] Additionally, there is a higher prevalence (up to 10.9%) and risk (2.69 times more likelihood) of FS in people diagnosed with thyroid problems.[22,33] Other musculoskeletal conditions such as Dupuytren's contracture of the hand are also characterized by tissue restriction and have been shown to be both associated with, and a risk factor for FS, but the exact relationship is unclear.[92,134] There also appear to be links between mental health and frozen shoulder but whether these have any causal link, influence outcomes, or are caused by FS is uncertain.[8,26,131]

Diagnosis

Making a diagnosis of FS can present problems to healthcare professionals perhaps because of the complex classification, wide spectrum of presentations, variable course of the condition and lack of blood tests or imaging confirmation. A Delphi process gained expert consensus on important diagnostic features of FS, but the identified factors were not validated clinically in a follow up study.[149,150] A survey of physical therapists (physiotherapists) in the UK attempted to identify clinically diagnostic features of FS, with only restrictive passive lateral (external) shoulder rotation having a high level of agreement for those that participated.[52,53]

Certain ultrasound and magnetic resonance imaging (MRI) findings such as thickening of the anterior capsule, capsule hyperintensity on MRI, coracohumeral ligament thickening, and rotator cuff interval synovitis, have been correlated with clinical tests and may form part of the diagnosis.[29,43,136,161] Imaging is important to exclude other conditions that may mimic FS such as glenohumeral osteoarthritis, avascular necrosis, osteosarcoma, or locked posterior shoulder dislocation, and for this reason is relevant in the assessment process. However, no imaging modality has currently emerged as a gold standard diagnostic test to rule in FS.[84,115] Even during arthroscopy, variations in FS presentation occur and some clinically diagnosed cases turn out to be falsely positive once under anesthetic.[59,60]

Box 18.1 Clinical findings to support the hypothesis that the presenting shoulder stiffness is due to frozen shoulder

- Age of patient at onset: approximately 50 years of age.
- Glenohumeral external rotation range (measured in adduction with elbow flexed) is equally limited actively and passively by at least 50% compared to the contralateral side (for suggested measurement technique see Valentine and Lewis[143]).
- Other glenohumeral movements are equally limited actively and passively compared to the contralateral side in one or more additional planes of movement (such as hand behind back/shoulder flexion/abduction/scaption).
- The symptoms have been present for at least one month.
- Red flags considered and nothing substantially abnormal being detected on routine radiographs.
- Subclassify according to Figure 18.1.

These findings call into question the certainty by which a definitive diagnosis may be achieved. As a result of these challenges, the diagnosis remains one largely made through the clinical reasoning process and importantly, when other possible diagnoses are excluded.[52,84,113] Box 18.1 details a suggestion to support the clinical hypothesis that the presenting shoulder stiffness is due to a frozen shoulder.

The patient's story

The patient voice is increasingly being recognized as an essential part of healthcare[109] however, a paucity of research has investigated the lived experiences of the individual diagnosed with FS. One qualitative study used interviews and thematic analysis to explore patients' priorities and perceptions when living with FS.[69] They identified four main themes: pain – severe pain on movement and sleep deprivation due to pain; confusion – difficulty obtaining diagnosis, contradictory advice, poor communication;

inconvenience – time with symptoms hugely disruptive, delays in getting (specialist) care; and treatment – hoping for earliest possible resolution, main priority pain-free movement.

Further work is being conducted to more fully appreciate the experiences of people living with FS. In addition to the key features identified by Jones et al.,[69] King[75,76] has identified other concerns, including the difficulty maintaining a normal life, and the detrimental effect on mental well-being. The findings from these qualitative studies[69,75,76] provide valuable insight and help support the development of a meaningful therapeutic alliance between the clinician and patient.

Management

Research efforts have focused on finding a safe, cost effective treatment for FS, especially as it is a long-term condition associated with substantial morbidity.[12,67,84-86,90,105,106,115,142] Systematic and narrative reviews investigating treatment for FS have investigated acupuncture, nonsteroidal anti-inflammatory drugs (NSAIDs), oral steroids, manual therapy, electrotherapy, exercises, corticosteroid injections, hyaluronic acid injections, hydrodistension injections, and surgical options.[11,13-15,42,47,67,79,94,98,99,103,130,137] Findings from a recent review on acupuncture efficacy suggested short-term benefit for pain and movement.[11] Reviews of acupuncture, NSAIDs and electrotherapy modalities have indicated there is little evidence to support any mid to long-term effect on FS pain, movement and function.[42,94,105] Other commonly prescribed nonsurgical treatment modalities include exercise and manual therapy. One systematic review suggested that a range of mobilization techniques are effective for FS[103] and two reviews have suggested physical therapy (physiotherapy) modalities are effective in the short to mid-term (up to six months).[94,98]

Various types of injections, at different anatomical locations using a variety of routes of administration, medicines, and dosages have been recommended in the treatment of FS. The most common of these involves corticosteroid (CS). As with most nonsurgical options, CS injections have shown short to mid-term benefit (up to six months) for FS.[79,94,107,130,137,156] Outcome effectiveness following injection therapy may not substantially be influenced by injection site (glenohumeral joint or subacromial), or method of delivery (landmark or ultrasound guided).[40,111,130] Hyaluronic acid injection has been shown to be effective and comparable, but not superior, to CS injections for FS.[107]

Platelet-rich plasma injections and suprascapular nerve block injections are used in clinical practice, but no comparative trials are currently available. Hydrodistension, an injection using a high volume of fluid (usually isotonic saline) placed intra-articularly (usually combined with a CS injection and analgesic) has also shown short-term improvements in pain and disability.[15,159] However, other authors have questioned whether the physical mechanism of hydrodistension can cause capsular stretching, and a recent meta-analysis concluded hydrodistension has only a small and possibly unimportant clinical effect in the treatment of FS.[122] More information on injection therapy in the management of FS is presented in Chapter 23.

When nonoperative treatments do not achieve the desired outcomes, surgery is often considered.[41] Two techniques have historically been advocated: surgical release of the contracted capsule (arthroscopic capsular release (ACR)) and manipulation under anesthetic (MUA). These techniques are effective and comparable over the mid to long term.[13,47] A recent high-quality trial concluded that MUA is the most cost-effective surgical treatment when compared to ACR in terms of quality added life years.[113]

There is a paucity of high-quality controlled trials with adequate follow-up times to better inform clinical practice and support management of this condition.[10] We recommend a watch and wait approach for patients who are able to tolerate their symptoms. They should receive advice and education and be encouraged to use their arm as able, use mental imagery and breathing exercises, and control the pain with appropriate over-the-counter and prescribed medications as required. They should be provided with a safety net and a fast track back into the clinic should their symptoms worsen or become intolerable.

Those patients in the pain > stiffness phase who are not able to tolerate the pain, have disrupted sleep, and severe pain on movement should be fast-tracked for CS injection therapy into the glenohumeral joint (± subacromial bursa) once the expected benefits and potential harms of injection therapy have been discussed, contraindications to injections excluded, and consent obtained. A post injection exercise program should be included in the management plan. Then finally, if injection therapy and exercise does not produce the desired outcome, capsular release, or manipulation under anesthetic should be considered, being guided by the findings of the most recent and best quality evidence.[113]

Frozen shoulder and diabetes mellitus

Diabetes mellitus (DM) is a lifelong metabolic condition, associated with high blood sugar. The global prevalence of DM is projected to almost double from 476 million in 2017 to 798 million in 2025.[72,87,145] DM is a persistent, systemic disease associated with myriad complications.[3,128,129] DM is associated with conditions such as Dupuytren's contracture, FS, carpal tunnel syndrome, tenosynovitis, trigger finger, and general limited joint mobility.[21,61,74,83,164] DM is the main risk factor for developing frozen shoulder, closely followed by thyroid disorders and increased body mass index.[92] The incidence of FS is estimated to be two to four times higher in people with diabetes when compared to people without diabetes,[139] with the prevalence of frozen shoulder ranging from 9% to 79%[61] in type 1 (previously known as insulin-dependent) DM, and 7%–30% in type 2 DM, compared to 2%–20% in a non-diabetic population.[2,49,139] Rai et al.[112] have recommended that patients diagnosed with FS should have appropriate blood screening to determine DM status.

For an individual living with DM, there is a daily challenge to control the glycemic (sugar) levels in the blood, as poor glycemic control increases blood levels of hemoglobin A_{1c} (HbA_{1c}) or glycated hemoglobin.[23,158] HbA_{1c} is reported in mmol/mol or as a percentage, and values less than 5.6% are considered normal; values between 5.6% and 6.5% (48mmol/mol) signals pre-diabetes and levels above 6.5% indicate diabetes. The HbA_{1c} value provides an average of how high blood glucose levels have been over a period of time, whereas blood glucose levels (mmol/L) represent the concentration of glucose in the blood at a given point in time, i.e., the time of the test.

Chan et al.[23] reported that a new measure of long-term glucose control, termed cumulative HbA_{1c}, was positively associated with FS, and that for each year HbA_{1c} was greater than 7%, there was an increase in the risk of developing FS. Yian et al.[158] demonstrated that individuals living with DM for more than 10 years had an increased risk of developing FS. DM is associated with generalized joint stiffness and loss of motion as evident in Dupuytren's contracture, trigger finger, cheiroarthropathy, as well as frozen shoulder, at higher rates than in people without DM. The development of these conditions has been attributed to biomechanical abnormalities related to the disturbance of glucose metabolism such as hyperglycemia (excess glucose). Hyperglycemia occurs when increased blood sugar or glucose at levels higher than 11.1 mmol/L are detected in the blood plasma.

As discussed, the etiology and pathophysiology of FS are not fully understood, as are the links with DM,[3,80] and remains an important area for future research. Although uncertainty persists, hypotheses have been proposed aiming to provide insight into the FS-DM relationship. One hypothesis proposes a link between extended periods of high blood glucose levels (hyperglycemia) and the physiological effects this has at a molecular level. Glycation is a random, nonenzymatic reaction that involves the covalent bonding of sugar to protein or lipid. A covalent bond is a chemical bond that involves two atoms sharing electrons.[97] Water (H_2O) is an example, where two hydrogen atoms are linked covalently to an oxygen atom and produces a stable covalent bond. This complex interaction leads to the formation of advanced glycation end products (AGEs). The normal physiological rate of AGE accumulation increases with advancing age but is markedly increased in a hyperglycemic environment such as occurs in DM. AGEs bind to AGE receptors (RAGEs) located on the cell membrane and transmit signals into the cell. This process produces reactive oxygen species (ROS) within the cell. Oxygen is abundant within cells and readily accepts electrons generated by normal metabolism within a cell. Examples of ROS include hydroxl radical (·OH) and superoxide ion (O_2^-).[4,97]

An imbalance between the production of ROS and the antioxidant defenses that normally protect cells leads to an increase in free radicals and oxidative stress, which can cause increased damage to proteins, lipids, and nucleic acid (DNA and RNA) resulting in disruption of normal cellular processes and cell death. Oxidative stress has been implicated in the pathogenesis of many diseases including cancer and asthma.[4,97] There is clear evidence that overproduction of ROS will result in cell and tissue injury and will also contribute to persistent inflammation underlying many neurodegenerative, cardiovascular, and metabolic diseases.[24,63] AGEs appear to accelerate vascular calcification through RAGE and resultant oxidative stress.[151] It is possible that this may be a mechanism that contributes to calcific deposits observed in rotator cuff calcific tendinopathy (see Chapter 27). Clearly this is a hypothesis and requires further investigation.

Aging, lifestyle (e.g., smoking, poor diet, inadequate physical activity as discussed in Chapter 5) and hyperglycemic conditions, such as in DM, results in an accumulation of AGEs. For people diagnosed with DM, AGEs have been implicated in diabetic retinopathy, nephropathy, and cardiomyopathy. AGEs can also accumulate in the skin, tendon, and ligament cells, as well as cells in capsular tissue. In these tissues, increased cross-linking between AGEs and the proteins in these tissues will alter their biological structure and function and will result in increased tissue stiffness and reduced movement, i.e., less elastic skin, alterations to normal tendon mechanics, and reduced joint motion due to excessive ligament and capsule stiffness. The effect may take a long time to resolve or may be irreversible,[46] although this is uncertain.[96]

AGEs will accumulate in everyone but will be more prevalent with increasing age, in response to certain lifestyle behaviors and significantly increase in hyperglycemic environments. Accumulation of AGEs with cross-linking and stabilization of collagen has been hypothesized to contribute to the higher incidence of frozen shoulder in diabetic patients. Importantly, an increase in AGEs may also play a role in the pathogenesis of FS in nondiabetic populations, with increased expression of AGEs contributing to the fibroblast proliferation seen in FS.[64]

Little is known about the best management for people diagnosed with secondary systemic frozen shoulder associated with DM. Due to the paucity of knowledge that exists, it is common for people in this subgroup of FS to be offered the same management as people with idiopathic FS. We currently do not know if this is best practice. For example, the use of CS injections for the management of FS in people with DM is likely to result in hyperglycemia[31,160] for a protracted time period,[9,156,160] without current knowledge of the long-term consequences. What is known is that prognosis and treatment outcomes are poorer and adverse events are greater for people with DM and FS,[13,25,48,125] and, it is likely that more treatment will be required.[68,155]

Osteoarthritis

Glenohumeral joint osteoarthritis (GHJ-OA) is a progressive and degenerative joint disease involving the hyaline articular cartilage, subchondral and periarticular bone, and the periarticular soft tissues – muscles, tendons, bursae, synovium, capsule, and ligaments.[65] Our understanding of the pathogenesis of GHJ-OA and the reason for symptoms is not complete. Symptoms include shoulder pain, stiffness (reduction in range of motion), and a reduction in function that may range from mild to incapacitating. After the hip and knee, the GHJ is the third most common joint affected with OA.[65,162] Although not as common, for many, it can be as debilitating due to the profound loss of upper limb function and physical independence. Etiology is multifactorial, with increasing age being one factor. Together with the rise in the average age of the world's population, there has been a concomitant increase in both the radiological signs of OA and symptoms.[55,65] In addition to age, other factors associated with the pathogenesis of GHJ-OA include trauma, recurrent GHJ instability, obesity, chronic inflammation (see Chapter 5), sex (more common in women), white European heritage, and genetics.[36] There is no cure for GHJ-OA.

The center of the humeral head and the periphery of the glenoid fossa (most notably in the inferior region) demonstrate the thickest hyaline cartilage. The upper two-thirds of the humeral head contacts the glenoid fossa in mid-range of shoulder abduction and in GHJ-OA this region demonstrates loss of articular cartilage and subchondral bone. GHJ-OA may, in part, be due to normal or excessive stress on normal or weakened cartilage. The reason for the experience of pain associated with GHJ-OA is multifactorial (see Chapter 7). Loss of cartilage does not completely explain pain – for example, the knee is subject to substantial weightbearing forces, and loss of cartilage thickness contributes minimally to pain.[6] Structurally, the subchondral bone, bursae, synovium, capsule and ligamentous tissues associated with the GHJ are more richly innervated than the cartilage and may have a greater role in the pain experienced by the individual.

Increased expression of inflammatory cytokines (see Chapter 5) can induce apoptosis of chondrocytes.[154] It is therefore likely that GHJ-OA results from a complex relationship of biochemical and biomechanical factors that are more likely to manifest in the presence of known risk factors. As discussed in Chapter 6, psychosocial and environmental factors must also be considered and as such GHJ-OA must be viewed as a biopsychosocial problem.[133] GHJ-OA changes are present in approximately one-third of adults over the age of 60 years,[71] and when symptomatic for some people, GHJ-OA has a detrimental impact on quality of life that is comparable to acute myocardial infarction, diabetes, and congestive heart failure.[45]

Two categorizes of GHJ-OA have been described: primary GHJ-OA is more common in elderly populations,[30] and secondary GHJ-OA is more common in younger people (aged <60 years). It is categorized as occurring secondary to trauma (e.g., fracture, dislocation), shoulder surgery, avascular necrosis (alcohol induced, corticosteroid therapy, cytotoxic drugs, Gaucher's disease, obesity, radiation, sickle cell disease), inflammatory arthritis (e.g., rheumatoid arthritis), reactive arthritis (e.g., Lyme), and previous infection (e.g., septic arthritis), and secondary to massive rotator cuff tears (rotator cuff arthropathy).[123] Rotator cuff arthropathy (RTA) affects 2.5% of the population over 70 years of age.[104] Classically RTA is described as GHJ-OA that occurs following a massive tear of the rotator cuff tendons. RTA commonly progresses through a continuum involving one of four types (type IA, IB, IIA, and IIB). Type IIA involves superior migration of the humeral head due to failure of the rotator cuff to dynamically stabilize the humerus, and the final stage, type IIB, is when the humeral head dislocates in an anterior superior direction.[118,127]

Diagnosis

Diagnosis of glenohumeral arthritis is made through careful and thorough assessment, involving an interview (see Chapter 11), consideration of red flags, and combination of clinical findings and radiological features. Typically, there will be pain, initially on movement, and then at rest that also may be present at night, and interrupt sleep. Movement will be restricted and there may be signs of muscle atrophy. Shoulder strength may be compromised, and this may be due to inactivity, structural compromise of the tendons, and/or inhibition of muscle performance due to pain.

Shoulder imaging helps support the clinical hypothesis and establish the diagnosis. Radiographic evaluation commonly involves an anteroposterior view, a Grashey view, and an axillary view. These three views not only help clinicians determine the presence, type and degree of OA but also help to rule out other possible conditions often related to trauma or other pathologies.[37] The purpose of a Grashey view (also known as an anteroposterior (AP) oblique internal rotation view), is to obtain a view parallel to the glenoid fossa, and to achieve this the patient is rotated 30°–45° so that the scapular body is against the radiographic plate. One benefit of the Grashey view is to infer the status of the rotator cuff.[37] This is achieved using the Hamada-Fukuda classification system that ranges from type I (normal joint morphology and an acromiohumeral distance >6 mm), to type 5 (acromiohumeral distance <5 mm, acetabularization of the acromion, narrowing of the GHJ space and collapse of the humeral head).[37,51] The Samilson-Prietro classification system is another method of describing the extent that GHJ-OA can be observed radiologically.[124] Other imaging investigations that help establish the diagnosis of GHJ-OA and support surgical planning include computed tomography (CT),[147] and magnetic resonance imaging (MRI).[62]

Management

With no known interventions that can "cure" GHJ-OA, treatment involves education, pain control, support for self-management and self-efficacy, maintenance and if possible, improving range of motion and function. Management falls into three main categories: watch and wait, nonsurgical, and surgical intervention.

Nonsurgical management

In the early stages, a watch and wait approach is underpinned by education, promotion of self-efficacy and self-management, and is supported as appropriate by activity modification, and reduction of unhealthy and integration of healthy lifestyle behaviors, together with pharmacological and nonpharmacological pain relief as and when required.

Pharmacological management

The UK National Institute for Health and Care Excellence (NICE) recommends the following pharmacological management (https://www.nice.org.uk/guidance/cg177/chapter/1-Recommendations#pharmacological-management):

- In addition to other nonsurgical management such as exercise and weight loss, healthcare professionals should consider paracetamol (acetaminophen) and topical nonsteroidal anti-inflammatory drugs (NSAIDs).

- Paracetamol and topical NSAIDs should be considered ahead of oral NSAIDs, cyclooxygenase 2 (COX-2) inhibitors or opioids.
- Where paracetamol or topical NSAIDs provide *insufficient* pain relief for people with osteoarthritis, then the addition of an oral NSAID/COX-2 inhibitor to paracetamol should be considered.
- Where paracetamol or topical NSAIDs are *ineffective* for pain relief for people with osteoarthritis, then substitution with an oral NSAID/COX-2 inhibitor should be considered.
- Use oral NSAIDs/COX-2 inhibitors at the lowest effective dose for the shortest possible period and co-prescribe a proton pump inhibitor (PPI).
- If a person with osteoarthritis needs to take low-dose aspirin, healthcare professionals should consider other analgesics before substituting or adding an NSAID or COX-2 inhibitor (with a PPI) if pain relief is *ineffective* or *insufficient*.
- All oral NSAIDs/COX-2 inhibitors have analgesic effects of a similar magnitude but vary in their potential gastrointestinal, liver and cardio-renal toxicity; therefore, when choosing the agent and dose, consider individual patient risk factors, including age.
- There is limited evidence for the use of nutritional supplements such as glucosamine and chondroitin,[146] and NICE do not recommend the use of glucosamine or chondroitin products in the management of OA.

Intra-articular injections for shoulder OA are discussed in detail in Chapter 23. They should only be considered as part of a package of care, and not as a standalone treatment. Corticosteroids are the most common injectable medication used in the management of GHJ-OA. Recommendations for the use of injectable corticosteroids in GHJ-OA are inconclusive, nevertheless, guidelines regarding type and dose of cortisone are similar to the knee joint.[73] Hyaluronic acid (HA) is a high molecular weight glycosaminoglycan, which is thought to have anti-inflammatory, analgesic, and chondro-protective effects.[66,135] Although insufficient evidence is available to draw definitive conclusions regarding its effectiveness in GHJ-OA, a recent randomized controlled trial evaluating the efficacy of HA with corticosteroid at 1, 3 and 6 months found that the HA group had improved pain and disability scores at all time points. The corticosteroid group, however, only saw improvements at 1 month.[91]

Fuggle et al.[44] recommend that oral opioids should only be prescribed for people with severe symptoms associated with OA. A relatively weak opioid should be prescribed for a short period and should be prescribed as the final pharmacological therapy prior to considering surgery.

Nonpharmacological management

Exercise therapy is commonly prescribed in the management of GHJ-OA. However, there is a paucity of research evidence to support both the use, and type of exercise for GHJ-OA.[138] This uncertainty must be shared with patients during discussions relating to management and anticipated outcomes.[58] Nonetheless, clinicians and patients should consider lifestyle factors, exercise therapy and possibly adjunct treatments for 12 weeks or longer to determine if acceptable improvements, or satisfactory maintenance of symptoms, have been achieved. Due to the largely unproven effect of exercise therapy for GHJ-OA, no specific program may currently be recommended. Millett et al. have suggested that surgery for GHJ-OA should be considered if the symptoms are unresponsive to nonsurgical intervention.[93] If nonsurgical management does not achieve the desired results, and following shared decision-making discussion with the patient, surgical intervention would typically be the next stage in management.

Surgery

The principal goal of surgical intervention for GHJ-OA is pain relief, as improved function is commonly less predictable. The most common surgical interventions related to GHJ-OA include hemiarthroplasty with glenoid resurfacing, total shoulder arthroplasty (TSA) and reverse total shoulder arthroplasty (rTSA). Indications and subsequent periods and magnitude of recovery vary with each type of procedure. Hemiarthroplasty with glenoid surfacing is performed when the humeral head requires replacing but the severity of OA on the glenoid surface does not warrant replacement. TSA is indicated when both the glenoid and humeral aspects are significantly effective and require replacement, but the rotator cuff is intact. Finally, the rTSA is reserved for those individuals with rotator cuff arthropathy. The purpose of the rTSA is to replace the concave glenoid with a convex component and the convex humeral head with a concave component, which shifts the center of rotation at the glenohumeral joint medially and inferiorly giving the deltoid a mechanical advantage to act more as a shoulder elevator.[120,121]

Due to the increase in the average age of the population, improved surgical techniques and expertise, the number of surgical procedures for GHJ-OA is increasing,[35,116] and although intraoperative and postoperative complications occur, the numbers appear to be relatively low in some patient populations and are higher in others.[35,102] Cowling et al.[34] reported a 2.5% intraoperative complication rate with the majority being fractures. The incidence of all complications was higher in women, and the risk of complications increased if the surgical procedure performed was a stemmed hemiarthroplasty or a reverse total shoulder arthroplasty. The incidence of all complications was less in patients undergoing a resurfacing arthroplasty.

Craig et al.[35] reported that the lifetime risks of revision surgery following elective shoulder replacement were approximately 25% (1 in 4) men aged 55–59 years, and approximately 3% (1 in 37) women aged 85 years and older. The risks of revision were highest during the first five years after surgery. The risk of any post-surgical serious adverse event was 3.5% (1 in 28 people) at 30 days post-surgery and 4.6% (1 in 22 people) at 90 days post-surgery. For patients aged 85 years and older, 1 in 9 women, and 1 in 5 men, experienced at least one serious adverse event within 90 days.[35] Adverse events included: an increase in all-cause death, pulmonary embolism, myocardial infarction, lower respiratory tract infection, acute kidney disease, urinary tract infection, and cerebrovascular events.[35] These data should be shared with patients considering surgery.

There are many important research questions to be answered regarding the role of surgical and nonsurgical management for people seeking care with GHJ-OA. One crucial question to address is to determine the effectiveness of education, exercise therapy and lifestyle management, with or without the treatments and modalities discussed in Chapters 31, 32, 33, and 34. Another is a comparison of surgical and nonsurgical treatments, in terms of short to medium and long-term clinical outcomes, health economics, and patient satisfaction. To address these gaps in our knowledge, a broad range of biopsychosocial outcome measures need be included in such a program of research.

Osteosarcoma

Osteosarcomas are malignant tumors of bone and are classified as either central or surface tumors. Each type can be further classified into different subtypes.[95] Osteosarcomas can develop in any bone in the body but are most common around the knee (34%), in either the lower femur or upper tibia. The second most common location is the proximal humerus (12%), with 8% occurring in the ribs, sternum, and clavicle. Osteosarcomas are slightly more common in males than females.[117] Osteosarcomas may occur at any age, but most commonly present in two distinct age categories. The incidence of osteosarcomas is highest (8 per million people) in childhood, adolescence, and early adulthood (peak age 15–19 years) and the second peak (6 per million people) between 65 to 85 years (peak age 75–79 years).[95]

Approximately 160 people are diagnosed with osteosarcomas each year in the UK (2.6 per million people) and 1,000 new cases are diagnosed in the US annually. The earliest symptoms of an osteosarcoma are pain and swelling (mass or lump) in the region of the tumor. The pain may be intermittent in the earlier stages, and may be worse with movement, mimicking a mechanical musculoskeletal presentation.[110] As they are more common in children, they may be misdiagnosed as "growing pains". When present near the shoulder, the combination of pain, swelling and increasing size of the osteosarcoma can lead to movement restriction. Other rarer symptoms include fever, malaise, weight loss, and anemia. Surgery, chemotherapy, and radiation therapy are the most common treatments, with physical therapy, occupational therapy, dietetics, orthotics, and prosthetics, also being required.

Locked posterior dislocations of the humeral head

The shoulder is the most commonly dislocated joint in the body. Three main types occur: anterior (95%), inferior (1%), and posterior (4%). Being rare, posterior dislocations pose a diagnostic challenge and diagnosis is often delayed. In up to 73% of cases,[157] the diagnosis is made only once the injury has become chronic, resulting in a locked posterior dislocation and is associated with a poorer prognosis.[5] Posterior dislocations may be caused by trauma (59%), epileptic, hypoglycemic, or drug-induced seizures (40%), or electric shocks (1%).[5] Seizures and electric shocks may cause the internal rotators to contract with substantial force leading to the posterior dislocation.[5] In addition to pain and weakness, shoulder stiffness is a prominent symptom and may mimic other shoulder conditions such as a frozen shoulder.[5] Management involves a combination of nonsurgical and surgical approaches.

Avascular necrosis of the humeral head

Avascular necrosis, also known as osteonecrosis, aseptic necrosis, or ischemic necrosis is a disease resulting in the death of bone cells due to insufficient blood supply.[140] It may have a traumatic or nontraumatic onset. Although it can occur in any bone, it most commonly affects the epiphysis of long bones with around 15,000 to 20,000 people being diagnosed with the condition each year in the US, most commonly between 30 and 50 years of age.[163] The humeral head is the second most common site for avascular necrosis.[56,82,140] The posterior humeral circumflex artery supplies most of the blood supply to the humeral head, with interosseous continuation of the ascending branch of the anterior circumflex artery, the arcuate artery, the suprascapular artery, and the circumflex scapular artery also contributing. Any disturbance of blood supply to the humeral head can predispose avascular necrosis.[56] Long-term high-dose systemic (oral or intravenous) corticosteroid use is a major risk factor, accounting for 35% of nontraumatic avascular necrosis. There appears to be little risk associated with infrequent use of corticosteroids, inhaled steroids, or steroid injections into joints. Other risk factors include human immunodeficiency virus, sickle cell anemia, diabetes, Gaucher's disease, systemic lupus erythematosus, pancreatitis, autoimmune disease, smoking, cancer and related treatments, and decompression sickness (Caisson's disease, the bends).[56,140] A four-part fracture-dislocation of the humeral head has an associated risk of developing avascular necrosis approaching 100%, and a displaced four-part fracture of approximately 45%. Radiographic findings may not be observed at the onset of the disease and magnetic resonance imaging is the preferred imaging modality. Symptoms involve pain, weakness, crepitus and increasing joint stiffness. Management involves a combination of nonsurgical and surgical procedures.[56,82,140]

References

1. Abrassart S, Kolo F, Piotton S, et al. 'Frozen shoulder' is ill-defined. How can it be described better? EFORT Open Rev. 2020;5:273-279.
2. Alsubheen SA, Nazari G, Bobos P, MacDermid JC, Overend TJ, Faber K. Effectiveness of nonsurgical interventions for managing adhesive capsulitis in patients with diabetes: a systematic review. Arch Phys Med Rehabil. 2019;100:350-365.
3. Arkkila PE, Gautier JF. Musculoskeletal disorders in diabetes mellitus: an update. Best Pract Res Clin Rheumatol. 2003;17:945-970.
4. Auten RL, Davis JM. Oxygen toxicity and reactive oxygen species: the devil is in the details. Pediatric Research. 2009;66:121-127.
5. Aydin N, Enes Kayaalp M, Asansu M, Karaismailoglu B. Treatment options for locked posterior shoulder dislocations and clinical outcomes. EFORT Open Rev. 2019;4:194-200.
6. Bacon K, LaValley MP, Jafarzadeh SR, Felson D. Does cartilage loss cause pain in osteoarthritis and if so, how much? Annals of the Rheumatic Diseases. 2020;79:1105-1110.
7. Baer W. Operative treatment of subdeltoid bursitis. Bull. Johns Hopkins Hosp. 1907;18:282-284.
8. Bagheri F, Ebrahimzadeh MH, Moradi A, Bidgoli HF. Factors associated with pain, disability and quality of life in patients suffering from frozen shoulder. Arch Bone Jt Surg. 2016;4:243-247.
9. Barbosa F, Swamy G, Salem H, et al. Chronic adhesive capsulitis (frozen shoulder): comparative outcomes of treatment in patients with diabetes and obesity. J Clin Orthop Trauma. 2019;10:265-268.
10. Bateman M, McClymont S, Hinchliffe SR. The effectiveness and cost of corticosteroid injection and physiotherapy in the treatment of frozen shoulder: a single-centre service evaluation. Clin Rheumatol. 2014;33:1005-1008.
11. Ben-Arie E, Kao P-Y, Lee Y-C, Ho W-C, Chou L-W, Liu H-P. The effectiveness of acupuncture in the treatment of frozen shoulder: a systematic review and meta-analysis. Evidence-Based Complementary and Alternative Medicine. 2020;2020:9790470.
12. Boudreault J, Desmeules F, Roy J-S, Dionne C, Fremont P, MacDermid JC. The efficacy of oral non-steroidal anti-inflammatory drugs for rotator cuff tendinopathy: a systematic review and meta-analysis. Journal of Rehabilitation Medicine. 2014;46:294-306.
13. Boutefnouchet T, Jordan R, Bhabra G, Modi C, Saithna A. Comparison of outcomes following arthroscopic capsular release for idiopathic, diabetic and secondary shoulder adhesive capsulitis: a systematic review. Orthopaedics &

Traumatology: Surgery & Research. 2019;105:839-846.

14. Buchbinder R, Green S, Youd JM, Johnston RV. Oral steroids for adhesive capsulitis. Cochrane Database of Systematic Reviews. 2006: CD006189.

15. Buchbinder R, Green S, Youd JM, Johnston RV, Cumpston M. Arthrographic distension for adhesive capsulitis (frozen shoulder). Cochrane Database of Systematic Reviews. 2008:CD007005.

16. Bunker T. Time for a new name for frozen shoulder-contracture of the shoulder. Shoulder & Elbow. 2009;1:4-9.

17. Bunker TD. Frozen shoulder: unravelling the enigma. Ann R Coll Surg Engl. 1997;79:210-213.

18. Bunker TD. Time for a new name for 'frozen shoulder'. Br Med J (Clin Res Ed). 1985;290:1233-1234.

19. Bunker TD, Anthony PP. The pathology of frozen shoulder. A Dupuytren-like disease. J Bone Joint Surg Br. 1995;77:677-683.

20. Burne G, Mansfield M, Gaida JE, Lewis JS. Is there an association between metabolic syndrome and rotator cuff-related shoulder pain? A systematic review. BMJ Open Sport & Exercise Medicine. 2019;5:e000544.

21. Cagliero E, Apruzzese W, Perlmutter GS, Nathan DM. Musculoskeletal disorders of the hand and shoulder in patients with diabetes mellitus. Am J Med. 2002;112:487-490.

22. Cakir M, Samanci N, Balci N, Balci MK. Musculoskeletal manifestations in patients with thyroid disease. Clin Endocrinol (Oxf). 2003;59:162-167.

23. Chan JH, Ho BS, Alvi HM, Saltzman MD, Marra G. The relationship between the incidence of adhesive capsulitis and hemoglobin A. J Shoulder Elbow Surg. 2017;26:1834-1837.

24. Chelombitko M. Role of reactive oxygen species in inflammation: a minireview. Moscow University Biological Sciences Bulletin. 2018;73:199-202.

25. Cho C-H, Jin H-J, Kim DH. Comparison of clinical outcomes between idiopathic frozen shoulder and diabetic frozen shoulder after a single ultrasound-guided intra-articular corticosteroid injection. Diagnostics. 2020;10:370.

26. Cho C-H, Jung S-W, Park J-Y, Song K-S, Yu K-I. Is shoulder pain for three months or longer correlated with depression, anxiety, and sleep disturbance? Journal of Shoulder and Elbow Surgery. 2013;22:222-228.

27. Cho C-H, Lee Y-H, Kim D-H, Lim Y-J, Baek C-S, Kim D-H. Definition, diagnosis, treatment, and prognosis of frozen shoulder: a consensus survey of shoulder specialists. Clinics in Orthopedic Surgery. 2020;12:60.

28. Cho C-H, Song K-S, Kim B-S, Kim DH, Lho Y-M. Biological aspect of pathophysiology for frozen shoulder. BioMed Research International. 2018;2018:7274517.

29. Choi Y-H, Kim DH. Correlations between clinical features and MRI findings in early adhesive capsulitis of the shoulder: a retrospective observational study. BMC Musculoskeletal Disorders. 2020;21:1-9.

30. Chong PY, Srikumaran U, Kuye IO, Warner JJ. Glenohumeral arthritis in the young patient. J Shoulder Elbow Surg. 2011;20:S30-40.

31. Choudhry MN, Malik RA, Charalambous CP. Blood glucose levels following intra-articular steroid injections in patients with diabetes: a systematic review. JBJS Rev. 2016;4:01874474-201603000-00002.

32. Codman E. The Shoulder: Rupture of the Supraspinatus Tendon and Other Lesions in or about the Subacromial Bursa. Boston: Thomas Todd Company; 1934.

33. Cohen C, Tortato S, Silva OBS, Leal MF, Ejnisman B, Faloppa F. Association between frozen shoulder and thyroid diseases: strengthening the evidences. Revista Brasileira de Ortopedia. 2020;55:483-489.

34. Cowling PD, Holland P, Kottam L, Baker P, Rangan A. Risk factors associated with intraoperative complications in primary shoulder arthroplasty. Acta Orthop. 2017;88:587-591.

35. Craig RS, Lane JC, Carr AJ, Furniss D, Collins GS, Rees JL. Serious adverse events and lifetime risk of reoperation after elective shoulder replacement: population based cohort study using hospital episode statistics for England. BMJ. 2019;364:l298.

36. Cushnaghan J, Dieppe P. Study of 500 patients with limb joint osteoarthritis. I. Analysis by age, sex, and distribution of symptomatic joint sites. Annals of the Rheumatic Diseases. 1991;50:8-13.

37. Dekker TJ, Steele J, Vinson E, Garrigues G. Current peri-operative imaging concepts surrounding shoulder arthroplasty. Skeletal Radiology. 2019;48:1485-1497.

38. Duplay S. De la périarthrite scapulo-humérale. Archives Générales de Médicine. November 1872.

39. Duplay S. De la périarthrite scapulo-humérale. La Semaine Médicale. 1896.

40. Erickson BJ, Shishani Y, Bishop ME, Romeo AA, Gobezie R. Adhesive capsulitis: demographics and predictive factors for success following steroid injections and surgical intervention. Arthroscopy, Sports Medicine, and Rehabilitation. 2019;1:e35-e40.

41. NICE. Scenario: Frozen Shoulder. Available at: https://cks.nice.org.uk/topics/shoulder-pain/management/frozen-shoulder/.

42. Favejee M, Huisstede B, Koes B. Frozen shoulder: the effectiveness of conservative and surgical interventions—systematic review. British Journal of Sports Medicine. 2011;45:49-56.

43. Fields BK, Skalski MR, Patel DB, et al. Adhesive capsulitis: review of imaging findings, pathophysiology, clinical presentation, and treatment options. Skeletal Radiology. 2019;1-14.

44. Fuggle N, Curtis E, Shaw S, et al. Safety of opioids in osteoarthritis: outcomes of a systematic review and meta-analysis. Drugs & Aging. 2019;36:129-143.

45. Gartsman GM, Brinker MR, Khan M, Karahan M. Self-assessment of general health status in patients with five common shoulder conditions. Journal of Shoulder and Elbow Surgery. 1998;7:228-237.

46. Gerrits EG, Landman GW, Nijenhuis-Rosien L, Bilo HJ. Limited joint mobility syndrome in diabetes mellitus: a minireview. World J Diabetes. 2015;6:1108-1112.

47. Grant JA, Schroeder N, Miller BS, Carpenter JE. Comparison of manipulation and arthroscopic capsular release for adhesive capsulitis: a systematic review. Journal of Shoulder and Elbow Surgery. 2013;22:1135-1145.

48. Gundtoft PH, Attrup ML, Kristensen AK, Vobbe JW, Sørensen L, Hölmich P. Diabetes mellitus affects the prognosis of frozen shoulder. Dan Med J. 2020;67:A02200071.

49. Gundtoft PH, Kristensen AK, Attrup M, et al. Prevalence and impact of diabetes mellitus on the frozen shoulder. South Med J. 2018;111:654-659.

50. Hall K, Mercer C. The stiff shoulder: a case study. Man Ther. 2015;20:884-889.

51. Hamada K, Fukuda H, Mikasa M, Kobayashi Y. Roentgenographic findings in massive rotator cuff tears. A long-term observation. Clinical Orthopaedics and Related Research. 1990;92-96.

52. Hanchard NC, Goodchild L, Thompson J, O'Brien T, Davison D, Richardson C. Evidence-based clinical guidelines for the diagnosis, assessment and physiotherapy management of contracted (frozen) shoulder: quick reference summary. Physiotherapy. 2012;98:117-120.

53. Hanchard NC, Goodchild L, Thompson J, O'Brien T, Davison D, Richardson C. A questionnaire survey of UK physiotherapists on the diagnosis and management of contracted (frozen) shoulder. Physiotherapy. 2011;97:115-125.

54. Hand C, Clipsham K, Rees JL, Carr AJ. Long-term outcome of frozen shoulder. J Shoulder Elbow Surg. 2008;17:231-236.

55. Harkness E, MacFarlane GJ, Silman A, McBeth J. Is musculoskeletal pain more common now than 40 years ago? Two population-based cross-sectional studies. Rheumatology. 2005;44:890-895.

56. Hernigou P, Hernigou J, Scarlat M. Shoulder osteonecrosis: pathogenesis, causes, clinical evaluation, imaging, and classification. Orthopaedic Surgery. 2020;12:1340-1349.

57. Hettrich CM, DiCarlo EF, Faryniarz D, Vadasdi KB, Williams R, Hannafin JA. The effect of myofibroblasts and corticosteroid injections in adhesive capsulitis. Journal of Shoulder and Elbow Surgery. 2016;25:1274-1279.

58. Hoffmann TC, Lewis J, Maher CG. Shared decision making should be an integral part of physiotherapy practice. Physiotherapy. 2020;107:43-49.

59. Hollmann L, Halaki M, Haber M, Herbert RD, Dalton S, Ginn KA. Determining the contribution of active stiffness to reduced range of motion in frozen shoulder. Physiotherapy. 2015;101:e585.

60. Hollmann L, Halaki M, Kamper SJ, Haber M, Ginn KA. Does muscle guarding play a role in range of motion loss in patients with frozen shoulder? Musculoskelet Sci Pract. 2018;37:64-68.

61. Holte KB, Juel NG, Brox JI, et al. Hand, shoulder and back stiffness in long-term type 1 diabetes: cross-sectional association with skin collagen advanced glycation end-products. The Dialong study. J Diabetes Complications. 2017;31:1408-1414.

62. Hopkins CM, Azar FM, Mulligan RP, Hollins AM, Smith RA, Throckmorton TW. Computed tomography and magnetic resonance imaging are similarly reliable in the assessment of glenohumeral arthritis and glenoid version. Archives of Bone and Joint Surgery. 2021;9:64.

63. Hussain T, Tan B, Yin Y, Blachier F, Tossou MC, Rahu N. Oxidative stress and inflammation: what polyphenols can do for us? Oxidative Medicine and Cellular Longevity. 2016;2016:7432797.

64. Hwang KR, Murrell GA, Millar NL, Bonar F, Lam P, Walton JR. Advanced glycation end products in idiopathic frozen shoulders. J Shoulder Elbow Surg. 2016;25:981-988.

65. Ibounig T, Simons T, Launonen A, Paavola M. Glenohumeral osteoarthritis: an overview of etiology and diagnostics. Scandinavian Journal of Surgery. 2020;1457496920935018.

66. Iwata H. Pharmacologic and clinical aspects of intraarticular injection of hyaluronate. Clin Orthop Relat Res. 1993;285-291.

67. Jain TK, Sharma NK. The effectiveness of physiotherapeutic interventions in treatment of frozen shoulder/adhesive capsulitis: a systematic review. J Back Musculoskelet Rehabil. 2014;27:247-273.

68. Jenkins EF, Thomas WJ, Corcoran JP, et al. The outcome of manipulation under general anesthesia for the management of frozen shoulder in patients with diabetes mellitus. Journal of Shoulder and Elbow Surgery. 2012;21:1492-1498.

69. Jones S, Hanchard N, Hamilton S, Rangan A. A qualitative study of patients' perceptions and priorities when living with primary frozen shoulder. BMJ Open. 2013;3:e003452.

70. Kelley MJ, Shaffer MA, Kuhn JE, et al. Shoulder pain and mobility deficits: adhesive capsulitis: clinical practice guidelines linked to the international classification of functioning, disability, and health from the Orthopaedic Section of the American Physical Therapy Association. Journal of Orthopaedic & Sports Physical Therapy. 2013;43:A1-A31.

71. Kerr R, Resnick D, Pineda C, Haghighi P. Osteoarthritis of the glenohumeral joint: a radiologic-pathologic study. American Journal of Roentgenology. 1985;144:967-972.

72. Khan MAB, Hashim MJ, King JK, Govender RD, Mustafa H, Al Kaabi J. Epidemiology of type 2 diabetes - global burden of disease and forecasted trends. J Epidemiol Glob Health. 2020;10:107-111.

73. Khazzam MS, Pearl ML. AAOS Clinical Practice Guideline: Management of Glenohumeral Joint Osteoarthritis. J Am Acad Orthop Surg. 2020;28:790-794.

74. Kiani J, Goharifar H, Moghimbeigi A, Azizkhani H. Prevalence and risk factors of five most common upper extremity disorders in diabetics. J Res Health Sci. 2014;14:92-95.

75. King W. The lived experience of frozen shoulder: and interpretative phenomenonological analysis. British Elbow and Soulder Society (BESS) Conference; 14 October 2020.

76. King W. The lived experience for frozen shoulder: and interpretative phenomenological analysis. VP-Virtual Physiotherapy Conference; 13-14 November 2020.

77. Kingston K, Curry EJ, Galvin JW, Li X. Shoulder adhesive capsulitis: epidemiology and predictors of surgery. Journal of Shoulder and Elbow Surgery. 2018;27:1437-1443.

78. Kobayashi T, Karasuno H, Sano H, et al. Representative survey of frozen shoulder questionnaire responses from the Japan Shoulder Society: what are the appropriate diagnostic terms for primary idiopathic frozen shoulder, stiff shoulder or frozen shoulder? Journal of Orthopaedic Science. 2019;24:631-635.

79. Koh KH. Corticosteroid injection for adhesive capsulitis in primary care: a systematic review of randomised clinical trials. Singapore Medical Journal. 2016;57:646.

80. Kraal T, Lübbers J, van den Bekerom M, et al. The puzzling pathophysiology of frozen shoulders–a scoping review. Journal of Experimental Orthopaedics. 2020;7:1-15.

81. Lamplot JD, Lillegraven O, Brophy RH. Outcomes from conservative treatment of shoulder idiopathic adhesive capsulitis and factors associated with developing contralateral disease.

Orthopaedic Journal of Sports Medicine. 2018;6:2325967118785169.

82. Le Coz P, Herve A, Thomazeau H. Surgical treatments of atraumatic avascular necrosis of the shoulder. Morphologie. 2021;105:155-161.

83. Lebiedz-Odrobina D, Kay J. Rheumatic manifestations of diabetes mellitus. Rheum Dis Clin North Am. 2010;36:681-699.

84. Lewis J. Frozen shoulder contracture syndrome - aetiology, diagnosis and management. Man Ther. 2015;20:2-9.

85. Lewis J, O'Sullivan P. Is it time to reframe how we care for people with non-traumatic musculoskeletal pain? Br J Sports Med. 2018;52:1543-1544.

86. Lewis JS, Cook CE, Hoffmann TC, O'Sullivan P. The elephant in the room: too much medicine in musculoskeletal practice. J Orthop Sports Phys Ther. 2020;50:1-4.

87. Lin X, Xu Y, Pan X, et al. Global, regional, and national burden and trend of diabetes in 195 countries and territories: an analysis from 1990 to 2025. Sci Rep. 2020;10:14790.

88. Lippmann RK. Frozen shoulder; periarthritis; bicipital tenosynovitis. Archives of Surgery. 1943;47:283-296.

89. Lundberg BJ. The frozen shoulder. Clinical and radiographical observations. The effect of manipulation under general anesthesia. Structure and glycosaminoglycan content of the joint capsule. Local bone metabolism. Acta Orthop Scand Suppl. 1969;119:1-59.

90. Maund E, Craig D, Suekarran S, et al. Management of frozen shoulder: a systematic review and cost-effectiveness analysis. Health Technol Assess. 2012;16:1-264.

91. Merolla G, Sperling JW, Paladini P, Porcellini G. Efficacy of hylan G-F 20 versus 6-methylprednisolone acetate in painful shoulder osteoarthritis: a retrospective controlled trial. Musculoskelet Surg. 2011;95:215-224.

92. Milgrom C, Novack V, Weil Y, Jaber S, Radeva-Petrova DR, Finestone A. Risk factors for idiopathic frozen shoulder. The Israel Medical Association Journal. 2008;10:361.

93. Millett PJ, Gobezie R, Boykin RE. Shoulder osteoarthritis: diagnosis and management. Am Fam Physician. 2008;78:605-611.

94. Minns Lowe C, Barrett E, McCreesh K, De Burca N, Lewis J. Clinical effectiveness of non-surgical interventions for primary frozen shoulder: a systematic review. Journal of Rehabilitation Medicine. 2019;51:539-556.

95. Misaghi A, Goldin A, Awad M, Kulidjian AA. Osteosarcoma: a comprehensive review. SICOT J. 2018;4:12.

96. Mueller MJ, Sorensen CJ, McGill JB, et al. Effect of a shoulder movement intervention on joint mobility, pain, and disability in people with diabetes: a randomized controlled trial. Phys Ther. 2018;98:745-753.

97. Nakamura A, Kawahrada R. Advanced glycation end products and oxidative stress in a hyperglycaemic environment. IntechOpen; 2021. 10.5772/intechopen.97234.

98. Nakandala P, Nanayakkara I, Wadugodapitiya S, Gawarammana I. The efficacy of physiotherapy interventions in the treatment of adhesive capsulitis: a systematic review. J Back Musculoskelet Rehabil. 2021;34:195-205.

99. Neviaser AS, Hannafin JA. Adhesive capsulitis: a review of current treatment. Am J Sports Med. 2010;38:2346-2356.

100. Neviaser J. Adhesive capsulitis of the shoulder. A study of the pathological findings in periarthritis of the shoulder. Journal of Bone and Joint Surgery (Am). 1945;27:211-222.

101. Neviaser RJ, Neviaser TJ. The frozen shoulder. Diagnosis and management. Clin Orthop Relat Res. 1987;59-64.

102. Neyton L, Kirsch JM, Collotte P, et al. Mid-to long-term follow-up of shoulder arthroplasty for primary glenohumeral osteoarthritis in patients aged 60 or under. Journal of Shoulder and Elbow Surgery. 2019;28:1666-1673.

103. Noten S, Meeus M, Stassijns G, Van Glabbeek F, Verborgt O, Struyf F. Efficacy of different types of mobilization techniques in patients with primary adhesive capsulitis of the shoulder: a systematic review. Archives of Physical Medicine and Rehabilitation. 2016;97:815-825.

104. Nove-Josserand L, Walch G, Adeleine P, Courpron P. Effect of age on the natural history of the shoulder: a clinical and radiological study in the elderly. Revue de Chirurgie Orthopedique et Reparatrice de L'appareil Moteur. 2005;91:508-514.

105. Page MJ, Green S, Kramer S, Johnston RV, McBain B, Buchbinder R. Electrotherapy modalities for adhesive capsulitis (frozen shoulder). Cochrane Database of Systematic Reviews. 2014;CD011324.

106. Page MJ, Green S, Kramer S, et al. Manual therapy and exercise for adhesive capsulitis (frozen shoulder). Cochrane Database of Systematic Reviews. 2014;CD011275.

107. Papalia R, Tecame A, Vadalà G, et al. The use of hyaluronic acid in the treatment of shoulder capsulitis: a systematic review. Journal of Biological Regulators and Homeostatic Agents. 2017;31:23-32.

108. Pietrzak M. Adhesive capsulitis: an age related symptom of metabolic syndrome and chronic low-grade inflammation? Medical Hypotheses. 2016;88:12-17.

109. Pomey M-P, Hihat H, Khalifa M, Lebel P, Néron A, Dumez V. Patient partnership in quality improvement of healthcare services: patients' inputs and challenges faced. Patient Experience Journal. 2015;2:29-42.

110. Prater S, McKeon B. Osteosarcoma. StatPearls. Treasure Island, FL: StatPearls Publishing; 2021. Available at: https://www.ncbi.nlm.nih.gov/books/NBK549868/.

111. Raeissadat SA, Rayegani SM, Langroudi TF, Khoiniha M. Comparing the accuracy and efficacy of ultrasound-guided versus blind injections of steroid in the glenohumeral joint in patients with shoulder adhesive capsulitis. Clinical Rheumatology. 2017;36:933-940.

112. Rai SK, Kashid M, Chakrabarty B, Upreti V, Shaki O. Is it necessary to screen patients with adhesive capsulitis of shoulder for diabetes mellitus? J Family Med Prim Care. 2019;8:2927-2932.

113. Rangan A, Brealey SD, Keding A, et al. Management of adults with primary frozen shoulder in secondary care (UK FROST): a multicentre, pragmatic, three-arm, superiority randomised clinical trial. The Lancet. 2020;396:977-989.

114. Rangan A, Gibson J, Brownson P, Thomas M, Rees J, Kulkarni R. Frozen shoulder. Shoulder & Elbow. 2015;7:299-307.

115. Rangan A, Hanchard N, McDaid C. What is the most effective treatment for frozen shoulder? BMJ. 2016;354:i4162.

116. Rasmussen JV, Amundsen A, Sørensen AKB, et al. Increased use of total shoulder arthroplasty for osteoarthritis and improved patient-reported outcome in Denmark, 2006–2015: a nationwide cohort study from the Danish Shoulder

Arthroplasty Registry. Acta Orthopaedica. 2019;90:489-494.

117. Rojas GA, Hubbard AK, Diessner BJ, Ribeiro KB, Spector LG. International trends in incidence of osteosarcoma (1988-2012). International Journal of Cancer. 2021;149:1044-1053.

118. Rugg CM, Gallo RA, Craig EV, Feeley BT. The pathogenesis and management of cuff tear arthropathy. Journal of Shoulder and Elbow Surgery. 2018;27:2271-2283.

119. Ryan V, Brown H, Minns Lowe CJ, Lewis JS. The pathophysiology associated with primary (idiopathic) frozen shoulder: a systematic review. BMC Musculoskelet Disord. 2016;17:340.

120. Salamh PA, Kolber MJ, Cheatham SW, Hanney WJ, Speer KP, Singh H. Postrehabilitation exercise considerations after reverse total shoulder arthroplasty. Strength & Conditioning Journal. 2014;36:23-33.

121. Salamh PA, Speer KP. Post-rehabilitation exercise considerations following total shoulder arthroplasty. Strength & Conditioning Journal. 2013;35:56-63.

122. Saltychev M, Laimi K, Virolainen P, Fredericson M. Effectiveness of hydrodilatation in adhesive capsulitis of shoulder: a systematic review and meta-analysis. Scandinavian Journal of Surgery. 2018;107:285-293.

123. Saltzman BM, Leroux TS, Verma NN, Romeo AA. Glenohumeral osteoarthritis in the young patient. Journal of the American Academy of Orthopaedic Surgeons. 2018;26:e361-e370.

124. Samilson R, Prieto V. Dislocation arthropathy of the shoulder. The Journal of Bone and Joint Surgery. 1983;65:456-460.

125. Sana'a AA, Nazari G, Bobos P, MacDermid JC, Overend TJ, Faber K. Effectiveness of nonsurgical interventions for managing adhesive capsulitis in patients with diabetes: a systematic review. Archives of Physical Medicine and Rehabilitation. 2019;100:350-365.

126. Sano H, Hatori M, Mineta M, Hosaka M, Itoi E. Tumors masked as frozen shoulders: a retrospective analysis. J Shoulder Elbow Surg. 2010;19:262-266.

127. Seebauer L. Biomecanical classification of cuff tear arthropaty. Global Shoulder Society Meeting. 2003:17-19.

128. Shah KM, Clark BR, McGill JB, Mueller MJ. Upper extremity impairments, pain and disability in patients with diabetes mellitus. Physiotherapy. 2015;101:147-154.

129. Shah KM, Ruth Clark B, McGill JB, Lang CE, Mueller MJ. Shoulder limited joint mobility in people with diabetes mellitus. Clin Biomech. 2015;30:308-313.

130. Shang X, Zhang Z, Pan X, Li J, Li Q. Intra-articular versus subacromial corticosteroid injection for the treatment of adhesive capsulitis: a meta-analysis and systematic review. BioMed Research International. 2019;2019:1274790.

131. Sharma SP, Moe-Nilssen R, Kvåle A, Bærheim A. Predicting outcome in frozen shoulder (shoulder capsulitis) in presence of comorbidity as measured with subjective health complaints and neuroticism. BMC Musculoskeletal Disorders. 2017;18:1-7.

132. Sheridan MA, Hannafin JA. Upper extremity: emphasis on frozen shoulder. Orthopedic Clinics. 2006;37:531-539.

133. Sheth MM, Morris BJ, Laughlin MS, Elkousy HA, Edwards TB. Lower socioeconomic status is associated with worse preoperative function, pain, and increased opioid use in patients with primary glenohumeral osteoarthritis. Journal of the American Academy of Orthopaedic Surgeons. 2020;28:287-292.

134. Smith SP, Devaraj VS, Bunker TD. The association between frozen shoulder and Dupuytren's disease. Journal of Shoulder and Elbow Surgery. 2001;10:149-151.

135. Strauss EJ, Hart JA, Miller MD, Altman RD, Rosen JE. Hyaluronic acid viscosupplementation and osteoarthritis: current uses and future directions. Am J Sports Med. 2009;37:1636-1644.

136. Suh CH, Yun SJ, Jin W, et al. Systematic review and meta-analysis of magnetic resonance imaging features for diagnosis of adhesive capsulitis of the shoulder. Eur Radiol. 2019;29:566-577.

137. Sun Y, Zhang P, Liu S, et al. Intra-articular steroid injection for frozen shoulder: a systematic review and meta-analysis of randomized controlled trials with trial sequential analysis. The American Journal of Sports Medicine. 2017;45:2171-2179.

138. Thomas M, Bidwai A, Rangan A, et al. Glenohumeral osteoarthritis. Shoulder & Elbow. 2016;8:203-214.

139. Tighe CB, Oakley WS. The prevalence of a diabetic condition and adhesive capsulitis of the shoulder. South Med J. 2008;101:591-595.

140. Tyrrell Burrus M, Cancienne JM, Boatright JD, Yang S, Brockmeier SF, Werner BC. Shoulder arthroplasty for humeral head avascular necrosis is associated with increased postoperative complications. HSS Journal. 2018;14:2-8.

141. Uitvlugt G, Detrisac DA, Johnson LL, Austin MD, Johnson C. Arthroscopic observations before and after manipulation of frozen shoulder. Arthroscopy. 1993;9:181-185.

142. Uppal HS, Evans JP, Smith C. Frozen shoulder: a systematic review of therapeutic options. World Journal of Orthopedics. 2015;6:263.

143. Valentine RE, Lewis JS. Intraobserver reliability of 4 physiologic movements of the shoulder in subjects with and without symptoms. Arch Phys Med Rehabil. 2006;87:1242-1249.

144. Van der Windt D, Koes BW, de Jong BA, Bouter LM. Shoulder disorders in general practice: incidence, patient characteristics, and management. Annals of the Rheumatic Diseases. 1995;54:959-964.

145. van Dieren S, Beulens JW, van der Schouw YT, Grobbee DE, Neal B. The global burden of diabetes and its complications: an emerging pandemic. Eur J Cardiovasc Prev Rehabil. 2010;17 Suppl 1:S3-8.

146. Vasiliadis HS, Tsikopoulos K. Glucosamine and chondroitin for the treatment of osteoarthritis. World Journal of Orthopedics. 2017;8:1.

147. Vo KV, Hackett DJ, Gee AO, Hsu JE. Classifications in brief: Walch classification of primary glenohumeral osteoarthritis. Clinical Orthopaedics and Related Research. 2017;475:2335-2340.

148. Walker-Bone K, Palmer KT, Reading I, Coggon D, Cooper C. Prevalence and impact of musculoskeletal disorders of the upper limb in the general population. Arthritis Rheum. 2004;51:642-651.

149. Walmsley S, Osmotherly PG, Rivett DA. Clinical identifiers for early-stage primary/idiopathic adhesive capsulitis: are we seeing the real picture? Physical Therapy. 2014;94:968-976.

150. Walmsley S, Rivett DA, Osmotherly PG. Adhesive capsulitis: establishing consensus on clinical identifiers for stage 1 using the Delphi technique. Physical Therapy. 2009;89:906-917.

151. Wei Q, Ren X, Jiang Y, Jin H, Liu N, Li J. Advanced glycation end products accelerate rat vascular calcification through RAGE/oxidative stress. BMC Cardiovasc Disord. 2013;13:13.

152. Wiley AM. Arthroscopic appearance of frozen shoulder. Arthroscopy. 1991;7:138-143.

153. Wong CK, Levine WN, Deo K, et al. Natural history of frozen shoulder: fact or fiction? A systematic review. Physiotherapy. 2017;103:40-47.

154. Woo C-H, Eom Y-W, Yoo M-H, et al. Tumor necrosis factor-α generates reactive oxygen species via a cytosolic phospholipase A2-linked cascade. Journal of Biological Chemistry. 2000;275:32357-32362.

155. Woods D, Loganathan K. Recurrence of frozen shoulder after manipulation under anaesthetic (MUA) the results of repeating the MUA. The Bone & Joint Journal. 2017;99:812-817.

156. Xiao RC, Walley KC, DeAngelis JP, Ramappa AJ. Corticosteroid injections for adhesive capsulitis: a review. Clin J Sport Med. 2017;27:308-320.

157. Xu W, Huang L-X, Guo JJ, Jiang D-H, Zhang Y, Yang H-L. Neglected posterior dislocation of the shoulder: a systematic literature review. Journal of Orthopaedic Translation. 2015;3:89-94.

158. Yian EH, Contreras R, Sodl JF. Effects of glycemic control on prevalence of diabetic frozen shoulder. J Bone Joint Surg Am. 2012;94:919-923.

159. Yoon JP, Chung SW, Kim J-E, et al. Intra-articular injection, subacromial injection, and hydrodilatation for primary frozen shoulder: a randomized clinical trial. Journal of Shoulder and Elbow Surgery. 2016;25:376-383.

160. Younes M, Neffati F, Touzi M, et al. Systemic effects of epidural and intra-articular glucocorticoid injections in diabetic and non-diabetic patients. Joint Bone Spine. 2007;74:472-476.

161. Zappia M, Di Pietto F, Aliprandi A, et al. Multi-modal imaging of adhesive capsulitis of the shoulder. Insights into Imaging. 2016;7:365-371.

162. Zhang Y, Jordan JM. Epidemiology of osteoarthritis. Clin Geriatr Med. 2010;26:355-369.

163. Zippelius T, Matziolis G, Röhner E, Windisch C, Lindemann C, Strube P. Psychological distress and health-related quality of life in patients with bone marrow edema syndrome. Annals of Translational Medicine. 2019;7:552.

164. Zreik NH, Malik RA, Charalambous CP. Adhesive capsulitis of the shoulder and diabetes: a meta-analysis of prevalence. Muscles, Ligaments and Tendons Journal. 2016;6:26.

165. Zuckerman JD, Rokito A. Frozen shoulder: a consensus definition. J Shoulder Elbow Surg. 2011;20:322-325.

19 The weak shoulder

Jeremy Lewis, Karen McCreesh, Kathryn Fahy, Jared Powell

Introduction

Although clinicians will often *diagnose* shoulder weakness and patients will frequently *report* that their shoulders are weak, this common shoulder impairment is difficult to describe in a clinically meaningful way. Definitions of weakness include: liable to "give way" under load, break under pressure, lacking in strength, not able to sustain or exert weight, force, or pressure, not able to resist external force, and lacking the power to perform physically demanding tasks.[58]

Weakness, if identified, is only the starting point, as the clinician then needs to determine if weakness is due to: substantial or partial loss of structural integrity (e.g., tear, fracture), pain inhibition, fear of pain, fear of further damage, red-flag pathology, neurological or vascular involvement, endocrine myopathies (e.g., thyroid dysfunction, pituitary dysfunction, diabetes), electrolyte disorders (e.g., hypokalemia), acute infection, long-term consequences of infection, autoimmune and inflammatory conditions (e.g., multiple sclerosis, amyotrophic lateral sclerosis, SARS-CoV-2, rheumatoid arthritis, lupus, Sjögren's syndrome), toxic causes (e.g., side effect of alcohol, statins, colchicine, antimalarial drugs, zidovudine), sarcopenia, vitamin D deficiency, or iron deficiency, to name only a few. Is the weakness local, bilateral, general symmetrical, or general asymmetrical, and how should the clinical findings be integrated into the clinical reasoning process? Identifying the underlying reason(s) for the presenting weakness is essential to implement the most appropriate management strategy. Suffice to say, strengthening programs are not a panacea for all forms of weakness, and suggesting that it is, is not evidence-based practice.

The etiology, assessment, and management of weakness is complex and cannot be reduced to how many repetitions and sets are required to redress the clinical findings. Neither can weakness be reduced to the need for surgical repair to restore structural integrity (e.g., rotator cuff tendon tear) followed by rehabilitation. Weakness is truly a biopsychosocial problem and is rarely attributable to one cause in isolation (see Figure 15.1). In this chapter we will address the more common neuromusculoskeletal causes of shoulder weakness. This chapter should be read together with Chapter 7 (Pain neuroscience), Chapter 8 (Red flags), Chapter 12 (Outcome measures), and Chapter 15 (Assessing and classifying musculoskeletal shoulder conditions).

What is shoulder weakness and how can it be assessed?

If strength is "the maximum voluntary resultant output that muscles can bring to bear on the environment under a specific set of conditions",[5] weakness would represent a significant reduction in the ability of a biological system (i.e., the shoulder) to voluntarily generate maximal force. It is important to clarify that strength testing is a measure of force output of a particular joint action (i.e., shoulder abduction), not a particular muscle (i.e., supraspinatus) due to the synergistic nature of muscles in a biological system. The shoulder often manifests weakness in specific direction, such as shoulder abduction and external rotation, and therefore it would be appropriate to describe the finding as reduced force output, or reduced muscle performance in these directions and not simply as a weak shoulder.

What objective tests are available to detect shoulder weakness? For practical reasons, we will focus on measurement techniques that are pragmatic and applicable to clinical practice. This includes: manual muscle tests, handheld dynamometry, functional tests, and hand-grip dynamometry.[5] It should be noted that isokinetic strength testing is viewed as the gold standard measure of strength[57] but due to high cost, lack of portability, and lack of widespread clinical availability, it will not be covered in this chapter.

Manual muscle testing (MMT) is a clinical method of measuring strength, where the clinician places the patient's body part to be tested in a predetermined position and instructs the patient to push that body part against the clinician's hand(s). Typically MMT is graded on a 0–5 scale, where 0 represents no detectable muscle action and 5 represents the ability to isometrically hold against a maximum break force.[5] While MMT may be a practical method of ascertaining approximate strength values, what of its reliability and validity? MMT demonstrates substantial intra- and interrater reliability[6] but it may have limited sensitivity as a precise measure of strength, especially in those without significant strength impairments.[5] MMT is suggested to be a valid measure of strength due to its correlation with functional activities,[19] for example sit to stand, but there is a paucity of research demonstrating this specifically for the clinical assessment of shoulder muscle strength.

There are many limitations of MMT in the clinical assessment of shoulder strength, including its dependence on the strength of the tester, confidence and willingness of the tester and patient to exert force, interpretation of the grading system, assigning the correct grade of strength following testing, detection of subtle side to side differences, and knowledge of minimal detectable differences for each testing position and direction of testing, and strength threshold at which differences between sides and between sessions may be detected. In summary, MMT is a subjective assessment of muscle strength.[6] Despite the many limitations of MMT, it may be considered as a relatively straightforward and inexpensive initial measure (impression) of shoulder strength in clinical practice.

Handheld dynamometry (HHD) is a method of measuring strength that is gaining in popularity due to its convenience, portability, and relative affordability. HHD uses a dynamometer in the hand of a tester, applied to the body of an individual, to measure the force output of a particular bodily action. HHD demonstrates good to high intra- and inter-rater reliability as a measure of shoulder strength.[15,27] HHD has demonstrated significant correlation to isokinetic testing when measuring shoulder strength.[27] Similar to MMT, the reliability and validity of HHD is limited by the strength of the tester. However, an advantage of testing shoulder strength, compared to the knee for example, is the inherent inability of the shoulder to produce relative high force, which may reduce the need of the tester having to be excessively strong.[66] While this is the case for many people seeking care for musculoskeletal shoulder complaints, it is acknowledged that HDD may not be appropriate for many athletes and others presenting with shoulder symptoms, where adaptations will be required.

HHD is a reliable and valid measure of shoulder strength and is a more sensitive measure of strength than MMT. Its portability, ease of use, clinical utility, and improving affordability positions HHD to be a useful measure of shoulder strength in clinical practice. Functional tests and grip strength are a proxy method of gauging shoulder strength and may be considered due to their clinical utility. A seated medicine ball throw demonstrates a moderate correlation with shoulder strength,[7] and hand grip strength is strongly correlated with shoulder strength.[28] If it is not possible to test the contralateral shoulder, or if both shoulders are symptomatic, testing hand grip strength may be of value.

It is arguable that the assessment of strength is only one component of the larger, over-arching, and more meaningful clinical assessment of muscle performance. Muscle performance, which includes strength testing, may be assessed using multifarious methods. For example, it may be of more value for the clinician to evaluate muscle performance by assessing the number of repetitions of an activity a patient can perform until the patient reports pain (or other relevant symptoms) and/or fatigue, than a single repetition maximum (1RM) contraction in isolation. As such it would be useful for researchers to assess the value of repetitions to fatigue and repetitions to pain as part of muscle performance testing.

"Strengthening" is a biopsychosocial, and not just a "bio" intervention

Observations of individuals with rotator cuff related shoulder pain (RCRSP) suggest the presence of shoulder weakness of the symptomatic side when compared to people without symptoms or to the unaffected shoulder of a person with symptoms. Specifically, shoulder abduction and external rotation strength have been shown to be reduced by up to 29% and 43%, respectively, in people with RCRSP.[12,37] Strength deficits have also been observed in movements that are suggested to bias scapulothoracic joint muscles, such as protraction and horizontal extension, but these deficits are not as profound as those observed during shoulder abduction and external rotation.[12] Strength deficits are a frequent characteristic of individuals with RCRSP, and it would be logical that if shoulder weakness is detected, a strengthening program would need to be implemented. Although appealing and intuitive to argue a strength deficit requires strengthening, the clinical reality is less clear-cut.

Clinical trials that utilized resistance exercise(s) as part of a rehabilitation regimen for RCRSP have observed clinically *unimportant* increases in shoulder strength, most commonly for the movements of shoulder abduction and external rotation.[35,39] Despite the modest increases in strength, there are significant improvements in shoulder pain and function. This clinical observation presents a direct challenge to our biomedical-based clinical reasoning and Newtonian understanding of cause and effect. More importantly, what does this mean for our clinical practice? Do we cease strengthening? Not quite, but it necessitates a nuanced approach to "strengthening".

The process of strengthening does not occur in a vacuum. The movements we are trying to strengthen are attached to a person with thoughts, feelings, and past experiences, who is also part of a broader sociocultural environment. This type of clinical thinking leads us inexorably to the biopsychosocial model of healthcare: a holistic and humanistic perspective of a person suffering with illness or injury.[18] If we were to apply a biopsychosocial model and not just a biological-biomechanical model to "strengthening" as an intervention to address "weakness", we can appreciate that resistance exercises may:

- Reduce pain (and the hypoalgesic effect may possibly reverse the impact of pain inhibition on muscles).
- Improve pain self-efficacy and confidence.
- Lead to a re-evaluation/reinterpretation of pain.
- Improve health-related quality of life.
- Divert attention away from pain to a specific task.
- Simply mark time while nature takes its course.
- Improve systemic and local inflammatory/biochemical markers.
- Improve mood and mental health.
- Increase strength and neuromuscular function.

Resistance training for a "weak and painful shoulder" is a cost-effective intervention that clinicians are encouraged to utilize. However, the clinical rationale for including strengthening exercises must be acknowledged as going beyond simply aiming to increase shoulder strength. The process of strengthening, when viewed through a biopsychosocial lens, becomes a versatile tool capable of influencing health, pain, and function on many levels. Strength deficits are an acknowledged risk factor for future shoulder disorders, especially in athletic populations,[11,24] and it is important to consider resistance exercises in most clinical encounters for people presenting with musculoskeletal shoulder conditions, if there are no contraindications and it is at the appropriate stage of the rehabilitation program.

For at least 100 years, clinicians from all health professions have informed people seeking care with shoulder problems that the reason for their symptoms is due to abnormal posture and that to fix the problem, the individual's posture needs improving. Current research suggests that there does not appear to be a consistent relationship between "abnormal posture" and symptoms. Furthermore, exercises prescribed to improve posture are associated with a reduction in symptoms but do not change static posture (see Chapter 20). Therefore, benefit derived from the exercises to "improve posture" may not relate to the belief that abnormal posture is the cause of the symptoms.

The same exercises are commonly prescribed as part of a shoulder strengthening program, and comparably the benefit may not be due to increased strength. Research informs us that although people with shoulder pain report improvement, their static posture does not improve with "postural" exercises and their strength doesn't improve with "strengthening" exercises. Therefore, the benefit of exercise is not due to improved posture or becoming stronger. As such, telling a patient their problem is caused by weak or deconditioned shoulder muscles and that they must get stronger to reduce their symptoms, may be the contemporary equivalent of saying their posture is at fault and all they need do is improve it.

It is important to acknowledge that improving and maintaining general body strength, being physically active and living a healthy lifestyle are valuable behaviors for current and future health, but currently available research does not support the contention that "weak" shoulders must get "strong" to reduce pain and disability, just as it doesn't support that posture must "improve" to reduce shoulder pains and disability. This is considered further in Chapters 20 and 36.

Musculoskeletal conditions involving the shoulder associated with weakness

Rotator cuff related shoulder pain

Clinicians and researchers continue to debate the most appropriate nomenclature to describe shoulder symptoms. One side of the debate is the call to retain current diagnoses such as subacromial impingement syndrome, subacromial bursitis, rotator cuff tendon tears, and rotator cuff tendinitis/tendinopathy. Those on the other side call to reject diagnostic labels, and adopt the diagnostic terminology used in the lumbar region when symptoms are not attributed to sinister (red flag) pathology or radiculopathy, e.g., aligning terms such as simple back pain, mechanical back pain, lumbago, or low back pain, with the shoulder equivalents: simple shoulder pain (± weakness), mechanical shoulder pain and weakness, or shoulder pain and weakness. There is both merit and concern on both sides of the debate.

As discussed in Chapter 15, most people presenting with shoulder symptoms seeking care will present with varying amounts of pain, weakness, stiffness, and instability (see Figure 15.1). The clinician working as a clinical detective puts together information gained during the interview and physical examination, supported as required by investigations (see Chapter 14), to make sense of presenting symptoms. For example, Person A, aged 50 years, presenting with an idiopathic onset of an extremely painful and weak nondominant-side shoulder with no signs of instability and nothing of concern detected on a radiograph, with multiplane restriction of active and passive movement, could be classified as having a painful, weak, and stiff shoulder. Alternatively, the clinician may consider that the combination of pain, weakness, and restricted movement fits into a known pattern and as such informs the patient that based on the assessment, it is *likely* that they have a frozen shoulder.

The value of classifying the combination of symptoms as a likely frozen shoulder is that it facilitates communication between health professionals, it permits research to be conducted to add much needed knowledge (see Chapter 10) to understanding pathology and management, and includes current evidence to offer best management. Those advocating for the rudimentary classification model of weak, pain, and stiff, may then suggest strengthening as the best option to address many of the symptoms, whereas in fact, current knowledge would suggest this is not best care, and although not without risk, injection therapy for an early-stage frozen shoulder is associated with better outcomes. This is not unlike a clinical diagnosis of Achilles tendinopathy or lateral elbow tendinopathy, where clinicians combine clinical reasoning, pattern recognition, patient history, and assessment, to make sense of the symptoms.

Clearly there are myriad possibilities for symptoms in these anatomical regions and a clinician could classify symptoms according to the anatomical region, such as lateral elbow pain or posterior heel pain. However, we argue, as with the term headache (head pain), findings from the history, interview, and physical examination, supported by investigations and clinical reasoning, permit clinicians to hypothesize and say, "based on our conversation and the assessment findings it is *likely* that you have lateral elbow tendinopathy/Achilles tendinopathy/migraine headaches." This should be followed by, "this is what we mean by the term", and "these are your management options."

In 2016 Lewis introduced the term rotator cuff related shoulder pain (RCRSP).[33] This is hypothesized to be present when referred pain to the shoulder (see Chapter 16) is (as best as possible) excluded, and when shoulder pain and weakness are identified, most commonly during shoulder elevation and external rotation. Another important feature suggestive of RCRSP is a history of increased muscle and tendon load preceding the onset of symptoms, or when the muscle and tendon load remains consistent but lifestyle factors that may detrimentally impact on the muscles and tendon such as poor sleep, stress, reduced physical activity, uptake of or increased smoking, or nutritional changes are identified. Since its introduction, the term RCRSP has gained increasing acceptance and has now been used in over 150 peer-reviewed publications.

The term RCRSP[33] was proposed to find middle ground in the debate between clinicians and researchers over retaining traditional diagnoses (such as partial and full thickness rotator cuff tears, subacromial impingement syndrome and subacromial bursitis), versus promoting a symptom-based classification system (painful and weak shoulder). The diagnosis of RCRSP is made based on a pattern of signs and symptoms, *and not* by referring to observed pathology, such as an acromial spur (subacromial impingement syndrome), and enlarged bursa (bursitis), or a rotator cuff tendon tear.

Informing a patient that their symptoms are due to a definitive structural problem (e.g., acromial impingement, bursitis, or tendon tear) may make the clinical process easier – this is the pathology, and the "fix" is an injection or surgery – however, this approach is no longer supported by the available research. There is also the potential for harm, wasted healthcare resources and unnecessary clinical risk if the patient is convinced that a structural pathology (that is likely to be a

Box 19.1 Clinical scenario

Clinician: *Based on our discussion and assessment it is likely that you have rotator cuff-related shoulder pain. The rotator cuff is made up of the muscles and tendons of the shoulder. They contribute to stability of the shoulder and help it to move, so you can reach up to the top of a cupboard, or throw a ball, or brush your teeth. What do you know about muscles?*

Patient: *Isn't exercise good for muscles?*

Clinician: *Absolutely, that's one of the best treatments available for RCRSP. However, before we make a final decision, I would like to discuss all the different treatment options you might like to consider, together with their benefits, and harms (risks), expected time course, what you will have to do, and expected outcomes.*

normal morphological variation) is causing symptoms and requires injection, repair, or removal. Equally, patients want to understand their symptoms. When asked by the clinician, "Why have you come to see me today?", the patient may respond, "My shoulder is sore, weak, I can't use it like I used to be able to, and I cannot sleep." Following investigations and clinical tests, if the clinician informs the patient that there doesn't appear to be anything seriously wrong with the shoulder (i.e., no red flags) and yet the shoulder is weak, stiff, and sore, they may not address all the patient's concerns.

The middle ground is to avoid an uncertain structural diagnosis and to help the patient make sense of their pain and weakness. A common clinical scenario is presented in Box 19.1.

Clearly the treatment options mentioned in the scenario above would include watch and wait, injections, surgery, and rehabilitation, all supported by advice and education. For the patient choosing rehabilitation a suggested program, Shape-Up-My-Shoulder is presented in Chapter 36.

Massive rotator cuff tears

Defining massive rotator cuff tears

Massive rotator cuff tears (RCTs) account for 10% to 40% of all RCTs and 80% of re-tears,[1,14] and fall within the spectrum of RCRSP. Although massive rotator cuff tears may result from trauma, the majority do not to have a definitive or substantial episode of trauma associated with onset of symptoms. The dimensions of large nontraumatic rotator cuff tears may increase over time and are commonly defined as massive tears when there is at least detachment of two tendons.[22] Massive tears may still respond well to surgery, although several hallmarks of massive tears, e.g., intramuscular fatty infiltration and muscular atrophy, may not improve post-surgery.[22]

As the size of a massive but repairable tear increases, or is associated with other factors, the tear may be classified as a massive inoperable rotator cuff tear, also known as an irreparable massive rotator cuff tear (iMRCT). Further common hallmarks of both repairable and irreparable rotator cuff tears are shoulder weakness and concomitant pain. The weakness may manifest as pseudoparesis, where weakness is such that there is limited active movement (i.e., less than 90° elevation, with substantially greater passive range of motion).[61] The terms pseudoparesis or pseudoparalysis were investigated in a systematic review[61] that included 16 studies, where nine did not use or define the term and seven used heterogeneous definitions. Further confusion was identified with heterogeneity relating to pain, stiffness, and arthritic changes. The findings suggest caution using these terms until the confusion is resolved. For those using pseudoparalysis to describe a clinical finding, it would be beneficial to clarify their definition.

Determining what constitutes and separates massive rotator cuff tears (MRCTs) from iMRCTs is difficult, and has resulted in confusion clinically, and in research investigations. The main reason for this is that several definitions have been proposed by different research groups and clinicians, with some definitions being used both for repairable and irreparable massive rotator cuff tears. Examples include authors who have defined massive rotator cuff tears according to tear size (≥ 5 cm/2 in),[13] number of tendons torn (≥ 2 rotator cuff tendons involved),[22] and amount of humeral head exposure.[44] In an attempt to improve clarity, Schumaier et al.[55] conducted a Delphi study that resulted in the following definition of a massive rotator cuff tear:

MRCTs should be defined as retraction of tendon(s) to the glenoid rim in either the coronal or axial plane and/or a tear with ≥67% of the greater tuberosity exposed measured in the sagittal plane. The measurement can be performed either with MRI [magnetic resonance imaging] or intraoperatively.

The Delphi study results did not incorporate the term pseudoparalysis in the final definition or include duration of symptoms.[55] The definition reached by Schumaier et al.[55] appears to be an overarching term for both massive tears where repairs might be attempted as well as irreparable tears, as they stated: "our goal was not to define whether the tear is repairable or the likelihood of healing following repair." In reality, a definition of an iMRCT would need to include tear-specific characteristics, patient-related factors, and surgical skill,[47] that would make a tear irreparable. An agreement on definitions would be beneficial to enhance clinical communication, research investigations, and patient education.

In summary, the term "massive" in relationship to rotator cuff tears is used extensively, but a definitive definition remains elusive, as does subcategorizing a massive tear as repairable or irreparable. The ongoing confusion regarding definitions requires multiprofessional consensus, as well as patient representatives to identify appropriate terminology. Future research designed to address the many areas of uncertainty relating to massive rotator cuff tears is needed.

The clinical picture is very complicated. Imaging may reveal a massive tear (retracted to the margins of the glenoid rim) that involves two or more tendons, that may or may not be associated with degenerative changes involving the glenohumeral joint and clinically will involve combinations of weakness (that may be structural and/or due to disuse atrophy and/or due to pain), stiffness (that may be due to aberrant joint biomechanics, and/or muscle guarding (due to pain and/or fear, and/or changes in sensory motor control), and pain (due to multifarious reasons). What remains clear is there are myriad possibilities for the clinical presentation.

Management of massive rotator cuff tears associated with combinations of weakness, movement restriction, and pain

The management of massive rotator cuff tears is principally divided into surgical and nonsurgical options. Surgical procedures include repair when viable, and when a repair is not viable, once the intended benefits and potential harms are evaluated and discussed with the patient, may include superior capsular reconstruction using a fascia lata autograft or acellular dermal allograft.[48,51] These procedures are more commonly considered in people with iMRCTs without advanced glenohumeral arthritis. Findings from a systematic review of superior capsular reconstruction reported good to excellent short-term clinical outcomes in pain and function in the management of iMRCTs. However, the conclusions were based upon studies that were poor to fair in quality, without long-term follow-up, and with some notable complications: retears, infections, severe fatty degeneration of infraspinatus, and postoperative shoulder stiffness.[3]

Other procedures that have been used include latissimus dorsi,[34] lower,[59] or middle[43] trapezius tendon transfers, and the arthroscopic insertion of a biodegradable subacromial spacer.[38] The majority of these procedures have not undergone rigorous placebo-controlled testing, supported by long-term outcomes. For older people with or without arthritis of the glenohumeral joint,[20,46,65] a reverse total shoulder arthroplasty is another surgical intervention for iMRCTs.

The nonsurgical management of massive (repairable or irreparable) rotator cuff tears is not supported by definitive evidence. The findings of one prospective randomized placebo-controlled trial investigated a dedicated exercise program for people diagnosed with massive >5 cm (2 in) rotator cuff tears.[2] Although subject to limitations (acknowledged by the authors), the findings suggested that greater improvement was recorded by those participating in the exercise group. (The program used in the investigation is available at: https://www.torbayandsouthdevon.nhs.uk/services/physiotherapy/support-videos/torbay-shoulder-exercise-programme/.)

Agout et al.[1] conducted a multicenter (n=12) cohort study that involved nonsurgical management for 71 people diagnosed with iMRCTs. Three patients underwent surgery in the first 3 months and 68 completed the program that included nonsteroidal anti-inflammatory medications, rehabilitation (not defined) and/or subacromial corticosteroid injections. Although at risk of substantial bias, they reported improvement in shoulder movement and function, and a reduction in pain that peaked at 6 months and remained stable at 12 months. What is clear is that the management of iMRCTs is not supported by well-designed robust clinical trials. Until these data are available the surgical and nonsurgical management of massive rotator cuff tears will remain informed by research associated with substantial bias and expert opinion.

Biceps tendinopathy

Pain in the long head of biceps (LHB) tendon may occur when the LHB tendon is subjected, in isolation or combination, to unaccustomed loads, inadequate rest after activity, and lifestyle factors. When symptomatic, the condition is diagnosed as LHB tendinopathy. As with most tendinopathies, LHB tendinopathy is associated with pain and concomitant weakness. The weakness is most likely due to inhibition of muscle performance because of pain. LHB tendinopathy is covered in detail in Chapter 26.

Calcific tendinopathy

There are myriad disorders that affect the rotator cuff tendons, one of which is calcific tendinopathy. It is characterized by the presence of calcium deposits in the rotator cuff tendons and are commonly observed in people without shoulder pain. When symptomatic, the condition is referred to as rotator cuff calcific tendinopathy (RCCT). The deposits appear to be symptomatic in approximately one-third of cases,[52] and RCCT manifests most frequently in middle-aged adults and more commonly in women.[36] Why some people remain asymptomatic, and others experience severe pain remains uncertain. When symptomatic, shoulder weakness (reduced force production) is extremely common, and the weakness is most commonly due to inhibition of muscle performance because of pain. RCCT is covered in detail in Chapter 27.

Early frozen shoulder

Frozen shoulder (FS) is a complex musculoskeletal condition affecting the shoulder in people predominantly in their sixth decade of life. Lewis[32] proposed that clinically the condition could be differentiated into two phases: shoulder pain predominant phase, and the second, shoulder stiffness predominant phase. Detectable weakness in the early phase is most probably due to inhibition of muscle performance because of pain. In the stiffness predominant phase, reduced ability to generate force may be due to many months of relative inactivity resulting in reduced muscle performance, and potentially ongoing fear of symptoms.[32] Frozen shoulder is covered in detail in Chapter 18.

Distal clavicular osteolysis

Distal clavicular osteolysis (DCO), colloquially known as weightlifter's shoulder, is an often overlooked pathology capable of contributing to the clinical presentation of a weak and painful shoulder. The mechanism underpinning the emergence of DCO can be atraumatic (ADCO), as a result of repetitive shoulder use (frequently observed with chronic weight training), or secondary to trauma.[53] Observational data reveal radiographic evidence of ADCO is present in 28% of long-term weight trained men, and, crucially, all who exhibited radiographic evidence of DCO reported experiencing shoulder pain.[53] This may suggest DCO is an important nociceptive contributor to the clinical presentation of a weak and painful shoulder.

The underlying pathoetiology of ADCO is suggested to result as an imbalance between cumulative external load and the inherent reparative capacity of the tissues within the acromioclavicular joint (ACJ).[9] Imaging may reveal widening of the ACJ, owing to lysis of the distal clavicle, subchondral fracture and a microcystic appearance of the distal clavicle.[30] Frequently, the pathology is limited to the distal clavicle, with no acromial involvement.[30] MRI is the gold standard imaging modality.

The clinical presentation of ADCO often involves pain of a dull quality local to the ACJ, which may also be tender to touch and swollen.[9] The pain location may represent an area greater than the ACJ, particularly as symptoms become more persistent, however the ACJ is often highlighted as the epicenter of the pain. Classically, pain is aggravated by pushing movements, e.g., bench pressing and push-ups, and throwing motions. Range of motion is mostly preserved, although may be painful depending on the irritability of the presentation. Pain will often worsen during a training session.

Differential diagnosis of ADCO is made clinically via history of repetitive shoulder loading and pain that is most prominent in the region of the ACJ that worsens during a training session. Physical examination may reveal sensitivity and swelling of the ACJ and pain may be reproduced by resisted pushing movements or throwing action. Weakness, if present, is often described as being generalized, and may be due to inhibition of muscle performance because of pain.

Other conditions involving the shoulder associated with weakness

The differential diagnosis of shoulder weakness should consider the possibility of a neurological cause, either from an upper or lower motor neuron source. Upper motor neuron sources could be neurological disorders such as multiple sclerosis, stroke, or motor neuron disease. Lower motor neuron sources of shoulder weakness include cervical radiculopathy, thoracic outlet syndrome, brachial neuritis, or injury to the peripheral nerves such as the long thoracic, axillary, spinal accessory, or suprascapular nerves. Cervical radiculopathy is one of the key differential diagnoses when determining the cause of shoulder weakness, particularly in the presence of radiating pain or paresthesia, or in older adults. A comprehensive assessment of the cervical spine and attendant nerve roots is essential. Thoracic outlet syndrome is similarly an important differential diagnosis in the presence of neurological signs (see Chapter 22). Less prevalent peripheral neurological causes of shoulder weakness are presented in the following section.

Brachial neuritis

Brachial neuritis, which is also known as Parsonage Turner syndrome, and neuralgic amyotrophy, are a spectrum of clinical presentations with core features of sudden onset of severe shoulder pain, which may radiate to the forearm and hand, followed by marked weakness of the shoulder, muscle atrophy, and sensory loss.[62] Causes include an interaction of genetic, mechanical, and autoimmune factors. Variations of neurological impact have been described. Commonly affected nerves include the long thoracic, anterior interosseus and suprascapular motor nerves and the lateral antebrachial cutaneous and superficial radial sensory nerves, resulting in weakness of rotator cuff and scapular stabilizing muscles.

Missed diagnosis is common and the diagnostic approach is one of exclusion, with MRI, and needle electromyography being useful investigations. It may be distinguished from cervical neuropathy (where only a single nerve root is affected) with careful neurological examination, and lack of exacerbation with neck movements.[40] Preservation of passive shoulder movement distinguishes it from frozen shoulder. Recovery of motor and sensory function occurs over a 2-year timescale, but up to 50% of patients may experience persistent, incapacitating symptoms of pain and weakness.[63] While the pain intensity usually subsides after the initial onset, persistent weakness, and resultant kinesiological changes in shoulder movement are a source of ongoing disability for many. Physical therapy (physiotherapy) input initially focuses on preservation of joint mobility, pain management and maintenance of power in non-affected musculature, according to the person's capacity. Once reinnervation has begun, a gradual, progressive exercise program may be implemented.

Peripheral nerve injury

Peripheral nerve injuries may be a feature of traumatic shoulder injury. Such nerve injuries range from neuropraxia, caused by transient ischemia and focal demyelination, where recovery occurs within 12 weeks, to complete axonal disruption where there is little capacity to recover without surgical intervention.[4] The incidence of *axillary nerve injury*, with resultant deltoid paralysis, has been reported in 13–21% of glenohumeral joint dislocations.[50,60] Up to 67% of proximal humeral fractures demonstrate various grades of traction-related nerve injury, most commonly affecting the axillary nerve.[64] The axillary nerve is also vulnerable to compression in the quadrilateral space of the posterior shoulder, presenting as a mild neuropraxia in throwing athletes.

While *long thoracic nerve palsy* may occur as part of a brachial neuritis presentation, it may also arise as an isolated occurrence. An identifiable history of nerve trauma, compression or stretch from occupational or athletic activities is present in some cases, while for others it appears to be idiopathic. Scapular winging will be observed, along with weakness of the serratus anterior muscle, with accompanying pain and limitation of active shoulder elevation. Manual stabilization of the scapula with the examiner's hand may result in an improved range of shoulder elevation, reduced pain, and improved muscle performance. Rehabilitation comprises an exercise program for the remaining scapular stabilizing muscles, and maintenance of shoulder range of motion. Scapular taping or bracing may provide some symptomatic relief. The majority of cases resolve over a 6–24-month timescale.[21] Surgical opinion should be sought for those not spontaneously resolving.[45] Other less commonly reported neuropathies are of the *suprascapular* and *spinal accessory nerves.*

Accessory nerve injury has been reported as a consequence of cervical lymph node biopsy.[42] The suprascapular nerve can be compressed by space-occupying lesions in the suprascapular notch such as cysts. Electrodiagnostic tests along with appropriate targeted MRI can supplement the clinical examination and support a diagnosis of nerve entrapment.[8]

In summary, knowledge of the neurological structure and function of the shoulder is necessary to understand the causes, impact, and prognosis of neurological shoulder weakness. A multidisciplinary approach should be employed including medical, radiological, surgical, and occupational therapy colleagues as required. The nature of these disorders necessitates a prolonged phase of rehabilitation, with unpredictable recovery trajectories, therefore a strong therapeutic alliance with the patient will be foremost in optimizing outcomes.

Osteomyelitis

Osteo (bone) myelitis (inflammation) is an infection of bone and has been present throughout human history, with discussion of the condition dating to the time of Hippocrates (460–370 BCE).[54]

There have been many terms used to describe the condition, with Nelaton acknowledged as introducing osteomyelitis in 1844.[54] The annual incidence of pediatric osteomyelitis is disproportionally higher in low-income countries (43–200 per 100,000 children)[17] when compared to high-income countries (2–13 per 100,000).[17,49] It appears to be more common in adults, and in a study from a highly economically developed country, the annual incidence in adults was reported as 90 individuals per 100,000, in comparison to 13 per 100,000 children.[49] The condition appears to be more common in males. *Staphylococcus aureus* is the most common bacteria which causes osteomyelitis, but it may be caused by other bacteria and more rarely by a fungal infection.

The most common sites for osteomyelitis are the vertebrae, pelvis, and long bones such as the clavicle[10] and humerus,[56] and has also been reported in the sternoclavicular joint,[29] and scapula.[23,26] The infection involves the bone and bone marrow and results in necrosis. The infection can be acute or persistent. When osteomyelitis involves the shoulder there will typically be considerable pain and weakness (due to pain and muscle atrophy),[31] but this will not occur in isolation. Acute osteomyelitis will develop over 7–10 days and symptoms include fever, fatigue, nausea, pain, warmth, swelling, and tenderness in the infected area. There will also be a loss of motion. Risk factors for osteomyelitis include diabetes, human immunodeficiency virus, peripheral vascular disease, sickle cell disease, rheumatoid arthritis, intravenous drug use, removal of the spleen, tuberculosis, joint replacement, alcoholism, smoking, long-term steroid use, immunosuppression, hemodialysis, trauma (such as a fracture), surgery including dental treatment, and vaccine administration.

Tumors and inflammatory arthropathies involving the shoulder

Benign and malignant tumors may also be a cause of shoulder pain and weakness. We can never exclude red flags, and must remain constantly vigilant for any changes in the patient's story and symptoms that may suggest the clinical presentation is not musculoskeletal, or not purely musculoskeletal, in origin. Rheumatoid arthritis is the most common type of inflammatory arthropathy involving the shoulder,[16] and will affect the shoulders of more than 90% of people who have had the condition for more than five years.[16] Rheumatoid arthritis has a prevalence of approximately 1% and affects women more than men (3:1).[16] Other and rarer inflammatory conditions affecting the shoulder that will also be associated with pain and weakness include psoriatic arthritis, polymyalgia rheumatica, Reiter's syndrome, Lyme disease, ankylosing spondylitis, and crystalline arthropathies (gout, pseudogout, and Milwaukee shoulder).[16]

Chapters 8, 14, 15, 16, 22, and 25 include discussions on red flag conditions such as tumors, inflammatory conditions, other pathologies, and structures that can refer to the shoulder, that may cause shoulder pain and associated weakness.

Traumatic presentations

Muscle weakness is an inevitable consequence of significant trauma to the shoulder such as fractures, traumatic tendon tears, or dislocation, and following shoulder surgery. Pain, tissue damage, fear of movement and disuse may all be mediators of the loss of strength. While immobilization is a common early management strategy to facilitate healing, it is important to consider its negative impact on shoulder strength.

Increasingly, post shoulder injury and surgery protocols encouraging early mobilization to counteract these potential negative effects and foster early restoration of shoulder strength and mobility are being seen as safe and effective.[25,41] Management of post-trauma weakness should be guided by a joint decision-making process between the medical and surgical team, physical therapist and patient, informed by imaging findings and known healing timescales. Further information is presented in Chapters 24, 29, and 41.

Summary

Shoulder weakness is one of the most common concerns for people presenting with shoulder complaints. It has also been shown to be a risk factor for future injury in athletic populations. Management of weakness requires a comprehensive approach, founded on knowledge of causes, proficiency in assessment techniques, and skilled planning and progression of rehabilitation programs, with patient education and shared decision-making at the center. The approach to rehabilitation will vary according to baseline neuromuscular function, concurrent symptoms, patient goals and capacity, and overall prognosis and recovery trajectory. It is important to emphasize that although it seems counterintuitive, the corollary of shoulder weakness is not always shoulder strengthening exercises.

References

1. Agout C, Berhouet J, Spiry C, et al. Functional outcomes after non-operative treatment of irreparable massive rotator cuff tears: prospective multicenter study in 68 patients. Orthopaedics & Traumatology: Surgery & Research. 2018;104:S189-S192.
2. Ainsworth R, Lewis J, Conboy V. A prospective randomized placebo controlled clinical trial of a rehabilitation programme for patients with a diagnosis of massive rotator cuff tears of the shoulder. Shoulder & Elbow. 2009;1:55-60.
3. Altintas B, Scheidt M, Kremser V, et al. Superior capsule reconstruction for irreparable massive rotator cuff tears: does it make sense? A systematic review of early clinical evidence. The American Journal of Sports Medicine. 2020;48:3365-3375.
4. Avis D, Power D. Axillary nerve injury associated with glenohumeral dislocation: a review and algorithm for management. EFORT Open Rev. 2018;3:70-77.
5. Bohannon RW. Considerations and practical options for measuring muscle strength: a narrative review. Biomed Res Int. 2019;2019:8194537.
6. Bohannon RW. Reliability of manual muscle testing: a systematic review. Isokinetics and Exercise Science. 2018;26:245-252.
7. Borms D, Maenhout A, Cools AM. Upper quadrant field tests and isokinetic upper limb strength in overhead athletes. J Athl Train. 2016;51:789-796.
8. Budzik JF, Wavreille G, Pansini V, Moraux A, Demondion X, Cotten A. Entrapment neuropathies of the shoulder. Magn Reson Imaging Clin N Am. 2012;20:373-391, xii.
9. Cahill B. Atraumatic osteolysis of the distal clavicle: a review. Sports Med. 1992;13:214-22.
10. Chen C, Yin Y, Xu H, Li Z, Wang F, Chen G. Personalized three-dimensional printed polyether-ether-ketone prosthesis for reconstruction after subtotal removal of chronic clavicle osteomyelitis: a case report. Medicine. 2021;100:e25703.
11. Clarsen B, Bahr R, Andersson SH, Munk R, Myklebust G. Reduced glenohumeral rotation, external rotation weakness and scapular dyskinesis are risk factors for shoulder injuries among elite male handball players: a prospective cohort study. Br J Sports Med. 2014;48:1327-1333.
12. Clausen MB, Witten A, Holm K, et al. Glenohumeral and scapulothoracic strength impairments exists in patients with subacromial impingement, but these are not reflected in the shoulder pain and disability index. BMC Musculoskelet Disord. 2017;18:302.
13. Cofield R. Subscapular muscle transposition for repair of chronic rotator cuff tears. Surgery, Gynecology & Obstetrics. 1982;154:667-672.
14. Denard PJ, Jiwani AZ, Lädermann A, Burkhart SS. Long-term outcome of arthroscopic massive rotator cuff repair: the importance of double-row fixation. Arthroscopy. 2012;28:909-915.
15. Dollings H, Sandford F, O'Conaire E, Lewis JS. Shoulder strength testing: the intra-and inter-tester reliability of routine clinical tests, using the PowerTrack II Commander. Shoulder & Elbow. 2012;4:131-140.
16. Duquin T, Sperling J. Inflammatory Arthropathies of the Shoulder. Cancer Therapy Advisor. Available at: https://www.cancertherapyadvisor.com/home/decision-support-in-medicine/shoulder-and-elbow/inflammatory-arthropathies-of-the-shoulder/.

17. Emeagui N, Obu G, Opara H, et al. Paediatric osteomyelitis in a tertiary hospital in South-South Nigeria: clinical experience at Federal Medical Centre Asaba. Journal of Advances in Medicine and Medical Research. 2020;57-64.

18. Engel GL. The need for a new medical model: a challenge for biomedicine. Science. 1977;196:129-136.

19. Eriksrud O, Bohannon RW. Relationship of knee extension force to independence in sit-to-stand performance in patients receiving acute rehabilitation. Physical Therapy. 2003;83:544-551.

20. Flynn L, Struk A, Wright TW. Reverse total shoulder arthroplasty for irreparable rotator cuff tears. Operative Techniques in Orthopaedics. 2018;28:238-243.

21. Friedenberg SM, Zimprich T, Harper CM. The natural history of long thoracic and spinal accessory neuropathies. Muscle Nerve. 2002;25:535-539.

22. Gerber C, Fuchs B, Hodler J. The results of repair of massive tears of the rotator cuff. JBJS. 2000;82:505.

23. Gerber N, Fawcett K, Bittman M, Beiner J. Osteomyelitis in an unusual location with an atypical presentation: a case report and review of the literature of scapular osteomyelitis in pediatric patients. Pediatric Emergency Care. 2021;37:e149-e151.

24. Hams AH, Evans K, Adams R, Waddington G, Witchalls J. Shoulder internal and external rotation strength and prediction of subsequent injury in water-polo players. Scand J Med Sci Sports. 2019;29:1414-1420.

25. Handoll H, Brealey S, Rangan A, et al. The ProFHER (PROximal Fracture of the Humerus: Evaluation by Randomisation) trial - a pragmatic multicentre randomised controlled trial evaluating the clinical effectiveness and cost-effectiveness of surgical compared with non-surgical treatment for proximal fracture of the humerus in adults. Health Technol Assess. 2015;19:1-280.

26. Hébert-Seropian S, Pelet S. Aspergillus osteomyelitis of the scapula: a case report. JBJS Case Connector. 2020;10:e0343.

27. Holt KL, Raper DP, Boettcher CE, Waddington GS, Drew MK. Hand-held dynamometry strength measures for internal and external rotation demonstrate superior reliability, lower minimal detectable change and higher correlation to isokinetic dynamometry than externally-fixed dynamometry of the shoulder. Phys Ther Sport. 2016;21:75-81. 10.1016/j.ptsp.2016.07.001

28. Horsley I, Herrington L, Hoyle R, Prescott E, Bellamy N. Do changes in hand grip strength correlate with shoulder rotator cuff function? Shoulder Elbow. 2016;8:124-129.

29. González Muñoz JI, Córdoba Peláez M, Tébar Boti E, Téllez Cantero JC, Castedo Mejuto E, Varela de Ugarte A. Surgical treatment of sternoclavicular osteomyelitis. Archivos De Bronconeumologia. 1996;32:541-543.

30. Kassarjian A, Llopis E, Palmer WE. Distal clavicular osteolysis: MR evidence for subchondral fracture. Skeletal Radiol. 2007;36:17-22.

31. Kendall J, McNally M. Septic arthritis of the shoulder with proximal humerus osteomyelitis, treated by Ilizarov shoulder arthrodesis. J Bone Jt Infect. 2017;2:90-95.

32. Lewis J. Frozen shoulder contracture syndrome: aetiology, diagnosis and management. Man Ther. 2015;20:2-9.

33. Lewis J. Rotator cuff related shoulder pain: assessment, management and uncertainties. Man Ther. 2016;23:57-68.

34. Li X. Editorial commentary: is it time to abandon the latissimus dorsi tendon transfer as a salvage procedure for patients with large irreparable rotator cuff tears that failed primary repair? Arthroscopy. 2020;36:95-98.

35. Lombardi I, Jr., Magri AG, Fleury AM, Da Silva AC, Natour J. Progressive resistance training in patients with shoulder impingement syndrome: a randomized controlled trial. Arthritis Rheum. 2008;59:615-622.

36. Louwerens JK, Sierevelt IN, van Hove RP, van den Bekerom MP, van Noort A. Prevalence of calcific deposits within the rotator cuff tendons in adults with and without subacromial pain syndrome: clinical and radiologic analysis of 1219 patients. Journal of Shoulder and Elbow Surgery. 2015;24:1588-1593.

37. MacDermid JC, Ramos J, Drosdowech D, Faber K, Patterson S. The impact of rotator cuff pathology on isometric and isokinetic strength, function, and quality of life. J Shoulder Elbow Surg. 2004;13:593-598.

38. Malahias M-A, Brilakis E, Avramidis G, Trellopoulos A, Antonogiannakis E. Arthroscopic partial repair with versus without biodegradable subacromial spacer for patients with massive rotator cuff tears: a case–control study. Musculoskeletal Surgery. 2020;1-9.

39. Malliaras P, Johnston R, Street G, et al. The efficacy of higher versus lower dose exercise in rotator cuff tendinopathy: a systematic review of randomized controlled trials. Arch Phys Med Rehabil. 2020;10:1822-1834.

40. Mamula CJ, Erhard RE, Piva SR. Cervical radiculopathy or Parsonage-Turner syndrome: differential diagnosis of a patient with neck and upper extremity symptoms. J Orthop Sports Phys Ther. 2005;35:659-664.

41. Mazuquin BF, Wright AC, Russell S, Monga P, Selfe J, Richards J. Effectiveness of early compared with conservative rehabilitation for patients having rotator cuff repair surgery: an overview of systematic reviews. Br J Sports Med. 2018;52:111-121.

42. Minami R, Ito E, Nishijima N. Trapezius palsy resulting from accessory nerve injury after cervical lymph node biopsy dramatically improved with conservative treatment. Prog Rehabil Med. 2016;1:20160006.

43. Moroder P, Akgün D, Lacheta L, et al. Middle trapezius transfer for treatment of irreparable supraspinatus tendon tears: anatomical feasibility study. Journal of Experimental Orthopaedics. 2021;8:5.

44. Nobuhara K, Hata Y, Komai M. Surgical procedure and results of repair of massive tears of the rotator cuff. Clinical Orthopaedics and Related Research. 1994;304:54-59.

45. Noland SS, Krauss EM, Felder JM, Mackinnon SE. Surgical and clinical decision making in isolated long thoracic nerve palsy. Hand (N Y). 2018;13:689-694.

46. Pandya J, Johnson T, Low AK. Shoulder replacement for osteoarthritis: a review of surgical management. Maturitas. 2018;108:71-76.

47. Plachel F, Siegert P, Moroder P, et al. Treatment of non-arthritic pseudoparetic shoulders with irreparable massive rotator cuff tears: arthroscopic procedures yield comparable midterm results to reverse arthroplasty. BMC Musculoskeletal Disorders. 2021;22:1-9.

48. Prinja A, Mohan H, Singh J, Walton M, Funk L, Monga P. Superior capsular

reconstruction for irreparable rotator cuff tears: a literature review and specialist practice report. Journal of Clinical Orthopaedics and Trauma. 2021;19:62-66.

49. Riise ØR, Kirkhus E, Handeland KS, et al. Childhood osteomyelitis-incidence and differentiation from other acute onset musculoskeletal features in a population-based study. BMC Pediatrics. 2008;8:1-10.

50. Robinson CM, Shur N, Sharpe T, Ray A, Murray IR. Injuries associated with traumatic anterior glenohumeral dislocations. J Bone Joint Surg Am. 2012;94:18-26.

51. Roth TS, Welsh ML, Osbahr DC, Varma A. Arthroscopic single-row superior capsular reconstruction for irreparable rotator cuff tears. Arthroscopy Techniques. 2020;9:e675-e681.

52. Sansone V, Consonni O, Maiorano E, Meroni R, Goddi A. Calcific tendinopathy of the rotator cuff: the correlation between pain and imaging features in symptomatic and asymptomatic female shoulders. Skeletal Radiology. 2016;45:49-55.

53. Scavenius M, Iversen, BF. Nontraumatic clavicular osteolysis in weight lifters. AJSM. 1992;20:463-7.

54. Schmitt SK. Osteomyelitis. Infectious Disease Clinics of North America. 2017;31:325-338.

55. Schumaier A, Kovacevic D, Schmidt C, et al. Defining massive rotator cuff tears: a Delphi consensus study. Journal of Shoulder and Elbow Surgery. 2020;29:674-680.

56. Smith SS, Lee Y, Wang L. Adolescent with osteomyelitis after intramuscular administration of a vaccine: a case report. Journal of the American Pharmacists Association. 2020;60:e357-e360.

57. Stark T, Walker B, Phillips JK, Fejer R, Beck R. Hand-held dynamometry correlation with the gold standard isokinetic dynamometry: a systematic review. PM R. 2011;3:472-479.

58. Stevenson A. Oxford Dictionary of English. Oxford University Press, USA; 2010.

59. Stoll LE, Codding JL. Lower trapezius tendon transfer for massive irreparable rotator cuff tears. Orthop Clin North Am. 2019;50:375-382.

60. te Slaa RL, Wijffels MP, Brand R, Marti RK. The prognosis following acute primary glenohumeral dislocation. J Bone Joint Surg Br. 2004;86:58-64.

61. Tokish JM, Alexander TC, Kissenberth MJ, Hawkins RJ. Pseudoparalysis: a systematic review of term definitions, treatment approaches, and outcomes of management techniques. Journal of Shoulder and Elbow Surgery. 2017;26:e177-e187.

62. van Alfen N. Clinical and pathophysiological concepts of neuralgic amyotrophy. Nat Rev Neurol. 2011;7:315-322.

63. van Alfen N, van Engelen BG. The clinical spectrum of neuralgic amyotrophy in 246 cases. Brain. 2006;129:438-450.

64. Visser CP, Coene LN, Brand R, Tavy DL. Nerve lesions in proximal humeral fractures. J Shoulder Elbow Surg. 2001;10:421-427.

65. Viswanath A, Bale S, Trail I. Reverse total shoulder arthroplasty for irreparable rotator cuff tears without arthritis: a systematic review. Journal of Clinical Orthopaedics and Trauma. 2021;17:267-272.

66. Wikholm J, Bohannon, RW. Hand-held dynamometer measurements: tester strength makes a difference. J Orthop Sports Phys Ther. 1991;13:191-198.

Posture 20

Jeremy Lewis, Filip Struyf

Introduction

Over the past century, considerable attention has been given to the relationship between upper body posture and the development and perpetuation of shoulder pain. Many logical and well-reasoned hypotheses supporting these relationships have been proposed, accepted, and integrated into clinical assessment and practice. Clinicians commonly identify one or more postural abnormalities, and people seeking an explanation for their shoulder symptoms are frequently informed that abnormalities in upper body posture and scapular position are at the heart of their symptoms. They are also informed that the key to reducing pain and disability is to improve their posture, which might entail decreasing the thoracic kyphosis, reducing a forward head posture, and repositioning the scapula into its correct position.

The purpose of this chapter is to investigate these beliefs. We will explore our understanding of posture from both historic and contemporary perspectives. We will present what is known about posture, and what is hypothesized. We will synthesize the available literature and discuss the value of assessing and treating suspected deviations of body posture and scapular position for people presenting with musculoskeletal problems of the shoulder.

What is it about posture?

The "perfect" upright standing posture that is considered "normal" and the benchmark to assess for postural abnormality in Western society appears to have originated in the late 16th century during military training drills.[34] The importance of good posture permeated into civilian life during the 19th century and became synonymous with good health, while poor posture became correspondingly associated with poor health, and inferior character. For example, Quasimodo the bell ringer in Victor Hugo's *The Hunchback of Notre-Dame* (1831) is described as wicked and ugly, and a physical monstrosity. German physician, Daniel Gottlob Moritz Schreber (1808–1861), concerned about the impact on health of the industrial revolution, developed a systematic remedial exercise program and devices to improve posture (Figure 20.1). German anatomist, Christian Wilhelm Braune (1831–1892) and physiologist, Otto Fischer (1861–1917) identified the body's center of gravity,[16] and their research added momentum to the medicalization of posture.

During the Victorian and Edwardian eras in the United Kingdom, deportment classes that encouraged good posture were popular among the more affluent – and good posture was proposed as a way of fighting consumption (tuberculosis). Stiff and wide collars (Figure 20.2) became part of fashion for men and women. Without doubt they would have made a forward-poking chin or slouched posture impossible but would also have restricted normal head movement and function.

Later, in the early to mid-20th century, women were taught to "improve" their postures by walking with books on their head.[117] And in the United States, based on a combination of clinical and radiological assessment, women could compete in the annual Miss Correct Posture competition, a competition run by chiropractors.[118]

The medicalization of posture and the assumption that good posture meant good health became integrated into clinical practice. For example, Braun and Amundson[15] stated that assessment of posture is an important component of the clinical examination and the findings will affect the design of the treatment program. This is based on the belief that deviations from normal posture subject the body to abnormal stress, potentially resulting in pain and a loss of function, thus leading to the clinical truism that correction of posture will reduce stress, decrease pain, and improve function.[48-50,53,54,86,104]

In the absence of an alternative explanation, many clinicians continue to inform patients that "your poor posture" is the underlying cause for their symptoms.[48,71] One specific example is that poor upper body posture, colloquially termed a "slouched" posture, has been commonly cited as a potential etiological factor in the pathogenesis of many upper body conditions, including those affecting the shoulder such as subacromial impingement syndrome.[4,39,97] Many authors refer to a slouched posture as a forward head posture (FHP). The FHP has been associated with an increase in the thoracic kyphosis, an anterior translation of

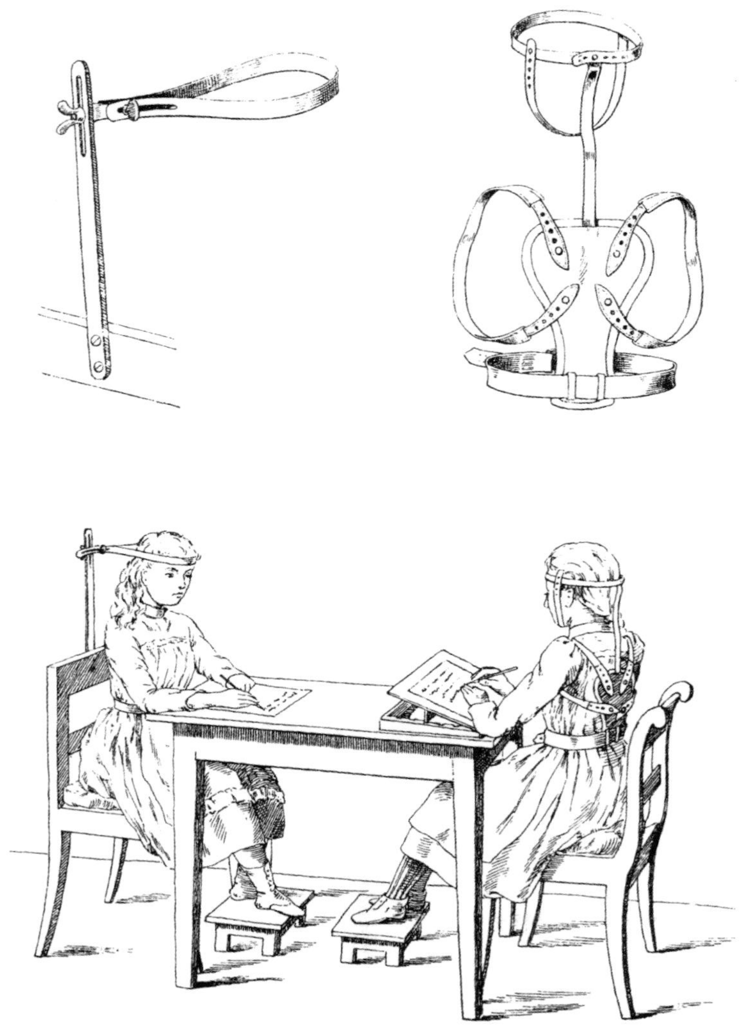

FIGURE 20.1
Moritz Schreber's devices to improve posture.
(Wikimedia Commons. https://commons.wikimedia.org/wiki/File:Geradhalter_(Schreber).png.)

the head on the neck (and body) and an altered scapular position.[4,48,50,89] In the shoulder, these changes are thought to compromise the subacromial structures leading to the development of subacromial impingement. The following is an example:

In a person with good postural alignment, elevation of the arm is free to proceed through a full 160° to 180° of motion without impingement of soft tissues in the subacromial space. In the patient with the classic forward head, rounded shoulders, and increased thoracic kyphosis, the scapula rotates forward and downward, depressing the acromial process and changing the direction of the glenoid fossa. Now as the patient attempts to elevate the arm, the supraspinatus tendon and/or the subdeltoid bursa may become impinged against the anterior portion of the acromion process.[39]

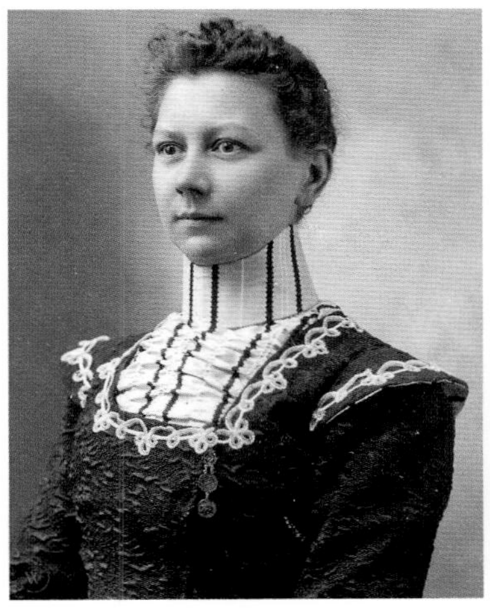

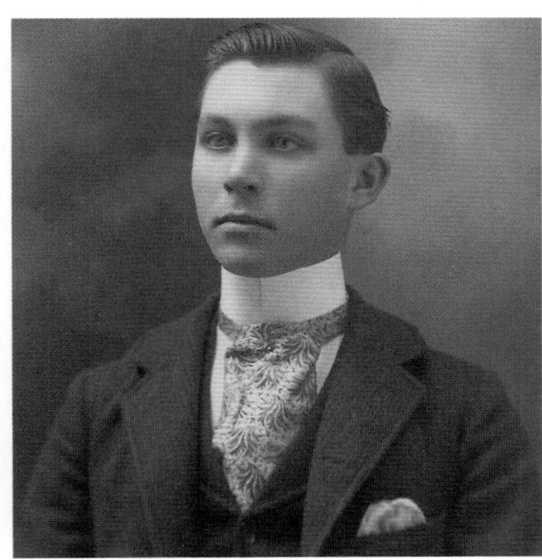

FIGURE 20.2
Collars to control head posture.
(Left: https://www.worthpoint.com/worthopedia/edwardian-woman-high-neck-collar-1852471947. Right: https://www.pinterest.co.uk/pin/316870523753655998/.)

Defining posture

Normal posture

Posture has been defined as *the relative position of parts of the body*[98] and *the attitude of the body.*[2] Kendall et al.[48,50] stated that good posture is dependent upon an ideal alignment of the body and a normal balance of the skeletal musculature. Ideal static standing posture has been defined by Kendall et al.[48] as the line passing through the points outlined in Table 20.1.

Table 20.1 The points a line should pass through in the sagittal plane in a person with ideal posture

Anatomical structures	Surface landmarks
• Slightly posterior to the apex of the coronal suture • External auditory meatus • The dens of the axis • The bodies of the cervical vertebrae • The bodies of the lumbar vertebrae • The sacral promontory • Slightly posterior to the center of the hip • Slightly anterior to the center of the knee • Slightly anterior to the lateral malleolus • Through the calcaneo-cuboid joint	• The lobe of the ear • Through the middle of the shoulder joint • Midway through the front and back of • the thorax • Midway through the back and abdomen • Through the greater trochanter of the femur • Slightly anterior to the midline of the knee • Slightly anterior to the lateral malleolus

Abnormal posture

The American Academy of Orthopaedic Surgeons (1947) stated that poor posture is a faulty relationship of the various parts of the body,[105] which produces increased strain on the supporting structures.[48] Turner[108] argued that pain is an almost inevitable consequence of a faulty posture, and, Kendall et al.[48,50] stated that poor posture is not merely an aesthetic enigma, as it may give rise to discomfort and disability. These concepts have permeated into clinical practice and the importance of postural assessment as an integral part of the clinical examination are found in medical,[19,53] physical therapy (physiotherapy),[4,39] and osteopathic[104] literature. Following these principles, an individual's posture is compared to an ideal norm and deviations are often considered to be the basis of pathology. These concepts of posture have been based primarily on extensive clinical observation and opinion. The following section introduces commonly observed postural presentations that are considered abnormal and believed to cause, contribute, or perpetuate symptoms.

Forward head posture

Forward head posture (FHP), is considered to be present when the head is held forward of the shoulders and has been cited as a potential etiologic factor in the pathogenesis of subacromial impingement syndrome.[39,89] This is because FHP has been associated with an increase in the thoracic kyphosis angle, a forward shoulder posture (FSP), and a scapula that is positioned in relatively more elevation, protraction, downward rotation, and anterior tilt.[19,39,48] The effect of these changes leads to a loss of glenohumeral flexion and abduction range,[19,39,53] compression and irritation of the uppermost (bursal) surface of the supraspinatus tendon, and a reduction in the range of glenohumeral elevation.[4,53,89]

Static scapular position and dyskinesis

Scapular position and movement may be clinically defined as normal or abnormal. Abnormal movement is termed scapular dyskinesis. Definitions of abnormal scapular posture and movement are multifarious, and the reliability and validity of many assessment methods appear equivocal. In a relaxed static position, the scapula may be classified as being "overly" elevated, depressed, protracted, retracted, rotated (upward or downward), and tilted (anteriorly or posteriorly). Scapular position is dependent upon the shape of the thorax and its connection to the trunk via the clavicle and the surrounding muscles that position it. Scapular position may be influenced by normal variations in body shape, bone shape, and muscle mass. It may also be influenced by multiple pathologies, including trauma, nerve damage, and the presence of osteochondromas.[13,94]

If the medial border and/or inferior angle of the scapula are posteriorly displaced away from the thorax, this is considered by many as abnormal scapular posture and is referred to as winging or scapular winging. However, from the clinical observation of static scapular position of an individual presenting with musculoskeletal shoulder symptoms, it is difficult to determine whether changes such as winging are within normal range, or are causing, contributing to, or resulting from symptoms. The complexity is further compounded as side-to-side asymmetries are common in people without symptoms.

The scapula provides a base of support for the humeral head. As discussed in Chapter 4, available research attests to a predictable relationship between the glenoid fossa and humeral head during most shoulder movements. Scapular movement and/or position are determined by the shape of the thorax, muscle control, lower limb energy transfer, presence of pain, and the biomechanics of the glenohumeral, acromio- and sternoclavicular joints.[101] Scapular movement is dependent upon the shape of the thorax and its connection to the trunk via the clavicle and the surrounding muscles that move and position it. An alteration in movement of the scapula, especially if it is erratic, not smooth, or excessive, is referred to as scapular dyskinesis. To standardize understanding between clinicians, we recommend the following classification of scapular dyskinesis:[70,102]

1. A premature or excessive elevation, depression, protraction, rotation, or tilt of the scapula, and/or,
2. An erratic or jerking motion of the scapular during arm elevation and/or return, and/or,
3. A rapid downward rotation of the scapula during arm return.

If none of the above is present, the clinician may document that no scapular dyskinesis was observed. If any of the above are observed individually or in combination, then scapular dyskinesis may be documented and classified as subtle or obvious. If any of the above are not consistent or just perceptible then the diagnosis is subtle. When consistent and clearly observed, the diagnosis is obvious dyskinesis. Although scapular dyskinesis may cause or contribute to symptoms, we again urge caution in implicating scapular dyskinesis as the cause of symptoms from observation alone, as it may be asymptomatic, or it may be a consequence of an underlying pathology.

Proximal crossed syndrome

Janda[43-45] proposed that muscle imbalance and subsequent posture abnormalities occurred within the musculoskeletal system due to characteristic differences in muscle types. Postural muscles, that tend to span more than one joint, become shortened, hyperactive, and lose their extensibility. Phasic muscles respond in an opposite fashion, becoming hypotonic and atrophy. In the upper body, Janda implicated pectoralis major, levator scapulae, sternocleidomastoid, scalenes, and upper trapezius as postural muscles, and the lower trapezius, rhomboids, and serratus anterior as phasic muscles.[43-45] An imbalance between the postural and phasic muscles results in a forward head and increased kyphotic posture with a concomitant change in scapular position. Janda called this imbalance upper crossed, or proximal crossed syndrome, and to improve posture, stretching the postural muscles was a principle focus of treatment.[43-45]

SICK scapula syndrome

The term SICK scapula was introduced by Burkhart et al.[18] to describe a pathological position of the scapula characterized by: *s*capular malposition, *i*nferior medial border prominence, *c*oracoid pain and malposition, and dys*k*inesis of scapular movement. Symptoms associated with SICK scapula include anterior and superior shoulder pain, posterosuperior scapular region pain, coracoid pain, and combinations of these pain presentations. Abnormalities of scapular position, i.e., when SICK, have been associated with subacromial impingement syndrome, reduced rotator cuff strength, tendinopathy, and generalized shoulder pain.[40] As described above, the muscles that position and move the scapulae are considered a primary target to treat the symptoms associated with this postural abnormality, and combinations of stretching, strengthening, and so called soft-tissue "release" techniques are recommended to achieve a better posture.[18,23]

The etiology of forward head posture

FHP is one of the most commonly observed postural abnormalities, and it has been associated with carpal tunnel syndrome,[116] cervical pain and radiculopathy,[4,41,67] headache,[113] myofascial pain syndrome,[107] temporomandibular joint dysfunction,[86] thoracic outlet syndrome,[104] thoracic pain,[43,45] shoulder pain,[14,19] and subacromial impingement syndrome.[39]

McKenzie[71] proposed that prolonged sitting may be a predisposing factor for FHP. Other causative factors that have been suggested include sedentary habits,[68] poorly equipped work sites, and lack of postural awareness.[37] Psychological factors such as anxiety, insecurity, fear, or despondency may be a cause of excessive thoracic kyphosis and FHP.[32] Calliet[19] suggested that structural change, emotions and bi- or trifocal spectacles may play a part in the development of FHP. Rasch and Burke[84] have suggested that injury, disease, muscular or nervous weakness, heredity, or improper clothing may be factors. Mouth breathing has also been considered a predisposing factor to FHP.[27] Neviaser[76] stated that the two main underlying causes of postural disturbances were poor occupational and sleeping habits. A relationship between the use of smartphones, FHP, and scapular dyskinesis has been reported.[1]

Abnormal posture and its relationship with shoulder pain and disability

With respect to musculoskeletal shoulder conditions, postural theorists have commonly described how abnormalities in posture cause, contribute, and lead to the perpetuation of subacromial impingement syndrome.[4,14,15,19,39,45,48,51,77,86,97] Clinical theorists have proposed how an FHP and an associated increase in the thoracic kyphosis can compromise shoulder function.[4,39,43,90] This combined postural abnormality will cause the scapulae to elevate, abduct (protract), downwardly rotate (glenoid fossa faces downwards and inferior angle moves towards the spine), and tilt anteriorly (acromion moves more anteriorly). This will be associated with an increased internal rotation of the humerus in the neutral position.[39,43,48]

Postural theorists argue that these changes occur concurrently with a lengthening and weakening of the deep neck flexors, major and minor rhomboids, middle and inferior trapezius, infraspinatus and teres minor, and a serratus anterior less capable of stabilizing the scapula on the thoracic wall during upper limb function. The pectoralis major and minor will shorten, as well as latissimus dorsi, subscapularis and teres major.[39,43,48,90] The elevated position of the scapula[48,86] has been associated with a shortened levator scapulae, which causes the downward rotation of the scapula.[21,43] In contrast, Darnell[27] described a weakening of the levator scapulae due to dorsal scapula nerve entrapment, and Calliet[19] proposed that the downward rotation of the scapula would elongate the levator scapulae, leading to irritation of its insertion.

The downwardly rotated, protracted, elevated, and anteriorly tilted scapula will alter the normal scapulohumeral mechanism. The loss of normal serratus anterior function implies a scapula that is unable to adequately upwardly rotate and act as a base of support for the humerus. Clinically, this may also be associated with a "winging scapula".[48] Due to its attachment on the coracoid process, a shortened pectoralis minor will pull the acromion anteriorly,[21,90] and the downwardly rotated and anteriorly tilted scapula will cause a mechanical block to elevation of the arm, causing compression of the subacromial contents by the acromion, leading to impingement symptoms.

Scapular elevation occurs due to weakness of the inferior trapezius and shortening of the levator scapulae as well as the upper trapezius. This will lead to an altered scapular movement pattern on the thoracic wall during arm elevation with the potential of compromise of the subacromial contents.[39] The shortened pectoralis major, subscapularis, teres minor and latissimus dorsi will internally rotate the humerus, stretching the supraspinatus, teres minor, and infraspinatus as well as the biceps tendon.[4,39,43,48,53,54] This will cause the anterior shoulder capsule to shorten.[4,39] This is confusing, as other authors have described a contracture of the posterior capsule[109] in association with the impingement process. Evidence to validate the existence of posterior or anterior joint capsule contraction, or information detailing different areas of contracture occurring in different pathological processes, is not available.

It has been argued that the internal rotation of the humerus will limit the range of glenohumeral external rotation, abduction and extension, during upper limb activity.[4,39] The pectoralis major acting on the humerus will pull the shoulder girdle into protraction, which together with weakened and lengthened retractors suggests that the scapula cannot be fully retracted prior to certain upper limb activities, such as throwing.[53,54] This loss of retraction range implies that the pectoralis major cannot be adequately stretched, reducing the energy and force the muscle has available to propel the arm forwards during throwing, or related activities.[53,54] The effect of this is a potential increase in demand on other shoulder muscles including the rotator cuff, which may lead to early fatigue and failure.

The loss of adequate retraction range and the inability for the retractors to slow the shoulder eccentrically after forceful forward movement, implies increased strain on the static shoulder stabilizers such as the capsule, glenohumeral ligaments and labrum, with the potential to cause injury to these structures.[53,54] The lack of thoracic extension due to the increased thoracic kyphosis will lead to a reduction in range of glenohumeral elevation, leading to compromise and impingement on the subacromial contents under the acromion.[19,53,54,97]

Ayub[4] also suggested that the protracted position of the scapulae may result in increased acromioclavicular joint compression, which may shorten the conoid ligament while lengthening the trapezoid ligament (see Figure 4.2). This would cause the clavicle to slide posteriorly on the sternum, which would shorten the anterior portion of the sternoclavicular joint capsule. As a result, the movement available at the clavicle would be reduced, limiting the available range of clavicular rotation and scapular rotation. The altered position of the scapula will increase traction on the coracoacromial ligament which may then result in the formation of traction spurs on the anterior and inferior aspects of the acromion and be another cause of impingement.

As with all the structures in the subacromial space, the long head of biceps is also considered to be at risk of impingement as a result of postural change. According to Ayub[4] and Grimsby and Gray,[39] since the sheath of the biceps tendon is a continuation of the shoulder joint's synovial lining, and as the synovium is related to the rotator cuff, an inflammatory process involving one of these structures has the potential to affect another.

Darnell[27] hypothesized that FHP would increase tension on the dorsal scapula nerve due to the effect the altered posture would have on the scalene muscles. The compromised nerve may lead to an entrapment neuropathy that could cause the rhomboids and levator scapulae to weaken and allow the shoulder girdle to protract. Darnell[27] also suggested that prolonged shoulder girdle protraction would stretch the suprascapular nerve, which would result in pain and weaken the infraspinatus.

Support for some of these hypotheses comes from studies that have reported a decrease in acromiohumeral distance in people with severe FHP compared to people with an FHP classified as normal.[28] Additionally, FHP appears to be associated with the thickness of the serratus anterior at rest, which although not yet established, may in time contribute to the development of shoulder symptoms.[52] Furthermore, FHP may be associated with reduced glenohumeral range of movement in people diagnosed with subacromial impingement syndrome,[55] reduced strength in people without symptoms (acting as their own controls),[80] and reduced shoulder movement and shoulder abduction strength in people with neck pain.[92] As with previous research on posture, many of these studies have substantial methodological concerns and small study populations. It is clear that more research is needed. Table 20.2 presents a summary of postural and functional changes associated with an FHP.

Muscles involved in postural theory

As detailed in Table 20.2, imbalances in cervical, axioscapular, and scapulohumeral muscles are associated with

Table 20.2 A summary of postural and functional changes associated with an FHP

Muscles that shorten	Muscles that lengthen and weaken	Consequences
• Suboccipital muscles • Levator scapulae • Upper trapezius • Sternocleidomastoid • Pectoralis major • Pectoralis minor • Subscapularis • Latissimus dorsi • Teres major	• Deep neck flexors • Supraspinatus • Infraspinatus • Teres minor • Rhomboids • Middle trapezius • Lower trapezius • Serratus anterior	Contraction of the anterior glenohumeral capsule Increased thoracic kyphosis Scapula • protraction • anterior tilt • downward rotation • elevation • ± winging

Adapted from Janda[43] and Chaitow.[21]

changes in posture and symptoms. Three of the muscles commonly implicated by postural theorists in the pathogenesis of posture-related symptoms and pain are trapezius, serratus anterior, and pectoralis minor.

In a systematic review comparing scapulothoracic muscle activity and recruitment timing in people with and without shoulder pain, Struyf et al.[99] reported that in people diagnosed with subacromial impingement syndrome (SIS) and glenohumeral instability, many variations in muscle activity were identified. In the SIS group, the lower trapezius and serratus anterior activity decreased, and upper trapezius activity increased. Findings in the instability group were less clear, and there was no consensus regarding muscle recruitment. Twelve articles were included in the review based upon studies that used electromyography (EMG) which, as discussed in Chapter 4, is not without limitations. In addition, this research cannot provide information on a causal relationship.

Trapezius

The spinal accessory nerve provides the most consistent motor innervation for the trapezius. The muscle is divided into an upper, middle, and lower part. The roles traditionally ascribed to the upper fibers of trapezius are elevation and upward rotation of the scapula. The middle and lower fibers retract the scapula, and the lower fibers also upwardly rotate the scapula.[11,84,114] These traditional roles have been challenged. Johnson et al.[46] examined the origin, insertion, and direction of the three sections of the trapezius in four shoulders, in two embalmed specimens. They concluded that the upper fibers (all fascicles above the level of the seventh cervical vertebra) were found to be mainly aligned in a horizontal direction. All these fibers inserted along the posterior border of the distal third of the clavicle. Fibers from the superior nuchal line were noted as the only fibers exhibiting a downward orientation.

Fibers from the seventh cervical vertebra (C7) and the first thoracic vertebra (T1) were found to pass transversely to attach to the inner border of the acromion and to the crest of the scapular spine. Fascicles from T2 to T5 converged to a common aponeurotic tendon that inserted into the deltoid tubercle on the medial aspect of the spine of the scapula. Fascicles from T6 to T10 inserted into the medial border of the deltoid tubercle, and those from T10 to T12 inserted into the lower edge of the tubercle. Fascicles from T6 to T12 were reported as not always being present. The largest fascicles were found to arise from C6 and T1. The uppermost fibers from the superior nuchal line and the upper ligamentum nuchae were structurally in the correct plane to elevate and upwardly rotate the scapula but were found to be thin and did not appear to have the capacity to produce these movements. Johnson et al.[46] reported their findings following examination of four elderly cadaver specimens. An investigation on a larger number of subjects covering a wider age distribution is necessary to further support their findings.

Camargo et al.[20] concluded that the trapezius and serratus anterior act synergistically to produce movement of the scapula and clavicle. The trapezius may be considered a dominant stabilizer of the scapula, while the serratus anterior a dominant mover of the scapula, although considerable overlap exists in function.

Serratus anterior

The serratus anterior is innervated by the long thoracic nerve and its primary actions are, stabilizing the medial border of the scapula against the thorax, protraction and upward rotation of the scapula.[75] The strong protraction function is based on the muscle's overall near horizontal line of force, coupled with its long moment arm relative to the sternoclavicular joint.[75] The uppermost fibers may assist in elevation of the scapula. During a push-up, the serratus anterior lifts the thorax posteriorly.

Pectoralis minor

The pectoralis minor originates from the third to fifth ribs and inserts on the medial inferior border of the coracoid process. Its actions include protraction and downward rotation of the scapula. It has also been ascribed the action of shoulder depression, as well as lifting the medial border and inferior angle of the scapula away from the ribs (winging of the scapula).[48,84,114] Traditionally it has been argued that pectoralis minor shortening will lead to an increased scapular anterior tilt, protraction, and downward rotation, and because of this triad of postural changes is commonly implicated as a cause of abnormal upper body and scapular posture, and is a primary target for treatment designed to improve posture and reduce symptoms.[19,21,39,54,89,90]

Sahrmann[89] has described several clinical syndromes that are associated with a shortening of pectoralis minor. These include thoracic outlet syndrome, scapular winging and tilting syndrome, scapular abduction syndrome, scapular depression syndrome, and scapular downward rotation syndrome. To identify a postural shortening of pectoralis minor in association with these and other upper quadrant syndromes, a test of the muscle's length has been proposed. Sahrmann[89] has described that when the pectoralis minor muscle is of normal length the distance between the treatment table and posterior aspect of the acromion (patient supine, arms by side, elbows flexed) should not exceed 2.5 cm (1 in). A distance greater than this would suggest a muscle imbalance had occurred and the muscle had shortened. Identifying a muscle imbalance involving a short pectoralis minor is then used within the context of the clinical reasoning process to inform and direct the clinician as regards appropriate therapeutic intervention.

Lewis and Valentine[65] assessed the intrarater reliability of this test in 45 people with and 45 people without shoulder pain. They reported that the pectoralis minor length test was found to have excellent intrarater reliability for the dominant and nondominant side of people without symptoms, and for the pain-free and painful side of people with symptoms. However, the values calculated for the sensitivity, specificity, positive and negative likelihood ratios suggest that the test lacks diagnostic credibility. One reason for this is that the 2.5 cm/1 in threshold described as the cut off for a normal distance from the table to the acromion was exceeded in all 90 participants (180 shoulders) with no difference between those with and without symptoms.

Struyf et al.[100] reported on another method suggested to assess the intra- and interrater reliability of an alternative pectoralis minor length test in 25 people with SIS and 25 people with no symptoms. The test involved measuring the distance between the inferomedial aspect of the coracoid process and the caudal edge of the fourth rib at the sternum. The distance was then divided by the patient's height to produce a normalized measurement called the pectoralis minor index (PMI). The reliability of the measurement was reported to be good to excellent. The validity of the measurement process and the differences between people with and without symptoms were not reported.

Force couples

A force couple involves two or more muscles or muscle groups that individually may have opposing actions, but when they work in unison, they produce synergistic movement around a joint. The trapezius and serratus anterior muscles have traditionally been considered to produce a force couple and when they work together, they produce rotation of the scapula around an axis that is found between the insertions of both muscles and, by doing so, create a stable base for the humeral head and support the function of the rotator cuff. The certainty of this has been challenged. The axis of rotation of the scapula has been described as initially the root of the spine of the scapula and then its deltoid tubercle, eventually migrating to the acromioclavicular joint.[5] The horizontal orientation of the C7 and T1 fibers pass through this axis and, according to Johnson et al.,[46] would not be able to rotate the scapula. The insertion of the lower fibers of the muscle onto the deltoid tubercle, implies that they act at the axis of rotation and not around it during various stages of scapular upward rotation. This suggests that the lower fibers might contribute more to scapular stabilization and less to scapular rotation. The transversely oriented upper and middle fibers can draw the clavicle and scapula backwards, as might occur in activities such as rowing. The axis of rotation of the clavicle is located at the sternoclavicular joint, and the transverse fibers of middle trapezius pass above and through this axis. These fibers are therefore able to maintain compression through the sternoclavicular joint, at the same time as rotating the clavicle on the sternoclavicular joint and thereby elevating its lateral end, which indirectly elevates the scapula.

In summary, Johnson et al.[46] concluded that the function of the trapezius was to transfer the load of the upper limb to the sternoclavicular joint and not the cervical spine. Other functions involve upward rotation of the lateral end of the clavicle, and to maintain a horizontal and vertical equilibrium to allow the serratus anterior to upwardly rotate the scapula. The trapezius was not thought to have a direct role in scapular elevation. Johnson et al.[46] reported their findings following examination of four elderly cadaver specimens. An investigation on a larger number of subjects covering a wider age distribution is necessary to further support their findings.

Assessment

Forward head posture

Depending on its extent, FHP may be classified as slight, moderate, or severe.[56] Methods commonly used to determine the presence of an FHP include visual assessment,[4,14,37] comparison to a plumb line,[15,48,50] and lateral photographs.[15,38,62,66,82,83,113] Using photography, two lines are drawn. One connects the tragus of the ear to the skin surface marking that corresponds with the seventh cervical spinous process (C7). From C7 a line is then drawn horizontally. The resultant angle is termed the FHP angle. Braun and Amundson[15] reported that the average resting head posture position in 20 male subjects to be 51.97°. This compares favorably with 51.9° reported by Raine and Twomey[83] who examined the angle in men and women. As the angle becomes smaller, the observed FHP becomes more pronounced. FHP has been defined as having an angle less than 48°–50°.[91]

Forward shoulder posture

FHP has been associated with protracted (rounded) shoulders known as a forward shoulder posture (FSP). To measure FSP from a lateral photograph, two lines are constructed: a horizontal line drawn at the level of C7, and a second line from C7 to the midpoint of the shoulder. The resulting angle is the FSP angle. The mean sagittal plane shoulder posture reported by Raine and Twomey[83] was 47.6°. The smaller the angle, the greater the FSP.

Measuring scapular posture

The resting position of the scapula has been measured using multiple methods. These have included visual observation, photography,[5,83] palpation,[5,95] goniometery,[29] radiological investigation,[30,33,72,81,88] tape measurements,[64] calipers,[106] and analogue and digital inclinometers.[64,106] Combinations of these techniques enable clinicians to measure scapular protraction, elevation, depression, upward and downward rotation, and anterior and posterior tilt. (For more detailed descriptions see Lewis and Valentine.[64])

Methods suggested to measure scapular posture during movement, also called dynamic scapular posture, include radiological investigations,[30,33,72,81,88] electromechanical tracking,[111] electromagnetic tracking,[7,26] palpation, and photography.[5] Measuring dynamic scapular posture is more problematic than measuring static posture, and is influenced by many confounding factors. One problem is that motion sensors, secured to the skin in fixed locations identified before movement starts, may not accurately track the motion of the scapula during movement. Another is the need to stop shoulder motion at selected angles and re-palpate the skin surface markings overlying the scapula to determine how it has moved between the selected angles of shoulder movement. The stop-start methodology used in this type of analysis of scapular motion may produce different results than the uninterrupted scapular movement during common daily activities. This method may also introduce fatigue, which may also influence the findings.

Thoracic kyphosis

O'Gorman and Jull[78] examined the thoracic kyphosis angle and thoracic mobility in 120 women without symptoms, grouped into 10-year age bands. The thoracic kyphosis was found to increase with age. The angles ranged from 41° (standard deviation [SD] = 9) in the youngest group (22–29 years old) to 66° (SD = 10) for the oldest group (more than 70 years old). For each 10-year increment, the angle of the kyphosis increased, most significantly after the fifth decade.

The study also found that the movement of thoracic extension significantly decreased with increasing age. There was a 68% decrease in the extension range from the youngest (37°, SD = 11) to the oldest (12°, SD = 7) group.

Crawford and Jull[25] investigated the relationship between bilateral shoulder flexion and thoracic extension in 60 women without symptoms, assigned into a younger group (18–30 years old) and an older group (50–75 years old). Mean bilateral arm elevation was 172° (SD = 12) with a mean kyphosis angle of 33° (SD = 10) for the younger group. Arm elevation in the older group was 157° (SD = 10) with an associated kyphosis angle of 52° (SD = 12). Their results suggested that the younger group used 15° thoracic extension during bilateral arm elevation, representing approximately 51% of the available thoracic extension range. In comparison, the older subjects used 13° representing a mean of 68% of the available extension.

Thoracic kyphosis may be measured in several ways, with a standing radiograph being the gold standard. Using this method, the Cobb, modified Cobb, computer assisted method for deriving radius of thoracic spine curvature, and thoracic vertebral centroid angles, may be measured and calculated.[17,35] Clinically, flexicurve[115] and inclinometers[63] have been recommended. The reliability of inclinometry has been demonstrated in several studies,[10,63,110] and is reported to be valid[42] and have greater validity than the flexicurve method.[9]

Managing scapular dyskinesis

Cools et al.[24] have published management suggestions for scapular dyskinesis that involves increasing both soft tissue flexibility and muscle performance. Flexibility should be restored to shortened muscles which may include pectoralis minor, levator scapulae, and upper trapezius. Other components of the program involve spinal posture correction, to reduce the FHP. Patients are encouraged to achieve a neutral lumbopelvic posture, followed by correction of the scapulothoracic and cervical postures with a subtle, gentle "occipital lift" maneuver to position the head in neutral position.[24] Improving muscle performance may involve addressing muscle strength and timing of the serratus anterior, and the upper, middle and lower parts of the trapezius. Sensory motor exercises may also be required.

Challenges to the postural theory

The definition of poor posture and lack of 95% confidence intervals

Posture is defined as perfect when a plumb line passes through the lobe of the ear, middle of the shoulder, and greater trochanter of the femur, and passes slightly anterior to the midline of the knee. It is therefore clear that the concept of ideal body posture has been given a binary status: there is one faultless body posture and one ideal scapular position and any deviation from this norm is classified as abnormal. However, this classification model, perfect or not, conflicts with most diagnostic criteria in healthcare. For example, when assessing glucose or iron levels in the blood, there is a minimum and maximum range, between which the result is considered normal. In science, the concept of a 95% confidence interval – the range of values between which we can be 95% certain the true mean of the population lies – is readily accepted. Surprisingly, however, with respect to posture there is no range of normal values and no 95% confidence interval: people are either classified as having perfect or abnormal posture, with no variation being accepted.

Another issue is that decisions are made on the presence or absence of normality based on a clinical assessment of external landmarks that are chosen to represent internal anatomical structures. There is a paucity of evidence that demonstrates a clear correlation between these variables, and body habitus and respiration are two factors that may confound assessment. Furthermore, research findings suggest that the interrater reliability of clinicians (chiropractors, physical therapists, physiatrists, rheumatologists, and orthopedic surgeons) to assess sagittal plane posture is poor.[31]

Does posture follow the rules?

Attempts have been made to provide evidence to better understand the relationship between so-called abnormal posture and shoulder symptoms, most of which has not been able to provide support for the relationship between the observation of static posture, loss of function, and symptoms.

Raine and Twomey[82,83] examined sagittal and coronal plane postural variables in 160 asymptomatic people and reported that no relationship existed between FHP, FSP and the curve of the thoracic kyphosis. Greenfield et al.[36] compared the posture of 30 people with subacromial impingement syndrome with 30 people without symptoms, matched for age and gender (age range 17–65 years). Their findings did not provide evidence to support the contention that a relationship between posture and shoulder pathology existed, as no difference between the two groups for scapular rotation, scapular protraction, and thoracic kyphosis angle were reported. Greenfield et al.[36] acknowledged their results were influenced by several confounding factors that included assessment of scapular posture only in one plane, uncertain diagnoses, possible muscular fatigue during the data collection for the study, and "improvement" in posture as most of those with impingement syndrome were undergoing treatment.

Lukasiewicz et al.[69] examined the orientation of the scapula in 20 people without symptoms and 17 people diagnosed with subacromial impingement syndrome. Participants were examined in constrained sitting with an electromechanical digitalizer. Taken from a graphical representation of their findings, their results suggest that there was no significant difference in the anterior to posterior tilt angle of the scapula at rest. There was also no significant difference in the amount of scapular internal rotation (around a vertical axis). Supporting postural theory that a weak lower trapezius influences scapular position, Lukasiewicz et al.[69] reported that when the arm was elevated (90° and maximal elevation), the scapula was more anteriorly tilted and elevated in the group with subacromial impingement.

In contrast, and in challenge to theories that have associated specific postures with pathology, the position of the scapula in the group with symptoms, was not more protracted or downwardly rotated than the group of people without symptoms. Confounding factors such as the need to hold arms in elevation for up to 60 seconds, respiration, slight postural adjustments, and measuring bony landmarks via the skin (especially as Lukasiewicz et al.[69] commented that muscular contraction at the site of digitization made palpatory confirmation difficult, especially at the inferior angle of the scapula and the posterior angle of the acromion), may have impacted on their findings.

Grimmer et al.[38] examined FHP in 427 randomly selected people without symptoms who were examined during unconstrained sitting using a custom-built device. None of the 427 asymptomatic participants demonstrated a head posture that conformed to the ideal head posture suggested by Kendall et al.,[48-50] which begs the question, is there such a thing as ideal posture?[62]

Lewis et al.[62] investigated static posture in 60 people without symptoms and 60 people with a clinical diagnosis of subacromial impingement syndrome. The purpose of this study was to investigate whether FHP was associated with an increased thoracic kyphosis, an altered position of the scapular and a reduction in glenohumeral elevation range. Their findings suggested that upper body posture did not follow the set patterns described extensively in the medical, physical therapy (physiotherapy), chiropractic, and osteopathic literature, and challenged the relationship between posture and subacromial impingement syndrome. Of note, subsequent research and syntheses have challenged the existence of impingement syndrome as a clinical condition.[12,57,58,60,79]

An important finding reported by Lewis et al.[62] is that people classified as having abnormal posture (based on historic definitions of ideal and abnormal posture) may be just as flexible, exhibit the same ranges of movement, and not have increased symptoms related to their static posture. Lewis et al.[62] argue that the clinical examination of static thoracic, scapular, head, and shoulder posture does not inform clinical decision-making for the vast majority of people seeking care. For example, an individual may be classified as having an FHP and concomitant thoracic kyphosis and anteriorly tilted scapula when observed in standing, but may have sufficient flexibility and muscle performance to function normally without symptoms. There is no argument that large and fixed postural variations in some people may lead to serious symptoms and loss of function.[59] However, Lewis et al.[62] argue that little could be derived from the static observation of upper body posture and subsequently have recommended that historic definitions of perfect posture, that most likely are medicalizing normality,[61] should no longer be used in clinical practice to inform clinical decision-making.

In a systematic review that aimed to establish if a relationship between subacromial impingement syndrome and scapular orientation existed, Radcliffe et al.[85] included ten studies that employed several methodologies to assess scapular position. They reported that considerable variation in findings existed, with some studies reporting patterns of reduced upward rotation of the scapula, increased anterior tilt of the scapula, and in contrast, other studies reported the opposite, while other studies did not identify a difference in scapular position when compared to people without symptoms. The conclusions of the review were that there is insufficient evidence to support a clinical belief that the scapula adopts a common and consistent posture in impingement syndrome. Furthermore, it raises the possibility that deviations from a hypothesized normal scapular posture may not contribute to impingement syndrome but may just represent normal variations in scapular position.

Barrett et al.[8] conducted a case series involving two groups of people diagnosed with shoulder pain. One group (n= 20) participated in a six-week exercise classes that involved shoulder exercises. The other group (n=19) participated in a six-week exercise class that consisted of both shoulder exercises and exercises to improve the thoracic posture, i.e., thoracic extension exercises. The primary outcome measure was the Disability of the Arm, Shoulder and Hand (DASH) score measured at six weeks and six months after the end of the classes. Although this was not a randomized controlled trial and no between-group comparison can be definitively made, both groups reported improvement at both timepoints. The effect sizes ranged from 0.78 to 1.16 in the group that performed shoulder exercises only, and in the group that performed additional thoracic exercises the effect size ranged from 0.85 to 1.88. The effect size in both groups may be considered as large. Importantly, the group that was given the thoracic extension exercises did not demonstrate any change in the thoracic resting posture at the end of the exercise intervention. This suggests that the improvement reported was not due to a change in the static thoracic spine posture.

The preceding studies suggesting resting posture may not change with rehabilitation were conducted in people who had reached skeletal maturity. In contrast, Ruivo et al.[87] randomized 130 adolescents (15–17 years old) to a 16-week resistance and stretching (n=84) or control group (n=46). Both groups participated in physical education classes at high school, with the experimental group performing the postural stretching and strengthening exercises in the last 15–20 minutes of the twice weekly physical education classes. At the end of the program, the authors reported significant changes in FHP and shoulder protraction in the postural group. At the final data collection, there was a decrease in FHP of 2.5° in the experimental group in comparison with 0.5° in the control group. There was a 2.0° difference in the shoulder angle in the control group compared with a 3.9° change in the postural group. The clinical importance of these changes is uncertain, but importantly for clinical practice, shoulder pain and function, measured with the ASES (American Shoulder and Elbow Surgeons Shoulder Assessment), did not demonstrate a difference between or within the groups during the clinical trial.[87]

Studies that have followed overhead athletes (e.g., tennis, volleyball, handball) have investigated the relationship between current asymptomatic scapular dyskinesia and the future occurrence of shoulder pain.[3,22,47,74,93,103] The findings were equivocal with studies reporting that scapular dyskinesis might be predictive of future shoulder symptoms. Møller et al.[73] reported that scapular dyskinesia may play a predictive role, but only in relation to load. They concluded that an individual with asymptomatic scapular dyskinesis who significant increases their exercise level (>60% increase per week), might increase the risk of shoulder injury in handball players, while scapular dyskinesia without increasing weekly load more than 60% was not associated with increased shoulder pain. This may be considered as an interactive risk factor: the faster the load is increased on the shoulder, the more likely a person who has scapular dyskinesia might experience shoulder pain. These studies suggest that the experience of shoulder pain will not always be the consequence of scapular dyskinesis. This uncertainty is compounded by findings from other studies that suggest scapular dyskinesis may be the consequence of shoulder pain or pathology.[6,96,112]

Synthesizing our understanding of posture

Posture has been afforded a binary status; perfect or abnormal, there is no middle ground, no 95% confidence intervals, and no range of "acceptable" postures. As such, it is likely that every person will, by definition, have abnormal posture. An alternative argument might be that if it is universal, perhaps it is not abnormal? There are approximately 600,000 physical therapists, osteopaths, and chiropractors practicing today, in addition to sports and conditioning coaches, athletic, and personal trainers, all of whom are potentially advising millions of people each year that their shoulder problems are due to abnormal posture. The magnitude of the problem, which is arguably medicalizing normality on an industrial scale, should not be undermined. Box 20.1 summarizes our thoughts, based on the current literature and knowledge.

Conclusions

In the absence of a specific or identifiable cause of symptoms, poor upper body posture, colloquially referred to as a "forward head posture", "slouched posture", "poking chin posture", or "rounded shoulder posture" has been cited as a potential etiological factor in the pathogenesis and perpetuation of many clinical syndromes involving the shoulder. Beliefs relating to posture have permeated into clinical practice and are frequently used to explain to patients the basis for symptoms and the rationale for rehabilitation.

Clinical theorists have defined ideal posture, the consequences of poor posture, and the importance of postural assessment and correction in the clinical examination and management of people seeking care with musculoskeletal shoulder pain. Postural examination is encouraged due to the belief that deviations from an ideal posture lead to numerous clinical syndromes and that improvement in posture will restore normal function and reduce pain. Although the assumed importance of postural assessment is evident in medical, physical therapy, physiotherapy and osteopathy literature, most claims concerning posture are made without definitive evidence.

One suggestion is to stop focusing on the patient's *static* head and shoulder posture and stop providing an unsubstantiated postural explanation for the presenting symptoms. Arguably, for most people presenting with shoulder symptoms, it would be much more appropriate to inform them that their posture is within a "normal" or acceptable range. Our assessment should be more focused on the frequency that people change their postures during the day than their current static posture. Maybe the answer to the uncertain relationship between upper body posture and shoulder pain is to be more like Quasimodo. Being the bell ringer of Notre-Dame de Paris Cathedral, he was physically active, climbing stairs, ringing heavy bells, and constantly changing his posture.

Box 20.1 Summary of current understanding of upper body posture

1. Substantial deviations of posture, especially ones that are fixed, may be directly related to symptoms and disability. However, this is not always the case (see https://en.wikipedia.org/wiki/Lamar_Gant).
2. More commonly, observations of posture, and assessment of muscle imbalances tell us very little, and we must be wary about drawing substantive conclusions from observation.
3. We cannot conclude from observation of static posture whether a deviation represents a variation of normal, is unrelated to symptoms, is the cause of the patient's symptoms, or is a way of "escaping" from, or reducing symptoms.
4. Reflect before you inform a patient that posture is the cause of their symptoms and that their posture needs to be improved to reduce symptoms. Ask yourself if you are telling the patient something that is evidence-based, or if you are perpetuating uncertainties, or perpetuating your own biases.
5. We recommend whenever possible, and unless proven otherwise, that we should inform the patient that their posture is within normal limits.
6. Giving exercises to correct or improve posture may not change static posture.
7. We do not yet know the effect that "postural" exercises have on dynamic movement, but until we do, we should still avoid suggesting that the prescribed exercises improve posture, and what the mechanism of symptom reduction is, until we really do know, one way or the other.
8. It may be that the only way we can determine if posture is involved, is by temporarily changing it and determining the patient's response. This may be achieved with visual cues, hands-on facilitation, taping, bracing, exercise programs, and postural reminders. However, even this is fraught with uncertainty, as all these interventions may produce a positive response for other reasons, such as movement confidence, fear reduction, placebo, and distraction.

References

1. Akodu AK, Akinbo SR, Young QO. Correlation among smartphone addiction, craniovertebral angle, scapular dyskinesis, and selected anthropometric variables in physiotherapy undergraduates. J Taibah Univ Med Sci. 2018;13:528-534.
2. Allen T. Dorland's Illustrated Medical Dictionary. Philadelphia: WB Saunders; 2003.
3. Andersson SH, Bahr R, Clarsen B, Myklebust G. Preventing overuse shoulder injuries among throwing athletes: a cluster-randomised controlled trial in 660 elite handball players. Br J Sports Med. 2017;51:1073-1080.
4. Ayub E. Posture and the upper quarter. In: Donatelli R (ed). Physical Therapy of the Shoulder, 2nd edition. Melbourne: Churchill Livingstone; 1991:81-90.
5. Bagg SD, Forrest WJ. A biomechanical analysis of scapular rotation during arm abduction in the scapular plane. Am J Phys Med Rehabil. 1988;67:238-245.
6. Bandholm T, Rasmussen L, Aagaard P, Diederichsen L, Jensen BR. Effects of experimental muscle pain on shoulder-abduction force steadiness and muscle activity in healthy subjects. Eur J Appl Physiol. 2008;102:643-650.
7. Barnett ND, Duncan RD, Johnson GR. The measurement of three dimensional scapulohumeral kinematics-a study of reliability. Clin Biomech. 1999;14:287-290.
8. Barrett E, Conroy C, Corcoran M, et al. An evaluation of two types of exercise classes, containing shoulder exercises or a combination of shoulder and thoracic exercises, for the treatment of nonspecific shoulder pain: a case series. J Hand Ther. 2018;31(3):301-307.
9. Barrett E, Lenehan B, O'Sullivan K, Lewis J, McCreesh K. Validation of the manual inclinometer and flexicurve for the measurement of thoracic kyphosis. Physiotherapy theory and practice. 2018;34:301-308.
10. Barrett E, McCreesh K, Lewis J. Intrarater and interrater reliability of the flexicurve index, flexicurve angle, and manual inclinometer for the measurement of thoracic kyphosis. Rehabilitation Research and Practice. 2013;2013:475870.
11. Basmajian JV, De Luca CJ. Muscles Alive: Their Function Revealed by Electromyography, 5th edition. Baltimore: Williams and Wilkins; 1985.
12. Beard DJ, Rees JL, Cook JA, et al. Arthroscopic subacromial decompression for subacromial shoulder pain (CSAW): a multicentre, pragmatic, parallel group, placebo-controlled, three-group, randomised surgical trial. Lancet. 2018;391:329-338.
13. Beauchamp-Chalifour P, Pelet S. Osteochondroma of the scapula with accessory nerve (XI) compression. Case Reports in Orthopedics. 2018;2018:7018109.
14. Bowling RW, Rockar PA, Jr., Erhard R. Examination of the shoulder complex. Phys Ther. 1986;66:1866-1877.
15. Braun BL, Amundson LR. Quantitative assessment of head and shoulder posture. Arch Phys Med Rehabil. 1989;70:322-329.
16. Braune W, Fischer O. On the Centre of Gravity of the Human Body: As Related to the Equipment of the German Infantry Soldier. Springer Science & Business Media; 2012.
17. Briggs A, Wrigley T, Tully E, Adams P, Greig A, Bennell K. Radiographic measures of thoracic kyphosis in osteoporosis: Cobb and vertebral centroid angles. Skeletal radiology. 2007;36:761-767.
18. Burkhart SS, Morgan CD, Kibler WB. The disabled throwing shoulder: spectrum of pathology. Part III: The SICK scapula, scapular dyskinesis, the kinetic chain, and rehabilitation. Arthroscopy. 2003;19:641-661.
19. Calliet R. Shoulder Pain, 3rd edition. Philadelphia: F.A. Davis Company; 1991.
20. Camargo PR, Neumann DA. Kinesiologic considerations for targeting activation of scapulothoracic muscles. Part 2: trapezius. Braz J Phys Ther. 2019;23:467-475.
21. Chaitow L. Muscle Energy Techniques. Edinburgh: Churchill Livingstone; 1996.
22. Clarsen B, Bahr R, Andersson SH, Munk R, Myklebust G. Reduced glenohumeral rotation, external rotation weakness and scapular dyskinesis are risk factors for shoulder injuries among elite male handball players: a prospective cohort study. Br J Sports Med. 2014;48:1327-1333.
23. Cools AM, Dewitte V, Lanszweert F, et al. Rehabilitation of scapular muscle balance: which exercises to prescribe? The American Journal of Sports Medicine. 2007;35:1744-1751.
24. Cools AM, Struyf F, De Mey K, Maenhout A, Castelein B, Cagnie B. Rehabilitation of scapular dyskinesis: from the office worker to the elite overhead athlete. Br J Sports Med. 2014;48:692-697.
25. Crawford HJ, Jull GA. The influence of thoracic posture and movement on range of arm elevation. Physiotherapy Theory and Practice. 1993;9:143-148.
26. Culham E, Peat M. Spinal and shoulder complex posture. I: Measurement using the 3Space Isotrak. Clinical Rehabilitation. 1993;7:309-318.
27. Darnell MW. A proposed chronology of events for forward head posture. J Craniomandibular Pract. 1983;1:49-54.
28. Dehqan B, Delkhoush CT, Mirmohammadkhani M, Ehsani F. Does forward head posture change subacromial space in active or passive arm elevation? J Man Manip Ther. 2020;1-8.
29. Doody SG, Waterland JC, Freedman L. Scapulo-humeral goniometer. Arch Phys Med Rehabil. 1970;51:711-713.
30. Dvir Z, Berme N. The shoulder complex in elevation of the arm: a mechanism approach. Journal of Biomechanics. 1978;11:219-225.
31. Fedorak C, Ashworth N, Marshall J, Paull H. Reliability of the visual assessment of cervical and lumbar lordosis: how good are we? Spine. 2003;28:1857-1859.
32. Feldenkrais M. Body and Mature Behaviour: A Study of Anxiety, Sex, Gravitation and Learning. New York: International University Press Incorporated; 1949.
33. Freedman L, Munro R. Abduction of the arm in the scapular plane: scapular and gleno-humeral movements. A roentgenographic study. The Journal of Bone and Joint Surgery. 1966;48A:1503-1510.
34. Gilman SL. "Stand Up Straight": notes toward a history of posture. Journal of Medical Humanities. 2014;35:57-83.
35. Goh S, Price R, Leedman P, Singer K. A comparison of three methods for measuring thoracic kyphosis: implications for clinical studies. Rheumatology. 2000;39:310-315.

36. Greenfield B, Catlin PA, Coats PW, Green E, McDonald JJ, North C. Posture in patients with shoulder overuse injuries and healthy individuals. J Orthop Sports Phys Ther. 1995;21:287-295.

37. Griegel-Morris P, Larson K, Mueller-Klaus K, Oatis CA. Incidence of common postural abnormalities in the cervical, shoulder, and thoracic regions and their association with pain in two age groups of healthy subjects. Phys Ther. 1992;72:425-431.

38. Grimmer K. An investigation of poor cervical resting posture. Aust J Physiother. 1997;43:7-16.

39. Grimsby O, Gray J. Interrelation of the spine to the shoulder girdle. In: Donatelli R (ed). Physical Therapy of the Shoulder, 3rd edition. New York: Churchill Livingstone; 1997:95-129.

40. Hickey D, Solvig V, Cavalheri V, Harrold M, McKenna L. Scapular dyskinesis increases the risk of future shoulder pain by 43% in asymptomatic athletes: a systematic review and meta-analysis. Br J Sports Med. 2018;52:102-110.

41. Horter TS. How to care for your neck. Physical Therapy. 1978;52:184-185.

42. Hunter DJ, Rivett DA, McKiernan S, Weerasekara I, Snodgrass SJ. Is the inclinometer a valid measure of thoracic kyphosis? A cross-sectional study. Braz J Phys Ther. 2018;22:310-317.

43. Janda V. Muscles and cervicogenic pain syndromes. In: Grant R (ed). Physical Therapy of the Cervical and Thoracic Spine. New York: Churchill Livingstone; 1988.

44. Janda V. Muscles and motor control in cervicogenic disorders. Grant R (ed). Physical Therapy of the Cervical and Thoracic Spine. Amsterdam: Elsevier Science; 2002.

45. Janda V. On the concept of postural muscles and posture in man. Australian Journal of Physiotherapy. 1983;29:83-84.

46. Johnson G, Bogduk N, Nowitzke A, House D. Anatomy and actions of the trapezius muscle. Clinical Biomechanics. 1994;9:44-50.

47. Kawasaki T, Yamakawa J, Kaketa T, Kobayashi H, Kaneko K. Does scapular dyskinesis affect top rugby players during a game season? J Shoulder Elbow Surg. 2012;21:709-714.

48. Kendall F, McCreary E, Provance P. Muscle Testing and Function, 4th edition. Baltimore: Williams and Wilkins; 1993.

49. Kendall FP, McCreary EK. Muscles: Testing and Function, 3rd edition. Baltimore: Williams and Wilkins; 1983.

50. Kendall H, Kendall F, Boynton D. Posture and Pain. Baltimore: The Williams and Wilkins Company; 1952.

51. Kessler RM, Hertling D. Management of common musculoskeletal disorders: physical therapy principles and methods. Philadelphia: Harper and Row; 1983.

52. Khosravi F, Peolsson A, Karimi N, Rahnama L. Scapular upward rotator morphologic characteristics in individuals with and without forward head posture: a case-control study. J Ultrasound Med. 2019;38:337-345.

53. Kibler WB. The role of the scapula in athletic shoulder function. Am J Sports Med. 1998;26:325-337.

54. Kibler WB. Shoulder rehabilitation: principles and practice. Med Sci Sports Exerc. 1998;30:S40-50.

55. Land H, Gordon S, Watt K. Clinical assessment of subacromial shoulder impingement - which factors differ from the asymptomatic population? Musculoskelet Sci Pract. 2017;27:49-56.

56. Lau HM, Chiu TT, Lam TH. Measurement of craniovertebral angle with electronic head posture instrument: criterion validity. J Rehabil Res Dev. 2010;47:911-918.

57. Lewis J. Bloodletting for pneumonia, prolonged bed rest for low back pain, is subacromial decompression another clinical illusion? Br J Sports Med. 2015;49:280-281.

58. Lewis J. The end of an era? J Orthop Sports Phys Ther. 2018;48:127-129.

59. Lewis J, O'Sullivan P. Is it time to reframe how we care for people with non-traumatic musculoskeletal pain? Br J Sports Med. 2018;52:1543-1544.

60. Lewis JS. Subacromial impingement syndrome: a musculoskeletal condition or a clinical illusion? Physical Therapy Review. 2011;16:388-398.

61. Lewis JS, Cook CE, Hoffmann TC, O'Sullivan P. The elephant in the room: too much medicine in musculoskeletal practice. J Orthop Sports Phys Ther. 2020;50:1-4.

62. Lewis JS, Green A, Wright C. Subacromial impingement syndrome: the role of posture and muscle imbalance. J Shoulder Elbow Surg. 2005;14:385-392.

63. Lewis JS, Valentine RE. Clinical measurement of the thoracic kyphosis. A study of the intra-rater reliability in subjects with and without shoulder pain. BMC Musculoskelet Disord. 2010;11:39.

64. Lewis JS, Valentine RE. Intraobserver reliability of angular and linear measurements of scapular position in subjects with and without symptoms. Archives of Physical Medicine and Rehabilitation. 2008;89:1795-1802.

65. Lewis JS, Valentine RE. The pectoralis minor length test: a study of the intra-rater reliability and diagnostic accuracy in subjects with and without shoulder symptoms. BMC Musculoskelet Disord. 2007;8:64.

66. Lewis JS, Wright C, Green A. Subacromial impingement syndrome: the effect of changing posture on shoulder range of movement. J Orthop Sports Phys Ther. 2005;35:72-87.

67. Lezberg S. Posture of the head: its relevance to the conservative treatment of cervicobrachial radiculitus. Journal of the American Physical Therapy Association. 1966;46:953-957.

68. Lu L, Robinson M, Tan Y, et al. Effective assessments of a short-duration poor posture on upper limb muscle fatigue before physical exercise. Front Physiol. 2020;11:541974.

69. Lukasiewicz AC, McClure P, Michener L, Pratt N, Sennett B. Comparison of 3-dimensional scapular position and orientation between subjects with and without shoulder impingement. J Orthop Sports Phys Ther. 1999;29:574-583; discussion 584-576.

70. McClure P, Tate AR, Kareha S, Irwin D, Zlupko E. A clinical method for identifying scapular dyskinesis, part 1: reliability. J Athl Train. 2009;44:160-164.

71. McKenzie R. Treat Your Own Neck. New Zealand: Spinal Publications; 1983.

72. Michiels I, Grevenstein J. Kinematics of shoulder abduction in the scapular plane. On the influence of abduction velocity and external load. Clin Biomech. 1995;10:137-143.

73. Møller M, Nielsen RO, Attermann J, et al. Handball load and shoulder injury rate: a 31-week cohort study of 679 elite youth handball players. Br J Sports Med. 2017;51:231-237.

74. Myers JB, Oyama S, Hibberd EE. Scapular dysfunction in high school baseball players sustaining throwing-related upper extremity injury: a prospective study. J Shoulder Elbow Surg. 2013;22:1154-1159.

75. Neumann DA, Camargo PR. Kinesiologic considerations for targeting activation of scapulothoracic muscles - part 1: serratus anterior. Braz J Phys Ther. 2019;23:459-466.

76. Neviaser J. Musculoskeletal disorders of the shoulder region causing cervicobrachial pain: differential diagnosis and treatment. Surgical Clinics of North America. 1963;43:1703-1714.

77. Nicholson G. Rehabilitation of common shoulder injuries. Clinics in Sports Medicine. 1989;8:633.

78. O'Gorman HJ, Jull GA. Thoracic kyphosis and mobility: the effect of age. Physiotherapy Theory and Practice. 1987;3:154-162.

79. Paavola M, Malmivaara A, Taimela S, et al. Subacromial decompression versus diagnostic arthroscopy for shoulder impingement: randomised, placebo surgery controlled clinical trial. BMJ. 2018;362:k2860.

80. Pheasant S, Haydt R, Gottstein T, Grasso A, Lombard N, Stone B. Shoulder external rotator strength in response to various sitting postures: a controlled laboratory study. Int J Sports Phys Ther. 2018;13:50-57.

81. Poppen NK, Walker PS. Normal and abnormal motion of the shoulder. J Bone Joint Surg Am. 1976;58:195-201.

82. Raine S, Twomey LT. Head and shoulder posture variations in 160 asymptomatic women and men. Arch Phys Med Rehabil. 1997;78:1215-1223.

83. Raine S, Twomey LT. Posture of the head, shoulder and thoracic spine in comfortable erect standing. Australian Journal of Physiotherapy. 1994;40:25-32.

84. Rasch PJ, Burke RK. Kinesiology and Applied Anatomy, 6th edition. Philadelphia: Febiger; 1978.

85. Ratcliffe E, Pickering S, McLean S, Lewis J. Is there a relationship between subacromial impingement syndrome and scapular orientation? A systematic review. Br J Sports Med. 2014;48(16):1251-1256.

86. Rocabado M. Arthrokinematics of the temporomandibular joint. Dental Clinics of North America. 1983;27:573-594.

87. Ruivo RM, Pezarat-Correia P, Carita AI. Effects of a resistance and stretching training program on forward head and protracted shoulder posture in adolescents. J Manipulative Physiol Ther. 2017;40:1-10.

88. Saha AK. Theory of Shoulder Mechanism: Descriptive and Applied. Springfield: Charles C. Thomas; 1961.

89. Sahrmann S. Diagnosis and Treatment of Movement Impairment Syndromes. London: Mosby; 2002.

90. Schenkman M, Rugo de Cartaya V. Kinesiology of the shoulder complex. Journal of Orthopedic and Sports Physical Therapy. 1987;8:438-450.

91. Shaghayegh Fard B, Ahmadi A, Maroufi N, Sarrafzadeh J. Evaluation of forward head posture in sitting and standing positions. Eur Spine J. 2016;25:3577-3582.

92. Shin YJ, Kim WH, Kim SG. Correlations among visual analogue scale, neck disability index, shoulder joint range of motion, and muscle strength in young women with forward head posture. J Exerc Rehabil. 2017;13:413-417.

93. Shitara H, Kobayashi T, Yamamoto A, et al. Prospective multifactorial analysis of preseason risk factors for shoulder and elbow injuries in high school baseball pitchers. Knee Surg Sports Traumatol Arthrosc. 2017;25:3303-3310.

94. Sivananda P, Rao BK, Kumar PV, Ram GS. Osteochondroma of the ventral scapula causing scapular static winging and secondary rib erosion. J Clin Diagn Res. 2014;8:LD03-LD05.

95. Sobush DC, Simoneau GG, Dietz KE, Levene JA, Grossman RE, Smith WB. The Lennie test for measuring scapular position in healthy young adult females: a reliability and validity study. J Orthop Sports Phys Ther. 1996;23:39-50.

96. Sole G, Osborne H, Wassinger C. Electromyographic response of shoulder muscles to acute experimental subacromial pain. Man Ther. 2014;19:343-348.

97. Solem-Bertoft E, Thuomas KA, Westerberg CE. The influence of scapular retraction and protraction on the width of the subacromial space. An MRI study. Clin Orthop Relat Res. 1993;99-103.

98. Stevenson A, Waite M (eds). Concise Oxford English Dictionary: Luxury Edition. Oxford University Press; 2011.

99. Struyf F, Cagnie B, Cools A, et al. Scapulothoracic muscle activity and recruitment timing in patients with shoulder impingement symptoms and glenohumeral instability. J Electromyogr Kinesiol. 2014;24:277-284.

100. Struyf F, Meeus M, Fransen E, et al. Interrater and intrarater reliability of the pectoralis minor muscle length measurement in subjects with and without shoulder impingement symptoms. Manual Therapy. 2014;19:294-298.

101. Struyf F, Nijs J, Baeyens JP, Mottram S, Meeusen R. Scapular positioning and movement in unimpaired shoulders, shoulder impingement syndrome, and glenohumeral instability. Scand J Med Sci Sports. 2011;21:352-358.

102. Struyf F, Nijs J, De Coninck K, Giunta M, Mottram S, Meeusen R. Clinical assessment of scapular positioning in musicians: an intertester reliability study. J Athl Train. 2009;44:519-526.

103. Struyf F, Nijs J, Meeus M, et al. Does scapular positioning predict shoulder pain in recreational overhead athletes? Int J Sports Med. 2014;35:75-82.

104. Sucher B. Thoracic outlet syndrome – a myofascial variant: Part 1. Pathology and diagnosis. Journal of the American Osteopathy Association. 1991;90:686-694.

105. American Academy of Orthopaedic Surgeons. Posture and its relationship to orthopaedic disabilities. A report of the posture committee. 1947.

106. Thomas SJ, Swanik KA, Swanik C, Huxel KC. Glenohumeral rotation and scapular position adaptations after a single high school female sports season. Journal of Athletic Training. 2009;44:230-237.

107. Travell JG, Simons DG. Myofascial Pain and Dysfunction: The Trigger Point Manual. Vol 1: The Upper Extremities. Baltimore: Williams and Wilkins; 1983.

108. Turner M. Posture and pain. Physical Therapy Review. 1957;37:294-297.

109. Tyler TF, Roy T, Nicholas SJ, Gleim GW. Reliability and validity of a new method of

measuring posterior shoulder tightness. J Orthop Sports Phys Ther. 1999;29:262-269; discussion 270-264.

110. Van Blommestein AS, MaCrae S, Lewis J, Morrissey M. Reliability of measuring thoracic kyphosis angle, lumbar lordosis angle and straight leg raise with an inclinometer. Open Spine Journal. 2012; 4: 10-15.

111. Wang CH, McClure P, Pratt NE, Nobilini R. Stretching and strengthening exercises: their effect on three-dimensional scapular kinematics. Arch Phys Med Rehabil. 1999;80:923-929.

112. Wassinger CA, Sole G, Osborne H. Clinical measurement of scapular upward rotation in response to acute subacromial pain. J Orthop Sports Phys Ther. 2013;43:199-203.

113. Watson DH, Trott PH. Cervical headache: an investigation of natural head posture and upper cervical flexor muscle performance. Cephalagia. 1993;13:272-284.

114. Williams P, Bannister L, Berry M, et al. (eds). Gray's Anatomy, 38th edition. Edinburgh: Churchill Livingstone; 1995.

115. Yanagawa TL, Maitland ME, Burgess K, Young L, Hanley D. Assessment of thoracic kyphosis using the flexicurve for individuals with osteoporosis. Hong Kong Physiotherapy Journal. 2000;18:53-57.

116. Zackarkow D. Posture: Sitting, Standing, Chair Design, and Exercise. Springfield: Charles C. Thomas; 1988.

117. Getty Images. Available at: https://www.gettyimages.co.uk/detail/video/models-walk-with-books-on-their-heads-during-a-deportment-news-footage/1B012404_0005.

118. Vintage Everyday. Available at: https://www.vintag.es/2017/10/miss-correct-posture-pictures-from.html.

Neurodynamics related to shoulder pain 21

Toby Hall, Michel Coppieters

A different perspective on neuropathies and neurodynamics

Neuropathies refer to damage, disease, or dysfunction of one or more nerves. Neuropathies are complex, and the underlying mechanisms of the different types of neuropathies, such as compression neuropathy, diabetic neuropathy, and cancer treatment-induced neuropathy, are very diverse. Clinically, we tend to assess and manage neuropathies as if the different types are all the same, and can be assessed and managed in a similar manner. For example, we apply neurodynamic tests when we assess compression neuropathy,[30] cancer treatment-induced neuropathy[21] and also diabetic neuropathy.[7] Similarly, electrodiagnostic tests are also used in each of these conditions. However, not only are the underlying pathomechanisms different across the various types of neuropathies, they also vary between different types of compression neuropathies, or between different types of cancer treatment-induced neuropathy, which will relate to the type of chemotherapy prescribed.[45] Moreover, the underlying mechanisms may differ between people with the same diagnosis. For example, the pathomechanisms that result in symptoms associated with carpal tunnel syndrome in two individuals may be very different.[4]

Nerve compression may be associated with multiple pathomechanisms, including local demyelination, axon degeneration, immune responses at the entrapment site and remote sites (such as the dorsal root ganglia, spinal cord, and regions of the brain), ion channel upregulation, impaired blood flow, intraneural edema, altered axonal transport, abnormal impulse generation, and blood–nerve barrier changes. These mechanisms may also be present in people presenting with shoulder pain occurring as a result of neuropathy.

The contemporary view of neurodynamics is that it is a clinical concept that uses movement to: 1) assess increased mechanosensitivity of the nervous system, and 2) restore homeostasis in and around the nervous system.[12] Increased mechanosensitivity of the nervous system is only one possible manifestation of a neuropathy. Other manifestations include paresthesia, numbness, hyperalgesia, allodynia, spontaneous pain, reduced strength, and reduced two-point discrimination threshold. This implies that neurodynamic tests are most likely relevant in conditions where increased mechanosensitivity of the nervous system is more common, and neurodynamic tests can help establish whether this mechanism is present or not.

The prevalence of increased mechanosensitivity likely varies for different types of neuropathies. It is likely to be less common in diabetic neuropathy and chemotherapy-induced neuropathy, and probably more common in acute radiculopathy due to a disc herniation, characterized by significant local inflammation. It also implies that neurodynamic tests do not assess many of the other characteristics of neuropathies, and neurodynamic tests are therefore likely to be negative in the absence of increased mechanosensitivity despite the presence of a neuropathy. This does not compromise the usefulness of neurodynamic tests. Each assessment method for neuropathies has limitations. Electrodiagnostic tests, for example, mainly assess the large-diameter nerve fibers, whereas many neuropathies are characterized or may commence as small-diameter nerve fiber pathologies.[11] Furthermore, electrodiagnostic tests are often negative in chemotherapy-induced peripheral neuropathy. Having an insight into the underlying mechanisms of neuropathies helps clinicians select and understand the results of clinical and technical investigations in people with peripheral neuropathies.

Whereas the diagnostic component of neurodynamics mainly focuses on increased mechanosensitivity, the indications for neurodynamic treatment are broader, and aim to restore homeostasis in and around the nervous system. "Altered homeostasis in and around the nervous system" may sound somewhat nebulous, but it relates to the mechanisms listed above, and includes increased edema, hypoxia, lower pH, demyelination, and increased concentrations of immune compounds locally at the entrapment and remote sites. This is supported by an increasing body of research conducted in animals that have revealed neurodynamic treatment reduces intraneural edema,[48] improves axon regeneration and remyelination,[18] and normalizes elevated concentrations of immune compounds and glial cells, not only at the local entrapment site[60] but also at the dorsal root ganglia and spinal cord.[29,46] Many of these desirable changes related to neurodynamic treatment are not dependent upon the presence of increased mechanosensitivity, and therefore, a positive neurodynamic test is not an essential prerequisite to implement neurodynamic management. Neurodynamic treatments may be considered as biologically plausible interventions in the management of neuropathies, provided that movement-based interventions would not be contraindicated.

Neurodynamics and shoulder pain

Shoulder pain is one of the most common of all musculoskeletal disorders. Much is written in this book about the uncertainty of a pathoanatomical diagnosis when evaluating an individual patient's shoulder pain. This is due to uncertainty in the relationships between structural change, the possible source(s) of nociception, and validity of the so-called gold standard diagnostic tests.[32] As discussed in Chapter 15, deriving a structural diagnosis and identification of the definitive cause of symptoms presents a diagnostic dilemma.

Respecting this uncertainty, nerve injuries and entrapment neuropathies in the shoulder region are potential sources of shoulder pain that need to be considered in differential diagnosis. Such nerve injuries may result from significant trauma associated with extreme force, such as may occur in certain sports, falls, or following motor vehicle accidents. Nerve injuries and consequent neuropathic pain may be associated with shoulder dislocations and subluxations, mishaps during shoulder surgery, and upper humeral fractures. Distinct clinical syndromes may develop after injuries to any of the nerves that traverse the shoulder including the axillary, suprascapular, long thoracic, and spinal accessory nerves.[36]

Shoulder region entrapment neuropathy is relatively uncommon but is increasingly recognized, and should be considered in athletes performing repetitive overhead arm activities, such as volleyball players or throwers see (Chapter 38).[54] The suprascapular nerve is the most likely to be affected, entrapped above or below the spine of the scapula. The clinical identification of nerve injury or entrapment neuropathy is through a comprehensive neurological examination with subsequent ongoing referral for electrodiagnostic tests and imaging where appropriate. Neurodynamic tests would not be particularly helpful in the diagnosis, as tests for these nerves have not been developed sufficiently with adequate research evidence regarding their reliability and validity.

Another potential source of shoulder pain is through compromise of the brachial plexus. True neurological thoracic outlet syndrome (TOS) is very rare. Nonspecific neurological TOS is considered the most common form of TOS but is a heavily disputed and controversial condition arising from dynamic compromise in the subcoracoid or costoclavicular space or interscalene triangle[3] that results in arm symptoms. However, compromise of the brachial plexus may also lead to shoulder pain, impaired mobility, and disability. A prime example of this is a Pancoast tumor, where the tumor compresses or invades the lower trunk of the brachial plexus, sensitizing the plexus to shoulder movements that elongate or compress the plexus. Pain may be felt in the shoulder region and may be associated with hand weakness and Horner's syndrome. While relatively rare, in our own clinical practice, we encountered patients eventually diagnosed with a Pancoast tumor who were referred by the patient's general practitioner (primary care doctor) for physical therapy (physiotherapy) for shoulder pain and movement limitations. The medical practitioner was unaware of the presence of a Pancoast tumor at the time of referral. Further investigations identified the presence of the tumor in the apex of the lung. In these individuals there were features of neural tissue mechanosensitivity with positive neurodynamic tests that were clearly associated with the presenting shoulder pain and movement impairment. In both cases, onset was insidious and there were no clinical signs of cervical or shoulder pathological features that might explain sensitization of the brachial plexus. In other words, no musculoskeletal origin for the patient's condition was identified.

Other conditions that may affect the brachial plexus and peripheral nervous system may be due to treatment for breast cancer. These include surgery and radiation therapy, as well as chemotherapy. Breast cancer survivors who undergo radiation therapy are more likely to develop a brachial plexus neuropathy.[22] There is evidence of increased neural mechanosensitivity on neurodynamic tests in breast cancer survivors:[20,52] for example, Smoot et al.[52] reported reduced movement during neurodynamic tests in breast cancer survivors who complained of upper limb pain around the shoulder compared to those survivors without pain. In another study of symptomatic breast cancer survivors, usual pain was provoked by neurodynamic testing and was altered by a sensitizing movement that involved cervical lateral flexion.[20] Shoulder range of motion was also impaired significantly in the symptomatic breast cancer survivor group, but that may not have been related to neuropathy. Negative neurodynamic tests do not rule out nerve involvement, as increased mechanosensitivity may not be a hallmark feature of chemotherapy-induced neuropathy.

One confounder in the challenge of shoulder pain diagnosis is the phenomenon of referred pain from the cervical spine. Clearly it is well accepted that the cervical spine can cause referred pain into the arm in a condition such as cervical radiculopathy (see Chapter 16). However, the concept of cervical-related shoulder pain is less well recognized in the literature.[59] Despite this evidence, many clinicians routinely screen the cervical spine in the examination of people with shoulder pain,[58] and clinical practice guidelines on the evaluation of frozen shoulder from the Orthopaedic Section of the American Physical Therapy Association recommends assessment of the cervical spine, including neurodynamic testing.[34] A survey of over 1000 people suggested a link between neck and shoulder pain and disability.[37] One explanation for cervical-related shoulder pain may be as a result of compromised cervical neural tissue.[31] Date and Gray[19] evaluated 33 people with a diagnosis of shoulder impingement and found electrodiagnostic test evidence for C5/6 radiculopathy in 2 out of 33 cases (6%), with a further 9 (27%) probable cases. Sensitization of neural tissue in the cervical spine has been postulated as a potential mechanism in some people with shoulder pain and impairment,[26] however, studies are lacking.

The term cervicobrachial pain syndrome has been suggested to describe the clinical situation where neural tissue mechanosensitivity, identified by neurodynamic tests, is the primary feature on clinical examination in patients presenting with shoulder/neck region pain.[27] The diagnosis in this case is based on clinical features as no medical investigative tests are definitive of this condition. One study evaluated 120 people with neck and shoulder region pain. Of these, 30 (25%) were found to have predominant features of neural tissue mechanosensitivity on neurodynamic tests over and above dysfunction of other musculoskeletal structures.[1] Similarly, Gangavelli et al.,[28] examined 361 people with cervicobrachial pain and found that 20% had definitive features of neural tissue mechanosensitivity. These findings suggest the presence of mechanosensitive neural tissue is an important consideration in shoulder pain evaluation.

Neurodynamic examination for shoulder pain

Neurodynamic tests, each with several variants, have been described to assess mechanosensitivity of upper limb peripheral nerves. The terminology used varies between authors but the base tests include the upper limb neurodynamic test (ULNT) 1 and 2A to test the median nerve, ULNT2B to test the radial nerve and ULNT3 to test the ulnar nerve.[9,25,50] These neurodynamic tests comprise a series of movements that apply mechanical stress to a component of the nervous system, to evaluate its mechanosensitivity. However, neurodynamic tests also impart mechanical stress on non-neural structures. Hence, structural differentiation is an important aspect of neurodynamic testing to identify symptoms arising from neural tissues.

The concept of structural differentiation is based on the continuity of the nervous system. The nervous system can be selectively loaded or unloaded by changing joint positions remotely. For example, wrist extension in a ULNT1 position increases strain in the cervical nerve roots,[40] but has no impact on local neck structures. Therefore, besides symptom reproduction, the ability to alter the reproduced symptoms with structural differentiation is an essential criterion for a positive neurodynamic test.[43] These criteria have fair to moderate reliability[47] and validity.[43] Range of motion during ULNTs is known to vary considerably between sides in healthy asymptomatic people[17,39,53] and cannot be relied on to indicate a positive test.[43] Muscle responses altering resistance to movement have not been well researched in terms of normal and abnormal responses, reliability or validity, and should not be considered criteria for a positive neurodynamic test. Table 21.1 describes and illustrates the test components for the neurodynamic tests of the median, ulnar, and radial nerves.

In the case of shoulder pain, neurodynamic testing of the median nerve (ULNT1) may reproduce the patient's shoulder symptoms during the elbow extension component of the test, with the shoulder in 90° abduction and 90° external rotation. However, this position places considerable stress on the local shoulder non-neural structures as well. Structural differentiation is required to confirm or deny a neural contribution to the symptoms. If wrist extension is added to the neurodynamic test movement, and consequently shoulder pain is increased, then this would support

TABLE 21.1 Components for neurodynamic tests of the median, ulnar and radial nerves

Neurodynamic test	Components of the base neurodynamic test	Typical end position of the test
ULNT1 (median)	Shoulder girdle fixation, 90° shoulder abduction and lateral rotation, elbow extension, forearm supination, wrist and finger extension.	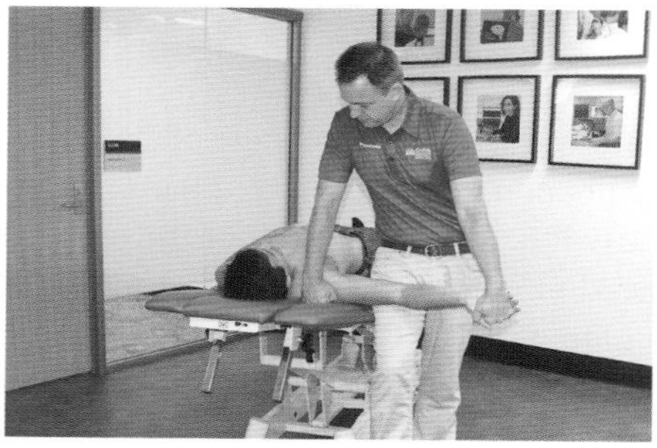
ULNT2A (median)	Shoulder girdle depression, shoulder external rotation and 20° to 30° abduction, elbow extension, forearm supination, wrist and finger extension.	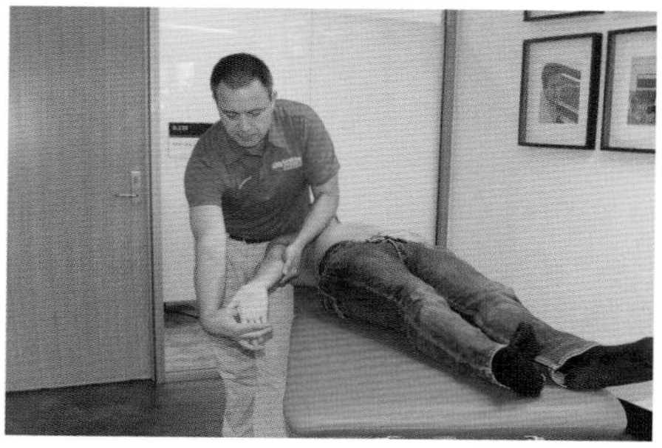
ULNT2B (radial)	Shoulder girdle depression, shoulder medial rotation and 20° to 30° abduction, elbow extension, forearm pronation, wrist and finger flexion.	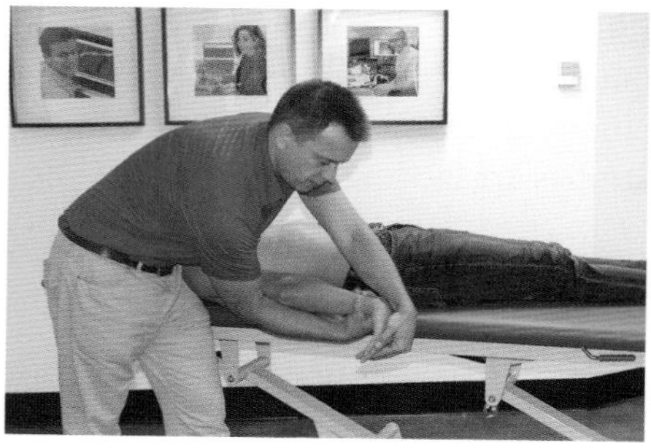
ULNT3 (ulnar)	Shoulder girdle depression, shoulder abduction and lateral rotation, elbow flexion, forearm pronation, wrist and finger extension.	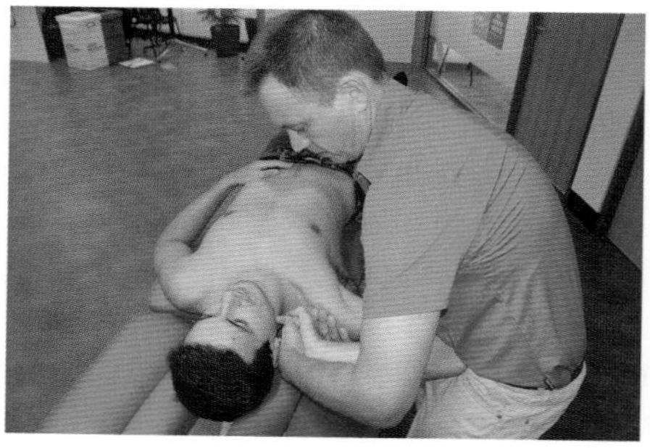

ULNT, upper limb neurodynamic testing.

the hypothesis that increased neural mechanosensitivity is a contributing factor to the patient's shoulder pain. In this case, contralateral lateral flexion of the neck may also be included to possibly increase the strain on the peripheral nervous system in the shoulder area. As mentioned, diagnosis is a challenge, and the responses to neurodynamic testing may help support or refute clinical hypotheses as part of the clinical reasoning process (see Chapter 13). A positive finding may suggest the presence of increased neural tissue mechanosensitivity which may be a contributing factor to the patient's shoulder pain and movement impairment. It also suggests that neural mobilization techniques may be considered as part of a management plan if no contraindications to movement-based intervention are present.

While the names used for each test implies some specificity to the nerve tested, the tests also place mechanical force on other nerves.[35,42] This is logical as the different tests share various components, for example, elbow extension is part of the test for the median nerve and the radial nerve. Cadaveric studies confirm this and show spread of force to the radial nerve during the application of the ULNT1.[35] It is therefore important to recognize that a positive test when considered in isolation does not necessarily indicate that the nerve tested is sensitized, nor does it indicate a problem of the neural tissue local to the shoulder. It would be important to evaluate responses to multiple tests before deciding which nerves are dominantly sensitized. Further tests, such as evaluation of hyperalgesic responses to nerve palpation, may also be indicated to support an understanding of nerve trunk mechanosensitivity.

The validity of neurodynamic tests have been investigated with respect to common upper limb neural pain disorders including cervical radiculopathy, carpal tunnel syndrome, and cubital tunnel syndrome.[43] One confounding factor associated with this type of research is that compression neuropathy (for example, cervical radiculopathy and carpal tunnel syndrome) does not always lead to increased neural tissue mechanosensitivity, and therefore compression neuropathy cannot always be detected by neurodynamic tests. Furthermore, the gold standard often used in these diagnostic accuracy studies include electrodiagnosis and/or advanced medical imaging, such as magnetic resonance imaging (MRI). It is important to recognize that electrodiagnosis, MRI, and neurodynamic tests assess different domains (electrodiagnosis: impulse conduction mainly of large-diameter myelinated fibres; MRI: anatomy; and ULNT: nerve mechanosensitivity). The use of electrodiagnosis and MRI as (part of) the gold standard to validate neurodynamic tests for a neuropathy is therefore debatable. For example, increased mechanosensitivity may occur even though electrodiagnostic tests are normal.[23]

Early validity studies[57] applied very lenient criteria for a positive neurodynamic test (e.g., reproduction of symptoms *or* (rather than *and*) changes with structural differentiation *or* a left-right difference of >10 degrees). The consequence of applying these lenient criteria was that ULNTs were believed to have extremely high sensitivity (valuable tests to rule out a neuropathy following a negative ULNT) and poor specificity (not useful to identify a neuropathy following a positive ULNT). The correct application of the criteria for a positive neurodynamic test (i.e., reproduction of symptoms that can be changed with structural differentiation) revealed that both the sensitivity and specificity of ULNTs are moderate.[2,51]

Although recent research has superseded the earlier findings, the incorrect beliefs that neurodynamic tests are good for ruling out, but not ruling in, a neuropathy still hold sway.[38] Vanti et al. reported that a subgroup of people with carpal tunnel syndrome did not have positive neurodynamic tests.[56] Similarly, Baselgia et al. found only 46% of people with electro-diagnostically confirmed carpal tunnel syndrome had positive neurodynamic tests based on symptom reproduction and structural differentiation.[4] When evaluated with quantitative sensory testing, patients with confirmed carpal tunnel syndrome and negative neurodynamic tests were found to have more severe nerve damage, particularly affecting small-diameter nerve fibers. The main purpose of neurodynamic testing is to evaluate nerve trunk mechanosensitivity. While the tests do point to a neural tissue disorder, they cannot be expected to be able to identify nerve compression disorders in the absence of nerve mechanosensitivity.

While standardization of testing is important for both clinical and research settings, the authors who originally developed neurodynamic tests[9,25,50] stressed the importance of variation in testing based on the individual patient's requirements and responses. Neurodynamic tests can only be carried out within the available range of passive movement, which is governed by the severity of pain associated with the disorder. In more severe cases of sensitized nerve trunks, the degree of movement impairment will be much greater, and performance of the base neurodynamic tests may not be possible. Therefore, it is unrealistic to have a standard form of neurodynamic test for all presentations, and the clinician is required to adjust test techniques for individual patients. An example would be for a patient with severe shoulder pain presenting with gross limitation of shoulder movement in abduction and external rotation. Standard neurodynamic tests for the median nerve (ULNT1) may not be possible. In this case, the test order and components may be altered, so that cervical lateral flexion is evaluated in different positions of shoulder abduction and external rotation with the elbow extended and wrist and fingers relaxed. Perhaps cervical lateral flexion may be tested with the arm by the side and then in 30° abduction and responses compared. In this way, even the most severely restricted patient may be evaluated for the presence of increased neural tissue mechanosensitivity.

It has been suggested that the sequence in which the various component movements are applied during neurodynamic tests is of importance, as it may provide information about the site of neural tissue pathology.[41,49] While this would be useful, it is unfortunately not supported by the literature[6,14,44] and it may be that responses to neurodynamic sequencing may simply be due to the attention placed on the first of a combination of movements.[10]

Management of shoulder pain using neurodynamics

If increased neural tissue mechanosensitivity, identified by neurodynamic tests, is seen to be a significant feature in a patient's presenting shoulder pain, then logically it would follow to address those neural components as part of the management plan. When neural tissue is sensitized, management may include manual techniques and exercise designed to desensitize neural tissues. However, management should not be isolated to just such an approach. It has been recommended in a recent review of physiotherapy for peripheral nerve disorders that physiotherapists should assess and monitor their patients' neuropathies and their wider health, educate them about their condition, coach them through a return to valued activity, and help them make sense of their predicament in addition to manual therapy and exercise.[33]

Neural mobilization incorporates movement between neural structures and their surrounding interface through movement and positioning of specific body parts. This includes "sliding" and "tensioning" nerve mobilization techniques that can be performed passively by the therapist or actively by the patient. To the authors' knowledge, no controlled studies have examined the effect of neural mobilization specifically in shoulder pain. However, a number of systematic reviews have investigated neural mobilization for musculoskeletal disorders.[5,24,55] The conclusion of the most recent and most comprehensive review [5] was that neural mobilization is effective for nerve-related neck pain and back pain, but that its effect remains unclear for most other conditions due to the limited research available.

Neural mobilization for cervicobrachial pain is the closest condition to shoulder pain where evidence is available. Four studies evaluated the cervical contralateral lateral glide technique, and all reported a significant improvement in pain for the groups receiving neural mobilization. In those studies, cervical mobilization was compared to waiting list, ultrasound, and advice to stay active. Meta-analysis revealed a reduction in pain intensity of 1.9 points (95%CI: 0.6–3.1) on a 0–10 scale.

The cervical contralateral lateral glide technique is a passive movement applied by the clinician with the patient lying supine. When the irritability is high, the patient's arm is positioned in such a way that their hand rests on their abdomen (Figure 21.5). The clinician stabilizes the shoulder girdle with one hand while supporting the patient's head and neck with the other. The affected cervical motion segment is targeted, and a lateral glide initiated. Once the nervous system becomes less sensitized, components of the most relevant neurodynamic test can be applied to position the arm so that the median, radial, or ulnar nerve is more loaded.

Gentle controlled lateral glide to the contralateral side is performed in a slow oscillating manner up to a point in range where resistance is felt. Oscillations may be performed in five sets, each of approximately 60 seconds. The cervical lateral glide technique not only mechanically influences neural tissue in the neck but also to some degree the median nerve in the arm.[8] The most obvious indicator of successful treatment following the application of the cervical lateral glide technique is an improvement in neurodynamic test response or shoulder movement together with a reduction in the severity of pain.

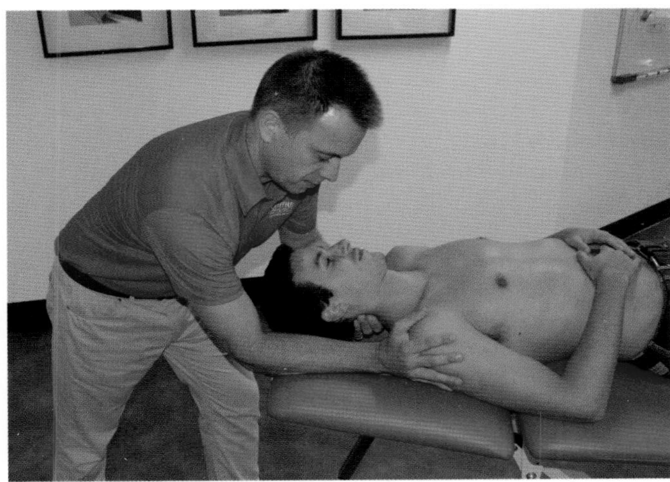

FIGURE 21.5
Cervical contralateral lateral glide.

Exercise should also be encouraged to continue to desensitize the neural tissue between treatment sessions. Sliding techniques are an appropriate first exercise, as they can be performed pain-free and promote desensitization. Tensioning techniques are typically avoided until the end stage of rehabilitation. The excursion and strain of peripheral nerves during tensioning and sliding exercises are vastly different.[13,15,16] Substantial increases in nerve strain that occur during tensioning techniques can be avoided during sliding techniques, and the excursion of the targeted nerve is approximately 2.5[13] to 5 times[16] larger with sliding techniques than with tensioning techniques. Evidence for the use of neural mobilization as an exercise is reported in studies using sliding and tensioning techniques.[5] Although studies were at a high risk of bias making conclusions less clear, this approach had a significant effect on pain. The amount of movement required during neurodynamic exercise is unclear, but it would be prudent to start at a low level and increase the volume of exercise progressively as the condition improves.

References

1. Allison GT, Nagy BM, Hall T. A randomized clinical trial of manual therapy for cervico-brachial pain syndrome: a pilot study. Man Ther. 2002;7:95-102.
2. Apelby-Albrecht M, Andersson L, Kleiva IW, Kvåle K, Skillgate E, Josephson A. Concordance of upper limb neurodynamic tests with medical examination and magnetic resonance imaging in patients with cervical radiculopathy: a diagnostic cohort study. J Manipulative Physiol Ther. 2013;36:626-632.
3. Balderman J, Abuirqeba AA, Eichaker L, et al. Physical therapy management, surgical treatment, and patient-reported outcomes measures in a prospective observational cohort of patients with neurogenic thoracic outlet syndrome. J Vasc Surg. 2019;70:832-841.
4. Baselgia LT, Bennett DL, Silbiger RM, Schmid AB. Negative neurodynamic tests do not exclude neural dysfunction in patients with entrapment neuropathies. Arch Phys Med Rehabil. 2017;98:480-486.
5. Basson A, Olivier B, Ellis R, Coppieters M, Stewart A, Mudzi W. The effectiveness of neural mobilization for neuromusculoskeletal conditions: a systematic review and meta-analysis. J Orthop Sports Phys Ther. 2017;47:593-615.
6. Boyd BS, Topp KS, Coppieters MW. Impact of movement sequencing on sciatic and tibial nerve strain and excursion during the straight leg raise test in embalmed cadavers. J Orthop Sports Phys Ther. 2013;43:398-403.
7. Boyd BS, Wanek L, Gray AT, Topp KS. Mechanosensitivity during lower extremity neurodynamic testing is diminished in individuals with type 2 diabetes mellitus and peripheral neuropathy: a cross sectional study. BMC Neurology. 2010;10:75.
8. Brochwicz P, von Piekartz H, Zalpour C. Sonography assessment of the median nerve during cervical lateral glide and lateral flexion. Is there a difference in neurodynamics of asymptomatic people? Man Ther. 2013;18:216-219.
9. Butler DS. Mobilisation of the Nervous System. Melbourne: Churchill Livingstone; 1991.
10. Butler DS, Coppieters MW. Neurodynamics in a broader perspective. Man Ther. 2007;12:e7-8.
11. Chao CC, Tseng MT, Lin YH, et al. Brain imaging signature of neuropathic pain phenotypes in small-fiber neuropathy: altered thalamic connectome and its associations with skin nerve degeneration. Pain. 2021;162:1387-1399.
12. Coppieters M, Nee B. Neurodynamic management of the peripheral nervous system. In: Jull G, Moore A, Falla D, Lewis J, McCarthy C, Sterling M (eds). Grieve's Modern Musculoskeletal Physiotherapy, 4th edition. Edinburgh: Elsevier; 2015:287-297.
13. Coppieters MW, Alshami AM. Longitudinal excursion and strain in the median nerve during novel nerve gliding exercises for carpal tunnel syndrome. Journal of Orthopaedic Research. 2007;25:972-980.
14. Coppieters MW, Alshami AM, Babri AS, Souvlis T, Kippers V, Hodges PW. Strain and excursion of the sciatic, tibial, and plantar nerves during a modified straight leg raising test. Journal of Orthopaedic Research. 2006;24:1883-1889.
15. Coppieters MW, Butler DS. Do 'sliders' slide and 'tensioners' tension? An analysis of neurodynamic techniques and considerations regarding their application. Man Ther. 2007;13:213-221.
16. Coppieters MW, Hough AD, Dilley A. Different nerve-gliding exercises induce

different magnitudes of median nerve longitudinal excursion: an in vivo study using dynamic ultrasound imaging. J Orthop Sports Phys Ther. 2009;39:164-171.

17. Covill LG, Petersen SM. Upper extremity neurodynamic tests: range of motion asymmetry may not indicate impairment. Physiother Theory Pract. 2012;28:535-41.

18. da Silva JT, Santos FM, Giardini AC, et al. Neural mobilization promotes nerve regeneration by nerve growth factor and myelin protein zero increased after sciatic nerve injury. Growth Factors. 2015;33:8-13.

19. Date ES, Gray LA. Electrodiagnostic evidence for cervical radiculopathy and suprascapular neuropathy in shoulder pain. Electromyography and Clinical Neurophysiology. 1996;36:333-339.

20. de la Rosa-Diaz I, Torres-Lacomba M, Acosta-Ramirez P, et al. Protective myoelectric activity at performing upper limb neurodynamic test 1 in breast cancer survivors. A cross-sectional observational study. Musculoskelet Sci Pract. 2018;36:68-80.

21. de la Rosa-Díaz I, Torres-Lacomba M, Acosta-Ramírez P, et al. Protective myoelectric activity at performing upper limb neurodynamic test 1 in breast cancer survivors. A cross-sectional observational study. Musculoskelet Sci Pract. 2018;36:68-80.

22. Delanian S, Lefaix JL, Pradat PF. Radiation-induced neuropathy in cancer survivors. Radiother Oncol. 2012;105:273-282.

23. Dilley A, Lynn B, Pang SJ. Pressure and stretch mechanosensitivity of peripheral nerve fibres following local inflammation of the nerve trunk. Pain. 2005;117:462-472.

24. Ellis RF, Hing WA. Neural mobilization: a systematic review of randomized controlled trials with an analysis of therapeutic efficacy. J Man Manip Ther. 2008;16:8-22.

25. Elvey R. Brachial plexus tension tests and the pathoanatomical origin of arm pain. In: Idczak R (ed). Aspects of Manipulative Therapy. Melbourne: Lincoln Institute of Health Sciences; 1979:105-110.

26. Elvey RL. Physical evaluation of the peripheral nervous system in disorders of pain and dysfunction. J Hand Ther. 1997;10:122-129.

27. Elvey RL, Hall TM. Neural tissue evaluation and treatment. In: Donatelli R (ed). Physical Therapy of the Shoulder, 3rd edition. Philadelphia: Churchill Livingstone; 1997:131-152.

28. Gangavelli R, Nair NS, Bhat AK, Solomon JM. Cervicobrachial pain: how often is it neurogenic? J Clin Diagn Res. 2016;10:YC14-16.

29. Giardini AC, Dos Santos FM, da Silva JT, de Oliveira ME, Martins DO, Chacur M. Neural mobilization treatment decreases glial cells and brain-derived neurotrophic factor expression in the central nervous system in rats with neuropathic pain induced by CCI in rats. Pain Res Manag. 2017;2017:7429761.

30. González Espinosa de Los Monteros FJ, Gonzalez-Medina G, Ardila EMG, Mansilla JR, Expósito JP, Ruiz PO. Use of neurodynamic or orthopedic tension tests for the diagnosis of lumbar and lumbosacral radiculopathies: study of the diagnostic validity. Int J Environ Res Public Health. 2020;17:7046.

31. Hall TM, Elvey RL. Nerve trunk pain: physical diagnosis and treatment. Man Ther. 1999;4:63-73.

32. Hegedus EJ, Goode AP, Cook CE, et al. Which physical examination tests provide clinicians with the most value when examining the shoulder? Update of a systematic review with meta-analysis of individual tests. Br J Sports Med. 2012;46:964-978.

33. Jesson T, Runge N, Schmid AB. Physiotherapy for people with painful peripheral neuropathies: a narrative review of its efficacy and safety. Pain Reports Online. 2020;5:e834.

34. Kelley MJ, Shaffer MA, Kuhn JE, et al. Shoulder pain and mobility deficits: adhesive capsulitis. J Orthop Sports Phys Ther. 2013;43:A1-31.

35. Kleinrensink GJ, Stoeckart R, Mulder PG, et al. Upper limb tension tests as tools in the diagnosis of nerve and plexus lesions. Anatomical and biomechanical aspects. Clin Biomech. 2000;15:9-14.

36. Kokkalis ZT, Pantzaris N, Iliopoulos ID, Megaloikonomos PD, Mavrogenis AF, Panagiotopoulos E. Nerve injuries around the shoulder. J Long Term Eff Med Implants. 2017;27:13-20.

37. Koller J, Bismarck C, Krebs S, Hitzl W, Mayer M, Koller H. Coexistence of neck and shoulder disability: results of a population-based cross-sectional study on normative scores and multifactorial risk factors for neck and shoulder problems. Asian Spine J. 2021;15:180-191.

38. Koulidis K, Veremis Y, Anderson C, Heneghan NR. Diagnostic accuracy of upper limb neurodynamic tests for the assessment of peripheral neuropathic pain: a systematic review. Musculoskelet Sci Pract. 2019;40:21-33.

39. Lohkamp M, Small K. Normal response to Upper Limb Neurodynamic Test 1 and 2A. Man Ther. 2011;16:125-130.

40. Lohman CM, Gilbert KK, Sobczak S, et al. 2015 Young Investigator Award Winner: cervical nerve root displacement and strain during upper limb neural tension testing. Part 1: a minimally invasive assessment in unembalmed cadavers. Spine (Phila PA 1976). 2015;40:793-800.

41. Maitland G. The Slump test: examination and treatment. Australian Journal of Physiotherapy. 1985;31:215-219.

42. Manvell N, Manvell JJ, Snodgrass SJ, Reid SA. Tension of the ulnar, median, and radial nerves during ulnar nerve neurodynamic testing: observational cadaveric study. Phys Ther. 2015;95:891-900.

43. Nee RJ, Jull GA, Vicenzino B, Coppieters MW. The validity of upper-limb neurodynamic tests for detecting peripheral neuropathic pain. J Orthop Sports Phys Ther. 2012;42:413-424.

44. Nee RJ, Yang CH, Liang CC, Tseng GF, Coppieters MW. Impact of order of movement on nerve strain and longitudinal excursion: a biomechanical study with implications for neurodynamic test sequencing. Man Ther. 2010;15:376-381.

45. Park SB, Goldstein D, Krishnan AV, et al. Chemotherapy-induced peripheral neurotoxicity: a critical analysis. CA Cancer J Clin. 2013;63:419-437.

46. Santos FM, Silva JT, Giardini AC, et al. Neural mobilization reverses behavioral and cellular changes that characterize neuropathic pain in rats. Molecular pain. 2012;8:57.

47. Schmid AB, Brunner F, Luomajoki H, et al. Reliability of clinical tests to evaluate nerve function and mechanosensitivity of the upper limb peripheral nervous system. BMC Musculoskelet Disord. 2009;10:11.

48. Schmid AB, Elliott JM, Strudwick MW, Little M, Coppieters MW. Effect of splinting and exercise on intraneural edema of the median nerve in carpal tunnel syndrome: an MRI study to reveal therapeutic

mechanisms. Journal of Orthopaedic Research. 2012;30:1343-1350.

49. Shacklock M. Clinical Neurodynamics. Edinburgh: Elsevier; 2005.

50. Shacklock M. Neurodynamics. Physiotherapy. 1995;81:9-16.

51. Sleijser-Koehorst MLS, Coppieters MW, Epping R, Rooker S, Verhagen AP, Scholten-Peeters GGM. Diagnostic accuracy of patient interview items and clinical tests for cervical radiculopathy. Physiotherapy. 2021;111:74-82.

52. Smoot B, Boyd BS, Byl N, Dodd M. Mechanosensitivity in the upper extremity following breast cancer treatment. J Hand Ther. 2014;27:4-11.

53. Stalioraitis V, Robinson K, Hall T. Side-to-side range of movement variability in variants of the median and radial neurodynamic test sequences in asymptomatic people. Man Ther. 2014;19:338-342.

54. Strauss EJ, Kingery MT, Klein D, Manjunath AK. The evaluation and management of suprascapular neuropathy. J Am Acad Orthop Surg. 2020;28:617-627.

55. Su Y, Lim EC. Does evidence support the use of neural tissue management to reduce pain and disability in nerve-related chronic musculoskeletal pain? A systematic review with meta-analysis. Clin J Pain. 2016;32:991-1004.

56. Vanti C, Bonfiglioli R, Calabrese M, et al. Upper Limb Neurodynamic Test 1 and symptoms reproduction in carpal tunnel syndrome. A validity study. Man Ther. 2011;16:258-263.

57. Wainner RS, Fritz JM, Irrgang JJ, Boninger ML, Delitto A, Allison S. Reliability and diagnostic accuracy of the clinical examination and patient self-report measures for cervical radiculopathy. Spine (Phila PA 1976). 2003;28:52-62.

58. Walker T, Cuff A, Salt E, Lynch G, Littlewood C. Examination of the neck when a patient complains of shoulder pain: a global survey of current practice (2019). Musculoskeletal Care. 2020;18:256-264.

59. Walker T, Salt E, Lynch G, Littlewood C. Screening of the cervical spine in subacromial shoulder pain: a systematic review. Shoulder Elbow. 2019;11:305-315.

60. Zhu GC, Tsai KL, Chen YW, Hung CH. Neural mobilization attenuates mechanical allodynia and decreases proinflammatory cytokine concentrations in rats with painful diabetic neuropathy. Phys Ther. 2018;98:214-222.

Hemodynamics and the shoulder 22

Alan J Taylor, Roger Kerry

Introduction

Hemodynamic or vascular factors are possible causes of shoulder symptoms. Although rare, their potential for serious complications requires clinicians to remain cognizant of presentations associated with hemodynamic compromise. It is accepted that involvement in repetitive and strenuous activity of the upper limb may expose individuals to shoulder pain.[21] Commonly these presentations involve, or are at least diagnosed as involving, the musculoskeletal, and less commonly, the neurological systems. More recently, there has been increased clinical understanding of the possibility of vascular involvement in clinical presentations involving the shoulder and upper limb.[19] Consideration of a vascular contribution to shoulder and upper limb symptoms should be considered in all people presenting with potential musculoskeletal shoulder conditions.

Due to their relative rarity, the index of suspicion for hemodynamic involvement such as flow limitation or embolic events may be low. As a result, upper limb vascular conditions may be misdiagnosed and the long-term consequences of this may be serious.[19] Early retirement from sport or professional occupations, through failed and misguided treatment has been reported as a potential consequence[2] and limb-threatening thromboembolic events are rare, but more serious sequalae.[25]

This chapter presents a range of vascular syndromes that all practitioners should consider in their differential diagnosis of upper limb conditions. The conditions are rare compared to musculoskeletal conditions, but nevertheless require consideration, as clinical reasoning, appropriate early recognition, and triage may improve outcomes for people seeking care. For simplicity, the conditions are divided into arterial and venous, and demarcated by their anatomical location or the common site of blood flow compromise. Box 22.1 lists the major hemodynamic conditions of concern.

Box 22.1 Shoulder and upper limb hemodynamic conditions of concern.

Arterial and venous thoracic outlet syndromes:

- Subclavian-axillary artery occlusion
- Subclavian-axillary artery aneurysms
- Paget-Schroetter syndrome (upper limb deep venous thrombosis)

Non-thoracic outlet syndromes:

- Subclavian steal syndrome
- Quadrilateral space syndrome

Vascular syndromes around the shoulder region

Arterial and venous thoracic outlet syndromes

The term thoracic outlet refers to the anatomical area of the shoulder below the clavicle and above the thorax. Figure 22.1 presents an overview of the key anatomical structures of the thoracic outlet. Technically it is a canal that carries the neurovascular bundle from the neck into the arm. The term thoracic outlet syndrome (TOS) is intentionally broad and covers neurogenic (nTOS), arterial (aTOS), and venous (vTOS) presentations. Arterial and venous TOS are rare disorders which are less common than neurogenic, but nonetheless essential to consider. They may affect individuals of all ages and both genders, and may present in young, active adults.[19] This chapter focuses on manifestations of aTOS and vTOS and considers the mechanisms, recognition, and management options.

CHAPTER TWENTY-TWO

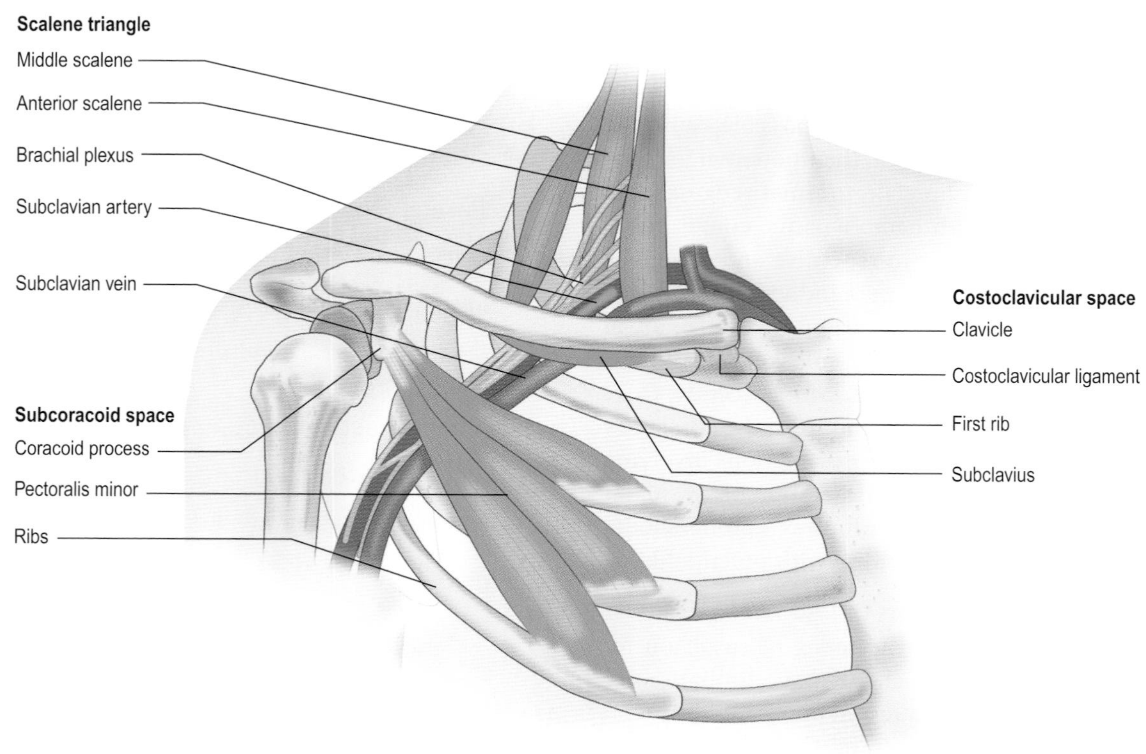

FIGURE 22.1
Thoracic outlet anatomy.

Subclavian-axillary arterial occlusion

Definition

Arterial occlusion in the subclavian-axillary region may be of an external or internal etiology. External occlusion involves compression of the artery from the surrounding musculoskeletal structures, leading to transient flow limitations. Within the region of the thoracic outlet the muscular structures that can cause compression are the anterior scalene, subclavius and pectoralis minor.[21] Hypertrophy or more subtle muscle imbalance dysfunctions may result in the occlusion of distal blood flow and create local and peripheral altered hemodynamics.[19] Bony structures associated with the costoclavicular space include the presence of a cervical rib, or an anomalous first rib.[2] Occlusion via these mechanisms may be a result of repetitive upper quadrant activity or direct trauma. Internal occlusion is related to atherosclerotic disease. Several case series regarding distal thrombosis from subclavian-axillary inducible occlusion (i.e., transient and as a result of the throwing action and glenohumeral instability) have been reported.[25]

Presentation

Pain in the region of the supraclavicular fossa and arm is seldom considered to have a vascular origin, especially in the younger population. The clinical presentation for arterial occlusion at this anatomical region mimics various neuromusculoskeletal conditions including ulna nerve injury, glenohumeral pathology, cervical dysfunction, “tennis elbow”, localized hand pathology, and nonvascular thoracic outlet syndrome. A description of distal symptoms including weakness, fatigue, coldness, and dysesthesia related to activity are common. A Raynaud's-type intolerance to cold should also raise the clinician's index of suspicion to an arterial cause.

Assessment

Vascular examination is normal at rest. Clinical examination must be performed in comparable positions as well as after effort. Examination may reveal reduced or absent distal pulses during positional change, therefore classic "thoracic outlet" tests, such as Adson's, Allen's, Halstead's maneuver, and the Roos Extension Abduction Stress Test (EAST) may or may not be positive. Negative positional tests do not exclude an arterial cause as the exertion component may be more relevant than the positional component in some cases. Further, the diagnostic utility and precise mechanisms behind provocative arm position tests is largely unknown, and care should be taken to consider test findings in line with the wider clinical picture.[28-32] Examination of the upper limb digits might reveal a prolonged capillary refill time in different positions/levels of exertion together with some cooling of the extremity. Arm to arm blood pressure examination (discussed below) forms part of the assessment and positional arteriography would confirm a diagnosis.

Management

Repetitive external trauma to a vessel may result in pathological changes to the intimal layer of the artery. Activity modifications or cessation of aggravating activities is important. Antiplatelet therapy may be required. In persistent cases that have failed to respond to previous intervention, surgical resection of the aberrant anatomical structures may become necessary. If surgical intervention is not indicated, physical therapy to address the underlying musculoskeletal dysfunction, together with a carefully planned rehabilitation and reloading program, with careful monitoring of arterial markers, should proceed.

Subclavian-axillary artery aneurysm

Definition

An increase in diameter of the arterial wall may be a result of repetitive trauma. Consequently, aneurysm formation may be a result of prolonged external forces related to mechanisms as described above. The risk of thrombosis and distal embolization (i.e., embolization into the hand) is significant in this pathology. The continual pressure of flow into the aneurysm during repetitive activity is a mechanism of thrombosis.

Presentation

Symptoms are commonly subtle, and a vascular hypothesis is rarely considered.[16] Clinical presentation is similar to occlusion problems described above. The clinician's threshold of suspicion should be increased if the patient reports cold in the fingers, loss of endurance during the activity, or a decrease in speed or control of the upper limb activity.

Assessment

Positional and post-exercise testing of distal pulses, capillary refill time, and blanching of the hand provide quick and easily obtainable measurements. Segmental systolic brachial, wrist, radial, and ulnar pressures will support or negate a vascular diagnosis.[21] Closer examination of the hand in terms of systolic finger pressures and Doppler measurements of finger pulses will contribute to assessing the extent of distal embolization into the palmar arch of the hand. On palpation, a pulsatile mass in the supraclavicular and infraclavicular region may be present depending on the size and location of the aneurysm.

Management

Catheter-driven thrombolysis has been reported as a method of dissolving clots in distal vessels.[19] Surgical resection of the aneurysm may be considered if return to high level activity is the goal. Physical therapy directed at rehabilitation and addressing the underlying biomechanical cause together with a carefully planned rehabilitation and reloading program should then be implemented.

Paget-Schroetter syndrome

Definition

Paget-Schroetter syndrome refers to the primary form of subclavian-axillary vein thrombosis and is also commonly referred to as "effort vein thrombosis", or "effort thrombosis", due to its association with physical effort and exertion.

The syndrome was first described following cases reported in 1875 by Sir James Paget and later in 1899 by Leopold van Schroetter. Paget-Schroetter syndrome is a deep vein thrombosis of the subclavian-axillary venous system, affecting the subclavian more commonly than the axillary vein. Due to misdiagnosis, the true incidence of Paget-Schrotter syndrome is unknown, and may account for approximately 3–7% of all deep vein thromboses. The risk of pulmonary embolism from Paget-Schroetter is around 12%.[26] The etiology of Paget-Schroetter syndrome is in keeping with the time-honored triad of Virchow, suggesting that stasis, vessel wall damage and a hypercoagulable state must exist in order for the development of a thrombus to occur.[33]

Sporting and non-sporting activities requiring either prolonged static postures combined with a high level of exertion are considered as risks factors for this syndrome. The effort component relates directly to the pathology and is associated with hypertrophy of surrounding muscle tissue, high physiological energy demand, and direct trauma to the vascular structures. Those involved in activities such as weightlifting and body building are particularly at risk. Direct pressure on the supraclavicular/brachial region can also be responsible for local stasis and vessel wall trauma. As such, load-bearing activities such as backpacking are considered risk factors. In extreme sports where intravenous infusions may be used for hydration, it is worth considering that needle insertion is a source of vessel wall damage.

Presentation

The typical clinical presentation of Paget-Schroetter syndrome is characterized by the youth and health of the individual.[35] The patient most commonly complains of a rapid insidious onset of arm pain with the possibility of associated supraclavicular fossa pain.[5,8,15,17,35] The onset may also be related to over-activity of the arm, unusual positioning or upper quadrant trauma. A thorough subjective history, considering past and family medical history, with focused special questions (linked to potential clotting disorders or other reasons for hypercoagulation, such as dehydration) is therefore required.[5,8] The correlation to a hypercoagulable state must be considered and as such the clinician must establish the nature of medications which the athlete may be taking. Oral contraceptives and hormone replacement therapies are two common groups of medication which may affect the hypercoagulable status of the patient.[26,35] The clinician must remain aware that the patient may be taking relevant medication which they may not be willing to reveal. Other risk factors include "traditional" thoracic outlet syndrome factors such as cervical rib, anomalous first rib, hypertrophy of anterior scalene, subclavius, or pectoralis minor as well as endogenous factors such as activated protein C resistance and anticardiolipin antibodies.[35]

Swelling and/or blueness of the arm is a common manifestation and may be the sole presentation.[5,8] More often though, pain and swelling accompany one another. As Paget-Schroetter syndrome is a condition of venous obstruction, pain and swelling are a result of muscular activity required to increase venous pressure. Pain and distal dysesthesia are related to repetitive activity of the upper limb. Other symptoms may include peripheral cyanosis. If pulmonary embolization has developed then there may be a description of shortness of breath, pleuritic chest pain, hemoptysis, and nonproductive cough.

Assessment

On examination edema, cyanosis, and superficial vein distension around the supraclavicular fossa and chest wall might be noticed.[5,8,15] Distal pulses are not affected, although some abnormality and discomfort around the supraclavicular pulse may be found. Signs and symptoms need to be recorded in relation to exertion of the upper extremity during the examination. The signs and symptoms associated with Paget-Schroetter syndrome may mimic patterns more commonly associated with adverse neural mechanics, and indeed neurodynamic testing may well be positive in this condition given the association with the subclavian vascular structure around the brachial plexus. A working diagnosis of reflex sympathetic dystrophy, or shoulder-hand syndrome might also be inaccurately given. Photoplethysmography and color duplex ultrasound imaging may reveal the presence of a thrombosis in the subclavian-axillary venous system.[5,8,15,17]

Management

Acute management may involve anticoagulation therapy together with the cessation of any relevant medication. Thrombolytic and surgical intervention have been reported as not being routinely indicated in the management of upper limb deep vein thrombosis.[5] The medical management will address only one component of Virchow's triad, i.e., the hypercoagulable state. The physical therapist may have a role in addressing the other two. For example, the localized stasis may be affected by a first rib dysfunction in a hockey player with excessive upper quadrant flexion/protraction during a period of exertion (i.e., while playing hockey). Likewise, vessel wall trauma could be a result of poor thoracic outlet mechanics, soft tissue hypertrophy, aberrant motor patterning during repetitive arm activity, etc. Successful management requires a harmonious combination of medical and therapeutic care.[8]

Non-thoracic outlet syndromes

Quadrilateral space syndrome

Definition

Anatomically the quadrilateral space is bounded superiorly by teres minor, inferiorly by teres major, medially by the long head of triceps, and laterally by the shaft of the humerus.[9] The axillary nerve and the posterior circumflex humeral artery (PCHA) pass through this area (Figure 22.2).

Mechanism

As the PCHA stretches around the neck of the humerus, upper limb activity can cause repetitive tension and mechanical stress to the PCHA wall, which may lead to thrombosis and aneurysmal degeneration.[7] The PCHA is a branch artery, coming off the distal third of the axillary artery. Injury to this site includes external compression, leading to potential thrombosis and aneurysm.[34] The PCHA is considerably larger than the anterior circumflex artery and winds around the surgical neck of the humerus.[12] Although the presenting symptoms may be similar, compression of the PCHA falls outside the anatomical region of the "thoracic outlet" and is usually associated with compression from the humeral head during elevation movements of the arm, most commonly abduction and external rotation. Due to

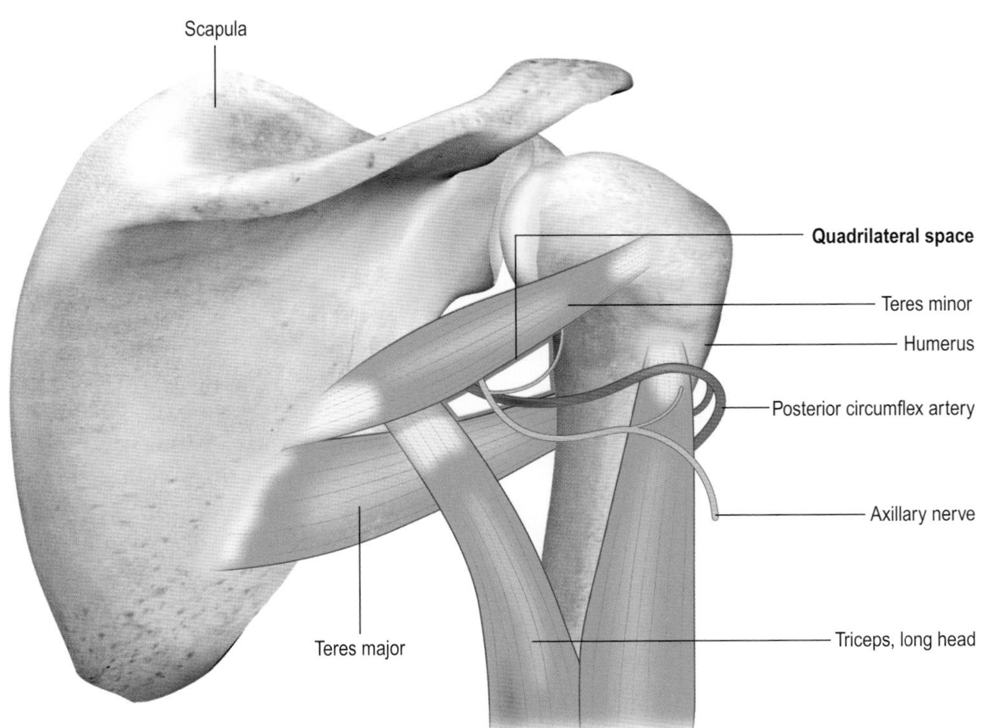

FIGURE 22.2
Quadrilateral space.

its relationship with the humeral head, the PCHA may become implicated in cases of glenohumeral instability. The clinician should therefore consider the presence of PCHA compromise when assessing glenohumeral instability in people who report unusual distal symptoms.

Presentation

Due to its association with true musculoskeletal dysfunction, e.g., glenohumeral instability, the clinical presentation will be of that dysfunction (e.g., localized glenohumeral intermittent pain, "clunking" of the joint etc.). Concomitantly there will be a report of transient weakness of the hand, classically during overhead activities such as swimming strokes and throwing. Sufferers commonly report an occasional odd feeling in the hand. The clinician needs to differentiate between a neural or vascular cause for these symptoms.

Assessment

Due to the distal site of this structure, the classic "thoracic outlet" features (e.g., anomalous first rib, cervical rib, anterior scalene hypertrophy etc.) need not be present or associated with this mechanism of injury. Rather, the nature and degree of glenohumeral instability should be assessed. When the patient's symptoms are reproduced, transient pulse obliteration may be noted. The use of arm to arm blood pressure measurements, may provide an objective measure relating to the degree of unilateral arterial compromise. However, clinicians should note that these may need to be taken in the positions of dysfunction e.g., arm overhead. Distal changes to the hand such as blanching, will also inform the extent of stenosis or thrombosis.

Management

Management of this injury will be dependent on the chronicity of the condition. It is known that repetitive external trauma to a vessel (i.e., repeated compression from the humeral head) may lead to pathological atherosclerotic changes on the intimal lining of the vessel.[26] There are no true indicators as to the time scale when these changes occur, and clinical judgement must be used to assess management priorities. Physical therapy addressing glenohumeral instability (i.e., the underlying cause of the injury or flow limitation) may be initiated with close monitoring of the arterial signs. If symptoms improve in line with improvement of other measures, then nonsurgical treatment may be successful. However, if arterial signs remain, or worsen, during the rehabilitation period as other measures are improving, then possible intimal pathology may have occurred, and surgical exploration/restructuring may be indicated.

Subclavian steal syndrome

Definition

Subclavian steal syndrome (SSS) is also known as subclavian-vertebral artery (VA) steal syndrome, since it can cause retrograde flow in the VA of the same side.[16,18,22 23] This occurs due to stenosis or occlusion of the subclavian artery, proximal to the origin of the VA. Peripheral demand of blood from upper limb activity can draw or "steal" blood from the ipsilateral vertebral artery, causing retrograde flow and transient signs and symptoms of hind-brain ischemia.[27] It may manifest in some patients with symptoms of vertebral artery insufficiency and in others as upper extremity insufficiency, usually associated with overhead movements or effort.

Mechanism

SSS (Figure 22.3) is commonly associated with atherosclerosis. It is most commonly seen on the left side, possibly due to the more acute origin of the left subclavian artery, which is thought lead to increased turbulence, causing accelerated atherosclerosis and stenosis of the vessel.[20] The subclavian stenosis leads to the phenomenon of flow reversal in the vertebral artery and resulting posterior circulation ischemia. This occurs when the demand increases for blood flow to the upper limb, but is impaired by the significantly narrowed subclavian or innominate artery and so steals from the vertebrobasilar system.[18,23]

Rare risk factors for SSS include mechanical subclavian artery compression in the thoracic outlet. This presentation usually occurs in overhead or throwing athletes like swimmers, cricket bowlers, and baseball pitchers, due to neuromuscular compression, as the subclavian artery crosses over the first rib. Additionally, the presence of anatomical anomalies, such as a cervical rib or congenital abnormalities like right aortic arch, may be a source of flow limitation.[18]

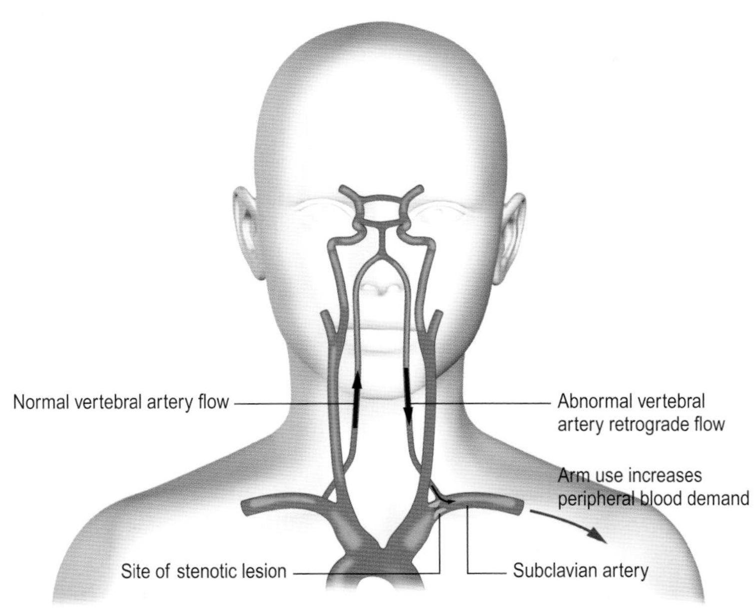

FIGURE 22.3
Subclavian steal syndrome mechanism.

Presentation

Those suffering SSS most commonly complain of transient dizziness/disequilibrium or associated symptoms of vertebrobasilar insufficiency such as drop attacks or double vision during overhead movements or efforts of the upper limb. Additionally, patients may complain of transient neurovascular symptoms in the upper limb such as numbness or weakness.[4]

Assessment

The index of suspicion for SSS is raised most by the patient's subjective history (interview) as described above. Providing the complaints are minor and transient, rather than more serious (e.g., drop attacks), then careful physical examination may proceed with pulse palpation (radial) and/or arm to arm blood pressures taken in neutral and or provocative positions as described by the patient. Findings may vary according to the exact mechanism or pathology at play. Those with underlying atherosclerotic stenosis may have reduced pulses and BP (affected arm) at rest, which is exacerbated by functional demonstrations, e.g., overhead activity. Healthy subjects with no underlying vascular pathology will only reveal their symptoms in the aggravating positions or activities where the mechanical flow limitation is reproduced.

Management

Subclavian stenosis is a marker of cardiovascular risk and patients will benefit from aggressive secondary prevention.[18,22-24] Medical therapy includes aspirin, β-blockade, angiotensin converting enzyme inhibition, and statins.[1] For patients with mild symptoms, medical therapy and observation may be appropriate, as symptomatic improvement without intervention has been described.

For patients with persistent symptoms, subclavian artery occlusion can be successfully treated either surgically or percutaneously.[3] Balloon angioplasty and stenting may be performed when stenting is unlikely to compromise the vertebral circulation. However, longer, or more distal occlusions may be better addressed surgically. Rehabilitation will be a consideration post-surgery.

Clinical assessment

It is important to appreciate that vascular examination at rest may be entirely normal. It is therefore easy to assume the absence of a vascular mechanism for the symptoms and attempt to fit the patient into a neuromusculoskeletal box. However, the timing of vascular diagnosis is of utmost importance and the longer the condition goes untreated, the worse the pathology may become. Numerous case reports demonstrate serious complications of vascular pathology that may have been avoided had the first contact clinician picked up the signs upon initial assessment. Simple clinical assessment techniques guide the clinician and attempt to refute a vascular hypothesis at an early stage.

Observation and hand examination

Blanching or whitening of the hand at rest or during function, is a sign of arterial occlusion of the upper extremity. In the case of positional flow limitations (in patients who are not expected to have serious pathology), this blanching will only be brought about by performing the activity to the onset of symptoms, e.g., overhead activity. During this performance, the clinician may observe the hand (being the most distal segment and therefore most sensitive indication to occlusion) for color changes. Nail bed capillary refill time is easily measured by squeezing the nail bed and recording the time it takes for color to return (which should be immediate). Non-pitting edema may be observed in severe venous obstructions (i.e., Paget-Schroetter syndrome). This is often associated with characteristic skin mottling and peripheral cyanosis, usually associated with a blue coloration of the hand or limb.[26] Figure 22.4 depicts an examination of the hand.

Pulse palpation

Palpation of relevant pulses is a simple and quick way of gaining an understanding of the vascular status early in the examination. The status of the brachial, radial, and ulnar pulses should be recorded on both arms. The reduction or obliteration of distal pulses during or immediately after effort or arm positioning indicates arterial occlusion but is nonspecific to location. In patients with vascular profile or higher risk for atherosclerosis, a pulsatile mass is characteristic of aneurysm formation and should be a consideration for examination around the supra- and infraclavicular pulses when subclavian aneurysm is suspected. A further consideration is auscultation, which may reveal a bruit.[14] Figure 25.5 depicts pulse palpation.

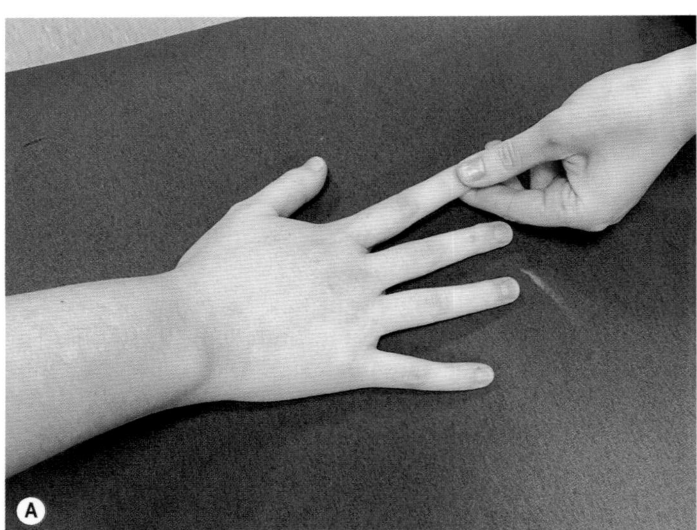

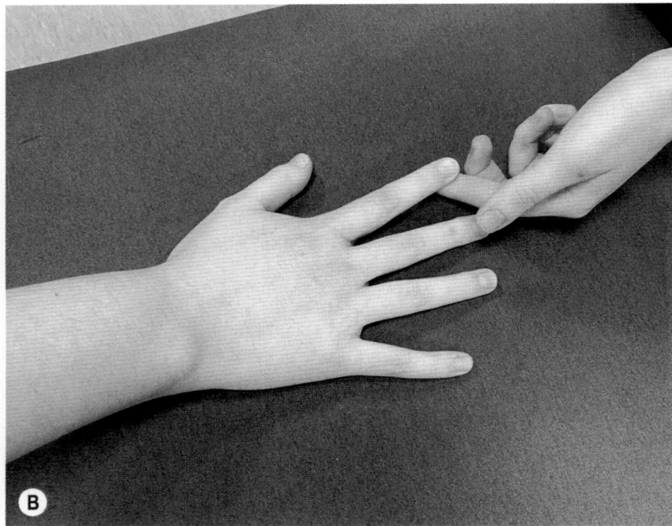

FIGURE 22.4
Hand examination. Capillary refill time is assessed by the clinician squeezing the nail bed for 2–3 seconds (A), releasing, and observing a return to normal color of the nail bed (B), which should be around 2 seconds.

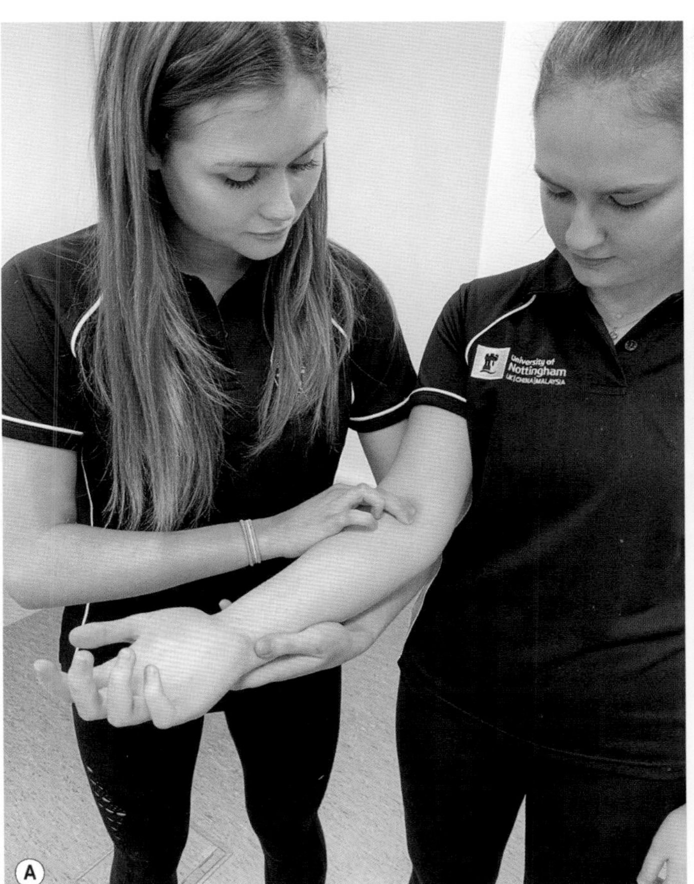

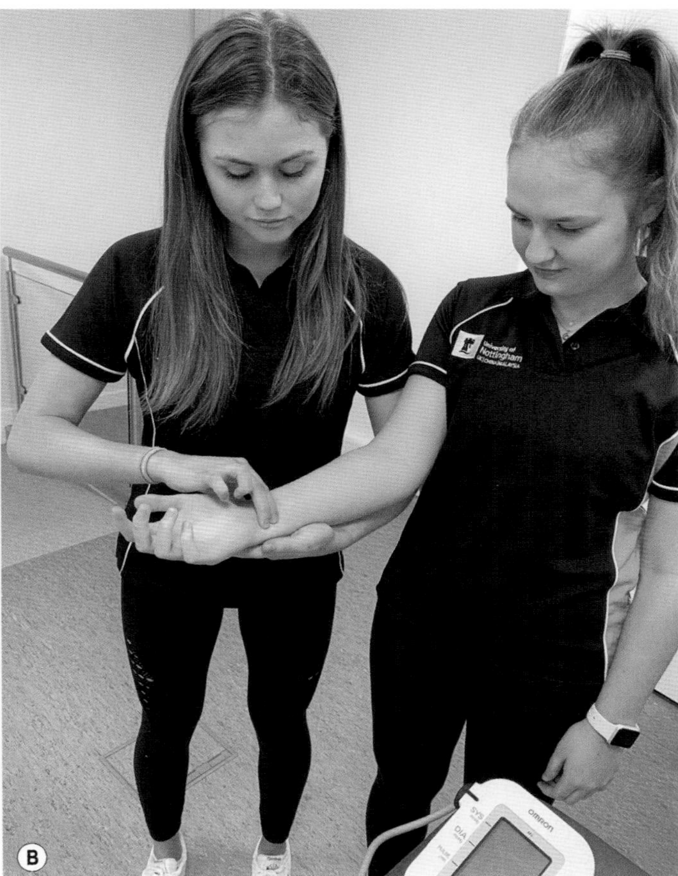

FIGURE 22.5
Pulse palpation. (A) Brachial and (B) radial pulses.

Arm to arm blood pressure testing

A blood pressure differential between arms of 20 mmHg may reveal a resting flow limitation. Side to side blood pressure recordings may be considered in the provocative positions (described by the patient) as an additional exploration of the presentation, where dynamic flow limitation is suspected.

Provocative maneuvers

There are a range of commonly used provocative maneuvers including the Extension Abduction Stress Test (EAST), and Adson's test. These provocative tests may add to the examination and perhaps raise the index of suspicion of a suspected diagnosis of arterial compromise. However, their utility is variable.[11] One study found that 58% of volunteers had at least one positive provocative test.[6] When used in isolation, Adson's test and the EAST test have specificity of 76% and 30%, respectively, but when the two tests are used in conjunction, diagnostic specificity rises to 82%. Despite this, it is suggested that magnetic resonance angiography appears to be the reference standard of choice to confirm a diagnosis of arterial involvement because it is able to evaluate the neurovascular bundle of the thoracic outlet in different provocative arm positions.[11] Figure 22.6 depicts the thoracic outlet syndrome functional tests. Table 22.1 details features that differentiate arterial and venous signs and symptoms.

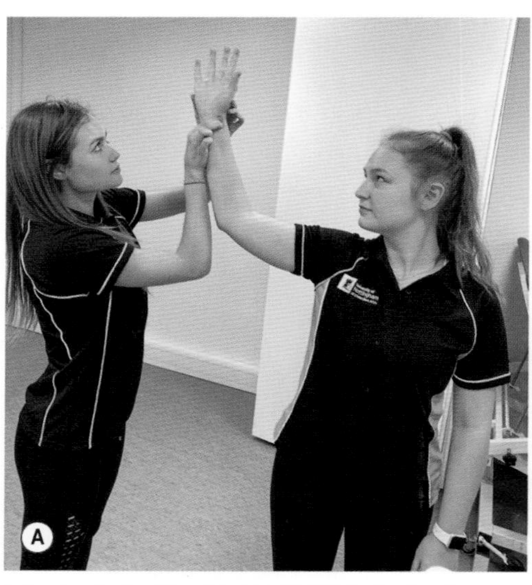

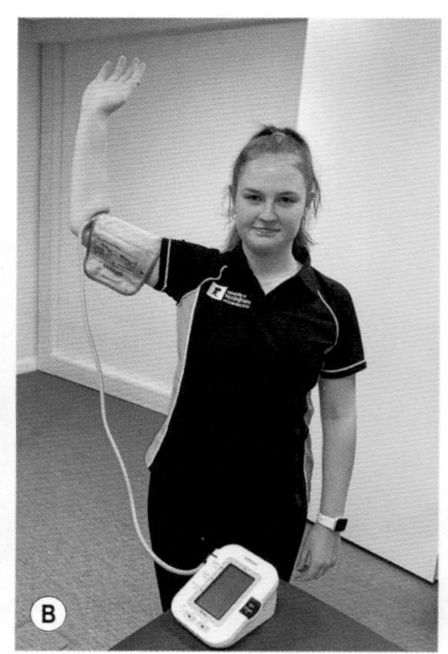

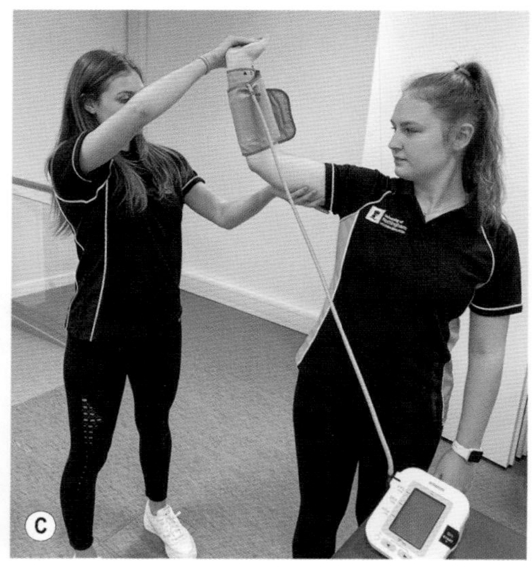

FIGURE 22.6
Thoracic outlet syndrome functional tests and pulse palpation. (A) Pulse palpation, (B) brachial blood pressure assessment, and (C) radial blood pressure assessment.

Management overview

Vascular flow limitations in the shoulder and upper limb remain a challenging and often misunderstood phenomenon, commonly not recognized due to a low index of suspicion. The key role of the clinician is initially to recognize and identify the arterial or venous flow limitation and apply appropriate examination techniques that which will expedite triage to appropriate services for further investigation. The urgency of referral will depend upon the suspected pathology and status of the patient. In short, worsening symptoms, a pulsatile mass, blanching of the limb or hand, or increasing limb swelling requires urgent action. However, most cases will likely present with much more transient and subtle symptoms which will ultimately only be elucidated via magnetic resonance angiography. Either way, appropriate and timely referral to a vascular team is the first step.

Nonsurgical and surgical management

While many identified upper limb cases will be referred for surgical decompression of anomalous ribs or structures, many cases may be adequately managed via nonsurgical measures to address musculoskeletal dysfunctions such as glenohumeral instability or other associated dysfunctions. A range of potential management options have been proposed. It is suggested that patient education is a key strategy which provides patients with an explanation for their (often prolonged) symptoms and offers hope that rehabilitation may be an option for management. Thereafter a range of potential interventions have been proposed, aiming to restore optimal joint kinematics, and address associated muscle and anatomical dysfunctions. These include relative rest, rehabilitation and graduated reloading, strengthening, stretching, and manual therapy techniques targeting the costoclavicular space, and first rib and posterior scalene triangle.[13] The efficacy of these techniques may vary from case to case. Failed nonsurgical measures may be followed by interventional surgical decompression.

Summary and conclusions

While vasculogenic causes of shoulder and arm dysfunction are rare, clinicians should be aware that they may occur across a range of ages. They are increasingly recognized in otherwise fit young adults, in the absence of vascular risk factors. It is suggested that the repetitive stresses and strains of high level sport may be a cause of vascular compromise and injury in susceptible individuals.[20] Combinations of

Table 22.1 Differentiating arterial and venous signs and symptoms

Syndrome	Symptom area	Symptom behavior	Symptom description	Clinical sign	Key clinical test/medical investigations
Subclavian-axillary artery occlusion	Supraclavicular fossa, upper limb	Related to effort and arm position	Pain, fatigue, weakness, coldness (distally)	Loss of distal pulses in provocative position, reduced systolic pressure on exertion, early onset fatigue	Contrast arteriography, MRA, duplex flow study
Subclavian aneurysm	Upper limb	Related to arm effort, general increase in activity (e.g., running)	Ache, pain, fatigue, weakness, coldness	Pulsatile supra-/infraclavicular mass. Loss of distal pulses in provocative position, reduced systolic pressure on exertion, early onset of fatigue	Contrast arteriography, MRA, duplex flow study, chest X-ray
Paget-Schroetter Syndrome (upper limb deep vein thrombosis)	Upper limb	Effort of upper quadrant, arm, shoulder complex position	Arm ache, swelling, coldness	Edematous arm, cyanosis, superficial venous distension on chest wall	Duplex ultrasound scan, venography
Subclavian steal syndrome	Transient hind-brain ischemia	Dizziness, feeling of fainting or actual fainting	Dizziness or syncope during upper limb activity or effort	Exercise-induced (upper limb) dizziness or fainting	Blood pressure with arm elevated
Quadrilateral space syndrome/posterior circumflex humeral artery injury	Upper limb/ shoulder	Effort-induced with abduction/ lateral rotation of the glenohumeral joint	Pain, transient weakness, early fatigue, distal dysesthesia	Transient loss of pulse inabduction/lateral rotation	Blood pressure with arm elevated, X-ray

MRA, magnetic resonance angiography.

training-related muscle hypertrophy, fatigue-induced joint translation and anatomical anomalies may combine to impact the vascular structures.[10]

Although rare, the consequences of misdiagnosis or delayed diagnosis of vascular conditions may be serious. It is essential that clinicians have an index of suspicion for vasculogenic mechanisms and are equipped with the necessary clinical reasoning skills to make appropriate physical examination and implement appropriate triage for these individuals.

References

1. Aboyans V, Kamineni A, Allison MA, et al. The epidemiology of subclavian stenosis and its association with markers of subclinical atherosclerosis: the Multi-Ethnic Study of Atherosclerosis (MESA). Atherosclerosis. 2010;211:266-270.
2. Adam G, Wang K, Demaree CJ, et al. A prospective evaluation of duplex ultrasound for thoracic outlet syndrome in high-performance musicians playing bowed string instruments. Diagnostics. 2018;8:11.
3. Babic S, Sagic D, Radak D, et al. Initial and long-term results of endovascular therapy for chronic total occlusion of the subclavian artery. Cardiovascular and Interventional Radiology. 2012;35:255-262.
4. Boettinger M, Busl K, Schmidt-Wilcke T, Bogdahn U, Schuierer G, Schlachetzki F. Neuroimaging in subclavian steal syndrome. Case Reports. 2009;2009:bcr1120081198.
5. Bosch FTM, Nisio MD, Büller HR, van Es N. Diagnostic and therapeutic management of upper extremity deep vein thrombosis. Journal of Clinical Medicine. 2020;9:2069.
6. Brantigan CO, Roos DB. Diagnosing thoracic outlet syndrome. Hand Clinics. 2004;20:27-36.
7. Brown S-AN, Doolittle DA, Bohanon CJ, et al. Quadrilateral space syndrome: the Mayo Clinic experience with a new classification system and case series. Mayo Clinic Proceedings. 2015:382-394.
8. Cook JR, Thompson RW. Evaluation and management of venous thoracic outlet syndrome. Thoracic Surgery Clinics. 2021;31:27-44.
9. Cothran Jr RL, Helms C. Quadrilateral space syndrome: incidence of imaging findings in a population referred for MRI of the shoulder. American Journal of Roentgenology. 2005;184:989-992.
10. de Mooij T, Duncan AA, Kakar S. Vascular injuries in the upper extremity in athletes. Hand Clinics. 2015;31:39-52.
11. Dessureault-Dober I, Bronchti G, Bussières A. Diagnostic accuracy of clinical tests for neurogenic and vascular thoracic outlet syndrome: a systematic review. Journal of Manipulative and Physiological Therapeutics. 2018;41:789-799.
12. Hangge PT, Breen I, Albadawi H, Knuttinen MG, Naidu SG, Oklu R. Quadrilateral space syndrome: diagnosis and clinical management. Journal of Clinical Medicine. 2018;7:86.
13. Hooper TL, Denton J, McGalliard MK, Brismée J-M, Sizer Jr PS. Thoracic outlet syndrome: a controversial clinical condition. Part 2: non-surgical and surgical management. Journal of Manual & Manipulative Therapy. 2010;18:132-138.
14. Illig KA, Donahue D, Duncan A, et al. Reporting standards of the Society for Vascular Surgery for thoracic outlet syndrome: executive summary. Journal of Vascular Surgery. 2016;64:797-802.
15. Jalota R, Soos MP. Subclavian Vein Thrombosis. StatPearls. Treasure Island: StatPearls Publishing; 2021.
16. Jordan SE, Ahn SS, Gelabert HA. Differentiation of thoracic outlet syndrome from treatment-resistant cervical brachial pain syndromes: development and utilization of a questionnaire, clinical examination and ultrasound evaluation. Pain Physician. 2007;10:441-452.
17. Karaolanis G, Antonopoulos CN, Koutsias SG, et al. A systematic review and meta-analysis for the management of Paget-Schroetter syndrome. Journal of Vascular Surgery. 2021;9:801-810.e5.
18. Kargiotis O, Siahos S, Safouris A, Feleskouras A, Magoufis G, Tsivgoulis G. Subclavian steal syndrome with or without arterial stenosis: a review. Journal of Neuroimaging. 2016;26:473-480.
19. Menon D, Onida S, Davies AH. Overview of arterial pathology related to repetitive trauma in athletes. Journal of Vascular Surgery. 2019;70:641-650.
20. Ochoa VM, Yeghiazarians Y. Subclavian artery stenosis: a review for the vascular medicine practitioner. Vascular Medicine. 2011;16:29-34.
21. Ohman JW, Thompson RW. Thoracic outlet syndrome in the overhead athlete: diagnosis and treatment recommendations. Current Reviews in Musculoskeletal Medicine. 2020;13:457-471.
22. Patel RAG, White CJ. Brachiocephalic and subclavian stenosis: current concepts for cardiovascular specialists. Progress in Cardiovascular Diseases. 2021; 65:44-48.
23. Potter BJ, Pinto DS. Subclavian steal syndrome. Circulation. 2014;129:2320-2323.
24. Rafailidis V, Li X, Chryssogonidis I, et al. Multimodality imaging and endovascular treatment options of subclavian steal syndrome. Canadian Association of Radiologists Journal. 2018;69:493-507.
25. Reutter D, Husmann M, Thalhammer C. The pitcher-syndrom: aneurysm of the posterior circumflex humeral artery-a rare source for upper limb ischemia. Vasa. 2010;39:113-114.
26. Saleem T, Baril DT. Paget Schroetter Syndrome. StatPearls. Treasure Island: StatPearls Publishing; 2021.
27. Shankar Kikkeri N, Nagalli S. Subclavian Steal Syndrome. StatPearls. Treasure Island: StatPearls Publishing; 2021.
28. Stapleton C, Herrington L, George K. Sonographic evaluation of the axillary artery during simulated overhead throwing arm positions. Phys Ther Sport. 2008;9:126-135.
29. Stapleton C, Herrington L, George K. Sonographic evaluation of the subclavian artery during thoracic outlet syndrome shoulder manoeuvres. Manual Therapy. 2009;14:19-27.
30. Stapleton CH, Elias J, Green DJ, Cable NT, George KP. Arterial compression during overhead throwing: a risk for arterial injury? Ultrasound in Medicine & Biology. 2010;36:1259-1266.
31. Stapleton CH, Green DJ, Cable NT, George KP. Flow-mediated dilation and intima-media thickness of the brachial and axillary

arteries in individuals with and without inducible axillary artery compression. Ultrasound in Medicine & Biology. 2009;35:1443-1451.

32. Stapleton CH, Herrington L, George K. Anterior translation at the glenohumeral joint: a cause of axillary artery compression? Am J Sports Med. 2008;36:539-544.

33. Stone J, Hangge P, Albadawi H, et al. Deep vein thrombosis: pathogenesis, diagnosis, and medical management. Cardiovasc Diagn Ther. 2017;7:S276-S284.

34. van de Pol D, Planken RN, Terpstra A, Pannekoek-Hekman M, Kuijer PPF, Maas M. Nonoperative management and novel imaging for posterior circumflex humeral artery injury in volleyball. Current Sports Medicine Reports. 2017;16:317-321.

35. Vemuri C, Salehi P, Benarroch-Gampel J, McLaughlin LN, Thompson RW. Diagnosis and treatment of effort-induced thrombosis of the axillary subclavian vein due to venous thoracic outlet syndrome. Journal of Vascular Surgery. 2016;4:485-500.

Injection therapy in the management of shoulder pain

23

Tim Cook, Christine Bilsborough Smith, Lorenzo Masci, Emma Salt, Stuart Wildman, Jeremy Lewis

Introduction

The shoulder is the third most common site of musculoskeletal symptoms with 1% of adults over the age of 45 years presenting to healthcare providers with a new episode of shoulder pain.[91] Injection therapy is one of several treatment options offered for a range of shoulder conditions including rotator cuff-related shoulder pain (RCRSP),[29] frozen shoulder,[70] glenohumeral and acromioclavicular osteoarthritis,[16] and calcific tendinopathy[73] (see Chapter 27). The shoulder is the most frequently injected region, accounting for one in every three musculoskeletal injections.[72] Approximately one in five people (22%) with shoulder pain receive an injection during their initial general practitioner (GP) consultation.[118] Despite the extensive utilization of injection therapy for the management of shoulder pain, evidence supporting its effectiveness as a treatment option is limited.[15,78] Considerable uncertainty regarding the dose, timing, frequency, substance injected, and technique used for the various procedures remains. There is also uncertainty as to what constitutes best post-injection advice.

The aim of this chapter is to synthesize existing knowledge relating to shoulder injections. We will refer to the use of injection therapy for common shoulder conditions namely, RCRSP, frozen shoulder, and osteoarthritis. For each condition we will describe the current consensus on which medications are most effective to inject and in what amounts. A description of the specific injection technique will be presented as well as suggestions for post-injection care. We will discuss the use of image-guided versus landmark-guided procedures, and the role of suprascapular nerve blocks. We will also identify deficits in our research knowledge, of which there are many, and we will make suggestions for future research in this area of clinical practice.

Injection therapy as a treatment for rotator cuff-related shoulder pain

Injection therapy (usually involving corticosteroid medication) is an established and prevalent treatment for the management of RCRSP.[63] RCRSP may be the most common musculoskeletal (MSK) condition to be treated with injection therapy, accounting for over a third of all injections.[72] This popularity appears to be supported by international guidelines that recommend corticosteroid injections as a viable treatment option to consider as part of the shared decision-making process.[1,14,67]

Although evidence informing patient suitability is sparse, it has been suggested that injection therapy might be most effective in certain subgroups of people with RCRSP. UK guidelines cite research supporting its effectiveness for patients in the acute stages of the pathology, particularly if pain levels are severe.[37] Other national guidelines suggest that injection therapy could be indicated when symptoms have persisted despite prior nonsurgical treatment,[120] and should be used in conjunction with other forms of nonsurgical management.[16,54] It has been recommended that patients are limited to a maximum of two injections, at least six weeks apart. Clinicians are advised not to offer repeat injections for those who have had little or no benefit from an initial injection.[14,67] The reasoning behind this guidance stems from a concern for potential tendon and cartilage damage as a result of repeated injections.[35]

Prior to any MSK injection and as part of a shared decision-making process, clinicians must obtain informed consent. This is an opportunity to discuss the anticipated benefits and likelihood of possible adverse effects associated with the procedure. Those considering an injection should be counselled on the signs, symptoms, and likelihood of any harm. Clinicians trained in injection therapy should be aware of the potential but rare side effects. A non-exhaustive list of side effects include post-injection flare of pain, anaphylaxis, subcutaneous atrophy or skin depigmentation, bruising, tendon rupture, infection, facial flushing, and deterioration of diabetic glycemic control.[72] Advice must be given on actions to take should any adverse effect be experienced. Good clinical practice involves taking written consent.

What to inject and why?

There is no conclusive evidence pertaining to the particular corticosteroid medication to inject and in what amount.[1] Several preparations are suggested in the British National Formulary (bnf.nice.org.uk),[11] but expert opinion suggests that triamcinolone and methylprednisolone are most commonly used.[1,72,108] Local anesthetic medications (such as lidocaine hydrochloride) are commonly injected in combination with a corticosteroid for pain relief and to help support the clinical diagnosis.[1,120] To date there is no strong evidence to support the use of other injectable substances such as platelet-rich plasma (PRP), hypertonic dextrose (otherwise known as prolotherapy), or sodium chloride (saline).[29]

The exact mechanisms of therapeutic effect by which corticosteroid injections (with or without anesthetic) act are unknown. Corticosteroids may play a role in reducing localized inflammation,[28] or overall tenocyte numbers,[18] and by inhibiting nociceptor activity.[62] It even has been suggested by some authors that any therapeutic benefit may be the result of a physical distension of the subacromial space[4] or via contextual "placebo" effects.[78] This ongoing uncertainty is in part due to a scarcity of research investigating the histological effects of injections. There is also a lack of clinical research comparing corticosteroid medication to an appropriate sham injection.[30] In particular, the popular use of saline as a sham injection has been questioned as it may indeed have a therapeutic effect that requires further investigation.[4,30]

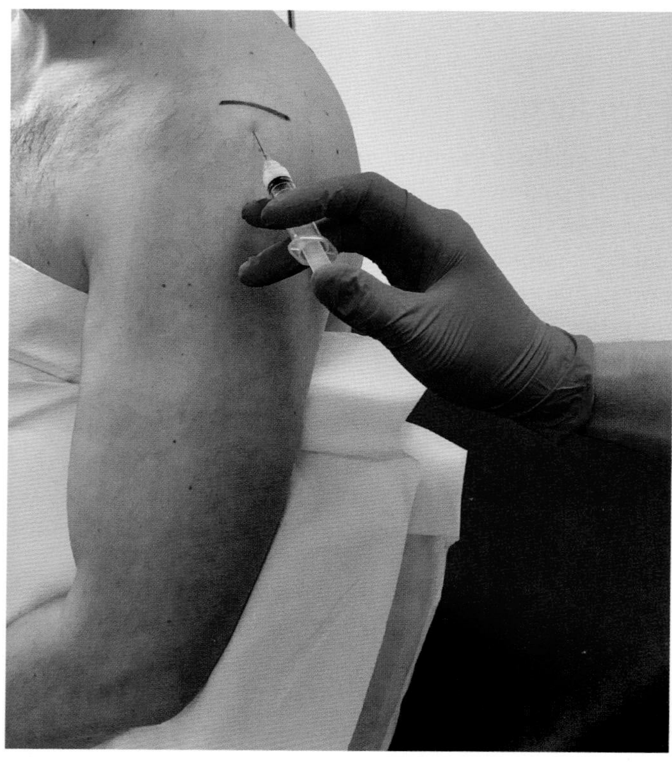

FIGURE 23.1
Landmark-guided injection into the subacromial space. The line drawn onto the skin represents the palpable lateral edge of the acromion.

Methods and post-injection advice

The preferred target for an injection is the subacromial-subdeltoid bursa within the subacromial space.[72,79] A 5 ml syringe is used with a 21-gauge needle of 30–40 mm (1.25–1.5 in) length.[72] Although there is no scientific consensus, a commonly recommended dose is 20 mg (0.5 ml) triamcinolone in combination with 45 mg (4.5 ml) 1% lidocaine (for a total volume of 5 ml).

The patient is usually advised to sit supported with their arm relaxed and hanging by their side, often with a pillow or rolled towel between their arm and body for comfort. To avoid vasovagal syncope, some clinicians prefer to perform the procedure with the patient in supine. The clinician will aim to insert the needle inferior to the middle of the lateral edge of the acromion. The path of the needle should follow an upwards direction attempting to position the tip underneath the acromion (Figure 23.1). The syringe must be drawn backwards to ensure the needle is not in a blood vessel. A bolus is then injected where no resistance is felt.[72] It is possible to perform this injection using both landmark- and ultrasound-guided techniques (discussed later). Following an injection, patients are advised to rest the injected shoulder as much as is practical for the next 24 hours, avoid strenuous exercise for the following week[41] and then very gradually reintroduce more demanding activities.

Summary and areas for future research

Despite the popularity of injection therapy as a treatment for RCRSP there is a lack of high-quality research supporting its use. Much of the research that has been conducted has been criticized as having a high risk of bias and only reporting short-term outcome measures, making it challenging to inform patients of their long-term prognosis.[30] Previous meta-analyses and systematic reviews suggest that injection therapy for this condition may provide minimal, short-term pain relief in a relatively small number of patients.[30,78]

Not only has the effectiveness of corticosteroid injections been questioned, but there is growing concern regarding their potential to induce negative effects on rotator cuff tendon tissue.[35,36,89,95] Local administration of corticosteroids appears to have toxic effects on tendon cells which result in a reduction in the mechanical properties of the tendon.[35,36] Although research in this area is limited, one prospective study reported a 17% incidence of full-thickness rotator cuff tears at 12-week follow-up in patients who received a corticosteroid injection.[95] Furthermore, limited evidence suggests a strong correlation between preoperative injections and poor outcomes following rotator cuff repair surgery.[121]

In light of these concerns, the continued practice of injection therapy for the treatment of RCRSP has been attributed by some to force of habit.[78] This is somewhat at odds with the concept of evidence based medicine (EBM), which demands that the effectiveness of clinical interventions be scrutinized and their usefulness proven prior to widespread use.[3] Despite this, clinicians still regard injection therapy as a viable treatment option for RCRSP if other nonsurgical measures have failed and the patient has been made aware of the possible risks involved as part of a shared decision-making process.

Injections for frozen shoulder

Frozen shoulder (FS) is a condition characterized by persistent and severe pain with a concomitant loss of passive shoulder movement.[64] The clinical stages of FS may be categorized into: 1) a painful greater than stiff phase, and 2) a stiff greater than painful phase.[70] Clinical, histopathological and arthroscopic findings broadly correlate through the phases, which are recognized as a continuum as opposed to well-delineated stages.[44] Injection therapy has been used as treatment for FS for almost 70 years.[33] Although initial results were poor,[33] the use of injection therapy for the management of FS is now a well-established treatment option.[97] Despite the growing popularity, there remains considerable conjecture regarding the optimal timing, method, and type of injection.

What to inject and why?

Corticosteroids are recognized chemical moderators and when injected into the shoulder joint of a patient with FS, have been shown to reduce fibromatosis, vascular hyperplasia, fibrosis and fibroblasts staining for α-smooth muscle actin.[56] This suggests an injection in the earlier phase of the condition may alter the course of the disease. Injections in this phase demonstrate a clinically meaningful difference in Shoulder Pain and Disability Index (SPADI) scores (see Chapter 12) and range of motion at 12 weeks compared to placebo.[124] Although inflammation is considered part of the pathogenesis of FS, the extent to which corticosteroids act on this process is uncertain. Substantial gaps in knowledge surrounding the pathogenesis of FS and action of corticosteroids remain.[32,56]

Although the exact mechanisms by which steroid injections seem to work are unknown, there appears to be strong evidence that their use can have a positive effect on symptoms of frozen shoulder. Systematic reviews report effectiveness up to six weeks,[20,45] and four months post injection.[45] Another systematic review,[115] involving eight randomized clinical trials (416 patients) reported intra-articular steroid injection to be safe and effective in the management of FS and improves function, increases range of motion and reduces pain. The benefits of corticosteroid injections were significant at 4–6 weeks, 12–16 weeks and may last up to 26 weeks.[115] It is important to add that improvement was not reported in all outcomes of interest, and although statistically significant differences were achieved in many of the outcome measures, the clinical benefit of some of the outcomes across all the time points was not demonstrated. Early physical therapy treatment combined with a steroid injection results in the same clinical outcome as surgery and physiotherapy. Subsequently, the former may be considered as the more practical first-line management option.[96]

Which drugs and what dose?

The two most injected corticosteroids used for the treatment of frozen shoulder are triamcinolone acetonide (TA) and methylprednisolone acetate (MP).[108] A survey of interventional radiologists showed TA was preferred over MP due to its longer-acting properties.[108] Despite this, there is little evidence to suggest a significant difference in functional outcomes or pain between medication types.[19]

Comparisons of 10 mg and 40 mg TA have been conducted. Greater improvements in pain and sleep were found at the higher dose, but differences did not last beyond six weeks.[34] A subsequent randomized, triple-blinded, placebo (5 ml of 1% lidocaine) controlled trial compared 20 mg and 40 mg injections. The authors reported significant improvements for both groups for pain, range of motion and SPADI scores, with no between-group differences beyond 12 weeks.[124] Similar studies comparing the same doses (20 mg and 40 mg) found no differences between groups for a range of outcomes up to six weeks post-injection.[19,66,124] In conclusion, most of the available evidence suggests no significant difference in outcome between low and high dose steroid injection.

Which site to inject?

Comparisons of glenohumeral intra-articular (IA) and subacromial (SA) injections suggest that there is a greater reduction in pain following an IA injection at 2–3 weeks,[82,111] with no differences between injections in terms of function and range of motion (except for internal rotation movement) at 12 weeks.[111] A recent meta-analysis reported greater reductions in pain following an IA injection compared to SA injection lasting up to three months.[24] Other studies comparing combined IA and SA injections report slightly better outcomes for internal rotation than an IA or SA injection alone.[25] It was hypothesized that this may be due to steroid seepage into the rotator interval from the SA space.[111] This remains uncertain as other studies have reported no differences in outcome between IA injection alone or in combination with an injection at the rotator interval.[92]

Hydrodilatation injection

Hydrodilatation (HD) (also known as arthro-distension) injections aim to increase shoulder joint range of motion by expanding the joint capsule using high-volume combinations of saline, steroid, and anesthetic injected into the glenohumeral joint. HD is a technically challenging procedure to perform. Short-term benefits compared to control groups have been found for pain, function and range of motion,[106,123] but the small and transient improvements for external rotation,[123] pain and range of motion,[106] may not be clinically important. Published evidence suggests repeating the procedure does not provide better outcomes compared to a single procedure.[106,123] HD may provide a better short-term effect at one month than an IA or SA injection, but by three months there are no discernable differences. A corticosteroid injection appears to be as effective as a combination of HD and steroid, and both are better than HD without steroid at three months.[94]

Future research

Available evidence supported by clinical practice guidelines suggests that injection therapy is well-established and has concomitant clinical benefit in the treatment of frozen shoulder.[97] Nonetheless, sizeable gaps in knowledge persist. As shared decision-making is at the heart of clinical practice,[58] the paucity of evidence poses a dilemma as to whether the benefits of an injection outweigh the harms. To better inform clinical practice, more knowledge on the best anatomical site(s) to inject, when to inject, mode of delivery (image- or landmark-guided), and adverse events, compared against natural history, would improve care.

Injection therapy for glenohumeral joint osteoarthritis

The glenohumeral (GH) joint is the third most commonly affected large joint to develop osteoarthritis after the knee and hip.[125] Etiology may be classified into two groups: primary and secondary osteoarthritis. Primary osteoarthritis is more common in elderly populations and is associated with posterior glenoid wear.[26] Secondary osteoarthritis is more common in younger people following trauma, previous recurrent dislocations, surgery, and atraumatic osteonecrosis. Shoulder joint prosthetic replacement may limit function which may have less impact on some more elderly people than those in younger age groups.[26] Specifically, in this younger patient group, nonsurgical options play a more important role in symptom reduction. In general, nonsurgical options include activity modification, education, exercise therapy,[31] oral pharmacotherapy, and intra-articular GH joint injections. Injection therapy may also be a consideration in older populations as well.

Technique

Injections into the GH joint can be performed with or without image guidance. Landmark-guided injections can be performed using various techniques.[12] Image-guided injections can be performed with ultrasound or fluoroscopy (see later for discussion). In general, landmark-guided injections for the GH joint are less accurate than image-guided, although accuracy depends on the approach, with the posterior approach being more accurate.[5,10,85,113] Ultrasound-guided injections are of equal accuracy to fluoroscopic-guided and are more often preferred by patients. They are also less expensive and there is no exposure to radiation.[52]

Injectable options

Corticosteroids are the most common injectable medication used in the management of GH joint osteoarthritis. Unlike other joints such as the knee, there is a lack of evidence of effectiveness, and most of the evidence supporting their use is anecdotal.[6] According to recent evidence, recommendations for the use of injectable corticosteroids in GH joint osteoarthritis are inconclusive. Nevertheless, guidelines regarding type and dose of cortisone are similar to those for the knee joint.[65]

Hyaluronic acid (HA) is a high molecular weight glycosaminoglycan, which is thought to have anti-inflammatory, analgesic, and chondro-protective effects in the exogenous form.[60,114] There is a paucity of high level research investigating HA injections for the treatment of GH joint osteoarthritis. A recent randomized controlled trial evaluating the efficacy of HA with corticosteroid at 1, 3 and 6 months found that the HA group had improved pain and disability scores at all time points. The corticosteroid group, however, only saw improvements at 1 month.[76]

Platelet-rich plasma (PRP) consists of a sample of blood with platelet concentrations above baseline values, which has been produced through the separation of whole blood by centrifugation.[68] Although the evidence for PRP injections in knee osteoarthritis is encouraging,[23] there is a lack of high-quality research from which to draw conclusions about their use in the treatment of GH joint osteoarthritis.

Injections for acromioclavicular and sternoclavicular joint osteoarthritis

Synovitis or osteoarthritis of the acromioclavicular (AC) joint is a common cause of shoulder pain often neglected by clinicians. Patients often report pain localized to the AC joint aggravated by shoulder movement especially into horizontal flexion (adduction).[48] X-ray or ultrasound imaging can confirm degenerative changes including subchondral cysts, joint space narrowing and osteophyte formation. Reduction in pain following injection of local anesthetic into the joint may support a clinical hypothesis that the AC joint is a source of nociception.[17,107] AC joint corticosteroid injections are considered a viable option when pain is severe[2] or when the patient has had a poor response to other nonsurgical intervention.[16]

Injections into the AC joint may be either landmark- or image-guided. Landmark-guided injections for the AC joint are accurate in less than 50% of cases. This is thought to be related to the relative small joint size, variable anatomy and the presence of osteophytes.[9] Image-guided injections are generally more accurate. Fluoroscopically-guided AC joint injection accuracy is 100%.[88] Similar accuracy has been demonstrated in ultrasound-guided injections with the added benefit of lack of ionizing radiation, portability and lower cost.[86]

It is unknown whether improved accuracy is important for a clinical effect. A study comparing intra-articular versus peri-articular corticosteroid injections both directed by ultrasound found no difference in pain or function between groups at short-term follow-up.[101] Moreover, there is little evidence for effectiveness of corticosteroid injections beyond the short-term, and no evidence that these injections alter the natural history of this pathology.[61]

Sternoclavicular (SC) joint injections are performed for osteoarthritis often presenting as medial shoulder or chest wall pain.[48] Accuracy of injections have been confirmed with CT-[87] and ultrasound-guidance.[90] There are no studies documenting effectiveness of injections for SC joint osteoarthritis.

In summary, corticosteroid injections for glenohumeral, acromioclavicular and sternoclavicular joint osteoarthritis are used for persistent pain unresponsive to nonsurgical management. There is a limited body of evidence to suggest whether corticosteroid injections are an effective treatment in these conditions. There is not enough research evidence to support the use of other injectable substances at this stage. National guidelines are currently based on limited data of studies deemed to be of high risk of bias[2,16] and more evidence is required to understand the precise clinical indication and effectiveness of injections for these conditions.

Ultrasound-guided shoulder injections

Ultrasound imaging was first used in the 1970s to guide medical procedures such as arthrocentesis and tissue biopsies.[75] It is now used to enhance the accuracy of injection therapy in the treatment of MSK disorders, and involves the real-time visualization of tracking a needle tip on an ultrasound image towards an anatomical target. Landmark-guided injections differ in that they involve the identification of anatomical landmarks using surface palpation to guide the location of an injection.[103]

Driven by a reduction in equipment costs and improved image resolution, the use of ultrasound to guide injections in MSK practice has increased.[7,51,80] In addition, with an expanding scope of practice, especially in the UK,[39,40] many nonmedical health professionals such as physiotherapists (physical therapists) are now performing injections using ultrasound guidance as part of their clinical practice.

Ultrasound-guided subacromial subdeltoid bursa injection

The subacromial subdeltoid bursa (SASD bursa) is a large synovium-lined structure,[22] and is a common injection site for people presenting with RCRSP.[71] The bursa will appear as an anechoic (black) or hypoechoic (dark gray) linear structure positioned superficial to the supraspinatus tendon and deep to the deltoid muscle. The linear appearance is generated by the hyperechoic borders of the adjacent peri-bursal fat layer. It is often injected via an "in-plane" technique, where the needle is parallel to the transducer, from a lateral approach with a green, 21-gauge 50 mm (2 in) needle (Figures 23.2A and 23.2B). No resistance should be felt and distension across the entire width of the bursa should be seen in real-time as the injection is performed. If there is local accumulation, then it is likely the needle tip is outside the bursal layer.

The accuracy of landmark injection techniques on cadaveric specimens report a rate of success varying between 63% and 80%.[84] If these data are further explored, injections of the SASD bursa alone, without infiltrating adjacent structures such as the rotator cuff tendons, deltoid and glenohumeral joint, suggest 20% accuracy. Injection research using cadavers has limitations due to the age of the tissue, with an increased prevalence of structural defects.[77] Studies evaluating magnetic resonance imaging immediately post-injection in people diagnosed with RCRSP have reported accuracy rates of 69–100% for landmark-guided techniques,[38,55,99] reducing to 24–31% when concomitant infiltration into adjacent structures are excluded.[55] In comparison, the accuracy of ultrasound-guided techniques is reported to range from 60% to 100%.[38,99] The wide range in

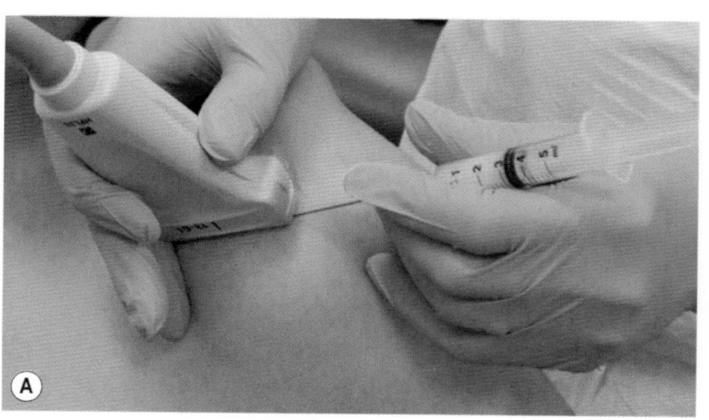

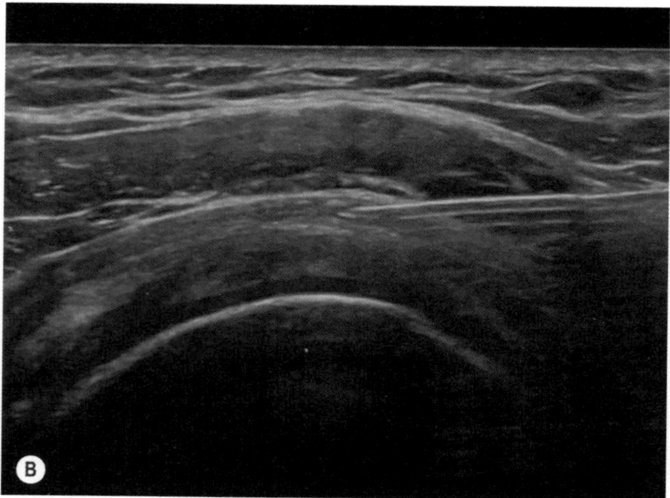

FIGURE 23.2

(A) Ultrasound-guided injection of the subacromial subdeltoid bursa. (B) An ultrasound image showing an ultrasound-guided injection into the hypoechoic subacromial subdeltoid bursal layer superficial to the supraspinatus tendon.

accuracy may reflect a high degree of variation in competency between clinicians, but may also reflect methodological differences such as ultrasound system quality and probe frequencies.

Outcomes from studies comparing the clinical efficacy of SASD bursal injection techniques continue to be mixed.[8,27,103] It is worth noting specifically that the target of the injection in studies is often termed the "subacromial space". The subacromial space includes many structures including the SASD bursa, bursal fat, rotator cuff tendons, capsule, and cartilage. Despite being distinctly different structures, the terms are used interchangeably, which may have implications for interpreting research findings. Sage et al.[103] reported a short-term improvement in both shoulder pain and shoulder abduction range of movement at six weeks for ultrasound-guided techniques of the subacromial region. Other studies have found no difference in clinical outcomes between ultrasound-guided and landmark-guided injection techniques for the SASD bursa and space.[8,99]

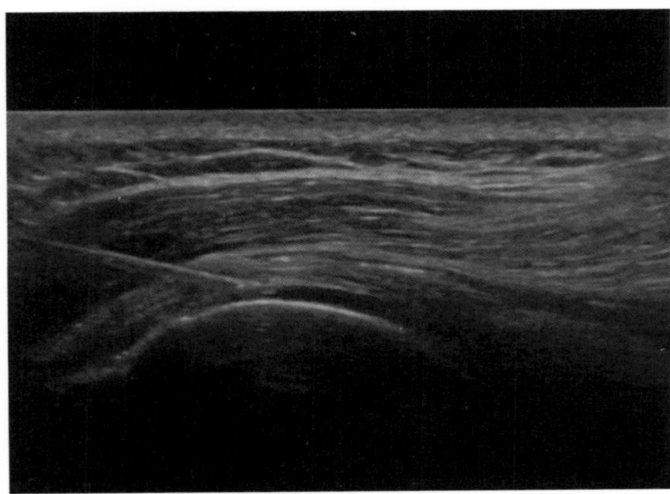

FIGURE 23.3
An ultrasound image showing an ultrasound-guided injection via an anterolateral approach into the glenohumeral joint, superficial to the hypoechoic articular cartilage on the humeral head.

Ultrasound-guided glenohumeral joint injection

Ultrasound guidance may be used for conditions affecting the glenohumeral (GH) joint such as frozen shoulder and osteoarthritis. A linear (or flat) probe with a frequency of 5–15 MHz is most commonly used together with a 21-gauge 50 mm (2 in) needle, and for people with larger body masses a curvilinear (or curved) probe may be required, together with a longer (spinal) needle. Several approaches are documented for injecting the GH joint under ultrasound guidance incorporating both "in-plane" and "out-of-plane" (when the needle is not parallel to the transducer) techniques. We will focus our discussions on two commonly performed posterior approaches. For both techniques, positioning the patient on their side, with the side to be injected uppermost, is recommended.

A posterior, anterolateral directed and almost "in-plane" approach (Figure 23.3) requires the needle tip to be advanced into the joint capsule, ensuring the bevel is facing down to flush the injectate into the joint accurately, with little resistance felt when injecting.[81] Ensuring that the location of entry is inferior to the infraspinatus tendon will usually improve the patient's comfort during the procedure. This is a technically demanding procedure requiring exacting needle angle of entry and visualization. Performance of this technique under ultrasound guidance raises an awareness of the challenges that are faced to inject accurately into this joint via a landmark approach, as the capsule can often be barely visible superficial to the anechoic layer of articular hyaline cartilage on the humeral head (Figure 23.4). If a joint effusion is present, it may be easier to approach the technique from a posteromedial approach, targeting the posterior recess of the glenohumeral joint (Figure 23.5).

Ultrasound-guided injections of the GH joint have reported high accuracy rates of 90–100% in patients undergoing the procedure[50,81,93] and 92.5% in cadavers.[85] Patel et al.[85] reported that landmark-guided procedures on cadaveric specimens are 72% accurate.

Ultrasound-guided acromioclavicular (AC) joint injection

The acromioclavicular (AC) joint is commonly injected for conditions such as osteoarthritis. The procedure is performed "in-plane" from the lateral side of the joint. The technique is challenging due to the presence of an intra-articular disc,[102] and adaptation of the needle and bevel position is often required to ensure an accurate procedure is performed (Figures 23.6A,B). Additional challenges include

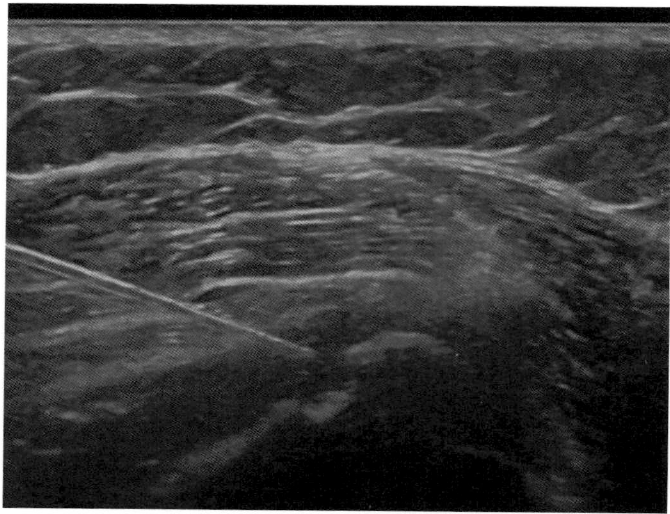

FIGURE 23.4

An ultrasound image showing an ultrasound-guided injection via a posteromedial approach into the effusion at the posterior aspect of a degenerative glenohumeral joint.

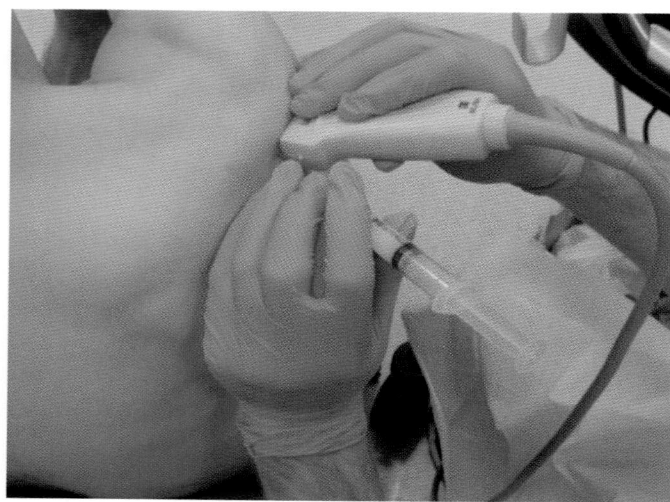

FIGURE 23.5

An ultrasound-guided injection via a posteromedial approach into the glenohumeral joint.

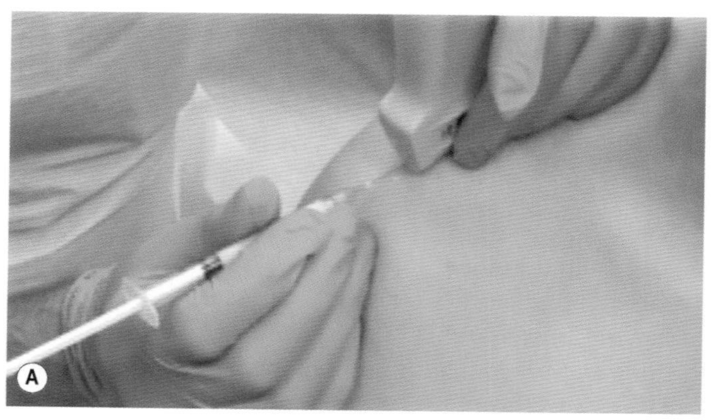

FIGURE 23.6

(A) Lateral approach to ultrasound-guided AC joint injection. (B) An ultrasound image showing an ultrasound-guided injection to the AC joint from a lateral, in plane approach.

large osteophytes located on the joint margins. A high-frequency linear probe is used due to the superficial position on the joint. A small, 23-gauge 25 mm (1 in) blue needle reduces the risk of blocking the needle tip and preventing the injectate being administered.

Ultrasound-guided injections of the AC joint have been shown to have an accuracy rate of 95–100% in cadavers.[86,100] Landmark-guided injections have reported accuracy of 39–50%.[9] In a clinical trial, accuracy of 96% for ultrasound-guided injections and 61% for landmark-guided injections was reported for people diagnosed with AC joint osteoarthritis.[83] Park et al.[83] reported a significantly greater improvement in SPADI scores, palpation and arm adduction test at 3 and 6 months in the ultrasound-guided injection group.

Ultrasound-guided long head of biceps tendon sheath injection

The long head of biceps tendon and its accompanying sheath may be a source of symptoms as a result of conditions such as tenosynovitis and tendinopathy.[53] Ultrasound-guided long head of biceps tendon sheath injections have a reported accuracy of 86.7%, with 26.7% accuracy reported for landmark-guided procedures.[53] The injection technique is often performed from a lateral approach, in-plane, ensuring avoidance of the arcuate branch of the anterior circumflex artery which is positioned on the lateral aspect of the bicipital groove.[49] Visualization of the needle tip is again important to ensure the injection is within the tendon sheath and not the tendon itself. A 21-gauge 50 mm (2 in) green needle is often required depending on the tissue depth of the patient. The clinical relevance of a biceps tendon sheath effusion is also important to reflect upon as it is rarely indicative of a localized tenosynovitis, and more often a reflection of either a glenohumeral joint effusion/synovitis or a rotator cuff tear.[83]

Are ultrasound-guided procedures worth the effort?

Despite the potential for improved accuracy with ultrasound-guided procedures,[47] there remains uncertainty whether therapeutic benefit over traditional landmark-guided injections is improved.[8,27] The time taken to train clinicians to perform ultrasound-guided procedures and the need for ongoing mentorship amplifies the uncertainty related to this practice. Despite this uncertainty there is now increasing demand for ultrasound-guided shoulder injection techniques.[59] With widespread use away from traditional radiology settings, patients are increasingly requesting that procedures are performed under ultrasound guidance. Patient satisfaction of ultrasound use has also been shown to be high.[74,122]

If a patient requires an injection into a joint, then there is an expectation that the injection goes into the joint, not the adjacent muscle or tendon. There is a growing awareness of the risks that steroid injections can pose, including subcutaneous fat atrophy, skin depigmentation, infection, and tendon and cartilage degeneration. Some of these risks may be heightened if an injection is placed outside the target structure. A significant proportion of musculoskeletal injection techniques are performed adjacent to tendinous structures, and corticosteroids have been shown to have a negative effect on tendon health.[36] Consequently, the use of guidance can provide clinical and medicolegal assurances that the technique was accurate and not within the tendon or the subcutaneous tissue in case an adverse event is encountered. It also enables the clinician to keep a definitive image of the location of the needle tip as further medicolegal evidence of treatment.

It is likely that the demand for ultrasound-guided injections will continue to rise as technology rapidly improves and the falling cost of equipment drives increased accessibility. Concomitant with this is the need to ensure this practice is necessary, cost-effective, safe, and beneficial.

Suprascapular nerve blocks

The suprascapular nerve (SSN) innervates a number of structures in and around the shoulder including the glenohumeral (GH) and acromioclavicular (AC) joints, supraspinatus and infraspinatus muscles, the subacromial bursa, and the coracoclavicular ligament.[42,112] Afferent information from one or more of these structures can relay sensory information to the central nervous system, potentially contributing to perception of pain in the shoulder (Figure 23.7).

A nerve block is a therapeutic injection that aims to reduce afferent input to the brain, thereby potentially helping to reduce the perception of pain. Suprascapular nerve blocks (SSNBs) have been used by clinicians for many years, and were first described by Wertheim and Rovenstine to treat chronic shoulder pain in 1941.[43]

Which patients are best suited to have a suprascapular nerve block?

Over the last decade, there has been an increased amount of published literature supporting the use of SSNBs to manage people with chronic musculoskeletal shoulder pain. Various types of shoulder pathology can be treated using

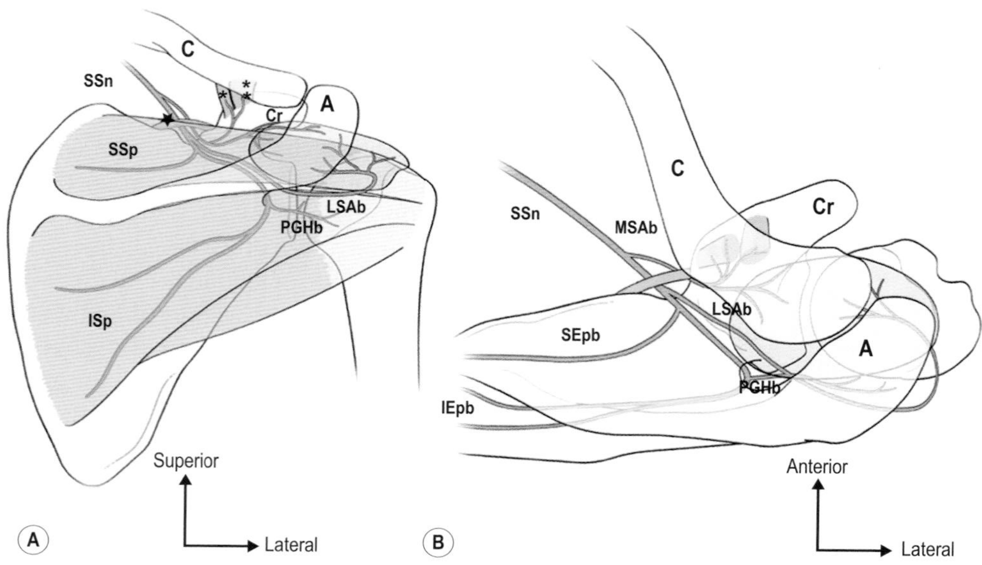

FIGURE 23.7

Diagram of the distal suprascapular nerve and its sensory branches (A, posterior view; B, superior view). The suprascapular nerve (SSN) has three sensory branches: a medial subacromial branch proximal to the suprascapular notch, a lateral subacromial branch (LSAb) at the level of the suprascapular notch, and a posterior glenohumeral branch (PGHb) distal to the spinal glenoid notch. The subacromial branches provide bipolar innervation to the subacromial bursa (in blue); the medial subacromial branch (MSAb) also innervates the coracoclavicular ligaments (conoid (*) and trapezoid (**) ligament). The PGHb provides sensory innervation to the posterior glenohumeral capsule. A, acromion; C, clavicle; Cr, coracoid process; ISp, branch to infraspinatus muscle; SSp, branch to supraspinatus muscle.[70]

(Reproduced with permission from Laumonerie P, Blasco L, Tibbo ME, et al. Sensory innervation of the subacromial bursa by the distal suprascapular nerve: a new description of its anatomic distribution. J Shoulder Elbow Surg. 2019;28:1788-1794.[70])

an SSNB, including GH and AC joint osteoarthritis, frozen shoulder, rotator cuff-related shoulder pain (RCRSP), and bursal-derived pain, or combinations of these.

National guidance from the British Elbow and Shoulder Society (BESS) and the British Orthopaedic Association (BOA) advocates considering SSNBs in the management of GH joint osteoarthritis and subacromial shoulder pain.[67,116] Evidence from systematic reviews suggest SSNBs may be effective in pain reduction for patients with frozen shoulder and persistent shoulder pain (derived from different musculoskeletal causes) when compared to sham or comparative treatments.[21,45] Furthermore, a survey of 492 physical therapists in 2019 reported that most respondents would consider an SSNB for patients with persistent shoulder pain. In particular, SSNBs were a popular treatment choice for patients with rotator cuff arthropathy, where shoulder surgery was not indicated.[104]

The likely mechanisms of action of a suprascapular nerve block

For a nerve to conduct an impulse and potentially contribute towards the perception of pain, sodium (Na) ions must enter the cell membrane. Through this mechanism, the nerve becomes depolarized and transmits an afferent impulse towards the brain. A change in the action potential of the nerve can therefore promote a pain-relieving effect. Therapeutic SSNBs typically use a combination of anesthetic and corticosteroid medication. The anesthetic interferes with Na ions, preventing depolarization in the short term (up to 24 hours).[117] The purpose of combining anesthetic with corticosteroid is to achieve a prolonged analgesic effect. The mechanism that leads to this effect is poorly understood. One theory is that corticosteroids directly reduce nociceptive

C-fiber transmission.[119] Another hypothesis is that the reduction in pain is a result of the corticosteroid's anti-inflammatory effects.[57]

Regardless of the mechanism, reducing nociceptive input to the central nervous system over time may result in modifying cortical networks innervating the shoulder, leading to long-term reduction in the perception of pain in the shoulder region.[13] Much of the research reports that participants who receive therapeutic SSNBs have pain relief at 12 weeks post intervention.[21] One service evaluation where SSNBs were used in conjunction with physical therapy rehabilitation reported a clinically meaningful and statistically significant reduction in pain from baseline at six months following the intervention.[104,105] Further research is required to substantiate time duration of effectiveness for therapeutic SSNBs and how this is achieved.

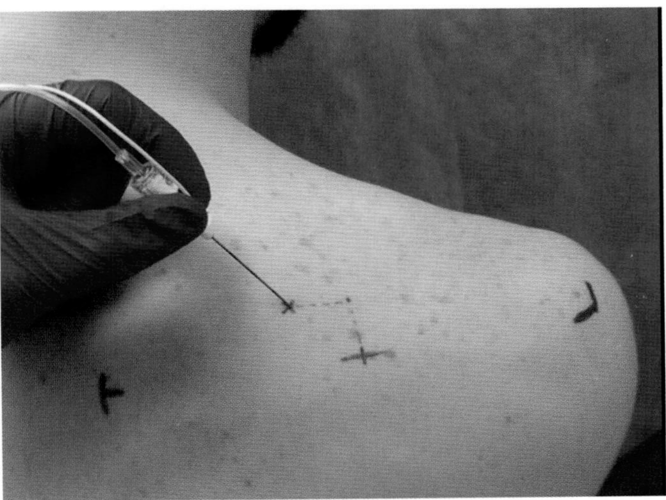

FIGURE 23.8
Suprascapular nerve block using the Meier landmark-guided method.

Methods to perform a suprascapular nerve block

Landmark-guided (Meier technique)

Bony landmarks are located at the medial end of the spine of the scapula and the lateral end of the acromion. The clinician locates the midpoint between these two points and measures 2 cm (0.8 in) up (cephalad) and 2 cm (0.8 in) medially. The needle is inserted at a 45-degree angle distal to the entry point until the end of the needle comes into contact with the supraspinatus fossa.[46] The needle is withdrawn a few millimeters. The practitioner draws back with the syringe checking for any backflow of blood to ensure as much as possible that the needle is not in the suprascapular artery. The injectate is delivered (Figure 23.8).

Electrostimulation-guided

This technique may help to confirm the accuracy of needle placement. Initially, the landmark-guided approach is used, however, at the point where the injectate is to be delivered, an electrical stimulator (the white cord attached to the needle in Figure 23.8) delivers an impulse to the nerve. If there is a twitch response of muscle contraction in the vicinity of the supraspinatus, the clinician gains a level of confidence that the nerve should be in the proximity of the needle before the injectate is delivered.

Ultrasound-guided

Ultrasound visualizes the target location of the needle which is as close to the suprascapular notch as possible without passing into the apex of the lung. The use of Doppler should reduce the likelihood of infiltrating the suprascapular artery which runs near to the nerve.

Fluoroscope-guided

This technique uses X-ray radiation to visualize where to direct the needle. Table 23.1 details the advantages and disadvantages of the different SSNB procedures. The landmark-guided approach is considered safe and effective.[109,110] However, for those who have been trained in musculoskeletal ultrasound scanning and injection therapy, it makes clinical sense to adopt the ultrasound-guided method as this is likely to be more accurate and potentially carries less risk of adverse events.[21]

It is unclear what the optimum dose of medication is when providing an SSNB, and whether a dose-response ratio exists. Most published research tends to use an anesthetic (such as 1% lidocaine or 0.5% bupivacaine) and a steroid (such as triamcinolone acetonide or methylprednisolone).

Table 23.1 Advantages and disadvantages between different suprascapular nerve block procedures

	Landmark-guided	Electrostimulation-guided	Ultrasound-guided	Fluoroscopy-guided
Advantages	• Little additional training required for clinicians who already inject. • No additional equipment required, therefore low cost.	• Gives some confidence that the needle is near the nerve.	• Good efficacy. • Theoretically a safer procedure than landmark approaches.	• Theoretically a safer procedure than landmark approaches.
Disadvantages	• Risk of causing damage to the nerve, infiltration to the blood vessel and pneumothorax.	• Risk of causing damage to the nerve, infiltration to the blood vessel, and pneumothorax. • Potentially an unpleasant experience for the patient to have nerve stimulated with needle in situ. • Some additional training and cost.	• Significant additional training and cost.	• Significant additional training and cost. • Radiation exposure.

Volumes for anesthetics range from 6–10 ml lidocaine or 10 ml bupivacaine. For corticosteroids, a dose of 0.5 ml (20 mg) triamcinolone acetonide or 1 ml (40 mg) methylprednisolone is frequently used.[21] It is unknown whether the dose should be adjusted for factors such as age and body mass index, or whether multiple SSNBs can safely be delivered across a specific period of time.

Suprascapular nerve ablation can be considered as a method of management if SSNBs are effective but short lasting. It is not known how the effectiveness of SSNBs compares to ablation techniques, and how harms compare between procedures. Future studies are required to help inform which procedures are the most effective, and which patient group is most likely to have a favorable response. In addition, researchers should consider whether SSNBs are effective in the long term if accompanied by other forms of treatment (such as a rehabilitation program).

How best to communicate the benefits and risks of the procedure to the patient

As with all injection therapy procedures, the aim for SSNBs is to reduce pain and disability. SSNBs may be a preferable option compared to taking medication, surgery, or committing to other forms of pain-relieving adjuncts such as acupuncture, which may require multiple visits. In addition, reducing pain might enable a patient to better participate in active rehabilitation exercises more effectively, potentially providing better long-term outcomes.[105]

It may be useful for patients to be informed that SSNBs do not work in the same way as other musculoskeletal injections that they may have received previously to treat their shoulder. This is particularly relevant if a patient has had several failed injections. Referring to the SSNB as a "procedure" (that involves an injection) rather than "another injection" may optimize patient engagement.

In considering whether to have an SSNB, patients should be encouraged to consider the possible benefits and harms to facilitate an informed decision. Table 23.2 summarizes possible harms, and advice clinicians can offer patients considering the procedure. SSNBs carry the same harms as the other forms of shoulder injections outlined earlier in this chapter. Additional harms associated with the SSNB procedure includes damage to the nerve leading to paralysis, infiltration to the blood vessel potentially leading to an adverse cardiovascular event, or piercing of the apex of the lung resulting in a pneumothorax. Patients will need to be informed that an SSNB is unlikely to be a long-term solution. In a similar manner to other injection procedures, SSNBs might provide respite from the pain and potentially enable patients to engage more effectively with other means of management such as exercise therapy. Patients should also be made aware that there is no guarantee that the block will work.

Table 23.2 Harms associated with suprascapular nerve block procedures and recommended guidance

Harm	On booking the SSNB appointment	What the patient needs to look out for	What action the patient needs to take
Nerve damage	• Make patients aware that the anesthetic could result in short-term loss of muscle power and altered sensation around the shoulder • Warn that there is a possibility that the needle could cause damage to the nerve resulting in paralysis • Advise patients to arrange for someone else to drive them home after the procedure	• Weakness in the arm (particularly into abduction) and numbness around the shoulder for 24 hours following the procedure	• Not to return to driving/operate machinery until pre-injection strength has returned • If weakness and numbness fail to resolve after a 24-hour period post procedure, the patient should contact the practitioner/department where the SSNB was provided
Cardiovascular (CVS) event	• Warn patients that due to the proximity of the nerve to a blood vessel, this procedure has a risk of introducing the injectates to the systemic circulation, which could result in an adverse CVS response. This risk is increased if the patient has an underlying cardiovascular condition or is taking medication that may interact with the injectates	• Development of any of the following: palpitations, feeling faint/fainting, chest pain, breathlessness, feeling generally unwell, slurred speech, droopy face or side of body	• Seek emergency help immediately
Pneumothorax	• Warn patients that due to the proximity of the nerve to the apex of the lung, there is a risk of a pneumothorax (punctured lung)	• Development of any of the following: increasing shortness of breath, pressure/tightness in chest/difficulty breathing	• Seek emergency help immediately

SSNB, suprascapular nerve block; CVS, cardiovascular system.

When discussing the potential harms associated with SSNBs, it is worth considering that other forms of treatment such as the prescription of analgesic medication and surgery are also not without risk. For people who are suffering severe and persistent shoulder pain who may have exhausted other treatment options, the potential benefits of the SSNB procedure may well outweigh the risks.

SSNBs may be an effective means of managing persistent shoulder pain especially when other treatment options are either not indicated or have been ineffective. Future research should aim to answer what constitutes an optimal dose, which adjuncts are preferable, which techniques are safer, when (in the management pathway) is a block most useful, and how SSNBs compare to other treatment options.

Conclusion

Is this chapter we have presented the indications for and methods involved in using injection therapy for the treatment of various common shoulder pathologies. As with all treatment modalities, healthcare practitioners are advised to consider their clinical experience, the available scientific evidence, and patient preference before deciding to use injection therapy. Although there are significant gaps within the current evidence base, it is difficult to deny that injection therapy is considered, an effective and popular nonsurgical treatment option for various shoulder conditions. As we have discussed, however, they are not without risk. Although adverse effects are difficult to quantify, and demands from patients for pain relief and improvements in function are often high, it is in a clinician's and the patient's best interest to discuss these risks as part of the shared decision-making process. What is clear from each section within this chapter is that there are myriad gaps in our knowledge that need be prioritized in future research.

References

1. National Institute for Health and Care Excellence. Scenario: Rotator cuff disorders. 2017. Available at: https://cks.nice.org.uk/topics/shoulder-pain/management/rotator-cuff-disorders/

2. National Institute for Health and Care Excellence. Scenario: Acromioclavicular joint disorders. 2017. Available at: https://cks.nice.org.uk/topics/shoulder-pain/management/acromioclavicular-joint-disorders/

3. Akobeng AK. Principles of evidence based medicine. Arch Dis Child. 2005;90:837-840.

4. Alvarez CM, Litchfield R, Jackowski D, Griffin S, Kirkley A. A prospective, double-blind, randomized clinical trial comparing subacromial injection of betamethasone and xylocaine to xylocaine alone in chronic rotator cuff tendinosis. Am J Sports Med. 2005;33:255-262.

5. Aly AR, Rajasekaran S, Ashworth N. Ultrasound-guided shoulder girdle injections are more accurate and more effective than landmark-guided injections: a systematic review and meta-analysis. Br J Sports Med. 2015;49:1042-1049.

6. Arroll B, Goodyear-Smith F. Corticosteroid injections for painful shoulder: a meta-analysis. Br J Gen Pract. 2005;55:224-228.

7. Bee WW, Thing J. Ultrasound-guided injections in primary care: evidence, costs, and suggestions for change. Br J Gen Prac. 2017;378-379.

8. Bhayana H, Mishra P, Tandon A, Pankaj A, Pandey R, Malhotra R. Ultrasound guided versus landmark guided corticosteroid injection in patients with rotator cuff syndrome: randomised controlled trial. J Clin Orthop Trauma. 2018;9:S80-s85.

9. Bisbinas I, Belthur M, Said HG, Green M, Learmonth DJ. Accuracy of needle placement in ACJ injections. Knee Surg Sports Traumatol Arthrosc. 2006;14:762-765.

10. Bloom JE, Rischin A, Johnston RV, Buchbinder R. Image-guided versus blind glucocorticoid injection for shoulder pain. Cochrane Database Syst Rev. 2012;CD009147.

11. British National Formulary. London: British Medical Association and Royal Pharmaceutical Society; 2020.

12. Borbas P, Eid K, Ek ET, Ricks M, Feigl G, Jeserschek JM. A cadaveric study of the three different palpation-guided techniques for glenohumeral joint injections. Shoulder Elbow. 2020;12:399-403.

13. Bradnam L, Shanahan EM, Hendy K, et al. Afferent inhibition and cortical silent periods in shoulder primary motor cortex and effect of a suprascapular nerve block in people experiencing chronic shoulder pain. Clin Neurophysiol. 2016;127:769-778.

14. BOA, RCS, CSP, BESS. Commissioning guide: subacromial shoulder pain. 2014. Available at: https://bess.ac.uk/subacromial-pain-2/.

15. Buchbinder R, Green S, Youd JM. Corticosteroid injections for shoulder pain. Cochrane Database Syst Rev. 2003;CD004016.

16. Burbank KM, Stevenson JH, Czarnecki GR, Dorfman J. Chronic shoulder pain: part II. Treatment. Am Fam Physician. 2008;77:493-497.

17. Buttaci CJ, Stitik TP, Yonclas PP, Foye PM. Osteoarthritis of the acromioclavicular joint: a review of anatomy, biomechanics, diagnosis, and treatment. Am J Phys Med Rehabil. 2004;83:791-797.

18. Carofino B, Chowaniec DM, McCarthy MB, et al. Corticosteroids and local anesthetics decrease positive effects of platelet-rich plasma: an in vitro study on human tendon cells. Arthroscopy. 2012;28:711-719.

19. Carroll MB, Motley SA, Smith B, Ramsey BC, Baggett AS. Comparing corticosteroid preparation and dose in the improvement of shoulder function and pain: a randomized, single-blind pilot study. Am J Phys Med Rehabil. 2018;97:450-455.

20. Challoumas D, Biddle M, McLean M, Millar NL. Comparison of treatments for frozen shoulder: a systematic review and meta-analysis. JAMA Network Open. 2020;3:e2029581.

21. Chang KV, Hung CY, Wu WT, Han DS, Yang RS, Lin CP. Comparison of the effectiveness of suprascapular nerve block with physical therapy, placebo, and intra-articular injection in management of chronic shoulder pain: a meta-analysis of randomized controlled trials. Arch Phys Med Rehabil. 2016;97:1366-1380.

22. Chang KV, Mezian K, Naňka O, Wu WT, Lin CP, Özçakar L. Ultrasound-guided interventions for painful shoulder: from anatomy to evidence. J Pain Res. 2018;11:2311-2322.

23. Chen P, Huang L, Ma Y, et al. Intra-articular platelet-rich plasma injection for knee osteoarthritis: a summary of meta-analyses. J Orthop Surg Res. 2019;14:385.

24. Chen R, Jiang C, Huang G. Comparison of intra-articular and subacromial corticosteroid injection in frozen shoulder: a meta-analysis of randomized controlled trials. International Journal of Surgery. 2019;68:92-103.

25. Cho CH, Kim du H, Bae KC, Lee D, Kim K. Proper site of corticosteroid injection for the treatment of idiopathic frozen shoulder: results from a randomized trial. Joint Bone Spine. 2016;83:324-329.

26. Chong PY, Srikumaran U, Kuye IO, Warner JJ. Glenohumeral arthritis in the young patient. J Shoulder Elbow Surg. 2011;20:S30-40.

27. Cole BF, Peters KS, Hackett L, Murrell GA. Ultrasound-guided versus blind subacromial corticosteroid injections for subacromial impingement syndrome: a randomized, double-blind clinical trial. Am J Sports Med. 2016;44:702-707.

28. Cole BJ, Schumacher HR. Injectable corticosteroids in modern practice. J Am Acad Orthop Surg. 2005;13:37-46.

29. Cook T, Lewis J. Rotator cuff-related shoulder pain: to inject or not to inject? J Orthop Sports Phys Ther. 2019;49:289-293.

30. Cook T, Minns Lowe C, Maybury M, Lewis JS. Are corticosteroid injections more beneficial than anaesthetic injections alone in the management of rotator cuff-related shoulder pain? A systematic review. Br J Sports Med. 2018;52:497-504.

31. Crowell MS, Tragord BS. Orthopaedic manual physical therapy for shoulder pain and impaired movement in a patient with glenohumeral joint osteoarthritis: a case report. J Orthop Sports Phys Ther. 2015;45:453-461, A451-453.

32. Cruz-Topete D, Cidlowski JA. One hormone, two actions: anti- and pro-inflammatory effects of glucocorticoids. Neuroimmunomodulation. 2015;22:20-32.

33. Cyriax J, Troisier O. Hydrocortone and soft-tissue lesions. Br Med J. 1953;2:966-968.

34. De Jong BA, Dahmen R, Hogeweg JA. Intra-articular triamcinolone acetonide injection in patients with capsulitis of

the shoulder: a comparative study of two dose regimens. Clinical Rehabilitation. 1998;12:211-215.

35. Dean BJ, Franklin SL, Murphy RJ, Javaid MK, Carr AJ. Glucocorticoids induce specific ion-channel-mediated toxicity in human rotator cuff tendon: a mechanism underpinning the ultimately deleterious effect of steroid injection in tendinopathy? Br J Sports Med. 2014;48:1620-1626.

36. Dean BJ, Lostis E, Oakley T, Rombach I, Morrey ME, Carr AJ. The risks and benefits of glucocorticoid treatment for tendinopathy: a systematic review of the effects of local glucocorticoid on tendon. Semin Arthritis Rheum. 2014;43:570-576.

37. Diercks RL. Practice guideline 'Diagnosis and treatment of the subacromial pain syndrome'. Ned Tijdschr Geneeskd. 2014;158:A6985.

38. Dogu B, Yucel SD, Sag SY, Bankaoglu M, Kuran B. Blind or ultrasound-guided corticosteroid injections and short-term response in subacromial impingement syndrome: a randomized, double-blind, prospective study. Am J Phys Med Rehabil. 2012;91:658-665.

39. Department of Health. Patients First and Foremost.2013. Available at: https://assets.publishing.service.gov.uk/government/uploads/system/uploads/attachment_data/file/170701/Patients_First_and_Foremost.pdf

40. Department of Health. The Musculoskeletal Services Framework. 2006. Available at: https://webarchive.nationalarchives.gov.uk/ukgwa/20130107105354/http:/www.dh.gov.uk/prod_consum_dh/groups/dh_digitalassets/@dh/@en/documents/digitalasset/dh_4138412.pdf

41. DTB. Articular and periarticular corticosteroid injections. Drug and Therapeutics Bulletin. 1995;33:67-70.

42. Ebraheim NA, Whitehead JL, Alla SR, et al. The suprascapular nerve and its articular branch to the acromioclavicular joint: an anatomic study. J Shoulder Elbow Surg. 2011;20:e13-17.

43. Elsharkawy HA, Abd-Elsayed AA, Cummings KC, Soliman LM. Analgesic efficacy and technique of ultrasound-guided suprascapular nerve catheters after shoulder arthroscopy. Ochsner J. 2014;14:259-263.

44. Faryniarz DA, Dicarlo EF, Hannafin JA. Adhesive capsulitis: a proposed clinical staging scheme with histological correlation. Available at: https://www.researchgate.net/publication/267772974_Adhesive_Capsulitis_A_Proposed_Clinical_Staging_Scheme_with_Histological_Correlation.

45. Favejee MM, Huisstede BM, Koes BW. Frozen shoulder: the effectiveness of conservative and surgical interventions: systematic review. Br J Sports Med. 2011;45:49-56.

46. Fernandes MR, Barbosa MA, Sousa AL, Ramos GC. Suprascapular nerve block: important procedure in clinical practice. Part II. Rev Bras Reumatol. 2012;52:616-622.

47. Finnoff JT, Hall MM, Adams E, et al. American Medical Society for Sports Medicine (AMSSM) position statement: interventional musculoskeletal ultrasound in sports medicine. PM R. 2015;7:151-168.e112.

48. Garretson RB, Williams GR. Clinical evaluation of injuries to the acromioclavicular and sternoclavicular joints. Clin Sports Med. 2003;22:239-254.

49. Gilbert GM, Nelson R. Anatomy, shoulder and upper limb, anterior humeral circumflex artery. StatPearls. Treasure Island: StatPearls Publishing; 2021.

50. Gokalp G, Dusak A, Yazici Z. Efficacy of ultrasonography-guided shoulder MR arthrography using a posterior approach. Skeletal Radiol. 2010;39:575-579.

51. Grassi W, Filippucci E, Busilacchi P. Musculoskeletal ultrasound. Best Pract Res Clin Rheumatol. 2004;18:813-826.

52. Gross C, Dhawan A, Harwood D, Gochanour E, Romeo A. Glenohumeral joint injections: a review. Sports Health. 2013;5:153-159.

53. Hashiuchi T, Sakurai G, Morimoto M, Komei T, Takakura Y, Tanaka Y. Accuracy of the biceps tendon sheath injection: ultrasound-guided or unguided injection? A randomized controlled trial. J Shoulder Elbow Surg. 2011;20:1069-1073.

54. Hazleman B. Shoulder problems in general practice. Reports on the Rheumatic Diseases Series 4. Arthritis Research Campaign. Versus Arthritis; 2005.

55. Henkus HE, Cobben LP, Coerkamp EG, Nelissen RG, van Arkel ER. The accuracy of subacromial injections: a prospective randomized magnetic resonance imaging study. Arthroscopy. 2006;22:277-282.

56. Hettrich CM, DiCarlo EF, Faryniarz D, Vadasdi KB, Williams R, Hannafin JA. The effect of myofibroblasts and corticosteroid injections in adhesive capsulitis. J Shoulder Elbow Surg. 2016;25:1274-1279.

57. Hewson D, Bedforth N, McCartney C, Hardman J. Dexamethasone and peripheral nerve blocks: back to basic (science). Br J Anaesth. 2019;122:411-412.

58. Hoffmann TC, Lewis J, Maher CG. Shared decision making should be an integral part of physiotherapy practice. Physiotherapy. 2020;107:43-49.

59. Innes S, Maybury M, Hall A, Lumsden G. Ultrasound guided musculoskeletal interventions: professional opportunities, challenges and the future of injection therapy. Sonography. 2015;2(4):84-91.

60. Iwata H. Pharmacologic and clinical aspects of intraarticular injection of hyaluronate. Clin Orthop Relat Res. 1993;285-291.

61. Jacob AK, Sallay PI. Therapeutic efficacy of corticosteroid injections in the acromioclavicular joint. Biomed Sci Instrum. 1997;34:380-385.

62. Johansson A, Hao J, Sjölund B. Local corticosteroid application blocks transmission in normal nociceptive C-fibres. Acta Anaesthesiol Scand. 1990;34:335-338.

63. Johansson K, Oberg B, Adolfsson L, Foldevi M. A combination of systematic review and clinicians' beliefs in interventions for subacromial pain. Br J Gen Pract. 2002;52:145-152.

64. Jones S, Hanchard N, Hamilton S, Rangan A. A qualitative study of patients' perceptions and priorities when living with primary frozen shoulder. BMJ Open. 2013;3:e003452.

65. Khazzam MS, Pearl ML. AAOS Clinical Practice Guideline: Management of Glenohumeral Joint Osteoarthritis. J Am Acad Orthop Surg. 2020;28:790-794.

66. Kim KH, Park JW, Kim SJ. High-vs low-dose corticosteroid injection in the treatment of adhesive capsulitis with severe pain: a randomized controlled double-blind study. Pain Medicine. 2018;19:735-741.

67. Kulkarni R, Gibson J, Brownson P, et al. Subacromial shoulder pain. Shoulder Elbow. 2015;7:135-143.

68. LaPrade RF, Dragoo JL, Koh JL, Murray IR, Geeslin AG, Chu CR. AAOS research symposium updates and consensus:

biologic treatment of orthopaedic injuries. J Am Acad Orthop Surg. 2016;24:e62-78.

69. Laumonerie P, Blasco L, Tibbo ME, et al. Sensory innervation of the subacromial bursa by the distal suprascapular nerve: a new description of its anatomic distribution. J Shoulder Elbow Surg. 2019;28:1788-1794.

70. Lewis J. Frozen shoulder contracture syndrome: aetiology, diagnosis and management. Manual Therapy. 2015;20:2-9.

71. Lewis J. Rotator cuff related shoulder pain: assessment, management and uncertainties. Man Ther. 2016;23:57-68.

72. Longworth S. Injection Techniques in Musculoskeletal Medicine: A Practical Manual for Clinicians in Primary and Secondary Care, 4th edition. Churchill Livingstone Elsevier; 2012.

73. Louwerens JK, Sierevelt IN, van Noort A, van den Bekerom MP. Evidence for minimally invasive therapies in the management of chronic calcific tendinopathy of the rotator cuff: a systematic review and meta-analysis. J Shoulder Elbow Surg. 2014;23:1240-1249.

74. Lumsden G, Lucas-Garner K, Sutherland S, Dodenhoff R. Physiotherapists utilizing diagnostic ultrasound in shoulder clinics. How useful do patients find immediate feedback from the scan as part of the management of their problem? Musculoskeletal Care. 2018;16:209-213.

75. McGahan JP. The history of interventional ultrasound. J Ultrasound Med. 2004;23:727-741.

76. Merolla G, Sperling JW, Paladini P, Porcellini G. Efficacy of Hylan G-F 20 versus 6-methylprednisolone acetate in painful shoulder osteoarthritis: a retrospective controlled trial. Musculoskelet Surg. 2011;95:215-224.

77. Minagawa H, Yamamoto N, Abe H, et al. Prevalence of symptomatic and asymptomatic rotator cuff tears in the general population: from mass-screening in one village. J Orthop. 2013;10:8-12.

78. Mohamadi A, Chan JJ, Claessen FM, Ring D, Chen NC. Corticosteroid injections give small and transient pain relief in rotator cuff tendinosis: a meta-analysis. Clin Orthop Relat Res. 2017;475:232-243.

79. Molini L, Mariacher S, Bianchi S. US guided corticosteroid injection into the subacromial-subdeltoid bursa: technique and approach. J Ultrasound. 2012;15:61-68.

80. Nazarian LN. The top 10 reasons musculoskeletal sonography is an important complementary or alternative technique to MRI. AJR Am J Roentgenol. 2008;190:1621-1626.

81. Ogul H, Bayraktutan U, Yildirim OS, et al. Magnetic resonance arthrography of the glenohumeral joint: ultrasonography-guided technique using a posterior approach. Eurasian J Med. 2012;44:73-78.

82. Oh JH, Oh CH, Choi JA, Kim SH, Kim JH, Yoon JP. Comparison of glenohumeral and subacromial steroid injection in primary frozen shoulder: a prospective, randomized short-term comparison study. J Shoulder Elbow Surg. 2011;20:1034-1040.

83. Park KD, Kim TK, Lee J, Lee WY, Ahn JK, Park Y. Palpation versus ultrasound-guided acromioclavicular joint intra-articular corticosteroid injections: a retrospective comparative clinical study. Pain Physician. 2015;18:333-341.

84. Partington PF, Broome GH. Diagnostic injection around the shoulder: hit and miss? A cadaveric study of injection accuracy. J Shoulder Elbow Surg. 1998;7:147-150.

85. Patel DN, Nayyar S, Hasan S, Khatib O, Sidash S, Jazrawi LM. Comparison of ultrasound-guided versus blind glenohumeral injections: a cadaveric study. J Shoulder Elbow Surg. 2012;21:1664-1668.

86. Peck E, Lai JK, Pawlina W, Smith J. Accuracy of ultrasound-guided versus palpation-guided acromioclavicular joint injections: a cadaveric study. PM R. 2010;2:817-821.

87. Peterson CK, Saupe N, Buck F, Pfirrmann CW, Zanetti M, Hodler J. CT-guided sternoclavicular joint injections: description of the procedure, reliability of imaging diagnosis, and short-term patient responses. AJR Am J Roentgenol. 2010;195:W435-439.

88. Pichler W, Weinberg AM, Grechenig S, Tesch NP, Heidari N, Grechenig W. Intra-articular injection of the acromioclavicular joint. J Bone Joint Surg Br. 2009;91:1638-1640.

89. Poulsen RC, Watts AC, Murphy RJ, Snelling SJ, Carr AJ, Hulley PA. Glucocorticoids induce senescence in primary human tenocytes by inhibition of sirtuin 1 and activation of the p53/p21 pathway: in vivo and in vitro evidence. Ann Rheum Dis. 2014;73:1405-1413.

90. Pourcho AM, Sellon JL, Smith J. Sonographically guided sternoclavicular joint injection: description of technique and validation. J Ultrasound Med. 2015;34:325-331.

91. Royal College of General Practitioners. Office of Populations, Censuses and Surveys. Third National Morbidity Survey in General Practice, 1980–1981. Department of Health and Social Security, series MB5 No 1. London: HMSO; 1980–1981.

92. Prestgaard T, Wormgoor ME, Haugen S, Harstad H, Mowinckel P, Brox JI. Ultrasound-guided intra-articular and rotator interval corticosteroid injections in adhesive capsulitis of the shoulder: a double-blind, sham-controlled randomized study. Pain. 2015;156:1683-1691.

93. Raeissadat SA, Rayegani SM, Langroudi TF, Khoiniha M. Comparing the accuracy and efficacy of ultrasound-guided versus blind injections of steroid in the glenohumeral joint in patients with shoulder adhesive capsulitis. Clin Rheumatol. 2017;36:933-940.

94. Raghavan R, Dwyer AJ. A systematic review of treatment of frozen shoulder by hydrodistension with or without steroid or intraarticular steroid injection. Current Orthopaedic Practice. 2019;30:377-384.

95. Ramírez J, Pomés I, Cabrera S, Pomés J, Sanmartí R, Cañete JD. Incidence of full-thickness rotator cuff tear after subacromial corticosteroid injection: a 12-week prospective study. Modern Rheumatology. 2014;24:667-670.

96. Rangan A, Brealey SD, Keding A, et al. Management of adults with primary frozen shoulder in secondary care (UK FROST): a multicentre, pragmatic, three-arm, superiority randomised clinical trial. The Lancet. 2020;396:977-989.

97. Rangan A, Hanchard N, McDaid C. What is the most effective treatment for frozen shoulder? BMJ. 2016;354:i4162.

98. Roddy E, Ogollah RO, Oppong R, et al. Optimising outcomes of exercise and corticosteroid injection in patients with subacromial pain (impingement) syndrome: a factorial randomised trial. Br J Sports Med. 2021;55:262-271.

99. Rutten MJ, Maresch BJ, Jager GJ, de Waal Malefijt MC. Injection of the subacromial-subdeltoid bursa: blind or ultrasound-guided? Acta Orthop. 2007;78:254-257.

100. Sabeti-Aschraf M, Lemmerhofer B, Lang S, et al. Ultrasound guidance improves the accuracy of the acromioclavicular joint infiltration: a prospective randomized study. Knee Surg Sports Traumatol Arthrosc. 2011;19:292-295.

101. Sabeti-Aschraf M, Stotter C, Thaler C, et al. Intra-articular versus periarticular acromioclavicular joint injection: a multicenter, prospective, randomized, controlled trial. Arthroscopy. 2013;29:1903-1910.

102. Saccomanno MF, De Ieso C, Milano G. Acromioclavicular joint instability: anatomy, biomechanics and evaluation. Joints. 2014; 2: 87-92.

103. Sage W, Pickup L, Smith TO, Denton ER, Toms AP. The clinical and functional outcomes of ultrasound-guided vs landmark-guided injections for adults with shoulder pathology: a systematic review and meta-analysis. Rheumatology. 2013;52:743-751.

104. Salt E, Van Der Windt D, Chesterton L, McRobert C, Foster N. Physiotherapists' use of suprascapular nerve blocks: an online survey. Physiotherapy. 2019;105:461-468.

105. Salt E, van der Windt DA, Chesterton L, Mainwaring F, Ashwood N, Foster NE. Physiotherapist-led suprascapular nerve blocks for persistent shoulder pain: evaluation of a new service in the UK. Musculoskeletal Care. 2018;16:214-221.

106. Saltychev M, Laimi K, Virolainen P, Fredericson M. Effectiveness of hydrodilatation in adhesive capsulitis of shoulder: a systematic review and meta-analysis. Scand J Surg. 2018;107:285-293.

107. Shaffer BS. Painful conditions of the acromioclavicular joint. J Am Acad Orthop Surg. 1999;7:176-188.

108. Shah A, Mak D, Davies AM, James SL, Botchu R. Musculoskeletal corticosteroid administration: current concepts. Can Assoc Radiol J. 2019;70:29-36.

109. Shanahan EM, Ahern M, Smith M, Wetherall M, Bresnihan B, FitzGerald O. Suprascapular nerve block (using bupivacaine and methylprednisolone acetate) in chronic shoulder pain. Ann Rheum Dis. 2003;62:400-406.

110. Shanahan EM, Smith MD, Wetherall M, et al. Suprascapular nerve block in chronic shoulder pain: are the radiologists better? Ann Rheum Dis. 2004;63:1035-1040.

111. Shang X, Zhang Z, Pan X, Li J, Li Q. Intra-articular versus subacromial corticosteroid injection for the treatment of adhesive capsulitis: a meta-analysis and systematic review. Biomed Res Int. 2019;2019:1274790.

112. Shi LL, Freehill MT, Yannopoulos P, Warner JJ. Suprascapular nerve: is it important in cuff pathology? Adv Orthop. 2012;2012:516985.

113. Sidon E, Velkes S, Shemesh S, Levy J, Glaser E, Kosashvili Y. Accuracy of non assisted glenohumeral joint injection in the office setting. Eur J Radiol. 2013;82:e829-831.

114. Strauss EJ, Hart JA, Miller MD, Altman RD, Rosen JE. Hyaluronic acid viscosupplementation and osteoarthritis: current uses and future directions. Am J Sports Med. 2009;37:1636-1644.

115. Sun Y, Zhang P, Liu S, et al. Intra-articular steroid injection for frozen shoulder: a systematic review and meta-analysis of randomized controlled trials with trial sequential analysis. Am J Sports Med. 2017;45:2171-2179.

116. Thomas M, Bidwai A, Rangan A, et al. BESS/BOA Patient Care Pathways. Glenohumeral osteoarthritis. Shoulder and Elbow. 2016;8:203-214.

117. Vadhanan P, Tripaty DK, Adinarayanan S. Physiological and pharmacologic aspects of peripheral nerve blocks. J Anaesthesiol Clin Pharmacol. 2015;31:384-393.

118. van der Windt DA, Koes BW, de Jong BA, Bouter LM. Shoulder disorders in general practice: incidence, patient characteristics, and management. Ann Rheum Dis. 1995;54:959-964.

119. Vieira PA, Pulai I, Tsao GC, Manikantan P, Keller B, Connelly NR. Dexamethasone with bupivacaine increases duration of analgesia in ultrasound-guided interscalene brachial plexus blockade. Eur J Anaesthesiol. 2010;27:285-288.

120. University of New South Wales. Clinical practice guidelines: management of rotator cuff syndrome in the workplace. University of New South Wales; 2013.

121. Weber AE, Trasolini NA, Mayer EN, et al. Injections prior to rotator cuff repair are associated with increased rotator cuff revision rates. Arthroscopy. 2019;35:717-724.

122. Wheeler P. What do patients think about diagnostic ultrasound? A pilot study to investigate patient-perceived benefits with the use of musculoskeletal diagnostic ultrasound in an outpatient clinic setting. International Musculoskeletal Medicine. 2010;32:68-71.

123. Wu WT, Chang KV, Han DS, Chang CH, Yang FS, Lin CP. Effectiveness of glenohumeral joint dilatation for treatment of frozen shoulder: a systematic review and meta-analysis of randomized controlled trials. Sci Rep. 2017;7:10507.

124. Yoon SH, Lee HY, Lee HJ, Kwack KS. Optimal dose of intra-articular corticosteroids for adhesive capsulitis: a randomized, triple-blind, placebo-controlled trial. Am J Sports Med. 2013;41:1133-1139.

125. Zhang Y, Jordan JM. Epidemiology of osteoarthritis. Clin Geriatr Med. 2010;26:355-369.

24 Shoulder trauma

Duncan Tennent, Ian Horsley, Yemi Pearse, Ben Ashworth

Introduction

Traumatic injury to the shoulder is common and results in damage to the soft tissues, bones, and joints, in isolation or in combination. Trauma may result in fractures and dislocations of the bones and joints that make up the shoulder region. Appreciation of the soft tissue anatomy is essential as the stabilizing structures and deforming forces will dictate outcome and management options. Clinical examination can be difficult and must be performed carefully. Many of the injuries may be treated nonsurgically but it is important to appreciate the limits of both nonsurgical and surgical treatment and the potential need for urgent intervention.

Proximal humeral fractures

The management of proximal humeral fractures remains controversial. There is infinite variability in terms of fracture configuration. However, in order to try to make sense of these injuries and produce a treatment algorithm, similar fracture patterns have been grouped together in classification systems with the assumption that fractures in the same group will: 1) have the same natural history if treated without an attempt to restore normal bony anatomy, and 2) respond to surgical treatment to restore normal bony anatomy in the same way.

The most used classification system is the Neer classification system[104] (Figure 24.1). It is based on the number of parts into which the proximal humerus is fractured and the degree of displacement of the fragments. When the fragments are not especially displaced, it is likely that they will heal without surgical intervention, and because they heal in near-normal positions, it is anticipated that the shoulder will function normally. The process of rehabilitation should begin as soon as possible, and outcome is better with a shorter period of immobilization.[61,84] The focus of rehabilitation is restoration of movement by preventing scarring and progressively restoring muscular activity without displacing the fragments as they heal.

When the fragments are widely displaced, they are less likely to heal and if they do, the relationship between them (and the muscles that attach to them) is substantially altered. The assumption is that this will have a negative effect on the biomechanics and therefore function of the shoulder. The amount of displacement deemed significant is arbitrary: initially Neer's classification was based on a displacement of 1 cm (0.4 in) (translation) or 45° (rotation). More recently, displacement of >5 mm (0.2 in) has been deemed significant.

The assumption is that when fragments are widely displaced, surgical restoration of bony anatomy will result in more normal shoulder mechanics and a better functional outcome.[45] Achieving perfect restoration of anatomy surgically is technically very difficult. Moreover, the implants that hold the fragments together must do so securely enough to resist the fragments being pulled apart once the muscles are activated during rehabilitation; however, due to the configuration of the fragments and the quality of the bone of the proximal humerus, this is not always possible. When this is not possible, the surgical option is to replace the proximal humerus with a prosthetic implant. A conventional prosthetic implant requires a functional rotator cuff and this is possible only if the tuberosity fragments maintain their anatomical relationship to the prosthetic humeral head.[17] Achieving anatomical healing of the tuberosities is very inconsistent and there is an increasing trend to use a reverse polarity shoulder replacement in people over 65 years of age, which does not rely on tuberosity healing or an intact rotator cuff.[27,137]

Several randomized controlled trials and systematic reviews have been published but have failed to show superiority of one treatment modality over any other,[54,112,122] however, this is probably due to the variability of fracture pattern, patient factors, and surgical intervention. Some authors have developed evidence-based treatment algorithms, but they have been selective in their use of the literature.[127] Most fractures are undisplaced, and should be treated nonsurgically with early mobilization.[61,84] If surgery is considered for displaced fractures then the following provides guidance:

- Function is better with restoration of anatomy.[17,60]
- Outcome is worse if patients have a complication such as failure of the metalwork, infection, or nerve damage.[78]

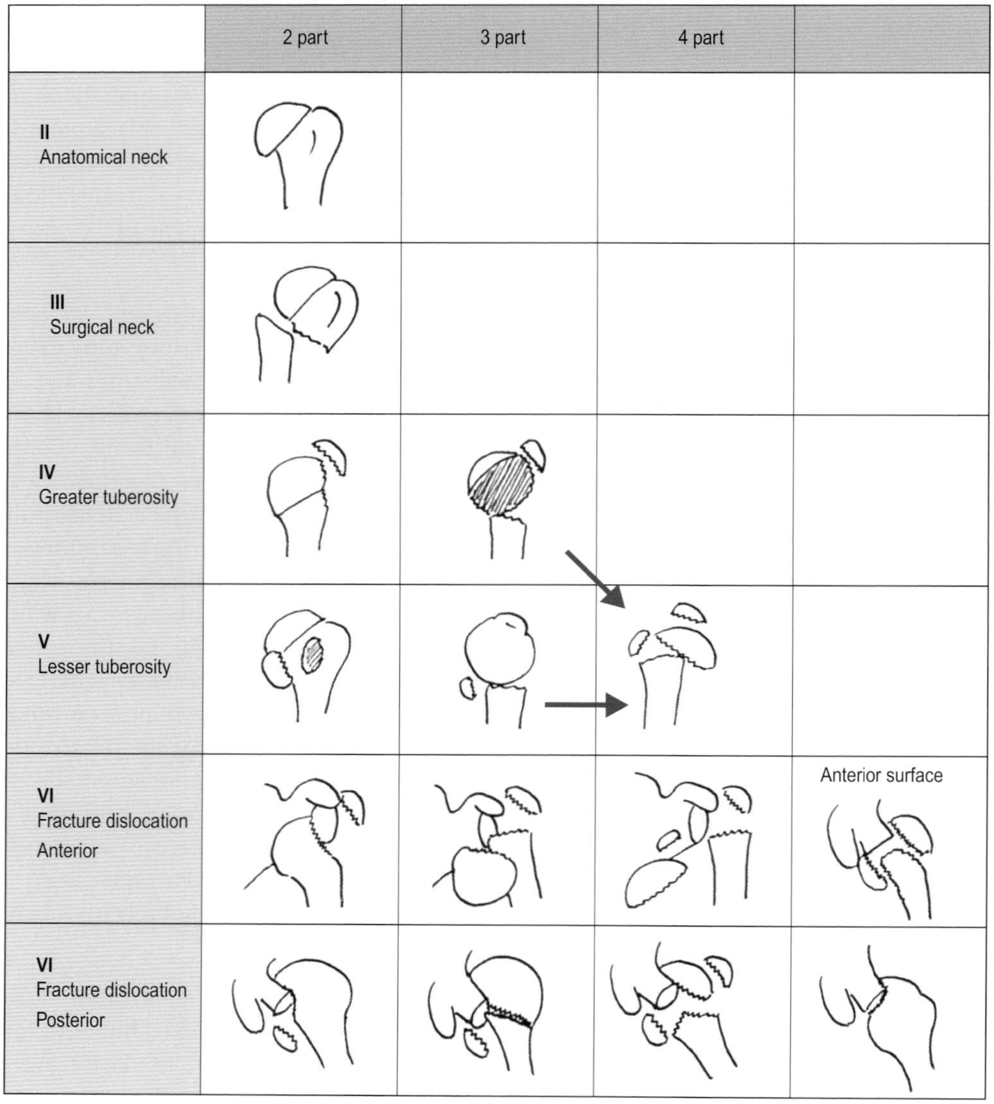

	2 part	3 part	4 part	
II Anatomical neck				
III Surgical neck				
IV Greater tuberosity				
V Lesser tuberosity				
VI Fracture dislocation Anterior				Anterior surface
VI Fracture dislocation Posterior				

FIGURE 24.1
The Neer classification of proximal humeral fractures.

- Outcome of reverse arthroplasty is more predictable than fixation or conventional arthroplasty in elderly patients.[137]
- Outcome of arthroplasty after failed fixation is worse than outcome of primary arthroplasty, and outcome of revising a failed hemiarthroplasty to a reverse arthroplasty is worse than primary reverse arthroplasty in the older patient.[37]
- Nothing is lost, other than time, trialing nonoperative management for elderly patients, as outcome of delayed reverse arthroplasty is equivalent to that of acute reverse arthroplasty.[130]

Glenohumeral dislocation

The shoulder is the most frequently dislocated joint in the body.[1,79,95] Exposure to high forces (e.g., 3400 N in rugby),[121] concomitant with vulnerable positions may result in dislocations and other traumatic injuries.[9,33] However, prognosis for shoulder dislocation is relatively good with an approximate return to pre-injury level within 3–6 months.[91]

Dislocations can be in an anterior (90%), posterior (2–5%), or less frequently inferior direction.[67,69,94,132,139] Shoulder hyperangulation or forced external rotation may result in anterior dislocation, whereas a posterior dislocation often results from forceful internal rotation, adduction, and flexion of the shoulder.[23,69]

Multiple factors that predispose the shoulder to dislocation and subsequent recurrence have been identified (Table 24.1).[109,131] Structural and functional contributions are classified in the Stanmore triangle,[65] a continuum that incorporates traumatic (TUBS) and atraumatic (AMBRII) mechanisms for shoulder instability.[11] A structurally "normal" shoulder can be destabilized due to a dysfunctional neuromuscular system ("muscle patterning"), requiring rehabilitation that addresses pathological activation patterns.[11,65,99]

Compressive force is a key component of stability. Dislocations occur when the active (functional) and passive (structural) constraints are unable to maintain normal joint congruency.[15] Alterations to bony and labral contributions to joint stability overwhelm the compressive capacity of the musculotendinous tissues.[65] The dislocating pull of dominant muscle groups needs counterbalancing by local stabilizers to reduce uncontrollable shear forces.[81] The position of the scapula and the concomitant function of rotator cuff are essential to prevent destabilization.[93] Proprioceptive feedback may be altered (Chapter 28) due to damage to capsule-labral tissues (mechanoreceptors) or neuromuscular fatigue.[25,59,65,83]

Shoulder assessment

Anterior and posterior shoulder instability tests (Table 24.2) are used by clinicians to determine appropriate intervention (e.g., a positive apprehension test increasing the likelihood of recommendations for surgery).[59] Systematic reviews have reported the sensitivity and specificity of these tests,[58,98] with poor outcomes for posterior instability.[65]

Table 24.1 Nonmodifiable and modifiable risk factors for first time and recurrent shoulder dislocations

Nonmodifiable
• Sex: males under 40 are three times more at risk than females[109]
• Age: younger population are more susceptible to first time dislocations, and elderly from falls. Higher recurrence rates (>50%) reported in males 15–20 years[109,130] (with those under 20 years 13 times more susceptible than those over the age of 20)[109]
• Bony morphology/anatomy: surface area of contact[69] (lack of bony surface congruence), shallow glenoid or other abnormal architectural position[8,49] (developmental), e.g., increased glenoid anteversion in recurrent anterior dislocation[8,11,49,65]
• Bone loss: meaningful bone loss (considered to be >13.5% of glenoid width). Humeral – Hill-Sachs; Glenoid – bony Bankart, reverse Bankart, or glenoid fracture[131]
• Genetic predisposition: hyperlaxity and hypermobility, reduced role of the periarticular soft tissue to act as passive restraints.[131] Men who suffered a shoulder dislocation were more likely to have ligamentous laxity, and as a result an objective increase in external rotation range of motion, compared with a control group.[25] However, both these factors have not been proven as risk factors for first time dislocations or as influencing likelihood of recurrence
• Past medical history of dislocation[29,110]
• Activity level: taking part in contact sports can not only predispose to injury but can also influence failure rates (e.g., 70% in male collision athletes under the age of 18) involved in collisions[92]
Modifiable*
• Strength: maximal force production
• Balanced, multidirectional force production (glenohumeral and scapulothoracic force couples)
• Stability: feedback, coordination and timing (rate of force development)

*Author's opinion.

Table 24.2 Shoulder testing for anterior and posterior shoulder instability

Anterior instability testing
• Apprehension test: highly influences whether surgery would be recommended, or generalized laxity[59,64]
• Subluxation/relocation test
• External rotation range of movement
Posterior instability testing[38,58]
• Kim "painful jerk" test[11,75]
• Wrightington posterior instability test (WPIT)[67]
• Posterior apprehension test[32]

Surgical management

Surgical intervention is usually necessary especially as nonsurgical management of anterior instability leads to high failure rates in collision sports,[134] particular in younger athletes (more than 70% failure in those under 18 years of age),[50,88,131] and may result in persistent instability episodes.[23] Arthroscopic repair resulted in better results than open stabilization for return to pre-injury level, and the Latarjet procedure significantly reduced likelihood of recurrent dislocation when compared to arthroscopic Bankart or open stabilization.[64,70] Modern arthroscopic techniques with suture anchors maybe as effective as an open surgical repair,[21] but more complex procedures are required to address more significant injuries (bony Bankart, large Hill-Sachs defect or humeral avulsion of the glenohumeral ligament (HAGL)). Posterior instability is treated effectively using similar surgical techniques.[38,47]

Rehabilitation and return to performance

Following surgery, rehabilitation should follow the key phases detailed in Figure 24.2. Progression should be based on quantifiable Return to Performance (RTP) criteria (e.g., force, stability, and mobility testing).[38,75] Prior to return to high-intensity actions, it is recommended to focus on exercises that specifically target the rate of force development, once ability to produce peak force has been restored.[7,32,38]

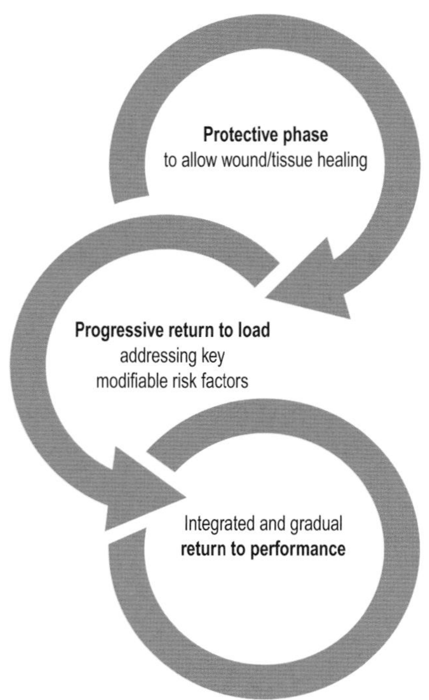

FIGURE 24.2
Return to play pathway.

Tears involving the glenoid labrum

Isolated trauma or, more frequently, repeated microtrauma, usually associated with sport or physically demanding occupations, may result in glenoid labrum damage. The incidence of superior labrum anterior to posterior (SLAP) lesions has been reported in the literature to range between 6% to 27% of all shoulder injuries evaluated arthroscopically,[68,135] although the values are much greater (55–93%) within people without shoulder symptoms.[68,119]

Anatomy

The glenoid labrum is the fibrocartilage of the shoulder joint, anchoring the joint capsule and shoulder ligaments[31] and forms approximately 50% of the total depth of the glenoid cavity. It is triangular in cross section,[55] and receives attachments from the long head of biceps superiorly and long head of triceps inferiorly. Additionally, the labrum acts like a valve block, sealing the joint from atmospheric pressure, maintaining the joint's negative intra-articular pressure, which if undermined may lead to adverse joint mechanics.[52]

Several different types (and subtypes) have been reported in literature (Table 24.3), but the most prevalent type is the SLAP lesion.

Traumatic causes may be dichotomized based on the presenting mechanism.[124] Compression-type injuries arise as the result of a fall onto an outstretched arm, with the shoulder positioned in abduction and slight forward flexion at the time of the impact. In addition to this, Funk[48] has described a mechanism in rugby players where the arm contacts an opponent or ground in a position of abduction and externally rotated position (ABER) which produces a high number of labral tears.

Traction-type injuries occur secondary to unexpected jerking movements such as when two people are carrying something and one person unexpectedly releases the object,[90] or following the repeated eccentric action of the long head of biceps acting at the elbow as is commonplace in overhead sports.[124]

Table 24.3 Classification of labral injuries

Labral Lesion		Anatomy	Mechanism	Symptoms
SLAP (superior labrum anterior to posterior)	Type 1	Labral-bicipital complex	• Repetitive use of the shoulder in throwing sports • Shoulder dislocation • Falling onto an outstretched arm • Falling onto the shoulder • Often following GHJ dislocation • Associated with ACJ injuries • "Peel back" mechanism in overhead sports	• Deep, aching pain • Popping, clicking, catching in the shoulder • Decreased range of motion • Feeling of instability • Loss of strength • Loss of range
	Type 2	Labrum and long head of the biceps tendon torn from the glenoid		
	Type 3	A "bucket-handle" detachment of superior labrum, not involving the labral insertion of long head of biceps		
	Type 4	Progression of type 3 extending to the long head of the biceps		
	Type 5	As type 2 but associated with anterior instability		
	Type 6	Large superior labral flaps without detachment of the biceps insertion		
	Type 7	As type 2 with middle and inferior glenohumeral ligament tear		
	Type 8	As type 2 with involvement of the cartilage adjacent to the biceps footplate		
Posterior labral tear (reverse Bankart tear)		Labral tear and partial tear of the rotator cuff at the supra/infraspinatus junction	• Repetitive microtrauma to the posterior capsulolabral complex • Posteriorly directed force with the arm flexed, internally rotated and adducted	• Ambiguous, nonspecific posterior shoulder pain exacerbated with posteriorly directed force
Bankart lesion		Anterior detachment of the capsule and labrum	• Repeated anterior shoulder subluxations or anterior dislocation	• Pain with movements into elevation • Pain at night • Feeling of instability • Repeated subluxation
Bony Bankart lesion		Anterior detachment of the capsule and labrum, with bone detachment	• Repeated anterior shoulder subluxations or anterior dislocation	
Perthe's lesion		Antero-inferior labrum detached	• Associated with anterior dislocation	
GLAD lesion (gleno-labral articular disruption)		Superficial detachment or fissuring of the anterior and inferior labrum, with adjacent cartilage defect	• Humeral head impaction on edge of glenoid cavity associated with dislocation forced adduction injury to the shoulder from an abducted and external rotated position	• Anterior shoulder pain main complaint • No signs of anterior instability are found on physical examination
GARD lesion (glenoid articular rim disruption)		Impaction injury affecting the posterior glenoid rim, glenoid cavity, or both	• Posterior instability following repeated axial loading in a flexed position	• Posterior shoulder pain NOT associated with instability
ALPSA (anterior labral periosteal sleeve avulsion)		Inferior glenohumeral ligament (IGHL) is expanded and labrum torn	• Following acute/chronic anterior instability	• Anterior shoulder pain • Feeling of instability • Pain at night • Pain with elevation
HAGL lesion (humeral avulsion glenohumeral ligament)		Avulsion of the IGHL from the medial humeral attachment	• Associated with anterior instability	• Anterior shoulder pain • Feeling of instability • Pain at night • Pain with elevation

Examination

Shoulder pain in active and overhead athletes poses a diagnostic challenge,[24,46] therefore clinical examination should be based on evidence-informed practice, as the most common presenting complaint is shoulder pain, which is similar for most shoulder conditions. A labral tear should be considered when the pain is on the posterior aspect of the joint when the arm is in the ABER position. Other considerations are summarized in Box 24.1.

Several orthopedic tests have been described in the literature to detect the presence of labral tears (Table 24.4), but the sensitivities and specificities of these tests are questionable.[39,56] It has been suggested that cluster testing (combining specific tests which have the highest combined sensitivity and specificity) may aid in the reliability of diagnosing pathologies.[57] Clark et al.[30] concluded that a combination of at least three positive SLAP lesion tests may be clinically useful in diagnosing a shoulder SLAP lesion with greater diagnostic accuracy than those reported for magnetic resonance imaging and arthrography. Previous clinical studies have produced varying reported sensitivity and specificity for diagnosing labral tears accurately. Fowler et al.[46] reported sensitivity of 94.74% and specificity of 14.67% for a combination of Jobe's and O'Brien's tests in recreationally active athletes as confirmed by arthroscopy who presented at a sports medicine clinic, and Oh et al.[108] reported a sensitivity of 22% and specificity of 95% within a general population presenting for arthroscopy at a general hospital, and Taylor et al.[129] proposed the "3-pack" examination (active compression test, throwing test, and bicipital tunnel palpation) as a critical screening tool for biceps-labrum disease. More recently, Hegedus et al.[56] stated that high quality clinical test clusters with powerful diagnostic characteristics for labral tears do not presently exist.

Box 24.1 Signs and symptoms of a glenoid labral tear

- Pain with overhead activities.
- Grinding, "popping", or catching in the shoulder joint.
- Pain at night.
- Reduced range of motion in the shoulder.
- Loss of shoulder strength.
- Subjective feeling of shoulder instability.
- Impingement pain with elevation.

Nonsurgical management

As the kinetic chain has a role in the optimal function of the shoulder girdle, it is important to identify suboptimal function of distal components and address these during management. Boyle[19] argued that mobility and stability of each region in the kinetic chain is important for optimum shoulder function. At a more local level there is often a reduction in the range of humeral internal rotation at 90° abduction, termed glenohumeral internal rotation deficit (GIRD)[22] when compared to the contralateral side. This loss of range may be due to tightness of the posterior shoulder capsule or shoulder muscles that may lead to superior translation of the humeral head when the shoulder is abducted and externally rotated. This may lead to strain on the long head of biceps tendon or the labrum, resulting in a SLAP lesion.[44] In this case, it is necessary to improve the endurance capacity of the glenohumeral external rotators both concentrically and eccentrically and obtain a balanced force production between the internal rotators and external rotators, as well as the desired functional length of the internal rotators.

Acromioclavicular joint injuries

Acromioclavicular (AC) joint injuries comprise 3–5% of injuries to the shoulder girdle.[115] They commonly arise because of direct trauma to the superior aspect of the acromion resulting in a vertical shearing force across the joint. The forces may cause disruption to the acromioclavicular or the coracoclavicular ligaments (conoid and/or trapezoid).

Typically, the injuries have been classified according to the degree of displacement of the clavicle with respect to the acromion as described by Rockwood[116] (Table 24.5). Type 6 arises as a result of a traction type injury and is associated with significant brachial plexus and vascular injuries.

More recently, the International Society of Arthroscopy, Knee Surgery and Orthopaedic Sports Medicine (ISAKOS)

Table 24.4 Diagnostic tests for labral tears		
Diagnostic test	**Pathology examined**	**Reference**
Yergason's test	SLAP lesion/labral lesion/long head of biceps pathology/ subacromial impingement	Yergason[138]
Crank test	SLAP/labral tear	Liu et al.[87]
Kim test	Posteroinferior labral tear	Kim et al.[75]
Jerk test	Posteroinferior labral tear	Kim et al.[76]
Pain provocation test	SLAP lesion	Mimori et al.[96]
Passive compression test	SLAP lesion	Kim et al.[77]
Apprehension test	SLAP/labral tear/anterior instability	Rowe and Zarins.[117]
Modified dynamic shear test	Labral tear	Speer et al.[125]
Modified relocation test	Labrum/anterior instability	Hamner et al.[53]
Supine flexion resistance test	Type 2 SLAP	Ebinger et al.[41]
Speed's test	SLAP/labral lesion/biceps pathology/subacromial impingement	Bennett.[14]
Forced shoulder abduction and elbow flexion test	Superior labrum	Nakagawa et al.[101]
O'Brien's test	SLAP/labrum/ACJ	O'Brien et al.[107]
Resisted supination external rotation test (RSERT)	SLAP lesion	Myers et al.[100]
Compression-rotation test	SLAP lesion	Snyder et al.[124]
Anterior slide	SLAP lesion	Kibler.[72]
Biceps load test	SLAP lesion	Kim et al.[74]
Biceps load II	SLAP lesion	Kim et al.[74]
Biceps tension test	SLAP lesion	Snyder et al.[124]
Upper cut test	Long head of biceps	Kibler et al.[73]
Ludington's test	SLAP lesion	Ludington.[89]
Dynamic labral shear	SLAP lesion	Kibler et al.[73]

ACJ, acromioclavicular joint; SLAP, superior labrum anterior to posterior.

have subdivided Rockwood type 3 injury into two subtypes:[13]

- IIIA: Stable
- IIIB: Additional horizontal instability on the axial view

Assessment

Following injury there will be tenderness in the region of the AC joint and the coracoclavicular ligaments. Inspection may reveal the relative inferior displacement of the glenohumeral joint with respect to the clavicle. Asking the patient to place the hand of the involved shoulder on the opposite shoulder may accentuate any posterior instability of the clavicle. Although uncommon, consideration of and assessment for associated neurological injuries is essential as the mechanism of injury may damage the brachial plexus. Associated glenohumeral joint injuries of labral tears, SLAP lesions and rotator cuff injuries have been reported in up to 42% of cases.[6]

Table 24.5 Classification of acromioclavicular joint injuries

Type	Acromioclavicular ligaments	Coracoclavicular ligaments	Radiographic appearance of clavicle	Radiograph
1	Sprain/partial tear	Intact	Normal	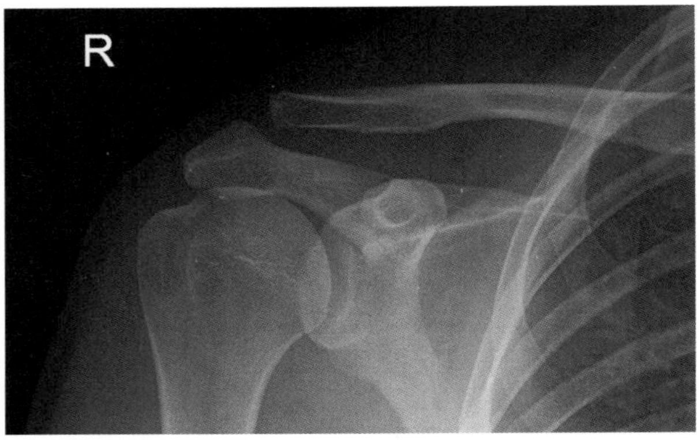
2	Ruptured	Sprain/partial tear	Superior displacement <100%	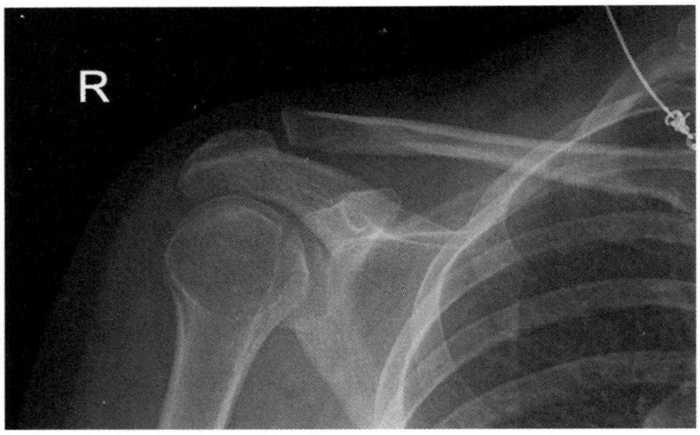
3	Ruptured	Ruptured	Superior displacement 100%	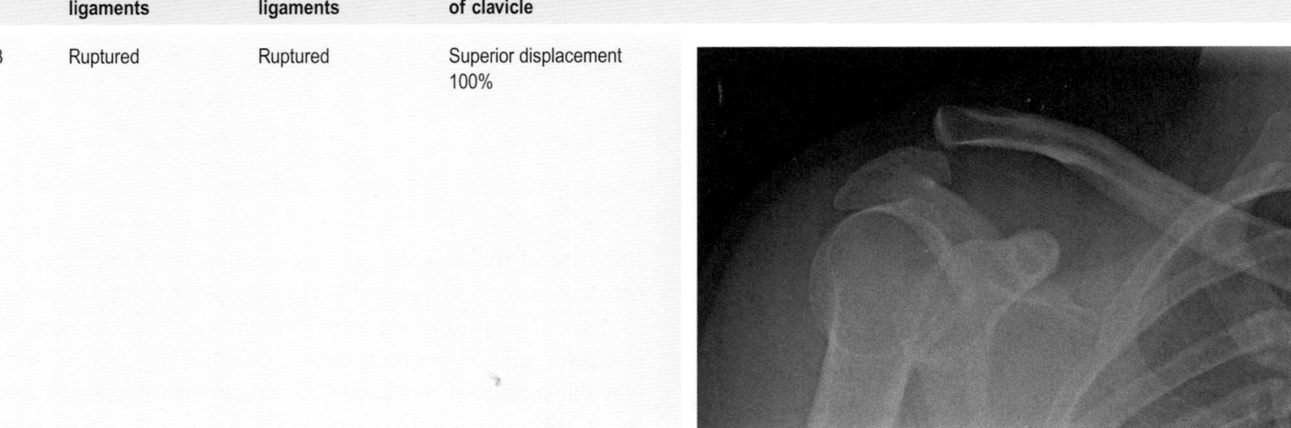

(Continued)

Table 24.5 *(Continued)*

Type	Acromioclavicular ligaments	Coracoclavicular ligaments	Radiographic appearance of clavicle	Radiograph 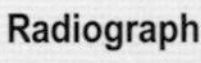
4	Ruptured	Ruptured	Posterior displacement on axial view	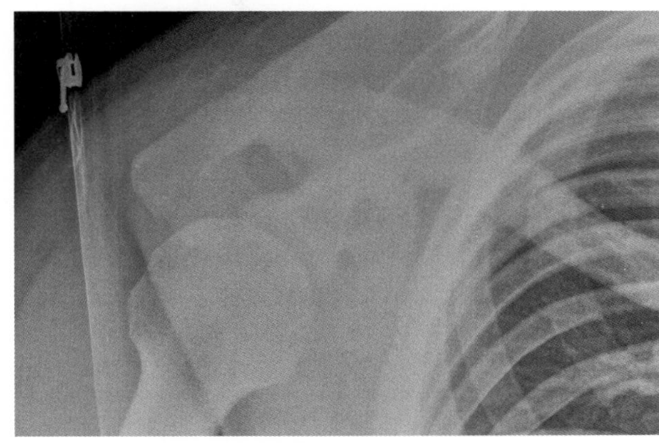
5	Ruptured	Ruptured	Superior displacement 100–300%	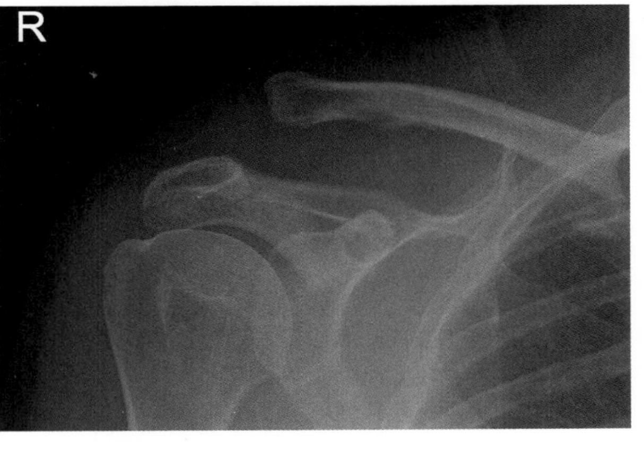
6	Ruptured	Ruptured	Inferior to coracoid	

Investigation

Anterior-posterior and axial radiographs of the AC joint are essential for diagnosis, giving both the relative superior and posterior displacement of the clavicle. Weightbearing films (in which the patient holds a 5 kg weight to accentuate the displacement) and contralateral radiographs (for comparison) are rarely indicated.[18] Further imaging such as ultrasound and magnetic resonance imaging is only required if more complex or associated soft tissue injuries are of concern.

Management

This is based largely on the radiological classification and may be implemented as follows:

- Grades 1 and 2: nonsurgical management; sling for comfort and early mobilization.[12]
- Grade 3: nonsurgical management; sling for comfort and early mobilization unless there are compelling reasons for surgical intervention.[113,118]

- Grade 4: usually surgical management as nonsurgical results are poor.[43]
- Grade 5: usually surgical although there is some evidence for good results with nonsurgical management.[80]
- Grade 6: this injury is very rare and is usually associated with significant trauma with neurovascular injuries, and emergency surgery is usually warranted.[10]

Surgical options

There are multiple surgical options, each with advantages and disadvantages.

Acute injury (less than 3 weeks)

The basic principle is for reduction of the AC joint with stabilization until ligament healing occurs. This may be achieved by suspensory devices (e.g., Tightrope) which may be performed arthroscopically or via open techniques, woven synthetic ligament cerclage (e.g., Surgilig type systems) or by plating (hook plate) with subsequent metalwork removal.

Persistent injury

With ongoing symptoms related to AC joint injury, the options are either to graft the ligaments (using coracoacromial ligament) or a graft (typically hamstring) looped around both coracoid and clavicle supplemented by a temporary device (as for the acute injuries) or a woven synthetic ligament. Regardless of the technique outcomes are generally good.

Sternoclavicular joint injuries

Sternoclavicular joint injuries are rare, comprising 0.9% of all shoulder girdle injuries,[16] and arise typically as a result of a fall on an outstretched hand. Although of uncertain value, the Allman classification[4] is the most widely used and is described as follows:

- Grade 1: sprain.
- Grade2: mild deformity.
- Grade 3: true dislocation, anterior or posterior direction.

In addition, physeal (growth plate) injuries need to be considered as the physis or growth plate, which is the translucent, cartilaginous disc separating the epiphysis from the metaphysis and is responsible for longitudinal growth of long bones, and does not fuse until the age of 25 years.

Assessment

Anterior dislocation is associated with visible anterior deformity and may be fixed or mobile.

Posterior dislocation is associated with brachial plexus injury,[63,66] pneumothorax and respiratory distress,[102] vascular injury, swallowing difficulties (dysphagia), and voice changes (raspy, strained, hoarseness).[97]

Investigation

Plain radiographs often do not identify the pathology and a computed tomography (CT) scan or CT angiogram is required if there is any doubt. MRI has a limited role.

Management

Anterior dislocation

- Grades 1/2: nonsurgical management.
- Grade 3: may be treated by either closed or open reduction techniques.
  - Closed reduction can be attempted but recurrence rates are 21–100%.[42,105]
  - Open reduction requires stabilization.

Acute stabilization

Several options are available including direct suture repair of the ligaments, with or without the use of suture anchors.[85] An alternative is the use of the medial portion of the sternomastoid tendon.[5]

Delayed reconstruction

Reconstruction of the anterior sternoclavicular ligament with the addition of a graft; fascia lata[3] or semitendinosis.[126]

Posterior dislocation

Closed reduction using the "abduction traction" technique with the possible addition of manipulation with a towel clip has been described with an overall 50–67% success rate.[51,82]

Open reduction

The anterior stabilization techniques have also been used for posterior dislocation although thoracic surgery support is advised. The case series are small, but the overall results are reported as good.

Physeal (growth plate) injuries

The medial clavicular physis does not fuse until age 25 years and therefore there should be a high index of suspicion in people under this age involved in trauma. Closed reduction has similar success rates to those for posterior dislocation in adults. Open reduction and stabilization with absorbable sutures has been described with good results.[130]

Nerve injuries to the shoulder

Twenty-six muscles are involved in the stabilization of movement of the scapula, clavicle, and humerus. The muscles can be subgrouped into axioscapular, axiohumeral, scapulohumeral, and others (Table 24.6). The nerve supply to the shoulder muscles is derived from the brachial plexus, which comprises the nerve roots of C5–T1, with the main nerve branches being the suprascapular, axillary, and lateral pectoral nerves.[86]

Nerve injuries around the shoulder occur mainly following motor vehicle accidents or sport, especially in contact

Table 24.6 Shoulder muscle classification and nerve supply

Muscle	Nerve supply	Classification
Trapezius	C2–4 (spinal accessory/cranial XI)	Axioscapular
Sternocleidomastoid	C2–4 (spinal accessory/cranial XI)	Other
Levator scapulae	C3–5 (dorsal scapular)	Axioscapular
Teres minor	C4–5 (axillary)	Scapulohumeral
Supraspinatus	C4–5 (suprascapular)	Scapulohumeral
Rhomboids	C4–5 (dorsal scapular)	Axioscapular
Infraspinatus	C4–6 (suprascapular)	Scapulohumeral
Deltoid	C5–6 (axillary)	Scapulohumeral
Teres major	C5–6 (lower subscapular)	Scapulohumeral
Biceps brachii	C5–6 (musculocutaneous)	Scapulohumeral
Subclavius	C5–6 (subclavian)	Other
Serratus anterior	C5–7 (long thoracic)	Axioscapular
Subscapularis	C5–8 (upper and lower subscapular)	Scapulohumeral
Pectoralis major	C5–T1 (medial and lateral pectoral)	Axiohumeral
Pectoralis minor	C6–C8 (medial pectoral)	Axioscapular
Coracobrachialis	C6–7 (musculocutaneous)	Scapulohumeral
Latissimus dorsi	C6–8 (thoracodorsal)	Axiohumeral

Table 24.7 Summary of commonly presenting nerve injuries around the shoulder

Nerve	Motor dysfunction	Sensory disturbance	Common cause
Suprascapular	Weakness of abduction and external rotation	Has no cutaneous branches. Supplies ACJ and GHJ	• Traction • Direct contusion • Repetitive trauma (ABER)
Axillary	Reduced external rotation strength. Reduced abduction strength May not be able to bend elbow	Loss of sensation over lateral shoulder "regimental badge" area	• Iatrogenic • Shoulder dislocation • Humeral fracture • Direct contusion
Long thoracic	Serratus anterior paralysis causing scapular dyskinesis	Pure motor nerve, no sensory branches	• Iatrogenic • Direct contusion • Traction
Brachial plexus	Inability to move the arm or wrist	No feeling in arm or hand	• Severe shoulder girdle trauma • Gunshot wounds • Penetrating injuries
Brachial plexus "stinger"	Transient weakness of • abduction • external rotation • elbow flexion • elbow extension • pronation • 5th digit abduction	Transient paresthesia in whole arm	• High-energy collision

ACJ, acromioclavicular joint; GHJ, glenohumeral joint.

sports including rugby,[36,106] American football,[28,35] or wrestling.[2,123] The mechanism occurs when extreme force is applied to the superior aspect of the shoulder, such as a fall onto the point of the shoulder, or whiplash-type incident at the cervical spine. Shoulder girdle nerve injuries can be associated with glenohumeral dislocation[71,114] and proximal humeral fractures.[133]

In addition to direct trauma, nerves of the brachial plexus can be injured due to repetitive overhead motion in such sports as volleyball,[62,136] tennis,[26] baseball,[34,94] and swimming,[94] in which the shoulder is repetitively positioned into abduction and external rotation.[20] A summary of the commonly presenting nerve injuries presenting around the shoulder is shown in Table 24.7.

The severity and extent of compression is related to the degree of the nerve injury.[103] There are several grading systems for nerve injury that aim to relate patients' symptoms with the pathophysiological status of the patient's injured nerve. Sunderland's classification stipulates five degrees of nerve injury[128] which correspond with Seddon's[120] more recent three-level classification:

- Neurapraxia (Class 1): experienced as a temporary incident of complete motor paralysis with minimal sensory or autonomic involvement. This is commonly referred to as a "stinger" or "burner" within sport.[91]
- Axonotmesis (Class 2): this is a more severe injury involving loss of continuity of the axon with conservation of the intact nerve sheath. There is complete motor, sensory, and autonomic paralysis, which causes muscle atrophy as time progresses. Recovery is possible and is dependent on the nerve

being decompressed. The time for recovery is dependent on the distance between the denervated muscle and the proximal regenerating axon. It is typically quoted that nerve regeneration occurs at 1.2 mm per day.[111]

- Neurotmesis (Class 3): this is the most serious level of injury, resulting in absolute loss of continuity of both the axon and nerve sheath. Recovery infrequently is incomplete, resulting in functional loss and total anesthesia of the nerve's cutaneous distribution.[40]

References

1. Abrams R, Akbarnia H. Shoulder Dislocations Overview. Treasure Island: StatPearls Publishing; 2020.
2. Afran MR. Nerve injury about the shoulder in athletes, part 2: long thoracic nerve, spinal accessory nerve, burners/stingers, thoracic outlet syndrome. Am J Sports Med. 2004;32(4):1063-76.
3. Allen AW. Living suture grafts in the repair of fractures and dislocations. Arch Surg. 1928;1;16(5):1007–1020.
4. Allman FL Jr. Fractures and ligamentous injuries of the clavicle and its articulation. J Bone Joint Surg Am. 1967;49(4):774-84.
5. Armstrong AL, Dias JJ. Reconstruction for instability of the sternoclavicular joint using the tendon of the sternocleidomastoid muscle. J Bone Joint Surg Br. 2008;90(5):610-3
6. Arrigoni P, Brady PC, Zottarelli L, Barth J, Narbona P, Huberty D, Koo SS, Adams CR, Parten P, Denard PJ, Burkhart SS. Associated lesions requiring additional surgical treatment in grade 3 acromioclavicular joint dislocations. Arthroscopy. 2014;30(1):6-10.
7. Ashworth B, Cohen DD. Force awakens: a new hope for athletic shoulder strength testing. Br J Sports Med. 2019;53(9):524.
8. Aygün Ü, Çalik Y, Işik C, Şahin H, Şahin R, Aygün DÖ. The importance of glenoid version in patients with anterior dislocation of the shoulder. J Shoulder Elbow Surg. 2016;25(12):1930-1936.
9. Badge R, Tambe A, Funk L. Arthroscopic isolated posterior labral repair in rugby players. Int J Shoulder Surg. 2009;3(1):4-7.
10. Balai E, Sabharwal S, Griffiths D, Reilly P. A type VI acromioclavicular joint injury: subcoracoid dislocation in a patient with polytrauma. Ann R Coll Surg Engl. 2020 Nov;102(9):e1-e3.
11. Bateman M, Jaiswal A, Tambe AA. Diagnosis and management of atraumatic shoulder instability. J Arthrosc Jt Surg. 2018;5(2):79-85.
12. Beitzel K, Cote MP, Apostolakos J, Solovyova O, Judson CH, Ziegler CG, Edgar CM, Imhoff AB, Arciero RA, Mazzocca AD. Current concepts in the treatment of acromioclavicular joint dislocations. Arthroscopy. 2013 Feb;29(2):387-97.
13. Beitzel K, Mazzocca AD, Bak K, Itoi E, Kibler WB, Mirzayan R, Imhoff AB, Calvo E, Arce G, Shea K; Upper Extremity Committee of ISAKOS. ISAKOS upper extremity committee consensus statement on the need for diversification of the Rockwood classification for acromioclavicular joint injuries. Arthroscopy. 2014;30(2):271-8.
14. Bennett WF. Specificity of the Speed's test: arthroscopic technique for evaluating the biceps tendon at the level of the bicipital groove. Arthroscopy. 1998;14(8):789-96.
15. Blanch P. Conservative management of shoulder pain in swimming. Phys Ther Sport. 2004;5(3):109-124.
16. Boesmueller S, Wech M, Tiefenboeck TM, Popp D, Bukaty A, Huf W, Fialka C, Greitbauer M, Platzer P. Incidence, characteristics, and long-term follow-up of sternoclavicular injuries: An epidemiologic analysis of 92 cases. J Trauma Acute Care Surg. 2016;80(2):289-95
17. Boileau P, Pennington SD, Ghassan A. Proximal humeral fractures in younger patients: fixation techniques and arthroplasty. J Shoulder Elbow Surg. 2011;20(2 Suppl):S47-60.
18. Bossart PJ, Joyce SM, Manaster BJ, Packer SM. Lack of efficacy of 'weighted' radiographs in diagnosing acute acromioclavicular separation. Ann Emerg Med. 1988;17(1):20-4.
19. Boyle MJ. Functional Training for Sports, 2nd edition. Human Kinetics Publishers; 2016.
20. Brown SA, Doolittle DA, Bohanon CJ, Jayaraj A, Naidu SG, Huettl EA, Renfree KJ, Oderich GS, Bjarnason H, Gloviczki P, Wysokinski WE, McPhail IR. Quadrilateral space syndrome: the Mayo Clinic experience with a new classification system and case series. Mayo Clin Proc. 2015;90(3):382-94.
21. Brownson P, Donaldson O, Fox M, et al. BESS/BOA Patient Care Pathways: Traumatic anterior shoulder instability. Shoulder Elb. 2015;7(3):214-226.
22. Burkhart SS, Morgan CD, Kibler WB. Shoulder injuries in overhead athletes. The "dead arm" revisited. Clin Sports Med. 2000;19(1):125-58.
23. Buss DD, Lynch GP, Meyer CP, Huber SM, Freehill MQ. Nonoperative management for in-season athletes with anterior shoulder instability. Am J Sports Med. 2004;32(6):1430-1433.
24. Calvert E, Chambers GK, Regan W, Hawkins RH, Leith JM. Special physical examination tests for superior labrum anterior posterior shoulder tears are clinically limited and invalid: a diagnostic systematic review. J Clin Epidemiol. 2009 May;62(5):558-63.
25. Chahal J, Leiter J, McKee MD, Whelan DB. Generalized ligamentous laxity as a predisposing factor for primary traumatic anterior shoulder dislocation. J Shoulder Elbow Surg. 2010;19(8):1238-1242.
26. Challoumas D, Dimitrakakis G. Insights into the epidemiology, aetiology and associations of infraspinatus atrophy in overhead athletes: a systematic review. Sports Biomech. 2017;16(3):325-341.
27. Chalmers PN, Slikker W 3rd, Mall NA, Gupta AK, Rahman Z, Enriquez D, Nicholson GP. Reverse total shoulder arthroplasty for acute proximal humeral fracture: comparison to open reduction-internal fixation and hemiarthroplasty. J Shoulder Elbow Surg. 2014;23(2):197-204.
28. Charbonneau RM, McVeigh SA, Thompson K. Brachial neuropraxia in Canadian Atlantic University sport football players: what is the incidence of "stingers"? Clin J Sport Med. 2012;22(6):472-7.
29. Ciccotti MC, Syed U, Hoffman R, Abboud JA, Ciccotti MG, Freedman KB. Return to play criteria following surgical stabilization

for traumatic anterior shoulder instability: a systematic review. Arthrosc J Arthrosc Relat Surg. 2018;34(3):903-913.

30. Clark RC, Chandler CC, Fuqua AC, Glymph KN, Lambert GC, Rigney KJ. Use of clinical test clusters versus advanced imaging studies in the management of patients with a suspected SLAP tear. Int J Sports Phys Ther. 2019;14(3):345-352.

31. Clavert P. Glenoid labrum pathology. Orthop Traumatol Surg Res. 2015;101(1 Suppl):S19-24.

32. Cotter EJ, Hannon CP, Christian D, Frank RM, Bach BR Jr. Comprehensive examination of the athlete's shoulder. Sports Health. 2018;10(4):366-375.

33. Crichton J, Jones DR, Funk L. Mechanisms of traumatic shoulder injury in elite rugby players. Br J Sports Med. 2012;46(7):538-542.

34. Cummins CA, Bowen M, Anderson K, Messer T. Suprascapular nerve entrapment at the spinoglenoid notch in a professional baseball pitcher. Am J Sports Med. 1999;27(6):810-2.

35. Daly CA, Payne SH, Seiler JG. Severe brachial plexus injuries in American football. Orthopedics. 2016;39(6):e1188-e1192.

36. de Beer J, Bhatia DN. Shoulder injuries in rugby players. Int J Shoulder Surg. 2009;3(1):1-3.

37. Dezfuli B, King JJ, Farmer KW, Struk AM, Wright TW. Outcomes of reverse total shoulder arthroplasty as primary versus revision procedure for proximal humerus fractures. J Shoulder Elbow Surg. 2016;25(7):1133–7.

38. Dhir J, Willis M, Watson L, Somerville L, Sadi J.. Evidence-based review of clinical diagnostic tests and predictive clinical tests that evaluate response to conservative rehabilitation for posterior glenohumeral instability: a systematic review. Sports Health. 2018;10(2):141-145.

39. Dinnes J, Loveman E, McIntyre L, Waugh N. The effectiveness of diagnostic tests for the assessment of shoulder pain due to soft tissue disorders: a systematic review. Health Technol Assess. 2003;7(29):iii, 1-166.

40. Ditty BJ ON, Rozelle CJ. Surgery for peripheral nerve trauma. In: Tubbs RS RE, Shoja MM, Loukas M, Barbaro N, Spinner RJ (eds). Nerves and Nerve Injuries. Amsterdam: Elsevier; 2015: 373-81.

41. Ebinger N, Magosch P, Lichtenberg S, Habermeyer P. A new SLAP test: the supine flexion resistance test. Arthroscopy. 2008;24(5):500-5.

42. Eskola A. Sternoclavicular dislocation. A plea for open treatment. Acta Orthop Scand. 1986;57(3):227-8.

43. Feichtinger X, Dahm F, Schallmayer D, Boesmueller S, Fialka C, Mittermayr R. Surgery improves the clinical and radiological outcome in Rockwood type IV dislocations, whereas Rockwood type III dislocations benefit from conservative treatment. Knee Surg Sports Traumatol Arthrosc. 2021;29(7):2143-2151.

44. Fitzpatrick MJ, Tibone JE, Grossman M, McGarry M H, Lee TQ. Development of cadaveric models of a thrower's shoulder. JSES. 2005;14:S49-S57.

45. Foruria AM, De Gracia MM, Larson DR, Munuera L, Sanchez Sotelo J. The pattern of the fracture and displacement of the fragments predict the outcome in proximal humeral fractures. J Bone Joint Surg [Br]. 2005;93-B(3):378-86.

46. Fowler EM, Horsley IG, Rolf CG. Clinical and arthroscopic findings in recreationally active patients. Sports Med Arthrosc Rehabil Ther Technol. 2010;2:2.

47. Funk L. Treatment of glenohumeral instability in rugby players. Knee Surg Sports Traumatol Arthrosc. 2016;24:430-439.

48. Funk L, Snow M. SLAP tears of the glenoid labrum in contact athletes. Clin J Sport Med. 2007;17(1):1-4.

49. Gauci M-O, Deransart P, Chaoui J, et al. Three-dimensional geometry of the normal shoulder: a software analysis. J Shoulder Elbow Surg. 2020;29(12):e468-e477.

50. Godin J, Sekiya JK. Systematic review of rehabilitation versus operative stabilization for the treatment of first-time anterior shoulder dislocations. Sports Health. 2010;2(2):156-65.

51. Groh GI, Wirth MA, Rockwood CA Jr. Treatment of traumatic posterior sternoclavicular dislocations. J Shoulder Elbow Surg. 2011;20(1):107-13.

52. Habermeyer P, Schuller U, Wiedemann E. The intra-articular pressure of the shoulder: an experimental study on the role of the glenoid labrum in stabilizing the joint. Arthroscopy. 1992;8(2):166-72.

53. Hamner DL, Pink MM, Jobe FW. A modification of the relocation test: arthroscopic findings associated with a positive test. J Shoulder Elbow Surg. 2000;9(4):263-7.

54. Handoll HH, Brorson S. Interventions for treating proximal humeral fractures in adults. Cochrane Database Syst Rev. 2015;(11):CD000434.

55. Hata Y, Nakatsuchi Y, Saitoh S, Hosaka M, Uchiyama S. Anatomic study of the glenoid labrum. J Shoulder Elbow Surg. 1992;1(4):207-14.

56. Hegedus EJ, Cook C, Lewis J, Wright A, Park JY. Combining orthopedic special tests to improve diagnosis of shoulder pathology. Phys Ther Sport. 2015;16(2):87-92.

57. Hegedus EJ, Goode AP, Cook CE, et al. Which physical examination tests provide clinicians with the most value when examining the shoulder? Update of a systematic review with meta-analysis of individual tests. Br J Sports Med. 2012;46(14):964-978.

58. Hegedus EJ, Goode A, Campbell S, Morin A, Tamaddoni M, Moorman CT 3rd, Cook C. Physical examination tests of the shoulder: a systematic review with meta-analysis of individual tests. Br J Sports Med. 2008;42(2):80-92; discussion 92.

59. Herrington L, Horsley I, Rolf C. Evaluation of shoulder joint position sense in both asymptomatic and rehabilitated professional rugby players and matched controls. Phys Ther Sport Off J Assoc Chart Physiother Sports Med. 2010;11(1):18-22.

60. Hirschmann MT, Quarz V, Audigé L, Ludin D, Messmer P, Regazzoni P, Gross T. Internal fixation of unstable proximal humerus fractures with an anatomically preshaped interlocking plate: a clinical and radiologic evaluation. J Trauma. 2007;63(6):1314-23.

61. Hodgson S. Proximal humerus fracture rehabilitaiton. Clin Orthop Relat Res. 2006;(442):131-138.

62. Holzgraefe M, Kukowski B, Eggert S. Prevalence of latent and manifest suprascapular neuropathy in high-performance volleyball players. Br J Sports Med. 1994;28(3):177-9.

63. Howard FM, Shafer SJ. Injuries to the clavicle with neurovascular complications. A study of fourteen cases. J Bone Joint Surg Am. 1965;47(7):1335-46.

64. Ialenti MN, Mulvihill JD, Feinstein M, Zhang AL, Feeley BT. Return to play following shoulder stabilization: a systematic review and meta-analysis. Orthop J Sports Med. 2017;5(9):2325967117726055.

65. Jaggi A, Lambert S. Rehabilitation for shoulder instability. Br J Sports Med. 2010;44(5):333-340.

66. Jain S, Monbaliu D, Thompson JF. Thoracic outlet syndrome caused by chronic retrosternal dislocation of the clavicle. Successful treatment by transaxillary resection of the first rib. J Bone Joint Surg Br. 2002;84(1):116-8.

67. Javed S, Gheorghiu D, Torrance E, Monga P, Funk L, Walton M. The incidence of traumatic posterior and combined labral tears in patients undergoing arthroscopic shoulder stabilization. Am J Sports Med. 2019;47(11):2686-2690.

68. Jost B, Zumstein M, Pfirrmann CW, Zanetti M, Gerber C. MRI findings in throwing shoulders: abnormalities in professional handball players. Clin Orthop Relat Res. 2005;(434):130-7.

69. Kammel KR, El Bitar Y, Leber EH. Posterior Shoulder Dislocations. StatPearls. Treasure Island: StatPearls Publishing; 2020.

70. Kavaja L, Lähdeoja T, Malmivaara A, Paavola M. Treatment after traumatic shoulder dislocation: a systematic review with a network meta-analysis. Br J Sports Med. 2018;52(23):1498-1506.

71. Kessler KJ, Uribe JW.Complete isolated axillary nerve palsy in college and professional football players: a report of six cases. Clin J Sports Med. 1994;4:272-274.

72. Kibler WB. Specificity and sensitivity of the anterior slide test in throwing athletes with superior glenoid labral tears. Arthroscopy. 1995;11(3):296-300.

73. Kibler W, Sciascia AD, Hester P, Dome D, Jacobs C. Clinical utility of traditional and new tests in the diagnosis of biceps tendon injuries and superior labrum anterior and posterior lesions in the shoulder. Am J Sports Med. 2009;37(9):1840-1847.

74. Kim SH, Ha KI, Ahn JH, Kim SH, Choi HJ. Biceps load test II: A clinical test for SLAP lesions of the shoulder. Arthroscopy. 2001;17(2):160-4.

75. Kim SH, Park JS, Jeong WK, Shin SK. The Kim test: a novel test for posteroinferior labral lesion of the shoulder: a comparison to the jerk test. Am J Sports Med. 2005;33(8):1188-92.

76. Kim SH, Park JC, Park JS, Oh I. Painful jerk test: a predictor of success in nonoperative treatment of posteroinferior instability of the shoulder. Am J Sports Med. 2004;32(8):1849-55.

77. Kim YS, Kim JM, Ha KY, Choy S, Joo MW, Chung YG. The passive compression test: a new clinical test for superior labral tears of the shoulder. Am J Sports Med. 2007;35(9):1489-94.

78. Klug A, Wincheringer D, Harth J, Schmidt-Horlohé K, Hoffmann R, Gramlich Y. Complications after surgical treatment of proximal humerus fractures in the elderly: an analysis of complication patterns and risk factors for reverse shoulder arthroplasty and angular-stable plating. J Shoulder Elbow Surg. 2019;28(9):1674-1684.

79. Kraeutler MJ, Currie DW, Kerr ZY, Roos KG, McCarty EC, Comstock RD. Epidemiology of shoulder dislocations in high school and collegiate athletics in the United States: 2004/2005 through 2013/2014. Sports Health. 2018;10(1):85-91.

80. Krul KP, Cook JB, Ku J, Cage JM, Bottoni CR, Tokish JM. Successful conservative therapy in Rockwood type V acromioclavicular dislocations. Orthop J Sports Med. March 2015. doi:10.1177/2325967115S00017.

81. Labriola JE, Lee TQ, Debski RE, McMahon PJ. Stability and instability of the glenohumeral joint: the role of shoulder muscles. J Shoulder Elbow Surg. 2005;14(1):S32-S38.

82. Laffosse JM, Espié A, Bonnevialle N, Mansat P, Tricoire JL, Bonnevialle P, Chiron P, Puget J. Posterior dislocation of the sternoclavicular joint and epiphyseal disruption of the medial clavicle with posterior displacement in sports participants. J Bone Joint Surg Br. 2010;92(1):103-9.

83. Lee JH, Park JS, Jeong WK. Which muscle performance can be improved after arthroscopic Bankart repair? J Shoulder Elbow Surg. 2020;29(8):1681-1688.

84. Lefevre-Colau MM, Babinet A, Fayad F, et al. Immediate mobilization compared with conventional immobilization for the impacted nonoperatively treated proximal humeral fracture: a randomized controlled trial. J Bone Joint Surg Am. 2007;89:2582-2590.

85. Lehmann W, Laskowski J, Grossterlinden L, Rueger JM. Refixation der sternoklavikulären Luxation mit einem Fadenankersystem [Refixation of sternoclavicular luxation with a suture anchor system]. Unfallchirurg. 2010;113(5):418-21.

86. Leinberry CF, Wehbé MA. Brachial plexus anatomy. Hand Clin. 2004;20(1):1-5.

87. Liu SH, Henry MH, Nuccion SL. A prospective evaluation of a new physical examination in predicting glenoid labral tears. Am J Sports Med. 1996;24(6):721-5.

88. Longo UG, Loppini M, Rizzello G, Ciuffreda M, Maffulli N, Denaro V. Management of primary acute anterior shoulder dislocation: systematic review and quantitative synthesis of the literature. Arthrosc J Arthrosc Relat Surg. 2014;30(4):506-522.

89. Ludington NA. Rupture of the long head of the biceps flexor cubiti muscle. Ann Surg. 1923;77(3):358-63.

90. Maffet MW, Gartsman GM, Moseley B. Superior labrum-biceps tendon complex lesions of the shoulder. Am J Sports Med. 1995;23(1):93-8.

91. Markey KL, Di Benedetto M, Curl WW. Upper trunk brachial plexopathy. The stinger syndrome. Am J Sports Med. 1993;21(5):650-5.

92. Mattern O, Funk L, Walton MJ. Anterior shoulder instability in collision and contact athletes. J Arthrosc Jt Surg. 2018;5(2):99-106.

93. Matthews PA, Scott M. Altering scapular position reduces isometric shoulder strength. Shoulder & Elbow. 2013;5: 266-270.

94. McClelland D, Hoy G. A case of quadrilateral space syndrome with involvement of the long head of the triceps. Am J Sports Med. 2008;36(8):1615-7.

95. Meixner C, Loder RT. The demographics of fractures and dislocations across the entire United States due to common sports and recreational activities. Sports Health. 2020;12(2):159-169.

96. Mimori K, Muneta T, Nakagawa T, Shinomiya K. A new pain provocation test for superior labral tears of the shoulder. Am J Sports Med. 1999;27(2):137-42.

97. Mirza AH, Alam K, Ali A. Posterior sternoclavicular dislocation in a rugby player as a cause of silent vascular compromise: a case report. Br J Sports Med. 2005;39(5):e28.

98. Mora MV, Ibán MÁR, Heredia JD, Gutiérrez-Gómez JC, Diaz RR, Aramberri M, Cobiella C. Physical exam and evaluation of the unstable shoulder. The Open Orthopaedics Journal. 2017;11:946-956.

99. Moroder P, Danzinger V, Maziak N, et al. Characteristics of functional shoulder instability. J Shoulder Elbow Surg. 2020;29(1):68-78.

100. Myers TH, Zemanovic JR, Andrews JR. The resisted supination external rotation test: a new test for the diagnosis of superior labral anterior posterior lesions. Am J Sports Med. 2005;33(9):1315-20.

101. Nakagawa S, Yoneda M, Hayashida K, Obata M, Fukushima S, Miyazaki Y. Forced shoulder abduction and elbow flexion test: a new simple clinical test to detect superior labral injury in the throwing shoulder. Arthroscopy. 2005;21(11):1290-5.

102. Nakayama E, Tanaka T, Noguchi T, Yasuda J, Terada Y. Tracheal stenosis caused by retrosternal dislocation of the right clavicle. Ann Thorac Surg. 2007;83(2):685-7.

103. Neal S, Fields KB. Peripheral nerve entrapment and injury in the upper extremity. Am Fam Physician. 2010;81(2):147-55.

104. Neer C. Displaced proximal humerus fractures. J Bone Joint Surg. 1970;52-A(6):1077-1089.

105. Nettles JL, Linscheid RL. Sternoclavicular dislocations. J Trauma. 1968;8(2):158-64.

106. Nicol A, Pollock A, Kirkwood G, Parekh N, Robson J. Rugby union injuries in Scottish schools. J Public Health (Oxf). 2011;33(2):256-61.

107. O'Brien SJ, Pagnani MJ, Fealy S, McGlynn SR, Wilson JB. The active compression test: a new and effective test for diagnosing labral tears and acromioclavicular joint abnormality. Am J Sports Med. 1998;26(5):610-3.

108. Oh JH, Kim JY, Kim WS, Gong HS, Lee JH. The evaluation of various physical examinations for the diagnosis of type II superior labrum anterior and posterior lesion. Am J Sports Med. 2008;36(2):353-9.

109. Olds M, Ellis R, Donaldson K, Parmar P, Kersten P. Risk factors which predispose first-time traumatic anterior shoulder dislocations to recurrent instability in adults: a systematic review and meta-analysis. Br J Sports Med. 2015;49(14):913-922.

110. Owens BD, Campbell SE, Cameron KL. Risk factors for anterior glenohumeral instability. Am J Sports Med. 2014;42(11):2591-2596.

111. Pfister BJ, Gordon T, Loverde JR, Kochar AS, Mackinnon SE, Cullen DK. Biomedical engineering strategies for peripheral nerve repair: surgical applications, state of the art, and future challenges. Crit Rev Biomed Eng. 2011;39(2):81-124.

112. Rangan A, Handoll H, Brealey S, Jefferson L, Keding A, Martin BC, et al. Surgical vs nonsurgical treatment of adults with displaced fractures of the proximal humerus the PROFHER randomized clinical trial. JAMA. 2015;313(10):1037-47.

113. Rawes ML, Dias JJ. Long-term results of conservative treatment for acromioclavicular dislocation. J Bone Joint Surg Br. 1996;78(3):410-2.

114. Robinson CM, Shur N, Sharpe T, Ray A, Murray IR. Injuries associated with traumatic anterior glenohumeral dislocations. J Bone Joint Surg Am. 2012;94(1):18-26.

115. Rockwood Jr CA, Matsen FA (eds). The Shoulder, 2nd edition. Philadelphia: WB Saunders; 1998.

116. Rockwood Jr CA, Young DC. Disorders of the acromioclavicular joint. In: Rockwood Jr CA, Matsen FA (eds). The Shoulder. Philadelphia: WB Saunders; 1990.

117. Rowe CR, Zarins B. Recurrent transient subluxation of the shoulder. J Bone Joint Surg. 1981;63(6):863-72.

118. Schlegel TF, Burks RT, Marcus RL, Dunn HK. A prospective evaluation of untreated acute grade III acromioclavicular separations. Am J Sports Med. 2001;29(6):699-703.

119. Schwartzberg R, Reuss BL, Burkhart BG, Butterfield M, Wu JY, McLean KW. High prevalence of superior labral tears diagnosed by MRI in middle-aged patients with asymptomatic shoulders. Orthop J Sports Med. 2016;4(1):2325967115623212.

120. Seddon HJ. Three types of nerve injuries. Brain. 1943;66:237.

121. Seminati E, Cazzola D, Preatoni E, Trewartha G. Specific tackling situations affect the biomechanical demands experienced by rugby union players. Sports Biomech. 2017;16(1):58-75.

122. Skou ST, Juhl CB, Hare KB, Lohmander LS, Roos EM. Surgical or non-surgical treatment of traumatic skeletal fractures in adults: systematic review and meta-analysis of benefits and harms. Systematic Reviews. 2020; 9:(179):1-17.

123. Snook GA. A survey of wrestling injuries. Am J Sports Med. 1980;8:450-3.

124. Snyder SJ, Karzel RP, Del Pizzo W, Ferkel RD, Friedman MJ. SLAP lesions of the shoulder. Arthroscopy. 1990;6(4):274-9.

125. Speer KP, Hannafin JA, Altchek DW, Warren RF. An evaluation of the shoulder relocation test. Am J Sports Med. 1994;22(2):177-83.

126. Spencer EE Jr, Kuhn JE. Biomechanical analysis of reconstructions for sternoclavicular joint instability. J Bone Joint Surg Am. 2004;86(1):98-105.

127. Spross C, Meester J, Mazzucchelli RA, Puskás GJ, Zdravkovic V, Jost B. Evidence-based algorithm to treat patients with proximal humerus fractures-a prospective study with early clinical and overall performance results. J Shoulder Elbow Surg. 2019;28(6):1022-1032.

128. Sunderland S. A classification of peripheral nerve injuries producing loss of function. Brain. 1951;74(4):491-516.

129. Taylor SA, Newman AM, Dawson C, et al. The "3-Pack" examination is critical for comprehensive evaluation of the biceps-labrum complex and the bicipital tunnel: a prospective study. Arthroscopy. 2017;33(1):28-38.

130. Tennent TD, Pearse EO, Eastwood DM. A new technique for stabilizing adolescent posteriorly displaced physeal medial clavicular fractures. J Shoulder Elbow Surg. 2012;21(12):1734-9.

131. Tokish JM, Kuhn JE, Ayers GD, et al. Decision making in treatment after a first-time anterior glenohumeral dislocation: A Delphi approach by the Neer Circle of the American Shoulder and Elbow Surgeons. Journal of Shoulder and Elbow Surgery. 2020;29(12):2429-2445.

132. Torchia MT, Austin DC, Cozzolino N, Jacobowitz L, Bell JE. Acute versus delayed reverse total shoulder arthroplasty for the treatment of proximal humeral fractures in the elderly population: a systematic review and meta-analysis. J Shoulder Elbow Surg. 2019;28(4):765-773.

133. Visser CP, Coene LN, Brand R, Tavy DL. Nerve lesions in proximal humeral fractures. J Shoulder Elbow Surg. 2001;10(5):421-7.

134. Wasserstein DN, Sheth U, Colbenson K, et al. The true recurrence rate and factors predicting recurrent instability after nonsurgical management of traumatic primary anterior shoulder dislocation: a systematic review. Arthroscopy. 2016;32(12):2616-2625.

135. Wilk KE, Reinold MM, Dugas JR, Arrigo CA, Moser MW, Andrews JR. Current concepts in the recognition and treatment of superior labral (SLAP) lesions. J Orthop Sports Phys Ther. 2005;35(5):273-91.

136. Witvrouw E, Cools A, Lysens R, Cambier D, Vanderstraeten G, Victor J, Sneyers C, Walravens M. Suprascapular neuropathy in volleyball players. Br J Sports Med. 2000;34(3):174-80.

137. Yahuaca BI, Simon P, Christmas KN, Patel S, Gorman RA, Mighell MA, Frankle MA. Acute surgical management of proximal humerus fractures: ORIF vs. hemiarthroplasty vs. reverse shoulder arthroplasty. J Shoulder Elbow Surg. 2020;29(7S):S32-S40.

138. Yergason J. Supination sign. J Bone Joint Surg. 1931;13:160-165.

139. Kardouni JR, McKinnon CJ, Seitz AL. Incidence of shoulder dislocations and the rate of recurrent instability in soldiers. Medicine and Science in Sports and Exercise. 2016;48(11):2150-2156.

The pediatric and adolescent shoulder 25

Mitchell Simpson, Keren Lewis, Maya Lewis, Rhiannon Joslin

Introduction

Shoulder problems are common in children and cover a wide range of etiologies including birth trauma, neoplasm, genetic and endocrine disorders, fractured growth plates, shoulder instability, and overuse injuries. Due to a child's vulnerability, nonaccidental injuries must also be considered in this population.

From the early neonatal period until late adolescence, the types of shoulder injuries differ greatly, making the approach and management of these conditions complex. This chapter aims to describe normal shoulder development throughout childhood and provide a framework to approach pediatric and adolescent shoulder injuries. The more common shoulder presentations will also be outlined, including diagnosis and basic management strategies.

Epidemiology

Traumatic shoulder injuries are commonly seen within accident and emergency departments. Fractures dominate shoulder injuries in children up to the age of 10 years old, with a similar incidence in both sexes.[24] Eighty-two percent of fractures in pediatrics involve the upper limb, with the clavicle and distal humerus frequently affected.[56,99] In younger children (0–2 years), the main cause of a fracture is falling off a bed or out of a cot.[113] In adolescence, fractures involving the shoulder occur most commonly during sport, with higher incidence (79%) in males.[21] Young males playing contact sports are also most at risk of traumatic dislocations of the shoulder,[106] an injury associated with high rates of ongoing instability in this age group.[27,87] Young females most commonly report acute soft tissue injuries of the shoulder in early adolescence (10–14 years).[24]

Nontraumatic shoulder pain is generally managed in primary care by the family doctor (primary care physician). Most pediatric patients presenting to primary care with musculoskeletal problems do so with conditions affecting their lower limb or spine. Problems involving the shoulder are the 12th most common musculoskeletal reason for a consultation.[118] Around 1–2% of children and adolescents present to tertiary multidisciplinary clinics with severe and disabling chronic pain.[15] These young people are more likely to be female adolescents[50] and again, the pain location is primarily the lower limb, with only 15% of children diagnosed with conditions having upper limb involvement such as complex regional pain syndrome.[68]

Normal shoulder development

During the fourth week of embryonic development limb buds start to develop.[29,74] During week five (Carnegie stage 15), the peripheral nerves grow from the brachial plexus into the mesenchyme of the upper limb bud, stimulating the development of the upper limb musculature. The humerus and scapula begin to chondrify at this time and the clavicle starts to ossify.[29] During the seventh week, the upper and lower limbs rotate in opposite directions, with the upper limbs rotating laterally, so that the elbow faces posteriorly. The shoulder joint is now well formed. Medial torsion of the humerus, important for forearm position and hand function, occurs during the second month. As the scapula moves from a lateral orientation to a more posterior position on the back of the rib cage, the torsion of the head of the humerus increases. It occurs to correspond with the more lateral orientation of the glenoid cavity. At this stage, the musculature of the upper limb is well defined; the shoulder joint has the adult form and the glenohumeral ligaments are visible.[74] The fibrous capsule of the glenohumeral joint and the glenoid labrum are observable from week seven (Carnegie stage 19).[40] In week 8 (Carnegie stages 20–23), rotator cuff tendons form and reinforce the capsule, and the long head of biceps tendon appears with the transverse humeral and coracohumeral ligaments.[40]

The fetal period commences from the end of the eighth week of intrauterine life and continues until term. Between weeks 12 to 16 there is rapid ossification of the skeletal elements, with the tendons, ligaments, epiphyses, and joint capsule around the shoulder penetrated by a rich vascular network. The subdeltoid, subcoracoid, and subscapularis bursae also develop during this period.[29] During fetal development, all the shoulder ligaments and the capsule become increasingly more fibrous. The rotator cuff muscles, present at the beginning of the fetal period, increase in size until term. The glenoid labrum, although present in the embryological period, develops markedly during the fetal period and is densely fibrous at term.[29]

Pediatric and adolescent shoulder development

The chronology of typical skeletal shoulder development follows a predictable course. The clavicle is both the first bone to ossify, around the fifth to seventh weeks in utero,[59] and the last bone to fully unite, around the 22nd to 25th year of life.[59] Ossification starts from one primary center in the body, appearing at eight weeks in utero, and from seven secondary centers: coracoid process (two centers, 12–18 months), glenoid (10–11 years), inferior angle, acromion (three centers) and medial border (all 14–20 years). The diaphysis of the proximal humerus appears at eight weeks in utero, the humeral head (1–6 months), greater tubercle (one year), and lesser tubercle (3–5 years).[59]

Variations in shoulder development may occur during maturation. A lack of descent of the scapula during embryological development results in Sprengel's deformity. The condition is associated with congenital elevation of the scapula and a detrimental impact on shoulder function. This rare congenital abnormality may be associated with scoliosis, torticollis, facial asymmetry, and Klippel-Feil syndrome. It is classified into four grades, depending on the extent of scapula elevation.[49]

Glenoid dysplasia (hypoplasia) is another developmental variation and involves bony deficiency of the postero-inferior glenoid and the adjacent scapular neck. Although often asymptomatic or mildly symptomatic in the pediatric population, it may be associated with symptoms in middle age or the elderly, including restricted shoulder range of motion, osteoarthritis, shoulder pain, and although rare, posterior glenoid instability.[4,5,7]

Infants with congenital pseudoarthrosis of the clavicle present with a clavicular protuberance, which usually becomes more prominent as the child develops. It is associated with no or minimal symptoms. It is a rare condition that occurs due to failure of fusion of the medial and lateral ossification centers of the clavicle. It mainly affects the lateral aspect of the right clavicle and has a female preponderance. It may be associated with scapular dyskinesis. Surgery is indicated if symptomatic.[18]

Assessment of a child with a musculoskeletal problem involving the shoulder

What are the differences between assessing a child and an adult?

Children are not little adults, and the pediatric assessment needs to be tailored accordingly. Children are continually developing physically, socially, and psychologically and it is important to reflect a child's age and developmental stage in the assessment. Developmental milestones (gross motor, fine motor, social, emotional, cognitive, language) become a major focus of assessment, with pediatric health professionals required to identify delays or regressions in a child's development.

Physically, the changes that occur within a child's musculoskeletal system through growth and puberty make this a susceptible period for injury. Additionally, the development of skeletal maturity brings a different range of musculoskeletal pathologies. Socially, there are huge changes that occur in childhood such as starting school, gaining independence, and establishing relationships. A protracted shoulder problem may stop a child from raising a hand in class to ask a question, they may not be able to participate in activities in school, such as art, music lessons, or sports, or take part in out of school activities or a valued hobby. At a sensitive age, these changes may affect how a young person interacts with the people around them and may detrimentally impact on their level of physical and emotional health. It is the duty of the clinician to remain cognizant of these issues and address them sensitively.

Adult patients choose to come to their hospital appointments, they can communicate their needs and wishes and have an expectation of what is required of them. Children are brought to appointments by their parents or carers, and it may be the first time they have encountered a health professional. It is vital to elicit and hear the child's voice by finding that personal connection. Healthcare professionals also have a duty of care to keep children safe. They need to be aware of common signs of nonaccidental injury such as incongruence of history or bruising in a nonambulant child, and escalate any safeguarding concerns. While the voice of the child must be heard, parents are not just observers – they offer a unique perspective of their child's presentation. When considering red flags for malignancy, infection, and inflammatory disease, parents can identify and report changes in their child's behavior that may indicate systemic illness, such as being more irritable, lethargic, or quiet. It is therefore essential to involve parents, listen to their story, and explain to parents as well as the child what is happening and why.

The interview

A large proportion of pediatric interviews will be conducted with someone other than the patient – typically the parents. As the child matures, and is old enough to contribute, it is best to direct questions to them. In adolescents, it may be appropriate to have parents leave the room during the interview. Discussing and maintaining an adolescent's confidentiality is important, as is the need to explain circumstances in which confidentiality may be broken. Traumatic and nontraumatic shoulder injuries may sometimes masquerade underlying social issues such as risk-taking behaviors, abuse, self-harm, and other reasons for distress.

Communicating with children and their parents is complicated and the topics discussed in Chapter 11 are relevant during the entirety of the clinician–child–parent interaction. Clinicians will need to address the history of the presenting complaint, and as discussed in Chapter 11, be mindful of language, and may need to use different skill sets when communicating with the child and the parents.

Antenatal/birth history

In most circumstances, especially when assessing newborns, a targeted antenatal or birth history is essential. This is particularly true for conditions that present soon after birth or in early childhood such as brachial plexus injuries, clavicle and humeral fractures, and neurodevelopmental disorders.

Box 25.1 details some key points to ascertain on maternal, antenatal, and birth history relevant to the shoulder.[30,31,39,70,95,116]

Box 25.1 Key points to ascertain on maternal, antenatal, and birth history relevant to the shoulder

- Maternal medical conditions: diabetes,[S] advanced maternal age (> 40 years),[S] alcohol or smoking during pregnancy.[N]
- Previous obstetric complications: history of shoulder dystocia.[S]
- Antenatal scans (morphology and growth): normal limb development, intrauterine growth restriction (IUGR) +/- head sparing.[N]
- Antenatal serology: TORCH screening (*T*oxoplasmosis; *O*ther – syphilis, parvovirus, hepatitis B; *R*ubella; *C*MV; *H*erpesviridae).[N]
- Antenatal testing: chorionic villus sampling (CVS), amniocentesis, non-invasive prenatal test (NIPT) (predisposed genetic/neurodevelopmental conditions).[N]
- Antenatal issues: antepartum hemorrhage or placental abruption (hypoxic insult to the fetal brain).[N]
- Birth gestation: premature[N] vs. term.
- Delivery method: vaginal delivery vs. elective/emergency cesarian section +/- instrumental.[S]
- Delivering part: cephalic vs. breech.
- Delivery complications: difficult extraction[S] (shoulder dystocia +/- need for cleidotomy), neonatal resuscitation.[N]
- Birth weight: macrosomic.[S]
- Associated neonatal intensive care unit/special care nursery stay.

[N]Risk of neurodevelopmental issues.

[S]Risk of shoulder dystocia and associated brachial plexus injuries.

Current history

Interviewing children is a challenge, not only in developing rapport with the child or adolescent, but also with the parents. A structured approach is important to ensure all relevant questions are asked; however, the interviewer must be flexible to tailor the questions and phrasing to match the child and responses. Recommendations made in Chapter 11 are relevant both for the child and the parent.

An approach to the interview for a child presenting with a shoulder problem is outlined below:

1. History of presenting complaint
    - Symptoms: pain, weakness, altered sensation, immobility.
    - Location/radiation.
    - Timeline: when it first started, how it has changed over time.
    - Aggravating and easing factors.
    - Associated features: numbness, tingling, clicking, weakness, other joint pain, rashes.
    - Loss of function: ability/inability to perform day to day activities.
2. Red flags
    - Fevers/sweats.
    - Increased lethargy.
    - Bruises/nonaccidental injury.
    - Bone pain.
    - History of serious illness (e.g., cancer).
3. Past medical history
    - Previous shoulder injuries: dislocations, fractures, overuse injuries.
    - Medical diagnoses: cancer, connective tissue disorders, neurodevelopmental disorders.
    - Hospital admissions: major trauma, relevant shoulder/joint issues.
    - Medications: drug type, dose, frequency.
4. Family history
    - Rheumatological conditions, connective tissue disorders.
    - Parental chronic pain.[14]
    - Relevant genetic conditions.
5. Developmental history
    - Milestones: fine and gross motor.[122]
    - Hand dominance.
6. Psychosocial history
    - Where the child lives and with whom.
    - Nursery/school/hobbies.
    - Sport/exercise.
    - HEEADSSS screen.[43,117]
    - Smoking/recreational drugs (parents, visitors, and child).
7. Other pediatric questions
    - Immunizations.
    - Allergies: drug, food, asthma, eczema, hayfever.
    - Diet.
    - Sleep.
    - Bowels/bladder.
    - Height/weight.

It is important to conclude the interview by summarizing the key pieces of information and ensuring that you and the family have a shared understanding of the main issues. Ask the family if they have any further questions or concerns before moving on to the physical examination.

Physical examination

The same components of a shoulder physical examination are involved in children and adults; however, young children may not offer the same willingness to follow instructions. Assessment measures such as the pediatric Gait Arms Legs and Spine (pGALs) offer a quick and evidence-based assessment to detect abnormal joints in school-aged children and young people.[26] In younger children, routine assessments can be more challenging. To engage young children, prepare the space with age-appropriate toys and allow free play when asking their parent questions. Constantly observe the child's movements, behaviors, and upper limb function and monitor for verbal and nonverbal indications of pain. When assessing active ranges of motion, use the play equipment and encourage reaching in different directions. To assess active and passive shoulder and other joint movements, coordination, muscle tone, and the kinetic chain, songs and rhymes that involve culturally and age-appropriate play such as "how big is…", "old MacDonald had a farm", or "row-row-row-your-boat" should be considered.

When assessing strength, asking a child to push you away and pretend they are so strong that you stumble will make the assessment entertaining and often children will want to do it again allowing repetition in different positions and directions. Consider asking the parent to participate in the assessment or perform the assessment first with the parent to reduce the child's anxiety. Use stickers and certificates as rewards when appropriate, as well as getting the favorite teddy "to help". The physical assessment is likely to include a review of other systems: e.g., neurological, vascular, respiratory. When assessing younger children, the clinician will need to be creative to appropriately examine the system(s) of interest – for example, "assess" the teddy or parent first.

Investigations

Investigating shoulder pathologies in children should be done in a manner that aims to prevent the child's exposure to any unnecessary, distressing, invasive, and potentially harmful tests. Depending on the pathology, variable investigations may be useful. These may include blood tests (either routine or specialized), radiological imaging, joint fluid aspiration, bone biopsies, and tests to assess neurological and neuromuscular function.

In children with suspected septic arthritis of the shoulder, blood tests identifying raised inflammatory markers such as white cell count, neutrophils, c-reactive protein, and erythrocyte sedimentation rate (ESR) are monitored. Peripheral blood cultures and joint aspirates are also often taken prior to starting systemic antibiotics to help determine a causative organism and rationalize antibiotic used.

Imaging includes, but is not limited to, radiographs, magnetic resonance imaging, ultrasound scans and computer tomography. In the pediatric population, imaging modalities that emit radiation should be limited where possible, to avoid the potentially damaging effects that these may have on radiosensitive developing structures.[25] However, the use of radiological imaging is useful in not only confirming a diagnosis, but to also permit classification. The use of X-ray imaging to investigate proximal humeral fractures is one such example of this. Both the Neer and Horwitz and the Salter-Harris classifications can be used in distinguishing between pediatric proximal humeral fracture subtypes.

These classification systems, which are based on radiological findings, provide an insight into the type of injury involved, and inform management algorithms.[60] Table 25.1 details the Neer and Horwitz classification for proximal humeral fractures.[80] Table 25.2 details the Salter-Harris classification for proximal humeral fractures and relates to the degree of physeal plate involvement.[105]

Table 25.1 Neer and Horwitz[80] classification for proximal humeral fractures

Type I	Minimally displaced (<5 mm)
Type II	Displaced <1/3 of shaft width
Type III	Displaced >1/3 and <2/3 of shaft width
Type IV	Displaced >2/3 of shaft width

Table 25.2 Salter-Harris[105] classification for proximal humeral fractures

Type I	Fracture through physis, causing separation of physis
Type II	Fracture goes through lateral aspect of physis and extends into the metaphysis
Type III	Fracture goes through the physis and epiphysis
Type IV	Fracture extends into metaphysis, physis, and epiphysis
Type V	Crush injury to physis

More specialized investigations, such as those that test the neurological and neuromuscular function, can be useful when investigating the presence and severity of brachial plexopathies.[88]

Principals of management

The management of pediatric shoulder injuries differs with presentation, pathology, and age. In general, children heal very well, with noninvasive management being preferred. Basic principles for shoulder management in the pediatric population are outlined below and discuss the importance of tailoring treatment for the individual.

Child development from the neonatal period to adulthood is a continuum that represents a transition to independence from parents/family. Knowing where a child is on the continuum is an important factor when managing their shoulder problem. For example, when considering pain relief following a clavicle fracture, a neonate is solely reliant on a parent to be observant of pain behavior and administer analgesics. A child can verbalize pain but the decision to give analgesics remains with the parent. In contrast, an older adolescent starts to make their own decisions on how they want to respond to pain, and despite their parents' suggestions may choose not to take analgesics, perceiving that they do not require them or preferring not to take tablets. Healthcare professionals have to sensitively facilitate children and adolescents to manage their own health, in their own time, tailoring management to their developmental stage as well as the pathology.

A clear explanation of the diagnosis and treatment plan is pivotal. The child or adolescent requires more than a diagnostic name to make sense of their symptoms. If they can understand why they feel pain, or have symptoms such as instability, then the treatment has meaning and they may visualize their recovery. Diagnostic uncertainty and unclear explanations of the health problem leads to confusion for both parent and child.[81,93,119] Diagnostic uncertainty may originate from mixed messages from medical professionals surrounding the injury, disease, or investigation findings or when a diagnosis is provided that does not fit the expectations or beliefs of the child and their family. However, if a diagnosis is accepted, parent narratives were found to have a more positive affect and show resilience.[82] It is therefore important to understand what the child and parent believe and understand about the shoulder problem, and address any concerns they may have regarding the cause of symptoms.

It is important that all treatment plans are tailored to the individual child and family.[123] The need for repeated hospital appointments are burdensome for families, while repetitive exercises may lead to child and parental boredom, adherence problems, and family conflict. Treatment plans that involve activities instead of exercises are more likely to be accepted, especially when incorporated into existing family life, school routines, or within social activities.[123] When a traumatic fracture has healed after immobilization, a child rarely requires formal rehabilitation, and instead could be encouraged to return to playing games and participating in valued hobbies, sports, and recreational activities. Activities such as swimming, flying kites, surfing, throwing frisbees, take the emphasis away from their injury and facilitates a return to normal life.

Children diagnosed with atraumatic or traumatic shoulder instability are more likely to require a formal nonsurgical rehabilitative program. This too needs to be meaningful. The child or adolescent needs to see how exercises link to activities they believe are important. An exercise that links to an overarm throw is going to create meaning for a cricketer or basketball player, whereas an exercise that works on stability in weightbearing will be meaningful to a gymnast. Without such purpose, exercises become onerous. Young people with persistent shoulder pain may require a multidisciplinary approach with medical, surgical, physical therapy, occupational therapy, and psychology involvement.

It is important to work with the young person and build confidence in their body and their own capabilities. Often when pain persists and treatments have been tried without success it is important to find solutions within the child's own narrative, guiding children and young people back to spontaneous activity that is enjoyable and requires less conscious thought. Whether the child's goal is to be able to pick up their rabbit, play the violin or guitar, throw a javelin, rock climb, or put on make-up, it is important to find activities that matter in their world, at that particular time.

Pediatric musculoskeletal shoulder presentations

There are a wide variety of pediatric shoulder conditions, ranging in presentation from the early neonatal period into adulthood. Some of the more common musculoskeletal shoulder complaints that clinicians should be aware of are discussed below.

Shoulder dystocia and long-term consequences

The fetal shoulder is exposed to complications during vaginal delivery, especially when the fetus is unable to traverse the female pelvis spontaneously. This obstetric emergency is called shoulder dystocia and occurs when vaginal cephalic birth requires additional obstetric maneuvers to assist the birth of the fetal body after gentle axial traction on the fetal occiput has failed.[13,100] Shoulder dystocia occurs when either the anterior shoulder or less commonly the posterior shoulder impacts on the maternal symphysis pubis or the sacral promontory, respectively.

Risk factors

Macrosomia, fetal weight greater than 4 kg (8.8 lb), maternal diabetes, maternal age greater than 40 years, gestational age greater than 40 weeks, and instrument-assisted vaginal delivery, are all risk factors known to increase the incidence of shoulder dystocia. A previous birth complicated by shoulder dystocia significantly increases the risk of recurrence in subsequent pregnancies.[33,37]

Immediate management

Upon recognition of a shoulder dystocia during vaginal delivery, the mother should immediately stop pushing, since this increases the shoulder impaction onto the pubic symphysis. The McRoberts maneuver involves assisting the mother to lie flat on her back and flexing her hips at the chest. This position increases the relative anteroposterior diameter of the pelvic inlet. If the maneuver does not allow the impacted shoulder to be delivered, other measures such as suprapubic pressure on the shoulder of the fetus should be attempted.[13,94] If this maneuver or others are unsuccessful, a cleidotomy (fracturing the clavicle) may be performed by applying digital pressure on the mid-portion of the fetal clavicle.[13,100]

Complications associated with shoulder dystocia

Shoulder dystocia may result in long-term complications involving the brachial plexus, including Erb's and Klumpke's palsies.[48,100] Predicting which neonates will experience long-term complications is difficult.[78]

Erb's palsy

Trauma to the fifth and sixth cervical nerve roots (C5/6) results in Erb's palsy, characterized by paralysis of the shoulder muscles, elbow flexor, bicep and forearm supinator muscles; the neonate's arm is often limp and extended, inwardly rotated towards the trunk and the wrist pronated. Extended Erb's palsy presents when trauma involves C7 and effects the neonate's wrist and finger extensor muscles.[124]

Klumpke's palsy

The risk of Klumpke's palsy increases when the mother is small and/or the fetus is large and is associated with injury to C8–T1 nerves. Klumpke's palsy is commonly characterized by a supinated forearm, extended wrist, and flexed fingers, giving the appearance of a "clawed hand".[124]

Shoulder instability

Shoulder instability is an overarching term used to describe a wide spectrum of disease that is usually classified in the same way as in adults according to the Stanmore triangle.[10,63] The majority (86%) of children under 16 years of age have a traumatic onset, with a smaller number developing multidirectional instability without a traumatic event.[57] Multidirectional instability is defined as the symptomatic subluxation or dislocation of the glenohumeral joint occurring in two or three directions, with symptoms that may include pain (musculoskeletal and neuropathic), apprehension, kinesiophobia, and neurovascular symptoms.[58,121] This is most likely to occur in younger children, with a mean age of onset of 10 years.[57]

Traumatic anterior dislocations are more common in older adolescents (>14 years) due to their closed humeral physis,[87] and are often complicated by recurrent instability (93%).[87] In this group, surgery is considered on an individual basis and has shown a lower rate of recurrence in comparison to nonoperative treatment.[66] Skeletally immature children appear less likely to sustain a traumatic dislocation, have lower recurrence rates (21.4%) and are less likely to present with labral tears.[16,57] While it is known that children display increased ligament laxity and higher prevalence of joint hypermobility (34%),[110] shoulder instability can occur without generalized ligamentous laxity,[23,77,109] and in one study of asymptomatic adolescents, over half demonstrated shoulder instability.[23]

Shoulder instability in the pediatric population is usually managed nonsurgically.[67] Rehabilitation usually follows similar recommendations used when treating adults with the same condition.[46] A small group require pediatric tertiary services with ongoing instability, pain, and worsening function despite seemingly appropriate rehabilitation. Studies have identified that previous pain experiences in children are good predictors of subsequent pain experiences, with those who have previously had negative pain experiences, experiencing increased pain over time.[83,84] It is therefore important in this group to take a different approach, to reduce the perceived threat and reframe pain memories into a more positive light. To do this, clinicians need to understand who, where, or what makes the young person feel more confident to move their body. Questions to ask the child that may help the clinician plan an appropriate and meaningful rehabilitation strategy include: "What's it like living with your shoulder problem now?", "When was the last time your shoulder was less of (or wasn't) a problem?", "Why was it less of a problem then?", "What will it take to get it back to that level of function?", "How can we achieve that together?", "What would give you confidence in your shoulder again?", and "What do you feel safe/confident to do today?" Incorporating other members of the multidisciplinary team such as psychologists may also help to challenge beliefs and thoughts about movement and allow the young person to put all their focus towards meaningful goals and the future.

Fractures

Clavicle fractures

The clavicle is one of the most common bones to fracture in children. These injuries may occur as early as the perinatal period associated with birth trauma, or later in adolescents with either a direct blow to the outer end of the shoulder during contact sports, or from falling with an outstretched arm.[42,111] Clavicle fractures can be very painful, associated with localized tenderness, swelling, and deformity on examination. Radiographs are used to confirm the fractures, which are generally classified by location.

Middle third (80%): Most pediatric clavicle fractures occur in the middle third or midshaft of the bone, with the outer segment most likely to displace inferiorly and the medial segment superiorly. Controversy exists regarding best practice for this group of fractures – nonoperative versus operative.[79,112] Nonsurgical management has traditionally been offered for most middle third clavicle fractures with good results. However, there is growing evidence to support surgical management of displaced fractures, with better functional outcomes, faster return to activity, and reduced complication rates of non-union and malunion.[28,34] Children with non-displaced or minimally displaced midshaft clavicle fractures that are otherwise uncomplicated may be appropriately managed with sling immobilization, analgesics and elbow range of motion exercises. While clinical union usually occurs by 6–12 weeks in adults, this occurs more quickly in children, usually between 3–6 weeks.[36] Radiographs are usually obtained at this point although callus may not appear for several more weeks. Children younger than 11 years with undisplaced clavicle fractures do not routinely require follow-up or X-ray, and can remove the sling and slowly return to normal function when the fracture site is no longer tender. Contact sports should be avoided for approximately six weeks after removing the sling.

Lateral third (15%): Distal or lateral third fractures of the clavicle are generally more problematic. They often involve the acromioclavicular or coracoclavicular ligaments and are more prone to non or delayed union. Surgical opinion should be considered in these cases.

Clavicle fractures of the neonatal period are most often associated with birth trauma and shoulder dystocia. These can occur spontaneously or as a result of a cleidotomy (deliberate clavicle fracture), a maneuver to allow the fetal passage through the birth canal.[95] The majority of these fractures heal with minimal intervention. Immobilization of the arm may be facilitated by fastening the sleeve of the neonate's clothing to the central section of the garment.

Complications associated with clavicle fractures include neurovascular compromise, non-/malunion, acromioclavicular joint instability, or loss of power of shoulder elevation.[36,87] Appropriate orthopedic and neurological opinion should be sought for injuries that include neurovascular damage, lateral third factures with instability or acromioclavicular joint incongruence, or non-union with loss of function or pain. Urgent orthopedic referral should be sought for children with clavicle fractures associated with signs of neurovascular compromise, open wounds, or skin tenting. Referral to the emergency department should occur if there any concerns for associated respiratory or hemodynamic compromise.[36]

Proximal humeral fractures

Proximal humeral fractures account for less than 5% of all pediatric fractures.[54] These fractures usually occur through the growth plate (physis) or through the metaphysis depending on the child's age and injury mechanism.

Most of these injuries occur from falls onto an outstretched hand where the humeral head is compressed against the glenoid, transmitting the force through the physeal or metaphyseal regions. Most physeal injuries occur during the late childhood and early adolescent period, aligning with a child's rapid growth phase and relative susceptibility to fracture. Prepubescent children are more likely to present with fractures through their metaphysis, although growth plate injuries still occur (Figure 25.1).

Initial treatment involves pain management, immobilization and radiographic evaluation. Basic paracetamol and ibuprofen may be useful for mild to moderate pain, with intranasal fentanyl appropriate for initial severe pain to assist with examination and radiographs.[104] For non-displaced proximal humeral fractures, clinical findings may be limited to tenderness and mild swelling.[51] For displaced fractures, more significant anterior swelling and shoulder deformity relative to the unaffected side may be seen.[51]

Basic anterior-posterior (AP) and lateral (axillary) radiographs are used to ascertain the degree of angulation or displacement of the humeral shaft relative to the humeral

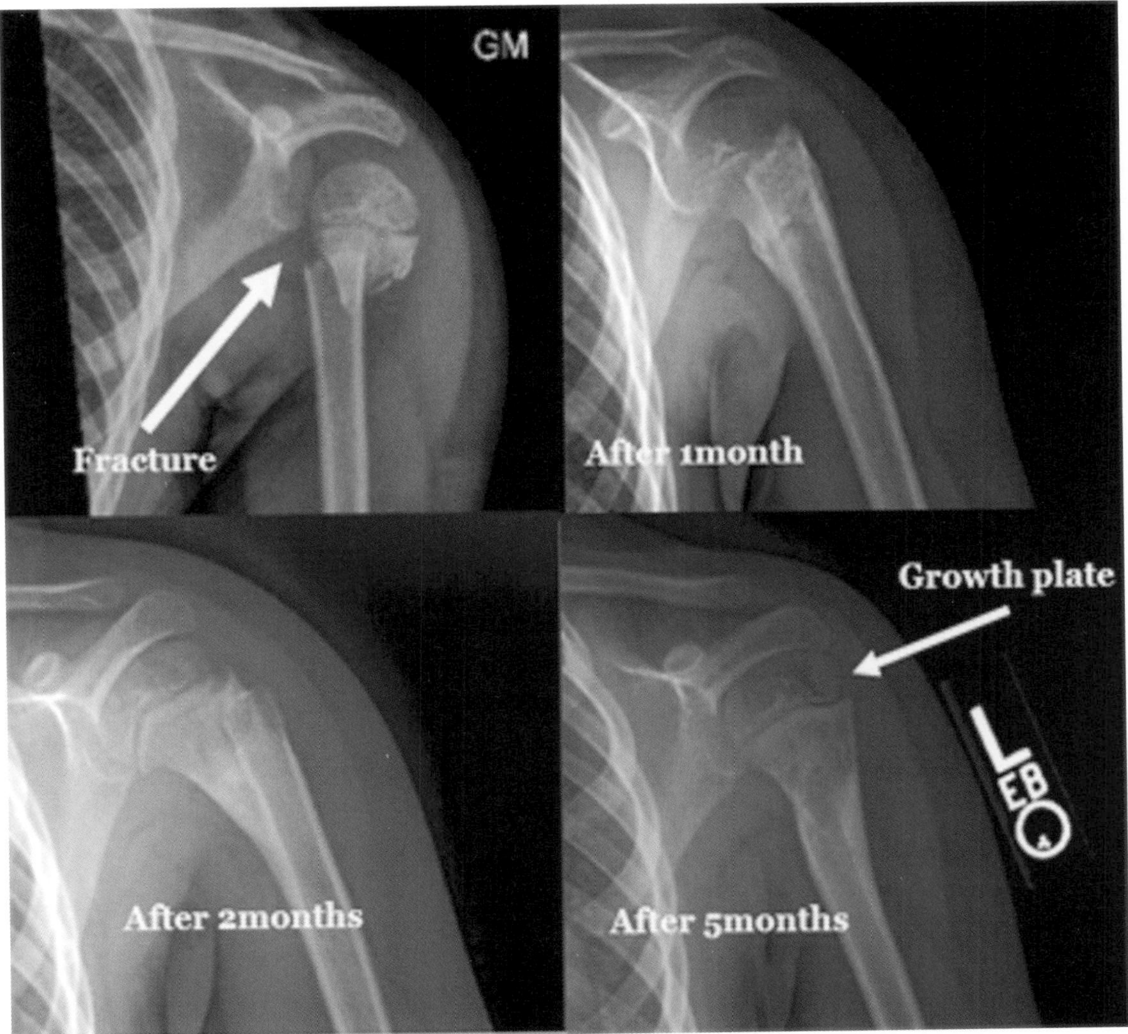

FIGURE 25.1

Radiographs of proximal humeral fractures.

(Reproduced with permission from Dr Joe Eichinger, MD. https://www.josefeichingermd.com/orthopaedic-surgeon-charleston-mount-pleasant-sc-patient-instruction-modules-pediatric-proximal-humerus-fractures.html)

head. Salter-Harris classification is also widely used to describe the fracture deformity when the growth plate is involved (see Table 25.2).

Approximately 80% of humeral growth is estimated to occur from the proximal humeral physis, which closes between the ages of 16 and 19 years.[96] Children have a greater ability than adults to remodel their bone, with most proximal humeral fractures in children successfully managed nonsurgically.[35,41] Rarely is reduction in the emergency department indicated. For marked displacement in older children (>12 years) operative management is recommended[35,41] (Table 25.3).

Children and adolescents with non-displaced or minimally displaced proximal humeral fractures are typically immobilized for several weeks for comfort, and then start gentle exercises between two and four weeks post injury, and active range of motion between four and six weeks. Most children recommence overhead activities after four to six weeks with almost normal function from two months post injury. Infants may only require four weeks' immobilization with sling or swathe, with early healing potential and often palpable callous already formed.[104,108]

Complications from proximal humeral fractures in children are rare. The most common complication is mild shortening of the humerus secondary to physeal damage and growth restriction, which may be more prevalent in older children.[80] This infrequently correlates to functional disability and is often not clinically apparent.[104] Radiographic malunion is similarly uncommon and is seldom associated with functional limitation. Occasionally axillary nerve injuries occur but most are temporary neuropraxias. In neonates, brachial plexus injuries can be an adjunct complication from birth trauma and therefore should be monitored closely with repeat neurological examinations to identify potential injury.[19]

Specialist orthopedic opinion should be sought for humeral head displacement of more than 50%; radiographic angulation of >60 degrees in a child older than 12 years or >30 degrees in a child younger than 12 years; pathological facture; associated neurovascular injuries (e.g., brachial plexus); or multi-trauma.[104]

Fracture in an otherwise healthy child younger than two years with a mechanism inconsistent with the injury should raise concern for nonaccidental injury.[102] Occasionally fractures occur through areas of bone cyst or tumor. These injuries require far less energy trauma to break and are termed pathological fractures.

Pathological fractures

Malignant cancers of the bone are defined as primary or secondary. Primary bone cancers originate from the bone itself, and metastatic spread to bone leads to secondary bone cancers.[6] Malignant bone tumors tend to have a male preponderance and are uncommon before the onset of puberty.[65] The malignant bone tumors that mainly affect children include osteosarcomas, Ewing sarcoma, and chondrosarcoma.

Table 25.3 Treatment algorithm adapted from Hohloch et al.[41]

Condition	Non or slightly displaced fractures	Displaced or severely displaced fractures		
Definition	Displacement <1/3 of shaft width <20° angulation	Displacement >1/3 of shaft width >20° angulation		
Management	All pediatric presentations	Children ≤10 years	Children >10 years	Children ≥13 years
	Nonsurgical: Desault bandage or sling With or without closed reduction	Nonsurgical If not successful: ESIN and K-wires	Attempt closed reduction and nonsurgical management Surgical option: ESIN for osteosynthesis	Prioritize surgical management ESIN for osteosynthesis

ESIN, elastic stable intramedullary nailing.

Ewing sarcoma

Ewing sarcoma (ES) primarily affects the bones of children and adolescents. While most ES occur in the long bones of the leg and at the pelvis, small percentages also occur around the shoulder joint (humerus 4.8%, scapula 3.8%, clavicle 1.2%).[17] ES should be considered in children and adolescents with localized swelling or pain, often presenting over weeks to months, associated with fever, fatigue, weight loss, or anemia.[73,103] Diagnostic workup usually begins with plain radiographs, escalating to computed tomography (CT) scans and magnetic resonance imaging (MRI) scans to further stage the disease, and tissue biopsy (CT-guided or open).

Osteosarcoma

Osteosarcomas represent the most common of the malignant bone cancers in the pediatric population, with an estimated 2.6 per 1,000,000 people being diagnosed each year.[3] Definitive etiology remains largely unknown. Pain is the most common symptom, and initially it may not be constant; swelling may also be present. Risk factors include inherited conditions (e.g., Li-Fraumeni syndrome, retinoblastoma, Werner's syndrome), pre-existing bone disease (e.g., Paget's disease), environmental exposure (e.g., previous radiotherapy, previous exposure to pesticides, previous exposure to chemotherapeutic agents), and being male, adolescent, and taller in stature.[3]

Ninety percent of osteosarcomas originate in the proximal humerus.[89] Possible clinical features of osteosarcomas include pain and swelling over the affected bone and/or joint, restricted movement of affected limbs, pathological fractures and/or dislocations, or with the symptoms of metastatic disease. Plain X-rays of the affected bone may show evidence of lytic lesions, new bone formation in soft tissue, or the characteristic "sun-burst" appearance that is commonly described with osteosarcoma. Subsequent imaging with CT or MRI can further assess the site and extent of the bone malignancy, and its possible metastatic spread.[52] Treatment usually involves chemotherapy given prior to surgical management, with limb amputation being avoided where possible.

Benign tumors of bone

Benign bone tumors may also occur in the pediatric population. One benign tumor is an osteoid osteoma, which usually affects the spine and the long bones. The age of presentation may range between 10 to 25 years, with the presenting clinical features correlating to the bone that is affected. When presenting in the proximal humerus, osteoid osteomas may present as shoulder pain, that is typically worse at night.[85] Osteoid osteoma is typically self-limiting although surgery is considered in patients with severe pain who do not respond to nonsteroidal anti-inflammatory medications.[85]

Distal clavicular osteolysis

Distal clavicular osteolysis (DCO) may occur following trauma, or from repetitive stress. MRI findings are consistent in both forms: bone marrow edema, subchondral cysts and, in advanced cases, periostitis at the distal clavicle. In adults, the most common mechanism of stress-induced DCO is weightlifting. DCO has also been reported in pediatric populations.[101] In a retrospective study of 1432 children, mean age 15.9 years (range 13–19 years) who had undergone shoulder MRIs with no history of trauma, 6.5% (n=93) were identified as having DCO. All had distal clavicular edema and 74% (69/93) had a subchondral fracture. A control group of 93 children without DCO was used as a comparison. Those with DCO were more likely to participate in overhead activity (tennis, swimming, basketball, and volleyball) and weight training.[101]

The two most significant predictors of DCO in this group were: 1) pain at the acromioclavicular joint/distal clavicle, and 2) participating in both overhead activity and weight training.[101] Significant improvement or resolution of symptoms was associated with relative rest for three months and graduated return to function in 93% of those with DCO. A long-term clinical and MRI follow-up (average 4.3 years) was reported in 28/93 with DCO and 34/93 in the control group. The average age at follow-up was 20.1 years. Osteoarthritic changes in the acromioclavicular joint were observed in 71% of the DCO group compared with 35% in the control group. Those with more moderate or severe changes were more likely to be clinically symptomatic.[101] The longer-term sequalae of DCO in a pediatric population are not yet established and recommendations, such as no more than 70 and 90 tennis matches per year for 14- and 16-year olds respectively should be considered. When weight training, the concomitant number of overhead sporting training sessions and competitions may need to be reduced.[101]

Os acromiale

The acromion usually ossifies by the 22nd to 25th year. It is formed from three separate centers termed the pre-acromion, meso-acromion, and meta-acromion (Figure 25.2). If these centers fail to unite, the ununited portion is called an os acromiale. Edelson et al.[20] reported an 8% incidence in an osteological examination of 270 scapulae, with the length of the unfused segment varying from 1.4 cm to 2.6 cm (0.5 to 1 in). Although it has been suggested that contraction of the deltoid may displace the loose portion of the acromion inferiorly leading to rotator cuff damage[76] there is no certainty that os acromiale is associated with symptoms.[64] Care must be taken not to confuse an acromial fracture and os acromiale with a section of the acromion yet to fuse,[126] and although the condition may be asymptomatic, it may be present in adolescents[126] and may be associated with symptoms including pain and instability.[126]

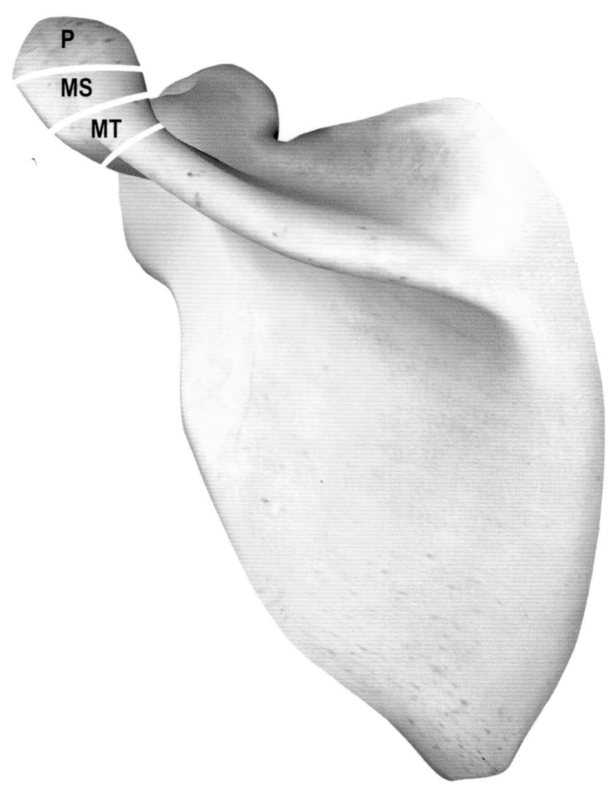

FIGURE 25.2

Os acromiale. The three ossification centers of the acromion: pre-acromion (P), meso-acromion (MS), and meta-acromion (MT). In most cases, os acromiale occurs between the meso and meta-acromion.

(Redrawn with permission of Jeremy Lewis.)

Connective tissue disorders

Shoulder pain in the pediatric population may be due to connective tissue disorders (CTDs), two of which, Ehlers-Danlos syndrome and Marfan syndrome, are described below.

Ehlers-Danlos syndrome

Ehlers-Danlos syndrome (EDS) is an umbrella term that encompasses a group of 13 subtypes that are characterized by joint hypermobility, skin extensibility and tissue fragility.[72] EDS subtypes (including classical, vascular, kyphoscoliotic) can either be inherited via an autosomal dominant or autosomal recessive pattern. In contrast, hypermobile EDS (hEDS) does not have a known genetic basis and has shown no clear connective tissue abnormality.[72] hEDS is a topic of debate within pediatrics,[8,32] however, a recent public position statement from the Royal College of Paediatrics and Child Health offers clear clinical guidance.[120] They recommended that pediatricians use the EDS 2017 consensus criteria[72] to correctly diagnose hEDS, and outline that clinical findings such as fractures, retinal hemorrhages and extensive bruising need to be investigated to safeguard children with a diagnosis of hEDS who at present, as evidence currently stands, cannot have these findings attributed to hEDS. Although studies have found no association between hypermobility and musculoskeletal pain,[62] the position statement also highlights that a diagnosis of persistent musculoskeletal pain (with or without joint laxity) can be associated with an array of symptoms that include dizziness, nausea, blurred vision, hypersensitivity, and a change in bowel habit.

Hypermobility is common in the shoulder, with approximately 85% of children with hEDS reporting shoulder pain as one of their symptoms. Recent evidence suggests that patients with hEDS may have a relatively large subacromial space compared with individuals without this condition. This may be associated with symptoms.[12]

Marfan syndrome

Marfan syndrome is an autosomal dominant CTD that has an incidence of 1 in 5000 people in the UK, making it one of the more common CTDs.[2] The syndrome is associated with a mutation in the protein fibrillin-1 which is responsible for skin, ligament, and blood vessel elasticity.[1] As such, Marfan syndrome affects many parts of the body including the musculoskeletal, cardiovascular, ocular, and respiratory systems, the spinal cord, and the skin. Above-average height, scoliosis, spondylolisthesis, arachnodactyly, high-arched palate, crowded teeth, pes planus, chest wall concavity and joint hypermobility are associated.[65] Seventy percent of people with Marfan syndrome will report joint pain. Joint hypermobility may lead to shoulder dislocations and pain. Children with Marfan syndrome may also present with visible stretch marks over their shoulders (as well as their hips and lower back) due to changes in the skin elasticity.[2]

Facioscapulohumeral dystrophy

Facioscapulohumeral dystrophy (FSHD) is a muscular dystrophy that is dominantly inherited and characterized by muscle weakness and wasting of muscles around the face and scapula. The age of onset varies widely from childhood to adulthood, with the mean age of onset being in the early twenties.[92] Those with FSHD demonstrate progressive muscle weakness that is usually slow and follows a descending pattern from the face and shoulder, to the trunk, pelvis and lower extremities.[71] During a shoulder assessment it is important to ask about family history of muscular dystrophy and to carefully examine scapulohumeral and fascial muscle strength. Young people with FSHD demonstrate difficulty squeezing their eyes shut, furrowing the brow, or puckering the lips. On observation, they usually have a characteristic winging of the scapula with limitation due to weakness moving the shoulder into abduction.[71,114] Children and adolescents with FSHD are managed by a pediatric neurologist and are regularly treated and monitored within specialist multidisciplinary muscular dystrophy clinics.

Overuse injuries

A consensus statement from The American Orthopedic Society for Sports Medicine stated there was no evidence that pre-pubertal children benefited from specializing in a single sport and that by doing so, they were subject to overuse injury and burnout.[55] Instead, children should participate in multiple sports with a focus on enjoyment.[9,75] Reasons for shoulder overuse injuries are multifactorial with intrinsic and extrinsic factors. Extrinsic factors include the intensity of play or level of sport, the training or match volume per week, and the amount of rest between play (e.g., days off between games, and length of off-season). Intrinsic factors include skeletal maturity, growth, and associated muscular support of the shoulder.

Growth periods may increase the susceptibility to injury. Children who mature younger are at higher risk than those maturing later.[47,98] Periods of growth can be established using growth charts; however, parents will often report a recent need for new shoes and clothes. If radiographs are not available, skeletal maturity can be guided by asking about parent height and asking girls if and when their menstruation began.[53] As a guide, a child should not be playing more hours of sport per week than their years of age.[97] They should play their primary sport for less than eight months in a year[97] and training should include specific neuromuscular injury prevention strategies[22] such as those used with success in youth football.[44]

Little Leaguer's Shoulder

Chapter 38 discuses throwing injuries and rehabilitation primarily for adults. Here we focus on throwing injuries in children, specifically "Little Leaguer's Shoulder". This condition is an overuse injury that results in a proximal humeral epiphysiolysis, which occurs when shear or stress on the proximal humeral growth plate (epiphyseal cartilage) exceeds its tensile strength and causes it to separate.[11] It has also been called osteochondrosis of the proximal humeral epiphysis and rotational stress fracture of the proximal humeral epiphyseal plate.

Rotational forces are thought to have a larger role than distraction force.[11,45] The repetitive microtrauma results in cartilage damage of the proximal humeral epiphysis. It occurs exclusively in athletes whose growth plate has not closed, most commonly between the ages of 11 and 16 years, although theoretically up to 21 years when the growth plate closes. The condition typically occurs in junior league baseball players and throwing athletes, and it has also been reported in gymnasts and tennis players.[45] The condition is associated with the substantial external rotation torque on the humeral shaft during late cocking (Chapter 38) just prior to the acceleration phase of pitching.[45] Typically pain gradually increases with more exposure to throwing but may eventuate in pain when lifting the arm and sometimes pain at rest. Clinically there may be tenderness over the lateral aspect of the proximal humerus and swelling may also be present.[61] Range of motion restriction and weakness are also common findings;[11] in rare cases, nerve injury may occur.[125] Radiographs (AP view with the shoulder in external rotation) may reveal widening of the proximal humeral physis, ultrasound may detect hypoechoic swelling not observed on the contralateral side and magnetic resonance imaging may detect edema around the physis. If detected early, relative rest and graduated return may allow resumption of sporting pursuits.[11] If detected late, a prolonged period of relative rest of up to six months may be indicated followed by a carefully planned and incremental return to play. Surgery is not indicated for this condition.[11]

In summary, shoulder overuse injuries are a frequent problem seen in the young overhead throwing athlete and Little League Shoulder is an example of an injury of the proximal humeral physis that occurs at this susceptible period of growth (normally around the ages of 11 to 16 years).[109] On examination, there can be tenderness and swelling over the anterolateral aspect of the shoulder with weakness into abduction and internal rotation.[61] Treatment involves rest and activity modification followed by a progressive program to return to throwing.[11,38]

Child abuse (nonaccidental injury)

Musculoskeletal presentations are common in pediatric populations; most are benign, self-limiting, and resolve relatively quickly. However, they may be associated with more serious conditions such as infection, malignancy, and physical abuse. Clinicians must consider red-flag conditions and physical abuse as differential diagnoses.

Abuse can clearly impact heavily on the psychological and physical well-being of a child. One in five children in the UK have been subjected to some form of abuse before reaching the age of 16 years, with many cases remaining hidden.[69] Nonaccidental injury (NAI), suspected physical abuse (SPA) and inflicted injury (II) are used to describe injury resulting from purposefully inflicted and direct physical abuse towards children. NAI or II are used to distinguish physical abuse from injuries caused by accidents such as falling off a bike, skateboard, out of a tree, or road traffic accidents.

Physical abuse is insidious and may not present in a predictable fashion, and occurs in approximately 20% of childhood abuse cases. Cutaneous injuries are most common followed by fractures; NAI/II may present as bruising, bite marks, cuts, and burns to the skin. NAI/II should be considered in the differential diagnosis in dependent and nonambulatory children who present with such injuries as retinal hemorrhage, torn frenulum, delay in seeking care, multiple co-existing fractures, and fractures of different chronological ages with no family history or clinical features of bone disease such as osteogenesis imperfecta, and fractures resulting from falls – falls being common while fractures are not.[90]

Deep cigarette burns and burns inflicted by irons may damage skin and underlying soft shoulder tissues. Metaphyseal lesions in infants are synonymous with NAI/II and the mechanism is a shearing or torsional force across the metaphysis. They are most likely in children less than a year old with the proximal humeri, distal femur, and proximal and distal tibia being the most common locations. Forceful shaking may also result in a metaphyseal lesion.[90] A humeral fracture in a child under 18 months raises the suspicion of an NAI/II, even more so if the child is less than 15 months old. Spiral, oblique, and bucket handle fractures (subacute metaphyseal fracture that forms an arc along the proximal margin of the metaphysis) are strongly associated with abuse. Fractures in usual locations, commonly referred to as the 3-Ss: scapula (including the acromion), sternum and spinous processes, should alert the clinician to the possibility of NAI/II. Scapular fractures are very unusual in children and require substantial force. They may occur following significant trauma such as a fall from a substantial height (tree), but in a young child when such activities would not be possible, NAI/II must be considered.[90,91,107,115]

Conclusion

Pediatric shoulder injuries include a broad range of conditions that occur at different stages of a child's life. Traumatic shoulder injuries are often first seen in accident and emergency departments with access to specialty consultation and imaging services. Shoulder injuries with slower, more insidious onset are often first seen in family practice where the diagnosis may be less obvious. A comprehensive history involving guardian and child, followed by a targeted physical examination will help guide subsequent investigation or management. Basic radiographs are particularly useful in identifying clavicle or humeral fractures, with ultrasound, MRI and nerve conduction studies sometimes required to differentiate between other conditions.

Most children heal quickly, and a large proportion of shoulder injuries can be managed nonsurgically with immobilization, analgesia, and exercises at the forefront of treatment. As a child matures skeletally, their body loses the ability to remodel bone as effectively, with surgical management more commonly required. Clinicians must remain cognizant that pain in the region of the shoulder may not be musculoskeletal in origin. For more complex neurological and developmental conditions, it is important to involve the larger multidisciplinary team including physiotherapy, psychology, occupational therapy, and multiple medical specialties. Given the social complexities and vulnerabilities of many children in the community, practitioners should be mindful of nonaccidental injuries, particularly in children otherwise well with an injury that does not correlate to the reported mechanism of insult.

References

1. MedlinePlus. FBN1 gene. Available at: https://medlineplus.gov/genetics/gene/fbn1/#resources.
2. NHS. Marfan syndrome. Available at: https://www.nhs.uk/conditions/marfan-syndrome/.
3. Bone Cancer Research Trust. Osteosarcoma. Available at: https://www.bcrt.org.uk/information/information-by-type/osteosarcoma/.
4. Abboud JA, Bateman DK, Barlow J. Glenoid dysplasia. Journal of the American Academy of Orthopaedic Surgeons. 2016;24:327-336.
5. Allen B, Schoch B, Sperling JW, Cofield RH. Shoulder arthroplasty for osteoarthritis secondary to glenoid dysplasia: an update. J Shoulder Elbow Surg. 2014;23:214-220.
6. Arinima P, Ishak A. Persistent shoulder pain in young male: osteosarcoma. Korean J Fam Med. 2018;39:266-269.
7. Baca MJ, King RW, Bancroft LW. Glenoid hypoplasia. Radiology Case Reports. 2016;11:386-390.
8. Bailey K, Debelle G. Comment on: the multisystemic nature and natural history of joint hypermobility syndrome and Ehlers-Danlos syndrome in children. Rheumatology. 2018;57:2248-2250.
9. Bergeron MF, Mountjoy M, Armstrong N, et al. International Olympic Committee consensus statement on youth athletic development. British Journal of Sports Medicine. 2015;49:843-851.
10. Brownson P, Donaldson O, Fox M, et al. BESS/BOA Patient Care Pathways: traumatic anterior shoulder instability. Shoulder and Elbow. 2015;7:214-226.
11. Casadei K, Kiel J. Proximal humeral epiphysiolysis (Little League Shoulder). StatPearls. Treasure Island: StatPearls Publishing; 2020.
12. Castori M, Camerota F, Celletti C, et al. Natural history and manifestations of the hypermobility type Ehlers-Danlos syndrome: a pilot study on 21 patients. American Journal of Medical Genetics. Part A. 2010;152a:556-564.
13. Chopra S. Management of pregnancy with a history of shoulder dystocia and difficult delivery. In: Rohilla M (ed). Recurrent Pregnancy Loss and Adverse Natal Outcomes. CRC Press; 2020.
14. Clementi MA, Faraji P, Poppert Cordts K, et al. Parent factors are associated with pain and activity limitations in youth with acute musculoskeletal pain: a cohort study. Clin J Pain. 2019;35:222-228.
15. Clinch J, Eccleston C. Chronic musculoskeletal pain in children: assessment and management. Rheumatology. 2009;48:466-474.
16. Cordischi K, Li X, Busconi B. Intermediate outcomes after primary traumatic anterior shoulder dislocation in skeletally immature patients aged 10 to 13 years. Orthopedics. 2009;32(9):orthosupersite.com/view.asp?rID=42855.
17. Cotterill SJ, Ahrens S, Paulussen M, et al. Prognostic factors in Ewing's tumor of bone: analysis of 975 patients from the European Intergroup Cooperative Ewing's Sarcoma Study Group. Journal of Clinical Oncology. 2000;18:3108-3114.
18. de Figueiredo MJPSS, Dos Reis Braga S, Akkari M, Prado JCL, Santili C. Congenital pseudarthrosis of the clavicle. Revista Brasileira de Ortopedia. 2015;47:21-26.
19. Drew SJ, Giddins GE, Birch R. A slowly evolving brachial plexus injury following a proximal humeral fracture in a child. J Hand Surg Br. 1995;20:24-25.
20. Edelson JG, Zuckerman J, Hershkovitz I. Os acromiale: anatomy and surgical implications. J Bone Joint Surg Br. 1993;75:551-555.
21. Ellis HB, Li Y, Bae DS, et al. Descriptive epidemiology of adolescent clavicle fractures: results from the FACTS (Function after Adolescent Clavicle Trauma and Surgery) prospective, multicenter cohort study. Orthopaedic Journal of Sports Medicine. 2020;8:2325967120921344.
22. Emery CA, Roy T-O, Whittaker JL, Nettel-Aguirre A, van Mechelen W. Neuromuscular training injury prevention strategies in youth sport: a systematic review and meta-analysis. British Journal of Sports Medicine. 2015;49:865-870.
23. Emery RJ, Mullaji AB. Glenohumeral joint instability in normal adolescents. Incidence and significance. The Journal of Bone and Joint Surgery. British volume. 1991;73:406-408.
24. Enger M, Skjaker SA, Melhuus K, et al. Shoulder injuries from birth to old age: a 1-year prospective study of 3031 shoulder injuries in an urban population. Injury. 2018;49:1324-1329.

25. FDA. Pediatric X-ray Imaging. Available at: https://www.fda.gov/radiation-emitting-products/medical-imaging/pediatric-x-ray-imaging.

26. Foster HE, Jandial S. pGALS - paediatric Gait Arms Legs and Spine: a simple examination of the musculoskeletal system. Pediatric Rheumatology. 2013;11:44.

27. Franklin CC, Weiss JM. The natural history of pediatric and adolescent shoulder dislocation. Journal of Pediatric Orthopaedics. 2019;39:S50-S52.

28. Gao B, Dwivedi S, Patel SA, Nwizu C, Cruz AI, Jr. Operative versus nonoperative management of displaced midshaft clavicle fractures in pediatric and adolescent patients: a systematic review and meta-analysis. J Orthop Trauma. 2019;33:e439-e446.

29. Gardner E. The prenatal development of the human shoulder joint. Surg Clin North Am. 1963;43:1465-1470.

30. Gherman RB, Chauhan S, Ouzounian JG, Lerner H, Gonik B, Goodwin TM. Shoulder dystocia: the unpreventable obstetric emergency with empiric management guidelines. American Journal of Obstetrics and Gynecology. 2006;195:657-672.

31. Ginsberg NA, Moisidis C. How to predict recurrent shoulder dystocia. American Journal of Obstetrics and Gynecology. 2001;184:1427-1429; discussion 1429-1430.

32. Grahame R. Comment on: the multisystemic nature and natural history of joint hypermobility syndrome and Ehlers-Danlos syndrome in children: reply. Rheumatology. 2018;57:2250-2251.

33. Grossman L, Pariente G, Baumfeld Y, Yohay D, Rotem R, Weintraub AY. Trends of changes in the specific contribution of selected risk factors for shoulder dystocia over a period of more than two decades. Journal of Perinatal Medicine. 2020;48:567-573.

34. Guerra E, Previtali D, Tamborini S, Filardo G, Zaffagnini S, Candrian C. Midshaft clavicle fractures: surgery provides better results as compared with nonoperative treatment: a meta-analysis. Am J Sports Med. 2019;47:3541-3551.

35. Hannonen J, Hyvönen H, Korhonen L, Serlo W, Sinikumpu JJ. The incidence and treatment trends of pediatric proximal humerus fractures. BMC Musculoskelet Disord. 2019;20:571.

36. Hatch RL, Clugston JR, Taffe J. Clavicle fractures. UpToDate. 2020. Available at: https://www.uptodate.com/contents/clavicle-fractures/print.

37. Heinonen K, Saisto T, Gissler M, Kaijomaa M, Sarvilinna N. Rising trends in the incidence of shoulder dystocia and development of a novel shoulder dystocia risk score tool: a nationwide population-based study of 800 484 Finnish deliveries. Acta Obstet Gynecol Scand. 2021;100:538-547.

38. Heyworth BE, Kramer DE, Martin DJ, Micheli LJ, Kocher MS, Bae DS. Trends in the presentation, management, and outcomes of little league shoulder. American Journal of Sports Medicine. 2016;44:1431-1438.

39. Hirvonen M, Ojala R, Korhonen P, et al. Cerebral palsy among children born moderately and late preterm. Pediatrics. 2014;134:e1584-1593.

40. Hita-Contreras F, Sanchez-Montesinos I, Martinez-Amat A, Cruz-Diaz D, Barranco RJ, Roda O. Development of the human shoulder joint during the embryonic and early fetal stages: anatomical considerations for clinical practice. J Anat. 2018;232:422-430.

41. Hohloch L, Eberbach H, Wagner FC, et al. Age- and severity-adjusted treatment of proximal humerus fractures in children and adolescents: a systematical review and meta-analysis. PloS One. 2017;12:e0183157.

42. The Royal Children's Hospital. Clavicle fractures – Emergency Department. Available at: https://www.rch.org.au/clinicalguide/guideline_index/fractures/Clavicle_fractures_Emergency_Department/

43. The Royal Children's Hospital. Engaging with and assessing the adolescent patient. Available at: https://www.rch.org.au/clinicalguide/guideline_index/Engaging_with_and_assessing_the_adolescent_patient/

44. Hyunmin K, Juseoung L, Junghoon K. The Impact of the FIFA 11+ program on the injury in soccer players: a systematic review. The Asian Journal of Kinesiology. 2020;22:55-61.

45. Ito A, Mihata T, Hosokawa Y, Hasegawa A, Neo M, Doi M. Humeral retroversion and injury risk after proximal humeral epiphysiolysis (Little Leaguer's Shoulder). The American Journal of Sports Medicine. 2019;47:3100-3106.

46. Jaggi A, Lambert S. Rehabilitation for shoulder instability. British Journal of Sports Medicine. 2010;44:333-340.

47. Johnson A, Doherty PJ, Freemont A, et al. Investigation of growth, development, and factors associated with injury in elite schoolboy footballers: prospective study. BMJ. 2009;338:694-696.

48. Johnson GJ, Denning S, Clark SL, Davidson C. Pathophysiologic origins of brachial plexus injury. Obstetrics and Gynecology. 2020;136:725-730.

49. Kadavkolan AS, Bhatia DN, Dasgupta B, Bhosale PB. Sprengel's deformity of the shoulder: current perspectives in management. International Journal of Shoulder Surgery. 2011;5:1-8.

50. King S, Chambers CT, Huguet A, et al. The epidemiology of chronic pain in children and adolescents revisited: a systematic review. Pain. 2011;152:2729-2738.

51. Kohler R, Trillaud JM. Fracture and fracture separation of the proximal humerus in children: report of 136 cases. Journal of Pediatric Orthopedics. 1983;3:326-332.

52. Kundu ZS. Classification, imaging, biopsy and staging of osteosarcoma. Indian Journal of Orthopaedics. 2014;48:238-246.

53. Lai EH-H, Chang JZ-C, Yao C-CJ, et al. Relationship between age at menarche and skeletal maturation stages in Taiwanese female orthodontic patients. Journal of the Formosan Medical Association. 2008;107:527-532.

54. Landin LA. Epidemiology of children's fractures. J Pediatr Orthop B. 1997;6:79-83.

55. LaPrade RF, Agel J, Baker J, et al. AOSSM Early Sport Specialization Consensus Statement. Orthopaedic Journal of Sports Medicine. 2016;4:2325967116644241.

56. Larsen A, Mundbjerg E, Lauritsen J, Faergemann C. Development of the annual incidence rate of fracture in children 1980–2018: a population-based study of 32,375 fractures. Acta Orthopaedica. 2020;91:593-597.

57. Lawton RL, Choudhury S, Mansat P, Cofield RH, Stans AA. Pediatric shoulder instability: presentation, findings, treatment, and outcomes. Journal of Pediatric Orthopedics. 2002;22:52-61.

58. Lawton RL, Choudhury S, Mansat P, Cofield RH, Stans AA. Pediatric

shoulder instability: presentation, findings, treatment, and outcomes. Journal of Pediatric Orthopedics. 2002;22:52-61.

59. LeBel ME. Clavicle fractures. In: Greiwe M (ed). Shoulder and Elbow Trauma and its Complications. Woodhead Publishing; 2015:191-213.

60. Lefèvre Y, Journeau P, Angelliaume A, Bouty A, Dobremez E. Proximal humerus fractures in children and adolescents. Orthopaedics & Traumatology: Surgery & Research. 2014;100:S149-S156.

61. Leonard J, Hutchinson M. Shoulder injuries in skeletally immature throwers: review and current thoughts. British Journal of Sports medicine. 2010;44:306-310.

62. Leone V, Tornese G, Zerial M, et al. Joint hypermobility and its relationship to musculoskeletal pain in schoolchildren: a cross-sectional study. Archives of Disease in Childhood. 2009;94:627-632.

63. Lewis A, Kitamura T, Bayley JIL. (ii) The classification of shoulder instability: new light through old windows! Current Orthopaedics. 2004;18:97-108.

64. Lewis J, Green A, Dekel S. The aetiology of subacromial impingement syndrome. Physiotherapy. 2001;87:458-469.

65. Lissauer T, Carroll W. Malignant disease. In: Illustrated Textbook of Paediatrics, 5th edition. Elsevier; 2017:396-397.

66. Longo UG, Coco V, Denaro V, Van Der Linde JA, Poolman RW, Loppini M. Surgical versus nonoperative treatment in patients up to 18 years old with traumatic shoulder instability: a systematic review and quantitative synthesis of the literature. Arthroscopy. 2016;32:944-952.

67. Longo UG, Salvatore G, Locher J, et al. Epidemiology of paediatric shoulder dislocation: a nationwide study in Italy from 2001 to 2014. International Journal of Environmental Research and Public Health. 2020;17:2834.

68. Low AK, Ward K, Wines AP. Pediatric complex regional pain syndrome. Journal of Pediatric Orthopedics. 2007;27:567-572.

69. Office for National Statistics. Child abuse extent and nature, England and Wales: year ending March 2019. Available at: https://www.ons.gov.uk/peoplepopulationandcommunity/crimeandjustice/articles/childabuseextentandnatureenglandandwales/yearendingmarch2019.

70. MacLennan AH, Thompson SC, Gecz J. Cerebral palsy: causes, pathways, and the role of genetic variants. American Journal of Obstetrics and Gynecology. 2015;213:779-788.

71. Mah JK, Chen Y-W. A pediatric review of facioscapulohumeral muscular dystrophy. Journal of Pediatric Neurology. 2018;16:222-231.

72. Malfait F, Francomano C, Byers P, et al. The 2017 international classification of the Ehlers-Danlos syndromes. American Journal of Medical Genetics. 2017;175:8-26.

73. Mendenhall CM, Marcus RB, Enneking WF, Springfield DS, Thar TL, Million RR. The prognostic significance of soft tissue extension in Ewing's sarcoma. Cancer. 1983;51:913-917.

74. Moore KL. The Developing Human. Philadelphia: WB Saunders; 1982.

75. Mostafavifar AM, Best TM, Myer GD. Early sport specialisation, does it lead to long-term problems? British Journal of Sports Medicine. 2013;47:1060-1061.

76. Mudge MK, Wood VE, Frykman GK. Rotator cuff tears associated with os acromiale. J Bone Joint Surg Am. 1984;66:427-429.

77. Muhammad AA, Jenkins P, Ashton F, Christopher MR. Hypermobility: a risk factor for recurrent shoulder dislocations. British Journal of Sports Medicine. 2013;47:4-5.

78. Narendran LM, Mendez-Figueroa H, Chauhan SP, et al. Predictors of neonatal brachial plexus palsy subsequent to resolution of shoulder dystocia. The Journal of Maternal-Fetal & Neonatal Medicine. 2021;1-7.

79. Nawar K, Eliya Y, Burrow S, et al. Operative versus non-operative management of mid-diaphyseal clavicle fractures in the skeletally immature population: a systematic review and meta-analysis. Curr Rev Musculoskelet Med. 2020;13:38-49.

80. Neer CS, 2nd, Horwitz BS. Fractures of the proximal humeral epiphysial plate. Clin Orthop Relat Res. 1965;41:24-31.

81. Neville A, Jordan A, Beveridge JK, Pincus T, Noel M. Diagnostic uncertainty in youth with chronic pain and their parents. The Journal of Pain. 2019;20:1080-1090.

82. Noel M, Beals-Erickson SE, Law EF, Alberts NM, Palermo TM. Characterizing the pain narratives of parents of youth with chronic pain. The Clinical Journal of Pain. 2016;32:849-858.

83. Noel M, Chambers CT, McGrath PJ, Klein RM, Stewart SH. The influence of children's pain memories on subsequent pain experience. Pain. 2012;153:1563-1572.

84. Noel M, Rabbitts JA, Fales J, Chorney J, Palermo TM. The influence of pain memories on children's and adolescents' post-surgical pain experience: a longitudinal dyadic analysis. Health Psychology. 2017;36:987-995.

85. Noordin S, Allana S, Hilal K, et al. Osteoid osteoma: contemporary management. Orthop Rev (Pavia). 2018;10:7496-7496.

86. O'Neill BJ, Molloy AP, Curtin W. Conservative management of paediatric clavicle fractures. Int J Pediatr. 2011;2011:172571-172571.

87. Olds M, Donaldson K, Ellis R, Kersten P. In children 18 years and under, what promotes recurrent shoulder instability after traumatic anterior shoulder dislocation? A systematic review and meta-analysis of risk factors. British Journal of Sports Medicine. 2016;50:1135.

88. Orozco V, Balasubramanian S, Singh A. A systematic review of the electrodiagnostic assessment of neonatal brachial plexus. Neurol Neurobiol (Tallinn). 2020;3:10.31487/j.nnb.2020.02.12

89. Ottaviani G, Jaffe N. The epidemiology of osteosarcoma. Cancer Treatment and Research. 2009;152:3-13.

90. Paddock M, Sprigg A, Offiah AC. Imaging and reporting considerations for suspected physical abuse (non-accidental injury) in infants and young children. Part 2: axial skeleton and differential diagnoses. Clin Radiol. 2017;72:189-201.

91. Pandya NK, Baldwin KD, Wolfgruber H, Drummond DS, Hosalkar HS. Humerus fractures in the pediatric population: an algorithm to identify abuse. Journal of Pediatric Orthopaedics B. 2010;19:535-541.

92. Pastorello E, Cao M, Trevisan CP. Atypical onset in a series of 122 cases with facioscapulohumeral muscular dystrophy. Clinical Neurology and Neurosurgery. 2012;114:230-234.

93. Pincus T, Noel M, Jordan A, Serbic D. Perceived diagnostic uncertainty

in pediatric chronic pain. Pain. 2018;159:1198-1201.

94. Polchleb C, Messenger H. Management of an obstetric emergency. O&G Magazine. 2020;22.

95. Politi S, D'Emidio L, Cignini P, Giorlandino M, Giorlandino C. Shoulder dystocia: an evidence-based approach. J Prenat Med. 2010;4:35-42.

96. Popkin CA, Levine WN, Ahmad CS. Evaluation and management of pediatric proximal humerus fractures. J Am Acad Orthop Surg. 2015;23:77-86.

97. Post EG, Trigsted SM, Riekena JW, et al. The association of sport specialization and training volume with injury history in youth athletes. American Journal of Sports Medicine. 2017;45:1405-1412.

98. Rejeb A, Johnson A, Farooq A, et al. Sports injuries aligned to predicted mature height in highly trained Middle-Eastern youth athletes: a cohort study. BMJ Open. 2019;9:e023284.

99. Rennie L, Court-Brown C, Mok J, Beattie T. The epidemiology of fractures in children. Injury. 2007;38:913-922.

100. Rodis J. Shoulder Dystocia: Intrapartum Diagnosis, Management, and Outcome. UpToDate; 2021. Available at: https://www.uptodate.com/contents/shoulder-dystocia-intrapartum-diagnosis-management-and-outcome?topicRef=4472&source=see_link.

101. Roedl JB, Nevalainen M, Gonzalez FM, Dodson CC, Morrison WB, Zoga AC. Frequency, imaging findings, risk factors, and long-term sequelae of distal clavicular osteolysis in young patients. Skeletal Radiology. 2015;44:659-666.

102. Rosado N, Ryznar E, Flaherty EG. Understanding humerus fractures in young children: abuse or not abuse? Child Abuse & Neglect. 2017;73:1-7.

103. Rud NP, Reiman HM, Pritchard DJ, Frassica FJ, Smithson WA. Extraosseous Ewing's sarcoma. A study of 42 cases. Cancer. 1989;64:1548-1553.

104. Ryan LM. Proximal Humeral Fractures in Children. UpToDate; 2020. Available at: https://www.uptodate.com/contents/proximal-humeral-fractures-in-children?_escaped_fragment_=.

105. Salter RB, Harris WR. Injuries involving the epiphyseal plate. JBJS. 1963;45:587–622.

106. Shah A, Judge A, Delmestri A, et al. Incidence of shoulder dislocations in the UK, 1995-2015: a population-based cohort study. BMJ Open. 2017;7:e016112.

107. Shaw BA, Murphy KM, Shaw A, Oppenheim WL, Myracle MR. Humerus shaft fractures in young children: accident or abuse? Journal of Pediatric Orthopaedics. 1997;17:293-297.

108. Shrader MW. Proximal humerus and humeral shaft fractures in children. Hand Clinics. 2007;23:431-435.

109. Smucny M, Kolmodin J, Saluan P. Shoulder and elbow injuries in the adolescent athlete. Sports Medicine and Arthroscopy Review. 2016;24:188-194.

110. Sobhani-Eraghi A, Motalebi M, Sarreshtehdari S, Molazem-Sanandaji B, Hasanlu Z. Prevalence of joint hypermobility in children and adolescents: a systematic review and meta-analysis. Journal of Research in Medical Sciences. 2020;25:104.

111. Solomon L, Warwick D, Nayagam S. Apley's System of Orthopaedics and Fractures, 9th edition. London: Hodder Arnold; 2010.

112. Song MH, Yun YH, Kang K, Hyun MJ, Choi S. Nonoperative versus operative treatment for displaced midshaft clavicle fractures in adolescents: a comparative study. J Pediatr Orthop B. 2019;28:45-50.

113. Soto F, Fiesseler F, Morales J, Amato C. Presentation, evaluation, and treatment of clavicle fractures in preschool children presenting to an emergency department. Pediatric Emergency Care. 2009;25:744-747.

114. Statland JM, Tawil R. Facioscapulohumeral muscular dystrophy. Continuum (Minneapolis, Minn.). 2016;22:1916-1931.

115. Strait RT, Siegel RM, Shapiro RA. Humeral fractures without obvious etiologies in children less than 3 years of age: when is it abuse? Pediatrics. 1995;96:667-671.

116. Streja E, Miller JE, Bech BH, et al. Congenital cerebral palsy and prenatal exposure to self-reported maternal infections, fever, or smoking. American Journal of Obstetrics and Gynecology. 2013;209:332.e331-332.e310.

117. Talley N, O'Connor S. The paediatric history and examination. In: Clinical Examination, 8th edition. Elsevier; 2018.

118. Tan A, Strauss VY, Protheroe J, Dunn KM. Epidemiology of paediatric presentations with musculoskeletal problems in primary care. BMC Musculoskeletal Disorders. 2018;19:1-6.

119. Tanna V, Heathcote LC, Heirich MS, et al. Something else going on? Diagnostic uncertainty in children with chronic pain and their parents. Children-Basel. 2020;7:165.

120. Royal College of Paediatrics and Child Health. Establishing a correct diagnosis of Ehlers Danlos Syndrome hypermobility type (hEDS) in children and adolescents – position statement. Available at: https://www.rcpch.ac.uk/resources/establishing-correct-diagnosis-ehlers-danlos-syndrome-hypermobility-type-heds-children.

121. Watson L, Warby S, Balster S, Lenssen R, Pizzari T. The treatment of multidirectional instability of the shoulder with a rehabilitation program: Part 1. Shoulder Elbow. 2016;8:271-278.

122. Williams DJ, Jaggi A, Douglas T. The association between crawling as a first mode of mobilisation and the presentation of atraumatic shoulder instability: a retrospective cohort study. Shoulder & Elbow. 2021;13:339-344.

123. World Health Organization. Web Annexes A to K. In: Guidelines on the management of chronic pain in children. Available at: https://apps.who.int/iris/bitstream/handle/10665/337644/9789240017894-eng.pdf

124. Yarfi C, Elekusi C, Banson AN, Angmorterh SK, Kortei NK, Ofori EK. Prevalence and predisposing factors of brachial plexus birth palsy in a regional hospital in Ghana: a five year retrospective study. The Pan African Medical Journal. 2019;32:211.

125. Zaremski JL, Wright TW, Herman DC. Humeral stress fracture with median nerve injury in a baseball player: a case report and discussion. Current Sports Medicine Reports. 2018;17:183-186.

126. Zember J, Vega P, Rossi I, Rosenberg ZS. Normal development imaging pitfalls and injuries in the pediatric shoulder. Pediatr Radiol. 2019;49:1617-1628.

Biceps tendinopathy 26

Angela Spontelli Gisselman, Jeremy Lewis

Introduction

Pathology of the long head of biceps brachii tendon (LHBT) may result in dysfunction and pain experienced predominantly in the anterior region of the shoulder. The pathogenesis of tendinopathy of the long head of the biceps (LHB) tendon describes the physiological response of the tendon under excessive physiological load that results in pain and dysfunction.[26,88] Tendinopathy includes a continuum of pathologies that may occur to the LHBT, ranging from reactive tendinopathy, inflammation, to degenerative tendinosis and full-thickness tears.[26,93] LHB tendinopathy may also occur when the tendon is subject to repetitive, submaximal loading without appropriately paired unloading and recovery.[79,88] Lifestyle factors (Chapter 5) may also contribute to the development of symptoms. While isolated structural lesions of the LHBT do occur, the overwhelming majority of LHBT pathologies appear to occur alongside rotator cuff tears.[91,101,117] This has led to uncertainty if symptoms occur with isolated LHBT pathology or only in combination with other pathological processes.

Adding to the confusion is the disputed role of the LHBT at the shoulder joint. Despite these uncertainties, surgical procedures to address lesions of the LHBT, such as biceps tenodesis, have increased substantially.[10] The aim of this chapter is to investigate disorders of the LHBT, and present suggestions for assessment and management of LHB tendinopathy.

Anatomy

The biceps brachii is a primary flexor at the elbow, with its short head originating proximally at the coracoid process and long head attaching at the supraglenoid tubercle of the scapula. Distally the muscle attaches to the bicipital tuberosity of the radius. Given its attachment sites, biceps brachii also assists with elbow supination, and minimally with shoulder flexion. Looking specifically at the LHB, the tendon originates from the supraglenoid tubercle of the scapula and the posterior aspect of the superior glenoid labrum. The tendon traverses through the glenohumeral joint before exiting at the bicipital groove and terminating at the bicipital tuberosity.[35] The bicipital groove is a relatively shallow bony channel located between the lesser and greater tuberosities of the humerus. The groove has a bottleneck formation from top to bottom.[113]

Variations in the width, depth, and angle of the groove have been hypothesized as mechanisms leading to LHB pathology such as LHB tendinitis and LHBT instability, but uncertainty persists.[1,17,29,35,124] Within the bicipital groove the LHBT is stabilized by an entwined network of capsular ligaments including the superior glenohumeral ligament, coracohumeral ligament, and fibers from subscapularis and supraspinatus (Figure 26.1).[46,50] Collectively, these soft tissues are referred to as the biceps reflective pulley.[81,82] Injuries to this soft tissue sling have been associated with common shoulder pathologies including rotator cuff tears, shoulder instability, and biceps tears.[46,82] Arterial supply to the LHBT is provided by the thoracoacromial and brachial arteries at its boney and muscular junctions.[23] The LHBT receives neural innervation from the musculocutaneous nerve and boasts a rich supply of sensory sympathetic fibers that may play a role in tendon pain.[6,115,127]

Function of the long head of the biceps tendon

The challenges encountered with diagnosing and treating LHBT tendinopathy may first be attributed to the lack of a universally accepted role of the LHBT in glenohumeral kinematics. Findings from cadaveric investigations suggest that the LHBT actively depresses the humeral head,[67,122] a role confirmed in more recent research.[64,85,125] Other studies have demonstrated that the LHBT provides stabilization in the anterior and posterior directions at the shoulder,[56,57,96,104] and limits external rotation in varying degrees of shoulder abduction.[37] These findings remain uncertain following electromyographic studies demonstrating minimal biceps activity at the shoulder when movements of the elbow and forearm were restricted,[71] therefore challenging the role the LHBT plays in glenohumeral stability and positioning. In the presence of glenohumeral instability, the LHBT appears to contribute to dynamic joint stability when the arm is in vulnerable positions such as abduction and external rotation.[55,57,65] These conclusions seemingly contradict findings that the LHBT is a vestigial structure, having a negligible role in shoulder

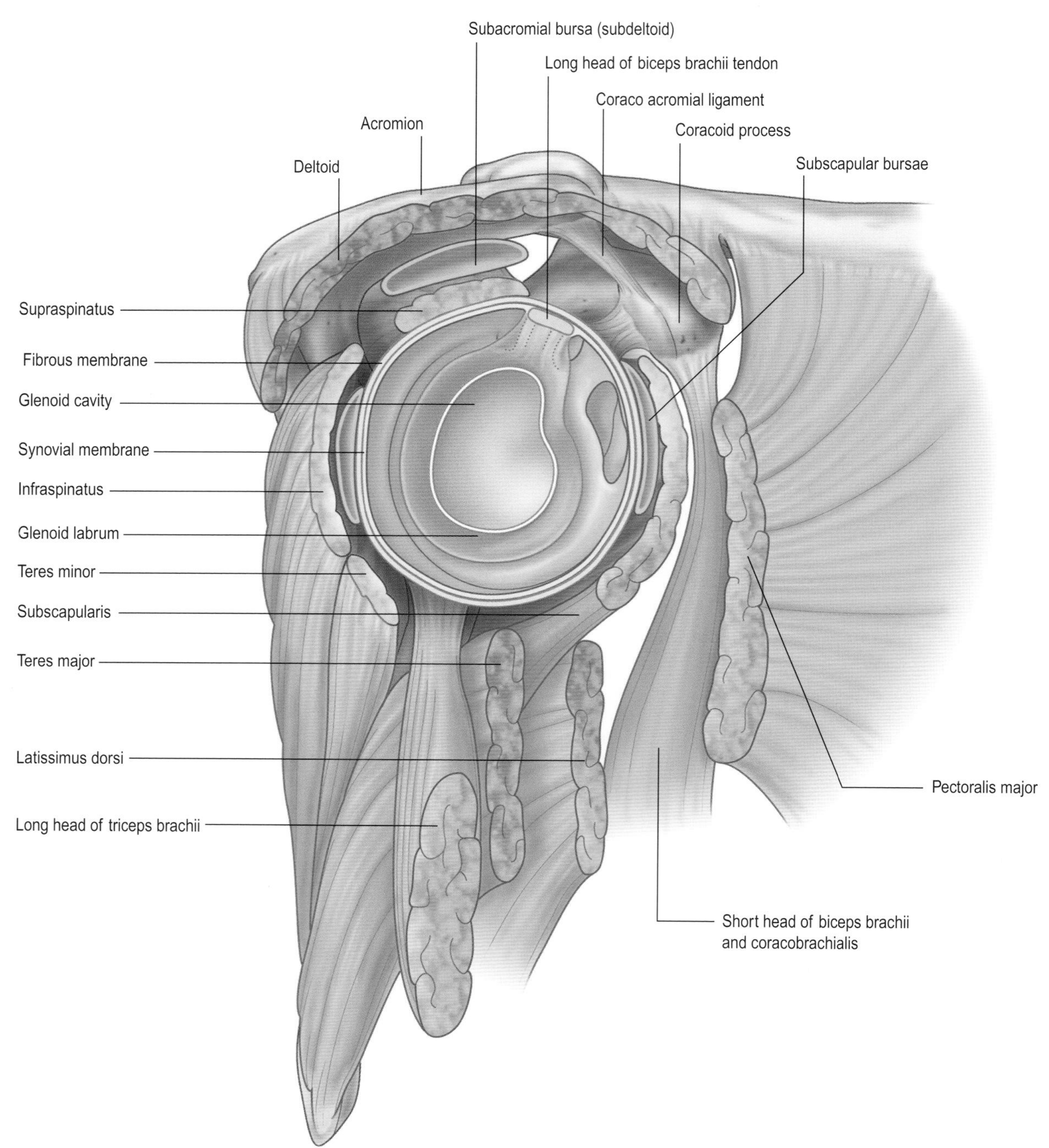

FIGURE 26.1
Lateral view of the right glenohumeral joint with humerus removed.
(Reproduced with permission from Drake R, Vogl AW, Mitchell A. Gray's Anatomy for Students, 4th edition. Elsevier; 2019.)

stability.[111] Biceps tenodesis involves surgically detaching the LHBT from the superior labrum and reattaching it below the humeral head to treat anterior shoulder pain attributed to LHB tendinopathy. Due to the contention that the LHBT plays a minimal role in glenohumeral stability, those recommending this procedure argue it may be performed with minimal consequences.

Our knowledge of the role of the LHBT at the shoulder is primarily based on in vitro experiments. The use of cadaver models present limitations that are important to evaluate. First, cadaveric models cannot account for the influence of muscular activity on the shoulder joint. Second, it is common in cadaveric studies that assess the effect of LHBT on glenohumeral motion to apply a weighted tension to the tendon prior to testing. While these may be considered appropriate biomechanical methods for the purposes of the research, the methods cannot mimic in vivo characteristics such as the role of energy transfer from the lower limb (Chapter 4), which may influence the study findings.[71]

In contrast to the preponderance of LHBT kinematic studies performed in vitro, relatively little research has been carried out in vivo. While there are in vivo studies [64,122] with results that corroborate previous in vitro findings, the external validity of their results is limited due to outdated imaging technology (i.e., use of anterior posterior radiographs that cannot capture three-dimensional movements or measurements). In fact, more recent investigations support the challenges made on the earlier hypothesized roles of the LHBT at the shoulder. One such study investigated the difference in glenohumeral position in patients who underwent unilateral and isolated biceps tenodesis with biplanar fluoroscopy.[43] Patients performed three dynamic shoulder positions and researchers compared glenohumeral motion of the operated and nonoperated shoulders. While a statistically significant difference in motion between the sides was reported, it never exceeded 1.5 mm (0.06 in) in any direction. Giphart et al.[43] concluded that this amount of motion change is unlikely to produce a clinically significant difference in patients following biceps tenodesis. Furthermore, it may support the contention that the LHBT is not a primary stabilizer of the humeral head. Ongoing research is required using more sophisticated techniques to measure musculoskeletal soft tissue strain and integrity such as implantable and biodegradable strain sensors to improve the reliability and validity of in vivo research,[130] but their current use is in its infancy.

The conflicting theories on the role of the LHBT may be explained by the fact that studying the tendon in isolation does not recognize its shared anatomy and relationship with the labrum. Given its intimate approximation with the labrum, some clinician researchers assert a more appropriate term to describe its anatomy is the biceps-labral complex.[82,114] Investigating the role of this complex versus its separate entities may provide a better understanding of the region's pathoanatomy and function. Another possible explanation for these contradicting findings is that the LHBT, much like stabilizing ligaments at the shoulder, may have a more prominent role as a passive stabilizer, especially in extreme shoulder positions.[68]

Pathophysiology

Clinically, LHB tendinopathy may range from a reactive tendinopathy to traumatic and degenerative full-thickness tears of the tendon.[26,84] The overwhelming majority of injuries to the LHBT, such as tendinopathy, coincide with rotator cuff pathologies.[21,28,91] In one study of 200 people who underwent subacromial decompression for shoulder pain and suspected "impingement" syndrome involving the LHBT, rotator cuff tears were identified in 91% of cases.[91] Furthermore, LHBT pathologies are even more prevalent in people with large to massive rotator cuff tears, with Chen et al. reporting 97% of patients with subscapularis tears had concomitant LHBT lesions.[21]

Isolated injuries of the LHBT are rare, but when they do occur, they are most common in middle aged individuals who experienced an abrupt eccentric force through the biceps.[19,41] Acute ruptures of the LHBT have been documented in younger overhead athletes when repeated overhead positioning and accumulating microtrauma to the tendon resulted in an LHBT tear.[76]

Since LHB tendinopathy is the predominant pathology reported, the remainder of this section will focus on the pathophysiology of tendinopathy. Our understanding of tendinopathy has evolved and will be presented before discussing management for people diagnosed with LHB tendinopathy.

Tendons are comprised primarily of type I collagen embedded in dense, regular connective tissue.[88] Due to their unique position between muscle belly and a bony attachment site, tendons are subject to large amounts of tensile or compressive strain.[32,79] Mechanical loading of a tendon contributes significantly to both the synthesis and degradation of collagen fibers.[32,79,94] Several cellular processes involved in tendon health are altered by mechanical loading, some of which include the release of metabolic and growth factors, changes in tendon blood flow, collagen synthesis, and proteolytic enzyme activity.[32,66,79,94] The manner by which a tendon responds to mechanical loading, known as mechanotransduction, is complex and is influenced by a number of intrinsic and extrinsic factors including the tendon's location and size;[121] the magnitude, direction, frequency, rate, and duration of the mechanical loading;[26,32,45] the history of tendon loading; age; and genetics.[26,87,88]

Several distinct theoretical models have been proposed to explain the course of tendinopathy and the relationship between tissue pathology and clinical presentation. Examples include theories that have focused on factors such as neuronal proliferation and collagen disruption, while other theories describe mechanical overload and tendon cell response to injury.[26,34,87,94] Although no single model can definitively accommodate all interactions between variables that determine tissue pathology and clinical presentation, researchers agree on two crucial factors in the development of tendon overuse injuries: the amount and type of load applied to the tendon and, critically, the tendon's physiological response to the load.[26,32,34,45,79,88]

In a healthy tendon under optimal loading, it is believed that an "ideal" inflammatory response occurs that maintains the balance between collagen degradation and collagen synthesis.[32,88,94,109] However, if the load exceeds the tendon's physiological capacity, excessive collagen degradation occurs, offsetting the balance between collagen breakdown and repair, leading to reduced tendon strength and function.[88,109,110] When normal tendon homeostasis is undermined, neuronal pathways within the tendon release inflammatory mediators, initiating an immunological cascade of events designed to address the damaged tissue.[109] These abnormal biological responses result in pathological, degenerative changes of the tendon that are also observed when a tendon is subject to repetitive, submaximal loading without appropriately paired unloading and recovery.[26,79,88]

Failure of the tendon's normal homeostatic responses results in early, or reactive, tendinopathy, and continued dysregulation of the tendon's repair processes can lead to persistent tendinopathy that is often observed in the LHBT.[26,88,110] Although the macrostructure of tendinopathy as observed with ultrasound or magnetic resonance imaging investigations appear similar in people with and without symptoms, it is possible that the pain may relate to biochemical imbalances within the tendon of people experiencing pain. This hypothesis requires investigation for LHB tendinopathy and for rotator cuff-related shoulder pain (Chapter 19).

Research comparing painful human tendinopathy with healthy controls suggests there is a significant change in the location and presence of autonomic, excitatory, and sensory neuromediators in an overused and painful tendon.[2,27,88] For example, in painful, tendinopathic Achilles tendons, a reduction of noradrenaline in vascular nerve fibers has been noted, whereas increases in acetylcholine are also observed.[2] Some of these inflammatory mediators released by the parasympathetic and sympathetic nervous systems are also believed to be responsible for activating nociceptors at the site of injury and subsequent pain associated with tendinopathy.[27,58,87] However, the origin of pain in tendinopathy remains a debated topic with opposing beliefs, incomplete information, and conflicting evidence.[75,88,100]

Assessment

A diagnosis of biceps tendinopathy is based on the combination of patient interview findings characteristic of tendinopathy, and pain-provoking examination procedures (i.e., physical examination tests). Due to the continuum of biceps tendinopathy, patients may present with distinct symptoms in early stages of reactive tendinopathy versus those in later stages of chronic, degenerative tendinopathy.[26,32,88] In either stage of the disease, patients' clinical symptoms mirror those with rotator cuff-related shoulder pain, and in some cases mimic symptoms associated with labral pathologies.[123] People with reactive tendinopathy may report shoulder pain that is localized to the anterior shoulder and sharp in nature. They may also report the pain is worse at night and can wake the patient when sleeping on the involved shoulder.[18] At later stages of tendinopathy, patients describe the pain as a deep, dull ache that is provoked with functional activities such as overhead movements, repetitive lifting or throwing, shoulder external rotation, and reaching behind the back.[18,88]

In either stage, patients may have pain that radiates down the anterior and/or lateral aspect of the shoulder and arm. This referral pain pattern warrants a thorough screening of the cervical spine and other regions that may refer pain to the shoulder (Chapter 16). When severe and in the early stages, the pain and movement guarding associated with LHB tendinopathy may mimic the presentation of an early frozen shoulder. In fact, Lippmann suggested that bicipital tenosynovitis may result in firm adhesions of the LHBT to the bicipital sheath and groove and be the cause of frozen shoulder.[74]

In contrast to patients with tendinopathy, those with an acute tear of the LHBT will likely present with a "Popeye" deformity (Figure 26.2) which may be accompanied by ecchymosis. The clinician will note palpable tenderness along the biceps muscle belly and the patient reports of significant pain with active elbow flexion and supination.[41] Unlike a traumatic rupture, biceps tendinopathy is not as easily diagnosed due to its frequent occurrence alongside other shoulder pathologies such as rotator cuff or labral pathologies.[93,117]

Numerous provocation tests have been developed for the shoulder, and several claim to isolate pathologies of the biceps tendon. Clinicians should be cautious when interpreting findings from any physical examination test which asserts that the maneuver can reliably discriminate between pain arising directly from LHBT versus pain arising from several structures that will also be stressed during testing (e.g., rotator cuff tendons, labrum, neural, vascular, capsular ligaments). Indeed, it is the intricate and intertwining anatomy of this region that is likely to blame for overall poor diagnostic accuracy of physical examination for biceps tendinopathy.

The most common physical examination tests used for biceps pathology are Speed's test, upper cut test, Yergason's test, and palpation of the bicipital groove. These tests have been referenced against the gold standard of diagnosis for

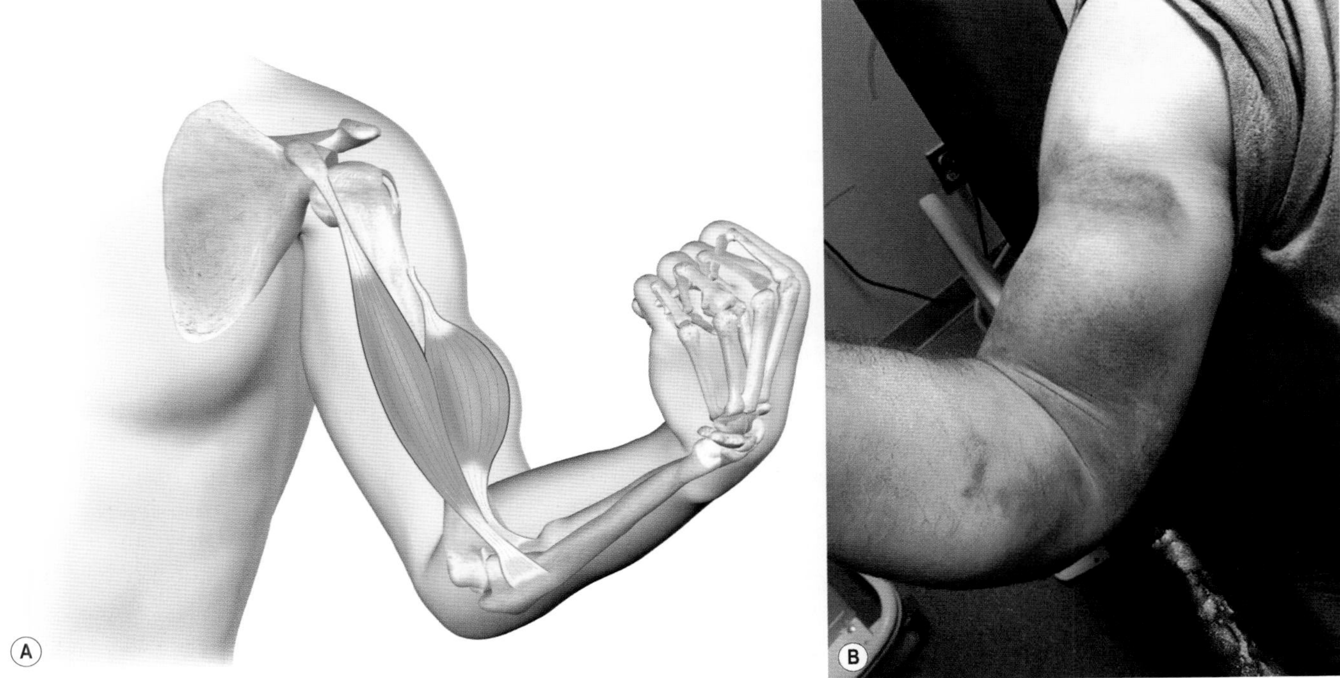

FIGURE 26.2

(A) Popeye deformity, named after the cartoon character created by Elzie Crisler Segar. (B) The deformity may be associated with ecchymosis after an acute tear.

(B, From Polvino DM, Wei G. Biceps tendon rupture. JETem. 2018. https://jetem.org/biceps_tendon_rupture/. Reproduced with permission from Grant Wei, MD.)

biceps tendinopathy (i.e., glenohumeral arthroscopy and/or magnetic resonance imaging), and have repeatedly demonstrated poor to moderate sensitivity, poor specificity, and low likelihood ratios.[9,18,44,51] For ruling in a diagnosis of LHBT pathology, the upper cut test is the most specific test available but provides only a small increase in probability of accurately diagnosing LHBT pathology (positive likelihood ratio (LR+) 3.38).[9,11]

Combining two physical examination tests, such as upper cut and Speed's test, or biceps palpation and Speed's test, improves the diagnostic accuracy, but again only marginally (LR+ 1.31).[42,51] Palpation of the biceps tendon does not provide any additional diagnostic accuracy, although it is commonly performed when attempting to confirm a diagnosis of LHBT pathology.[42] A recent study highlighted disappointing interrater reliability and poor accuracy (<50% accuracy rate) of experienced clinicians who aimed to palpate LHBT in asymptomatic participations.[83] The results of this study indicate that the most optimal position to palpate the LHBT remains unknown, and that examination findings derived from palpation alone should be interpreted with great caution. Table 26.1 details the clinical tests suggested to assess the LHBT.

Table 26.1 Clinical tests to assess the long head of biceps tendon

Test name	Description from original paper	Labral injury (No labral injury)	+LR (-LR)	Study population and notes
O'Brien's active compression[95]	Patient asked to forward flex the affected arm 90° with the elbow in full extension. The patient then adducted the arm 10° to 15° medial to the sagittal plane of the body. The arm was internally rotated so that the thumb pointed downward. The examiner then applied a uniform downward force to the arm. With the arm in the same position, the palm was then fully supinated, and the maneuver was repeated. The test was considered positive if pain was elicited with the first maneuver and was reduced or eliminated with the second maneuver. Pain localized to the acromioclavicular joint or on top of the shoulder was diagnostic of acromioclavicular joint abnormality. Pain or painful clicking described as inside the glenohumeral joint itself was indicative of labral abnormality.	53 (203)	∞ (0.02)	318 consecutive patients at the Hospital for Special Surgery New York – 50 with no shoulder pain, 50 subsequently excluded for "incorrect testing". Note: "...patient can distinguish between pain 'on top' of the shoulder (that is, at the acromioclavicular joint) and pain 'deep inside' the shoulder joint with or without a click."
Speed's test [12, 62]	Speed's test was performed with the patient's arm elevated to 90° of forward flexion, the elbow extended, and the forearm supinated. The examiner applied resistance distal to the elbow in the direction of arm extension. A positive test was indicated by localized pain over the bicipital groove.	10 (36)	1.05 (0.70)	Forty-six shoulders in 45 patients, 31 men (average age, 53 years; range, 16 to 76 years) and 14 women (average age, 64 years; range, 30 to 80 years) with 26 dominant and 20 nondominant extremities.
Upper cut test[11]	This maneuver was performed with the involved shoulder in a neutral position, the elbow flexed to 90°, the forearm supinated, and the patient making a fist. The patient was asked to rapidly bring the hand up and toward the chin – a boxing "upper cut" punch. The examiner placed his hand over the patient's fist and resisted the motion as the hand came up to the chin. A positive test was pain or a painful pop over the anterior portion of the involved shoulder during the resisted movement.	48 (101)	3.38 (0.34)	A total of 325 consecutive patients (age, 43.2 ± 12.6 years; 232 men and 93 women) who were seen at our center for shoulder pain...Of the 325 patients evaluated for shoulder pain, 101 patients (59 male, 42 female; mean age, 49 ± 15 years; age range, 28–64 years) underwent surgical intervention.
Yergason's test [11]	With the patient's elbow flexed to 90°, stabilized against the thorax, and forearm pronated, the examiner manually resisted supination while the patient also externally rotated the arm against resistance. A positive result was pain over the bicipital groove and/ or subluxation of the long head of the biceps brachii.	48 (101)	1.94 (0.74)	A total of 325 consecutive patients (age, 43.2 ± 12.6 years; 232 men and 93 women) who were seen at our center for shoulder pain...Of the 325 patients evaluated for shoulder pain, 101 patients (59 male, 42 female; mean age, 49 ± 15 years; age range, 28–64 years) underwent surgical intervention.

(Continued)

Table 26.1 *(Continued)*

Test name	Description from original paper	Labral injury (No labral injury)	+LR (-LR)	Study population and notes
Palpation of biceps tendon[42]	Eliciting point tenderness by palpation of the biceps tendon in the biceps groove 3–6 cm below the anterior acromion with the arm in approximately 10° of internal rotation…As the arm is moved through an internal-external range of rotation, the area of point tenderness should move with the arc of motion. A positive test result for bicipital groove tenderness was pain elicited in the bicipital groove to deep pressure in the involved shoulder compared with no pain elicited with similar pressure to the bicipital groove of the opposite shoulder.	5 (842)	1.13 (0.87)	Study population consisted of 847 patients who underwent diagnostic arthroscopy of the shoulder by the senior author…Because our study was designed to evaluate the clinical effectiveness of the examination only for partial tears of the biceps tendon and not for a wide variety of biceps injuries, no patient in this study had surgery to repair complete tears of the biceps tendon, SLAP lesions, or biceps dislocations.

∞, infinity; -LR, negative likelihood ratio; +LR, positive likelihood ratio; SLAP, superior labrum anterior to posterior.

Overall, the use of diagnostic imaging for biceps tendinopathy is not supported by the literature because pathological changes related to early and degenerative stages of tendinopathy are not easily identified on imaging.[9] Alternatively, diagnostic imaging of the LHBT may be useful when a partial or full-thickness tear of the tendon is suspected. Ultrasound provides high diagnostic accuracy for full-thickness tears and dislocations of the biceps tendon, but this relies heavily on a clinician with adequate experience in ultrasound imaging (Figures 26.3 and 26.4).[52] There is some evidence to suggest that ultrasound may assist in the diagnosis of reactive tendinopathy although the evidence for this is limited and debated.[52] Radiographs are limited in their direct evaluation of soft tissue but can provide a suitable evaluation of the bicipital groove and boney abnormalities such as osteophytes that may suggest LHBT pathology.[127] And while magnetic resonance arthrography is the most advanced imaging option, it has demonstrated conflicting validity and

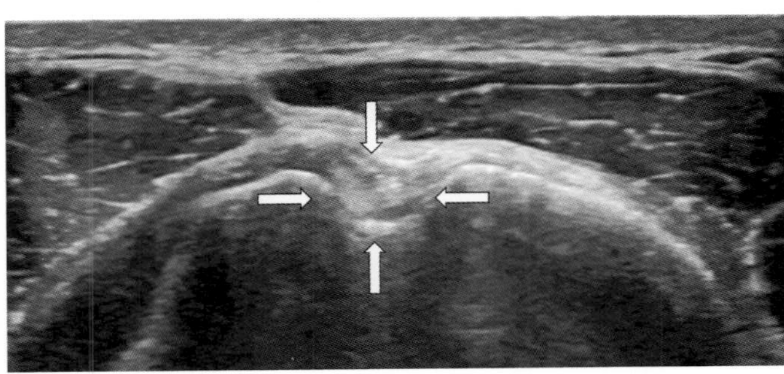

FIGURE 26.3

Ultrasound image of a healthy, intact long head of the biceps tendon in its normal position (arrows) within the intertubercular groove.

(Figure used with the kind permission of Mark Maybury, Research physiotherapist/sonographer, NIHR BRC Birmingham, University Hospitals Birmingham NHS Foundation Trust, UK.)

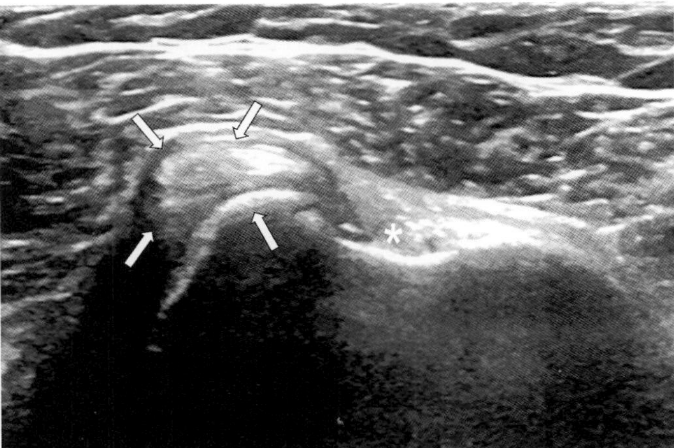

FIGURE 26.4

Ultrasound image of a long head of the biceps tendon (arrows) that has dislocated out of the intertubercular groove (asterisk).

(Figure used with the kind permission of Mark Maybury, Research physiotherapist/sonographer, NIHR BRC Birmingham, University Hospitals Birmingham NHS Foundation Trust, UK.)

reliability to identify pathological changes seen in biceps tendinopathy.[60,78,105]

Management

Nonsurgical

In contrast to the preponderance of treatment protocols for rotator cuff-related shoulder pain, currently there are no published protocols for the nonsurgical treatment of LHB tendinopathy. This paucity of evidence should come as no surprise given the entanglement of rotator cuff lesions and biceps tendon pathologies as previously discussed. Treatment of proximal biceps tendon pathology will vary according to patient presentation and the pathophysiology phenotype. Due to the concomitant presence of rotator cuff abnormalities with LHBT lesions, nonsurgical treatment of biceps tendinopathy commonly mirrors that of rotator cuff tendinopathy or rotator cuff-related shoulder pain[72,123] (this is presented in more detail in Chapter 36).

For people presenting with clinical signs and symptoms of reactive biceps tendinopathy, the initial phase of rehabilitation aims to minimize pain and protect the tendon from further aggravation. This is achieved by relative rest with discussion around keeping pain to a tolerable level and avoiding any activity-related increase in night pain or pain the following day. Adjunct treatments such as modalities, taping, direct dry needling, or injections should only be considered following a review of the research literature, and as part of a shared decision-making process where all anticipated benefits, timescales, and possible harms have been discussed.[53,88,106]

Injection therapies

Prescription of nonsteroidal anti-inflammatory drugs may be considered within the shared decision-making model for short-term pain control and reduction of inflammation.[5] While corticosteroid injections may be considered, it may be sensible to avoid direct injections to the LHBT and instead consider injecting in the subacromial space for an indirect benefit from the corticosteroid.[88,106]

Research on the efficacy of corticosteroid injections for LHB tendinopathy is sparse but studies investigating its use in rotator cuff tendinopathy support the consideration of injections for short-term pain relief (<8 weeks).[73,89] Ultrasound-guided injection of the LHBT is recommend for greater accuracy and reductions in pain compared to a landmark-guided approach.[49,83,128] Clinicians should exercise caution when performing repeated corticosteroid injections, especially for patients with persistent biceps tendinopathy due to documented adverse outcomes (i.e., tendon rupture) when injecting steroid directly at the LHBT.[24,99] Dry needling to the LHBT and biceps muscle belly may help reduce pain,[123] as may manual therapies if included in the early stages and embedded within an exercise program.[98]

The use of biologics, such as platelet rich plasma (PRP) injections, for the treatment of tendinopathy has grown exponentially in sports medicine but its clinical efficacy remains highly disputed.[15,36] The basic science of PRP asserts that its autologous whole-blood product promotes tendon healing and repair following injury.[15,129] The clinical outcomes of PRP on tendinopathy, however, are far from definitive.[15,22,77,86,88,90] There is a notable paucity of studies investigating PRP use in LHBT pathologies, with only one pilot study identified that enrolled eight participants and presented inadequate results.[54] Although there is evidence to support improvements in pain and function when using PRP for pathologies in other tendons (e.g., rotator cuff, Achilles, and patellar), these outcomes are primarily based on nonrandomized cohort studies or case series and need to be interpreted with caution.[30,36,86,90,112]

Most PRP studies to date have suffered from significant heterogeneity in research design and lack of a comparator to PRP.[22,36,90,112] Well-designed randomized clinical control trials have shown limited to no additional improvements in pain reduction or function when compared to placebo injection[61] or exercise interventions.[70] Indeed, these conflicting results have been repeatedly shown in over 20 systematic reviews and meta-analyses investigating PRP use for musculoskeletal conditions.[16,20,38,59,90,112,116] Taken together, the literature is insufficient to suggest the use of PRP for patients with bicipital tendinopathy.

Rehabilitation exercises

A critical component of rehabilitation for LHB tendinopathy, regardless of the tendinopathy phenotype, is loading of the tendon through exercise intervention.[26,32,79,88]

As mentioned, mechanotransduction is a principal physiological process responsible for tendon injury *and* subsequent repair.[79,94] At the cellular level, tendons require mechanical loading and unloading for normal adaptation and growth.[32,79,80] The challenge for clinicians is prescribing the appropriate type and dosage of progressive loading and unloading that promotes healthy, and not pathological, changes in the tendon. The role of tendon loading has become very well recognized in the research literature.[26,32,63] Cellular studies have reinforced understanding that complete rest leads to immediate and significant cessation of protein signaling and therefore tissue synthesis in injured tendons.[13,31,79] For this reason, a progressive loading program that is tailored to the individual should be introduced as promptly as possible[26,32] (see Chapter 36 for more information).

While numerous studies have reinforced the role of exercise for rotator cuff tendinopathy,[48] little empirical work has been done on exercise interventions specific to LHB tendinopathy. The exercise recommendations that follow represent an aggregation of evidence for rotator cuff tendinopathy, subacromial impingement syndrome, Achilles tendinopathy, and patellar tendinopathy that can be considered when treating bicipital tendinopathy. It is important to recognize, however, that there are limitations when applying literature related to Achilles and rotator cuff tendinopathy interventions given the distinctly different anatomical roles of various tendons throughout the body.

An exercise regimen for bicipital tendinopathy should address local and regional muscle performance deficits identified on examination. Exercises targeting the biceps tendon and its actions at both the shoulder and elbow should be incorporated alongside exercise for surrounding shoulder and periscapular musculature. Isolated resistance training of the biceps brachii may be best reserved for later stages of treatment when irritability is under control.[26,123]

Exercises that require rotator cuff muscle activation and dynamic stability of the glenohumeral joint will require increasing demands of the LHBT and are appropriate to incorporate in early stages of rehabilitation. Weight-bearing exercises may also be used to stimulate mechanoreceptors and address altered proprioception that may be present following injury.[123] Examples of weight-bearing exercises include wall or table push-ups, quadruped exercises (e.g., "bird-dog", single arm rows, single arm reverse fly), and prone planks. The mode, type, and dosage of exercise will vary and should be adjusted according to the stage of tendinopathy and the patient's clinical presentation.

Eccentric strengthening is often recommended as an early treatment option for tendinopathy due to the theory that eccentrics have a positive effect on neovascularization of a damaged tendon.[79] Eccentric exercise has shown to be beneficial in Achilles and patellar tendinopathies[108,126] but its role for shoulder tendinopathies remains unclear. More recently, literature has emerged that offers contradictory findings on the effects of eccentric exercise on rotator cuff tendinopathy.[69] When compared to other exercise, eccentric exercise provided a minimally improved effect on pain, but this did not reach the threshold for a statistically significant difference.[69] Additionally, eccentric exercise was not superior to any other form of exercise for improving function in patients with rotator cuff tendinopathy.[69] These results are not surprising when considering literature that highlights the similarities of cellular response to concentric and eccentric contractions.[39] Eccentric exercise remains useful for treating tendinopathy given that some respond well to eccentric exercise with less pain.[97] In summary, eccentric exercises should be considered, but not as the only intervention, and must be embedded within a graduated rehabilitation program (see Chapter 36).

Evidence from experimental studies has established the possible analgesic effects of isometric exercise on patients with tendinopathy.[40,102,103,120] However, systematic reviews indicate that isometric exercises are not superior to isotonic exercises in reduction of pain both immediately following the activity and at short-term follow-up.[25] In fact, ice therapy may be just as effective as isotonic exercise for short-term pain relief.[14,25] Although they may have a small role in symptom management, nonactive adjuncts, such as ice therapy and manual therapy, will not induce mechanotransduction and therefore do not result in tissue turnover or repair.[79]

Taken together, the evidence suggests there is no superior form of exercise (i.e., isometric versus isotonic) for pain reduction and/or improved function in patients with LHB tendinopathy. The research does indicate the importance of designing individualized and progressive exercise programs through a clinician–patient therapeutic alliance.[88] The alliance is critical to identify the patient's expectations and priorities for rehabilitation, and to foster optimal patient adherence. Tendon healing is a slow, gradual process that can take 6–12 months for full recovery. Clinicians should focus efforts on selecting exercises that those seeking care are willing to perform for at least 12 weeks.[88] Further, clinicians should remain cognizant to adjust exercise variables according to patient presentation.

Surgical

If nonsurgical management does not achieve the desired outcome, then surgery may be considered. Commonly, this involves biceps tenotomy or tenodesis. During a biceps tenotomy, the LHBT is detached from its origin and allowed to naturally retract through the bicipital groove. During tenodesis, after detaching the LHBT at its origin, it is reattached distally either above or below pectoralis major on the humeral shaft. An updated analysis of the American Board of Orthopedic Surgery Database revealed that the annual number of surgical interventions performed on patients with LHBT pathologies is significantly increasing.[10] This same study identified that while bicep tenotomy is on the decline, biceps tenodesis has become the predominant approach for LHB tendinopathy since 2008.[10] Given the association between rotator cuff and LHBT pathologies, it is unsurprising that men aged 50–60 years are most likely to receive surgical intervention for LHBT lesions.[10]

Recommending LHB tenodesis needs to be informed by the available research literature. Schrøder et al. randomized people with anterior shoulder pain attributed to a type II SLAP lesion into one of three arms: 40 people received a type II SLAP repair, 39 received a biceps tenodesis, and 39 received sham surgery involving insertion of a diagnostic arthroscope and a skin incision to mimic a labral repair.[107] All groups were immobilized after the procedure and received the same post-surgical rehabilitation. The mean age of participants was 40 years. At two-year follow-up, the findings of this three-arm, randomized, double-blinded, sham-controlled trial reported no difference between the groups. This important finding suggests that biceps tenodesis for anterior shoulder pain may not provide greater benefit than natural history or an exercise-based rehabilitation program. We therefore strongly recommend an exercise-based program (see Chapter 36) for a minimum of 12 weeks before considering surgery.

Currently, there is no consensus on which surgical approach, tenotomy or tenodesis, produces superior patient outcomes for patients with LHBT pathologies, or if surgery is required at all.[131] Compared with tenodesis, tenotomy is a less complex procedure with a shorter rehabilitation timeline. Adverse outcomes following a tenotomy include Popeye deformity, residual arm cramping, and perceived arm weakness,[119] but there is evidence which suggests that patients do not view these outcomes as unfavorably as previously reported.[3,33] These surgical complications may also occur following tenodesis, although patient-reported weakness and new or residual anterior shoulder pain are more commonly reported following tenodesis.[119] Tenodesis is a technically complex procedure with numerous surgical techniques to choose from such as determining the anatomic location of the tenodesis, or selecting the fixation method.[118] Tenodesis requires longer recovery time and has an increased risk of severe consequences such as humeral fractures, implant failure, reflex sympathetic dystrophy, and infection.[7,50,119]

Despite their disparate surgical methods, there are high-quality systematic reviews that state minimal difference in patient outcomes between the two procedures.[47,92,131] Whereas other reviews with meta-analyses suggest that tenodesis is the superior approach due to slightly improved functional outcomes at two years follow-up,[4,8] and less frequency of adverse outcomes such as Popeye deformity and arm cramping.[92] As with any surgical procedure, the decision to select a tenotomy versus tenodesis is best made when the patient and clinician use a shared decision-making model and engage in open dialogue focused on the patient's injury status, beliefs, and goals.

Conclusion

Despite the long-assumed role of the LHBT in anterior shoulder pain, there remain many unanswered questions and contradictions surrounding its biomechanical role, pathophysiology, and injury management. The findings of this chapter suggest there are three key points related to LHB tendinopathy. First, anatomy at the shoulder and the LHBT is integrated and complex, but our biomechanical studies to date do not reflect this complexity. An undisputed fact is the LHBT does not function in isolation and works alongside the rotator cuff and glenohumeral ligaments to provide active and passive stability at the shoulder joint. Most biomechanical investigations have failed to investigate the LHBT in coordination with other passive and dynamic stabilizers at the shoulder, therefore producing results that do not accurately reflect its true, in vivo function at the shoulder.

Second, the precise role of the LHBT in anterior shoulder pain remains disputed despite an increasingly popular notion that surgical removal of the LHBT (i.e., tenodesis or tenotomy) is an efficacious approach to managing LHB tendinopathy and related anterior shoulder pain. This trend should be concerning in light of emerging evidence that questions the clinical efficacy of surgery for LHBT pathologies where sham surgery produced equivalent outcomes in pain and function compared to patients who received biceps tenodesis.[107]

Third, and likely due to its close relationship with rotator cuff pathologies, there is a remarkable lack of research on nonsurgical rehabilitation protocols and best practice guidelines for managing LHB tendinopathy. The findings in this chapter draw our attention to the importance of adopting a more holistic and regional versus local approach to investigating LHB pathologies. To develop a holistic picture of the LHBT and improve our understanding of how to best manage pain related to the LHBT, it may be worthwhile to approach LHB tendinopathy alongside of, and not separate from, pathologies related to the rotator cuff.

References

1. Abboud JA, Bartolozzi AR, Widmer BJ, DeMola PM. Bicipital groove morphology on MRI has no correlation to intra-articular biceps tendon pathology. J Shoulder Elbow Surg. 2010;19:790-794.
2. Ackermann PW, Franklin SL, Dean BJ, Carr AJ, Salo PT, Hart DA. Neuronal pathways in tendon healing and tendinopathy: update. Front Biosci (Landmark Ed). 2014;19:1251-1278.
3. Aflatooni JO, Meeks BD, Froehle AW, Bonner KF. Biceps tenotomy versus tenodesis: patient-reported outcomes and satisfaction. J Orthop Surg Res. 2020;15:56.
4. Ahmed AF, Toubasi A, Mahmoud S, Ahmed GO, Al Ateeq Al Dosari M, Zikria BA. Long head of biceps tenotomy versus tenodesis: a systematic review and meta-analysis of randomized controlled trials. Shoulder & Elbow. 2020;1758573220942923.
5. Aicale R, Bisaccia RD, Oliviero A, Oliva F, Maffulli N. Current pharmacological approaches to the treatment of tendinopathy. Expert Opinion on Pharmacotherapy. 2020;21:1467-1477.
6. Alpantaki K, McLaughlin D, Karagogeos D, Hadjipavlou A, Kontakis G. Sympathetic and sensory neural elements in the tendon of the long head of the biceps. J Bone Joint Surg Am. 2005;87:1580-1583.
7. AlQahtani SM, Bicknell RT. Outcomes following long head of biceps tendon tenodesis. Curr Rev Musculoskelet Med. 2016;9:378-387.
8. Anil U, Hurley ET, Kingery MT, Pauzenberger L, Mullett H, Strauss EJ. Surgical treatment for long head of the biceps tendinopathy: a network meta-analysis. Journal of Shoulder and Elbow Surgery. 2020;29:1289-1295.
9. Bélanger V, Dupuis F, Leblond J, Roy JS. Accuracy of examination of the long head of the biceps tendon in the clinical setting: A systematic review. J Rehabil Med. 2019;51:479-491.
10. Belk JW, Jones SD, Thon SG, Frank RM. Trends in the treatment of biceps pathology: an analysis of the American Board of Orthopaedic Surgery Database. Orthop J Sports Med. 2020;8:2325967120969414.
11. Ben Kibler W, Sciascia AD, Hester P, Dome D, Jacobs C. Clinical utility of traditional and new tests in the diagnosis of biceps tendon injuries and superior labrum anterior and posterior lesions in the shoulder. Am J Sports Med. 2009;37:1840-1847.
12. Bennett WF. Specificity of the Speed's test: arthroscopic technique for evaluating the biceps tendon at the level of the bicipital groove. Arthroscopy. 1998;14:789-796.
13. Boesen AP, Dideriksen K, Couppé C, et al. Tendon and skeletal muscle matrix gene expression and functional responses to immobilisation and rehabilitation in young males: effect of growth hormone administration. J Physiol. 2013;591:6039-6052.
14. Bonello C, Girdwood M, De Souza K, et al. Does isometric exercise result in exercise induced hypoalgesia in people with local musculoskeletal pain? A systematic review. Phys Ther Sport. 2021;49:51-61.
15. Bowers RL, Troyer WD, Mason RA, Mautner KR. Biologics. Techniques in vascular and interventional radiology. 2020;23:100704.
16. Cai Y-Z, Zhang C, Lin X-J. Efficacy of platelet-rich plasma in arthroscopic repair of full-thickness rotator cuff tears: a meta-analysis. Journal of Shoulder and Elbow Surgery. 2015;24:1852-1859.
17. Cardoso A, Ferreira JN, Viegas R, et al. Radiographic evaluation of the bicipital groove morphology does not predict intraarticular changes in the long head of biceps tendon. Radiologia. 2020:S0033-8338(20)30162-4.
18. Carr RM, Shishani Y, Gobezie R. How accurate are we in detecting biceps tendinopathy? Clin Sports Med. 2016;35:47-55.
19. Carter AN, Erickson SM. Proximal biceps tendon rupture: primarily an injury of middle age. Phys Sportsmed. 1999;27:95-101.
20. Chahal J, Van Thiel GS, Mall N, et al. The role of platelet-rich plasma in arthroscopic rotator cuff repair: a systematic review with quantitative synthesis. Arthroscopy. 2012;28:1718-1727.
21. Chen C-H, Hsu K-Y, Chen W-J, Shih C-H. Incidence and severity of biceps long-head tendon lesion in patients with complete rotator cuff tears. Journal of Trauma and Acute Care Surgery. 2005;58:1189-93.
22. Chen X, Jones IA, Togashi R, Park C, Vangsness CT. Use of platelet-rich plasma for the improvement of pain and function in rotator cuff tears: a systematic review and

meta-analysis with bias assessment. Am J Sports Med. 2019;48:2028-2041.

23. Cheng NM, Pan W-R, Vally F, Le Roux CM, Richardson MD. The arterial supply of the long head of biceps tendon: anatomical study with implications for tendon rupture. Clinical Anatomy. 2010;23:683-692.

24. Childress MA, Beutler A. Management of chronic tendon injuries. Am Fam Physician. 2013;87:486-490.

25. Clifford C, Challoumas D, Paul L, Syme G, Millar NL. Effectiveness of isometric exercise in the management of tendinopathy: a systematic review and meta-analysis of randomised trials. BMJ Open Sport & Exercise Medicine. 2020;6:e000760.

26. Cook JL, Rio E, Purdam CR, Docking SI. Revisiting the continuum model of tendon pathology: what is its merit in clinical practice and research? Br J Sports Med. 2016;50:1187.

27. Dean BJ, Gwilym SE, Carr AJ. Why does my shoulder hurt? A review of the neuroanatomical and biochemical basis of shoulder pain. Br J Sports Med. 2013;47:1095-1104.

28. Desai SS, Mata HK. Long head of biceps tendon pathology and results of tenotomy in full-thickness reparable rotator cuff tear. Arthroscopy. 2017;33:1971-1976.

29. Deurzen DFP, Garssen FL, Kerkhoffs GMMJ, Bleys RLAW, Have I, Bekerom MPJ. Clinical relevance of the anatomy of the long head bicipital groove, an evidence-based review. Clinical Anatomy. 2021;34(2):199-208.

30. Di Matteo B, Filardo G, Kon E, Marcacci M. Platelet-rich plasma: evidence for the treatment of patellar and Achilles tendinopathy: a systematic review. Musculoskeletal Surgery. 2015;99:1-9.

31. Dideriksen K, Boesen AP, Reitelseder S, et al. Tendon collagen synthesis declines with immobilization in elderly humans: no effect of anti-inflammatory medication. J Appl Physiol. 2017;122:273-282.

32. Docking SI, Cook J. How do tendons adapt? Going beyond tissue responses to understand positive adaptation and pathology development: a narrative review. J Musculoskelet Neuronal Interact. 2019;19:300-310.

33. Duff SJ, Campbell PT. Patient acceptance of long head of biceps brachii tenotomy. Journal of Shoulder and Elbow Surgery. 2012;21:61-65.

34. Durgam S, Stewart M. Cellular and molecular factors influencing tendon repair. Tissue Engineering Part B: Reviews. 2017;23:307-317.

35. Elser F, Braun S, Dewing CB, Giphart JE, Millett PJ. Anatomy, function, injuries, and treatment of the long head of the biceps brachii tendon. Arthroscopy. 2011;27:581-592.

36. Engebretsen L, Steffen K, Alsousou J, et al. IOC consensus paper on the use of platelet-rich plasma in sports medicine. Br J Sports Med. 2010;44:1072.

37. Eshuis R, De Gast A. Role of the long head of the biceps brachii muscle in axial humeral rotation control. Clin Anat. 2012;25:737-745.

38. Fu C-J, Sun J-B, Bi Z-G, Wang X-M, Yang C-L. Evaluation of platelet-rich plasma and fibrin matrix to assist in healing and repair of rotator cuff injuries: a systematic review and meta-analysis. Clinical Rehabilitation. 2016;31:158-172.

39. Garma T, Kobayashi C, Haddad F, Adams GR, Bodell PW, Baldwin KM. Similar acute molecular responses to equivalent volumes of isometric, lengthening, or shortening mode resistance exercise. J Appl Physiol. 2007;102:135-143.

40. Gatz M, Betsch M, Dirrichs T, et al. Eccentric and isometric exercises in Achilles tendinopathy evaluated by the VISA-A score and shear wave elastography. Sports Health. 2020;12:373-381.

41. Geaney LE, Mazzocca AD. Biceps brachii tendon ruptures: a review of diagnosis and treatment of proximal and distal biceps tendon ruptures. The Physician and Sportsmedicine. 2010;38:117-125.

42. Gill HS, El Rassi G, Bahk MS, Castillo RC, McFarland EG. Physical examination for partial tears of the biceps tendon. Am J Sports Med. 2007;35:1334-1340.

43. Giphart JE, Elser F, Dewing CB, Torry MR, Millett PJ. The long head of the biceps tendon has minimal effect on in vivo glenohumeral kinematics: a biplane fluoroscopy study. Am J Sports Med. 2011;40:202-212.

44. Gismervik SØ, Drogset JO, Granviken F, Rø M, Leivseth G. Physical examination tests of the shoulder: a systematic review and meta-analysis of diagnostic test performance. BMC Musculoskelet Disord. 2017;18:41.

45. Glasgow P, Phillips N, Bleakley C. Optimal loading: key variables and mechanisms. Br J Sports Med. 2015;49:278.

46. Godenèche A, Nové-Josserand L, Audebert S, Toussaint B, Denard PJ, Lädermann A. Relationship between subscapularis tears and injuries to the biceps pulley. Knee Surgery, Sports Traumatology, Arthroscopy. 2017;25:2114-2120.

47. Gurnani N, van Deurzen DFP, Janmaat VT, van den Bekerom MPJ. Tenotomy or tenodesis for pathology of the long head of the biceps brachii: a systematic review and meta-analysis. Knee Surgery, Sports Traumatology, Arthroscopy. 2016;24:3765-3771.

48. Hanratty CE, McVeigh JG, Kerr DP, et al. The effectiveness of physiotherapy exercises in subacromial impingement syndrome: a systematic review and meta-analysis. Semin Arthritis Rheum. 2012;42:297-316.

49. Hashiuchi T, Sakurai G, Morimoto M, Komei T, Takakura Y, Tanaka Y. Accuracy of the biceps tendon sheath injection: ultrasound-guided or unguided injection? A randomized controlled trial. Journal of Shoulder and Elbow Surgery. 2011;20:1069-1073.

50. Hassan S, Patel V. Biceps tenodesis versus biceps tenotomy for biceps tendinitis without rotator cuff tears. Journal of Clinical Orthopaedics and Trauma. 2019;10:248-256.

51. Hegedus EJ, Goode AP, Cook CE, et al. Which physical examination tests provide clinicians with the most value when examining the shoulder? Update of a systematic review with meta-analysis of individual tests. Br J Sports Med. 2012;46:964.

52. Henderson REA, Walker BF, Young KJ. The accuracy of diagnostic ultrasound imaging for musculoskeletal soft tissue pathology of the extremities: a comprehensive review of the literature. Chiropr Man Therap. 2015;23:31-31.

53. Holshouser C, Jayaseelan DJ. Multifaceted exercise prescription in the management of an overhead athlete with suspected distal biceps tendinopathy: A case report. J Funct Morphol Kinesiol. 2020;5:56.

54. Ibrahim VM, Groah SL, Libin A, Ljungberg IH. Use of platelet rich plasma for the treatment of bicipital tendinopathy in

spinal cord injury: a pilot study. Top Spinal Cord Inj Rehabil. 2012;18:77-78.

55. Itoi E, Kuechle DK, Newman SR, Morrey BF, An KN. Stabilising function of the biceps in stable and unstable shoulders. J Bone Joint Surg Br. 1993;75:546-550.

56. Itoi E, Motzkin NE, Morrey BF, An K-N. Stabilizing function of the long head of the biceps in the hanging arm position. Journal of Shoulder and Elbow Surgery. 1994;3:135-142.

57. Itoi E, Newman SR, Kuechle DK, Morrey BF, An KN. Dynamic anterior stabilisers of the shoulder with the arm in abduction. J Bone Joint Surg Br. 1994;76:834-836.

58. Jewson JL, Lambert EA, Docking S, Storr M, Lambert GW, Gaida JE. Pain duration is associated with increased muscle sympathetic nerve activity in patients with Achilles tendinopathy. Scandinavian Journal of Medicine & Science in Sports. 2017;27:1942-1949.

59. Johal H, Khan M, Yung S-hP, et al. Impact of platelet-rich plasma use on pain in orthopaedic surgery: a systematic review and meta-analysis. Sports Health. 2019;11:355-366.

60. Kang Y, Lee JW, Ahn JM, Lee E, Kang HS. Instability of the long head of the biceps tendon in patients with rotator cuff tear: evaluation on magnetic resonance arthrography of the shoulder with arthroscopic correlation. Skeletal Radiology. 2017;46:1335-1342.

61. Keene DJ, Alsousou J, Harrison P, et al. Platelet rich plasma injection for acute Achilles tendon rupture: PATH-2 randomised, placebo controlled, superiority trial. BMJ. 2019;367:l6132.

62. Kibler B, Sciascia AD, Hester P, Dome D, Jacobs C. Clinical utility of traditional and new tests in the diagnosis of biceps tendon injuries and superior labrum anterior and posterior lesions in the shoulder. Am J Sports Med. 2009;37:1840-1847.

63. Kibler WB, Chandler TJ, Stracener ES. Musculoskeletal adaptations and injuries due to overtraining. Exerc Sport Sci Rev. 1992;20:99-126.

64. Kido T, Itoi E, Konno N, Sano A, Urayama M, Sato K. The depressor function of biceps on the head of the humerus in shoulders with tears of the rotator cuff. The Journal of Bone and Joint Surgery. 2000;82-B:416-419.

65. Kim SH, Ha KI, Kim HS, Kim SW. Electromyographic activity of the biceps brachii muscle in shoulders with anterior instability. Arthroscopy. 2001;17:864-868.

66. Kjaer M, Bayer ML, Eliasson P, Heinemeier KM. What is the impact of inflammation on the critical interplay between mechanical signaling and biochemical changes in tendon matrix? Journal of Applied Physiology. 2013;115:879-883.

67. Kumar VP, Satku K, Balasubramaniam P. The role of the long head of biceps brachii in the stabilization of the head of the humerus. Clin Orthop Relat Res. 1989;172-175.

68. Landin D, Thompson M, Jackson MR. Actions of the biceps brachii at the shoulder: a review. J Clin Med Res. 2017;9:667-670.

69. Larsson R, Bernhardsson S, Nordeman L. Effects of eccentric exercise in patients with subacromial impingement syndrome: a systematic review and meta-analysis. BMC Musculoskelet Disord. 2019;20:446.

70. Lee H-W, Choi K-H, Kim J-Y, Yang I, Noh K-C. Prospective clinical research of the efficacy of platelet-rich plasma in the outpatient-based treatment of rotator cuff tendinopathy. Clin Shoulder Elbow. 2019;22:61-69.

71. Levy AS, Kelly BT, Lintner SA, Osbahr DC, Speer KP. Function of the long head of the biceps at the shoulder: electromyographic analysis. J Shoulder Elbow Surg. 2001;10:250-255.

72. Lewis J. Rotator cuff related shoulder pain: assessment, management and uncertainties. Manual Therapy. 2016;23:57-68.

73. Lin M-T, Chiang C-F, Wu C-H, Huang Y-T, Tu Y-K, Wang T-G. Comparative effectiveness of injection therapies in rotator cuff tendinopathy: a systematic review, pairwise and network meta-analysis of randomized controlled trials. Archives of Physical Medicine and Rehabilitation. 2019;100:336-349.e315.

74. Lippmann RK. Frozen shoulder; periarthritis; bicipital tenosynovitis. Archives of Surgery. 1943;47:283-296.

75. Littlewood C, Malliaras P, Bateman M, Stace R, May S, Walters S. The central nervous system – an additional consideration in 'rotator cuff tendinopathy' and a potential basis for understanding response to loaded therapeutic exercise. Manual Therapy. 2013;18:468-472.

76. Liu X, Tan AHC. Rupture of the long head of the biceps brachii tendon near the musculotendinous junction in a young patient: a case report. World J Orthop. 2020;11:123-128.

77. Loiacono C, Palermi S, Massa B, et al. Tendinopathy: Pathophysiology, therapeutic options, and role of nutraceutics. A narrative literature review. Medicina (Kaunas). 2019;55:447.

78. Loock E, Michelet A, D'Utruy A, et al. Magnetic resonance arthrography is insufficiently accurate to diagnose biceps lesions prior to rotator cuff repair. Knee Surgery, Sports Traumatology, Arthroscopy. 2019;27:3970-3978.

79. Magnusson SP, Kjaer M. The impact of loading, unloading, ageing and injury on the human tendon. The Journal of Physiology. 2019;597:1283-1298.

80. Magnusson SP, Langberg H, Kjaer M. The pathogenesis of tendinopathy: balancing the response to loading. Nature Reviews Rheumatology. 2010;6:262-268.

81. Martetschläger F, Tauber M, Habermeyer P. Injuries to the biceps pulley. Clin Sports Med. 2016;35:19-27.

82. Martetschläger F, Zampeli F, Tauber M, Habermeyer P. Lesions of the biceps pulley: a prospective study and classification update. JSES International. 2020;4:318-323.

83. McDevitt AW, Cleland JA, Strickland C, et al. Accuracy of long head of the biceps tendon palpation by physical therapists; an ultrasonographic study. Journal of Physical Therapy Science. 2020;32:760-767.

84. McFarland EG, Borade A. Examination of the biceps tendon. Clinics in Sports Medicine. 2016;35:29-45.

85. McGarry MH, Nguyen ML, Quigley RJ, Hanypsiak B, Gupta R, Lee TQ. The effect of long and short head biceps loading on glenohumeral joint rotational range of motion and humeral head position. Knee Surgery, Sports Traumatology, Arthroscopy. 2016;24:1979-1987.

86. Milano G, Sánchez M, Jo CH, Saccomanno MF, Thampatty BP, Wang JHC. Platelet-rich plasma in orthopaedic sports medicine: state of the art. Journal of ISAKOS. 2019;4:188.

87. Millar NL, Murrell GAC, McInnes IB. Inflammatory mechanisms in tendinopathy

– towards translation. Nature Reviews Rheumatology. 2017;13:110-122.

88. Millar NL, Silbernagel KG, Thorborg K, et al. Tendinopathy. Nature Reviews Disease Primers. 2021;7:1.

89. Mohamadi A, Chan JJ, Claessen FMAP, Ring D, Chen NC. Corticosteroid injections give small and transient pain relief in rotator cuff tendinosis: a meta-analysis. Clinical Orthopaedics and Related Research. 2017;475:232-243.

90. Moraes VY, Lenza M, Tamaoki MJ, Faloppa F, Belloti JC. Platelet-rich therapies for musculoskeletal soft tissue injuries. Cochrane Database of Systematic Reviews. 2014;CD010071.

91. Murthi AM, Vosburgh CL, Neviaser TJ. The incidence of pathologic changes of the long head of the biceps tendon. J Shoulder Elbow Surg. 2000;9:382-385.

92. Na Y, Zhu Y, Shi Y, et al. A meta-analysis comparing tenotomy or tenodesis for lesions of the long head of the biceps tendon with concomitant reparable rotator cuff tears. J Orthop Surg Res. 2019;14:370.

93. Nho SJ, Strauss EJ, Lenart BA, et al. Long head of the biceps tendinopathy: diagnosis and management. JAAOS. 2010;18:645-656.

94. Nourissat G, Berenbaum F, Duprez D. Tendon injury: from biology to tendon repair. Nature Reviews Rheumatology. 2015;11:223-233.

95. O'Brien SJ, Pagnani MJ, Fealy S, McGlynn SR, Wilson JB. The active compression test: a new and effective test for diagnosing labral tears and acromioclavicular joint abnormality. Am J Sports Med. 1998;26:610-613.

96. Pagnani MJ, Deng X-H, Warren RF, Torzilli PA, O'Brien SJ. Role of the long head of the biceps brachii in glenohumeral stability: a biomechanical study in cadavera. Journal of Shoulder and Elbow Surgery. 1996;5:255-262.

97. Peterson M, Butler S, Eriksson M, Svärdsudd K. A randomized controlled trial of eccentric vs. concentric graded exercise in chronic tennis elbow (lateral elbow tendinopathy). Clin Rehabil. 2014;28:862-872.

98. Pieters L, Lewis J, Kuppens K, et al. An update of systematic reviews examining the effectiveness of conservative physical therapy interventions for subacromial shoulder pain. J Orthop Sports Phys Ther. 2020;50:131-141.

99. Puzzitiello RN, Patel BH, Nwachukwu BU, Allen AA, Forsythe B, Salzler MJ. Adverse impact of corticosteroid injection on rotator cuff tendon health and repair: a systematic review. Arthroscopy. 2020;36:1468-1475.

100. Raney EB, Thankam FG, Dilisio MF, Agrawal DK. Pain and the pathogenesis of biceps tendinopathy. Am J Transl Res. 2017;9:2668-2683.

101. Redondo-Alonso L, Chamorro-Moriana G, Jiménez-Rejano JJ, López-Tarrida P, Ridao-Fernández C. Relationship between chronic pathologies of the supraspinatus tendon and the long head of the biceps tendon: systematic review. BMC Musculoskelet Disord. 2014;15:377.

102. Rio E, Kidgell D, Purdam C, et al. Isometric exercise induces analgesia and reduces inhibition in patellar tendinopathy. Br J Sports Med. 2015;49:1277.

103. Rio E, van Ark M, Docking S, et al. Isometric contractions are more analgesic than isotonic contractions for patellar tendon pain: an in-season randomized clinical trial. Clin J Sport Med. 2017;27:253-259.

104. Rodosky MW, Harner CD, Fu FH. The role of the long head of the biceps muscle and superior glenoid labrum in anterior stability of the shoulder. Am J Sports Medicine. 1994;22:121-130.

105. Rosenthal J, Nguyen ML, Karas S, et al. A comprehensive review of the normal, abnormal, and post-operative MRI appearance of the proximal biceps brachii. Skeletal Radiol. 2020;49:1333-1344.

106. Schickendantz M, King D. Nonoperative management (including ultrasound-guided injections) of proximal biceps disorders. Clinics in Sports Medicine. 2016;35:57-73.

107. Schrøder CP, Skare Ø, Reikerås O, Mowinckel P, Brox JI. Sham surgery versus labral repair or biceps tenodesis for type II SLAP lesions of the shoulder: a three-armed randomised clinical trial. Br J Sports Med. 2017;51:1759.

108. Sprague AL, Couppé C, Pohlig RT, Snyder-Mackler L, Silbernagel KG. Pain-guided activity modification during treatment for patellar tendinopathy: a feasibility and pilot randomized clinical trial. Pilot and Feasibility Studies. 2021;7:58.

109. Steinmann S, Pfeifer CG, Brochhausen C, Docheva D. Spectrum of tendon pathologies: triggers, trails and end-state. Int J Mol Sci. 2020;21:844.

110. Streit JJ, Shishani Y, Rodgers M, Gobezie R. Tendinopathy of the long head of the biceps tendon: histopathologic analysis of the extra-articular biceps tendon and tenosynovium. Open Access J Sports Med. 2015;6:63-70.

111. Szabó I, Boileau P, Walch G. The proximal biceps as a pain generator and results of tenotomy. Sports Med Arthroscopy Rev. 2008;16:180-6.

112. Taylor DW, Petrera M, Hendry M, Theodoropoulos JS. A systematic review of the use of platelet-rich plasma in sports medicine as a new treatment for tendon and ligament injuries. Clin J Sport Med. 2011;21:344-352.

113. Taylor SA, Fabricant PD, Bansal M, et al. The anatomy and histology of the bicipital tunnel of the shoulder. Journal of Shoulder and Elbow Surgery. 2015;24:511-519.

114. Taylor SA, O'Brien SJ. Clinically relevant anatomy and biomechanics of the proximal biceps. Clinics in Sports Medicine. 2016;35:1-18.

115. Tosounidis T, Hadjileontis C, Triantafyllou C, Sidiropoulou V, Kafanas A, Kontakis G. Evidence of sympathetic innervation and α1-adrenergic receptors of the long head of the biceps brachii tendon. J Orthop Sci. 2013;18:238-244.

116. Vavken P, Sadoghi P, Palmer M, et al. Platelet-rich plasma reduces retear rates after arthroscopic repair of small- and medium-sized rotator cuff tears but is not cost-effective. Am J Sports Med. 2015;43:3071-3076.

117. Vestermark GL, Van Doren BA, Connor PM, Fleischli JE, Piasecki DP, Hamid N. The prevalence of rotator cuff pathology in the setting of acute proximal biceps tendon rupture. Journal of Shoulder and Elbow Surgery. 2018;27:1258-1262.

118. Virk MS, Cole BJ. Proximal biceps tendon and rotator cuff tears. Clinics in Sports Medicine. 2016;35:153-161.

119. Virk MS, Nicholson GP. Complications of proximal biceps tenotomy and tenodesis. Clinics in Sports Medicine. 2016;35:181-188.

120. Vuvan V, Vicenzino B, Mellor R, Heales LJ, Coombes BK. Unsupervised isometric exercise versus wait-and-see for lateral elbow tendinopathy. Medicine & Science in Sports & Exercise. 2020;52:287-295.

121. Wang JHC, Guo Q, Li B. Tendon biomechanics and mechanobiology: a minireview of basic concepts and recent

advancements. Journal of Hand Therapy. 2012;25:133-141.

122. Warner JJ, McMahon PJ. The role of the long head of the biceps brachii in superior stability of the glenohumeral joint. J Bone Joint Surg Am. 1995;77:366-372.

123. Wilk KE, Hooks TR. The painful long head of the biceps brachii: nonoperative treatment approaches. Clinics in Sports Medicine. 2016;35:75-92.

124. Yoo JC, Iyyampillai G, Park D, Koh KH. The influence of bicipital groove morphology on the stability of the long head of the biceps tendon. J Orthop Surg. 2017;25:2309499017717195.

125. Youm T, ElAttrache NS, Tibone JE, McGarry MH, Lee TQ. The effect of the long head of the biceps on glenohumeral kinematics. Journal of Shoulder and Elbow Surgery. 2009;18:122-129.

126. Young MA, Cook JL, Purdam CR, Kiss ZS, Alfredson H. Eccentric decline squat protocol offers superior results at 12 months compared with traditional eccentric protocol for patellar tendinopathy in volleyball players. Br J Sports Med. 2005;39:102-105.

127. Zappia M, Chianca V, Di Pietto F, et al. Imaging of long head biceps tendon. A multimodality pictorial essay. Acta Biomed. 2019;90:84-94.

128. Zhang J, Ebraheim N, Lause GE. Ultrasound-guided injection for the biceps brachii tendinitis: results and experience. Ultrasound in Medicine and Biology. 2011;37:729-733.

129. Zhang J, Wang JHC. Platelet-rich plasma releasate promotes differentiation of tendon stem cells into active tenocytes. Am J Sports Med. 2010;38:2477-2486.

130. Zhang Q, Adam NC, Hosseini Nasab SH, Taylor WR, Smith CR. Techniques for in vivo measurement of ligament and tendon strain: a review. Annals of Biomedical Engineering. 2021;49:7-28.

131. Zhou P, Liu J, Deng X, Li Z. Biceps tenotomy versus tenodesis for lesions of the long head of the biceps tendon: a systematic review and meta-analysis of randomized controlled trials. Medicine (Baltimore). 2021;100:e23993-e23993.

27 Calcific tendinopathy

Mitchell Simpson, Jeremy Lewis

Introduction

Many symptomatic shoulder conditions are associated with the rotator cuff tendons, one of which is calcific tendinopathy. This condition is characterized by the presence of calcium deposits of varying sizes within the tendons. Calcium deposits are commonly seen in people without shoulder pain, and when associated with symptoms, the condition is diagnosed as rotator cuff calcific tendinopathy (RCCT). The deposits appear to be symptomatic in approximately 30–50% of cases;[52,73] RCCT manifests most frequently in middle-aged adults,[7,18,46,84] and is more common in women.[46,60] Why some people remain asymptomatic and others experience severe pain and morbidity remains uncertain.

Asymptomatic calcifications are generally identified incidentally on imaging. When symptoms are present, RCCT is commonly associated with often substantial pain, tenderness near the greater tuberosity of the humerus, nocturnal discomfort and reduced shoulder range of motion.[7,32,62] Three stages of the condition have been defined – pre-calcific, calcific and post-calcific – with symptoms thought to peak during the calcium resorption that occurs in the latter phases of the calcific stage.[80]

Diagnosis of RCCT requires imaging confirmation, with calcific deposits having been observed in radiographs for over a century.[3] For many, ultrasound (US) has become the imaging modality of choice, due to its ability to identify and measure the size of the deposits, identify the presence of neovascularity, detect changes over time, and is not associated with ionizing radiation.[13,41] Ultrasound imaging may also be useful in differentiating other rotator cuff pathologies or be used to classify and help stage the RCCT process.[7,18,26,27,56] It is not definitive in guiding symptom prognosis, given the uncertain relationship between calcification and symptoms.

The pathoetiology of RCCT remains equivocal and may be self-limiting.[62,80] Nonsurgical intervention is therefore typically recommended as the first stage of management for RCCT.[60,80] The majority of interventions aim at reducing the calcium deposit, with an assumption that by reducing the calcification, the symptoms will resolve.[82] Other noninvasive interventions focus on reducing pain and increasing shoulder function.[30,47,78]

Nonsurgical interventions include rest, nonsteroidal anti-inflammatory drugs (NSAIDs), resistance-based exercise programs, transcutaneous electrical nerve stimulation (TENS), acetic-acid iontophoresis (AAI), and pulsed ultrasound.[30,47,78] For those with more prolonged or severe symptoms, minimally invasive nonsurgical interventions such as subacromial steroid injections (SAI), ultrasound-guided percutaneous irrigation of the calcific deposits (US-PICT) such as needling and lavage (barbotage), and extracorporeal shockwave therapy (ESWT) have been recommended.[2,39,48,78,86]

Surgical intervention is rarely indicated, but may be effective in improving shoulder function in those for whom nonsurgical management has previously failed.[82] Three main surgical options exist: acromioplasty with removal of calcium deposits, acromioplasty without removal of calcium deposits, and removal of calcium deposits alone.[82] As with the nonsurgical interventions, recommendations for surgery should be given cautiously due to insufficient research, and the uncertain relationship between symptoms and presence of calcification.

Epidemiology

RCCT is a relatively common musculoskeletal condition that is typically seen in adults between the ages of 30 and 60 years.[7,18,46,84] The presence of calcific deposits is reported to range from 2.7% to 10.3% in shoulder radiographs of adults.[7] The actual prevalence of calcific tendinopathy may be far higher than this, with US and magnetic resonance imaging (MRI) studies respectively reporting 24.4% and 17.1%.[73,75] When calcification is observed, multifocal calcific deposits are estimated to exist in 28.2% of cases,[73] with up to 50% of those who have observed calcifications going on to develop symptoms.[52] Factors associated with increased odds of RCCT include female sex, hypothyroidism, and insulin-dependent diabetes.[33,46,51,71] Heavy lifting or more active lifestyles do not appear to be associated with an increased incidence of RCCT.[63,80] Calcifications occur in the mid-substance or insertion of the rotator cuff tendons, most commonly of supraspinatus (80%), with infraspinatus (15%) and subscapularis (5%) less frequently involved.[54,73]

Nomenclature

There are several terms commonly used to describe the multifocal, cell-mediated calcification and resorption process occurring in rotator cuff tendons, with the term calcific tendinopathy possibly the most appropriate.[80] Previous terms have included "calcific tendinitis", "calcific periarthritis", "tendinosis calcarea", and "periarticular apatite deposit".[19,49,62]

Radiological studies have observed calcific tendinopathy occurring both within the tendon body and at the tendon insertion. Studies investigating lower limb tendinopathy have described different disease processes between insertional and intratendinous pathologies and this may also be true for rotator cuff tendons, and the location of the calcification may need to be considered differently.[62] Further research is required to better understand these differences and their relationship, if any, with symptoms.

Etiology

The etiology of RCCT remains uncertain.[2,12,62,74] Theories dating back to the early 1900s have been proposed, but the answer remains elusive. Codman[14] was among the first to describe the presence of calcium within the rotator cuff tendons and proposed an early theory of degenerative calcification.[14,15] This theory was supported by several authors through subsequent observations of repetitive trauma and hyaline degeneration,[6,7] local ischemia, and vascular change,[72] and the necrosis of tenocytes resulting in intracellular accumulation of calcium.[55] Furthermore, age may contribute to tendon degeneration, with RCCT rarely seen to affect people before their fourth decade of life.[7] However, the degenerative theory alone fails to account for tendon repair and calcium resorption, which has been observed in recent longitudinal cohort studies and trials.[29,37,60]

Perhaps the most accepted theory of calcification at present is the reactive hypothesis of Uhthoff and Loehr.[80] Although not without limitations, the model proposes the transition of a tendon between stages, and the ability of the tendon to repair and return to normal structure. Recent investigations into tendon stem cells and role of a tendon's extracellular matrix support this theory.[5,88] Under normal circumstances tendon stem cells can differentiate into tenocytes allowing for tendon regeneration and repair. However, under altered conditions, tendon stem cells may differentiate into chondrocytes and osteoblasts instead of tenocytes, possibly mediated by prostaglandin E2.[87] Activity of these non-tenocytes leads to chondrometaplasia and ossification, leading to the formation of calcific deposits within the tendon structure. Additionally, there appears to be an association with RCCT and people with diabetes, suggesting that exposure to high-glucose environments may precipitate the glycosylation of several matrix proteins further disrupting the tendon's extracellular matrix (ECM).[51,71] There may be a similar relationship between diabetes and frozen shoulder (see Chapter 18).

Coinciding with advances in genomic sequencing, the possibility of genetic predisposition to RCCT needs consideration. Studies have observed an increased frequency of human leukocyte antigen serotype class A1 (HLA-A1) in people with RCCT,[77] although this has not been consistent across studies.[25] Murine studies have identified a mutation in the ANK gene (progressive ankylosing locus) as a possible predisposing factor to calcification development.[35] The ANK gene codes for a transmembrane protein, essential for the transport of inorganic pyrophosphate (PPi) – a major inhibitor to calcification formation. Mutation to this gene is believed to cause a marked decrease in PPi, subsequently producing a favorable environment for calcification formation.[35] In the clinical setting, variants in the ANK gene have been associated with rotator cuff tears, however, the clinical significance in RCCT is yet to be ascertained.[65]

Pathogenesis

Based on cellular mediation, a cyclical model of calcification pathogenesis was proposed by Uhthoff and Loehr.[80] According to the authors, the calcific deposits undergo three distinct stages of pathology: pre-calcific, calcific, and post-calcific (Figure 27.1).

The pre-calcific stage is thought to be asymptomatic, and characterized by the presence of chondrocyte-like cells that may derive from the metaplasia of tenocytes.[12,62,80] The calcific stage is subdivided into a formative phase, resting phase, and resorptive phase, and may last for several months to several years.[80] These phases are thought to involve a period of calcium deposition and foci formation,

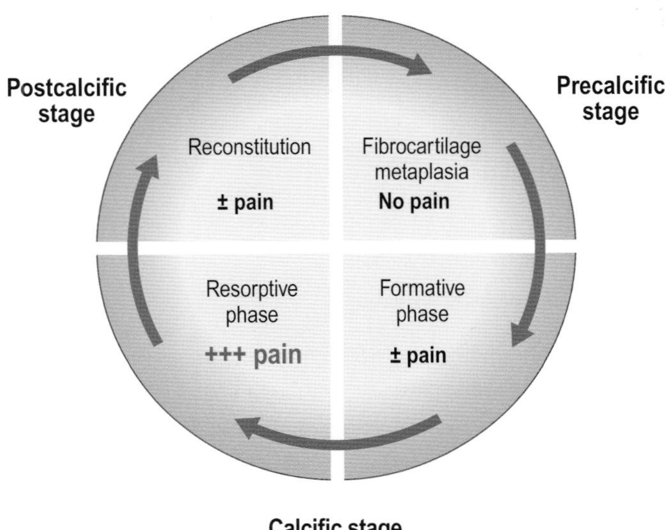

FIGURE 27.1

Adaptation of the reactive calcification cyclical model originally proposed by Uhthoff et al.[81]

a variable period of cellular inactivity indicated by fibrocollagenous tissue bordering the calcific foci, and a final phase involving the spontaneous resorption of calcium that has been most associated with pain.[12,80] The post-calcific stage is also regarded as asymptomatic, and involves the remodeling of the previously occupied space with young fibroblasts and granulation tissue.[12,80]

Increased cellular activity and granulation tissue have been linked to pain in tendinopathy,[1,61] and have recently been hypothesized to contribute to the pain derived from calcifications at the rotator cuff.[32] Increased vascularity and neuronal ingrowths have been observed in people with RCCT, but before any definitive conclusions may be derived, these studies need be conducted on the calcific deposits in people without symptoms to identify if differences exist.[32] The calcific material may induce an inflammatory response within the tendon and stimulate the formation of new blood vessels and nerves known to contribute to pain. Neovascularization and neoinnervation are proposed as a potential source of RCCT pain, but this cannot be determined until both symptomatic and asymptomatic populations are investigated. Furthermore, it is still unknown whether the calcific deposits are in themselves the source of pain.

Sonographic studies have attempted to investigate the relationship between pain and pathology.[12,41] In a study by Le Goff et al.,[41] a positive power Doppler signal within the calcific deposit was reported to be strongly associated with pain when comparing people with and without symptoms in the presence of observed calcification. Moreover, it was reported that larger calcific deposits had greater association with symptoms than smaller deposits. This is consistent with earlier findings.[7]

Radiological studies have attempted to classify calcific morphology but have not attempted to correlate morphology to symptoms. Instead, as detailed in Table 27.1, authors have classified calcific morphology based on size, density, and shape of deposits. The Gärtner et al.[26] classification is the most commonly used.

Assessment and diagnosis

Diagnosing RCCT involves a thorough history and clinical assessment, followed by imaging to confirm the presence of calcific pathology within the rotator cuff tendon.

Diagnosing RCCT is complicated by the uncertainty between the observed calcification and symptoms, as at least 50% or more rotator cuff calcifications are believed to be asymptomatic.[7] As such, if a relationship is hypothesized, the clinician at best should tell the patient it is *likely* that their symptoms are associated with the deposits of calcium observed in their tendon. The explanation must include qualifying information such as the uncertainty of the relationship, as the deposits are just as, if not more, common in people without symptoms.

Clinical presentation

The clinical presentation of calcific tendinopathy is highly variable.[11,12,80] Studies by Uhthoff and Loehr[80] and Chiou et al.[12] report that pain is most significant during calcium resorption, suggesting that a person may not present clinically until after the calcification process has occurred. Pain may be relatively short-term (acute) or may be more protracted (persistent), lasting for several months.[12,41,60] Manifestations of a symptomatic tendon may include tenderness over the rotator cuff insertion, nocturnal discomfort, reduced shoulder range of motion, and localized edema.[7,9,32,62]

Table 27.1 Imaging classifications of calcific tendinopathy

Study	Year	Imaging type	Classification	Description
Bosworth[7]	1941	Radiological	Small	< 0.5 cm
			Medium	0.5–1.5 cm
			Large	1.5 cm
DePalma and Kruper[18]	1961	Radiological	Type I	Fluffy, amorphous and ill-defined
			Type II	Defined and homogenous
Molé et al.[56]	1993	Radiological	Type A	Dense, rounded, sharply delineated
			Type B	Multi-nodular, radio-dense, sharp
			Type C	Radiolucent, heterogeneous, irregular outline
			Type D	Dystrophic calcific deposit
Gärtner and Heyer[26]	1995	Radiological	Type I	Well demarcated, dense
Gärtner and Simons[27]	1990		Type II	Soft contour/dense or sharp/transparent
			Type III	Soft contour/translucent and cloudy

There are currently no recommendations for specific shoulder tests to contribute to a diagnosis of RCCT. Pain mapping may be considered as an adjunct to clinical examination, with one study reporting calcific tendinopathy pain as generally sharp and localized around the shoulder joint (with no radiation below). However, these recommendations are not definitive due to the small sample size.[4]

Imaging

Calcific tendinopathy is characterized by the presence of calcification within the tendon, with current practice requiring observation of this process for a formal diagnosis of RCCT irrespective of the clinical relevance of the deposits.[53,73] Conventional radiology involves standard anterior-posterior (AP), outlet and axillary radiographs (Figure 27.2). Calcium depositions in the supraspinatus tendon are observed on films obtained in neutral rotation, whereas calcifications in the infraspinatus and teres minor tendons are best observed when the shoulder is placed in internal rotation.[23,80] When available, other imaging options include US and MRI.

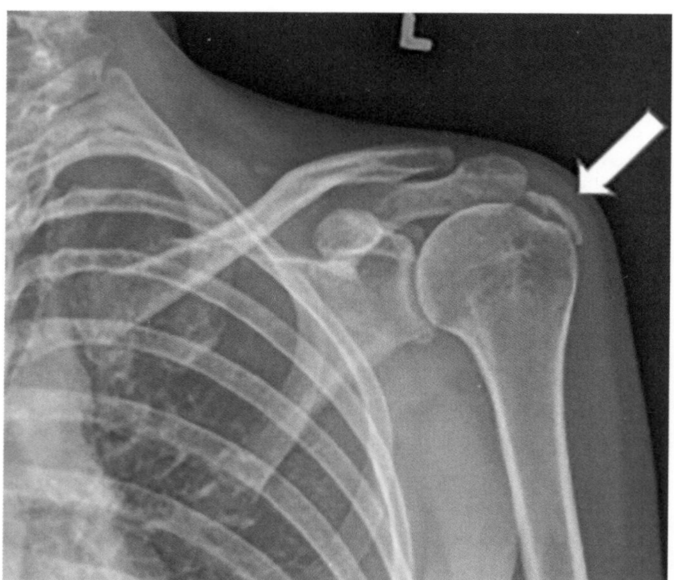

FIGURE 27.2

Radiographic image of a calcific deposit (arrow).

(Reproduced with permission from Orthopaedia – Collaborative Orthopaedic Knowledgebase. © Association of Bone and Joint Surgeons. https://www.orthopaedicsone.com/display/MSKMed/Calcific+tendonitis+of+the+shoulder)

Ultrasound is a validated, practical form of shoulder imaging that is currently the preferred method of RCCT investigation.[13,24,64] In the hands of a skilled sonographer,

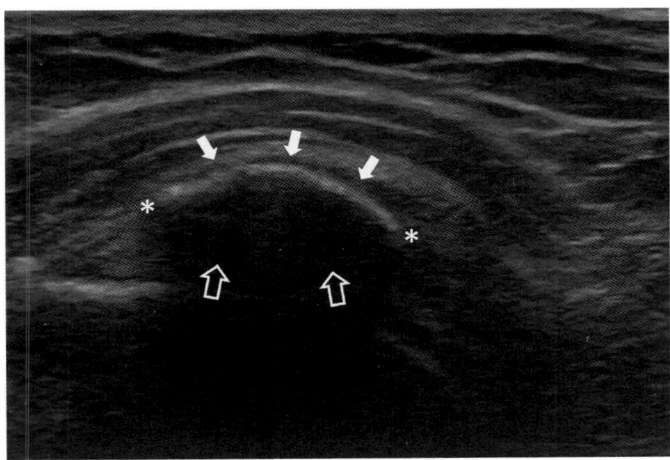

FIGURE 27.3

Diagnostic ultrasound scan image of a calcific deposit. Solid arrows represent the superior aspect of the calcific deposit in the tendon. The two asterisks (*) are the medial and lateral ends of the calcification. The two open arrows inferior to the calcification indicate an ultrasound artefact known as an acoustic shadow (black urea under the calcification). The shadow occurs because the ultrasound waves are unable to pass through the calcification.

(Figure used with the kind permission of Mark Maybury, Research physiotherapist/sonographer, NIHR BRC Birmingham, University Hospitals Birmingham NHS Foundation Trust, UK.)

US imaging can clearly identify the morphological structure and shape of calcium deposits (arc, fragmented/punctuate, nodular, and cystic).[12,41,43] Figure 27.3 demonstrates an US image of a calcific deposit.

While the presence or absence of calcification may be determined, the clinical importance of these deposits remains uncertain. Therefore, clinicians should be mindful of over-investigating without the clinical reasoning to do so.[8] Furthermore, the implications to treat based on the investigative findings should be considered, as they may result in unnecessary intervention. As such, we strongly recommend translating the available research and starting with the least invasive options before considering more invasive procedures associated with greater potential harms.

Management

The current best evidence recommends nonsurgical intervention for up to the first six months. Ultrasound-guided percutaneous irrigation of RCCT (US-PICT) and extracorporeal shockwave therapy (ESWT) are two modalities that are supported by favorable evidence when compared to placebo and other management options. However, there are large variations in their clinical application (e.g., radial versus focused shockwave therapy, one versus two needle ultrasound-guided irrigation) and dosage parameters (e.g., shockwave intensity, duration, frequency).[78] Surgical intervention is rarely indicated, but may be considered if symptoms persist.

Nonsurgical management

Noninvasive interventions

Current nonsurgical interventions include paracetamol (acetaminophen), nonsteroidal anti-inflammatory medications, therapeutic ultrasound, pulsed electromagnetic field (PEMF), and physiotherapy-based progressive exercises to improve muscle and tendon performance and movement.[30,31] The evidence to support these methods, however, is largely anecdotal, with only a limited number of clinical trials comparing these methods to placebo.[30] Furthermore, while clinical practice regularly involves a combination of nonsurgical treatment methods, few studies have investigated these combinations.[30,78]

In the presence of symptoms that may relate to calcification observed in the rotator cuff tendons, the following methods of nonsurgical management may be considered:

1. Watch and wait, supported by relative rest, empathy, education, and advice. Most cases of RCCT resolve within six months of nonsurgical intervention and may be self-limiting.[80,85] Clinicians should therefore tailor their management accordingly and focus on supporting the patient emotionally as well as guiding physical recovery.
2. Paracetamol (acetaminophen) and nonsteroidal anti-inflammatory drugs. Several case studies (level V evidence) reported the use of nonsteroidal anti-inflammatory drugs in calcific tendinitis, although few are specific to the rotator cuff.[38,79,89] Most cases were associated with retropharyngeal calcific (periarthritis) of longus coli and found that generally the pain resolved in less than two weeks with the use of nonsteroidal anti-inflammatory drugs. Anecdotally, paracetamol and other non-opioid medications may also be

beneficial at controlling pain in the short term, although this has not been studied in an RCCT population.

3. Supervised exercise program: while there have been no known studies comparing exercise programs to placebo in the RCCT population, there is strong evidence that a supervised exercise program improves function and range of motion in musculoskeletal shoulder conditions in both short- and long-term follow-ups and, therefore, may be beneficial in RCCT.[30]
4. Therapeutic US: the largest known randomized controlled trial reported a statistically significant improvement in favor of pulsed US over sham treatment immediately post six weeks of treatment for pain and quality of life, however, there were no significant differences between groups at nine months follow-up.[21,22]

There is currently a paucity of high-quality randomized controlled trials investigating nonsurgical interventions in the RCCT population.[78] Consequently, there is great variation in the treatment methods prescribed. There is limited evidence to support the use of pulsed US over placebo, and no evidence to support the use of transcutaneous electrical nerve stimulation (TENS) or acetic-acid iontophoresis (AAI) in the treatment of RCCT.[78] Prescribing exercises may be considered, but cannot be recommended with confidence due to inadequate research supporting this intervention.[78]

Minimally invasive procedures

Ultrasound-guided percutaneous irrigation of calcific tendinopathy (US-PICT)

Unlike more noninvasive, nonsurgical techniques, US-PICT aims to treat RCCT by targeting the calcification directly, despite the unknown relationship between calcifications and RCCT symptoms. Several terms have been used to describe the procedure in the past (e.g., needling, lavage, barbotage), with the acronym US-PICT aiming to uniquely describe the method for future reporting.[40] It may be performed under local anesthetic, with or without steroid injection,[28,40,78] and aims to irrigate the region of calcification. There are no known serious side effects or long-term complications (one year follow-up), with the main side effects being discomfort during and after the procedure.[48,78]

The most recent systematic review of nonsurgical interventions for RCCT concluded that the use of US-PICT may be superior to ESWT for pain and calcification reduction in the long term; however, US-PICT is yet to be compared adequately to placebo.[78] Large variation in US-PICT techniques also exist, with no clinically significant difference between single and double needle lavage, warm and room temperature saline, or between puncture-aspiration and puncture alone.[78] The more minimally invasive techniques of single needle and no aspiration may be preferred. Patients undergoing US-PICT should be monitored for mild vagal reactions, which may occur in up to 5% of patients.[17]

Injectables

The evidence for injectable therapies in musculoskeletal practice is contentious, ranging from more traditional subacromial corticosteroid injections (SAI) through to the hypothesized benefits of platelet rich plasma (PRP) and stem cell therapy. Recent attempts to summarize the evidence of SAI in RCCT treatment pooled data from a small number of low methodological randomized controlled trials.[2] While the use of SAI as an adjunct to US-PICT may be safe and more effective than other modalities (combined US-PICT and ESWT, ESWT alone, and SAI alone), these conclusions were weak. The use of SAI in RCCT needs to be compared more rigorously to placebo and to US-PICT alone to deem the combined injectable therapy effective.

Other injectable therapies (e.g., platelet rich plasma (PRP) and stem cell therapy) lack sufficient evidence from high-quality prospective trials conducted on humans. While injectable therapies may become effective adjuncts or alternate treatment modalities for RCCT in the future, the current level of evidence is insufficient.

Shockwave therapy

Extracorporeal shockwave therapy (ESWT) is commonly used in the treatment of RCCT, with conjecture over the mechanism of action and effectiveness across the different application methods. Applying similar principles to shockwave lithotripsy for renal calculi, ESWT is believed to involve the fragmentation and subsequent phagocytosis of the tendon calcifications,[44,57] with disintegration of calcium deposits reported in in vivo studies.[16,66] In contrast, some authors have proposed absorption of deposits through a molecular mechanism involving enhanced neovascularization and circulation.[83] Secondary analgesic effect may occur through denervation of pain receptors,[34,57] and in the absence of a relationship between calcific pathology and symptoms, this theory may best explain the positive effects from ESWT on patient symptoms. Further research is required to determine the exact mechanism of ESWT across the different application methods.

The main two methods of ESWT application are focused ESWT (fESWT) and radial ESWT (rESWT).[76] They apply distinctly different methods of shockwave, yet are often not distinguished accurately in the literature.[58,76] Focused ESWT uses an acoustic lens to angle and concentrate the sound onto a small area, which allows for a more penetrating and targeted point of treatment. Radial ESWT instead uses a divergent transducer that disperses the shockwave throughout the tissue, with maximum intensity felt at the skin. Both have been compared to placebo, and both appear to be effective treatments of RCCT, although there have been more studies on fESWT.[2,20,81,86] Research on rESWT is promising, with a randomized controlled trial[10] reporting that rESWT effectively reduces pain and improves shoulder function when compared to sham treatment in RCCT. Moreover, the study concluded that these results were maintained for at least six months. Malliaropoulos et al.[50] reported similar findings in a retrospective cohort suggesting greater benefit and few recurrences in individualized rESWT treatment programs. Further research is required to compare the effectiveness between the two application methods and there is also a need to clarify the different dosage parameters that exist within each application method.

Energy flux density (EFD) is used to further subdivide fESWT, and although not universally agreed upon, is often classified into low (below 0.08 mJ/mm^2), medium (0.08–0.28 mJ/mm^2), and high (0.28–0.6 mJ/mm^2).[70] Studies that have accurately distinguished between EFD suggest that high-energy focused shockwave (H-FSW) is be more effective than low-energy focused shockwave (L-FSW) in the treatment of RCCT.[29,37,67] The most recent systematic review of nonsurgical interventions for RCCT[78] revealed moderate evidence that high-energy ESWT was favored over placebo for shoulder function in the first six months,[36,66,69] and moderate evidence that higher energy ESWT was favored over lower energy ESWT for pain and function between three and six months of treatment. The review[78] also supported earlier conclusions[47,86] that high-energy ESWT is more effective than low-energy ESWT, however, deemed the level of evidence to be only moderate given the current quality of randomized controlled trials available.

Side effects of shockwave therapy are minimal, with most resolving either immediately post treatment or within a few days. They include reddening of skin, soft tissue swelling, small hematomas, and pain.[57] Rarely do these occur with L-FSW and because of this they may be dose related.[57] Repeated low EFD sessions of ESWT have been trialed to minimize these side effects and have been found to be effective.[68] Researchers and clinicians have also trialed regional anesthesia prior to H-FSW treatment in an attempt to avoid pain,[69] although there is currently no consensus. Administering anesthesia or sedation according to pain tolerance may be appropriate,[59] however, the peripheral nervous system may play a role in mediating the shockwave effects on the musculoskeletal system and therefore prophylactic anesthesia may reduce this effect.[76] More research in a RCCT-specific population is required.

Surgical

Surgical intervention for RCCT is contentious and is usually only considered after a six-month trial of nonsurgical intervention. There is definitive lack of placebo-controlled surgical trials comparing each surgical method, and this needs to be conveyed to patients during the shared decision-making process. Subsequently there is a need for further research.

Based on current literature, the main three surgical options used for RCCT include: acromioplasty with removal of calcific deposits, acromioplasty without removing the deposits, and removal of calcium deposits with preservation of the acromion.[82] Each have varying degrees of evidence, with a recent systematic review unable to recommend a preferred treatment option.[82] This may be contributed to by a lack of high-quality studies (two randomized controlled trials, one quasi-randomized controlled trial and three comparative cohort studies). Alternatively, the parallel recovery from each surgical method may be explained by placebo or post-surgical relative rest.[42]

The rationale for several of the RCCT surgical methods is also debatable. There appears to be a lack of correlation between calcific tendinopathy and findings associated with subacromial impingement and therefore this surgery may not be effective in people with RCCT.[45] Similarly, surgical removal of calcific deposits may prove to be an effective RCCT treatment, however, it is still uncertain whether calcifications contribute to patient symptoms and therefore the rationale for this surgery remains uncertain.

Comparisons between surgical and nonsurgical interventions are also inconclusive and lack randomized controlled trial level evaluation. The best available evidence found no clinical difference in persistent RCCT outcomes between arthroscopic surgery and low-energy focused shockwave therapy (L-FSW).[68] In the absence of any clear benefit to surgical intervention compared to nonsurgical intervention for RCCT, and the lack of certainty surrounding the surgical treatment methods in RCCT, the less invasive management options should be considered first.

Summary

Calcific tendinopathy of the rotator cuff is a complex condition that is yet to be fully understood. The pathoetiology of RCCT remains uncertain but is believed to be multifactorial and may be self-limiting. Clarification of the pathoetiology and the relationship between calcific pathology and clinical symptoms will ultimately guide future diagnosis and management of this condition that is frequently associated with substantial pain and morbidity. Currently no gold standard for either diagnosis or treatment exist. Observation of tendon calcifications are best seen on ultrasound imaging, while clinical signs are nonspecific. Six months of nonsurgical treatment should be recommended first, and this may involve watch and wait, supported by pharmacological pain relief. Progressive exercises may be considered but the research evidence supporting this is very poor. If further intervention is considered, then evidence of varying quality supports ultrasound-guided percutaneous irrigation of calcific tendinopathy (US-PICT) and extracorporeal shockwave therapy (ESWT).

References

1. Alfredson H, Ohberg L, Forsgren S. Is vasculo-neural ingrowth the cause of pain in chronic Achilles tendinosis? An investigation using ultrasonography and colour Doppler, immunohistochemistry, and diagnostic injections. Knee Surg Sports Traumatol Arthrosc. 2003;11:334-338.
2. Arirachakaran A, Boonard M, Yamaphai S, Prommahachai A, Kesprayura S, Kongtharvonskul J. Extracorporeal shock wave therapy, ultrasound-guided percutaneous lavage, corticosteroid injection and combined treatment for the treatment of rotator cuff calcific tendinopathy: a network meta-analysis of RCTs. European Journal of Orthopaedic Surgery and Traumatology. 2017;27:381-390.
3. Baer W. Operative treatment of subdeltoid bursitis. Bull Johns Hopkins Hosp. 1907;18:282-284.
4. Bayam L, Arumilli R, Horsley I, Bayam F, Herrington L, Funk L. Testing shoulder pain mapping. Pain Medicine. 2017;18:1382-1393.
5. Bi Y, Ehirchiou D, Kilts TM, et al. Identification of tendon stem/progenitor cells and the role of the extracellular matrix in their niche. Nature Medicine. 2007;13:1219.
6. Bishop WA. Calcification of the supraspinatus tendon: cause, pathologic picture and relation to the scalenus anticus syndrome. Arch Surg. 1939;39:231-246.
7. Bosworth B. Calcium deposits in the shoulder and subacromial bursitis: a survey of 12,122 shoulders. JAMA. 1941;116:2477-2482.
8. Brun S. Shoulder injuries: management in general practice. Aust Fam Physician. 2012;41:217-220.
9. Brunner U, Habermeyer P, Krueger P. Clinical symptoms and classification of periarticular diseases of the glenohumeral joint. A retrospective study on 183 patients. [German]. Der Unfallchirurg. 1985;88:495-499.
10. Cacchio A, Paoloni M, Barile A, et al. Effectiveness of radial shock-wave therapy for calcific tendinitis of the shoulder: single-blind, randomized clinical study. Phys Ther. 2006;86:672-82.
11. Cacchio A, Rompe JD. US-guided percutaneous treatment of shoulder calcific tendonitis: some clarifications are needed. Radiology. 2010;254:990.
12. Chiou H, Hung S, Lin S, Wei Y, Li M. Correlations among mineral components, progressive calcification process and clinical symptoms of calcific tendonitis. Rheumatology. 2010;49:548-555.
13. Chiou HJ, Chou YH, Wu JJ, Hsu CC, Huang DY, Chang CY. Evaluation of calcific tendonitis of the rotator cuff: role of color Doppler ultrasonography. J Ultrasound Med. 2002;21:289-295; quiz 296-287.
14. Codman EA. On stiff and painful shoulders: the anatomy of the sub-deltoid and sub-acromial bursa and its clinical importance. Sub-deltoid bursitis. Boston Med Surg J. 1906;154: 613–616.
15. Codman EA. The Shoulder: Rupture of the Supraspinatus Tendon and Other Lesions in Or about the Subacromial Bursa. T Todd Company; 1934.
16. Daecke W, Kusnierczak D, Loew M. Long-term effects of extracorporeal shockwave therapy in chronic calcific tendinitis of

the shoulder. J Shoulder Elbow Surg. 2002;11:476-480.

17. Del Castillo-Gonzalez F, Ramos-Alvarez JJ, Rodriguez-Fabian G, Gonzalez-Perez J, Jimenez-Herranz E, Varela E. Extracorporeal shockwaves versus ultrasound-guided percutaneous lavage for the treatment of rotator cuff calcific tendinopathy: a randomized controlled trial. Eur J Phys Rehabil Med. 2016;52:145-151.

18. DePalma AF, Kruper JS. Long-term study of shoulder joints afflicted with and treated for calcific tendinitis. Clinical Orthopaedics. 1961;20:61-72.

19. Dickson JA, Crosby EH. Periarthritis of the shoulder: an analysis of two hundred cases. JAMA. 1932;99:2252-2257.

20. Dimitrios S. Extracorporeal shock-wave therapy: can it be used for the management of any calcific tendinopathy? Hong Kong Physiotherapy Journal. 2016;34:47-48.

21. Ebenbichler G, Erdogmus C, Resch K, et al. Ultrasound therapy for calcific tendinitis of the shoulder. N Engl J Med. 1999;340(20):1533-8.

22. Ebenbichler GR, Pieber K, Kainberger F, Funovics M, Resch KL. Long-term outcome of ultrasound therapy for calcific tendinitis of the shoulder: results of a RCT. PM and R. 2016;8 (9 Supplement):S156.

23. ElShewy MT. Calcific tendinitis of the rotator cuff. World Journal of Orthopedics. 2016;7:55-60.

24. Farin PU, Jaroma H. Sonographic findings of rotator cuff calcifications. J Ultrasound Med. 1995;14:7-14.

25. Gartner J. [Is tendinosis calcarea associated with HLA-A1?]. Zeitschrift fur Orthopadie und ihre Grenzgebiete. 1993;131:469.

26. Gärtner J, Heyer A. Calcific tendinitis of the shoulder. Orthopade. 1995;24:284-302.

27. Gärtner J, Simons B. Analysis of calcific deposits in calcifying tendinitis. Clin Orthop. 1990;111-120.

28. Gatt DL, Charalambous CP. Ultrasound-guided barbotage for calcific tendonitis of the shoulder: a systematic review including 908 patients. Arthroscopy. 2014;30:1166-1172.

29. Gerdesmeyer L, Wagenpfeil S, Haake M, et al. Extracorporeal shock wave therapy for the treatment of chronic calcifying tendonitis of the rotator cuff: a randomized controlled trial. JAMA. 2003 Nov 19;290:2573-80.

30. Green S, Buchbinder R, Hetrick S. Physiotherapy interventions for shoulder pain. Cochrane Database of Systematic Reviews. 2003;CD004258.

31. Greis AC, Derrington SM, McAuliffe M. Evaluation and nonsurgical management of rotator cuff calcific tendinopathy. Orthop Clin North Am. 2015;46:293-302.

32. Hackett L, Millar NL, Lam P, Murrell GA. Are the Symptoms of calcific tendinitis due to neoinnervation and/or neovascularization? J Bone Joint Surg Am. 2016;98:186-192.

33. Harvie P, Pollard TC, Carr AJ. Calcific tendinitis: natural history and association with endocrine disorders. J Shoulder Elbow Surg. 2007;16:169-173.

34. Haupt G. Use of extracorporeal shock waves in the treatment of pseudarthrosis, tendinopathy and other orthopedic diseases. The Journal of Urology. 1997;158:4-11.

35. Ho AM, Johnson MD, Kingsley DM. Role of the mouse ank gene in control of tissue calcification and arthritis. Science. 2000;289:265-270.

36. Ioppolo F, Tattoli M, Di Sante L, et al. Extracorporeal shock-wave therapy for supraspinatus calcifying tendinitis: a randomized clinical trial comparing two different energy levels. Physical Therapy. 2012;92:1376-1385.

37. Ioppolo F, Tattoli M, Sante L, et al. Extracorporeal shock-wave therapy for supraspinatus calcifying tendinitis: a randomized clinical trial comparing two different energy levels. Phys Ther. 2012;92:1376-85.

38. Khurana B. Calcific tendinitis mimicking acute prevertebral abscess. J Emerg Med. 42:e15-e16.

39. Lafrance S, Doiron-Cadrin P, Saulnier M, et al. Is ultrasound-guided lavage an effective intervention for rotator cuff calcific tendinopathy? A systematic review with a meta-analysis of randomised controlled trials. BMJ Open Sport & Exercise Medicine. 2019;5:e000506.

40. Lanza E, Banfi G, Serafini G, et al. Ultrasound-guided percutaneous irrigation in rotator cuff calcific tendinopathy: what is the evidence? A systematic review with proposals for future reporting. Eur Radiol. 2015;25:2176-2183.

41. Le Goff B, Berthelot JM, Guillot P, Glemarec J, Maugars Y. Assessment of calcific tendonitis of rotator cuff by ultrasonography: comparison between symptomatic and asymptomatic shoulders. Joint, Bone, Spine: Revue du Rhumatisme. 2010;77:258-263.

42. Lewis J. Rotator cuff related shoulder pain: assessment, management and uncertainties. Man Ther. 2016;23:57-68.

43. Lin CH, Chao HL, Chiou HJ. Calcified plaque resorptive status as determined by high-resolution ultrasound is predictive of successful conservative management of calcific tendinosis. Eur J Radiol. 2012;81:1776-1781.

44. Loew M, Daecke W, Kusnierczak D, Rahmanzadeh M, Ewerbeck V. Shock-wave therapy is effective for chronic calcifying tendinitis of the shoulder. Journal of Bone & Joint Surgery. 1999;81:863-867.

45. Loew M, Sabo D, Wehrle M, Mau H. Relationship between calcifying tendinitis and subacromial impingement: a prospective radiography and magnetic resonance imaging study. J Shoulder Elbow Surg. 1996;5:314-319.

46. Louwerens JK, Sierevelt IN, van Hove RP, van den Bekerom MP, van Noort A. Prevalence of calcific deposits within the rotator cuff tendons in adults with and without subacromial pain syndrome: clinical and radiologic analysis of 1219 patients. J Shoulder Elbow Surg. 2015;24:1588-1593.

47. Louwerens JK, Sierevelt IN, van Noort A, van den Bekerom MP. Evidence for minimally invasive therapies in the management of chronic calcific tendinopathy of the rotator cuff: a systematic review and meta-analysis. J Shoulder Elbow Surg. 2014;23:1240-1249.

48. Louwerens JKG, Veltman ES, Van Noort A, Van Den Bekerom MPJ. The effectiveness of high-energy extracorporeal shockwave therapy versus ultrasound-guided needling versus arthroscopic surgery in the management of chronic calcific rotator cuff tendinopathy: a systematic review. Arthroscopy. 2016;32:165-175.

49. Maffulli N, Wong J, Almekinders LC. Types and epidemiology of tendinopathy. Clin Sports Med. 2003;22:675-692.

50. Malliaropoulos N, Thompson D, Meke M, et al. Individualised radial extracorporeal shock wave therapy (rESWT) for symptomatic calcific shoulder

tendinopathy: a retrospective clinical study. BMC Musculoskelet Disord. 2017;18:513.

51. Mavrikakis ME, Drimis S, Kontoyannis DA, Rasidakis A, Moulopoulou ES, Kontoyannis S. Calcific shoulder periarthritis (tendinitis) in adult onset diabetes mellitus: a controlled study. Ann Rheum Dis. 1989;48:211-214.

52. McKendry RJ, Uhthoff HK, Sarkar K, Hyslop PS. Calcifying tendinitis of the shoulder: prognostic value of clinical, histologic, and radiologic features in 57 surgically treated cases. Journal of Rheumatology. 1982;9:75-80.

53. Merolla G, Singh S, Paladini P, Porcellini G. Calcific tendinitis of the rotator cuff: state of the art in diagnosis and treatment. Journal of Orthopaedics & Traumatology. 2016;17:7-14.

54. Meroni R, Piscitelli D, Valerio S, et al. Ultrasonography of the shoulder: asymptomatic findings from working-age women in the general population. Journal of Physical Therapy Science. 2017;29:1219-1223.

55. Mohr W, Bilger S. Basic morphologic structures of calcified tendopathy and their significance for pathogenesis. Z Rheumatol. 1990;49:346-355.

56. Molé D, Kempf JF, Gleyze P, Rio B, Bonnomet F, Walch G. Results of endoscopic treatment of non-broken tendinopathies of the rotator cuff. 2. Calcifications of the rotator cuff. Revue de Chirurgie Orthopedique et Reparatrice de L'Appareil Moteur. 1993;79:532-541.

57. Mouzopoulos G, Stamatakos M, Mouzopoulos D, Tzurbakis M. Extracorporeal shock wave treatment for shoulder calcific tendonitis: a systematic review. Skeletal Radiol. 2007;36:803-811.

58. Moya D, Ramon S, d'Agostino MC, et al. Incorrect methodology may favor ultrasound-guided needling over shock wave treatment in calcific tendinopathy of the shoulder. J Shoulder Elbow Surg. 2016;25:e241-243.

59. Moya D, Ramon S, Guiloff L, Gerdesmeyer L. Current knowledge on evidence-based shockwave treatments for shoulder pathology. Int J Surg. 2015;24:171-178.

60. Ogon P, Suedkamp NP, Jaeger M, Izadpanah K, Koestler W, Maier D. Prognostic factors in nonoperative therapy for chronic symptomatic calcific tendinitis of the shoulder. Arthritis Rheum. 2009;60:2978-2984.

61. Ohberg L, Alfredson H. Ultrasound guided sclerosis of neovessels in painful chronic Achilles tendinosis: pilot study of a new treatment. Br J Sports Med. 2002;36:173-175; discussion 176-177.

62. Oliva F, Via AG, Maffulli N. Physiopathology of intratendinous calcific deposition. BMC Med. 2012;10:95.

63. Olsson O. Degenerative changes of the shoulder joint and their connection with shoulder pain; a morphological and clinical investigation with special attention to the cuff and biceps tendon. Acta Chirurgica Scandinavica. Supplementum. 1953;181:1-130.

64. Papatheodorou A, Ellinas P, Takis F, Tsanis A, Maris I, Batakis N. US of the shoulder: rotator cuff and non-rotator cuff disorders. Radiographics. 2006;26:e23.

65. Peach CA, Zhang Y, Dunford JE, Brown MA, Carr AJ. Cuff tear arthropathy: evidence of functional variation in pyrophosphate metabolism genes. Clin Orthop Relat Res. 2007;462:67-72.

66. Peters J, Luboldt W, Schwarz W, Jacob V, Herzog C, Vogl TJ. Extracorporeal shock wave therapy in calcific tendinitis of the shoulder. Skeletal Radiology 2004;33(12):712-718.

67. Pleiner J, Crevenna R, Langenberger H, et al. Extracorporeal shockwave treatment is effective in calcific tendonitis of the shoulder. A randomized controlled trial. Wien Klin Wochenschr. 2004;116:536-41.

68. Rebuzzi E, Coletti N, Schiavetti S, Giusto F. Arthroscopy surgery versus shock wave therapy for chronic calcifying tendinitis of the shoulder. Journal of Orthopaedics and Traumatology. 2008;9:179-185.

69. Rompe JD, Bürger R, Hopf C, Eysel P. Shoulder function after extracorporal shock wave therapy for calcific tendinitis. J Shoulder Elbow Surg. 1998;7:505-509.

70. Rompe JD, Kirkpatrick CJ, Kullmer K, Schwitalle M, Krischek O. Dose-related effects of shock waves on rabbit tendo Achillis. A sonographic and histological study. J Bone Joint Surg Br. 1998;80:546-552.

71. Rosenthal AK, Gohr CM, Mitton E, Monnier V, Burner T. Advanced glycation end products increase transglutaminase activity in primary porcine tenocytes. J Invest Med. 2009;57:460.

72. Sandstrom C. Peridentinis calcarea: common disease of middle life. Its diagnosis, pathology and treatment. Am J Roentgenol. 1938;40:1-21.

73. Sansone V, Consonni O, Maiorano E, Meroni R, Goddi A. Calcific tendinopathy of the rotator cuff: the correlation between pain and imaging features in symptomatic and asymptomatic female shoulders. Skeletal Radiol. 2016;45:49-55.

74. Sansone V, Maiorano E, Galluzzo A, Pascale V. Calcific tendinopathy of the shoulder: clinical perspectives into the mechanisms, pathogenesis, and treatment. Orthopedic Research and Reviews. 2018;10:63-72.

75. Sansone VC, Meroni R, Boria P, Pisani S, Maiorano E. Are occupational repetitive movements of the upper arm associated with rotator cuff calcific tendinopathies? Rheumatol Int. 2015;35:273-280.

76. Schmitz C, Csaszar NBM, Milz S, et al. Efficacy and safety of extracorporeal shock wave therapy for orthopedic conditions: a systematic review on studies listed in the PEDro database. British Medical Bulletin. 2015;116:115-138.

77. Sengar DP, McKendry RJ, Uhthoff HK. Increased frequency of HLA-A1 in calcifying tendinitis. Tissue Antigens. 1987;29:173-174.

78. Simpson M, Pizzari T, Cook T, Wildman S, Lewis J. Effectiveness of non-surgical interventions for rotator cuff calcific tendinopathy: a systematic review. J Rehabil Med. 2020;10.2340/16501977-2725.

79. Tagashira Y, Watanuki S. Acute calcific retropharyngeal tendonitis. Canadian Medical Association Journal. 2015;187:995-995.

80. Uhthoff HK, Loehr JW. Calcific tendinopathy of the rotator cuff: pathogenesis, diagnosis, and management. The Journal of The American Academy of Orthopaedic Surgeons. 1997;5:183-191.

81. Verstraelen F, In den Kleef NJ, Jansen L, Morrenhof J. High-energy versus low-energy extracorporeal shock wave therapy for calcifying tendinitis of the shoulder: which is superior? A meta-analysis. Clin Orthop Relat Res. 2014;472:2816-25.

82. Verstraelen FU, Fievez E, Janssen L, Morrenhof W. Surgery for calcifying tendinitis of the shoulder: a systematic review. World J Orthop. 2017;8:424-430.

83. Wang CJ, Wang FS, Yang KD, et al. Shock wave therapy induces neovascularization at the tendon-bone junction. A study in rabbits. J Orthop Res. 2003;21:984-989.

84. Welfling J, Kahn M, Desroy M, Paolaggi J, de Sèze S. [Calcifications of the shoulder. II. The disease of multiple tendinous calcifications]. Rev Rhum Mal Osteoartic. 1965;32:325-334.

85. Wölk T, Wittenberg RH. [Calcifying subacromial syndrome--clinical and ultrasound outcome of non-surgical therapy]. Zeitschrift fur Orthopadie und ihre Grenzgebiete. 1997;135:451-457.

86. Wu Y-C, Tsai W-C, Tu Y-K, Yu T-Y. Comparative effectiveness of nonoperative treatments for chronic calcific tendinitis of the shoulder: a systematic review and network meta-analysis of randomized controlled trials. Arch Phys Med Rehabil. 2017;98:1678-1692.e1676.

87. Zhang J, Wang JH-C. Production of PGE2 increases in tendons subjected to repetitive mechanical loading and induces differentiation of tendon stem cells into non-tenocytes. Journal of Orthopaedic Research. 2010;28:198-203.

88. Zhang J, Wang JH. Platelet-rich plasma releasate promotes differentiation of tendon stem cells into active tenocytes. Am J Sports Med. 2010;38:2477-2486.

89. Zibis AH, Giannis D, Malizos KN, Kitsioulis P, Arvanitis DL. Acute calcific tendinitis of the longus colli muscle: case report and review of the literature. Eur Spine J. 2013;22:434-438.

Reconsidering assessment and management of proprioceptive impairment of the shoulder

28

Gisela Sole, Craig Wassinger

Introduction

Sensorimotor control is critical to maintain the body's equilibrium, balance, stability, and safety, to respond to perturbations, and to create awareness of the surrounding space. Such control refers to all sensory (somatosensation) and motor control of a segment (from the brain to the muscle and other tissues).[1] The somatosensory system relays information from sensory stimuli to the central nervous system (CNS) for interpretation and integration. Shoulder function requires coordinated responses from the spine, scapulothoracic segment, glenohumeral, acromioclavicular and sternoclavicular joints, as well as the elbow, wrist, and hand joints. The position of the trunk and lower limbs, as well as power generated by those segments, substantially influences the outputs of the shoulder. As the glenohumeral joint is essential for upper limb mobility, precision, and speed, it is highly reliant on a well-organized sensorimotor system to control joint stability while facilitating upper limb function for daily and recreational activities.[2]

Proprioception is part of the somatosensory system and relates to the ability to sense where the limbs and joints are in relation to the body and to the surrounding environment and space.[3] Proprioception entails processes from multifaceted systems that regulate motor control and behavior.[4,5] Studies have explored shoulder proprioception related to injury and pain,[3,6] fatigue,[7,8] work-related repetitive movements,[9] throwing performance,[10] and following surgery for recurrent anterior glenohumeral dislocations, where it has been shown to improve.[11] "Proprioceptive training", with or without the addition of vibration, has formed part of clinical guidelines following shoulder injury, with goals to "enhance" or "restore" proprioception.[12-14] Adjuncts, such as manual therapy, taping, and bracing are also suggested to improve proprioception, albeit with conflicting evidence.[14] In this chapter, we explore current concepts of proprioception as part of the somatosensory system and its responses to shoulder pain, focusing on the glenohumeral joint. We use a narrative form to explore various evidence-based findings as well as theoretical concepts and clinical approaches for assessment and rehabilitation.

The context of proprioception within the somatosensory system

Considering proprioception in isolation from other sensory input, neural networks, as well as psychosocial domains, is challenging and perhaps futile from a clinical perspective. Proprioception involves both peripheral and central systems.[15] Sensations are generated by our own movements and contribute to generation of our body image.[16] Proprioceptive sensations are subconscious during routine movements, and are accessible using internal foci of attention, for example, when thinking about where the arm is positioned.[16] Proprioception forms part of the complex afferent somatosensory system, in addition to thermoception, nociception, equilibrioception, and mechanoreception.[15]

The somatosensory system, described as the "sixth sense" by Sir Charles Bell in the 1830s, complements the primary senses: visual, vestibular (including orientation and speed of movement, equilibrium, and balance), tactile (touch), auditory (hearing), gustatory (taste), and olfactory (smell) senses.[17] Somatosensation includes sub-modalities of kinesthesia or movement sense (interpretation of joint motions), joint position sense (interpretation of information concerning orientation in space), and sensation of force (interpretation of force generated within a joint), sense of heaviness and others.[16,18-20] Proprioceptive signals are integrated with visual, vestibular, and other sensory information, and used by the CNS to determine an appropriate motor response. Thus, the sensorimotor system involves three main steps: 1) afferent somatosensory signaling (input), 2) central interpretation and integration of all sensory inputs (analysis), and 3) efferent motor responses (output).[21]

The result of a well-functioning sensorimotor system is neuromuscular control that includes the continuous unconscious activation of dynamic restraints (motor responses) in response to joint motion and loading (feedback mechanisms) in anticipation of what will happen next and correction of movement errors (feedforward mechanisms).[18] The feedforward process occurs after the task is practiced and mastered to permit correct sequencing, timing, and adjustments.

Assessment of proprioception for people with shoulder pain

Shoulder proprioception has been measured using goniometers or inclinometers and laser pointers,[8,22,23] smartphone apps,[24,25] custom-made equipment,[10,26] electromagnetic tracking devices,[27] and most commonly, isokinetic dynamometers.[28,29] Current research is exploring the use of virtual reality (see Chapter 40) to assess shoulder proprioception.

The most common methods to assess proprioception are to determine the angular Threshold To Detect Passive Movement (TTDPM) for the sense of movement or kinesthesia (Figure 28.1), the repositioning error for joint (re-) position sense (JPS),[30,31] and force matching error for force perception. Larger errors for JPS and force sense, as well as larger TTDPM are considered to indicate impaired proprioceptive sense. Assessment of these are described in Table 28.1. Related sensorimotor assessments include time to stabilization following a perturbation, response time, and electromyographic activity.

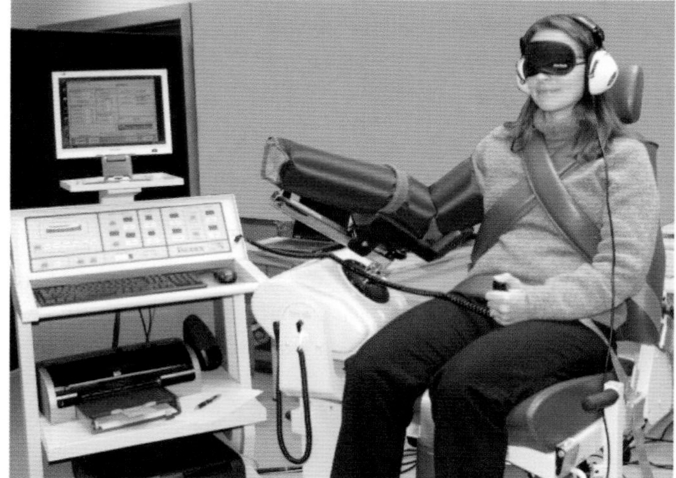

FIGURE 28.1
Assessment of threshold to detection of passive motion (TTDPM).

Proprioception has been explored in people with subacromial pain syndrome (impingement),[34,35] rotator cuff tendinopathy,[36,37] nonspecific shoulder pain,[38] frozen shoulder,[39] and glenohumeral instability (post-dislocation).[40] Although active and passive JPS appear to be the most commonly assessed sub-modality, such findings do not consistently differentiate participants with shoulder pain or injury from those without symptoms.[3,6] Moderate evidence describes group differences for TTDPM (kinesthesia),[3,6] and low evidence for impaired sense of force.[3] Mean differences between people with shoulder pain and people without shoulder pain are generally below 3° for joint position error and less for TTDPM.[8,36,41]

To interpret such findings, an understanding of reliability of the measurement is needed. Acceptable to high *relative reliability*, defined with intraclass correlation coefficients (ICCs), has been reported.[4,39] Assessment protocols for internal and external rotation in positions of 90° abduction appear to be most reliable for passive JPS and kinesthesia (TTDPM).[4] *Absolute reliability* includes calculating standard error of measurement (SEM) and smallest detectable differences (SDD).[42] A difference with a value smaller than the SEM is likely to be the result of "measurement noise". For differences that range between the SEM and the SDD, it is ambiguous whether these are due to measurement noise or are "real" differences. A difference or change greater than the SDD is 95% likely to be a real difference.[42]

Assessing reliability for internal and external rotation JPS (in modified neutral glenohumeral position) with an isokinetic dynamometer in asymptomatic participants, SEMs of 0.5–1° and SDD of 1–2.7° have been calculated.[39,43] For TTDPM for external/internal rotation (also a modified neutral position), we defined a SEM of 0.15°, equating to a SDD of 0.42°.[43] Small differences of around 1–3° can thus be confidently determined for passive joint position error, and 0.5° for TTDPM when using an isokinetic dynamometer.

The SDD for active JPS using inclinometers and smartphone apps may range from 1.5° for internal and external rotation when measured at 90° abduction[22] to 12° for active flexion.[24] Vafadar et al.[23] reported good reliability (ICC 0.86) for mean joint position errors for shoulder flexion using a laser pointer for people with no shoulder pain, and SDDs ranging between 1.8° and 3.1°. Such SDDs are large when considering that differences found between people with shoulder pain and asymptomatic people when using laser pointers or smartphone apps can be smaller. For example, Boarati et al.[8] reported a mean difference of 1.6° between a group of people with subacromial pain syndrome and asymptomatic people when using a laser pointer to 90° shoulder flexion, smaller than SDDs (1.8–3.1°)

Table 28.1 Proprioceptive sub-modalities and assessments processes

Sub-modality	Assessment
Kinesthesia or movement sense	**Threshold to detect passive movement (TTDPM):** The arm is placed in a pneumatic sleeve to decrease tactile sensation, and to stabilize the distal joints to minimize proprioceptive input, and visual input is blocked using blindfolds. Headphones with white noise are used to occlude aural cues (Figure 28.1). The person is usually in a seated or lying position and the arm placed on the device lever. The arm is then passively moved by the device at slow speeds (0.25–5°/s) and the participant is instructed to press a stop button at the first instance that they feel the motion and the direction of the movement. The angular threshold and movement direction for detecting movement is recorded.[11,30]
Joint position sense	**Joint position sense (JPS):** A pneumatic sleeve is used, if available, and the person is blindfolded. • *Isokinetic dynamometer:* The limb or joint is passively moved to a target angle and returned to the starting position. – *Passive JPS:* The limb is then again moved passively by the device and the participant indicates with a stop button when the perceived target position is replicated. – *Active JPS:* The participant actively moves the limb back to the target angle. The angular error between the target and the replicated position is determined.[30] • *Laser pointer:* The person stands facing a wall, at a distance of their arm length plus 10 cm (3.9 in). A tape measure is fixed to the wall to determine error (in cm). A laser pointer is fixed to the distal upper arm. The person is asked to flex (or abduct) the shoulder keeping elbow in extension and wrist in neutral to a specified target. The participant resumes a resting posture and actively aims the pointer at the target position (without visual feedback). The linear distance error between the target and final position is measured. (Trigonometry can be used to calculate the angular error.)[23] • *Inclinometer or smartphone apps:* A similar process as for the laser pointer is used. The angular positions for the target and replicated positions are measured and errors are calculated.[23,25,32]
Force sense	**Force matching error:** Using an isokinetic dynamometer, the maximum voluntary isometric contraction (MVIC) is first assessed. Then a target force is set, such as 60% of the MVIC. Participants are then asked to produce the "target force" alternately with and without visual feedback on the computer screen and maintain for a few seconds. The error between the target force and the observed force generated without visual feedback is calculated.[22,33]

calculated from reliability studies.[23,32] It may thus be difficult to differentiate a deficit for JPS in an individual person from measurement noise, specifically when using the clinically based assessment procedures with laser pointers, smartphone apps, or inclinometers.

Considering individual studies, differences between people with and without symptomatic shoulders are often small in comparison to documented absolute reliability (such as SEM and SDDs). Such clear differentiation between groups is partly due to large variability, evident in large standard deviations compared to mean differences. Thus, while some people with shoulder pain may have a measurable proprioceptive deficit, others with similar shoulder pain or disorders may not. To understand individual variability of assessments, we also need to consider models underlying proprioception. Early proprioceptive theories were focused on contemporary knowledge of peripheral anatomical models, and advances in neurosciences have reframed our understanding. These concepts are considered in the next section.

Peripheral anatomical model for proprioception

Mechanoreceptors located within most anatomical structures of the shoulder are sensitive to mechanical deformation of the tissue.[44] Table 28.2 outlines the mechanoreceptors and their locations in the shoulder girdle. Mechanoreceptors in the joint and skin (non-musculotendinous) are more likely to contribute towards JPS at the *end ranges* of motion.[4,14,43] The joint mechanoreceptors were historically considered the most important proprioceptive organs in the joints.[44] More recent understanding suggests that muscle spindles and Golgi tendon organs (GTOs) are the primary proprioceptors, signaling *throughout the*

Table 28.2 Primary mechanoreceptors of the shoulder[48,49]

Receptor type	Responsive forces	Location in shoulder
Ruffini ending (corpuscle)	Tension, compression, rotation Limit detectors	Labrum – sustained compression Capsular/ligament junctions (capsulolabral and capsulohumeral) Skin
Pacinian (Krause) corpuscle	Compression, tension, rate of loading, vibration	Labrum–compression Capsule/ligaments Skin
Golgi tendon organ (GTO)	Tension	Capsule/ligaments Tendons
Muscle spindle (nuclear bag fiber and nuclear chain fiber)	Tension and rate of tensile loading	Muscles (gamma system)
Free nerve ending	Noxious stimuli	Labrum, capsule, ligaments, muscle, skin, bursa

joint range of motion.[45] Direction throughout the range of motion is perceived based on muscle length changes and anticipation in muscle length changes.[15] This is achieved by detecting changes in muscle length and velocity of contraction which contribute to sense of force and effort.[16,44,46,47] Importantly, muscle spindles and GTOs also have adaptable thresholds. That is, their sensitivity can be modified with active movement and exercise.[44]

Movements or postures initiate action potentials within proprioceptive primary afferents emanating from the mechanoreceptors, muscle spindles and GTOs. These action potentials have fast conduction velocities; transmission entails minimal synapses and accurate somatotopic organization (a specific part of the body is associated with a distinct location in the CNS). Proprioceptive action potentials ascend ipsilaterally via the posterior column-medial lemniscal system in the spinal cord to the nucleus cuneatus in the medulla. Here the fibers cross the midline, project to the thalamus (relay station for motor and sensory signals to the cerebral cortex), and ultimately terminate in the anterior parietal cortex (primary sensory cortex). The primary sensory cortex is responsible for integration and interpretation of somatosensory information.[50-52]

The descending motor system comprises three relevant areas: 1) the primary motor cortex, 2) the pre-motor cortex, and 3) supplemental motor cortex.[53,54] Both the primary and pre-motor cortex have direct inputs from the primary sensory cortex.[53,54] Descending motor commands are adapted within the cerebellum and basal ganglia, and terminate in both alpha (α) and gamma (γ) motor neurons which respond to sensory inputs.[54] This completes the cycle of planning and modification of motor activities.

Theories over the past decades considered proprioception from a peripheral and anatomical model, i.e., injury led to impairment of the local mechanoreceptors in the capsule or ligaments (Ruffini ending or Pacinian corpuscle) and, thereby, the afferent signaling.[21] An injury to either the muscle–tendon units (such as rotator cuff) or capsule (as in dislocations) of the glenohumeral joint was suggested to lead to impaired mechanical stability and sensory signaling.[18,55] Disruption of the capsule impairs passive joint stability in the dislocation direction. Furthermore, the mechanoreceptors responsible for providing proprioceptive information regarding tension of the joint capsule were believed to respond to altered tension loads within the stretched or torn capsule.[2,40,56] Loss of proprioceptive input from mechanoreceptors of the injured joint would change the afferent signaling, and thereby influence motor programs or neuromuscular control.[26] This loss in proprioceptive afferent information was suggested to lead to further joint stability compromises. Thus, the focus was on the peripheral injury to the shoulder and damage to the capsule and ligaments with the embedded mechanoreceptors, leading to disruption of normal neuromuscular reflex joint stabilization.[57]

Neuromatrix model for proprioception

To advance understanding of proprioception as a sensation, and implications for assessment and rehabilitation, more recent neuroscientific concepts need to be incorporated into the previous peripheral-dominant mechanisms. CNS interpretation and processing of proprioception input are influenced by a multitude of factors.

As described above, defined neuroanatomical regions of the brain are responsible for receiving afferent proprioceptive input, process that input, and determine an appropriate motor response or output, as for example, during an assessment of JPS or kinesthesia. Functional neurophysiological processes that extend across different brain regions and systems influence movement outputs. The model of a neuromatrix and neurotags has been used to illustrate the complexity of such influences (Figure 28.2).[3,58,59]

The neuromatrix represents the complex connections of cells, nerve impulses, and chemical reactions within and

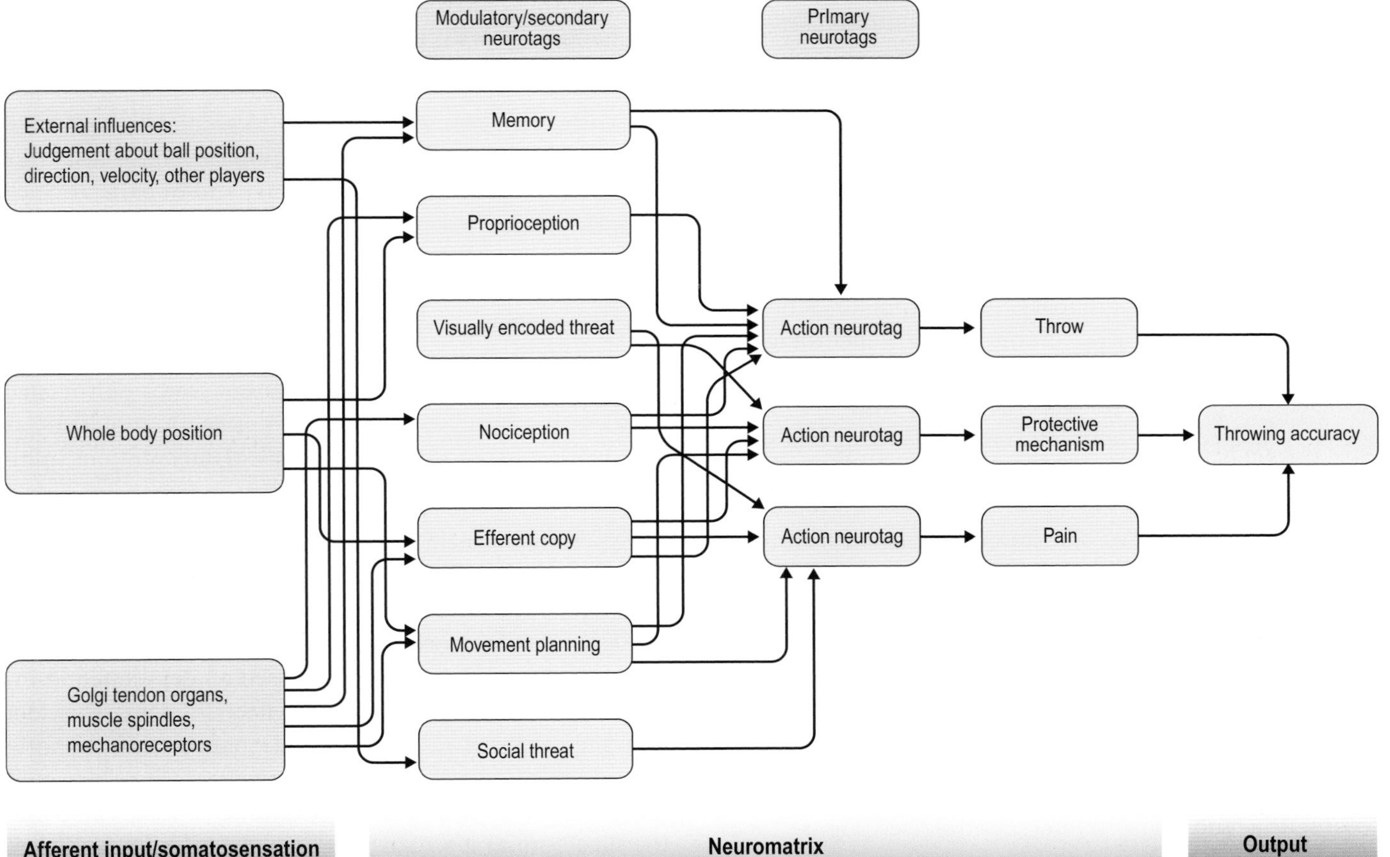

FIGURE 28.2

Theoretical model for integrating a peripheral-dominant model with that of the neuromatrix. The neuromatrix boxes in the middle present central pathways, whereas boxes on the left represent overlapping external factors and proprioceptive receptors within the shoulder joint, muscles, and tendons. Multiple arrows represent complex, modifiable pathways that can influence throwing accuracy and the experience of pain (or the lack thereof). An arrow from the right side back to the left would complete the feedback mechanisms.

(Modified with permission from Wallwork SB, Bellan V, Moseley GL. Applying current concepts in pain-related brain science to dance rehabilitation. J Dance Med Sci. 2017;21(1):13-23.[59])

between regions of the brain. Besides the regions mentioned above, it also includes the frontal lobes (thought and emotion), limbic system (experience and expression of emotion), and pituitary gland (hormonal control), and others. Thus, thoughts, emotions, memory, and whether we are feeling relaxed or stressed can influence how we move and how accurate the movements are. Such influences can be understood with the concept of neurotags within the neuromatrix.

Neurotags are networks of anatomically and physiologically linked neurons across the brain regions that, at a particular time, lead to and influence movement.[60] In essence, a neurotag is a group of neurons across brain regions that are active (or "fire") at the same time. Larger and more frequently used neurotags are likely to have greater influence than smaller or less used ones. The influences of the neurotags are not constant and may change over time. This is known as neuroplasticity.[58,60]

A primary neurotag may act on motor units that lead to the desired output or action, such as an accurate throw.[58] Secondary neurotags influence that output or action by modulating the precision of the primary neurotags.[58,59] Proprioception can be seen as one of a number of secondary neurotags influencing the accuracy of a throw, along with memory, nociceptive input, movement planning and social threat (e.g., another player on the sports field). Thus, within a sensorimotor context, a specific shoulder movement or a throw are the result of activation of a primary neurotag, which is modulated by secondary neurotags. Similarly, the TTDPM assessed as illustrated in Figure 28.1, is not only influenced by the proprioception neurotag, but also by the participant's familiarity with the task, potential nociceptive input, and attention.[55,56,61]

In the neuromatrix model, proprioception is one of a multitude of mechanisms used by the CNS for somatosensation and sensorimotor control (see Figure 28.2). Proprioceptive input is continuously integrated with inputs from the visual, auditory, vestibular, and olfactory systems,[3] to update internal predictions and modify desired or required outputs.[58] Thus, changes in other secondary neurotags, such as nociception,[62] or a slightly different body position, interact with the proprioception neurotag, leading to changes in the movement outcome. Such interaction can change the outcomes of a proprioceptive assessment, contributing towards high variability and, thereby, measurement error.

Findings of impaired motion and position sense in study participants with stroke support a significant mechanism of the CNS to underlie proprioceptive changes.[63] Patients with stroke exhibit *bilateral deficits* in movement detection and repositioning tests for the shoulder compared to healthy participants.[64] When comparing TTDPM for external and internal rotation (in 90° abduction) of people with stroke to people without stroke, mean differences were around 7° for the contralateral and 3° for the ipsilateral stroke side.[64] In these people, changes in proprioception are thus evident despite no damage or injury to the peripheral mechanoreceptors. Thus, afferent proprioceptive signaling from the mechanoreceptors is likely to be normal, but CNS processing of afferent information has changed post-stroke.[63,64]

Central processing changes due to secondary neurotags may also influence the results of proprioceptive tests (the output) in people with shoulder injury and/or pain.[65,66] Such central changes may occur in addition to potential changes in the shoulder mechanoreceptors and muscle spindle system, adding to individual-specific changes. Such complex systems explain, in part, the challenge with comparing proprioceptive measures in people with the same shoulder condition (such as frozen shoulder or rotator cuff-related shoulder pain) to people with asymptomatic shoulders, as well as when exploring whether clinical interventions influence proprioception.

Experimental pain models permit the impact of pain to be assessed when administered to individuals without tissue injury. Methods include injecting hypertonic saline into muscle and other anatomical structures, creating transient local or referred pain.[67] We have used an experimental-induced pain model to investigate effects of acute shoulder pain on isokinetic external and internal rotation strength, throwing accuracy,[68] and proprioception.[43] Shoulder pain was generated in response to hypertonic saline injected into the subacromial space. In the experimental pain condition, participants had 20% decreased peak torque for external and internal rotation and throwing accuracy compared to the control condition, validating the model.[68]

In terms of proprioception, no differences were found for passive joint reproduction error when comparing the pain condition to baseline and follow-up (no pain). However, for TTDPM, enhanced kinesthesia was evident for the pain condition compared to baseline and recovery control conditions.[43] While the differences were small (0.5°), the

TTDPM was reduced on average by 30% for the experimental pain condition compared to the control conditions. Decreased thresholds, thus "improved" movement sense, were unexpected and contrasted to those expected for patients with shoulder pain and concomitant injury.

This study demonstrated that injection of hypertonic saline into the subacromial space produced shoulder pain associated with enhanced movement sense, while having no significant effect on passive JPS across the group of particpiants.[43] The enhanced movement sense may reflect a central protective mechanism. When considering the neuromatrix model, in this case, a nociceptive modulatory neurotag (facilitated by the noxious stimulus of the saline) may have had a facilitatory influence on the kinesthesia neurotag during the specific test.

Pain is an indicator for danger, and one role of the CNS is to protect the body from further harm.[69,70] The experimental pain rendered the shoulder more sensitive to movement, which may be protective. Whether such heightened sensitivity to movement (as assessed with TTDPM) is due to enhanced muscle spindle activity via the fusiform system, due to changes in processing (central mechanisms), and as part of a response to a specific neurotag, needs further investigations. These findings further challenge the specificity of the assessments for proprioception and provide a strong direction towards CNS processes influencing such measurements.

Recent realization is that proprioceptive afferents are integrated across several muscles and at different joints of the kinetic chain, rather than from one isolated joint segment.[44] The proprioceptive mechanisms are thus complex at the levels of input, processing, as well as output. Adaptations occur due to neuroplasticity, compensating at any level for influences of injury, pain, or other factors (secondary neurotags). In summary, movement planning and execution are influenced by complex, modifiable interactions between afferent signals and neural networks in the brain (neurotags), and are not isolated to specific areas of sensory and motor matrices.[58]

Exercise and shoulder proprioception

Exercise can disturb or enhance proprioception. Current understanding suggests that exercise enhances function of the muscle spindle and Golgi tendon organs via enhanced sensitivity of the α and γ systems, rather than the mechanoreceptors of joints.[5,16,44] Disturbances to proprioception can be as an acute response to fatigue related to exercise. Laboratory-based studies can assess a defined modality before and after a fatigue protocol. For example, repetitive, rapid external and internal rotation can be performed on an isokinetic dynamometer until the torque drops to a predefined level relative to initial or maximal levels.[71-73] Contrasting post-fatigue findings have been reported, ranging from no differences[73] to increases of up to 0.8° [72] to 3.3° [71] for active joint position error, and 0.5° for TTDPM.[74]

More recently, Sadler and Cressman[75] used a repetitive reaching task, paced with a metronome, until the participant reported a defined rate of perceived exertion or could no longer maintain the pace of movement. The study explored the influence of unilateral shoulder fatigue (right side) on acuity of hand position sense of both sides using a computer-assisted device. The results indicated that both the fatigued right and the non-fatigued left sides had decreased hand position acuity.[75] Thus, fatigue of one shoulder led to bilateral hand proprioceptive deficits.

A series of studies outlined by Proske[16] suggest it is less likely that post-exercise changes in proprioceptive sense involve peripheral receptors, but that the exercise (fatigue) effects are more likely to occur within the brain.[75] Future studies may explore how fatigue protocols influence proprioceptive measures for people with shoulder pain.

An important question is whether deficits in proprioceptive measures, assessed in a laboratory or clinic, are associated with function- and performance-related deficits. What is the relevance of a deficit of 0.5° for TTDPM or 3° for joint position error, even if found to be statistically significant in experimental conditions? Exploring a potential relationship between proprioception and sports-related performance, Dover et al.[76] showed that overhead female athletes had larger external rotation active joint position errors (measured with inclinometers) compared to non-athletes, and for the throwing compared to non-throwing shoulders. Thus, contradicting expectations, the athletes had less accurate JPS compared to non-athletes.

Those findings contrast with a more recent study using an active movement extent discrimination assessment (AMEDA) of the shoulder[29] in 22 baseball players, finding no difference in positional acuity between the throwing and non-throwing arm.[10] Furthermore, proprioception was not correlated with speed and accuracy of throwing.[10] That contrasts with findings by Hams et al.,[77] that coach-rated throwing mechanics of water polo players were strongly correlated with active joint position sense assessed with an AMEDA in the water. In another study by the same research group, higher mean proprioceptive acuity of three joints, the shoulder, ankle and spine, was found to be associated with higher levels of performance of elite athletes.[78] Findings of those studies need to be considered under the limitation of cross-sectional designs.[29,76,78]

In a randomized clinical trial with healthy participants, Salles et al.[79] reported that an eight-week shoulder strengthening exercise program led to improved proprioception (mean decrease of 3.5° for absolute error of active joint position sense internal and external rotation in 90° abduction) in healthy participants.[79] Distinction may need to be made between chronic repetitive, lower intensity exercises versus strengthening exercises at higher intensity.

Overall, investigators have explored differences in proprioceptive acuity between overhand athletes and non-athletes, with conflicting findings. A shoulder muscle strengthening program was shown to enhance proprioception in non-athletes. Contrasting findings have been found, or have not yet been explored, between proprioceptive deficits of the shoulder and athletic performance (such as throwing accuracy), functional or performance capacity, or other measures of impairment (such as muscle weakness).

Clinical considerations

Assessment

Assessment of proprioception is required in laboratory-based experimental studies to explore consequences of injury and diseases, as well of efficacy of interventions. Such studies are critical to advance the scientific basis for clinical interventions. In clinical practice, assessments should be relevant and specific for the individual patient, and should influence decision-making for the intervention, rehabilitation, and functional retraining. As suggested above, clinical assessments of proprioceptive sub-modalities may not be sufficiently sensitive nor relevant in clinical practice for individual patients with musculoskeletal disorders. That contrasts with assessments for patient groups where proprioceptive deficits are well-defined, such as in people with stroke or other neurological disorders.[63,64]

Construct validity of the proprioceptive assessment for people with shoulder pain remains unclear as differences are not consistently found, or are very small when comparing groups of people with shoulder pain to those with asymptomatic shoulders.[3,6] The ecological validity of the proprioceptive assessments can be challenged as the proprioceptive testing environment is unlikely to be comparable to usual daily, work, and sporting activities.[29]

An isolated assessment of proprioception may not be meaningful to guide rehabilitation. It may, however, be helpful as part of a holistic assessment within the World Health Organization International Classification of Functioning, Health and Disability (ICF) Model (Figure 28.3).[80] In short, the ICF model expands the view of disease from one specific entity towards a more global perspective of the individual. Proprioceptive impairments fit under the 'Body Function and Structure' component, and may overlap with those of motor control, such as of the scapula.[81,82]

Assessment, and subsequent treatment, must also consider 'Activity' limitations and 'Participation' restrictions, as well environmental and personal factors. Examples of assessments at Activity level are the Closed Kinetic Chain Upper Extremity Stability Test,[83] the Athletic Shoulder Test,[84] the Shoulder Endurance Test,[85] and the Shoulder Arm Return to Sport Test Battery.[86] The outcomes of these assessments all depend on somatosensation (including proprioception), central integration and the motor output. The clinician can then use outcomes of the proprioceptive assessment (Body Function and Structure) in the context of the assessments targeting the Activity and Participation limitations, and combined, these may offer clinicians a clearer starting point for rehabilitation.

Rehabilitation

A number of studies have explored whether nonsurgical interventions influence proprioceptive variables for the shoulder;[13] it is evident that exercises improve the sensorimotor system related to shoulder function.[13] Practice guidelines and commentaries have promoted exercises which improve proprioception in the rehabilitation of a variety of shoulder-related conditions.[12,14] Although joint

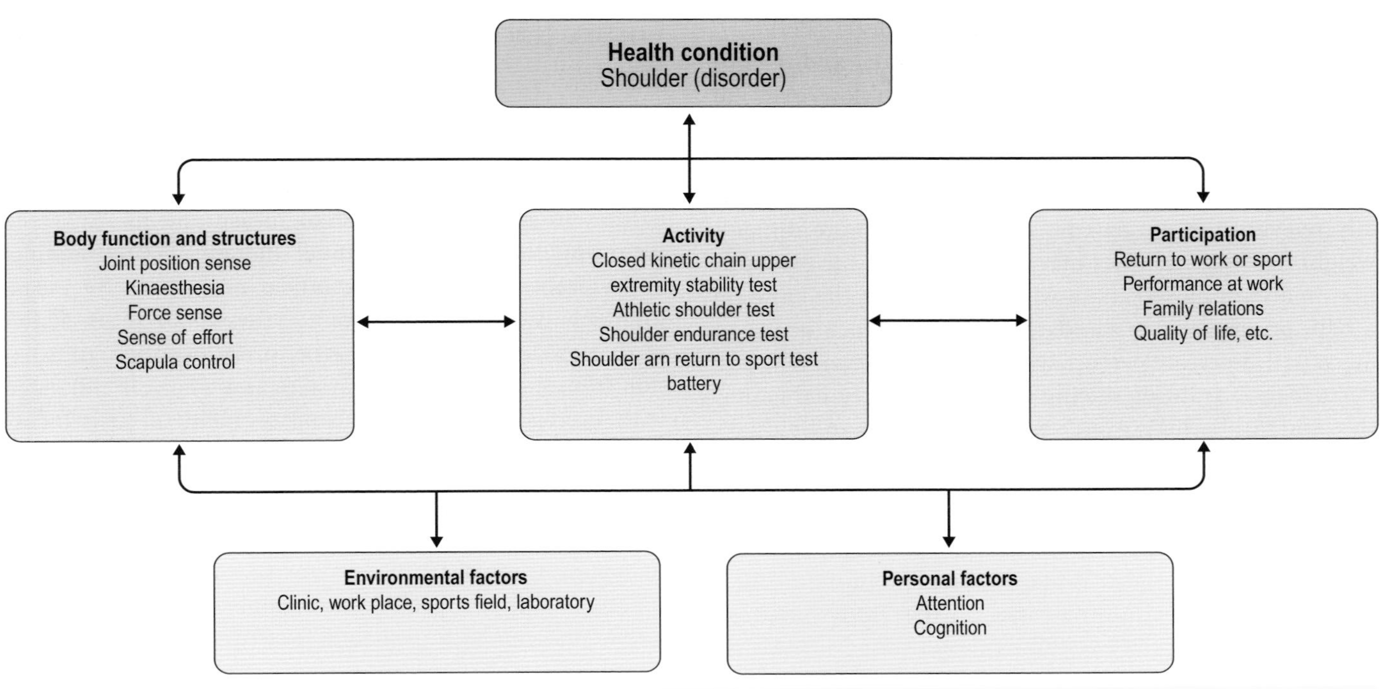

FIGURE 28.3
International Classification of Functioning, Health and Disability (ICF) Model applied to integration of proprioceptive or sensorimotor assessments into clinical practice for people with shoulder pain. Examples for assessments of Body Function and Structure, Activity Limitations, and Participation Restrictions are provided.

repositioning exercises with eyes closed have been proposed following shoulder injury,[12,87] evidence of their efficacy and effectiveness is lacking. The best, or most appropriate, exercises to improve sensorimotor system function are unknown.

In reality, all exercises can appropriately be described as 'proprioceptive' given that all active movements will initiate afferent action potentials from mechanoreceptors, muscle spindles and GTOs in and around the involved joints, irrespective of classification of exercise.[14] Principles of exercises to target proprioception are, in essence, based on principles of motor relearning[88] to improve motor control and coordination.[14] Proprioceptive exercises described in the past also have overlapping principles with those of "graded exposure" activities.[89] From clinical perspectives, graded exposure interventions are behavioral approaches used to decrease fear of pain or reinjury, using a progressive approach.[89]

Exercises purporting to have a specific focus on proprioception should consider multilevel aspects of training. Firstly, an internal focus of attention is initially used, where attention is directed to the action itself. Using an internal focus, the person's attention (cognition) is on the movement or position, such as during scapula setting exercises or low-intensity rotator cuff exercises.[81] The focus is then shifted to an external focus as part of the progressive program, for example on accuracy or direction of a throw. Secondly, the exercises are initiated with slow controlled movements at low loads. They are progressed by increasing velocity, load, variability in movement pattern, and unpredictability.[14] Thirdly, weight-bearing exercises have been recommended under the premise that articular surface compression stimulates articular receptors and co-contraction of surrounding muscles, so that the muscle spindle and GTO complex might be facilitated.[12,14,81]

The early phase of rehabilitation may entail slow reversals and dynamic stabilization, within the concept of

Proprioceptive Neuromuscular Facilitation (PNF).[12,90] Local, conscious exercises of the scapula and glenohumeral joint can be included, such as slow external and internal rotation movements with or without elasticated resistance bands or a ball in the hand,[81] progressing from a neutral shoulder position to those more functionally relevant for the patient. Progressively more difficult weight-bearing exercises may be performed, for example, first in a semi-closed chain while seated with the hand on a ball, progressing to hands placed on balance board or Swiss balls to create perturbations.[81] The program may add perturbation training during simulated functional activities, and fast ballistic exercises specific for the individual's requirements.[14]

We can use the ICF and the neuromatrix models to rationalize the exercise prescription. For example, localized exercises for the scapula or the glenohumeral joint movement and positioning focus on the 'Body Function & Structure' component. Considering that new scientific insights suggest that the CNS processes proprioceptive afferent information from a number of muscles across various joints (thus, the kinetic chain),[44] the exercise program should progress to multi-joint exercises specific for the individual person. Examples are whole arm exercises with cables or elasticated resistance bands that also include trunk rotation or weight shifts. For people who engage in sports, drills used as part of their routine warm-ups and warm-downs can form part of the proprioceptive training, initially focusing on slow, controlled drills, progressively increasing in speed, complexity, and unpredictability.

Such exercise would be in line with the concept that proprioceptive information is used for a body image and body schema, rather than for an isolated joint.[44] With reference to the neuromatrix model, perhaps such exercises establish neurotags that become used more frequently during daily life, work or sports, with less modulation or interference by secondary nociceptive neurotags. With such considerations, the exercise focus would move towards the 'Activity' and 'Participation' components of the ICF, merging with individual- and function-specific exercises, relevant for the person's daily, work- and sports-related activities and contexts. We suggest that clinical decision-making for rehabilitation can be guided by using these concepts, rather than by specific prescriptive protocols.

Future perspectives

There are many factors which influence the outcomes of, what should be termed, sensorimotor system tests. Shoulder injury,[3,6] experimental pain,[43] muscle fatigue,[16] and thermal modalities[91] have all shown changes in specific sub-modalities of sensorimotor system measurements. Evidence regarding the effect of manual therapy, taping/bracing, and vibration training on shoulder proprioceptive measurements is equivocal.[8,13] Twenty years ago, Ashton-Miller et al.[5] posed the question whether proprioception, in isolation from the sensorimotor system as a whole, is enhanced with exercise, and whether improvement of such measures predict enhanced outcomes. This question remains unanswered.

Influences on somatosensation and motor responses from the spine, scapula, trunk and lower limbs, thus the entire kinetic chain, also provide directions for future research. Based on currently available measurements, the contribution of changes in proprioception to the sensorimotor system and performance is still unclear.[13,14] Longitudinal studies are needed to determine if proprioceptive deficits following shoulder injury influence recovery of functional capacity and physical or sports performance.

Consideration of the neuromatrix model, interconnectivity between neurotags and how neuroplasticity compensates for loss or to improve function and performance, particularly following injury, provides directions for future clinical interventions, and needs further exploration. Studies utilizing neuroimaging such as fMRI,[66,92] merging fields of neuroscience, neuropsychology, ageing, neurological disorders, and musculoskeletal injury, will add further insights into how the somatosensory system changes, and the efficacy of interventions.

Conclusion

Proprioception, as part of the somatosensory system, is a critical element of providing sensation of body movement, position, and image. Currently, accurate clinical measurement of proprioception may not be feasible nor valid when performed in isolation. Sensorimotor system tests which focus on functional performance are advocated for clinical use. Principles of exercise that have targeted proprioception are similar to those targeting skills-based motor learning, motor control, and graded exposure interventions. Within current knowledge, we should consider the clinical assessments and influence of interventions and exercises within the ICF model and the neuromatrix model. It may be more appropriate to consider how active exercises (and other interventions) influence the CNS processing and outputs, and potential modulation by various neurotags, tying into the biopsychosocial model of health.

References

1. Hodges PW, Barbe MF, Loggia ML, Nijs J, Stone LS. Diverse role of biological plasticity in low back pain and its impact on sensorimotor control of the spine. J Orthop Sports Phys Ther. 2019;49:389-401.
2. Myers JB, Lephart SM. The role of the sensorimotor system in the athletic shoulder. J Athl Train. 2000;35:351-63.
3. Ager AL, Borms D, Deschepper L, Dhooghe R, Dijkhuis J, Roy J-S, et al. Proprioception: how is it affected by shoulder pain? A systematic review. J Hand Ther. 2020;33:507-16.
4. Ager AL, Roy J-S, Roos M, Belley AF, Cools A, Hébert LJ. Shoulder proprioception: how is it measured and is it reliable? A systematic review. J Hand Ther. 2017;30:221-31.
5. Ashton-Miller JA, Wojtys EM, Huston LJ, Fry-Welch D. Can proprioception be trained? Knee Surg Sports Traumatol Arthrosc. 2001;9:128-36.
6. Fyhr C, Gustavsson L, Wassinger C, Sole G. The effects of shoulder injury on kinaesthesia: a systematic review and meta-analysis. Man Ther. 2015;20:28-37.
7. Freeston J, Adams R, Ferdinands RE, Rooney K. Indicators of throwing arm fatigue in elite adolescent male baseball players: a randomized crossover trial. J Strength Cond Res. 2014;28:2115-20.
8. Boarati EdL, Hotta GH, McQuade KJ, de Oliveira AS. Acute effect of flexible bar exercise on scapulothoracic muscles activation, on isometric shoulder abduction force and proprioception of the shoulder of individuals with and without subacromial pain syndrome. Clin Biomech. 2020;72:77-83.
9. Haik MN, Camargo PR, Zanca GG, Alburquerque-Sendin F, Salvini TF, Mattiello-Rosa SM. Joint position sense is not altered during shoulder medial and lateral rotations in female assembly line workers with shoulder impingement syndrome. Physiother Theory Pract. 2013;29:41-50.
10. Freeston J, Adams RD, Rooney K. Shoulder proprioception is not related to throwing speed or accuracy in elite adolescent male baseball players. J Strength Conditioning Res. 2015;29:181-7.
11. Rokito AS, Birdzell MG, Cuomo F, Di Paola MJ, Zuckerman JD. Recovery of shoulder strength and proprioception after open surgery for recurrent anterior instability: a comparison of two surgical techniques. J Shoulder Elbow Surg. 2010;19:564-9.
12. Wilk K, Meister K, Andrews J. Current concepts in the rehabilitation of the overhead throwing athlete. Am J Sports Med. 2002;30:136-51.
13. Ager AL, Borms D, Bernaert M, Brusselle V, Claessens M, Roy J-S, et al. Can a conservative rehabilitation strategy improve shoulder proprioception? A systematic review. J Sport Rehabil. 2021;30:136-51.
14. Clark NC, Röijezon U, Treleaven J. Proprioception in musculoskeletal rehabilitation. Part 2: Clinical assessment and intervention. Man Ther. 2015;20:378-87.
15. Hillier S, Immink M, Thewlis D. Assessing proprioception: a systematic review of possibilities. Neurorehabil Neural Repair. 2015;29:933-49.
16. Proske U. Exercise, fatigue and proprioception: a retrospective. Exp Brain Res. 2019;237:2447-59.
17. McCloskey DI. Kinesthetic sensibility. Physiol Rev. 1978;58:763-820.
18. Riemann BL, Lephart SM. The sensorimotor system, part I: the physiologic basis of functional joint stability. J Athl Train. 2002;37:71-9.
19. Myers JB, Wassinger CA, Lephart SM. Sensorimotor contribution to shoulder stability: effect of injury and rehabilitation. Man Ther. 2006;11:197-201.
20. Aman JE, Elangovan N, Yeh I-L, Konczak J. The effectiveness of proprioceptive training for improving motor function: a systematic review. Front Hum Neurosci. 2015;8:1-18.
21. Lephart SM, Fu FH. Proprioception and Neuromuscular Control in Joint Stability. Champaign: Human Kinetics; 2000.
22. Dover G, Powers ME. Reliability of joint position sense and force-reproduction measures during internal and external rotation of the shoulder. J Athl Train. 2003;38:304-10.
23 Vafadar AK, Cote J, Archambault PS. Interrater and intrarater reliability and validity of 3 measurement methods for shoulder-position sense. J Sport Rehabil. 2016;25:2014-0309.
24. Ramos MM, Carnaz L, Mattiello SM, Karduna AR, Zanca GG. Shoulder and elbow joint position sense assessment using a mobile app in subjects with and without shoulder pain - between-days reliability. Phys Ther Sport. 2019;37:157-63.
25. Edwards E, S., Lin Y-L, King J, H., Karduna A, R. Joint position sense – there's an app for that. J Biomech. 2016;49:3529-33.
26. Lephart SM, Myers JB, Bradley JP, Fu FH. Shoulder proprioception and function following thermal capsulorraphy. Arthrosc. 2002;18:770-8.
27. Tripp BL, Boswell L, Gansneder BM, Shultz SJ. Functional fatigue decreases 3-dimensional multi-joint position reproduction acuity in the overhead-throwing athlete. J Athl Train. 2004;39:316-20.
28. Voight ML, Hardin JA, Blackburn TA, Tippett S, Canner GC. The effects of muscle fatigue on and the relationship of arm dominance to shoulder proprioception. J Orthop Sports Phys Ther. 1996;23:348-52.
29. Han J, Waddington G, Adams R, Anson J, Liu Y. Assessing proprioception: a critical review of methods. J Sport Health Sci. 2016;5:80-90.
30. Riemann BL, Myers JB, Lephart SM. Sensorimotor system measurement techniques. J Athl Train. 2002;37:85-98.
31. Fortier S, Basset FA. The effects of exercise on limb proprioceptive signals. J Electromyogr Kinesiol. 2012;22:795-802.

32. Suprak DN, Osternig LR, van Donkelaar P, Karduna AR. Shoulder joint position sense improves with elevation angle in a novel, unconstrained task. J Orthop Res. 2006;24:559-68.

33. Proske U, Gregory JE, Morgan DL, Percival P, Weerakkody NS, Canny BJ. Force matching errors following eccentric exercise. Hum Mov Sci. 2004;23:365-78.

34. Jerosch J, Wüstner P. [Effect of a sensorimotor training program on patients with subacromial pain syndrome]. Der Unfallchirurg. 2002;105:36-43.

35. Machner A, Merk H, Becker R, Rohkohl K, Wissel H, Pap G. Kinesthetic sense of the shoulder in patients with impingement syndrome. Acta Orthop Scandin. 2003;74:85-8.

36. Anderson VB, Wee E. Impaired joint proprioception at higher shoulder elevations in chronic rotator cuff pathology. Arch Phys Med Rehabil. 2011;92:1146-51.

37. Gumina S, Camerota F, Celletti C, Venditto T, Candela V. The effects of rotator cuff tear on shoulder proprioception. Int Orthop. 2019;43:229-35.

38. Mörl F, Matkey A, Bretschneider S, Bernsdorf A, Bradl I. Pain relief due to physiotherapy doesn't change the motor function of the shoulder. J Bodywork Mov Ther. 2011;15:309-18.

39. Fabis J, Rzepka R, Fabis A, Zwierzchowski J, Kubiak G, Stanula A, et al. Shoulder proprioception – lessons we learned from idiopathic frozen shoulder. BMC Musculoskel Disord. 2016;17:123.

40. Smith RL, Brunolli J. Shoulder kinesthesia after anterior glenohumeral joint dislocation. Phys Ther. 1989;69:106-12.

41. Keenan KA, Akins JS, Varnell M, Abt J, Lovalekar M, Lephart S, et al. Kinesiology taping does not alter shoulder strength, shoulder proprioception, or scapular kinematics in healthy, physically active subjects and subjects with Subacromial Impingement Syndrome. Phys Ther Sport. 2017;24:60-6.

42. Carter RE, Lubinsky J, Domholdt E. Rehabilitation Reseach: Principles and Applications, 4th edition. St Louis: Elsevier; 2011.

43. Sole G, Osborne H, Wassinger C. The effect of experimentally-induced subacromial pain on proprioception. Man Ther. 2015;20:166-70.

44. Proske U, Gandevia SC. The proprioceptive senses: their roles in signaling body shape, body position and movement, and muscle force. Physiol Rev. 2012;92:1651-97.

45. Proske U. Kinesthesia: the role of muscle receptors. Muscle and Nerve. 2006;34:545-58.

46. Erickson RIC, Karduna AR. Three-dimensional repositioning tasks show differences in joint position sense between active and passive shoulder motion. J Orthop Res. 2012;30:787-92.

47. Gandevia SC, McCloskey DI, Burke D. Kinaesthetic signals and muscle contraction. Trends Neurosci. 1992;15:62-5.

48. Laumonerie P, Dalmas Y, Tibbo ME, Robert S, Faruch M, Chaynes P, et al. Sensory innervation of the human shoulder joint: the three bridges to break. J Shoulder Elbow Surg. 2020;29:e499-e507.

49. Witherspoon JW, Smirnova IV, McIff TE. Neuroanatomical distribution of mechanoreceptors in the human cadaveric shoulder capsule and labrum. J Anat. 2014;225:337-45.

50. Delhaye BP, Long KH, Bensmaia SJ. Neural basis of touch and proprioception in primate cortex. In: Pollock DM (ed). Comprehensive Physiology. New York: John Wiley & Sons Inc; 2018: 1575-602.

51. ten Donkelaar HJ, Broman J, van Domburg P. The Somatosensory System. In: ten Donkelaar HJ (ed). Clinical Neuroanatomy. Cham: Springer; 2020: 171-255.

52. Röijezon U, Clark NC, Treleaven J. Proprioception in musculoskeletal rehabilitation. Part 1: Basic science and principles of assessment and clinical interventions. Man Ther. 2015;20:368-77.

53. Mihailoff G, Haines D. Motor system II: corticofugal systems and the control of movement. In: Fundamental Neuroscience. New York: Churchill Livingstone; 1997: 335-46.

54. Wolpert D, Pearson K, Ghez C, Kandel E. Principles of Neural Science. The Organization and Planning of Movement, 5th edition. New York: McGraw-Hill; 2013: 475-97.

55. Riemann BL, Lephart SM. The sensorimotor system, part II: the role of proprioception in motor control and functional joint stability. J Athl Train. 2002;37:80-4.

56. Myers JB, Lephart SM. Sensorimotor deficits contributing to glenohumeral instability. Clin Orthop Rel Res. 2002;400:98-104.

57. Lephart S, Warner JJ, Borsa PA, Fu FH. Proprioception of the shoulder joint in healthy, unstable and surgically repaired shoulder. J Shoulder Elbow Surg. 1994;3:371-80.

58. Wallwork SB, Bellan V, Catley MJ, Moseley GL. Neural representations and the cortical body matrix: implications for sports medicine and future directions. Br J Sports Med. 2016;50:990-6.

59. Wallwork SB, Bellan V, Moseley GL. Applying current concepts in pain-related brain science to dance rehabilitation. J Dance Med Sci. 2017;21:13-23.

60. Butler D, Moseley L. Explain Pain. NOI Publishers; 2003.

61. Elangovan N, Herrmann A, Konczak J. Assessing proprioceptive function: evaluating joint position matching methods against psychophysical thresholds. Phys Ther. 2014;94:553-61.

62. Nijs J, Daenen L, Cras P, Struyf F, Roussel N, Oostendorp RAB. Nociception affects motor output: a review on sensory-motor interaction with focus on clinical implications. Clin J Pain. 2012;28:175-81.

63. Niessen MH, Veeger DH, Meskers CG, Koppe PA, Konijnenbelt MH, Janssen TW. Relationship among shoulder proprioception, kinematics, and pain after stroke. Arch Phys Med Rehabil. 2009;90:1557-64.

64. Niessen MH, Veeger DH, Koppe PA, Konijnenbelt MH, van Dieën J, Janssen TW. Proprioception of the shoulder after stroke. Arch Phys Med Rehabil. 2008;89:333-8.

65. Sanchis MN, Lluch E, Nijs J, Struyf F, Kangasperko M. The role of central sensitization in shoulder pain: a systematic literature review. Sem Arthr Rheumat. 2015;44:710-6.

66. Li J-L, Yan C-Q, Wang X, Zhang S, Zhang N, Hu S-Q, et al. Brain functional alternations of the pain-related emotional and cognitive regions in patients with chronic shoulder pain. J Pain Res. 2020;13:575-83.

67. Olesen AE, Andresen T, Staahl C, Drewes AM. Human experimental pain models for assessing the therapeutic efficacy of analgesic drugs. Pharmacol Rev. 2012;64:722-79.

68. Wassinger CA, Sole G, Osborne H. The role of experimentally-induced subacromial pain on shoulder strength and throwing accuracy. Man Ther. 2012;17:411-5.

69. Bank PJ, Peper CE, Marinus J, Beek PJ, van Hilten JJ. Motor consequences of experimentally induced limb pain: a systematic review. Eur J Pain. 2013;17:145-57.

70. Hodges PW, Tucker K. Moving differently in pain: a new theory to explain the adaptation to pain. Pain. 2011;152:S90-8.

71. Voight ML, Hardin JA, Blackburn TA, Tippett S, Canner GC. The effects of muscle fatigue on and the relationship of arm dominance to shoulder proprioception. J Orthop Sports Phys Ther. 1996;23:348-52.

72. Myers JB, Guskiewicz KM, Schneider RA, Prentice WE. Proprioception and neuromuscular control of the shoulder after muscle fatigue. J Athl Train. 1999;34:362-7.

73. Sterner RL, Pincivero DM, Lephart SM. The effects of muscular fatigue on shoulder proprioception. Clin J Sport Med. 1998;8:96-101.

74. Carpenter JE, Blasier RB, Pellizzon GG. The effects of muscle fatigue on shoulder joint position sense. Am J Sports Med. 1998;26:262-5.

75. Sadler CM, Cressman EK. Central fatigue mechanisms are responsible for decreases in hand proprioceptive acuity following shoulder muscle fatigue. Hum Mov Sci. 2019;66:220-30.

76. Dover GC, Kaminski TW, Meister K, Powers ME, Horodyski M. Assessment of shoulder proprioception in the female softball athlete. Am J Sports Med. 2003;31:431-7.

77. Hams AH, Evans K, Adams R, Waddington G, Witchalls J. Throwing performance in water polo is related to in-water shoulder proprioception. J Sports Sci. 2019;37:2588-95.

78. Han J, Waddington G, Anson J, Adams R. Level of competitive success achieved by elite athletes and multi-joint proprioceptive ability. J Sci Med Sport. 2015;18:77-81.

79. Salles JI, Velasques B, Cossich V, Nicoliche E, Ribeiro P, Amaral MV, et al. Strength training and shoulder proprioception. J Athl Train. 2015;50:277-80.

80. World Health Organisation. International Classification of Functioning, Disability and Health (ICF) 2001. Available at: https://www.who.int/standards/classifications/international-classification-of-functioning-disability-and-health.

81. Magarey ME, Jones MA. Dynamic evaluation and early management of altered motor control around the shoulder complex. Man Ther. 2003;8:195-206.

82. Willmore EG, Smith MJ. Scapular dyskinesia: evolution towards a systems-based approach. Shoulder Elbow. 2015;8:61-70.

83. Tucci HT, Martins J, Sposito GdC, Camarini PMF, de Oliveira AS. Closed Kinetic Chain Upper Extremity Stability test (CKCUES test): a reliability study in persons with and without shoulder impingement syndrome. BMC Musculoskel Disord. 2014;15:1.

84. Ashworth B, Hogben P, Singh N, Tulloch L, Cohen DD. The Athletic Shoulder (ASH) test: reliability of a novel upper body isometric strength test in elite rugby players. BMJ Open Sport Exerc Med. 2018;4:e000365.

85. Declève P, Van Cant J, Attar T, Urbain E, Marcel M, Borms D, et al. The shoulder endurance test (SET): a reliability and validity and comparison study on healthy overhead athletes and sedentary adults. Phys Ther Sport. 2021;47:201-7.

86. Olds M, Coulter C, Marant D, Uhl T. Reliability of a shoulder arm return to sport test battery. Phys Ther Sport. 2019;39:16-22.

87. Helgeson K, Stoneman P. Shoulder injuries in rugby players: mechanisms, examination, and rehabilitation. Phys Ther Sport. 2014;15:218-27.

88. Krakauer JW, Mazzoni P. Human sensorimotor learning: adaptation, skill, and beyond. Curr Opinion Neurobiol. 2011;21:636-44.

89. George SZ, Giorgio Zeppieri J. Physical therapy utilization of graded exposure for patients with low back pain. J Orthop Sports Phys Ther. 2009;39:496-505.

90. Knott M, Voss P. Proprioceptive Neuromuscular Facilitation, 3rd edition. New York: Harper & Row; 1985.

91. Wassinger CA, Myers JB, Gatti JM, Conley KM, Lephart SM. Proprioception and throwing accuracy in the dominant shoulder after cryotherapy. J Athl Train. 2007;42:84-9.

92. Landelle C, Anton J-L, Nazarian B, Sein J, Gharbi A, Felician O, et al. Functional brain changes in the elderly for the perception of hand movements: a greater impairment occurs in proprioception than touch. NeuroImage. 2020;220:117056.

When to consider surgery 29

Ruth Delaney, Edel Fanning, Simon Lambert

Introduction

When suggesting to an individual seeking care that an operation should be considered, a surgeon is placed in a privileged position of trust. That privilege needs to be respected by the surgeon, and a decision to offer surgery should only be made based on the research evidence, the surgeon's skill, and most importantly, on the individual's presentation, circumstances, and values. Surgery should be considered when nonsurgical intervention has not achieved desired and realistic goals, and surgical intervention is considered likely to achieve the goal. Surgery must be considered when research outcomes have demonstrated better results than other interventions, such as with certain fractures, specific consequences of trauma, infections, and tumors.

Shoulder surgery should be considered when clinical reasoning suggests that operating on a structure will lead to meaningful clinical improvement. The decision to perform surgery is complex, and, as is applicable in all healthcare, should only be made when the benefits are judged to outweigh the harms. It is equally important to consider when not to perform surgery, and adopt a watch and wait approach.

Ultimately, the aim of surgery is to reduce disability. It is not acceptable to deem surgery successful because a tendon or labrum was repaired, or bone spur removed, in the presence of a patient who says the symptoms are the same or have worsened. The most meaningful outcome measure to consider for any patient is that patient's perception of their shoulder, and to maximize the patient's Subjective Shoulder Value.[9] The Subjective Shoulder Value is defined as a patient's subjective shoulder assessment expressed as a percentage of a normally functioning shoulder, which would score 100%.[9]

In this chapter, we outline the principles used to make the decision to offer surgery to a patient, illustrating these principles with case examples.

The hypothetico-deductive model

Figure 29.1 shows a schema of the hypothetico-deductive method as developed for the treatment of musculoskeletal shoulder problems, that will be used throughout this chapter. A primary working diagnosis – or hypothesis – is generated, and a treatment plan developed. Here, nonoperative management, as currently recommended by several sources, is pursued for a period sufficient to determine whether a durable outcome has been reached. Four questions (Q1–4) are then answered to understand the outcome for the treatment. After determining the outcome for the treatment, the important question of whether the goals or aims of the patient have been reached is posed. If they have, then coaching and mentoring to a point of sustainable improvement is offered.

If either the responses to Q1–4 and their summation demonstrates that the outcome has not been as expected, or the patient's goals have not been met, then a reassessment is required. A secondary working hypothesis is generated, investigated, and subsequently tested. This loop is repeated until a diagnosis (or diagnoses) has been reached that best explains the patient's symptoms and response to treatment.

If the overall response to the four questions is "YYYN" then it would be reasonable to consider a surgical intervention at this stage. However, the likely response to surgery then needs to be predicted and, for informed consent to be meaningful, the risk of an insufficient outcome must be considered. It is recognized, for example, that the outcome of arthroscopic subacromial decompression is not universally satisfactory in unselected cases.

When contemplating surgery, the patient is the key consideration: the beliefs, concerns, and understanding of the purpose for the procedure, expected outcomes, time frames, anticipated benefits, potential harms and, critically, the specific life circumstances of the individual will all influence the decision whether to proceed. Shared decision-making (see Chapter 13) is therefore important.[3] Patients, supported by their family, caregivers, or friends, may wish to place the decision to operate solely with the surgeon. This may be due to a patient's preference or expectation of a paternalistic approach to healthcare ("the doctor knows best") that may be due to culture or age. *All* patients, of *all* ages and in *all* societies should at the very least be informed of the main treatments for their condition: watch and wait, injections, nonsurgical intervention, and surgery with the concomitant anticipated benefits, harms, time

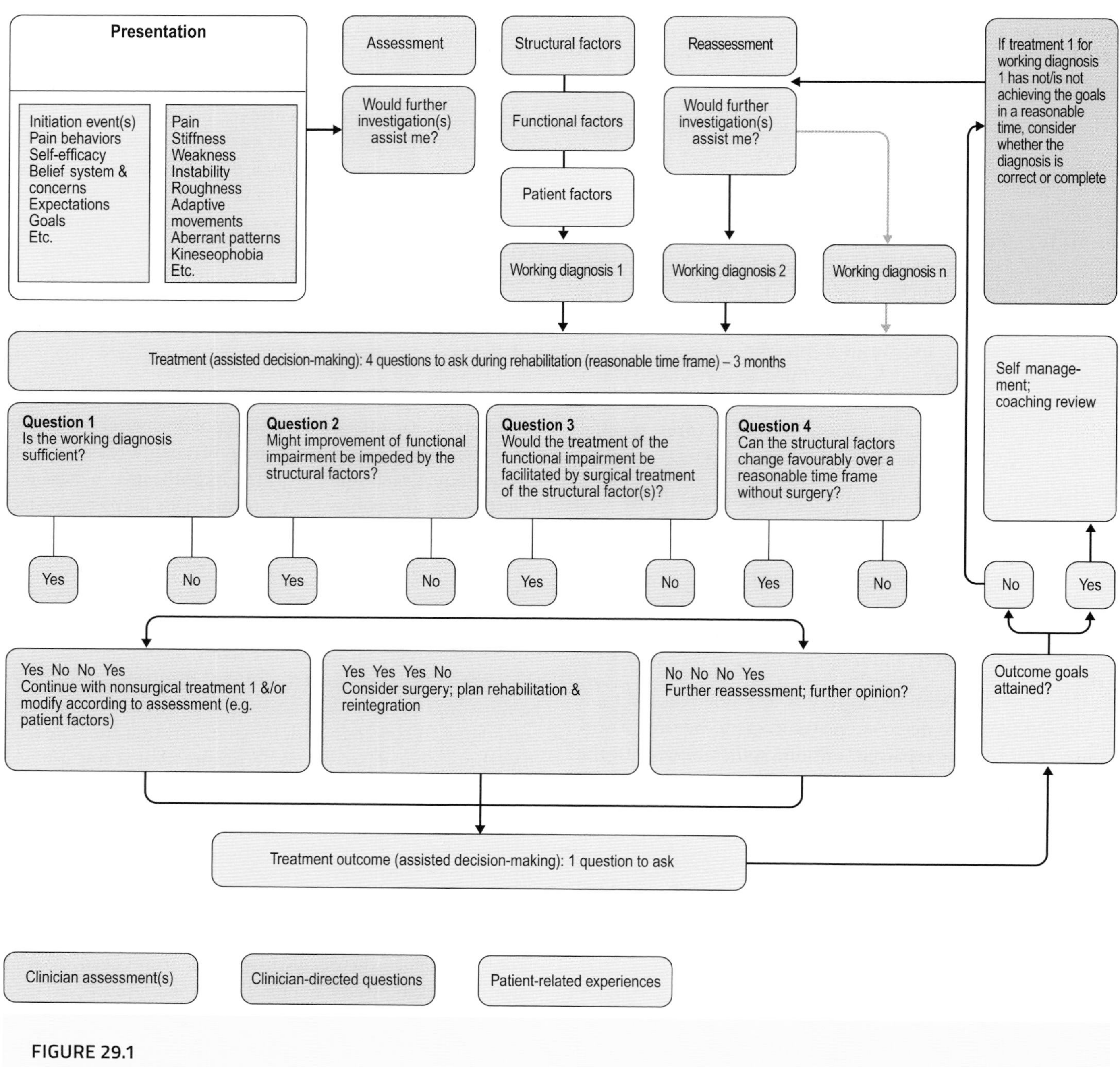

FIGURE 29.1
Schema of the hypothetico-deductive method as developed for the treatment of musculoskeletal shoulder problems.

scales and commitment required after the intervention. By using this approach there will be a greater translation of research evidence into practice and all health professionals will speak with "one voice", reducing patient confusion and frustration. Using this approach, the paternalistic model of healthcare will be relegated to history, and patients, who will be more informed, will become more invested in the process of their care. If surgery is the chosen option, the patient should understand its purpose, time frames, their contribution, and required commitment to rehabilitation and anticipated outcomes.

Once a decision has been made on *whether* to consider elective surgery, *when* to consider surgery is a question of timing. The decision to proceed with surgery is based on a harm–benefit analysis at that time in that patient's life. Surgeons have a responsibility to gain informed consent from the patient or advocate by explaining the harms versus benefits, without over- or understating either, in a manner which is understood. Asking the patient to explain back to the surgeon (see Chapter 11) may provide confidence that what was explained was understood, and together with adequate time to decide, will facilitate informed decision-making.

Although there are multiple time points at which a patient may choose to undergo surgery, it is critical that they understand that surgery is never the last point on their timeline, because postoperative rehabilitation will be essential. In the following sections, we discuss when to consider surgery along the timeline for common presenting shoulder symptoms: pain, stiffness, weakness, and instability.

Pain

Subacromial impingement syndrome is a common diagnosis given to people presenting with shoulder pain. Historically, the pain associated with this condition was considered to be due to a structural problem caused by stenosis (narrowing) of the supraspinatus outlet, leading to impingement on the structures located beneath the lateral end of the acromion, and therefore amenable to surgery.[18] Other mechanisms producing the same symptoms were suggested in the literature, with examples including changes in scapular position and rotator cuff tendinopathy, leading some authors to classify structural stenotic subacromial impingement as primary impingement, and the other mechanisms as leading to secondary impingement.

Knowledge of the innervation of the shoulder joint and subacromial space (see Chapter 4) permits a greater understanding of the potential anatomical basis for pain syndromes around the shoulder (see Chapter 7). One explanation for the incomplete resolution of pain attributed to subacromial impingement after apparently competent surgery and appropriate rehabilitation has been to invoke the concept of "central sensitization" without a clear description of what this means.[16] The following example (Case study 29.1) sets out a pathway of thinking about such a diagnosis that might avoid such pitfalls and puts surgery in its rightful place, as part of the pathway to restoration of functional competence to the shoulder, sometimes as the necessary initial event, sometimes as an adjunct to rehabilitation.

Case study 29.1

A 55-year-old female right-handed cleaner presents with nontraumatic onset of intermittent right shoulder pain of more than six months' duration, without recollection of an event related to onset. Pain disturbs sleep, even in supine. Arm movement is restricted: when reaching with a straight arm above mid-chest level she feels a dull, aching lateral brachialgia, relieved by returning her arm to the side. When sitting or standing, she avoids moving the arm to a position above shoulder level: if she does, she experiences sharp anterior brachialgia. When sitting, if she then brings her hand across to her opposite shoulder, there is a sudden sharp superior pain, and she specifically indicates the region of the acromioclavicular joint. She reports that she has lost endurance in the shoulder when working at her job. Over the last year she has noticed some tingling in the index finger of her right hand when stretching to clean above shoulder level, especially if she must extend her neck to do so. She does not report neck stiffness. She has no other musculoskeletal problems and has no other comorbidities or medical history. She has had no treatment at the time of presentation.

Examination: atrophy without fasciculation of the infraspinatus is noted; the shoulder is held slightly protracted; the thoracic spine is flattened and there is hyperlordosis of the cervical spine. Adverse neural signs for the upper trunk are provoked by posturing of the neck, and she reports that these reflect her experience of the index finger tingling, but there are no alterations in the pulses, and reflexes are present and of normal quality. There is restriction of shoulder internal rotation in elevation and the end-range of the available motion reproduces her experience of lateral brachialgia. Provocative tests of the long head of biceps tendon are unremarkable. Provocative tests for the function of any part of the rotator cuff do not provoke her lateral or anterior brachialgia, but greater effort is needed to resist downward pressure in both empty- and full-can tests.[13] However, when gently pushing the arm at shoulder level into cross-body adduction she reports a replication of her superior shoulder pain and specifically points to the acromioclavicular joint, and the area is tender to palpation but not enlarged.

During testing of motion and rotator cuff strength, crepitation and discomfort are provoked at the superior pole of the scapula, and this is relieved by encouraging scapular "setting", while resisting external rotation of the arm held in at waist level. At the end of the examination, she complains of a recurrence of her lateral brachialgia with the arm resting on her lap and this does not settle during the remainder of the consultation.

Clinical reasoning (by the hypothetico-deductive method) follows. A process of attempted confirmation of the possible diagnoses and the treatment relevant to each is considered. The deductive method involves analyzing the clinical presentation through a sequence of questions and applying similar "what ifs?" to each question. The rationale for surgery becomes a positive clinical decision rather than an event that occurs when other treatment has not delivered the desired end-result.

Two important diagnoses are considered:

- Does the patient have an infection?
- Does the patient have a tumor?

If either of these diagnoses appears possible, referral for an urgent and immediate expert opinion takes priority over all other considerations. If neither appear to be the case, the hypothetico-deductive process continues:

- On the timeline of the natural history for their condition, where is the patient now? In the absence of an injury, which might be expected to follow a resolving natural history over three to six months, is there a progressive degenerative condition or conditions, with or without a non-nociceptive component?
- Is the lateral brachialgia a direct manifestation of a possible cervicogenic neuropathy, or a consequence of the weakening of the rotator cuff due to cervicogenic neuropathy?
- Is the scapular dyskinesia a manifestation of cervicogenic neuropathy (affecting the dorsal scapular nerve that innervates the rhomboid muscles and levator scapulae), leading to poor rotator cuff recruitment through scapular protraction and lateral tilt?
- Is the scapular dyskinesia a result of the loss of internal rotation of the shoulder joint, with a possible cause in acromioclavicular joint pathology, or is a degenerative "silent" lesion of the rotator cuff causing contracture of the posterosuperior capsule[23] with subsequent glenohumeral internal rotation deficit (GIRD)?
- Is the acromioclavicular joint tender because of an upregulation of nociception in the superior aspect of the shoulder, due to a cervicogenic neuropathy?
- If the patient presents more than three weeks into the natural history of the condition, does this patient's pain experience have features that suggest a "central" component (i.e., is it now "chronic")?
- What do we expect to happen without any form of treatment? Is the outlook favorable (in the patient's terms) if left alone to fulfill the natural history of the condition?
- What aspects of the presentation are likely to have a structural basis which *cannot* be altered by nonoperative treatment?
- How can we visualize one or more structural contributors to the presentation of pain?
- How can we be clear whether a structural lesion seen on imaging is in fact the generator of the patient's pain?
- How can we test this?
- Should an early surgical intervention be considered?
- What aspects of the presentation (that we understand might have a structural basis) *can* be altered by nonoperative treatment?
- Might an early surgical intervention amplify the beneficial effect of nonsurgical interventions?
- Could an early surgical intervention modify the pain perception sufficiently to influence the nonsurgical restoration of a functional "normality"?

- What aspects of the presentation have a functional basis? Is this based in the structural problem(s)?
- How can we test this?
- What can't we explain or understand?
- Is there a quantum of non-nociceptive pain that has not been recognized?
- How can we find out?

A set of diagnoses or hypotheses may be formulated, and placed in a hierarchy of probability:

1. There are features suggesting pain generators in the superior compartment, including the subacromial space and acromioclavicular joint.
2. There are features consistent with posterosuperior contracture. This acts as a check rein on internal rotation in elevation motion (GIRD) with secondary obligate anterior glenohumeral translation[11] causing tertiary subacromial pain due to conflict between the superior surface of the rotator cuff and the undersurface of the coracoacromial arch, including the inferior capsule of the acromioclavicular joint.
3. There are features to suggest cervicogenic neuropathy affecting the upper trunk of the brachial plexus or its constituent roots (C5/6), resulting in rotator cuff weakness, and possibly also related to both the scapular dyskinesia and to an alteration in the threshold for nociception in the shoulder girdle.
4. There are features that might be consistent with a lateral thoracic outlet syndrome due to scapular dyskinesia.
5. The rotator cuff appears structurally intact but weak and fatigues rapidly.
6. There might be pain-provoked or anticipatory muscular guarding during internal rotation of the shoulder thus resisting this movement.

Each of these components of the overall diagnosis may comprise structural and functional elements. Structural elements may comprise nociceptive and/or non-nociceptive components. In deciding whether surgery has a role in this case we should dissect the features individually and then construct a working diagnosis or hypothesis for each, which can then be tested.

Generation of the working hypothesis: when does surgery have a role, if at all?

Using the schema depicted in Figure 29.1, a primary working diagnosis is generated, in this case, superior compartment syndrome or subacromial impingement syndrome. Relevant nonsurgical treatment, as currently advocated for this syndrome, is initiated and the response to treatment is monitored over time that reflects the likely period for which improvement might be expected, usually 12 weeks. In addition, cross-sectional imaging is considered, but at this stage it is not clear which modality might be the most revealing of the diagnosis(es). Each of the putative diagnoses in this case is amenable to nonsurgical treatment, especially if the seemingly adverse effect of occupational activities is temporarily removed. However, if there was a safe, effective, and individualized surgical treatment that might reduce the duration of symptoms, then this is clearly worth considering. In helping the patient make her decision, we should have evidence at our disposal that a surgical intervention is likely to be beneficial.

Evolution of Case study 29.1

The patient has had appropriate nonsurgical management for the working diagnosis of subacromial impingement syndrome, together with anti-inflammatory medication and occupation modification, but has persistent pain as previously described. Further investigations are considered to review and reframe the diagnosis.

An ultrasound examination of the shoulder is reported as showing: an articular surface partial thickness anterior supraspinatus tear of less than 50% of the thickness of the tendon, without long head of biceps instability; a marked thickening of the subacromio-subdeltoid bursa with a large, septated effusion; acromioclavicular degenerative arthropathy with intra-articular disc fragmentation, synovitis,

Box 29.1

Principle: surgery has a role in restoring the patient to the anticipated or expected recovery timeline, particularly if the progression of recovery is not as expected, or other factors intervene during recovery.

Box 29.2

Principle: the working diagnosis should be based on the clinical reasoning applied to each symptom and should be reasonable.

and effusion. The radiologist notes that there is excessive posterior laxity in the acromioclavicular joint when palpated with the probe, and that this provokes lateral, as well as anterior, brachialgia, and tingling in the index finger of the ipsilateral hand. There is now an evolved working diagnosis including acromioclavicular joint arthropathy.

Standard-of-care treatment for this diagnosis comprised guided intra-articular acromioclavicular joint injection with cortisone and local anesthetic, and the continuation of physiotherapy focusing on the scapular dynamics. The injection reduces the lateral and anterior brachialgia by over 50% as estimated using a numeric rating scale, and the patient reported fewer instances of tingling in the hand. Treatment is pursued for an additional three months, and the same four questions reapplied (Q1–4, Figure 29.1). The summation of the responses is now "YYYN" referring to the structural changes in the acromioclavicular joint. At this juncture, one option would be to continue with a sequence of intra-articular injections if benefit from injection is experienced. Another option is to leave matters alone if the patient is content with a diagnosis and understands the limitations her condition places on her occupation. A further consideration is to undertake surgical management of the acromioclavicular arthropathy.

The persisting tingling in the index finger remains, and there is now reason to investigate the cervical spine (with the potential option of relevant nerve root blockade after further imaging of the neck), or to consider whether the acromioclavicular joint is the primary cause of pain with secondary subacromial bursopathy (the range of active motion of the shoulder is insufficient to determine with certainty whether the acromioclavicular joint is clinically involved and passive motion is resisted in elevation with the same result). Equally the posture of the scapula may be responsible for the establishment and maintenance of the cervicogenic pain and peripheral neuropathic symptom.

Box 29.3

Principle: the diagnosis of pain is not static. A working diagnosis is a clinical impression at a point in time and needs to be modified according to evidence from natural history progression, investigations, and results of treatment.

Box 29.4

Principle: surgery may be of undoubted benefit in specific diagnoses. The more usual complex presentations may not be as susceptible to surgery for the reasons discussed above, related to non-nociceptive pain mechanisms.

The question of whether there is also a contribution to the overall burden of pain by non-nociceptive pain is now relevant due to the time elapsed after the onset of symptoms. This is important since prolonged residual pain is a common feature after surgery for a long-term pain condition. The post-surgical pain may take longer to reduce than the pain of recovery from the acute trauma of surgery.

At this stage treatment for the first working diagnosis is ongoing, and treatment for the evolved diagnosis has been started: the patient and clinician now need to decide again how the patient's response to treatment is helping them reach their goal of pain-free function. The four questions are posed again (see Figure 29.1). If the overall impression remains uncertain then the diagnosis remains opaque, and surgery should not be undertaken until the diagnosis is clarified.

The difficulty of unravelling this syndrome can be eased by four further interventions: 1) selective (image-guided) local anesthetic injections (into the subacromial bursa); 2) cervical nerve root blockade; 3) examination under anesthetic (thus eliminating the possible protective muscle activation effect which can disguise some diagnoses) combined with option 1; and 4) the so-called pentothal test (see below), often combined with options 1 and 3.

Box 29.5

Principle: surgery may offer a "window of opportunity" for the re-establishment of an appropriate rehabilitation timeline. In the case of subacromial "decompression" this may be through a denervation of the afferent field or a large part of it, thus reducing "unhelpful" nociception and reducing the central re-presentation of pain that may inhibit postural and muscular strengthening therapies. The subacromial space will, of course, reinnervate over several weeks following surgery. As this occurs, the rehabilitation program must include strategies to re-establish afferent feedback from the subacromial space to the shoulder girdle.

Pentothal tests

Pentothal, or thiopentone (sodium thiopental/pentothal), is a short-acting lipid-soluble anesthetic induction agent. Pentothal can be used to titrate the patient to a stage of anesthesia in which they are aware of a nociceptive stimulus (a squeeze of the trapezius muscle, a sternal rub, or a rub of the supraorbital margin) but have no memory of it. Pentothal tests are performed with an anesthetist controlling the patient's airway and are usually an adjunct to examination under anesthetic, diagnostic injections, and diagnostic arthroscopy of the shoulder.

In this ongoing case example, the awake, and therefore aware, recumbent patient actively elevates the arm until she reports onset of her pain, which is determined to be at 60°, with another 30° of painful movement, and at 90° the increase in pain inhibits any further motion. Passive motion of the arm does not alter these observations. Pentothal is administered until an ipsilateral trapezius squeeze response produces a grimace or withdrawal reflex but there is no response to gently stimulating the eyelashes, confirming pre-unconscious anesthesia. The patient's arm is then moved passively through the same motion (flexion) until the facial expression of pain (a grimace) is provoked (a withdrawal reflex of the upper extremity, and head turning to the side of the stimulus are also noted). If the grimace happened with the arm at 130° (but not before) and persisted through higher ranges of elevation, we can deduce:

- There is nociceptive pain generated at 130°.
- The pain experienced between 60° and 130° does not appear to be nociceptive in origin.
- Whatever the findings of the ultrasound examination, the patient's painful arc (60–130°) does not appear to be nociceptive, and structural "lesions" seen in the subacromial bursa and rotator cuff do not appear to account for the crescendo pain.
- The subacromial bursa does not appear to be the source of pain in this case.

The conclusions that can be drawn from the pentothal test are that: 1) the acromioclavicular joint appears to be the major source of symptoms, and 2) importantly it also suggests that a subacromial bursectomy is unlikely to provide pain relief if undertaken as the sole procedure, and may not be a useful part of any procedure that may be performed, including acromioclavicular joint surgery. The test "saves" the patient from potentially unnecessary surgery.

Interestingly, if the trapezius squeeze response on the ipsilateral side is more readily provoked than the same response on the contralateral side, this suggests an upregulation of nociception in the entire ipsilateral shoulder girdle, which again fits with the overall presentation. It does not necessarily imply a cervical cause for the hyperalgesia, but this should be considered. It does not imply a fabrication of pain either, but rather the maladaptation of a basic guarding or protective response over the course of the prolonged experience of pain.

Adjunctive tests: local anesthetic challenge tests

A local anesthetic injection is given into the acromioclavicular joint under image guidance and while under general anesthesia to confirm this hypothesis. The selective basis of the injection has been supported by the findings of the pentothal test, so that the probability that the test will be positive (and therefore useful in confirming the diagnosis) should be high. Like all tests, the pentothal test should be considered as part of the overall work-up, not a definitive test for the quantum of non-nociceptive pain present in a chronic pain presentation. The test is a guide but is not unequivocal in its interpretation.

Box 29.6 The corollary of the pentothal test

The patient's total pain experience can be described by the equation:

Total experience of pain = {[nociceptive pain] + [non-nociceptive pain]} + {psychosocial factors} + {change over time}

Surgery can probably offer a relief of, at best, 90% of nociceptive pain, and may contribute, if it does so at all, to the relief of non-nociceptive pain through a placebo effect. Thus, the overall relief of pain is 90% of nociceptive pain and 0% of non-nociceptive pain (other than through a placebo effect, which at best might amount to a 30% positive effect). If, after the pentothal test, the deduction in the example case is that nociceptive pain amounts to approximately 20% of the overall pain experience (the high-range grimace versus the awake patient's experience) then surgery will, at best, give a benefit of 90% of 20% (18%) of the overall pain burden while non-nociceptive pain may be, at best, relieved by the placebo effect (30% of 80%, thus approximately 37%). The overall benefit due to a surgical effect might be as little as 55% (18% + 37%) of the overall pain burden. This patient might not consider surgery of enough value to undergo a procedure under these circumstances.

Summary

A patient rarely has a single source or generator of pain: each potential source must be weighed up and both the nociceptive and non-nociceptive elements of each source of pain given a value in the overall diagnostic equation. The decision to offer a surgical approach for the relief of pain is made after considering all possible diagnoses and subjecting each element to clinical and interventional tests to determine the relevance of each to the overall diagnosis. The proportion of non-nociceptive pain can be deduced from clinical observation and specific tests. Surgery can offer improved outcomes for diagnoses when the diagnoses have been made as specifically as feasible, but can never completely restore the status ante (most surgery offers between 85% and 90% improvement after the *repair* of soft tissue lesions, and less sustained improvement after *reconstruction* of similar lesions). The non-nociceptive element of pain is not helped directly by surgery. The patient can make an informed decision about whether to have surgery for a particular diagnosis if they are counselled about the proportion of their experience which can be explained by non-nociceptive mechanisms, what proportion is nociceptive, and what the likelihood is of surgery being beneficial in the latter.

Stiffness

Patients may often underestimate their shoulder stiffness, and when stiffness is associated with another symptom, usually pain, it is common that this other symptom is what prompts presentation. Particularly in long-standing stiffness, compensatory patterns that have developed will often result in less awareness of the shoulder stiffness. Difficulty in performing specific daily tasks may draw attention to the shoulder stiffness, for example lack of internal rotation to pull up trousers or to do up a bra, or lack of external rotation resulting in difficulty brushing hair. Stiffness that has plateaued or failed to respond to nonsurgical intervention may warrant consideration of surgery.

Case study 29.2

A 45-year-old, right-hand dominant woman presents with a stiff right shoulder of eight months' duration, associated with pain on certain movements. She was having difficulty sleeping at night but this has recently improved. Active and passive shoulder external rotation ranges are recorded to be 20°, associated with end range pain. Flexion and internal rotation are also limited, 140° and thumb to L1, respectively. Shoulder strength is intact. She experienced discomfort on shoulder impingement tests. The region of the long head of biceps is tender to palpation. Magnetic resonance imaging (MRI) would be unlikely to influence clinical management, and plain radiographs would be sufficient. In this case, nothing abnormal was identified on the X-ray. Therefore, a diagnosis of frozen shoulder (adhesive capsulitis) is made and nonsurgical treatment, consisting of glenohumeral and subacromial corticosteroid injections combined with a gentle exercise program, is commenced.

This is a very common clinical scenario and in most cases the patient experiences resolution of symptoms, sometimes requiring repeat injections. If, after two sets of injections and an exercise program, the patient reports that she is still struggling with shoulder stiffness, this may lead to consideration of surgery, specifically an arthroscopic capsular release. That intervention at that time point in this patient's journey would be performed to achieve the aim of hastening her recovery.

An alternative scenario to consider is that this patient may have early arthritis at a time point before glenohumeral degenerative changes are seen on X-ray. In this scenario, her management would be different. The corticosteroid injections may afford temporary relief and the same decision, to proceed to arthroscopy, might still be made, but during the procedure, the more likely diagnosis would become apparent. The procedure would be similar in both instances: glenohumeral debridement, capsular release and subacromial bursectomy, possibly adding biceps tenodesis, but during the conversation after surgery, the patient would need be informed of the findings and her expectations reset as per the change in prognosis.

The management has still been appropriate up to this point, but the patient journey is now more complex, as it is likely that further interventions will be needed later in the timeline to manage the glenohumeral arthritis. Physiotherapy management post arthroscopy will also be different. Rather than an aggressive range of motion program for frozen shoulder, the approach will be gentler and more graduated. This patient's future timeline may include further injections – corticosteroid or viscosupplementation – and at an appropriate time point, consideration might be given to an arthroplasty procedure.

When to consider arthroplasty for a young person with arthritis is difficult, especially as the viability of total shoulder arthroplasty prostheses is generally 15–20 years.[22] In a younger person, activity levels will usually be higher, and this may compromise durability, particularly of the glenoid component of the prosthesis. It is likely that when a younger person experiences the significant pain relief associated with total shoulder arthroplasty, they may return to activities that will lead to deterioration of the prosthesis earlier than in a less active person. Therefore, the timing of the initial decision to consider an arthroplasty is crucial.

This timing will be driven by the patient's ability to live with their symptoms and the impact the symptoms are having on their life. Factors that often lead to a patient deciding to go ahead with arthroplasty, even at a younger age, include sleep disturbance, need for daily oral analgesia (and associated side-effects) and difficulty with simple daily activities such as driving, dressing, and self-care. On rare occasions, the surgeon may try to influence timing of the surgery if there is severe glenoid erosion where delaying surgery might mean that ongoing erosion would create technical difficulties or make it impossible to place a standard anatomic glenoid component.

Because of the above concerns, when a younger person arrives at the point that they want and would benefit from an arthroplasty procedure, consideration may be given to using a hemiarthroplasty rather than a total shoulder arthroplasty, and to using alternative bearing surfaces such as pyro-carbon. Consideration should be given to anatomic total shoulder replacement, which has been shown to have superior functional and subjective outcomes to hemiarthroplasty.[5,19]

This scenario has highlighted that the timeline of the individual with shoulder stiffness may involve surgery at more than one point, and this will depend on the underlying etiology.

Figure 29.2 illustrates the decision-making schema, this time as applied to the example of adhesive capsulitis.

Box 29.7

Principles:

- Stiffness is often associated with other symptoms and may not be the main complaint on presentation.
- Underlying diagnosis determines the prognosis of a stiff shoulder.
- Surgery for stiffness goes hand in hand with postoperative rehabilitation to avoid recurrent stiffness.

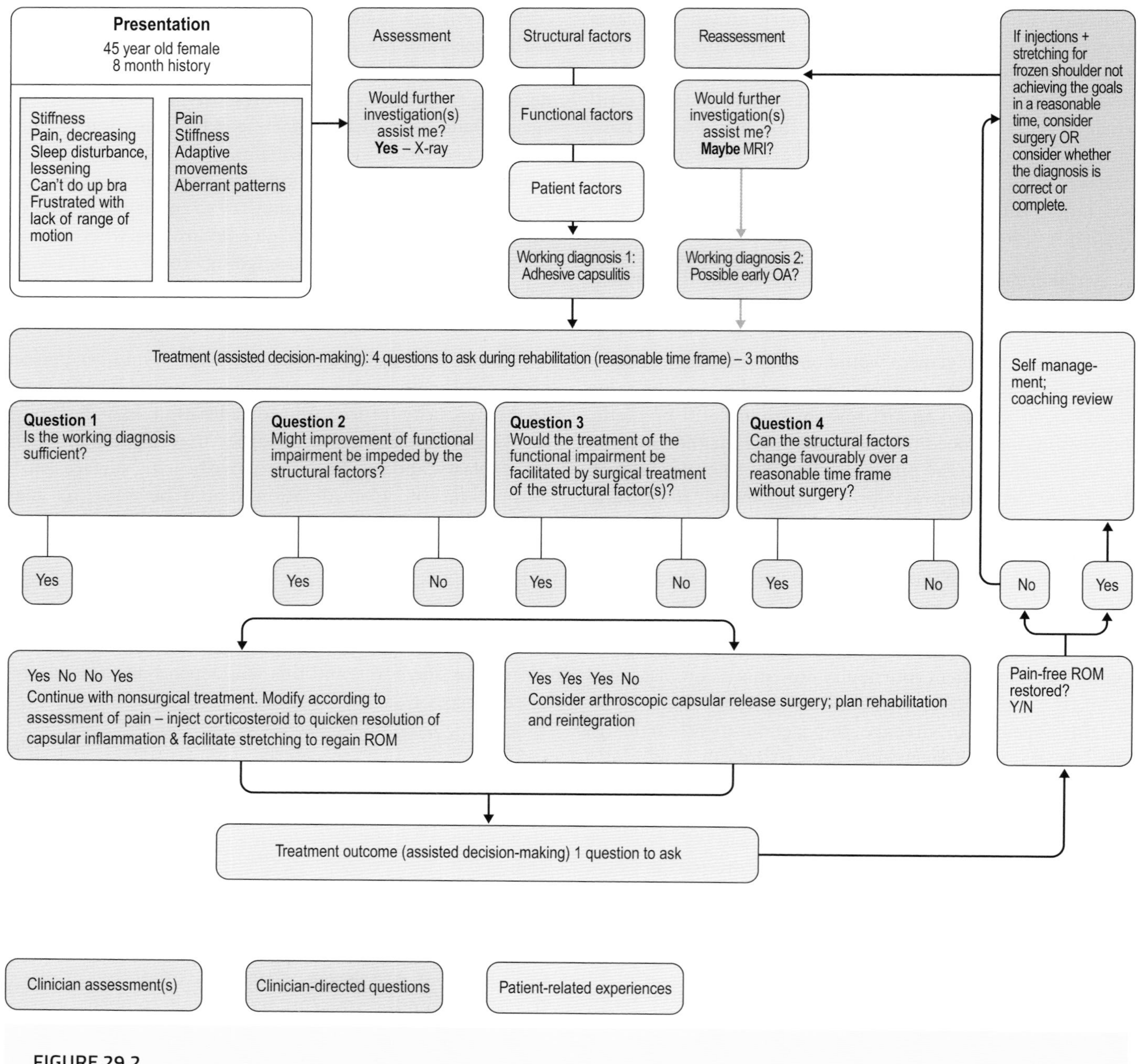

FIGURE 29.2
Schematic illustration of the decision-making process for a patient presenting with stiffness as the primary symptom.

Weakness

Acute shoulder weakness will often improve dramatically without surgical intervention. For example, a 65-year-old person with a full thickness but asymptomatic rotator cuff tear who falls and presents with acute pseudoparalysis may still respond favorably to nonsurgical intervention. It is possible that the clinical picture may be one of substantial improvement two months later with rehabilitation.[1,17]

Therefore, it is often advisable to wait before considering surgical intervention (a reverse shoulder arthroplasty), even if the tear is massive and irreparable, as rehabilitation may reduce the requirement for surgery.

Weakness may also present secondary to pain. Even in the presence of a confirmed full-thickness rotator cuff tear, weakness may substantially improve as pain diminishes. Injections for pain relief should not be considered if surgery will be performed within a month after the injection due to increased infection risk.[8] A more challenging presentation of weakness is presented in Case study 29.3.

Case study 29.3

A 58-year-old farmer presents with a two- to three-year history of weakness of his right, dominant-sided shoulder. He experiences anterior shoulder pain and there is no history of trauma. Examination reveals no shoulder stiffness, and tenderness to palpation in the bicipital groove and subcoracoid regions. When resistance is applied to the arm during shoulder abduction, pain is reported with a concomitant reduction in strength. No other weakness is recorded. A high-grade (more than 50% is torn) partial tear of supraspinatus is identified on MRI. He has not yet had any management for his symptoms.

Choosing the best management option here is challenging. It is tempting to intervene surgically to repair the tendon, aiming to reduce pain and weakness and prevent further deterioration. Surgical intervention would also allow the biceps and subcoracoid pain to be addressed, but he would not be able to lift for 12 weeks post-surgery and it would be up to six months before he could resume his full physical farming activities. Shared decision-making is essential in this context, and if surgery is not considered as the most appropriate current intervention, this man would require monitoring to identify any deterioration of symptoms. Although he is physically active, a graded shoulder rehabilitation program should be considered (see Chapter 36) together with any lifestyle changes (see Chapter 5).

The dilemma is that if we do not intervene now to prevent a full-thickness tear, surgery may be required later for that eventuality. This may be an acceptable course provided the full-thickness tear is repairable. The chances of and speed of cuff tear progression are difficult to predict.[15] In the worst-case scenario, the patient progresses to an irreparable cuff tear with significant weakness requiring a reverse shoulder arthroplasty. During shared decision-making, if the patient expresses that he cannot currently stop his farm work for the time required to operate and rehabilitate but would consider a reverse shoulder arthroplasty when it becomes necessary, then not operating now is an acceptable decision. In this case, patient-specific factors and preferences are essential in the decision whether to operate or not.

In Figure 29.3, the hypothetico-deductive model as previously described is applied to the case example of shoulder weakness.

When passive shoulder flexion is substantially greater than active, with a concomitant prominence of the humeral head anteriorly, known as anterosuperior escape, this shoulder may be considered pseudoparalytic. Attempts to define pseudoparalysis have generated controversy and debate.[6] Regardless of definition, pseudoparalysis involves profound shoulder weakness, usually due to a massive rotator cuff tear, that may or may not be repairable. Acute versus chronic pseudoparalysis is an important distinction to make. A patient who has been unable to actively raise their arm for several months is less likely to improve with ongoing nonsurgical management and surgical intervention should be considered. In people over 65–70 years of age, the surgery decision would be to offer a reverse shoulder arthroplasty because this is the only procedure that may reverse the profound weakness. However, in younger people in whom direct repair is not possible, other interventions, such as superior capsule reconstruction or tendon transfers, may be more appropriate, although it should be noted that results of these procedures are variable when pre-operative pseudoparalysis is present.[7]

True paralysis is a less common type of weakness seen in orthopedic clinics. An example would be an individual with a brachial plexus palsy post anterior shoulder dislocation. These neurapraxias may resolve with time and do not require surgical intervention for the weakness, but require careful monitoring clinically and neurophysiologically.

Case study 29.4

A 21-year-old, right-hand dominant, professional rugby player sustains a first-time anterior dislocation of his right

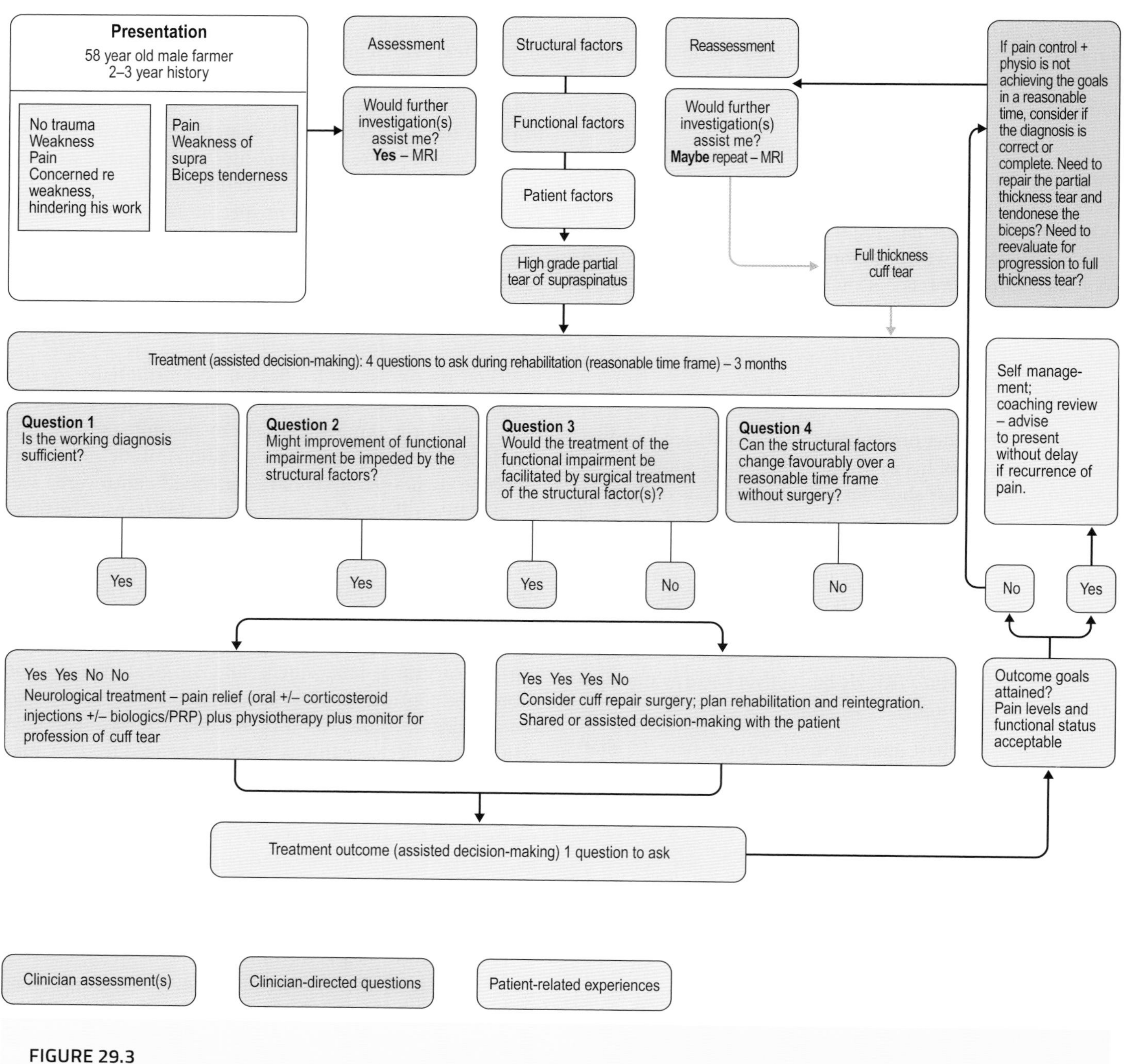

FIGURE 29.3
Schematic illustration of the decision-making process for a patient presenting with weakness as the primary symptom.

shoulder, which is reduced on the pitch. He has no previous history of shoulder instability but has a history of "stingers", which occur when nerves are stretched or compressed after impact. He presents one week post injury with weakness affecting his triceps, wrist extensors and digital extensors. He has a complete wrist drop. Nerve conduction and electromyography (EMG) were performed and a postganglionic injury to the posterior cord of the brachial plexus and the radial nerve, with some background chronic changes are reported. The player and coach have decided that he will go ahead with shoulder surgery for his instability and express a wish for minimal delay. The neurologist prefers surgery to be delayed until there is less weakness and neurologic improvement.

Initially, treatment involved steroids for neural edema and a resting splint for his wrist and digits. Neurophysiologic testing was repeated six weeks later. EMG demonstrated improvement and clinically he was stronger, and the neurologist considered it appropriate to operate. A labral and humeral avulsion of the glenohumeral ligament (HAGL) repair were performed. At 16 weeks postoperative, his radial nerve palsy had resolved, and isokinetic testing revealed no difference in shoulder strength between sides. He was cleared to return to contact training and had no further problems with weakness or recurrent instability.

This case of weakness was unusual in that it affected the posterior cord/radial nerve rather than the axillary or musculocutaneous nerves which are more commonly affected, but this may relate to his history of so-called "stingers" in that same limb prior to his shoulder dislocation. He improved quickly, which is typical in younger people.

Box 29.8

Principles:

- Weakness may be acute or persistent. Acute weakness often responds to rehabilitation.
- Structural injury underlying the weakness may merit consideration of surgery, depending on individual patient factors.
- The only surgical intervention to reliably reverse true pseudoparalysis is a reverse shoulder arthroplasty.
- True paralysis may indicate cervical spine pathology or brachial plexus injury. Cervical spine MRI and/or neurophysiology testing may form an important part of evaluation.

Instability

Confusion exists as to what causes instability of the shoulder. A combination of structural (traumatic and atraumatic) and neurological system disturbances may coexist.[14] All patients are individual people with their own stories to tell, their own circumstances, concerns, and ambitions and, even if symptoms of instability are similar, the routes that lead them to consider surgery may not be.

Case study 29.5

A 22-year-old male professional athlete involved in high-contact sport presents for rehabilitation post bilateral open Latarjet procedures, associated with considerable bone loss on the glenoid and humerus. His only concern was when he would be ready to return to competitive play. His father and medical team hoped for 12 weeks post-surgery so he could play in the first round of the championship.

His mother and brother also had shoulder problems, as had his father who also was a professional footballer and had won many awards. Since his teen years, the patient had suffered numerous dislocations of his left shoulder. He could not recall when he suffered his first dislocation and was always able to self-relocate. He had his first surgery at age 16 years, a left shoulder arthroscopic stabilization procedure. He followed all his rehabilitation diligently, but the shoulder continued to dislocate, and he had a second left shoulder arthroscopic stabilization a year later. He managed to return to football, however, only months later the right shoulder became problematic and at the age of 18 years he underwent a right open shoulder soft tissue stabilization (Bankart procedure).

He excelled in his football career despite his left shoulder continuing to dislocate; he would self-reduce the shoulder and hide his dislocations from his parents to avoid being taken to see the shoulder surgeon again. He returned to championship football nine months after his bilateral Latarjet procedures. His case is a reminder that "success is not linear". He reported that his shoulders felt very different than after previous shoulder surgery. He now reports hearing clunking and feelings of shoulder stiffness, intermittent posterior shoulder pain and episodes of the left shoulder "wobbling out the back".

Glenohumeral dislocations in adolescent contact athletes are highly significant injuries. An accurate history and examination are key. A good history should reveal the patient's beliefs, concerns, expectations, and goals as well as any accompanying diagnosis. Understanding the mechanism of injury is important. There is more likely to be a structural element to the instability if significant trauma occurred, while insidious onset or less significant trauma may indicate a non-structural cause.[14] A thorough examination should include tests for laxity and for neurological involvement.

Often it is necessary to investigate the unstable shoulder to rule out a structural cause. However, there is a delicate balance in the investigation of benign-sounding dislocations. Upon discovering a lesion on imaging, how does one then proceed? Evidence suggests a high incidence of labral pathology in asymptomatic athletes.[10] Therefore, it is imperative radiological investigations are used in the framework of an athlete's clinical examination, symptoms, and goals.

Other risk factors for recurrence need also to be considered in the surgical decision-making process. Research shows young age as the single most important prognostic factor in the development of recurrent traumatic anterior dislocations.[24] Patients with bony Bankart lesions are more likely to have recurrent instability. The rate of bone loss is significantly greater in adolescents versus older athletes. Fear of injury and self-reported pain may also increase the risk of recurrent shoulder instability.[21]

Immediate operative stabilization, where structural damage is present, may be a prudent approach for young individuals involved in contact or high-risk sports, although current evidence is not overwhelming.[12] Despite surgical reconstruction of injured structures, there can still be a relatively high frequency of further shoulder instability, most notably in young athletes in contact sports (5.9% to 51%).[2,24] Currently there is limited evidence from randomized controlled trials to infer conclusions as to whether surgery is more beneficial over rehabilitation for this cohort.[21] However, conditions that allow a true blinded randomized controlled trial design are extremely difficult to replicate for the vast majority of clinical situations.

Ultimately, a patient-focused benefit–risk analysis is required when contemplating whether to manage a case surgically or not. The decision to operate can have significant implications ranging from the safety of the athlete, to performance factors and litigation issues. Some risks associated with surgical repair for anterior dislocations include infection, nerve damage,[4] decreased range of motion, and pain. The major risks associated with managing a shoulder nonsurgically are a potential higher risk of recurrent instability, further structural damage sustained by subsequent dislocations, and an increased risk of instability arthropathy.[12] Patients may conclude that the higher risk of subsequent episodes of instability is unacceptable and elect for early stabilization through surgery.

The evidence to support the effectiveness of one method over another and the timing of surgical treatment remains limited. Clinicians must be prepared to reconsider the causes of symptoms that have initially been decided upon (Figure 29.4).

Case study 29.6

A 25-year-old female who works in a supermarket presents with right shoulder pain and instability after an injury at work. She was stacking shelves when the accident occurred. She was lifting a box from the top shelf when it slipped and fell on her. When she got home her shoulder was painful and warm, and her mother noticed that it was not sitting right. She went to an osteopath who did some manipulation and it felt slightly better. She took a few days off to rest the shoulder, however, when she tried to return to work the pain became unbearable and she struggled to lift the arm without it subluxating.

Over the course of three years, she saw several medical practitioners. All investigations including X-rays, MR arthrogram, brain scans, and nerve conduction studies were reported as normal. More recently she had reported the onset of back pain which resulted in severe weakness of the right leg. She described incidents where she was walking and felt some pain in her back and her ankles collapsed, resulting in her falling, and knocking out her front tooth.

Cases like this can be difficult to manage and often have a spectrum of underlying causes. A careful assessment is key in patients who present with a non-structural cause to their shoulder instability. A multidisciplinary team assessment is both appropriate and useful to identify what could be driving this type of shoulder instability and to guide management. For example, surgery often results in a poor outcome for patients with obvious muscle patterning,[20] and

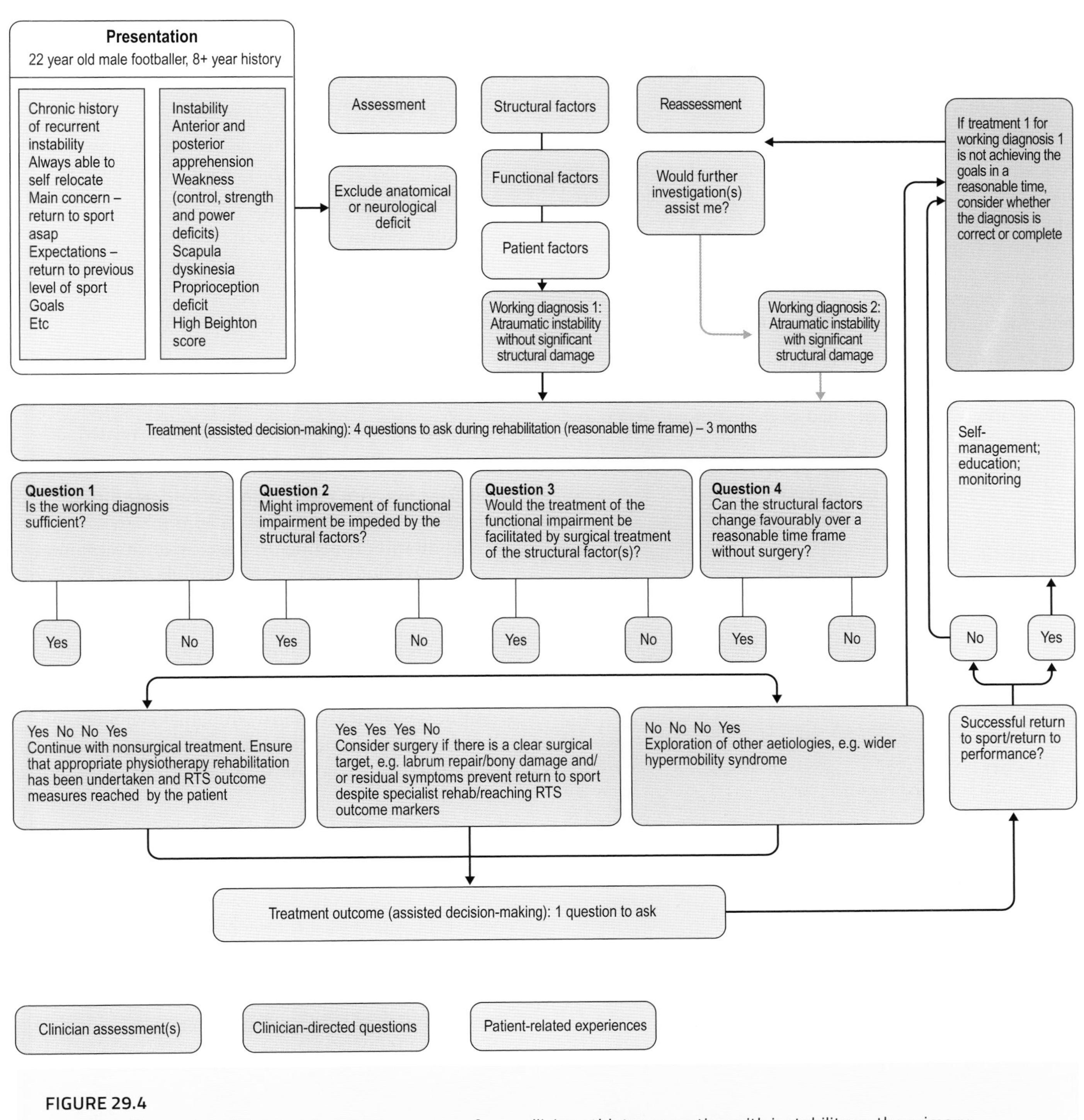

FIGURE 29.4

Schematic illustration of the decision-making process for a collision athlete presenting with instability as the primary symptom.

those with a strong underlying psychological component, evidence of central sensitization, hyperlaxity that may represent a collagen disorder, or childhood motor developmental issues.

Surgery should always be approached with caution and following discussion with an experienced multidisciplinary team. Surgical intervention is sometimes considered along the timeline of the patient's journey, as an adjunct to those not responding to nonsurgical treatment. If considered, there should be a clear target for surgical intervention such as a significant underlying lesion (e.g., labral, capsular, bony, or neurological) or capsular shift (Figure 29.5).

The patient in the above example had a chronically painful, unstable shoulder extending beyond a nociceptive presentation. Her journey had been one of confusion and frustration. A multidisciplinary approach was required and the willingness to talk to a psychiatrist was a key component in her journey to recovery.

Conclusions

In conclusion, some of the guiding principles when making the decision to consider surgery are as follows:

- Surgery has a role in restoring the patient to the expected recovery timeline for rehabilitation back to a level at which the patient's subjective shoulder value is optimal for them at that time, if the recovery progression is not as expected or other factors intervene in recovery.
- The working diagnosis should be based on the clinical reasoning applied to each symptom and should be reasonable.
- The diagnosis of pain is not static. A working diagnosis is a clinical impression at a point in time and needs to be modified according to evidence from natural history progression, investigations, and results of treatment.
- Surgery is not always appropriate. The more usual complex presentations may not be as susceptible to surgery for the reasons discussed above, related to non-nociceptive pain mechanisms.
- Surgery may offer a "window of opportunity" for the re-establishment of an appropriate rehabilitation timeline. In the case of subacromial decompression, this may be through a denervation of the afferent field or a large part of it, thus reducing unhelpful nociception and reducing the central re-presentation of pain which negatively impact on rehabilitation.
- Stiffness is often associated with other symptoms and may not be the main complaint on presentation, and the underlying diagnosis determines the prognosis of a stiff shoulder.
- Surgery for stiffness goes hand in hand with postoperative rehabilitation to avoid recurrent stiffness.
- Weakness may be acute or persistent. Acute weakness often responds to rehabilitation.
- Structural injury underlying the weakness may merit consideration of surgery, depending on individual patient factors.
- The only surgical intervention to reliably reverse true pseudoparalysis is a reverse shoulder arthroplasty.
- True paralysis may indicate cervical spine pathology or brachial plexus injury.

Box 29.9

Principles:

- Following a traumatic shoulder dislocation, surgery may have an important role in restoring stability, particularly where structural lesions are present and associated with significant risk factors for recurrence: young (under 25 years of age), male sex, and high-contact sport participation.
- In cases of atraumatic shoulder instability, surgery may have a role for patients for whom rehabilitation has failed, and present with structural pathology.
- In all cases, communication between a multidisciplinary team is essential.

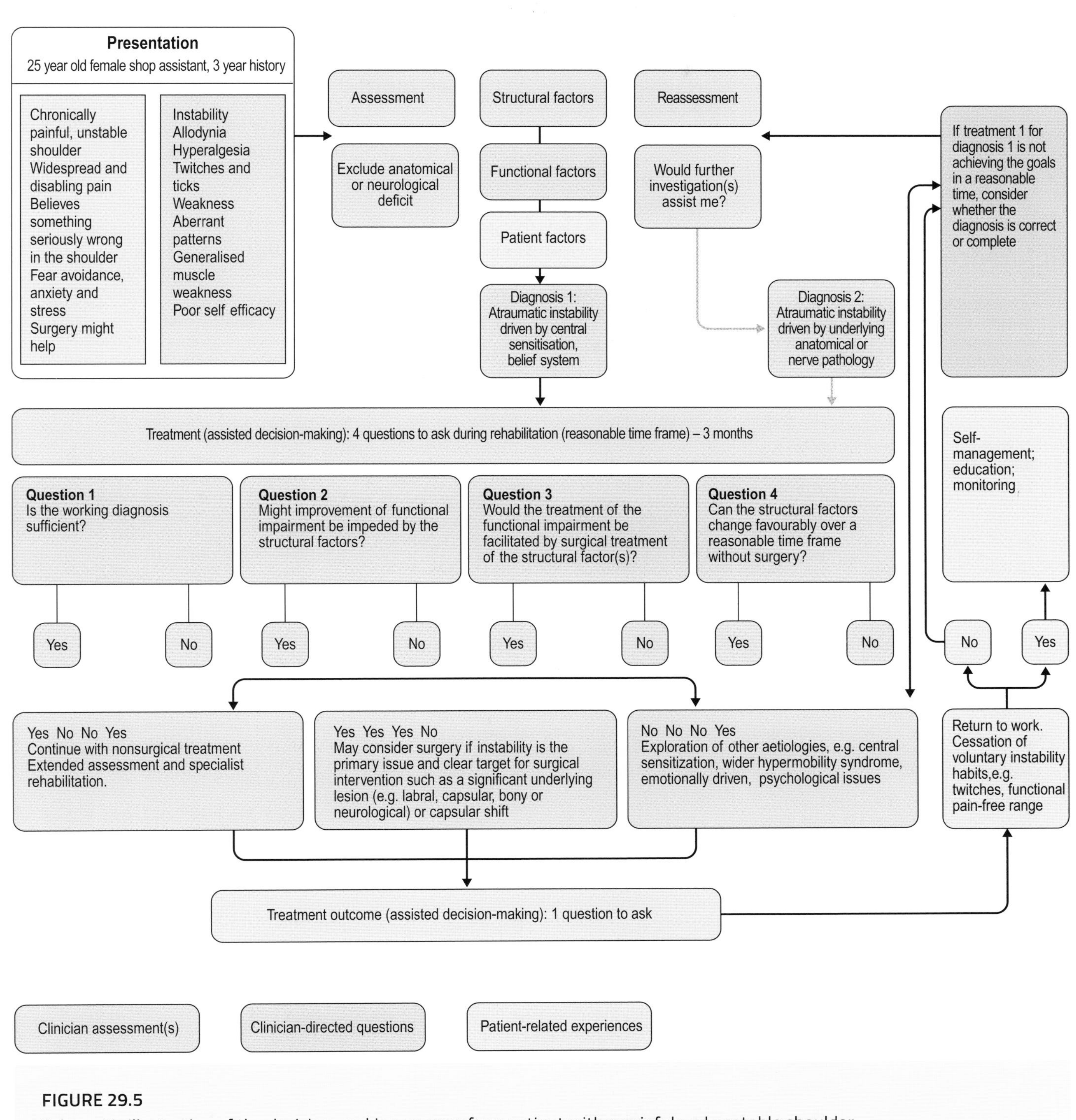

FIGURE 29.5

Schematic illustration of the decision-making process for a patient with a painful and unstable shoulder.

- Following a traumatic shoulder dislocation, surgery may have an important role in restoring stability, particularly where structural lesions are present with significant risk factors for recurrence such as in younger males involved in high-contact sport.
- In cases of atraumatic shoulder instability, surgery may have a role for patients for whom specialized rehabilitation input has failed, and who present with structural pathology or persistent symptoms despite appropriate rehabilitation.
- In all cases, communication between a multidisciplinary team is essential in optimizing the outcome.

References

1. Ainsworth R, Lewis JS, Conboy V. A prospective randomized placebo controlled clinical trial of a rehabilitation programme for patients with a diagnosis of massive rotator cuff tears of the shoulder. Shoulder & Elbow. 2009;1:55-60.
2. Alkaduhimi H, van der Linde JA, Willigenburg NW, Pereira NRP, van Deurzen DF, van den Bekerom MP. Redislocation risk after an arthroscopic Bankart procedure in collision athletes: a systematic review. J Shoulder Elbow Surg. 2016;25:1549-1558.
3. Bossen JK, van der Weijden T, Driessen EW, Heyligers IC. Experienced barriers in shared decision-making behaviour of orthopaedic surgery residents compared with orthopaedic surgeons. Musculoskeletal Care. 2019;17:198-205.
4. Delaney RA, Freehill MT, Janfaza DR, Vlassakov KV, Higgins LD, Warner JJ. 2014 Neer Award paper: neuromonitoring the Latarjet procedure. J Shoulder Elbow Surg. 2014;23:1473-1480.
5. Eichinger JK, Miller LR, Hartshorn T, Li X, Warner JJ, Higgins LD. Evaluation of satisfaction and durability after hemiarthroplasty and total shoulder arthroplasty in a cohort of patients aged 50 years or younger: an analysis of discordance of patient satisfaction and implant survival. J Shoulder Elbow Surg. 2016;25:772-780.
6. Fahey CJ, Delaney RA. Exploring expert variability in defining pseudoparalysis: an international survey. J Shoulder Elbow Surg. 2021;30:e237-e244.
7. Ferrando A, Kingston R, Delaney RA. Superior capsular reconstruction using a porcine dermal xenograft for irreparable rotator cuff tears: outcomes at minimum two-year follow-up. J Shoulder Elbow Surg. 2021;30:1053-1059.
8. Forsythe B, Agarwalla A, Puzzitiello RN, Sumner S, Romeo AA, Mascarenhas R. The timing of injections prior to arthroscopic rotator cuff repair impacts the risk of surgical site infection. JBJS. 2019;101:682-687.
9. Gilbart MK, Gerber C. Comparison of the subjective shoulder value and the Constant score. J Shoulder Elbow Surg. 2007;16:717-721.
10. Hacken B, Onks C, Flemming D, et al. Prevalence of MRI shoulder abnormalities in asymptomatic professional and collegiate ice hockey athletes. Orthopaedic Journal of Sports Medicine. 2019;7:2325967119876865.
11. Harryman DT, 2nd, Sidles JA, Clark JM, McQuade KJ, Gibb TD, Matsen FA, 3rd. Translation of the humeral head on the glenoid with passive glenohumeral motion. J Bone Joint Surg Am. 1990;72:1334-1343.
12. Hurley ET, Manjunath AK, Bloom DA, et al. Arthroscopic Bankart repair versus conservative management for first-time traumatic anterior shoulder instability: a systematic review & meta-analysis. Arthroscopy. 2020;36:2526-2532.
13. Itoi E, Kido T, Sano A, Urayama M, Sato K. Which is more useful, the "full can test" or the "empty can test," in detecting the torn supraspinatus tendon? Am J Sports Med. 1999;27:65-68.
14. Jaggi A, Lambert S. Rehabilitation for shoulder instability. British Journal of Sports Medicine. 2010;44:333-340.
15. Keener JD, Patterson BM, Orvets N, Chamberlain AM. Degenerative rotator cuff tears: refining surgical indications based on natural history data. The Journal of the American Academy of Orthopaedic Surgeons. 2019;27:156.
16. Latremoliere A, Woolf CJ. Central sensitization: a generator of pain hypersensitivity by central neural plasticity. The Journal of Pain. 2009;10:895-926.
17. Levy O, Mullett H, Roberts S, Copeland S. The role of anterior deltoid reeducation in patients with massive irreparable degenerative rotator cuff tears. J Shoulder Elbow Surg. 2008;17:863-870.
18. Neer CS, 2nd. Impingement lesions. Clin Orthop Relat Res. 1983;70-77.
19. Neyton L, Kirsch JM, Collotte P, et al. Mid- to long-term follow-up of shoulder arthroplasty for primary glenohumeral osteoarthritis in patients aged 60 or under. J Shoulder Elbow Surg. 2019;28:1666-1673.
20. Noorani A, Goldring M, Jaggi A, et al. BESS/BOA patient care pathways: atraumatic shoulder instability. Shoulder & Elbow. 2019;11:60-70.
21. Olds M, Ellis R, Donaldson K, Parmar P, Kersten P. Risk factors which predispose first-time traumatic anterior shoulder dislocations to recurrent instability in adults: a systematic review and meta-analysis. British Journal of Sports Medicine. 2015;49:913-922.
22. Raiss P, Bruckner T, Rickert M, Walch G. Longitudinal observational study of total shoulder replacements with cement: fifteen to twenty-year follow-up. JBJS. 2014;96:198-205.
23. Saini SS, Shah SS, Curtis AS. Scapular dyskinesis and the kinetic chain: recognizing dysfunction and treating injury in the tennis athlete. Current Reviews in Musculoskeletal Medicine. 2020;13:748-756.
24. Torrance E, Clarke CJ, Monga P, Funk L, Walton MJ. Recurrence after arthroscopic labral repair for traumatic anterior instability in adolescent rugby and contact athletes. The American Journal of Sports Medicine. 2018;46:2969-2974.

The role of virtual reality in the management of shoulder conditions

Niamh Brady, Beate Dejaco, Jeremy Lewis

Introduction

Virtual reality (VR) is a computer-generated environment that allows an individual to interact with the virtual surroundings using vision, sound, touch, and movement. VR is best known in the gaming and entertainment industry where gamers can play independently or interact with people around the world, and users can visit museums and art galleries, attend concerts and "visit the world" in ways that were previously unknown. The popularity of VR is increasing due to its accessibility, affordability and increasing simplicity.

More recently VR technology has become integrated into education, military training, and healthcare. There is evidence to support the use of VR in pain management, neurological rehabilitation, and treatment of mental health disorders.[22,26,39] The use of VR in musculoskeletal practice is relatively new and is an exciting area for research and development. In this chapter, we will explore the history of VR, the application of VR in various aspects of healthcare, and the potential role of VR interventions in the management and rehabilitation of musculoskeletal shoulder pain.

The history of virtual reality

Virtual reality may have its origins in art. The development of perspective art in Renaissance Europe (15th and 16th centuries) creating an illusion of three-dimensional (3D) environments on two-dimensional (flat) surfaces was an early example of virtual reality that aimed to immerse the viewer into a virtual world. Examples include Raphael's "The School of Athens" and da Vinci's "The Last Supper". M.C. Escher's (1898–1972) graphical art that immerses viewers into virtual worlds that depict impossible 3D scenes is a further example.

In the 1920s, a flight simulator developed by Edwin Link is probably the first example of technology that may be considered as VR. The simulator was initially used in amusement parks but became adopted by the United States Air Force who required a method of training pilots to fly in poor weather conditions. In 1940, Link sold approximately 10,000 Link Trainers to the Air Force and every American World War II fighter or bomber pilot trained with this technology before flying.[53]

In 1957, the Sensorama™ (also known as "The Cinema of the Future") was developed by Morton Heilig as the first interactive theatre experience.[26] The Sensorama™ was a little larger than a modern-day photo booth and one person could use it at a time. The viewer sat with their head and faces inside the device and held onto handlebars in a simulated motorcycle ride around New York City and experienced 3D motion images, stereo sound (engine and city sounds), odors (exhaust fumes and the smell of pizza), fan-generated wind, and a vibrating seat. In total, the Sensorama™ offered six VR experiences, including a dune buggy, and a helicopter ride.

The Philco Corporation developed Headsight in 1961 as a system for the military to remotely look at hazardous situations. Although heavy and large and suspended from the ceiling, it was the first-time a head-mounted display (HMD) was used. In 1965 Ivan Sutherland foresaw a future involving virtual reality, HMDs, eye tracking, haptics, and speech recognition. In 1968 he introduced the "Ultimate Display" also known as the "Sword of Damocles" because of the sword-like projection connecting the HMD to the ceiling. Sometimes referred to as the godfather of VR or the godfather of computer graphics, Sutherland's most important contribution was linking the HMD to the computer. In the 1990s the term "Virtual Reality" was introduced by Jaron Lanier who envisaged a future where VR would be widely used across the entertainment industry as well as in other areas, including healthcare.[21]

The technology

The "Virtual Reality" Lanier envisioned was an immersive multisensory experience, requiring an HMD in combination with other types of hardware designed to make the virtual environment as realistic as possible. The different forms of VR will be discussed in the following section.

Non-immersive VR technology

Non-immersive VR involves the user observing a computer-generated image of a virtual environment on a screen, but the real world is visible outside of the screen. Therefore, the user is not immersed completely in the virtual world. Non-immersive VR systems include Nintendo Wii™ and Microsoft Kinect™.

Semi-immersive VR technology

Semi-immersive VR uses more advanced visual displays such as panoramic or curved screens to create a greater sense of immersion than is used in non-immersive VR. Like non-immersive technology, the user can see the real world either side of the screen. However, in certain environments, such as a darkened room, the user will feel more immersed in the virtual world. Semi-immersive VR is popular for training purposes such as flight simulation devices for trainee pilots and for gait rehabilitation.

Immersive VR technology

Immersive VR involves the use of an HMD display unit that offers a multisensory experience for the user. The HMD is often complemented by additional equipment including hand-held devices, gloves, and vibrotactile platforms which provide sensory feedback to the user, enabling them to explore and interact with the virtual environment as an avatar (a computer-generated figure that represents the user in the virtual environment). The immersive VR market is growing and competitive, with Sony Playstation™, Samsung™, HTC™, PICO Neo™, and Oculus™ all developing and promoting VR equipment.

Applications in healthcare

Pain management

There is a growing body of research demonstrating the effectiveness of VR interventions for pain management.[25,33,52] For individuals experiencing pain due to burn injury, VR has been used as an alternative or adjunct to analgesic medication, particularly in pediatric settings.[20] Schmitt et al.[40] reported that for children aged 6–19 years who received VR intervention along with standard analgesia, significantly less pain was experienced compared to those who received analgesia alone. In addition to pain reduction, individuals with burn injuries experience reduced levels of stress and anxiety during wound care procedures compared to those who received standard care.[7]

Snow World™ was the first immersive VR intervention, designed specifically for individuals with burn injury. The success of Snow World™ demonstrated that context is also relevant, as the user is immersed in a virtual world of snow, where they can glide through icy canyons, throwing virtual snowballs at snowmen, penguins, and igloos. Snow World™ immerses the user into an environment that is symbolically cold, as opposed to images associated with burn injuries, heat, and fire. Functional magnetic resonance imaging studies have demonstrated reduced activity in regions of the brain associated with pain (thalamus, insula) during VR use,[12] which may be a potential mechanism for experiencing reduced pain when using software such as Snow World™.

The analgesic effect associated with VR use may be due in part to distraction. In other words, it may be possible that one's own attention is being shifted away from the painful region to focus on a virtual image or task while immersed in the virtual environment. Hoffman et al.[13] argued that humans have a limited amount of conscious attention available and that pain requires conscious attention. VR provides a computer-generated multisystem input that may reduce the conscious attention available to focus on pain. They suggest that more immersive high-tech VR providing a greater illusion and taking more conscious attention may lead to a greater reduction in pain than low-tech VR. They investigated whether the dose-response relationship between high-tech VR (high sense of presence) and low-tech VR (no multisensory feedback, less illusion) would influence the experience of pain. The high-tech group used an immersive, multisensory feedback system where physical reality was shut out by wearing a helmet and earphones, and head tracking was used to allow participants to see all around them in the virtual world when they moved their heads. The low-tech system elicited a less compelling illusion (see-through glasses, no earphones, no head tracking). Thirty-nine asymptomatic psychology students were quasi-randomized into one of the two groups. Each participant received a noxious thermal stimulus. The participants then played the Snow World™ game.

Participants in the high-tech VR group reported significantly greater "fun" and a stronger sense of illusion (presence). Post-VR pain thresholds correlated with the level of presence, suggesting a greater sense of presence (high-tech VR) limits conscious attention and decreases pain more effectively than a lower sense of presence (low-tech VR). The researchers postulated that painful thermal stimuli and VR compete for attention, suggesting that the more attention that is directed towards VR, the greater the reduction in pain experienced. The findings suggest that VR analgesia may work via a distraction or attentional mechanism and this needs to be tested in people experiencing shoulder pain to determine if the response is similar.

Synthesizing the findings of a systematic review, Triberti et al.[45] concluded that emotional responses are fundamental for the effectiveness of VR on pain management. Importantly, the effect is associated with the sense of presence in the virtual world – the greater the sense of being present in the VR world, the greater the effect. Furthermore, they postulated that the sense of fun when in the VR world may correlate with the sense of presence and may be related to the reduction in pain experienced.

Jones et al.[19] reported significant reductions in pain intensity when using immersive VR for individuals (n=30) with different types of persistent pain (e.g., musculoskeletal pain, neuropathic pain, connective tissue disorder, interstitial cystitis, chest wall pain, and abdominal pain). Pain was reduced from pre-session to post-session by 33%, and from pre-session to during-session by 60%. It is also theorized that the mechanisms underpinning the effect of VR in acute pain (e.g., distraction) may be different in persistent pain conditions. VR may offer a more attractive environment for rehabilitation and graded exposure for those with persistent pain and fear avoidance behavior.[2]

Exposure therapy

Virtual Reality Exposure Therapy (VRE) is a well-established intervention for people who suffer from phobias.[26] VRE acts as a controlled and safe environment for exposure to feared and potentially stressful situations such as fear of flying, heights, or spiders. VRE has been shown to be just as effective as in vivo exposure and significantly more effective than no intervention for symptom reduction, such as reduced anxiety and behavioral change in those who fear flying. Post treatment, 76% of participants in both the VRE and Standard In-Vivo Exposure groups took a flight compared to 20% in the waiting list control group. Importantly, the benefits were maintained at one- and three-year follow-ups.[36,51] VRE is practical, safe, and effective as an intervention for people with phobias and may provide similar beneficial effects for individuals with musculoskeletal pain who display fear avoidance behavior.

In a small RCT (n=52), Thomas et al.[44] demonstrated safety and the feasibility of using a VR dodgeball game as a method of graded exposure to lumbar spine flexion in individuals with persistent low back pain. The intervention group completed three 15-minute virtual dodgeball games where they were required to either duck to avoid balls or block balls. A scoreboard was visible in the virtual gym where participants could see their progress and their cash rewards. Participants in the control group received no intervention. Participants enjoyed the game, reported it was easy to use and it distracted them from their pain, attesting to the acceptability of the game. Although Thomas et al.[44] were testing the feasibility of the VR dodgeball game, it is worth noting that participants in the intervention group demonstrated increases in lumbar flexion for tasks that required bending between each level of gameplay.

Education

Virtual reality has the potential to act as a method to deliver healthcare education. This was demonstrated in the Oculus Study, where participants were invited to watch an educational movie through VR that discussed atrial fibrillation (AF) and stroke prevention strategies such as pharmacological treatments.[4] In this study, participants' awareness of AF and stroke increased from 22% at baseline to 83% immediately following the intervention. Unfortunately, there was no control group for comparison, but the outcomes suggest VR may be useful to provide condition-specific information as well as related management strategies, including lifestyle and behavioral change. The participants reported that they enjoyed the VR education and were able to recall information up to one year after the study. Participants also reported that the knowledge gained in the movie influenced their behavior in relation to their use of oral anticoagulant medication.

Saab et al.[37] demonstrated a similar result when using VR to educate men about testicular disorders. In this case, knowledge scores (12-item questionnaire) and testicular awareness scores (5-item scale) increased significantly between baseline and immediately post-test. Significant improvements were maintained at one-month follow-up. This demonstrates that VR may act as an effective tool for improving health literacy, particularly for persistent musculoskeletal conditions.

Rehabilitation and physical activity

Virtual reality has become popular in neurological rehabilitation, and research evidence to support its role in these fields is increasing.[22] Neurological rehabilitation is intensive and often requires extensive repetition of tasks. Research suggests that VR can motivate individuals to engage with rehabilitation by making exercise more stimulating.[46,50] In a systematic review, Miller et al.[31] evaluated the effect of VR use on home-based physical activity levels, physical impairments, emotional and cognitive well-being, and quality of life in adults over the age of 45 years, including those with neurological conditions and intellectual disabilities. The authors included 14 studies, only two of which were randomized controlled trials, the remaining 12 studies being a mix of study designs. Despite the weak evidence and high risk of bias in most studies, Miller et al.[31] found good adherence (63–100%) to VR rehabilitation and suggested that there is potential for VR to be used to promote physical activity in the home setting. Figure 30.1 depicts an individual using a non-tethered immersive VR game that involves whole body movement.

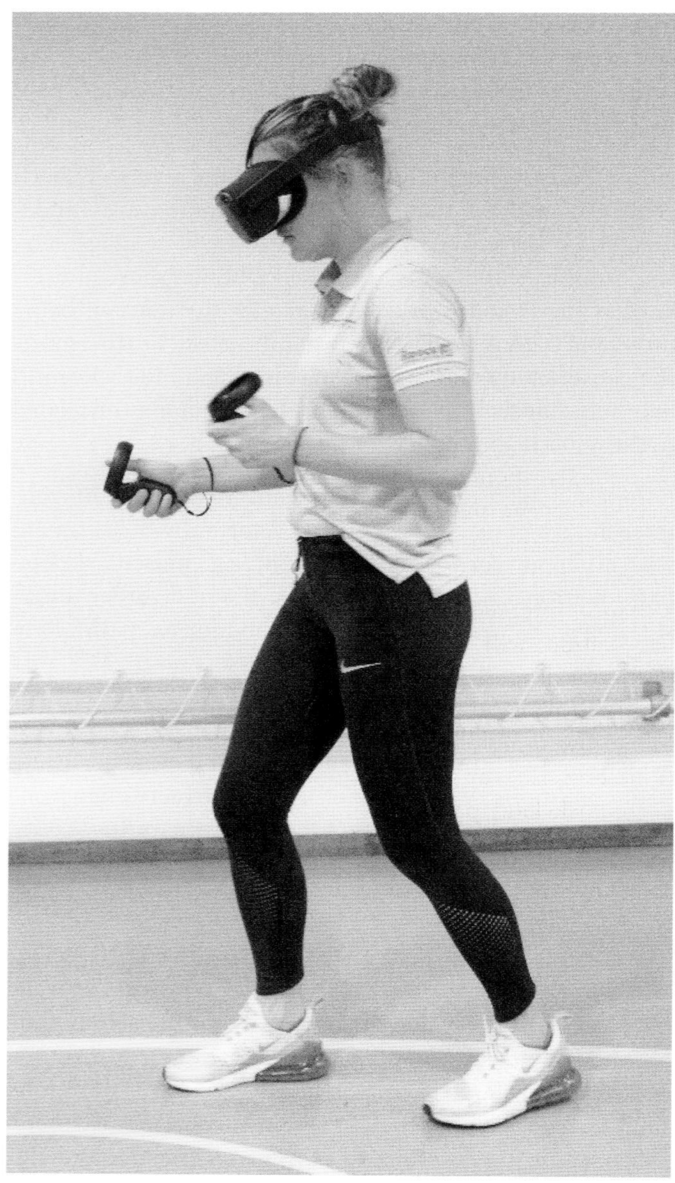

FIGURE 30.1
Using immersive VR gaming to promote physical activity that involves whole body movement.

Deutsch et al.[8] utilized a VR augmented cycling kit to assess feasibility of VR cycling in promoting cardiovascular fitness in people following stroke. In this small study, four participants completed two training sessions per week for 8 weeks. Participants cycled for 20–30 minutes in the initial session, eventually increasing to 60 minutes cycling by week eight. On average, participants completed between 90 and 125 minutes of cycling per week. Aerobic capacity increased in all participants, with mean improvement of 13% in submaximal VO_2 (range 6.0–24.5%).

Active gaming that combines VR with physical activity may facilitate physical activity and decrease sedentary behavior in healthy individuals.[49] Active gaming involves whole body exercise at a moderate-to-vigorous intensity.[48] There is evidence to suggest that active gaming leads to greater enjoyment, adherence, and metabolic requirements compared to traditional cycle-based training.[35] The Gamebike™ exercise was compared to traditional cycling and demonstrated that the VR game exercise had a significant impact on affective attitude (assessed by a three-item scale) and intention (two-item scale).[35]

The Theory of Planned Behavior suggests that an individual's behavior is predicted by one's intention and their perceived behavioral control. Intention is influenced by affective (e.g., enjoyment associated with the behavior) and instrumental (perceived benefit of the behavior) attitudes and social norms (e.g., perceived social approval). Potentially, immersive active gaming might distract users from boredom, pain, and fatigue when exercising. An advantage of active gaming is that it may be adapted to a wide variety of settings and for a wide range of physical and cognitive abilities.

Virtual reality in the management of musculoskeletal pain

Persistent musculoskeletal pain is multifactorial, associated with long-term disability. In isolation, pathoanatomical diagnoses do not adequately explain symptoms,[24] and musculoskeletal conditions require a biopsychosocial approach to management.[6] It is important to educate individuals about their condition and involve them in shared-decision making[14,17] ensuring they understand the available management options, their benefits and potential harms. There should not be an assumption that rehabilitation interventions, injections, or surgical procedures, in isolation, will "cure" symptoms, but there need be an understanding that lifestyle changes, including participating in physical activity, will contribute to reducing the impact of symptoms.[24] As with many healthcare conditions, exercise is an essential component of management for musculoskeletal pain.[41,42] Unfortunately, poor adherence with management, including exercise, is an acknowledged barrier to successful outcomes.[30] VR may be a useful tool in overcoming this barrier.

The use of VR for management of musculoskeletal pain is emerging and VR companies have produced software to facilitate musculoskeletal assessment and rehabilitation. VR has been shown to be a useful platform for facilitation of pain management, education, and exercise, which are key aspects of current musculoskeletal care.[24] VR has a positive influence on adherence to graded-exposure therapy and rehabilitation programs due to a reduction in pain and psychological distress, while using the technology.[25,26] VR may provide a more stimulating environment for patients to engage with activity and exercise than traditional rehabilitation programs, and may improve adherence to the program.[35,50]

Recent advances in VR technology designed to connect people may allow individuals to be present in the same virtual space such as a virtual clinic or gym where they can interact with one another as avatars or holograms. All those present will be able to observe the same scene, share experiences and interact without having to be in the same physical space. This may provide opportunities for virtual consultations that allow the clinician to assess the individual presenting to physiotherapy and provide more specific exercise prescription and feedback than would be possible via videocall consultation. Another potential use of such technology might be virtual exercise classes, where several participants could be synchronously present and physically active with the clinician or trainer in the same virtual space. Research findings support group exercise in the management of musculoskeletal shoulder pain.[5]

Research evidence suggests that there is potential for VR to support musculoskeletal rehabilitation of spinal pain,[1] orthopedic conditions,[10] and persistent pain conditions.[9,29] For people with pain in the cervical region, immersive VR was as effective as standard rehabilitation for pain intensity[43] and neck disability. Harvie et al.[11] demonstrated that VR may be used to manipulate somatosensory input and therefore pain-related movement in patients with mechanical neck pain. In their study, VR was used to create a visual illusion that either decreased or increased the user's actual movement. This led to an increase or decrease in movement performed by 6% and 7%, respectively.

Following total knee replacement, immersive VR was found to be effective during rehabilitation. The patients who used a VR rowing game in addition to standard rehabilitation demonstrated significantly greater improvements in range of movement and function compared to the standard rehabilitation group, although it is uncertain whether the difference between the groups was clinically important.[18] A single case report by Hong and Lee[15] demonstrated that an immersive VR intervention could be successfully added to standard rehabilitation following total knee replacement. The intervention was well tolerated and within two weeks the patient showed a 32% increase in muscle strength, a 45% increase in proprioception and a return of walking speed to baseline level.

Gulsen et al.[9] used immersive VR as an adjunct to rehabilitation in people with fibromyalgia and found that the VR group demonstrated reduced pain, kinesiophobia and fatigue compared to the standard rehabilitation group. Evidence suggests that VR interventions may provide a feasible and attractive platform for the rehabilitation of a variety of musculoskeletal conditions, but further research is needed to demonstrate efficacy and to guide clinical

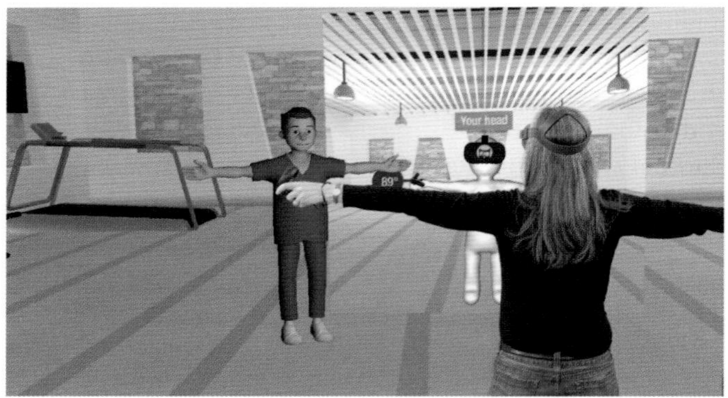

FIGURE 30.2
Using VR to assess shoulder range of motion.
(Reproduced with the kind permission of XRHealth.com.)

application. Figure 30.2 depicts an individual undergoing a shoulder range of motion assessment in VR.

Virtual reality and embodiment

Immersive VR seems to be more promising in musculoskeletal rehabilitation because of its ability to immerse participants into a computer-generated 3D environment, with a high sense of presence. This sense of presence may activate brain mechanisms that underlie sensorimotor integration, and therefore might play an important role in reducing pain and regaining function in the rehabilitation of musculoskeletal disorders. Presence is the sense of being embodied in a virtual body, meaning that the user feels the ownership of a virtual body. Vision, touch, proprioception, motor control, and vestibular sensations, all contribute to the sense of embodiment. Embodiment or "ownership" of a virtual body allows manipulation of body perception which may have clinical implications for conditions such as persistent pain.[28]

The sense of presence, or embodiment, in an immersive virtual environment has been the subject of multiple studies investigating pain mechanisms and experimental pain reduction in healthy people as well as in patients with persistent musculoskeletal pain.[12,27,28] Immersive VR allows for a controlled manipulation of the virtual environment, affecting visual, aural, tactile, and sensorimotor feedback. The visual manipulation is provided within the virtual environment by creating a world that differs from the real world including interactive sports fields, rollercoasters, train stations and many more scenes depending on the goals of the game. Aural and tactile feedback is provided using earphones and hand-held devices such as gloves and controllers. This manipulation of the immersive virtual environment combined with a sense of ownership of a virtual body and the effect this has on pain perception and function is the focus of on-going research.[27,28,47]

Virtual reality and rehabilitation of upper limb pain

The benefits of VR modalities in musculoskeletal upper limb rehabilitation and especially for people with shoulder symptoms have not been studied in detail, but some promising evidence is emerging in specific populations where VR technology is being used to facilitate pain management. Martini et al.[27] investigated the effect of virtual body ownership on pain threshold when heat was applied to the hands of 24 healthy participants. In this experiment participants received painful thermal stimuli under four conditions: 1) in the control condition, participants did not use VR and instead looked at a marker placed on a foam cover that prevented them from seeing their arms, 2) participants were immersed in VR using an HMD but did not see any avatar representing their own body (instead they saw a virtual cylinder placed on a table in front of them), 3) participants observed an avatar representing their own body where their own index finger was passively moved asynchronously with that of the avatar, and 4) participants observed an avatar representing their own body and their own index finger was passively moved synchronously (in time) with that of the avatar. In the final condition, moving the finger in time with that of the avatar was intended to increase the sense of ownership of the virtual limb. Indeed, it was in this condition alone that significant improvements in pain threshold were seen. These observations suggest that changes in pain threshold using VR are not due to distraction alone, as this experiment required attention to be focused on the painful region rather than being drawn away from it.

The ability of VR to reduce persistent arm and hand pain has been investigated in people diagnosed with complex regional pain syndrome (CRPS) type 1 (n=9 without nerve injury) and in people with peripheral nerve injury (PNI) (n=10).[29] In this study participants wore an HMD, and a life-size virtual arm and hand were projected at the same location where their painful arm and hand were positioned in the real world. The participants experienced a high sense of embodiment and ownership of the virtual arm, as if it was their own body part. The investigation involved varying the level of transparency and size of the virtual arm. Initially, the virtual arm was observed normally and then at 25%, 50%, and 75% transparency. At 75% it could still be observed but only faintly. In the following test, the size of the virtual arm was presented as normal, larger than normal, and smaller than normal.

For those with CRPS, greater transparency led to reduced pain which was opposite to the finding in people with PNI. In the size experiment, pain rating remained the same for people diagnosed with PNI in all three conditions and, in contrast, those with CRPS experienced slightly more pain when the virtual arm was bigger than the real arm and less pain when the virtual arm was smaller than life-size. The findings of this study suggest that manipulation of the body in the virtual environment for people with CRPS can modulate pain perception. In the group diagnosed with CRPS, disturbances in body representation in the primary somatosensory cortex may influence pain perception and therefore, increasing the transparency of the virtual arm may reduce afferent input from the affected arm.

It would be useful to conduct similar investigations (transparency and size) in people experiencing the often-unbearable pain associated with frozen shoulder (see Chapter 18) and calcific tendinopathy (see Chapter 27). The finding that the experience of pain did not change for those diagnosed with PNI raises further questions: are different VR strategies required to reduce pain in different conditions, and are there conditions that VR can lead to a reduction in pain, and others where it is not beneficial?

House et al.[16] investigated the feasibility of Bright Arm Duo therapy for postsurgical chronic pain and associated disability in breast cancer survivors. Post-mastectomy pain syndrome (PMPS) may lead to reduced range of motion in the shoulder, weakness, reduced function, sleep disorders, and depression. The Bright Arm Duo Rehabilitation System consisted of a robotic rehabilitation table, computerized forearm supports, a display and virtual rehabilitation games. The games were developed for motor function, cognitive, and emotive focus training. After 16 training sessions, pain intensity as reported by the Numeric Rating Scale (NRS) had decreased by 20%. Furthermore, an improvement was seen in both shoulder range of motion and strength. A very important finding was a significant improvement in depression. These findings suggests that VR may have a positive effect on emotional well-being, which may be linked to reductions in pain and improvements in function.

Virtual reality and functional rehabilitation of musculoskeletal shoulder pain

Only a few studies have investigated the effects of VR on pain and functional outcomes for people with musculoskeletal shoulder complaints. In a cohort study with pre- and post-test comparison, Lee et al.[23] investigated the effects of a goal-directed non-immersive VR system (GDSR) for people diagnosed with frozen shoulder. In this study, 16 participants received heat and interferential therapy and a 40-minute exercise session twice weekly for four weeks. The exercises involved range of movement, and arm, trunk and leg strengthening. Primary outcome measures were the Constant Murley Score (CMS), active and passive shoulder range of movement, and upper arm muscle strength. Other outcomes included task performance, defined as the ability to complete the VR tasks in the GDSR system, and motor indices defined as angular velocity, number of interruptions during joint rotation and varying rate of muscle strength. After four weeks of training, all participants demonstrated significant improvement in the CMS, range of movement, and upper arm muscle strength, as well as increased task performance and angular velocity. The findings suggest that non-immersive GDSR may be useful in the rehabilitation of people diagnosed with frozen shoulder. However, as there was no control group and other important features of low risk of bias interventions (randomization, allocation concealment, blinding, intention to treat analysis), the results should be interpreted with caution.

Pekyavas et al.[32] compared the short-term effects of a home exercise program and VR exercise-gaming in people diagnosed with subacromial pain syndrome. In their trial, 30 participants were randomized into two groups. One group performed exercises with a non-immersive Nintendo Wii™ device, the other group were instructed to participate in a home-based exercise program. Both groups exercised twice weekly for 45 minutes for a period of six weeks. Outcome measures included measuring pain using a visual analogue scale for pain at rest, pain during the day and pain at night, and the Shoulder Pain and Disability Index (SPADI). Other outcome measures included the Neer sign, the Hawkins test, the lateral scapular slide test (LSST), the scapular assistance test (SAT), and the scapular retraction test (SRT). The control group exercise program consisted of stretching exercises, bilateral shoulder elevation, and scapular mobility exercises. The VR exercise-gaming group performed stretching exercises, bilateral shoulder elevation, boxing, bowling, and tennis games. Pain intensity decreased significantly in both groups, which may have been a result of changes in symptoms over time, placebo, or the benefit of exercise.

Although the clinical relevance is uncertain, a statistically significant improvement was found for the pain response in the Neer sign, the SAT, and the SRT for the exercise-gaming group, but not for the control group. SPADI results demonstrated a significant improvement at all time factors (before treatment, after treatment, one-month post treatment) for the Nintendo Wii™ group, but only showed significant improvement one month after intervention in the control group. The authors postulated that the faster improvements in the VR group might be attributed to the multisensory feedback modalities of the VR technology enhancing sensorimotor feedback and response.[32]

In summary, using a VR system during shoulder and arm rehabilitation may reduce the experience of pain and increase function. Mechanisms are poorly understood, but may be attributed to different properties of VR, such as drawing attention away from the painful body part by attracting the user's attention into the virtual environment, reordering the somatosensory cortex via illusions, and stimulating positive emotions such as fun and thereby modulating patients' pain perception.

High-tech virtual environments where subjects are fully immersed in a virtual environment where they can interact with the VR world based on multisensorial feedback seem to be more promising than semi- or augmented immersion. The high correlation between embodiment or the sense of presence in the immersive virtual world and reduction in pain and improvement in function may be relevant in the musculoskeletal rehabilitation of the upper extremity. We speculate that patients suffering from persistent arm or shoulder pain who have altered somatosensory cortex processing and therefore altered motor control and pain perception may experience clinically important improvements using high-tech immersive VR. Figure 30.3 depicts an individual experiencing fully immersive VR gaming that involves functional upper limb movement.

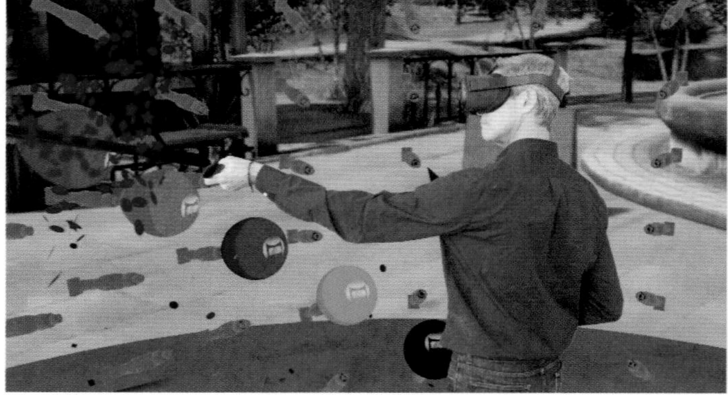

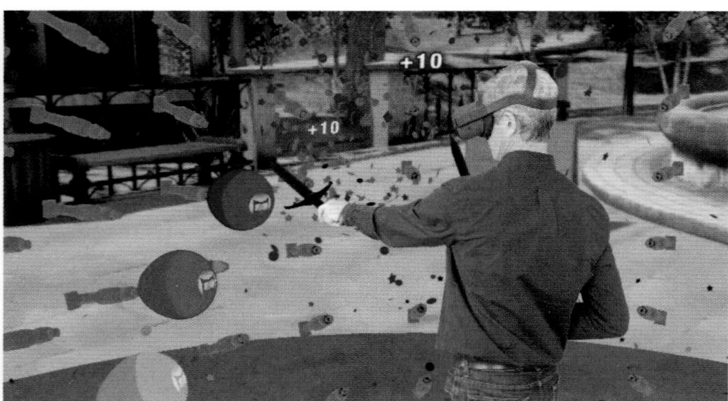

FIGURE 30.3

An immersive VR game that incorporates shoulder movement, concentration, fun, competition, distraction, and a progressive challenge. The individual is holding a virtual sword and is cutting through virtual targets. "Noise" (distraction) is generated by a popping sound, confetti, and verbal instruction, and challenge, by an increase in score for each target hit. Range of movement, speed, and complexity can be manipulated through the software. The software can also produce myriad data associated with the required tasks.

(Reproduced with the kind permission of XRHealth.com.)

Although VR may offer an exciting new platform for rehabilitation of musculoskeletal shoulder pain, there is much to be considered. The integration of VR into musculoskeletal practice requires careful introduction and substantial monitoring to ensure that it is practical, affordable, tolerable, and engaging. Adverse effects such as motion sickness are infrequent due to improving technology.[3,38] However, where there is reduced accuracy of motion tracking, symptoms of nausea and dizziness may occur.[34] Visual fatigue may also occur following long periods of use, since the virtual image presented through an HMD is very close to the user. Advice regarding time spent using VR may be an important consideration in clinical practice.

Safety is a priority for modern VR units that are designed for use at home, and users create virtual boundaries that correspond to the environments in which they use the VR equipment. Warnings are provided to the user when they get close to the VR boundaries to prevent contact between the virtual and real worlds. The same concerns pertaining to safety must be maintained when using VR in clinical practice.

Conclusion

Virtual reality as we think of it today has its origins in early flight simulators approximately 100 years ago. Modern VR provides a unique platform for manipulation of somatosensory input, thereby having the potential to reduce pain. VR is also a platform for education, which may be beneficial in explaining pain, injury and supporting self-management strategies. VR has the potential to make rehabilitation and exercise more challenging and engaging, by introducing a gaming element, which may improve participation and adherence. These features require further exploration and there are many other questions that need to be addressed. Future research needs to harness the thoughts, ideas, goals, values, and beliefs of patients, clinicians, and software and hardware engineers. Combining current shoulder pain research, exercise science, and behavioral science in the development of advanced VR technology is an exciting challenge that may change how we assess and manage musculoskeletal shoulder conditions in the future.

References

1. Ahern MM, Dean LV, Stoddard CC, et al. The effectiveness of virtual reality in patients with spinal pain: a systematic review and meta-analysis. Pain Pract. 2020;20:656-675.
2. Ariza-Mateos MJ, Cabrera-Martos I, Ortiz-Rubio A, Torres-Sanchez I, Rodriguez-Torres J, Valenza MC. Effects of a patient-centered graded exposure intervention added to manual therapy for women with chronic pelvic pain: a randomized controlled trial. Archives of Physical Medicine and Rehabilitation. 2019;100:9-16.
3. Bahat HS, Croft K, Carter C, Hoddinott A, Sprecher E, Treleaven J. Remote kinematic training for patients with chronic neck pain: a randomised controlled trial. European Spine Journal. 2018;27:1309-1323.
4. Balsam P, Borodzicz S, Malesa K, et al. OCULUS study: virtual reality-based education in daily clinical practice. Cardiology Journal. 2019;26:260-264.
5. Barrett E, Hayes A, Kelleher M, et al. Exploring patient experiences of participating in a group exercise class for the management of nonspecific shoulder pain. Physiotherapy Theory and Practice. 2018;34:464-471.
6. Booth J, Moseley GL, Schiltenwolf M, Cashin A, Davies M, Hubscher M. Exercise for chronic musculoskeletal pain: a biopsychosocial approach. Musculoskeletal Care. 2017;15:413-421.
7. Brown NJ, Kimble RM, Rodger S, Ware RS, Cuttle L. Play and heal: randomized controlled trial of Ditto intervention efficacy on improving re-epithelialization in pediatric burns. Burns. 2014;40:204-213.
8. Deutsch JE, Myslinski MJ, Kafri M, et al. Feasibility of virtual reality augmented cycling for health promotion of people poststroke. JNPT. 2013;37:118-124.
9. Gulsen C, Soke F, Eldemir K, et al. Effect of fully immersive virtual reality treatment combined with exercise in fibromyalgia patients: a randomized controlled trial. Assistive Technology. 2020;1-8.
10. Gumaa M, Rehan Youssef A. Is virtual reality effective in orthopedic rehabilitation? A systematic review and meta-analysis. Phys Ther. 2019;99:1304-1325.
11. Harvie DS, Broecker M, Smith RT, Meulders A, Madden VJ, Moseley GL. Bogus visual feedback alters onset of movement-evoked pain in people with neck pain. Psychological Science. 2015;26:385-392.
12. Hoffman HG, Richards TL, Bills AR, et al. Using fMRI to study the neural correlates of virtual reality analgesia. CNS Spectrums. 2006;11:45-51.
13. Hoffman HG, Sharar SR, Coda B, et al. Manipulating presence influences the magnitude of virtual reality analgesia. Pain. 2004;111:162-168.
14. Hoffmann TC, Lewis J, Maher CG. Shared decision making should be an integral part of physiotherapy practice. Physiotherapy. 2020;107:43-49.
15. Hong S, Lee G. Effects of an immersive virtual reality environment on muscle strength, proprioception, balance, and gait of a middle-aged woman who had total knee replacement: a case report. Am J Case Rep. 2019;20:1636-1642.

16. House G, Burdea G, Grampurohit N, et al. A feasibility study to determine the benefits of upper extremity virtual rehabilitation therapy for coping with chronic pain post-cancer surgery. Br J Pain. 2016;10:186-197.

17. Hutting N, Johnston V, Staal JB, Heerkens YF. Promoting the use of self-management strategies for people with persistent musculoskeletal disorders: the role of physical therapists. The Journal of Orthopaedic and Sports Physical Therapy. 2019;49:212-215.

18. Jin C, Feng Y, Ni Y, Shan Z. Virtual reality intervention in postoperative rehabilitation after total knee arthroplasty: a prospective and randomized controlled clinical trial. International Journal of Clinical and Experimental Medicine. 2018;11:6119-6124.

19. Jones T, Moore T, Choo J. The Impact of virtual reality on chronic pain. PloS One. 2016;11:e0167523.

20. Kipping B, Rodger S, Miller K, Kimble RM. Virtual reality for acute pain reduction in adolescents undergoing burn wound care: a prospective randomized controlled trial. Burns. 2012;38:650-657.

21. Lanier J. Dawn of the New Everything: A Journey Through Virtual Reality. Random House; 2017.

22. Laver KE, Lange B, George S, Deutsch JE, Saposnik G, Crotty M. Virtual reality for stroke rehabilitation. The Cochrane Database of Systematic Reviews. 2017;11:CD008349.

23. Lee SH, Yeh SC, Chan RC, Chen S, Yang G, Zheng LR. Motor ingredients derived from a wearable sensor-based virtual reality system for frozen shoulder rehabilitation. Biomed Res Int. 2016;2016:7075464.

24. Lewis J, O'Sullivan P. Is it time to reframe how we care for people with non-traumatic musculoskeletal pain? British Journal of Sports Medicine. 2018;52:1543-1544.

25. Mallari B, Spaeth EK, Goh H, Boyd BS. Virtual reality as an analgesic for acute and chronic pain in adults: a systematic review and meta-analysis. Journal of Pain Research. 2019;12:2053-2085.

26. Maples-Keller JL, Bunnell BE, Kim SJ, Rothbaum BO. The use of virtual reality technology in the treatment of anxiety and other psychiatric disorders. Harvard Review of Psychiatry. 2017;25:103-113.

27. Martini M, Perez-Marcos D, Sanchez-Vives MV. Modulation of pain threshold by virtual body ownership. European Journal of Pain. 2014;18:1040-1048.

28. Maselli A, Kilteni K, López-Moliner J, Slater M. The sense of body ownership relaxes temporal constraints for multisensory integration. Sci Rep. 2016;6:30628.

29. Matamala-Gomez M, Diaz Gonzalez AM, Slater M, Sanchez-Vives MV. Decreasing pain ratings in chronic arm pain through changing a virtual body: different strategies for different pain types. J Pain. 2019;20:685-697.

30. Meade LB, Bearne LM, Sweeney LH, Alageel SH, Godfrey EL. Behaviour change techniques associated with adherence to prescribed exercise in patients with persistent musculoskeletal pain: systematic review. British Journal of Health Psychology. 2019;24:10-30.

31. Miller KJ, Adair BS, Pearce AJ, Said CM, Ozanne E, Morris MM. Effectiveness and feasibility of virtual reality and gaming system use at home by older adults for enabling physical activity to improve health-related domains: a systematic review. Age and Ageing. 2014;43:188-195.

32. Pekyavas NO, Ergun N. Comparison of virtual reality exergaming and home exercise programs in patients with subacromial impingement syndrome and scapular dyskinesis: short term effect. Acta Orthopaedica et Traumatologica Turcica. 2017;51:238-242.

33. Pourmand A, Davis S, Marchak A, Whiteside T, Sikka N. Virtual reality as a clinical tool for pain management. Current Pain and Headache Reports. 2018;22:53.

34. Regan C. An investigation into nausea and other side-effects of head-coupled immersive virtual reality. Virtual Reality. 1995;1:17-31.

35. Rhodes RE, Warburton DE, Bredin SS. Predicting the effect of interactive video bikes on exercise adherence: an efficacy trial. Psychology, Health & Medicine. 2009;14:631-640.

36. Rothbaum BO, Hodges L, Anderson PL, Price L, Smith S. Twelve-month follow-up of virtual reality and standard exposure therapies for the fear of flying. Journal of Consulting and Clinical Psychology. 2002;70:428-432.

37. Saab MM, Landers M, Cooke E, Murphy D, Davoren M, Hegarty J. Enhancing men's awareness of testicular disorders using a virtual reality intervention: a pre-post pilot study. Nursing Research. 2018;67:349-358.

38. Sarig Bahat H, Takasaki H, Chen X, Bet-Or Y, Treleaven J. Cervical kinematic training with and without interactive VR training for chronic neck pain – a randomized clinical trial. Manual Therapy. 2015;20:68-78.

39. Scapin S, Echevarria-Guanilo ME, Junior PRBF, Goncalves N, Rocha PK, Coimbra R. Virtual reality in the treatment of burn patients: a systematic review. Burns. 2018;44:1403-1416.

40. Schmitt YS, Hoffman HG, Blough DK, et al. A randomized, controlled trial of immersive virtual reality analgesia, during physical therapy for pediatric burns. Burns. 2011;37:61-68.

41. Searle A, Spink M, Ho A, Chuter V. Exercise interventions for the treatment of chronic low back pain: a systematic review and meta-analysis of randomised controlled trials. Clinical rehabilitation. 2015;29:1155-1167.

42. Shire AR, Stæhr TA, Overby JB, Dahl MB, Jacobsen JS, Christiansen DH. Specific or general exercise strategy for subacromial impingement syndrome–does it matter? A systematic literature review and meta analysis. BMC Musculoskeletal Disorders. 2017;18:158.

43. Tejera DM, Beltran-Alacreu H, Cano-de-la-Cuerda R, et al. Effects of virtual reality versus exercise on pain, functional, somatosensory and psychosocial outcomes in patients with non-specific chronic neck pain: a randomized clinical trial. Int J Environ Res Public Health. 2020;17:5950.

44. Thomas JS, France CR, Applegate ME, Leitkam ST, Walkowski S. Feasibility and safety of a virtual reality dodgeball intervention for chronic low back pain: a randomized clinical trial. The Journal of Pain. 2016;17:1302-1317.

45. Triberti S, Repetto C, Riva G. Psychological factors influencing the effectiveness of virtual reality-based analgesia: a systematic review. Cyberpsychol Behav Soc Netw. 2014;17:335-345.

46. Tsekleves E, Paraskevopoulos IT, Warland A, Kilbride C. Development and preliminary evaluation of a novel low cost VR-based upper limb stroke rehabilitation platform using Wii technology. Disability and Rehabilitation: Assistive Technology. 2016;11:413-422.

47. Vecchiato G, Tieri G, Jelic A, De Matteis F, Maglione AG, Babiloni F. Electroencephalographic correlates of sensorimotor integration and embodiment during the appreciation of virtual architectural environments. Front Psychol. 2015;6:1944.

48. Warburton D, Sarkany D, Johnson M, et al. Metabolic requirements of interactive video game cycling. Medicine and Science in Sports and Exercise. 2009;41:920-926.

49. Warburton DE. The health benefits of active gaming: separating the myths from the virtual reality. Current Cardiovascular Risk Reports. 2013;7:251-255.

50. Warland A, Paraskevopoulos I, Tsekleves E, et al. The feasibility, acceptability and preliminary efficacy of a low-cost, virtual-reality based, upper-limb stroke rehabilitation device: a mixed methods study. Disability and Rehabilitation. 2019;41:2119-2134.

51. Wiederhold BK, Jang DP, Gevirtz RG, Kim SI, Kim I-Y, Wiederhold MD. The treatment of fear of flying: a controlled study of imaginal and virtual reality graded exposure therapy. IEEE Transactions on Information Technology in Biomedicine. 2002;6:218-223.

52. Won AS, Bailey J, Bailenson J, Tataru C, Yoon IA, Golianu B. Immersive virtual reality for pediatric pain. Children. 2017;4:52.

53. Original Link Flight Trainer at the MOST in Syracuse. Available at: https://www.youtube.com/watch?v=yAlcVOl2x1c.

Part 3

Manual therapy, needling, modalities, and taping

3

Hands-on (manual) therapy in the management of shoulder conditions

31

César Fernández-de-las-Peñas, Neil Langridge, Roger Kerry, Toby Hall, Joel Bialosky, Joshua Cleland

Introduction

The term manual therapy includes many different treatment approaches where the clinician's hands provide the intervention. Unsurprisingly, this type of intervention is also referred to as therapeutic touch and hands-on therapy. Manual therapy techniques used in the management of musculoskeletal pain disorders range from passive joint-biased interventions (joint mobilizations or manipulations) or soft tissue-biased interventions (muscle stretching or trigger point pressure release) to active joint mobilization.[1] In addition, nerve-biased interventions, referred to as neurodynamic treatment (see Chapter 21), should be also included in this umbrella term of hands-on interventions. The term passive refers to the clinical situation where a technique is performed by the clinician to the patient.

The shoulder complex includes multifarious structures, e.g., acromioclavicular, sternoclavicular, scapulothoracic, glenohumeral joint, that can be potentially targeted with manual therapy techniques. As discussed in Chapter 16, hands-on interventions may also be applied to the cervical and/or thoracic region when warranted in the management of musculoskeletal shoulder conditions. Each articulation and its surrounding soft tissues, including its concomitant neurovascular supply, contributes to shoulder movement and function. Dysfunction of any articulation around the shoulder may contribute to the generation of symptoms during movement or may lead to impairment of movement resulting in shoulder stiffness. The primary aims of hands-on interventions are to contribute to a reduction in pain and disability, to restore mobility, and thereby to restore normal function.

Different hands-on concepts use seemingly different, but probably complementary, clinical reasoning approaches for their application. For example, the Maitland approach uses symptom reproduction when identifying the most appropriate treatment technique to apply,[36] whereas the Mulligan approach (mobilization-with-movement (MWM)) uses an opposing clinical reasoning process, i.e., symptom reduction[37] (see Chapter 16). In addition, the principle of progressive tissue loading during symptom-free movement is performed using hands-on therapy, e.g., MWM. Symptom and movement modification approaches are currently proposed as one method to overcome the difficulties relating to diagnosis and treatment selection in individuals with shoulder problems.[50] There is substantial heterogeneity in the dosage, repetitions, and number of treatments to be applied by the different hands-on methods and no one method has demonstrated superiority over another.

Historic and current understanding of manual therapy

Historically, clinicians who practiced manual therapy believed that the basis for the procedures were mechanical and only influenced joints.[5,35] This is supported by the findings of one survey, where the majority of physical therapists advocated passive vertebral motion assessment in their clinical decision-making process.[2] Furthermore, physical therapy educators identify acquisition of manual joint assessment skills as a requirement for clinical competence.[81] Similar approaches and explanations persist in the manual therapy management of patients with shoulder conditions. For example, over 70% of 660 surveyed physical therapists indicated considering arthrokinematic motion at the shoulder as important in directing and validating manual therapy interventions.[42] Movement analysis, motion palpation, tissue resistance, and pain provocation have been proposed as hallmarks of manual therapy assessment.[43,55,89,92]

The hypothesis underpinning the manual evaluation of resistance of soft tissue and joint movement is in part based on mechanisms (nociceptive or other) that produce a local motor response, such as a sustained muscle contraction.[39,44] The sustained contraction is considered to reduce joint movement and soft tissue compliance. A sustained muscle contraction may also lead to a reduction in vascular supply, and this may further lead to chemical sensitization of the tissues, contributing to the pain experience. The associated sustained muscle spindle activity may negatively affect kinesthesia and proprioception.[8,65]

Research assessing the reliability and validity of motion palpation in the cervical, thoracic, and lumbar spine demonstrates poor validity (identifying the spinal level involved) and concomitant poor intertester and moderate intratester reliability. As such, there is support for arguments not to use these techniques in the assessment of spinal levels, passive joint movement, or tissue compliance.[34,88] The history of healthcare has been a continuous evolution of belief, experience, and especially in the past decades, an increase in research knowledge. All clinicians are obliged to be cognizant of new and emerging research to ensure their clinical practice is ethical, appropriate, and informed by evidence.[51]

Manual therapies may be defined as passive techniques applied to tissues,[1] and amongst other potential psychological and physiological responses, a mechanical effect accompanies manual therapy interventions. Research supports this hypothesis, as movement of the glenohumeral joint is observed with joint mobilization forces, both in vivo[84,91] as well as in cadaver studies.[38,59] Despite the associated mechanical force accompanying manual therapy interventions, an isolated mechanical explanation for improvement in symptoms is unlikely for multiple reasons: interrater reliability of manual assessment of the shoulder is generally poor,[24,46] common theories driving the mechanical explanation are proving questionable when subjected to research,[7] variability exists across clinicians in the application of the techniques,[27] and outcomes are similar across manual therapy techniques of different mechanical parameters.[17,28,48] Furthermore, manual therapy directed at the thoracic spine[70] and cervical spine[56] may both result in a decrease in shoulder pain with small to no changes in shoulder kinematics.[33,40,62] Subsequently, while a mechanical force accompanies manual therapy interventions, clinical outcomes are likely attributed to multiple factors. The mechanical force associated with manual therapy appears to result in neurophysiological responses[4,72] that may better represent the underlying mechanisms through which manual therapy is effective for some individuals presenting with shoulder problems. The neurophysiological responses to the mechanical force of a manual therapy intervention represent an interaction of the peripheral nervous system as well as the central nervous system at the level of the spinal cord and supraspinal structures.[4]

A systematic review summarizing current animal research regarding neurophysiological responses to manual therapy[52] reported:

1. Changes in nociceptive response and inflammatory profile, gene expression, neurotransmitter release, receptor activation, and enzymatic activity following joint mobilization.
2. Changes in muscle spindle response, nociceptive reflex response, neuronal activity, electromyography, and immunologic response following spinal manipulation.
3. Changes in autonomic, circulatory, lymphatic, and immunologic functions, visceral response, gene expression, neuroanatomy, function, and pathology, as well as cellular response following massage.[52]

Collectively, these findings support neurophysiological responses to the mechanical forces accompanying manual therapy interventions as indicated by direct observation of the nervous system as allowed by the animal models. Direct observation of the nervous system is typically not possible in human research participants requiring indirect assessment often through behavioral outcome measures. As such, extrapolating findings from animal studies to humans may not be appropriate and should be considered with caution. As an example, pharmacological research has shown that interventions effective in altering nociceptive responses in animals often perform poorly in treating pain in humans.[61] Furthermore, the clinical importance of these physiological responses to manual therapy is yet to be determined.[47]

Manual therapy has a hypoalgesic effect,[18,25,60] and increases in pressure pain threshold, suggesting a lessening of pain sensitivity, are associated with MWMs in individuals with anterior shoulder pain.[86] Additionally, increases in pressure pain threshold have been further observed at distal sites in response to anteroposterior mobilization of the glenohumeral joint suggesting a generalized rather than region-specific response.[23] Therefore, neurophysiological responses may be part of the reason for clinical responses observed after the application of manual therapies.

Peripherally mediated neurophysiological mechanisms of manual therapy

Proinflammatory mediators are a normal response to injury and suggest a nociceptive pain mechanism resulting in peripheral sensitization. Changes in the concentration of these proinflammatory mediators may reflect a peripheral neurophysiological response to manual therapy. Such responses have been observed following different manual therapy approaches. For example, a study considered such a response following exercise-induced muscle damage to the quadriceps in healthy men.[19] Eleven participants received a 10-minute massage to one leg with the other leg serving as the no-treatment control following an exercise protocol resulting in delayed onset of muscle soreness.[19] The authors observed a decrease in inflammatory biomarkers coupled with enhanced markers of cellular repair in the leg following massage and not observed in the control leg.[19] Additionally, a pilot study observed changes in circulatory biomarkers in 10 individuals with low back pain 24 hours following a treatment regimen including joint mobilization, muscle energy techniques, soft tissue mobilization, and strain-counterstrain.[20] Similar changes in circulatory biomarkers have been observed in women with neck pain immediately following cervical thrust manipulation,[53] and in subjects with low back pain receiving six sessions of spinal manipulation over two weeks.[85]

A systematic review concluded that spinal manipulative therapy may modulate substance P, neurotensin, oxytocin, and interleukin levels, and may influence cortisol levels post-intervention.[47] Collectively, this body of literature suggests changes in peripheral circulatory biomarkers in response to different types of manual therapy supporting a peripherally mediated neurophysiological mechanism.

Spinal cord-mediated neurophysiological mechanisms of manual therapy

Autonomic nervous system

Changes in skin temperature, skin conduction, and heart rate represent indirect measures of autonomic responses to manual therapy. A review and meta-analysis concluded spinal manipulation to the cervical or thoracic spine resulted in a sympathetic nervous system excitatory response as indicated by increased skin conductance and decreased skin temperature.[14] Furthermore, a systematic review of spinal mobilization concluded strong evidence existed for significant changes in skin conduction and heart rate in healthy participants following spinal mobilization, and limited evidence for changes in skin conduction and skin temperature in symptomatic participants.[41] The observed changes consistently supported an excitatory effect and occurred regardless of the manual therapy intervention, i.e., cervical, thoracic, or lumbar spine.[41]

Neuromuscular response

Manual therapy interventions result in detectable input to the central nervous system including afferent discharge from sensory neurons, including the muscle spindle and golgi tendon organ with the potential to influence clinical outcomes.[73] Direct observation of the nervous system in animal studies have reported responses to spinal manipulation-type forces which differ from non-manipulative-type forces,[74,75] and these are independent of the direction of the force.[77] One in vivo case study design investigated this in anesthetized humans (n=9) with lumbar radiculopathy undergoing surgery and observed positive compound action potential responses to spinal manipulation at the first sacral (S1) spinal nerve roots at the level of the dorsal root ganglia exceeding a sham manipulation.[15]

Changes in the Hoffman reflex (H-reflex) in response to manual therapy imply a mechanism related to spinal cord-mediated modulation of alpha motoneuron excitability. A study randomly assigned 66 adults without symptoms and 45 people with subacute low back pain to receive either positioning for a side-lying high velocity low amplitude lumbar thrust manipulation; joint preloading with no thrust for the same technique; or the side-lying high velocity low amplitude lumbar spine thrust manipulation.[22] An inhibitory effect was observed in both groups that was greatest in response to the side-lying high velocity, low amplitude lumbar thrust manipulation.[22]

Changes in muscle activation accompany manual therapy interventions. Specific to the shoulder, the findings are variable in strength and direction. A study of "manual muscle release" techniques combined with heat for people with frozen shoulder observed an immediate increase in the upper and lower trapezius muscle activation during functional tasks.[80] Additionally, a study of shoulder joint mobilization in healthy participants reported reduced muscle activity in the infraspinatus, deltoid, and serratus anterior during the eccentric phase of shoulder abduction.[69] Specific to thoracic spine thrust manipulation, small but significant increases in middle trapezius activity were observed in one trial of people with rotator cuff tendinopathy[62] while another study observed decreased activity of the middle trapezius, lower trapezius, and serratus anterior not differing from a sham manipulation in participants with shoulder impingement.[32] Furthermore, increased scapulothoracic muscle power was noted in 22 people with neck pain immediately following cervical spine manipulation and neck range of motion exercises.[71] Collectively, these findings suggest that spinal cord-mediated neuromuscular responses to manual therapy occur.

Supraspinal-mediated neurophysiological mechanisms of manual therapy

Manual therapy interventions are associated with neurophysiological responses at the supraspinal level.[30,31,66] For example, cortical responses in the medial parts of the postcentral gyrus (S1) bilaterally, the secondary somatosensory cortex (S2), posterior parts of the insular cortex, different parts of the cingulate cortex, and the cerebellum are observed during posterior to anterior glides to the lumbar spine.[58] Manual therapy is associated with a lessening of pain sensitivity and this response in individuals without symptoms following a thrust manipulation to the thoracic spine is associated with decreased activity in the sensorimotor cortices S1, S2, anterior cingulate cortex, cerebellum, and insular cortices.[82]

Thrust and non-thrust manual therapy interventions are associated with decreased coupling of cortical activity between sensory discriminant and affective regions (primary somatosensory cortex and posterior insular cortex), with increased coupling between affective regions (posterior cingulate and anterior insular cortices) and affective and descending pain modulatory regions (insular cortex and periaqueductal gray).[26] Collectively, these studies support supraspinal-mediated responses to manual therapy including changes in the resting state interactions of the cortical nociceptive processing networks.

In conclusion, it is more likely that the underlying mechanisms of hands-on therapy are neurophysiological rather than biomechanical. All these mechanisms should be integrated into a model integrating the patient–therapist interaction as presented in Figure 31.1.

Efficacy and effectiveness of hands-on therapy for the shoulder

Systematic reviews and meta-analyses investigating the effectiveness of hands-on interventions for the management of shoulder pain have been published; however, there are differences in the hands-on interventions investigated and the conclusions reached. For example, a meta-analysis was not possible in a Cochrane systematic review because of the heterogeneity or incomplete outcome reporting in the clinical trials included.[67] Desjardins-Charbonneau et al. found low to moderate quality evidence supporting a positive effect of manual therapy for decreasing pain in individuals with rotator cuff tendinopathy, but they were not able to determine the effects of manual therapy on function.[21]

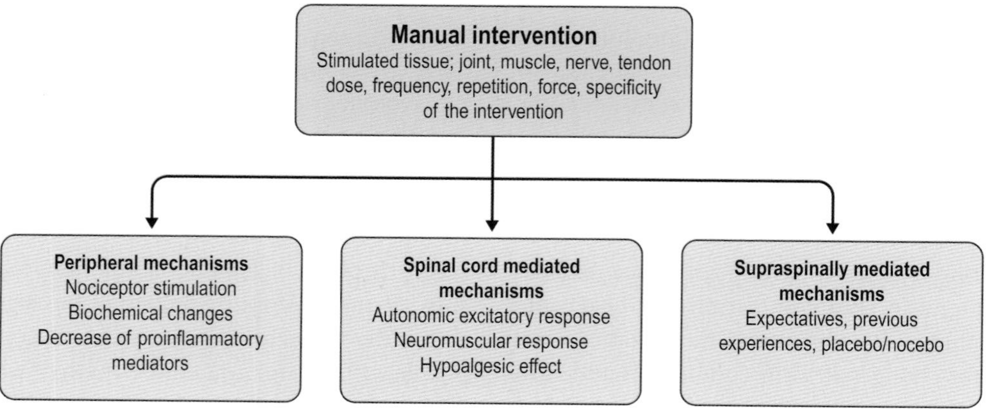

FIGURE 31.1
Integrative model explaining peripheral, spinal cord and supraspinally mediated mechanisms of manual therapy interventions.

A meta-analysis reported that manual therapy was superior to placebo (standardized mean difference (SMD) -0.35; 95% confidence interval (CI) -0.69 to -0.01) for improving pain in shoulder conditions, and when combined with exercise, manual therapy was superior to exercise alone, but only at the short-term follow-up (SMD -0.32; 95% CI -0.62 to -0.01).[83] These findings have been recently confirmed by the updated review of systematic reviews by Pieters et al. who have made strong recommendation for the inclusion of manual therapy as an additional therapy to exercise in the early stages of management for improving pain and related function in patients with shoulder pain.[76] It is important to acknowledge that the term "strong recommendation" was determined a priori and did not relate to the effect size of the intervention.

Bizzarri et al. reported from evidence deemed to be low quality, an immediate and beneficial effect of a single session of thoracic manual therapy when compared with placebo in people with shoulder dysfunction.[6] Similarly, the effects of scapular-based treatment approaches, although statistically significant, were not clinically relevant when compared with more generalized treatment regimens for reducing pain and related disability in people with shoulder problems.[10] Systematic reviews specifically assessing the efficacy of MWMs in shoulder conditions reported varying amounts of short-term benefit on shoulder range of motion, pain and function.[57]

Massage is another form of hands-on therapy. Meta-analyses investigating the effectiveness of massage for people with shoulder pain reported positive effects for reducing shoulder pain at short (SMD -1.08; 95% CI -1.51 to -0.65) and long (SMD -0.47; 95% CI -0.71 to -0.23) terms when compared with an inactive therapy,[93] but no better than active therapies (SMD 0.88; 95% CI -0.74 to 2.51).[45] However, the level of evidence was low.[87]

Risk of adverse events of hands-on therapy for the shoulder

Intervention choice should always be made by balancing both effectiveness and possible harm, and needs to be based on analysis of the research evidence, shared decision-making and gaining appropriate consent prior to commencing the intervention.[49] Adverse events (AEs) in manual therapy are typically rare, and usually relate to interventions directed to the spinal regions.[13] Defining AEs in manual therapy is difficult due to the complex nature of musculoskeletal pain and dysfunction.[11,13] However, it is practical to consider AEs in their simplest form as "any untoward medical occurrence that may present during treatment...but which does not necessarily have a causal relationship with this treatment".[12] Clinicians must be aware, however, of the multifactorial nature of AEs in manual therapy, especially considering the patient's understanding of what they are.[11]

The challenge is that there are no specific data available to provide a statistical commentary on the risk of manual therapy for *people with shoulder pain* with regards to AEs. This could be due to either the fact that there are no AEs to report, or poor reporting of AEs in manual therapy trials. A recent review focusing on AE reporting highlighted that only one clinical trial out of 16 studies reported AEs (in the case, there was just a single AE related to an "increase in back spasticity after treatments", which was attributed to spinal manual therapy). A recent Cochrane report on shoulder trials also did not report on AEs.[68] A survey of 1082 osteopathy clinicians and 1387 patients did not identify any adverse events related to manual therapy of the shoulder.[90] AEs that were recorded typically were associated with spinal manual therapy, and typically were largely an immediate and transient increase in pain or discomfort around the treated area.[90] Further, the known number of people not continuing treatment due to AEs in manual therapy is no different to AE-related discontinuation associated with comparator interventions (e.g., exercise, gabapentin).[78]

Risk associated with all proposed treatment options should also be considered in the shared decision-making and consent process.[16,49] For example, the absolute risk of having an AE when taking nonsteroidal anti-inflammatory drugs (NSAIDs) is up to 8%.[3,54,94] In comparison, the highest estimate of serious AEs associated with manual therapy is 1:20,000,[63] which equates to a fraction over 0% (0.00005%) for absolute risk – far lower than comparator interventions. Again, caution should be taken with these estimates as most of the data relate to spinal manual therapy. The risk is likely to be lower for shoulder therapy, and the response to the risk likely to be mild and acceptable.

From a practical perspective, the most rational way to mitigate against adverse events is to ensure proper safe, comfortable execution of therapeutic interventions to the right person, at the right time. Prior to choosing the intervention, competent reasoning should be displayed to ensure the nature of the person's pain and disability is of a musculoskeletal nature. This would involve ensuring the exclusion of non-musculoskeletal and pathological presentations. In summary, manual therapy with people who have shoulder pain and disability appears to have a very low risk of adverse events.

Integration of hands-on manual therapy into multimodal management

There is no clinical or scientific evidence supporting the sole use of manual therapy in the management of shoulder conditions. As part of the shared decision-making process where anticipated benefits, possible harms, treatment commitment (e.g., number and duration of treatments, requirements of travel for treatment) and timeframes are discussed, manual hands-on therapy may be considered as part of the multimodal management for people with shoulder complaints, with the patient's consent. Similar to other interventions for shoulder conditions, the effect size, or the anticipated benefit of hands-on therapy when compared with a control or usual treatment group, is small. For some people living with shoulder pain the expected benefit of hands-on therapy would not impact on their disability, for others, any change, even if short-lived may have meaning to them. Those patients who report previous benefit from manual therapy and are eager to receive it again should be counselled that the provision of manual therapy may be considered for a short period of time, early in management, but needs to be embedded within an exercise-based program.

Clinicians should no longer use outdated biomechanical explanations to explain the purpose of manual therapy in assessment or management. More research – qualitative, quantitative, and economic – is required to determine the contribution of manual therapy in the management of people with musculoskeletal shoulder conditions, across the different conditions it is commonly used for. Table 31.1 provides examples of manual therapy in the management of shoulder conditions, including techniques, duration of treatment, outcomes, and clinical relevance.

Table 31.1 Examples of manual therapy in the management of shoulder conditions, including techniques, duration of treatment, outcomes, and clinical relevance.

Shoulder condition	Study type	Number of research participants	Techniques investigated	Duration and number of treatments	Outcomes	Clinical relevance	Author, year, country
Frozen shoulder stage II	Systematic review & meta-analysis	655	MWM	Short to mid-term (3 months)	Significant improvement in ROM, pain, and disability	Improvement in ROM greater than the MCID for flexion and abduction ROM. Predominantly treated with AP glide	Satpute et al. 2021[79] India
Frozen shoulder	Systematic review	362	Maitland mobilization	Short to long term (2 years)	Meta-analysis was not undertaken. All but 1 study showed significant improvement in pain and ROM	High grade Maitland mobilization (grade III and IV) were more effective than low grade (II)	Noten et al. 2016[64] Belgium
Frozen shoulder	RCT	40	Cyriax deep friction massage and manipulation compared with usual care	Short term; 6 1-hour sessions of deep friction massage and manipulation	Recovery rate to achieve 80% of normal ROM significantly better compared with control at 2 weeks	The Cyriax method of rehabilitation provides a faster and better response than the conventional physical therapy methods in the early phase of treatment in adhesive capsulitis	Guler-Uysal & Kozanoglu 2004[29] Turkey
Frozen shoulder following glenohumeral joint distension	RCT	156	Manual therapy and exercise compared with placebo ultrasound	Short to mid-term (6 months); 8 visits over 6 weeks comprising muscle stretching, spine mobilization, glenohumeral mobilization, strength, coordination and proprioceptive exercise	No difference in pain, function or QoL, but significant improvement in ROM and patient-perceived success in experimental group	Interventions result in sustained greater active range of shoulder movement and participant-perceived improvement up to 6 months	Buchbinder et al. 2007[9] Australia
Shoulder pain with movement dysfunction	Systematic review & meta-analysis	329	Capsular mobilization or manipulation	Short term	Significant improvement in pain	Mean difference in pain compared with a sham or other intervention favored MT but may not be clinically relevant	Desjardins-Charbonneau et al. 2015[21] Canada
Shoulder pain with movement dysfunction	Systematic review & meta-analysis	349	MWM	Short term	Significant improvement in ROM, pain, and disability	Improvement in ROM greater than the MCID for flexion and abduction ROM. Predominantly treated with AP glide MWM for elevation and caudal glide MWM for hand-behind-back	Satpute et al. 2021[79] India

(Continued)

Table 31.1 *(Continued)*

Shoulder condition	Study type	Number of research participants	Techniques investigated	Duration and number of treatments	Outcomes	Clinical relevance	Author, year, country
Shoulder pain with movement dysfunction	Systematic review & meta-analysis	635	Soft tissue massage	Short to mid-term (14 weeks)	Significant improvement in pain	Wide variety of traditional and Western massage. Localized trigger point, shoulder region, or whole-body massage	Yeun et al. 2017[93] Korea
Shoulder pain with movement dysfunction	Systematic review & meta-analysis	247	Thoracic manipulation	Immediate effects	Significant improvement in pain	Seated and prone thoracic spine manipulation as well as scapula manipulation	Bizzarri et al. 2018[6] Italy
Rotator cuff-related shoulder pain	Systematic review & meta-analysis	406	Manual therapy	Short term	Significant improvement in pain that may be clinically relevant	A wide variety of MT techniques including MWM, mobilization, manipulation, and cervical spine mobilization used in 10 different studies	Desjardins-Charbonneau et al. 2015[21] Canada
Rotator cuff- related shoulder pain	Systematic review & meta-analysis	190	Scapula-focused intervention (including exercise therapy, stretches and/or manual therapy) compared with usual care	Short term	Significant improvement in pain but not disability	Interventions were focused on changing biomechanics of the scapula including position, movement, strength, motor control, and/or muscle length	Bury et al. 2016[10] UK

AP, anterior-posterior; MCID, minimal clinically important difference; MT, manual therapy; MWM, mobilization with movement; QoL, quality of life; ROM, range of movement.

References

1. APTA. Guide to Physical Therapist Practice. Available at: http://guidetoptpractice.apta.org/.

2. Abbott JH, Flynn TW, Fritz JM, Hing WA, Reid D, Whitman JM. Manual physical assessment of spinal segmental motion: intent and validity. Manual Therapy. 2009;14:36-44.

3. Bally M, Beauchamp ME, Abrahamowicz M, Nadeau L, Brophy JM. Risk of acute myocardial infarction with real-world NSAIDs depends on dose and timing of exposure. Pharmacoepidemiol Drug Saf. 2018;27:69-77.

4. Bialosky JE, Beneciuk JM, Bishop MD, et al. Unraveling the mechanisms of manual therapy: modeling an approach. The Journal of Orthopaedic and Sports Physical Therapy. 2018;48:8-18.

5. Bialosky JE, Simon CB, Bishop MD, George SZ. Basis for spinal manipulative therapy: a physical therapist perspective. Journal of Electromyography and Kinesiology. 2012;22:643-647.

6. Bizzarri P, Buzzatti L, Cattrysse E, Scafoglieri A. Thoracic manual therapy is not more effective than placebo thoracic manual therapy in patients with shoulder dysfunctions: a systematic review with meta-analysis. Musculoskeletal Science & Practice. 2018;33:1-10.

7. Brandt C, Sole G, Krause MW, Nel M. An evidence-based review on the validity of the Kaltenborn rule as applied to the glenohumeral joint. Manual Therapy. 2007;12:3-11.

8. Brumagne S, Cordo P, Lysens R, Verschueren S, Swinnen S. The role of paraspinal muscle spindles in lumbosacral position sense in individuals with and without low back pain. Spine. 2000;25:989-994.

9. Buchbinder R, Youd JM, Green S, et al. Efficacy and cost-effectiveness of physiotherapy following glenohumeral joint distension for adhesive capsulitis: a randomized trial. Arthritis Rheum. 2007;57:1027-1037.

10. Bury J, West M, Chamorro-Moriana G, Littlewood C. Effectiveness of scapula-focused approaches in patients with rotator cuff related shoulder pain: a systematic review and meta-analysis. Manual Therapy. 2016;25:35-42.

11. Carlesso LC, Cairney J, Dolovich L, Hoogenes J. Defining adverse events in manual therapy: an exploratory qualitative analysis of the patient perspective. Manual Therapy. 2011;16:440-446.

12. Carlesso LC, MacDermid JC, Santaguida LP. Standardization of adverse event terminology and reporting in orthopaedic physical therapy: application to the cervical spine. Journal of Orthopaedic & Sports Physical Therapy. 2010;40:455-463.

13. Carnes D, Mullinger B, Underwood M. Defining adverse events in manual therapies: a modified Delphi consensus study. Manual Therapy. 2010;15:2-6.

14. Chu J, Allen DD, Pawlowsky S, Smoot B. Peripheral response to cervical or thoracic spinal manual therapy: an evidence-based review with meta analysis. The Journal of Manual & Manipulative Therapy. 2014;22:220-229.

15. Colloca CJ, Keller TS, Gunzburg R. Biomechanical and neurophysiological responses to spinal manipulation in patients with lumbar radiculopathy. Journal of Manipulative and Physiological Therapeutics. 2004;27:1-15.

16. Copnell G. Informed consent in physiotherapy practice: it is not what is said but how it is said. Physiotherapy. 2018;104:67-71.

17. Coronado RA, Bialosky JE, Bishop MD, et al. The comparative effects of spinal and peripheral thrust manipulation and exercise on pain sensitivity and the relation to clinical outcome: a mechanistic trial using a shoulder pain model. The Journal of Orthopaedic and Sports Physical Therapy. 2015;45:252-264.

18. Coronado RA, Gay CW, Bialosky JE, Carnaby GD, Bishop MD, George SZ. Changes in pain sensitivity following spinal manipulation: a systematic review and meta-analysis. J Electromyogr.Kinesiol. 2012;22(5):752-67.

19. Crane JD, Ogborn DI, Cupido C, et al. Massage therapy attenuates inflammatory signaling after exercise-induced muscle damage. Sci Transl Med. 2012;4:119ra113.

20. Degenhardt BF, Darmani NA, Johnson JC, et al. Role of osteopathic manipulative treatment in altering pain biomarkers: a pilot study. J Am Osteopath Assoc. 2007;107:387-400.

21. Desjardins-Charbonneau A, Roy JS, Dionne CE, Fremont P, MacDermid JC, Desmeules F. The efficacy of manual therapy for rotator cuff tendinopathy: a systematic review and meta-analysis. The Journal of Orthopaedic and Sports Physical Therapy. 2015;45:330-350.

22. Dishman JD, Burke JR, Dougherty P. Motor neuron excitability attenuation as a sequel to lumbosacral manipulation in subacute low back pain patients and asymptomatic adults: a cross-sectional H-reflex study. Journal of Manipulative and Physiological Therapeutics. 2018;41:363-371.

23. Lluch E, Pecos-Martín D, Domenech-García V, Herrero P, Gallego-Izquierdo T. Effects of an anteroposterior mobilization of the glenohumeral joint in overhead athletes with chronic shoulder pain: a randomized controlled trial. Musculoskeletal Science & Practice. 2018;38:91-98.

24. Ellenbecker TS, Bailie DS, Mattalino AJ, et al. Intrarater and interrater reliability of a manual technique to assess anterior humeral head translation of the glenohumeral joint. J Shoulder Elbow Surg. 2002;11:470-475.

25. Gay CW, Alappattu MJ, Coronado RA, Horn ME, Bishop MD. Effect of a single session of muscle-biased therapy on pain sensitivity: a systematic review and meta-analysis of randomized controlled trials. Journal of Pain Research. 2013;6:7-22.

26. Gay CW, Robinson ME, George SZ, Perlstein WM, Bishop MD. Immediate changes after manual therapy in resting-state functional connectivity as measured by functional magnetic resonance imaging in participants with induced low back pain. Journal of Manipulative and Physiological Therapeutics. 2014;37:614-627.

27. Gorgos KS, Wasylyk NT, Van Lunen BL, Hoch MC. Inter-clinician and intra-clinician reliability of force application during joint mobilization: a systematic review. Manual Therapy. 2014;19:90-96.

28. Grimes JK, Puentedura EJ, Cheng MS, Seitz AL. The comparative effects of upper thoracic spine thrust manipulation techniques in individuals with subacromial pain syndrome: a randomized clinical trial. The Journal of Orthopaedic and Sports Physical Therapy. 2019;49:716-724.

29. Guler-Uysal F, Kozanoglu E. Comparison of the early response to two methods of rehabilitation in adhesive capsulitis. Swiss Med Wkly. 2004;134:353-358.

30. Haavik-Taylor H, Murphy B. Cervical spine manipulation alters sensorimotor integration: a somatosensory evoked potential study. Clin Neurophysiol. 2007;118:391-402.

31. Haavik Taylor H, Murphy B. The effects of spinal manipulation on central integration of dual somatosensory input observed after motor training: a crossover study. Journal of Manipulative and Physiological Therapeutics. 2010;33:261-272.

32. Haik MN, Alburquerque-Sendín F, Camargo PR. Short-term effects of thoracic spine manipulation on shoulder impingement syndrome: a randomized controlled trial. Archives of Physical Medicine and Rehabilitation. 2017;98:1594-1605.

33. Haik MN, Alburquerque-Sendín F, Silva CZ, Siqueira-Junior AL, Ribeiro IL, Camargo PR. Scapular kinematics pre- and post-thoracic thrust manipulation in individuals with and without shoulder impingement symptoms: a randomized controlled study. The Journal of Orthopaedic and Sports Physical Therapy. 2014;44:475-487.

34. Haneline MT, Young M. A review of intraexaminer and interexaminer reliability of static spinal palpation: a literature synthesis. Journal of Manipulative and Physiological Therapeutics. 2009;32:379-386.

35. Henderson CN. The basis for spinal manipulation: chiropractic perspective of indications and theory. Journal of Electromyography and Kinesiology. 2012;22:632-642.

36. Hengeveld HBK. Maitland's Peripheral Manipulation, 4th edition. London: Butterworth-Heinemann; 2010.

37. Hing W, Hall T, Mulligan B. The Mulligan Concept of Manual Therapy: Textbook of Techniques, 2nd edition. Elsevier; 2019.

38. Hsu AT, Chiu JF, Chang JH. Biomechanical analysis of axial distraction mobilization of the glenohumeral joint: a cadaver study. Manual Therapy. 2009;14:381-386.

39. Johansson H, Sojka P. Pathophysiological mechanisms involved in genesis and spread of muscular tension in occupational muscle pain and in chronic musculoskeletal pain syndromes: a hypothesis. Med Hypotheses. 1991;35:196-203.

40. Kardouni JR, Pidcoe PE, Shaffer SW, et al. Thoracic spine manipulation in individuals with subacromial impingement syndrome does not immediately alter thoracic spine kinematics, thoracic excursion, or scapular kinematics: a randomized controlled trial. The Journal of Orthopaedic and Sports Physical Therapy. 2015;45:527-538.

41. Kingston L, Claydon L, Tumilty S. The effects of spinal mobilizations on the sympathetic nervous system: a systematic review. Manual Therapy. 2014;19:281-287.

42. Kirby K, Showalter C, Cook C. Assessment of the importance of glenohumeral peripheral mechanics by practicing physiotherapists. Physiother Res Int. 2007;12:136-146.

43. Knutson GA. The role of the gamma-motor system in increasing muscle tone and muscle pain syndromes: a review of the Johansson/Sojka hypothesis. Journal of Manipulative and Physiological Therapeutics. 2000;23:564-572.

44. Knutson GA, Owens EF, Jr. Active and passive characteristics of muscle tone and their relationship to models of subluxation/joint dysfunction: Part I. J Can Chiropr Assoc. 2003;47:168-179.

45. Kong LJ, Zhan HS, Cheng YW, Yuan WA, Chen B, Fang M. Massage therapy for neck and shoulder pain: a systematic review and meta-analysis. Evid Based Complement Alternat Med. 2013;2013:613279.

46. Konieczka C, Gibson C, Russett L, et al. What is the reliability of clinical measurement tests for humeral head position? A systematic review. J Hand Ther. 2017;30:420-431.

47. Kovanur-Sampath K, Mani R, Cotter J, Gisselman AS, Tumilty S. Changes in biochemical markers following spinal manipulation: a systematic review and meta-analysis. Musculoskeletal Science & Practice. 2017;29:120-131.

48. Land H, Gordon S, Watt K. Effect of manual physiotherapy in homogeneous individuals with subacromial shoulder impingement: a randomized controlled trial. Physiother Res Int. 2019;24:e1768.

49. Lee A. 'Bolam' to 'Montgomery' is result of evolutionary change of medical practice towards 'patient-centred care'. Postgraduate Medical Journal. 2017;93:46-50.

50. Lewis J. Rotator cuff related shoulder pain: assessment, management and uncertainties. Man Ther. 2016;23:57-68.

51. Lewis J, O'Sullivan P. Is it time to reframe how we care for people with non-traumatic musculoskeletal pain? British Journal of Sports Medicine. 2018;52:1543-1544.

52. Lima CR, Martins DF, Reed WR. Physiological responses induced by manual therapy in animal models: a scoping review. Front Neurosci. 2020;14:430.

53. Lohman EB, Pacheco GR, Gharibvand L, et al. The immediate effects of cervical spine manipulation on pain and biochemical markers in females with acute non-specific mechanical neck pain: a randomized clinical trial. The Journal of Manual & Manipulative Therapy. 2019;27:186-196.

54. Masclee GM, Valkhoff VE, Coloma PM, et al. Risk of upper gastrointestinal bleeding from different drug combinations. Gastroenterology. 2014;147:784-792.e789; quiz e713-784.

55. McCarthy CJ. Spinal manipulative thrust technique using combined movement theory. Manual Therapy. 2001;6:197-204.

56. McClatchie L, Laprade J, Martin S, Jaglal SB, Richardson D, Agur A. Mobilizations of the asymptomatic cervical spine can reduce signs of shoulder dysfunction in adults. Man Ther. 2009;14:369-374.

57. Meena V, Varghese JG. Effectiveness of Mulligans mobilisation with movement on shoulder dysfunction: a systematic review. Journal of Clinical & Diagnostic Research. 2020;14:YE01-YE05.

58. Meier ML, Hotz-Boendermaker S, Boendermaker B, Luechinger R, Humphreys BK. Neural responses of posterior to anterior movement on lumbar vertebrae: a functional magnetic resonance imaging study. Journal of Manipulative and Physiological Therapeutics. 2014;37:32-41.

59. Melloni C, Alexander KP, Ou FS, et al. Predictors of early discontinuation of evidence-based medicine after acute coronary syndrome. Am J Cardiol. 2009;104:175-181.

60. Millan M, Leboeuf-Yde C, Budgell B, Amorim MA. The effect of spinal manipulative therapy on experimentally induced pain: a systematic literature review. Chiropr Man Therap. 2012;20:26.

61. Mogil JS. Animal models of pain: progress and challenges. Nat Rev Neurosci. 2009;10:283-294.

62. Muth S, Barbe MF, Lauer R, McClure PW. The effects of thoracic spine manipulation in subjects with signs of rotator cuff tendinopathy. J Orthop Sports Phys Ther. 2012;42:1005-1016.

63. Nielsen SM, Tarp S, Christensen R, Bliddal H, Klokker L, Henriksen M. The risk associated with spinal manipulation: an overview of reviews. Systematic Reviews. 2017;6:64.

64. Noten S, Meeus M, Stassijns G, Van Glabbeek F, Verborgt O, Struyf F. Efficacy of different types of mobilization techniques in patients with primary adhesive capsulitis of the shoulder: a systematic review. Archives of Physical Medicine and Rehabilitation. 2016;97:815-825.

65. O'Sullivan PB, Burnett A, Floyd AN, et al. Lumbar repositioning deficit in a specific low back pain population. Spine. 2003;28:1074-1079.

66. Ogura T, Tashiro M, Masud M, et al. Cerebral metabolic changes in men after chiropractic spinal manipulation for neck pain. Altern Ther Health Med. 2011;17:12-17.

67. Page MJ, Green S, McBain B, et al. Manual therapy and exercise for rotator cuff disease. Cochrane Database Syst Rev. 2016;CD012224.

68. Page MJ, Huang H, Verhagen AP, Gagnier JJ, Buchbinder R. Outcome reporting in randomized trials for shoulder disorders: literature review to inform the development of a core outcome set. Arthritis Care & Research. 2018;70:252-259.

69. Patterson A, Dickerson CR, Ribeiro DC. The effect of shoulder mobilization on scapular and shoulder muscle activity during resisted shoulder abduction: a crossover study of asymptomatic individuals. Journal of Manipulative and Physiological Therapeutics. 2020;43:832-844.

70. Peek AL, Miller C, Heneghan NR. Thoracic manual therapy in the management of non-specific shoulder pain: a systematic review. The Journal of Manual & Manipulative Therapy. 2015;23:176-187.

71. Petersen S, Domino N, Postma C, Wells C, Cook C. Scapulothoracic muscle strength changes following a single session of manual therapy and an exercise programme in subjects with neck pain. Musculoskeletal Care. 2016;14:195-205.

72. Pickar JG. Neurophysiological effects of spinal manipulation. Spine J. 2002;2:357-371.

73. Pickar JG, Bolton PS. Spinal manipulative therapy and somatosensory activation. Journal of Electromyography and Kinesiology. 2012;22:785-794.

74. Pickar JG, Sung PS, Kang YM, Ge W. Response of lumbar paraspinal muscles spindles is greater to spinal manipulative loading compared with slower loading under length control. Spine J. 2007;7:583-595.

75. Pickar JG, Wheeler JD. Response of muscle proprioceptors to spinal manipulative-like loads in the anesthetized cat. Journal of Manipulative and Physiological Therapeutics. 2001;24:2-11.

76. Pieters L, Lewis J, Kuppens K, et al. An update of systematic reviews examining the effectiveness of conservative physical therapy interventions for subacromial shoulder pain. The Journal of Orthopaedic and Sports Physical Therapy. 2020;50:131-141.

77. Reed WR, Long CR, Kawchuk GN, Sozio RS, Pickar JG. Neural responses to physical characteristics of a high-velocity, low-amplitude spinal manipulation: effect of thrust direction. Spine. 2018;43:1-9.

78. Rehman Y, Ferguson H, Bozek A, Blair J, Allison A, Johnston R. Dropout associated with osteopathic manual treatment for chronic noncancerous pain in randomized controlled trials. J Osteopath Med. 2021;121:417-428.

79. Satpute KH, Reid SA, Mitchell T, Mackay G, Hall T. Efficacy of mobilisation with movement (MWM) for shoulder conditions: a systematic review and meta-analysis. Journal of Manual and Manipulative Therapy. 2021;1-20. Online ahead of print. doi: 10.1080/10669817.2021.1955181.

80. Shih YF, Liao PW, Lee CS. The immediate effect of muscle release intervention on muscle activity and shoulder kinematics in patients with frozen shoulder: a cross-sectional, exploratory study. BMC Musculoskeletal Disorders. 2017;18:499.

81. Sizer PS, Jr., Felstehausen V, Sawyer S, Dornier L, Matthews P, Cook C. Eight critical skill sets required for manual therapy competency: a Delphi study and factor analysis of physical therapy educators of manual therapy. J Allied Health. 2007;36:30-40.

82. Sparks C, Cleland JA, Elliott JM, Zagardo M, Liu WC. Using functional magnetic resonance imaging to determine if cerebral hemodynamic responses to pain change following thoracic spine thrust manipulation in healthy individuals. The Journal of Orthopaedic and Sports Physical Therapy. 2013;43:340-348.

83. Steuri R, Sattelmayer M, Elsig S, et al. Effectiveness of conservative interventions including exercise, manual therapy and medical management in adults with shoulder impingement: a systematic review and meta-analysis of RCTs. Br J Sports Med. 2017;51:1340-1347.

84. Talbott, Nr, Witt DW. In vivo measurements of humeral movement during posterior glenohumeral mobilizations. The Journal of Manual & Manipulative Therapy. 2016;24:269-276.

85. Teodorczyk-Injeyan JA, McGregor M, Triano JJ, Injeyan SH. Elevated production of nociceptive CC chemokines and sE-Selectin in patients with low back pain and the effects of spinal manipulation: a nonrandomized clinical trial. The Clinical Journal of Pain. 2018;34:68-75.

86. Teys P, Bisset L, Vicenzino B. The initial effects of a Mulligan's mobilization with movement technique on range of movement and pressure pain threshold in pain-limited shoulders. Man Ther. 2008;13:37-42.

87. van den Dolder PA, Ferreira PH, Refshauge KM. Effectiveness of soft tissue massage and exercise for the treatment of non-specific shoulder pain: a systematic review with meta-analysis. British Journal of Sports Medicine. 2014;48:1216-1226.

88. van Trijffel E, Anderegg Q, Bossuyt PM, Lucas C. Inter-examiner reliability of passive assessment of intervertebral motion in the cervical and lumbar spine: a systematic review. Manual Therapy. 2005;10:256-269.

89. Vickers A, Zollman C. ABC of complementary medicine. Massage therapies. BMJ (Clinical research ed.). 1999;319:1254-1257.

90. Vogel S, Mars T, Keeping S, et al. Clinical Risk Osteopathy and Management Scientific Report. 2013.

91. Witt DW, Talbott NR. In-vivo measurements of force and humeral movement during inferior glenohumeral mobilizations. Man Ther. 2016;21:198-203.

92. Wytrazek M, Huber J, Lisinski P. Changes in muscle activity determine progression of clinical symptoms in patients with chronic spine-related muscle pain. A complex clinical and neurophysiological approach. Funct Neurol. 2011;26:141-149.

93. Yeun YR. Effectiveness of massage therapy for shoulder pain: a systematic review and meta-analysis. J Phys Ther Sci. 2017;29:936-940.

94. Zheng SL, Roddick AJ. Association of aspirin use for primary prevention with cardiovascular events and bleeding events: a systematic review and meta-analysis. JAMA. 2019;321:277-287.

Needling in the management of musculoskeletal shoulder conditions 32

Mike Cummings, Panos Barlas, César Fernández-de-las-Peñas

Introduction

Therapeutic needling techniques may date back more than 5000 years. Ötzi, the Tyrolean iceman, is the most well-persevered human mummified body ever found in Europe.[1,2] He was discovered to have 61 tattoos that may have been applied for acupuncture-like therapeutic purposes, possibly pain relief, three millennia before the first recorded use in China. They were produced by superficially piercing the skin with a needle made from bone followed by the application of charcoal. Several locations of these tattoos were in areas where Ötzi may have suffered pain from degenerative joint disease.

Such high-threshold stimulation techniques have developed independently in different human communities across the globe. For instance, children learn from adults to massage directly over an area where they are experiencing pain to reduce the noxious sensation. In the case of more persistent discomfort, many cultures use local and regional massage applied deeply and vigorously even though doing so may temporarily exacerbate the discomfort. This is likely to be conditioned behavior resulting from the analgesic effect of somatic sensory stimulation.

With the development of stone tools, it is easy to hypothesize a progression of therapeutic techniques that resulted ultimately in piercing the skin, fascia, and muscle at a site of persistent pain. It may be that pressing and piercing the body at the location of symptoms became recognized and accepted as a method of treating pain considered to be associated with myofascial tissues. Over time, these locations were given names such as acupressure points, acupuncture points, myofascial trigger points, tender points, and muscle knots. In some parts of the world, people developed superficial techniques of scratching or cauterizing the skin, whereas in the Far and Middle East the technique of acupuncture developed.[3]

Traditional Chinese Acupuncture (TCA)

Acupuncture techniques became part of the medical system in China around 2000 years ago when they were quite rapidly adopted and documented, together with the techniques and remedies that had been handed down within families and communities for many generations.[4,5]

It is uncertain where acupuncture using metal needles first developed, but it seems not to have developed in China before 168 BCE, according to the silk scrolls found in the Han Tomb No. 3 at Mawangdui, Changsha in the early 1970s.[6] The Mawangdui scrolls describe meridians and the use of moxibustion, but do not mention acupuncture points or needling. However, within 200 years, a comprehensive system of needle therapy had been documented and interwoven into the culture and philosophy of ancient China.[5]

The *bian shi* or sharpened stones claimed by some to represent the earliest forms of acupuncture needles may have been used therapeutically to prick the body,[7] but it seems unlikely that the sophisticated acupuncture system developed in the Han dynasty grew out of these primitive roots.[7A] A system of lines running from the chest to the hand, the hand to the face, the face to the foot and the foot back to the chest were developed. It has been argued that these meridians, or channels, were based on early anatomical studies of blood vessels.[8,9] Some 2000 years later, in the early 20th century, an influential Chinese physician, Cheng Dan'an, rejected the point positions based on blood vessels in favor of nerves.[10] Whether the lines were based on blood vessels, nerves, or another system, the locations (points) where needles were inserted occurred along these meridians.

Dry needling

Dry needling (DN) was developed as a therapeutic technique that focused on the importance of the needle effect rather than that of an injected substance. Karel Lewit was the first to recognize and write about the needle effect in myofascial pain.[11] Prior to this, the accepted treatments for myofascial pain consisted of manual therapy (therapeutic touch) or injection.[12–14] With the advent of systematic reviews of evidence, it became clear that injected substances did not seem to affect the outcome of treatment, and the use of a needle may have been the key component of either dry needling or injection.[15] While dry needling initially utilized hypodermic needles,[16] the much less traumatic filiform acupuncture needles are now used. The main targets for dry needling are myofascial trigger points (MTrPs), however, more contemporary practice has seen a potential overlap between dry needling and some acupuncture techniques, although several differences are also observed.

Western medical acupuncture

The term Western medical acupuncture (WMA) was first introduced over 20 years ago to differentiate a developing system of needle therapy with a basis in Western medical science from its traditional philosophical roots that happened to be in the East.[17] WMA is defined as: "a therapeutic modality involving the insertion of fine needles; it is an adaptation of Chinese acupuncture using current knowledge of anatomy, physiology and pathology, and the principles of evidence based medicine."[18] WMA principally focuses on trigger point needling or dry needling of local tissues, together with segmental or regional acupuncture,[19] but also takes into account the central and systemic effects of acupuncture needling.[20,21]

Theoretical overlaps between these approaches

Dry needling is a practice that appears to have developed independently from the popularity and acceptance of TCA in the West. WMA developed out of a scientific evaluation of TCA, and then adopted MTrPs as a target for needling.[22–25] The use of filiform needles in WMA may have hastened their adoption for use in DN instead of hypodermic needles.

As for the points, while there is some overlap between MTrPs and acupuncture points (APs),[26] and a strong similarity between meridian paths and pain referral patterns from MTrPs,[27] it is difficult to equate TCA with DN. Indeed, DN techniques distinct from TCA have been adopted in China, particularly in Shanghai,[28] and some intriguing and novel research on MTrPs is currently being published from this part of the world. WMA spans the conceptual divide between TCA and DN, by combining both MTrPs and APs as sites for therapeutic needling.

Acupuncture and dry needling

Mechanisms of needling

The acute analgesic effects of acupuncture are mediated principally through stimulation of the peripheral nervous system, and thus can be abolished by local anesthetic block of the relevant nerves.[29,30] In particular, stimulation of A-delta or type III afferent nerve fibers has been implicated as the key component in producing acupuncture-related analgesia.[31] The therapeutic effects of needling interventions are divided into three categories based on the area influenced: local (peripheral), segmental (spinal cord), and general (brainstem).

Local (peripheral) effects

Local effects are mediated through antidromic stimulation of high-threshold afferent nerves, in the same way as the "triple response". Release of trophic and vasoactive neuropeptides including neuropeptide Y (NPY), calcitonin gene-related peptide (CGRP) and vasoactive intestinal peptide (VIP) have been found following acupuncture in patients with xerostomia.[32,33] It is likely that the release of CGRP and VIP from peripheral nerves stimulated by acupuncture results in enhanced circulation and wound healing in rats,[34,35] and equivalent sensory stimulation has proved effective in humans.[36]

Increased circulation resulting from nerve stimulation is probably one of the most important local effects of acupuncture, and in rats, it appears to be principally mediated by the release of CGRP.[37] The effect of acupuncture on muscle blood flow, however, may not rely solely on nerve stimulation.[38] Under normal circumstances in healthy subjects, blood flow in muscle and skin is increased by needling muscle points and less affected by needling skin.[39] But this situation may be reversed if the subject is very sensitive, for example, in patients with fibromyalgia.[40] The increase in muscle and skin blood flow following local needling of muscles in patients with work-related trapezius myalgia appears to be lower than in healthy individuals, and this may reflect the degree of sympathetic activation and hypersensitivity of these patients.[41] Since hypoxia is thought to be one of the key components in chronic myalgia, and it is hypothesized that it also plays a role in the pathophysiology of myofascial pain,[42] any increase in blood flow caused by needling muscle may contribute to therapeutic responses.

Goldman et al. demonstrated (including data from multiple experiments in rodent models of inflammatory and neuropathic pain) a unilateral distal antinociceptive effect of acupuncture needling with manual stimulation via release of adenosine.[43] Moré et al. went on to show that a similar antinociceptive effect could be abolished by high levels of caffeine consumption in a rodent model.[44] The release of adenosine by acupuncture needling has also been demonstrated in humans using microdialysis.[45]

Segmental (spinal cord) effects

Through stimulation of high-threshold ergoreceptors in muscle tissue, needling can have an influence on sensory modulation within the dorsal horn at the relevant segmental level. C fiber pain transmission is inhibited via enkephalinergic interneurons in lamina II, the substantia gelatinosa.[44,45] Segmental stimulation appears to have a more powerful effect than an equivalent stimulus from a distant segment in modulating pain,[48–50] local autonomic activity, [51] and itch.[52] A-delta or type III afferent nerve fibers can be stimulated by superficial needling as well as by needling deeper tissues, but it seems that segmental stimuli from the latter (usually muscle) have a more powerful effect.[49,50,52,53]

General (brainstem) effects – heterosegmental

While segmental stimulation appears to be the more powerful effect, needling anywhere in the body can influence afferent processing throughout the spinal cord. The needle stimulus travels from the segment of origin to the ventral posterior lateral nucleus of the thalamus, and projects from there to the sensory cortex. Collaterals in the midbrain synapse in the periaqueductal gray (PAG), from where inhibitory fibers descend, via the nucleus raphe magnus, to influence afferent processing in the dorsal horn at every level of the spinal cord. Serotonin is the prominent neurotransmitter in the caudal stages of this descending pain pathway, and the fibers synapse with the enkephalinergic interneurons in lamina II. A second descending system from the PAG travels via the nucleus raphe gigantocellularis; its fibers are noradrenergic, and their influence is mediated directly on lamina II cells, rather than via enkephalinergic interneurons. Diffuse noxious inhibitory control (DNIC) is the term introduced by Le Bars et al. to define a third analgesic system, which is induced by a noxious stimulus anywhere in the body.[54,55] Heterosegmental needling exerts influence through all three mechanisms to different degrees,[46,47] and possibly through others, as yet undefined.

Recent evidence has shown that strong electroacupuncture (EA) (>2.0mA) applied daily to patients (n=301) with knee osteoarthritis is able to significantly increase descending inhibition as measured by conditioned pain modulation (CPM) compared with a milder form of EA (<0.5mA).[56] Clinically relevant changes in pain and functional outcomes were apparent at one week, after five treatment sessions, but significant changes in CPM were only apparent after two weeks (10 treatment sessions).

General (brainstem) effects – systemic

Systemic effects are more difficult to define, and there is clearly some overlap with heterosegmental effects. The term is used here to denote effects mediated at every segment of the spinal cord, as opposed to effects mediated by humeral means or by influence on higher centers in the central nervous system controlling general responses. Acupuncture needling has proven efficacy in the treatment of nausea and vomiting,[57–60] and this effect is likely to be mediated centrally. There is a substantial body of work that indicates the importance of beta-endorphin and other endogenous opioids in acupuncture-related analgesia,[50,61–63] and correlations have been identified between the endorphin-releasing effect of acupuncture and that of prolonged exercise.[64] Further correlations in terms of neuropeptide release have been also noted,[65] and it has been suggested that activation of opioid systems by exercise, or potentially by acupuncture, may mediate enhanced immunity.[66]

Functional magnetic resonance imaging (fMRI) studies indicate general effects on limbic structures,[67] and indicate the importance of the nature of the needle stimulus in achieving this effect.[68–70] The meta-analysis by Chae et al. concluded that acupuncture is able to activate several areas located in the sensorimotor cortical network, including the insula, thalamus, anterior cingulate cortex, and primary and secondary somatosensory cortices, but also is able to deactivate the limbic-paralimbic neocortical network, including the medial prefrontal cortex, caudate, amygdala, posterior cingulate cortex, and parahippocampus.[71]

While target-directed expectation may theoretically play a role in the mechanism of acupuncture under some circumstances,[72] the effects of acupuncture do not appear to be explained entirely by expectation.[73,74] In clinical practice, context-driven effects are considered important in acupuncture analgesia,[75] and areas of affective and cognitive processing are also consistently activated by acupuncture needling,[76] so in this environment it is challenging to untangle the direct effects of acupuncture needling on central nervous system structures from the indirect effects related to the context of treatment.[20]

Mechanisms of trigger point dry needling

The mechanisms by which dry needling exerts its analgesic effects share similar and common aspects with acupuncture, but additional factors related to a direct effect of dry needling into MTrPs are also considered.[77,78] In addition to the neurophysiological mechanisms explaining dry needling-related analgesia, it is possible that the more vigorous and fast insertion of the needling has a mechanical effect on endplates, muscle spindles, or nerve fibers themselves. Donnelly et al.[42] suggested that the therapeutic factor of needling interventions is produced by the mechanical effect of the needle, consisting of disruption of dysfunctional endplates, an increase of sarcomere length, and a reduction of the overlapping between actin and myosin filaments. The potential mechanical effects are supported by studies showing that dry needling decreased spontaneous electrical activity and acetylcholine levels of the MTrP area.[79] (A more extensive discussion of possible mechanisms of trigger point dry needling can be found in the textbook *Trigger Point Dry Needling*,[80] and in a pain model proposed by Fernández-de-Las-Peñas & Nijs.[81])

Safety aspects of needling interventions

Safety aspects of therapeutic needling with filiform needles have been studied extensively,[82–84] primarily reported in the acupuncture literature, but the principles apply equally to dry needling.[85,86] The most important adverse event to consider in the shoulder region is pneumothorax. This is particularly relevant to needling points in the shoulder girdle muscles overlying the thorax such as trapezius, rhomboid major and minor, levator scapulae, latissimus dorsi, and pectoralis major and minor. It is estimated that the incidence of clinically apparent pneumothorax after needling in at-risk areas is 1.75 per million treatments.[84]

The other main categories of adverse events are infection and trauma. In the past, the most prevalent infection related to needling was hepatitis B, but with widespread use of disposable needles, avoidance of needlestick injuries and implementation of contaminated sharps disposal, hepatitis B cases related to therapeutic needling have almost disappeared in modern medical environments.

Inoculation of bacteria from the skin surface is a very rare cause of infection related to needling with fine filiform needles because of the size and shape of the needle tip.[87] The risk is likely to be greatest where there are surgical implants close to the skin surface, and this may be the case following surgical repair after shoulder trauma. There is one known case report of glenohumeral joint infection following acupuncture.[88]

Safety is often used as a reason for employing imaging techniques during needling, however, this may give a false sense of security since fine needles cannot be visualized at all times. One report of cardiac tamponade following ultrasound-guided trigger point injection of pectoralis major perhaps illustrates this.[89] Nevertheless, it should be considered that most adverse events from dry needling and acupuncture are minor, and serious adverse events are rare.

Point selection

The two main approaches to point selection in WMA are dry needling of trigger points and segmental acupuncture.[20] The latter is defined as the technique of needling an area of the tissue innervated by the same spinal segment as the disordered structure under treatment.[17] In this way, the nerve signals created by needling travel into the same segments of the spinal cord as the nociceptive signals from the area of the body being treated, and thus the potential for sensory modulation is maximized.

Based on neurophysiological and clinical evidence,[46–49,51–53] the principle in point selection is to stimulate the tissue as close as is practical to the seat of the pathology, or at least within the same innervated-related segment. Trigger points, tender points, or acupuncture points can be chosen for treatment according to the needling approach. Figure 32.1 illustrates commonly used acupuncture points for the shoulder region, and Tables 32.1 to 32.3 provide details of the acupuncture points illustrated in the anterior, posterior, and paraspinal areas, respectively.

If the key element of the somatic pathology is an MTrP, this is arguably the only point necessary to treat. Figure 32.2

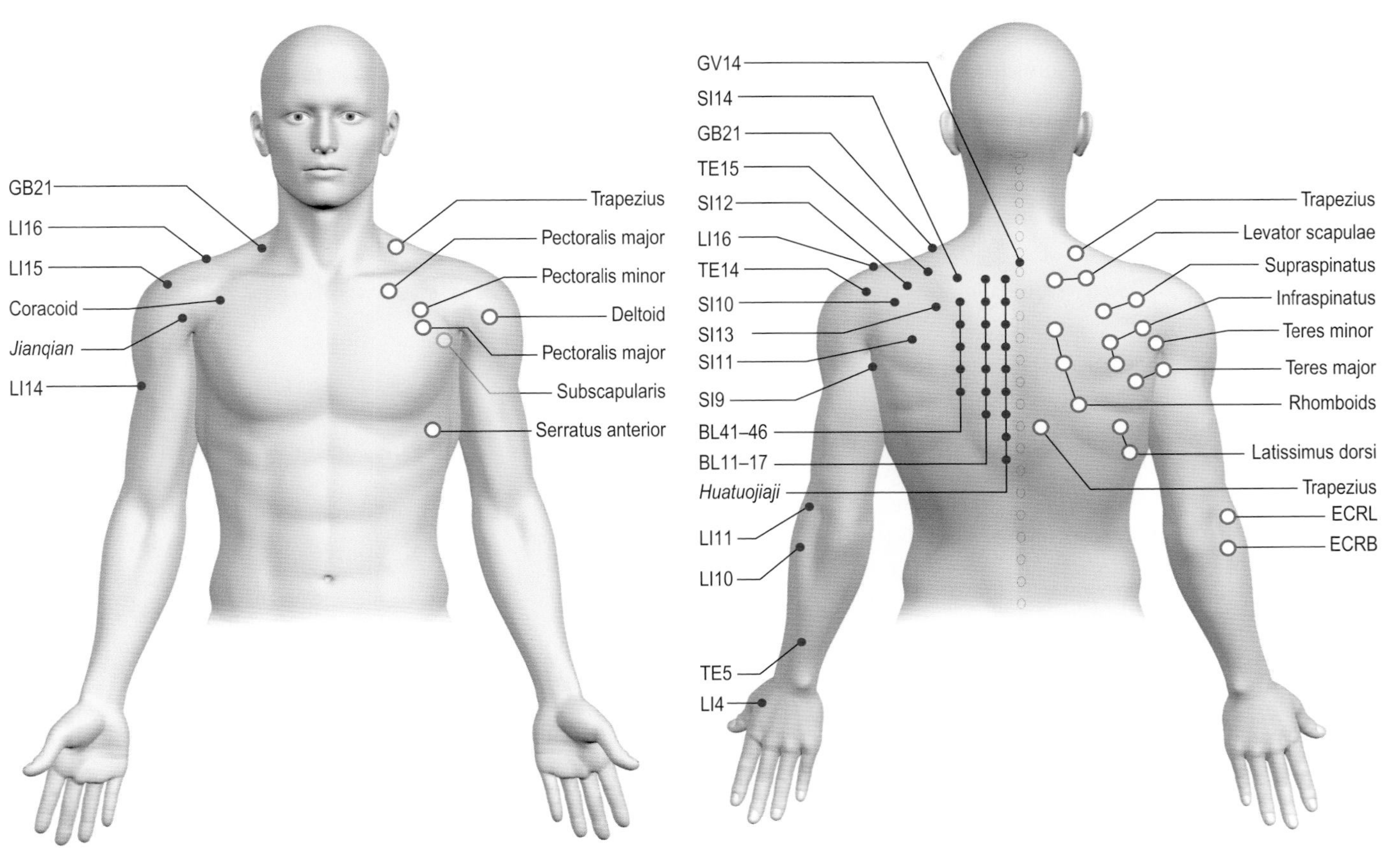

FIGURE 32.1
Commonly used acupuncture points for the shoulder region.

shows a selection of muscles related to the shoulder that may be affected by MTrPs with their associated referred pain patterns. In most cases, the analgesia afforded by local needling may be enhanced by using one or more points at a distance from the pathology, in addition to the relevant local points. Distant points are chosen because they stimulate the appropriate related segment, or because they are conveniently located and from clinical experience are known to generate a strong needling sensation in most subjects (heterosegmental acupuncture). In individual cases, point selection may be modified by the need to avoid local conditions, e.g., skin infection, ulceration, moles and tumors, varicosities; or to avoid regional conditions such as hydrostatic edema, lymphedema, anesthetic or hyperesthetic areas, or ischemia. As a rule, therapeutic needling should be performed in healthy tissue.

Needle technique

Sterile, single-use, disposable needles should always be used. In most cases, acupuncture needling involves stimulation of muscle tissue. Needling of muscle and possibly fascial planes between muscle tissue produces a characteristic sensation, often described as a dull, diffuse ache, pressure, swelling, or numbness, which can be referred some distance from the point of stimulation. Needling of other tissues of the soma, such as skin, ligament, tendon, periosteum, and the fascial covering of muscle, produces relatively localized and often sharp sensations, although there appear to be differences with age, particularly with periosteal needling. If the aim is to stimulate a muscle, a rapid insertion through the skin and superficial layers minimizes discomfort for the patient. Practitioners who are learning

Table 32.1 Shoulder and arm: anterior aspect

Point	Location, target, *indications, cautions*		Segments
GB21	Midway between GV14 and tip of the acromion at the highest point of trapezius		D C3
	Angulation: tangential to ribs, posteriorly	Target: upper trapezius	M C3–4
	Headache, neck pain and stiffness, anxiety		S (n/a)
	CAUTION – note the proximity of the pleura between the 1st and 2nd ribs		
LI16	In the depression medial to the acromion and between the lateral extremities of the clavicle and scapular spine		D C3
	Angulation: perpendicular	Target: supraspinatus	M C3–6
	Shoulder and arm pain		S C5–6
LI15	Anterolateral and inferior to the anterior tip of the acromion, in the groove between the anterior and middle fibers of deltoid		D C4
	Angulation: perpendicular	Target: supraspinatus insertion	M C5
	Shoulder and arm pain		S C5
Coracoid	Anterior to the glenohumeral joint, between the fibers of deltoid and pectoralis major		D C4
	Angulation: perpendicular	Target: coracoid	M C5–6
	Shoulder and arm pain		S C5
	CAUTION – avoid angulation towards the ribcage		
Jianqian	Midway between LI15 and the upper end of the anterior axillary fold		D C4
	Angulation: perpendicular	Target: deltoid or bicipital groove	M C5
	Shoulder and arm pain		S C5
LI14	Between the distal attachment of deltoid and the long head of biceps, in a tender depression, 3/5 of the distance on a line from LI11 to LI15		D C5–6
	Angulation: perpendicular	Target: connective tissue plane	M C5–6
	Shoulder and arm pain		S C5–6

D, dermatome; M, myotome; n/a, not applicable; S, sclerotome.

the technique find that the use of an introducer facilitates a rapid, often painless insertion. If an introducer is not used, the practitioner will stretch the skin over the point during insertion. Once through the skin, the needle should be carefully advanced to the desired position or muscle layer and is then stimulated by rotation back and forth combined with a varying degree of "lift and thrust" (slight withdrawal and reinsertion) until the desired sensation is achieved. If constant stimulation of the needle is required, an electrical stimulator can be also used. For the latter technique, usually a minimum of two needles are inserted, and different designed electroacupuncture devices can be used to deliver the electrical current.

Dry needling of MTrPs involves a very similar procedure, although the practitioner will often lift and thrust the needle (fast-in and fast-out technique) to a greater degree and with a variation in needle direction, aiming to hit the MTrP precisely. When the needle directly impinges on an MTrP, a local twitch response is often seen or felt in the associated taut band of muscle, and the symptoms derived from that point are usually reproduced.

In clinical practice, a wide variety of needling techniques have been described. These range from superficial needling to periosteal needling, with a variety of intermediate depths in muscle. Superficial needling of acupuncture

Table 32.2 Shoulder and arm: posterior aspect

Point	Location, target, *indications, cautions*		Segments
GV14	Between spinous processes C7 and T1		D C4–5/T1
	Angulation: transverse	Target: interspinous ligament	M C8
	Spinal neck pain, headache of cervical origin		S C8
	CAUTION – deep needling could reach the spinal cord		
SI14	3 *cun* lateral to spinous process of T1		D C3–4
	Angulation: tangential towards scapula	Target: levator scapulae	M C3–5
	Shoulder pain, neck pain and stiffness		S C5
	CAUTION – note the proximity of the pleura in slim patients		
TE15	Midway between the points GB21 and SI13 at the superior angle of the scapula (SI13 – tender depression superior to medial end of scapular spine)		D C3
	Angulation: perpendicular	Target: trapezius	M C3–4
	Shoulder pain, neck pain and stiffness		S (n/a)
	CAUTION – note the proximity of the pleura in slim patients		
LI16	In the depression medial to the acromion and between the lateral extremities of the clavicle and scapular spine		D C3
	Angulation: perpendicular	Target: supraspinatus	M C3–6
	Shoulder and arm pain		S C5–6
TE14	Posterolateral and inferior to the posterior tip of the acromion, in the depression between the middle and posterior fibers of deltoid		D C3–4
	Angulation: perpendicular	Target: infraspinatus insertion	M C5–6
	Shoulder and arm pain		S C6
SI13	In the tender depression superior to the medial end of the scapular spine		D C4/T1
	Angulation: towards suprascapular fossa	Target: supraspinatus	M C3–6
	Shoulder and arm pain		S C5
	CAUTION – do not needle deeply unless over suprascapular fossa		
SI12	Directly above SI11 in the middle of the suprascapular fossa, about 1 *cun* above the middle of the superior border of the scapular spine		D C3–4
	Angulation: towards suprascapular fossa	Target: supraspinatus	M C3–6
	Shoulder and arm pain		S C5
	CAUTION – do not needle deeply unless over suprascapular fossa		
SI11	1/3 down a line from the midpoint of the scapular spine to the inferior angle of the scapula		D C4/T1–2
	Angulation: perpendicular	Target: infraspinatus	M C5–6
	Shoulder and arm pain		S C5–6

(Continued)

Table 32.2 *(Continued)*

Point	Location, target, *indications, cautions*		Segments
SI10	In the depression below the spine of the scapula, directly superior to the posterior axillary crease when the arm hangs by the side of the body		D C3–4
	Angulation: perpendicular	Target: infraspinatus	M C5–6
	Shoulder and arm pain		S C6
SI9	1 *cun* superior to the posterior axillary crease when the arm hangs by the side of the body		D T3–4
	Angulation: perpendicular	Target: teres major	M C5–7
	Shoulder and arm pain		S C7
LI11	At the radial end of the antecubital crease, halfway between the biceps tendon and the lateral epicondyle		D C5–6
	Angulation: perpendicular	Target: ECRL	M C5–6
	Lateral epicondylalgia, forearm pain; immunomodulation		S C6–7
LI10	2 *cun* distal to LI11, on the line connecting LI11 with LI5 (the center of the anatomical snuff box)		D C5–6
	Angulation: perpendicular	Target: ECRB or supinator	M C5–7
	Lateral epicondylalgia, forearm pain		S C6–7
TE5	On the dorsal surface of forearm, 2 *cun* proximal to wrist joint, between radius and ulna, and between extensor indicis and extensor pollicis longus		D C6–8
	Angulation: perpendicular	Target: connective tissue plane	M C7–8
	Local pain; strong point for central effects		S C7–8
LI4	On the dorsal aspect of the hand, in the middle of the 1st web space, halfway along the second metacarpal bone		D C6–7
	Angulation: perpendicular	Target: 1st dorsal interosseous	M T1
	General point for pain; strong point for central effects		S (n/a)
	CAUTION – the radial artery is at the apex of the 1st web space		

D, dermatome; ECRB, extensor carpis radialis brevis; ECRL, extensor carpis radialis longus; M, myotome; n/a, not applicable; S, sclerotome.

points is common in Japanese forms of acupuncture, and Baldry described a superficial needling technique exclusively over MTrPs.[90] Periosteal needling was first described by Mann,[91,92] although he, as most Western practitioners who came after him, uses a variety of techniques. As suggested above, muscle is the most common site of stimulation. Depth and strength of needling in this tissue ranges from brief, superficial stimulation of the muscle surface to deep, repetitive intramuscular stimulation. The latter is not uncommon in Chinese acupuncture, but is also promoted by some practitioners in the West, in particular by Gunn,[93,94] who favored targeting motor points and paraspinal muscles.

Clinical aspects

There is a range of different responses to WMA or dry needling treatment: from no effect in 5–10% of the population, to profound analgesia and improved well-being, in a similar proportion. Patient selection will clearly influence success, and a healthy patient with a short-lived myofascial pain syndrome is much more likely to have a beneficial outcome than a debilitated patient with a chronic, ill-defined, and complex chronic pain problem.

It is difficult to define a “dose” for needling,[95] because on many occasions a judicious single needle insertion may have the same effect as ten or more needles left in place

Table 32.3 Paraspinal points in shoulder girdle region

Point	Location, target, *indications*, cautions		Segments
Bladder line: outer	3 *cun* lateral to the midline, on a vertical line joining the medial edge of the scapula and the outer border of the lumbar erector spinae		D C4/T2–5
	Angulation: oblique towards spine	Target: iliocostalis thoracis	M C4/T2–6
	Dorsal back pain, shoulder girdle pain		S T2–6
	CAUTION – note proximity of chest cavity and lung		– rib level
BL41	Level with the lower border of T2		
BL42	Level with the lower border of T3		
BL43	Level with the lower border of T4		
BL44	Level with the lower border of T5		
BL45	Level with the lower border of T6		
BL46	Level with the lower border of T7		
Bladder line: inner	1.5 *cun* lateral to the midline, halfway between the Outer Bladder Line and the spine		D C4/T2–5
	Angulation: oblique towards spine	Target: longissimus thoracis	M C4/T1–6
	Back pain		S T1–7
	CAUTION – note proximity of chest cavity and lung		– rib level
BL11	Level with the lower border of T1		
BL12	Level with the lower border of T2		
BL13	Level with the lower border of T3		
BL14	Level with the lower border of T4		
BL15	Level with the lower border of T5		
BL16	Level with the lower border of T6		
BL17	Level with the lower border of T7		
Huatuojiaji	A series of 17 extra points, 0.5 *cun* lateral to the lower border of the spinous processes of T1 to L5, T1 to T9 (see Fig 32.1)		D T1–7
	Angulation: perpendicular Target: multifidus		M T1–9
	Segmental acupuncture		S T1–9
	CAUTION – note proximity of chest cavity and lung		

D, dermatome; M, myotome; n/a, not applicable; S, sclerotome.

for 20 minutes, and similar strength sequential treatments often have increasing potency in early stages of a course of treatment. Experimental work does appear to support a type of dose–response relationship for sensory stimulation[96] but it is unlikely to be linear, and recent meta-analysis has not been able to identify exceptional acupuncture responders within a very large dataset drawn from clinical trials.[97] There is probably a stepwise increase in potency from 1 to 5 in the following sequence:

1. Superficial, heterosegmental needling with minimal sensation.
2. Superficial, segmental needling with minimal sensation.

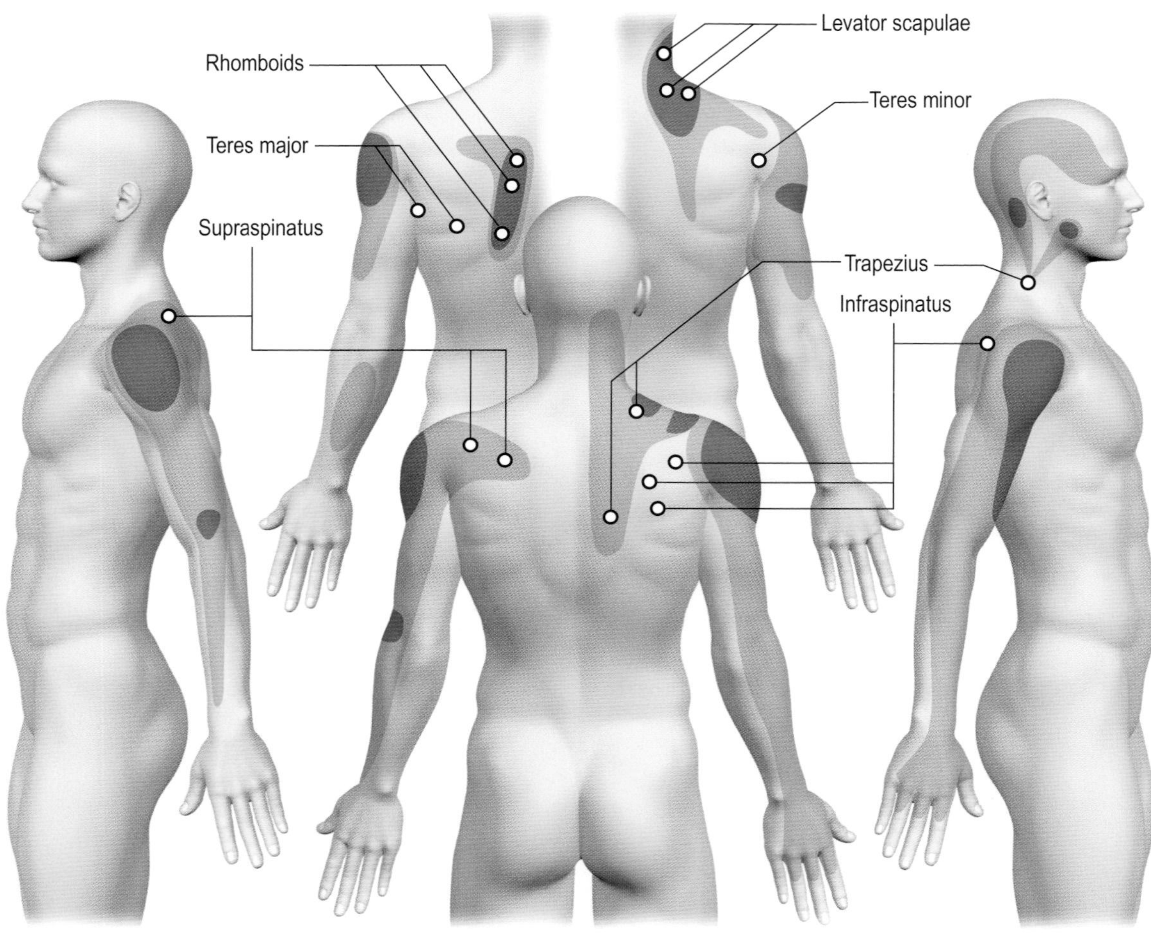

3. Deep, heterosegmental needling with strong sensation.
4. Deep, segmental needling with strong sensation.
5. Deep, segmental needling with electrical stimulation sufficient to cause muscle contraction.

While needling is likely to do more than simply offer pain relief, the standard pattern of effect from treatment is most easily appreciated in terms of analgesia. There may be little or no effect after the first session, as the practitioner will usually start with gentle treatment. This is to avoid aggravation of symptoms in people sensitive to needling. The initial response is seen within the first 72 hours after treatment, and its onset is often not perceived until the day after needling. Repeat treatments are performed either bi-weekly or weekly, and the interval can be lengthened with the response. Typically, there is a progressive increase in the quality and duration of the effect following repeated sessions, and in chronic pain states, symptom control can be maintained for some patients with relatively infrequent treatments, perhaps every four to six weeks.

Efficacy and effectiveness of acupuncture for shoulder pain conditions

The Acupuncture Trialists Collaboration (ATC) update of their individual patient data meta-analysis (IPDM) of acupuncture for chronic pain in 2018 included a category for shoulder pain for the first time.[98] They included four RCTs with a total of 766 patients.[99–102] Acupuncture was superior to sham acupuncture with a moderate effect size (standardized mean difference) of 0.57. Two of the four RCTs

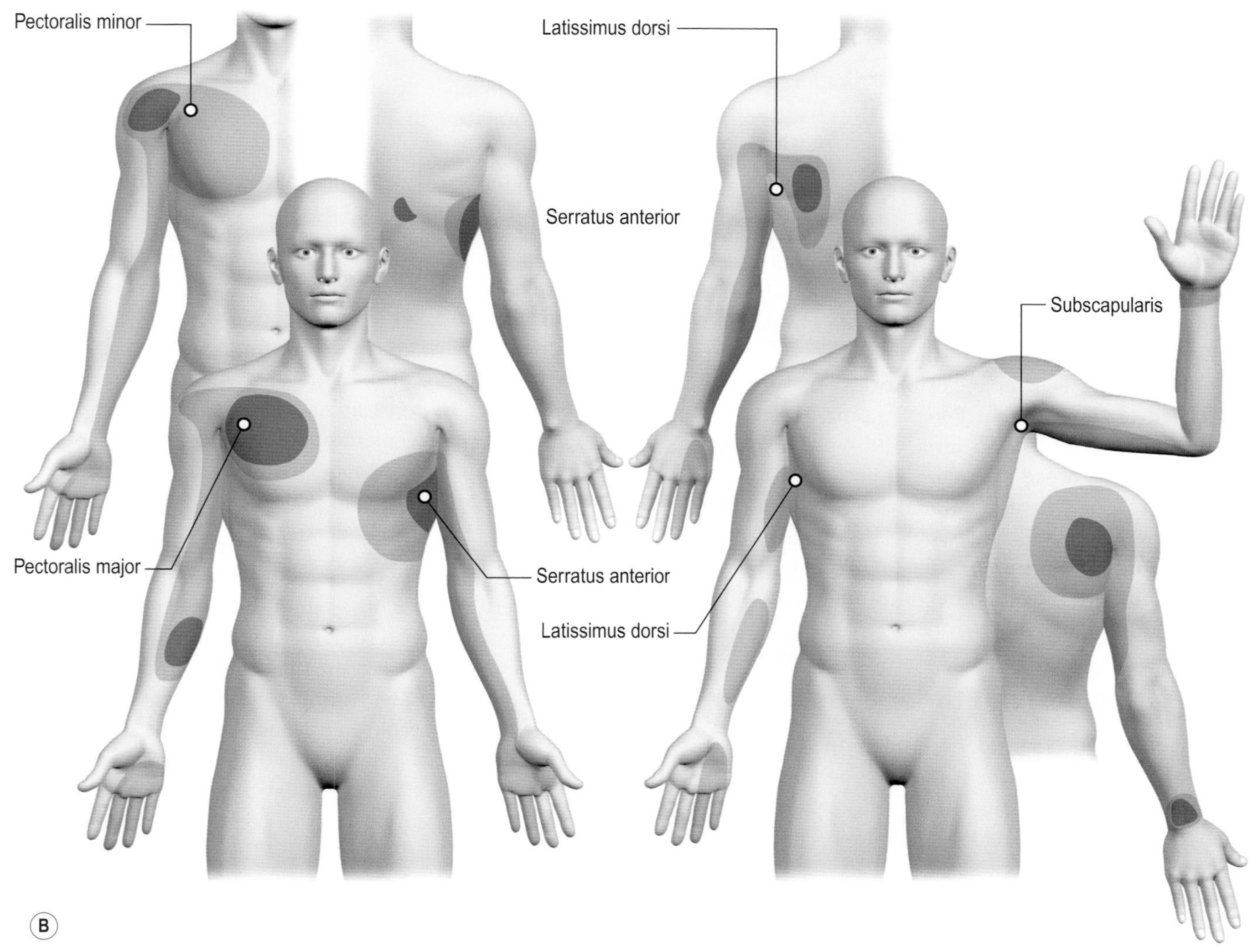

FIGURE 32.2
Myofascial trigger points (A), and referral patterns (B).

measured outcomes at 6 months,[100,102] and both demonstrated highly significant and clinically relevant benefits at this time point. It should be noted that while three out of four of these RCTs principally applied needling in the region of the shoulder in the active groups, one paper used a distant point technique in the lower leg combined with mobilization of the affected shoulder, and followed by physiotherapy, including graduated thermotherapy, recentering the humeral head with active and passive maneuvers, dynamic control of the scapula and cryotherapy.[101] In this situation, the needling may act as a heterotopic conditioning stimulus to reduced pain perception at the shoulder and facilitate a greater range of movement during simultaneous mobilization. Other authors have not found significant benefits of acupuncture or EA when compared with exercise in individuals with subacromial pain.[103] The most recent meta-analysis of acupuncture versus sham in musculoskeletal disorders demonstrates efficacy for pain, function, and quality of life, and for pain the effect is still apparent in the longer term.[104]

Efficacy and effectiveness of dry needling for shoulder pain conditions

Evidence related to dry needling in shoulder pain is conflicting. For instance, Arias-Buría et al. reported that the combination of dry needling with exercise was more effective than exercise alone for improving disability assessed with the DASH questionnaire at six and 12 months (large effect size >1.1), but both interventions were equally effective at decreasing pain intensity.[105] In contrast, Pérez-Palomares et al. observed that dry needling did not offer benefits when added to a multimodal physical therapy treatment at three months in individuals with nonspecific shoulder pain.[106] Discrepancies between these studies can be related to the fact that Pérez-Palomares et al. did not specify MTrP diagnostic criteria, and their inclusion criteria comprised a broad spectrum of patients with shoulder pain syndromes.[106] Two meta-analyses have reported moderate to low quality evidence suggesting a positive effect of dry needling for pain intensity (small effect) and pain-related disability (large effect) in nontraumatic shoulder pain, mostly with short-term outcomes.[107,108]

Integration into multimodal management

Clinicians should consider acupuncture or dry needing as part of the treatment plan for people seeking care for shoulder pain of a musculoskeletal origin, rather than isolated treatments. Treating shoulder conditions with only needling interventions is unlikely to be as effective as integrating these approaches into a multimodal management approach.[105,109,110] This is an important message, since passive treatments, such as needling therapies, can improve pain and related disability in the short term, but their isolated effects in the longer term may be limited. In such a scenario, active interventions such as exercise programs should be integrated into a comprehensive pain management approach to contribute to prolonged effects. While exercise approaches appear very promising in certain types of shoulder pain,[111] not all specific exercise approaches are beneficial.[112] Clinicians may apply dry needling or acupuncture in patients with persistent pain aiming to modulate the experience of pain, which may facilitate participation in an active intervention. This combined approach to management has been described by Vas et al.[101]

We feel that the ideal approach could include the early use of acupuncture or dry needling for rapid (non-pharmacological) pain relief in combination with physical therapy, exercise, and movement retraining, with perhaps the targeted monitoring of markers of psychosocial functioning to pick up those most at risk of developing chronic pain. As with all management approaches, the use of needling should be underpinned by sound clinical reasoning and shared decision-making as presented in Chapter 13.

Despite both the mechanistic and clinical evidence in favor of acupuncture and dry needling techniques, and their good safety profile, other more conventional approaches still dominate. Nonsteroidal anti-inflammatory drugs have a comparable effect size to that of acupuncture in osteoarthritis,[113] but a safety profile that appears to be considerably worse.[114] Steroid injections have been a mainstay of treatment both in physical medicine and rheumatology, however, evidence is accumulating to suggest that long-term outcomes are worse with steroid than without.[115,116] We know that local effects of corticosteroid on tendon are negative both in vitro and in vivo,[117] and considering the anatomical vulnerability of the supraspinatus tendon and its propensity to wear with age,[118] it may be appropriate to consider dry needling before considering steroid injections for shoulder pain. As always, more research is needed to help address uncertainties in clinical practice.

References

1. Dorfer L. 5200-year-old acupuncture in Central Europe? Science. 1998;282:242–3.

2. Dorfer L, Moser M, Bahr F, et al. A medical report from the stone age? Lancet. 1999;354:1023–5.

3. Cummings M. Acupuncture and trigger point needling. In: Hazelman B, Riley G, Speed C (eds). Soft Tissue Rheumatology. Cambridge: Oxford University Press; 2004:275–82.

4. Buck C. Acupuncture and Chinese Medicine: Roots of Modern Practice. London: Singing Dragon; 2015.

5. Unschuld PU. Huang Di Nei Jing Ling Shu: The Ancient Classic on Needle Therapy. Oakland, California: University of California Press; 2016.

6. Bai X, Baron RB. Acupuncture: Visible Holism. Butterworth-Heinemann; 2001.

7. Ma K-W. The Roots and Development of Chinese Acupuncture: From Prehistory to Early 20Th Century. Acupunct Med 1992;10:92–9. doi:10.1136/aim.10.Suppl.92

7A. Unschuld PU. Personal communication. 2018.

8. Shaw V. Chōng meridian an ancient Chinese description of the vascular system? Acupunct Med. 2014;32:279–85.

9. Shaw V, Mclennan AK. Was acupuncture developed by Han Dynasty Chinese anatomists? Anat Rec. 2016;299:643–59.

10. Andrews B. The Making of Modern Chinese Medicine, 1850–1960. Vancouver: University of British Columbia Press; 2014.

11. Lewit K. The needle effect in the relief of myofascial pain. Pain. 1979;6:83–90.

12. Steindler A. The interpretation of sciatic radiation and the syndrome of low-back pain. J Bone Jt Surg Am. 1940;22:28–34.

13. Travell J, Rinzler SH. The Myofascial Genesis of Pain. Postgrad Med. 1952;11:425–34.

14. Lewit K, Simons DG. Myofascial pain: relief by post-isometric relaxation. Arch Phys Med Rehabil. 1984;65:452–6.

15. Cummings TM, White AR. Needling therapies in the management of myofascial trigger point pain: a systematic review. Arch Phys Med Rehabil. 2001;82:986–92.

16. Hong C-Z. Lidocaine injection versus dry needling to myofascial trigger point. The importance of the local twitch response. Am J Phys Med Rehabil. 1994;73:256–63.

17. Filshie J, Cummings M. Western medical acupuncture. In: Ernst E, White A (eds). Acupuncture: A Scientific Appraisal. Oxford: Butterworth Heinemann; 1999:31–59.

18. White A, Editorial Board of Acupuncture in Medicine. Western medical acupuncture: a definition. Acupunct Med. 2009;27:33–5.

19. Macdonald AJR. Segmental acupuncture therapy. Acupunct Electrother Res. 1983;8:267–82.

20. Cummings M. Western medical acupuncture: the approach to treatment. In: Filshie J, White A, Cummings M (eds). Medical Acupuncture: A Western Scientific Approach. London: Elsevier; 2016:100–24.

21. White A, Cummings M, Filshie J. An Introduction to Western Medical Acupuncture, 2nd edition. London: Elsevier; 2018.

22. Melzack R. Myofascial trigger points: relation to acupuncture and mechanisms of pain. Arch Phys Med Rehabil. 1981;62:114–7.

23. Macdonald AJ, Macrae KD, Master BR, et al. Superficial acupuncture in the relief of chronic low back pain. Ann R Coll Surg Engl. 1983;65:44–6.

24. Lapeer GL, Monga TN. Myofascial trigger-point acupuncture in relieving chronic pain after endarterectomy. Can Fam Physician. 1986;32:1955–8.

25. Travell JG, Simons DG. Myofascial Pain & Dysfunction. The Trigger Point Manual. Volume 1. The Upper Extremities. Baltimore: Williams & Wilkins; 1983.

26. Melzack R, Stillwell DM, Fox EJ. Trigger points and acupuncture points for pain: correlations and implications. Pain. 1977;3:3–23.

27. Dorsher PT. Myofascial referred-pain data provide physiologic evidence of acupuncture meridians. J Pain. 2009;10:723–31.

28. Jin F, Guo Y, Wang Z, et al. The pathophysiological nature of sarcomeres in trigger points in patients with myofascial pain syndrome: a preliminary study. Eur J Pain. 2020:ejp.1647.

29. Chiang CY, Chang CT, Chu HL, et al. Peripheral afferent pathway for acupuncture analgesia. Sci Sin. 1973;16:210–7.

30. Dundee JW, Ghaly G. Local anesthesia blocks the antiemetic action of P6 acupuncture. Clin Pharmacol Ther. 1991;50:78–80.

31. Chung JM, Fang ZR, Hori Y, et al. Prolonged inhibition of primate spinothalamic tract cells by peripheral nerve stimulation. Pain. 1984;19:259–75.

32. Dawidson I, Angmar-Månsson B, Blom M, et al. The influence of sensory stimulation (acupuncture) on the release of neuropeptides in the saliva of healthy subjects. Life Sci. 1998;63:659–74.

33. Dawidson I, Angmar-Månsson B, Blom M, et al. Sensory stimulation (acupuncture) increases the release of vasoactive intestinal polypeptide in the saliva of xerostomia sufferers. Neuropeptides. 1998;32:543–8.

34. Jansen G, Lundeberg T, Samuelson UE, et al. Increased survival of ischaemic musculocutaneous flaps in rats after acupuncture. Acta Physiol Scand. 1989;135:555–8.

35. Jansen G, Lundeberg T, Kjartansson J, et al. Acupuncture and sensory neuropeptides increase cutaneous blood flow in rats. Neurosci Lett. 1989;97:305–9.

36. Lundeberg T, Kjartansson J, Samuelsson U. Effect of electrical nerve stimulation on healing of ischaemic skin flaps. Lancet. 1988;2:712–4.

37. Sato A, Sato Y, Shimura M, et al. Calcitonin gene-related peptide produces skeletal muscle vasodilation following antidromic stimulation of unmyelinated afferents in the dorsal root in rats. Neurosci Lett. 2000;283:137–40.

38. Shinbara H, Okubo M, Sumiya E, et al. Effects of manual acupuncture with sparrow pecking on muscle blood flow of normal and denervated hindlimb in rats. Acupunct Med. 2008;26:149–59.

39. Sandberg M, Lundeberg T, Lindberg LG, et al. Effects of acupuncture on skin and muscle blood flow in healthy subjects. Eur J ApplPhysiol. 2003;90:114–9.

40. Sandberg M, Lindberg L-G, Gerdle B. Peripheral effects of needle stimulation (acupuncture) on skin and muscle blood flow in fibromyalgia. Eur J Pain. 2004;8:163–71.

41. Sandberg M, Larsson B, Lindberg L-G, et al. Different patterns of blood flow response in the trapezius muscle following needle stimulation (acupuncture) between healthy subjects and patients with fibromyalgia and work-related trapezius myalgia. Eur J Pain. 2005;9:497–510.

42 Donnelly JM, Fernández-de-las-Peñas C, Finnegan M, et al. (eds). Travell, Simons & Simons' Myofascial Pain & Dysfunction. The Trigger Point Manual, 3rd edition. Philadelphia: Wolters Kluwer; 2019.

43. Goldman N, Chen M, Fujita T, et al. Adenosine A1 receptors mediate local anti-nociceptive effects of acupuncture. Nat Neurosci. 2010;13:883–8.

44. Moré AO, Cidral-Filho FJ, Mazzardo-Martins L, et al. Caffeine at moderate doses can inhibit acupuncture-induced analgesia in a mouse model of postoperative pain. J Caffeine Res. 2013;3:143–8.

45. Takano T, Chen X, Luo F, et al. Traditional acupuncture triggers a local increase in adenosine in human subjects. J Pain. 2012;13:1215–23.

46. Bowsher D. Mechanisms of acupuncture. In: Filshie J, White A, (eds). Medical Acupuncture: A Western Scientific Approach. Edinburgh: Churchill Livingstone; 1998:69–82.

47. White A. Neurophysiology of acupuncture analgesia. In: Ernst E, White A (eds). Acupuncture: A Scientific Appraisal. Oxford: Butterworth Heinemann; 1999:60-92.

48. Chapman CR, Chen AC, Bonica JJ. Effects of intrasegmental electrical acupuncture

on dental pain: evaluation by threshold estimation and sensory decision theory. Pain. 1977;3:213–27.

49. Lundeberg T, Eriksson S, Lundeberg S, et al. Acupuncture and sensory thresholds. Am J Chin Med. 1989;17:99–110.

50. Zhao Z-Q. Neural mechanism underlying acupuncture analgesia. Prog Neurobiol. 2008;85:355–75.

51. Sato A, Sato Y, Suzuki A, et al. Neural mechanisms of the reflex inhibition and excitation of gastric motility elicited by acupuncture-like stimulation in anesthetized rats. Neurosci Res. 1993;18:53–62.

52. Lundeberg T, Bondesson L, Thomas M. Effect of acupuncture on experimentally induced itch. Br J Dermatol. 1987;117:771–7.

53. Ceccherelli F, Gagliardi G, Visentin R, et al. Effects of deep vs. superficial stimulation of acupuncture on capsaicin- induced edema. A blind controlled study in rats. Acupunct Electrother Res. 1998;23:125–34.

54. Le Bars D, Dickenson a H, Besson JM. Diffuse noxious inhibitory controls (DNIC). I. Effects on dorsal horn convergent neurones in the rat. Pain. 1979;6:283–304.

55. Le Bars D, Dickenson AH, Besson JM. Diffuse noxious inhibitory controls (DNIC). II. Lack of effect on non-convergent neurones, supraspinal involvement and theoretical implications. Pain. 1979;6:305–27.

56. Lv Z, Shen L, Zhu B, et al. Effects of intensity of electroacupuncture on chronic pain in patients with knee osteoarthritis: a randomized controlled trial. Arthritis Res Ther. 2019;21:120.

57. Vickers AJ. Can acupuncture have specific effects on health? A systematic review of acupuncture antiemesis trials. J R Soc Med. 1996;89:303–11.

58. Lee A, Done ML. Stimulation of the wrist acupuncture point P6 for preventing postoperative nausea and vomiting. Cochrane Database Syst Rev. 2004:CD003281.

59. Lee A, Fan LT. Stimulation of the wrist acupuncture point P6 for preventing postoperative nausea and vomiting. Cochrane Database of Syst Rev. 2009:CD003281.

60. Lee A, Chan SK, Fan LT. Stimulation of the wrist acupuncture point PC6 for preventing postoperative nausea and vomiting. Cochrane Database Syst Rev. 2015:CD003281.

61. Han JS, Terenius L. Neurochemical basis of acupuncture analgesia. Annu Rev Pharmacol Toxicol. 1982;22:193–220.

62. Han JS. Acupuncture and endorphins. Neurosci Lett. 2004;361:258–61.

63. Han J-S. Acupuncture analgesia: areas of consensus and controversy. Pain. 2011;152:S41-8.

64. Thoren P, Floras JS, Hoffmann P, et al. Endorphins and exercise: physiological mechanisms and clinical implications. Med SciSports Exerc. 1990;22:417–28.

65. Bucinskaite V, Theodorsson E, Crumpton K, et al. Effects of repeated sensory stimulation (electro-acupuncture) and physical exercise (running) on open-field behaviour and concentrations of neuropeptides in the hippocampus in WKY and SHR rats. Eur J Neurosci. 1996;8:382–7.

66. Jonsdottir IH. Physical exercise, acupuncture and immune function. Acupunct Med. 1999;17:50–3.

67. Hui KK, Liu J, Makris N, et al. Acupuncture modulates the limbic system and subcortical gray structures of the human brain: evidence from fMRI studies in normal subjects. Hum Brain Mapp. 2000;9:13–25.

68. Hui KK, Nixon EE, Vangel MG, et al. Characterization of the 'deqi' response in acupuncture. BMC Complement Altern Med. 2007;7:33.

69. Hui KK, Marina O, Claunch JD, et al. Acupuncture mobilizes the brain's default mode and its anti-correlated network in healthy subjects. Brain Res. 2009;1287:84–103.

70. Hui KKS, Marina O, Liu J, et al. Acupuncture, the limbic system, and the anticorrelated networks of the brain. Auton Neurosci. 2010;157:81–90.

71. Chae Y, Chang D-S, Lee S-H, et al. Inserting needles into the body: a meta-analysis of brain activity associated with acupuncture needle stimulation. J Pain. 2013;14:215–22.

72. Benedetti F, Arduino C, Amanzio M. Somatotopic activation of opioid systems by target-directed expectations of analgesia. J Neurosci. 1999;19:3639–48.

73. Kong J, Kaptchuk TJ, Polich G, et al. Expectancy and treatment interactions: a dissociation between acupuncture analgesia and expectancy evoked placebo analgesia. Neuroimage. 2009;45:940–9.

74. Kong J, Kaptchuk TJ, Polich G, et al. An fMRI study on the interaction and dissociation between expectation of pain relief and acupuncture treatment. Neuroimage. 2009;47:1066–76.

75. Finniss DG, Kaptchuk TJ, Miller F, et al. Biological, clinical, and ethical advances of placebo effects. Lancet. 2010;375:686–95.

76. Huang W, Pach D, Napadow V, et al. Characterizing acupuncture stimuli using brain imaging with fMRI – a systematic review and meta-analysis of the literature. PLoS One. 2012;7:e32960.

77. Cagnie B, Dewitte V, Barbe T, et al. Physiologic effects of dry needling. Curr Pain Headache Rep. 2013;17:348.

78. Chou L-W, Kao M-J, Lin J-G. Probable mechanisms of needling therapies for myofascial pain control. Evidence-Based Complement Altern Med. 2012;2012:1–11.

79. Liu Q-G, Liu L, Huang Q-M, et al. Decreased spontaneous electrical activity and acetylcholine at myofascial trigger spots after dry needling treatment: a pilot study. Evidence-Based Complement Altern Med 2017;2017:1–7.

80. Dommerholt J, Fernández-de-las-Peñas C. Proposed mechanisms and effects of trigger point dry needling. In: Dommerholt J, Fernández-de-las-Peñas C (eds). Trigger Point Dry Needling. Elsevier; 2018:21–30.

81. Fernández-de-Las-Peñas C, Nijs J. Trigger point dry needling for the treatment of myofascial pain syndrome: current perspectives within a pain neuroscience paradigm. J Pain Res. 2019;12:1899–911.

82. White A. A cumulative review of the range and incidence of significant adverse events associated with acupuncture. Acupunct Med. 2004;22:122–33.

83. Witt CM, Pach D, Brinkhaus B, et al. Safety of acupuncture: results of a prospective observational study with 229,230 patients and introduction of a medical information and consent form. Forsch Komplementmed. 2009;16:91–7.

84. Lin S-K, Liu J, Hsu R, et al. Incidence of iatrogenic pneumothorax following acupuncture treatments in Taiwan. Acupunct Med. 2019;37:332–9.

85. Brady S, McEvoy J, Dommerholt J, et al. Adverse events following trigger point dry needling: a prospective survey of chartered physiotherapists. J Man Manip Ther. 2014;22:134–40.

86. Boyce D, Wempe H, Campbell C, et al. Adverse events associated with therapeutic dry needling. Int J Sports Phys Ther. 2020;15:103–13.

87. Hoffman P. Skin Disinfection and acupuncture. Acupunct Med. 2001;19:112-6.

88. Kirschenbaum AE, Rizzo C. Glenohumeral pyarthrosis following acupuncture treatment. Orthopedics. 1997;20:1184–6.

89. Jung J-W, Kim SR, Jeon SY, et al. Cardiac tamponade following ultrasonography-guided trigger point injection. J Musculoskelet Pain. 2014;22:389–91.

90. Baldry PE. Acupuncture, Trigger Points & Musculoskeletal Pain, 2nd edition. Edinburgh: Churchill Livingstone; 2005.

91. Mann F. Reinventing Acupuncture: A New Concept of Ancient Medicine. Oxford: Butterworth Heinemann; 1992.

92. Mann F. A new system of acupuncture. In: Filshie J, White A (eds). Medical Acupuncture: A Western Scientific Approach. Edinburgh: Churchill Livingstone; 1998:61–6.

93. Gunn CC. Treating Myofascial Pain: Intramuscular Stimulation (IMS) for Myofascial Pain Syndromes of Neuropathic Origin. Seattle: University of Washington; 1989.

94. Gunn CC. Acupuncture and the peripheral nervous system. In: Filshie J, White A (eds). Medical Acupuncture: A Western Scientific Approach. Edinburgh: Churchill Livingstone; 1998:137–50.

95. White A, Cummings M, Barlas P, et al. Defining an adequate dose of acupuncture using a neurophysiological approach – a narrative review of the literature. Acupunct Med. 2008;26:111–20.

96. Lundeberg T, Lund I. Peripheral components of acupuncture stimulation – their contribution to the specific clinical effects of acupuncture. In: Filshie J, White A, Cummings M (eds). Medical Acupuncture: A Western Scientific Approach. London: Elsevier; 2016:22–58.

97. Foster NE, Vertosick EA, Lewith G, et al. Identifying patients with chronic pain who respond to acupuncture: results from an individual patient data meta-analysis. Acupunct Med. 2021;39:83-90.

98. Vickers AJ, Vertosick EA, Lewith G, et al. Acupuncture for chronic pain: update of an individual patient data meta-analysis. J Pain. 2018;19:455–74.

99. Kleinhenz J, Streitberger K, Windeler J, et al. Randomised clinical trial comparing the effects of acupuncture and a newly designed placebo needle in rotator cuff tendinitis. Pain. 1999;83:235–41.

100. Guerra de Hoyos JA, Andrés Martín MDC, Bassas y Baena de Leon E, et al. Randomised trial of long term effect of acupuncture for shoulder pain. Pain. 2004;112:289–98.

101. Vas J, Ortega C, Olmo V, et al. Single-point acupuncture and physiotherapy for the treatment of painful shoulder: a multicentre randomized controlled trial. Rheumatology. 2008;47:887–93.

102. Molsberger AF, Schneider T, Gotthardt H, et al. German Randomized Acupuncture Trial for Chronic Shoulder Pain (GRASP): a pragmatic, controlled, patient-blinded, multi-centre trial in an outpatient care environment. Pain. 2010;151:146–54.

103. Lewis J, Sim J, Barlas P. Acupuncture and electro-acupuncture for people diagnosed with subacromial pain syndrome: a multicentre randomized trial. Eur J Pain 2017;21:1007–19.

104. Lenoir D, De Pauw R, Van Oosterwijck S, et al. Acupuncture versus sham-acupuncture. Clin J Pain. 2020;36:533–49.

105. Arias-Buría JL, Fernández-de-las-Peñas C, Palacios-Ceña M, et al. Exercises and dry needling for subacromial pain syndrome: a randomized parallel-group trial. J Pain. 2017;18:11–8.

106. Pérez-Palomares S, Oliván-Blázquez B, Pérez-Palomares A, et al. Contribution of dry needling to individualized physical therapy treatment of shoulder pain: a randomized clinical trial. J Orthop Sport Phys Ther. 2017;47:11–20.

107. Navarro Santana M, Gómez Chiguano G, Cleland J, et al. Effects of trigger point dry needling for non-traumatic shoulder pain of musculoskeletal origin: a systematic review and meta-analysis. Phys Ther. 2021;101(2):pzaa216.

108. Hall ML, Mackie AC, Ribeiro DC. Effects of dry needling trigger point therapy in the shoulder region on patients with upper extremity pain and dysfunction: a systematic review with meta-analysis. Physiotherapy. 2018;104:167–77.

109. Arias-Buría JL, Martín-Saborido C, Cleland J, et al. Cost-effectiveness evaluation of the inclusion of dry needling into an exercise program for subacromial pain syndrome: evidence from a randomized clinical trial. Pain Med. 2018;19:2336–47.

110. Arias-Buría JL, Valero-Alcaide R, Cleland JA, et al. Inclusion of trigger point dry needling in a multimodal physical therapy program for postoperative shoulder pain: a randomized clinical trial. J Manipulative Physiol Ther. 2015;38:179–87.

111. Pieters L, Lewis J, Kuppens K, et al. An update of systematic reviews examining the effectiveness of conservative physical therapy interventions for subacromial shoulder pain. J Orthop Sport Phys Ther. 2020;50:131–41.

112. Hotta GH, Gomes de Assis Couto A, Cools AM, et al. Effects of adding scapular stabilization exercises to a periscapular strengthening exercise program in patients with subacromial pain syndrome: a randomized controlled trial. Musculoskelet Sci Pract. 2020;49:102171.

113. Birch S, Lee MS, Robinson N, et al. The U.K. NICE 2014 Guidelines for Osteoarthritis of the Knee: lessons learned in a narrative review addressing inadvertent limitations and bias. J Altern Complement Med. 2017;23:242–6.

114. Hatt KM, Vijapura A, Maitin IB, et al. Safety considerations in prescription of NSAIDs for musculoskeletal pain: a narrative review. PM R. 2018;10:1404–11.

115. McAlindon TE, LaValley MP, Harvey WF, et al. Effect of intra-articular triamcinolone vs saline on knee cartilage volume and pain in patients with knee osteoarthritis: a randomized clinical trial. JAMA. 2017;317:1967–75.

116. Coombes BK, Bisset L, Brooks P, et al. Effect of corticosteroid injection, physiotherapy, or both on clinical outcomes in patients with unilateral lateral epicondylalgia: a randomized controlled trial. JAMA. 2013;309:461–9.

117. Dean BJF, Lostis E, Oakley T, et al. The risks and benefits of glucocorticoid treatment for tendinopathy: a systematic review of the effects of local glucocorticoid on tendon. Semin Arthritis Rheum. 2014;43:570–6.

118. Vincent K, Leboeuf-Yde C, Gagey O. Are degenerative rotator cuff disorders a cause of shoulder pain? Comparison of prevalence of degenerative rotator cuff disease to prevalence of nontraumatic shoulder pain through three systematic and critical reviews. J Shoulder Elb Surg. 2017;26:766–73.

Electrophysical modalities in the management of shoulder conditions 33

Tim Watson

Introduction

Electrophysical modalities or electrophysical agents (EPAs) have an established role in therapy practice, though their mode and rationale of application has certainly changed with the passage of time; their utilization in current practice has substantially changed over the past two decades.

The principles underpinning evidence-based practice have had a major role to play in this change of emphasis, combined with the even more recent tendency to move away from the so-called "passive" modalities – in which the therapist delivers a treatment to the patient rather than the patient being an active participant in the treatment protocol. Several authors argue that EPAs are a passive form of treatment.[15,67,72] However, if a so-called passive treatment contributes to improved function, the basis of the argument may be moot.

The evidence for the use of EPAs in shoulder conditions is substantial, with at least 1500 papers across the modalities, though the quality of that evidence varies considerably. Making an evidence-based selection of the modality that might be optimally employed for a patient with a particular presentation is critical, and is central in clinical decision-making.[65] Having made a modality selection based on the strongest available evidence, the treatment parameters, including dose, are also important: an effective modality, employed at an ineffectual dose is unlikely to result in a useful clinical benefit. This is clearly not confined to EPAs – the same would apply when selecting an exercise program, when considering manual therapy, or prescribing medication.

The general model through which electrophysical modalities may achieve their effect is detailed elsewhere.[62,63,65] In the context of this chapter, suffice it to say that the delivery of energy to the tissues will instigate a physiological response, whether the energy in question is electrical stimulation, ultrasound, laser, shortwave, or shockwave. For example, shockwave is known to stimulate cells to increase their expression of cytokines and chemical mediators.[62,66] The enhanced expression of these messengers will, in turn, stimulate responses in other cells, and these responses can have an overt effect on the gross tissue response in, for example, persistent tendinopathy.[62] The evidence clearly identifies which modalities instigate a particular tissue response. The evidence further identifies the amount of the applied energy necessary to make the magnitude of the response sufficient to be worthwhile (meaningful) in the therapy environment: this is the "dose" factor.

The issue of dose-response has been discussed in detail by numerous authors. Bjordal et al.[8] were among the first to make a serious dose-response analysis of laser therapy in tendinopathy. This work was expanded[9] in relation to the use of laser in acute pain presentations, and laser use in shoulder impingement syndrome.[8] Chow et al. also considering laser-based therapies, employ a strong dose-response argument to challenge published guidelines,[12] while both Sluka et al.[54] and Johnson[33] consider the same issues for TENS and pain management. These authors have identified an important issue: that there is a dose-response relationship associated with EPAs, and that if a trial fails to identify benefit, it is possible that suboptimal parameters have been employed.

In the management of most shoulder conditions, it is common to recommend a treatment plan that involves several interventions: for example, shoulder arthroplasty would involve advice and education, surgery, and rehabilitation, supported with analgesic medications, as required. This also applies to EPAs. Most of the research cited in this chapter has attempted to evaluate the effect of a modality in isolation, however, more recent work has tried, as much as possible, to evaluate the modality in the context of the treatment package – something that is likely to become more commonplace in future studies and publications.

Lastly, by way of introductory comments, a few words on systematic reviews and meta-analyses – though linked to the forgoing commentary. If a trial scores highly on a systematic review checklist (RCT, blinding, fully described randomization and such like) but delivers an ineffective dose, it is likely to be included in the review. For whatever reason, "dose appropriateness" does not feature on systematic review selection criteria or checklists commonly employed. It is probably assumed that those conducting the research will have identified and selected the optimal dose, which may or may not be the case. Reviews (considered in this chapter) can fail to reach a conclusion on the efficacy or effectiveness of a modality employed as a treatment option for a particular clinical condition. If six studies pass the inclusion/exclusion filtering (for example) and three of them failed to demonstrate clinically important benefit, it is almost inevitable to conclude that either it is not possible to draw a conclusion or simply that the therapy is ineffective. If those trials employed clinically inappropriate doses or treatment protocols, it does not appear to influence the conclusions reached by the reviewers: trial quality matters – appropriate doses appear to matter less.

In this chapter, the available evidence on the use of various electrophysical modalities will be presented alongside reviews and meta-analyses where available. The best evidence will be summarized as objectively as possible.

Pain relief

Of all the clinical issues for which EPAs are studied, pain, pain relief, pain management, and associated terms remain the most prevalent. Of the 70 or so most popular modalities, each has supportive clinical research for a beneficial effect on pain – from the more established and longstanding ultrasound[69] and laser,[26] through to the more recent innovations of radiofrequency electric currents[57] and scrambler therapy.[36] They may not all be equal in the size or duration of their effects, nor the clinical value of these effects, but unquestionably supportive research exists.

Modalities such as transcutaneous electrical nerve stimulation (TENS) has a primary objective of reducing perceived pain.[34] Similarly, interferential therapy is commonly applied with a primary intention of reducing pain. Gunay Ucurum et al.[28] compared several interventions in this regard (interferential, TENS and ultrasound), all added to an exercise and hot pack treatment program in 79 people diagnosed with shoulder impingement. All three modalities added significant pain relief compared with heat and exercise alone and, thus, their inclusion in treatment may provide a significant advantage to the patient. The authors reported that interferential therapy alone achieved significant additional benefits for quality-of-life measures.[28] Dewan and Sharma[14] also compared the effectiveness of TENS and interferential therapy in 50 people with adhesive capsulitis. Both were shown to be clinically effective for pain, movement, and function, and like Gunay Ucurum et al., they identified an advantage to the interferential-based approach.

It is the electrical stimulation modalities that are most likely to be employed to achieve symptomatic pain relief, TENS, and interferential being the most prevalent for musculoskeletal presentations. TENS and neuromuscular electrical nerve stimulation (NMES) are also employed in post-stroke shoulder syndrome.[74] While the application of TENS may achieve significant immediate (short-term) reduction in perceived pain and discomfort, it is less often strongly evidenced as having a longer-term benefit as a primary consequence of the therapy. However, if TENS reduces pain, and consequently enables the patient to undertake a greater level of activity, it may contribute to longer-term gains.

TENS and similar stimulation modalities achieve pain reduction by either stimulating Aβ sensory nerve fibers and thus activating gate control mechanisms or by stimulating (via Aδ sensory fibers) some combination of opioid pathways in the CNS.[34] Sluka et al. have published several critical papers that identify an *immediate* effect of TENS on pain relief.[54,59] Measuring the effect of one dose of a nonsteroidal anti-inflammatory medication 24 hours after administration would be inappropriate, as would measuring the effect of a TENS-mediated pain response, one day after application. Available pain data almost certainly fail to reflect the immediacy of the TENS-mediated response. This is a critical issue for both research planning and clinical application.

Simpson et al.[53] systematically reviewed a range of nonsurgical interventions for rotator cuff tendinopathy. TENS was supported as an appropriate intervention for this patient group (as were other modalities considered in subsequent sections). Haik et al.[29] suggest that there was some support for the use of TENS as a means to achieve pain relief in their review of therapy options in subacromial pain, while Hurley et al.[31] similarly included TENS as a supported intervention following shoulder arthroscopy with significant pain reduction and reduced analgesia requirement. Vrouva et al.[60] compared TENS and a microcurrent treatment option in 42 people with partial rotator cuff tears. Both TENS and microcurrent therapies (as delivered) were effective in achieving a significant reduction in pain, improved function, and quality of life.

Multiple studies have included TENS within their standard or conventional treatment group. For example, Pasin et al.[46] added TENS to an ultrasound and hot pack program for people with subacromial impingement in a study primarily evaluating platelet rich plasma and corticosteroid injections. The conventional treatment program was clinically effective, and the authors suggest that it would constitute a preferable first-line intervention given its inexpensive and noninvasive nature. Clearly it is not possible to directly attribute proportional benefit to any individual treatment component.

A person with shoulder pain who is given TENS as a component of their treatment package can, very reasonably, expect to experience a short-term reduction in perceived pain and, thus, it has a potential value in their treatment. It will not "cure" their underlying problem – but it is not aiming to do so. If the reduction in perceived pain enables other aspects of rehabilitation to be undertaken; this alone may be sufficient justification for it being considered. Interferential therapy, though supported by a smaller volume of research, will similarly achieve a short-term reduction in perceived pain. The success of both modalities is dependent on appropriate stimulation parameters and electrode positioning.[34,35]

An alternative approach to the application of modalities to achieve symptomatic pain relief is to utilize a modality which targets a change in the underlying tissue pathology, such as laser, ultrasound, or shockwave-based therapies. Most trials which have evaluated the use of these EPAs for shoulder-related problems have included some clinical pain measure, and a high percentage of the published trials have reported significant reduction of pain – at least in the short term. Kim et al.[37] evaluated a deep-heating option and ultrasound for (established) shoulder pain, with both demonstrating significant reduction in pain post-treatment, and four weeks later. This is not a new treatment approach – Echternach[23] claimed clinically useful pain reduction in a cohort of 73 people with (mixed) shoulder pain.

The use of shockwave therapy (for example) is not normally undertaken with a primary aim of reducing pain.[19] Its purpose is to change the state of the underlying tissue, most commonly tendon. The fact that pain reduction occurs is by no means a negative outcome – just that it is not the primary intention of the treatment. The same argument can be made with the modalities in the "non-thermal" group such as ultrasound, laser (photobiomodulation), radiofrequency applications, pulsed shortwave, and various magnetic therapy interventions, discussed below.

Influencing the underlying tissue

Multiple EPA interventions are employed with the primary purpose of influencing the state of musculoskeletal tissue – whether in a degenerative, pathological, or post-injury state. Classically these would include ultrasound, laser, pulsed shortwave, and various magnetic therapies. More recent additions include microcurrent therapies, shockwave (focused and radial), and other radiofrequency applications, all of which have evidence of benefit in shoulder-related clinical problems. A clinical rather than a modality-based approach is adopted in this chapter.

Frozen shoulder/adhesive capsulitis

Zhang et al.[73] considered a range of nonsurgical treatment options for frozen shoulder. Both shockwave and laser therapy (photobiomodulation (PBM)) are supported as being modalities that provide significant pain relief and subsequent improved function. This was a wide-scoped review (32 nonsurgical interventions). Both shockwave and laser benefits (for both pain and function) were highly significant and compared very strongly against other options. After capsular distension, these two EPAs were highest ranked of 18 therapy options.

Page et al.[44] produced a Cochrane review covering electrotherapy (now electrophysical agents) for adhesive capsulitis. Nineteen trials were included in their analysis; laser was the only one with any support from the reviewers. Interestingly, of the modalities covered in this review, shockwave (focused or radial) was not mentioned at all and not included in the search criteria, even though there were over 100 studies published between 2000 and their 2014 cutoff date in which shockwave was employed as a treatment for shoulder presentations. Jain et al.[32] published a systematic review of a wide range of therapy interventions for adhesive capsulitis. Exercise and manual therapy were the strongest supported intervention options. In keeping with the other reviews cited in this section, laser-based therapies attracted the strongest support from the EPA groups – both for pain relief and enhanced function. Deep heat (various modes) was supported for function and range of movement. Ultrasound did not receive support under any evaluated outcome.

Beyond the systematic reviews and meta-analyses, there is a raft of primary studies. Ebadi et al.[20] included ultrasound therapy alongside exercise and mobilization for 50 people with frozen shoulder. The addition of ultrasound failed to achieve a clinically significant benefit when compared with a sham intervention. A similar study[16] also failed to demonstrate clinical benefit. The use of ultrasound at 3MHz (as in these studies) is very unlikely to reach the affected tissues, and thus the failure to demonstrate benefit is expected from the "dose" employed in this pilot study. Ultrasound was not supported in the reviews (above), and to a large extent, this is expected given the nature of the lesion, the depth of the tissue being targeted, and the suboptimal doses often employed.

Thu et al.[58] evaluated ultrasound-guided platelet rich plasma (PRP) injection compared with an exercise program and shortwave diathermy to generate significant tissue heating. The treatments were found to be equal in their clinical effectiveness. While PRP injections are considered elsewhere in this text (see Chapter 23), the clinical value of providing significant tissue heating as a valid treatment option should not be overlooked. Page et al.[44] reported the benefits of adding heat (continuous shortwave) to an exercise program in this patient group. Their findings do not devalue the benefit of exercise, but show that adding continuous shortwave to the exercise program is able to achieve significant additional benefit. Shortwave is only one of many methods of achieving tissue heating, and although the popularity of shortwave in current therapy practice may have declined in recent years,[51] the evidence would support its application as a valid, thermal-based intervention. Jain and Sharma[32] attributed significant benefits from deep heating to gains in function and range of motion. Deep heating applications are clearly more advantageous than superficial heating methods in adhesive capsulitis.[27,41]

Heat (hot pack) and interferential therapy were components of a virtual reality exercise-based program for people with frozen shoulder.[40] The overall pre-post test results were strongly positive, but given that all patients were in receipt of the same treatment package, it is not possible to disaggregate the contribution made by either the heat or the interferential components. Similarly, Elhfez et al.[24] evaluated the contribution of ultrasound and laser-based therapies alongside an exercise program for 45 people with shoulder adhesive capsulitis. All groups demonstrated significant benefit in range of movement and pain. As previously, the trial design gives some insight into the value of the treatment package, and while the group analysis enables some evaluation of the ultrasound and laser contribution, their individual effects cannot be fully dissociated from the overall treatment gains.

Given a significant number of studies along similar lines (e.g., Alptekin et al.[4] evaluating a combination of interferential, hot pack, ultrasound, and exercise therapies), the clinician is faced with the position that combination packages of care have evidence of significant benefit, but that at the present time, it is not clear which of these modalities is most likely to have made a significant contribution to the positive outcome. Recent studies involving a detailed and robust evaluation of a single modality appear to be lacking in the published literature.

In a recent complex network meta-analysis (alongside a systematic review), Zhang et al.[73] identified both shockwave and laser therapy as the most strongly supported adjunctive therapies for this clinical presentation: the combination of capsular distension, shockwave, and laser was identified as top rank and most likely to achieve pain relief and functional improvement. The use of laser therapy is also supported in other reviews.[32,44]

In the management of frozen shoulder, modalities with the strongest evidence include laser-based therapy, shockwave, and heat (preferably employing continuous shortwave or other deep-heating modality). There are a broad range of other modalities with limited supportive evidence, but whichever approach is employed, utilization of the modality alongside an exercise program (rather than as a replacement for it) is the most appropriate approach.

Subacromial pain syndrome (rotator cuff-related shoulder pain)

Over recent decades, multiple EPA-based interventions have been employed as a management option for this clinical presentation. In the more recent literature, laser-based therapies (photobiomodulation) and shockwave (both radial and focused) have garnered most attention. Historically, ultrasound was widely employed, but given the nature of the underlying tissue problem, it is unlikely to achieve significant clinical benefit.[61,64] This has been confirmed by clinical trials[10,17,43,70] and reviews.[43,50] It remains possible that with adequate treatment doses, sufficient energy can be delivered to enable a clinical benefit.[71]

Shockwave therapy: radial vs. focused

Shockwave is a relatively new treatment option amongst EPAs for shoulder problems. It has an established role in the management of tendinopathy, but several trials have attempted to evaluate its clinical value in subacromial pain syndrome. Kvalvaag et al.[38,39] conducted a double-blind RCT involving 143 people, employing a radial shockwave versus sham treatment, combined with a supervised exercise program. Shockwave was delivered once weekly over four sessions. Using the Shoulder Pain and Disability Index (SAPDI) as a primary outcome, both groups demonstrated significant improvement at 24 weeks, but there was no effective difference between the shockwave and sham group results. The situation was unchanged at one year. Interestingly, a subgroup of patients presenting with calcification in the rotator cuff did demonstrate significant improvement in SPADI scores. The application of shockwave for patients with tendon calcification is considered elsewhere in this chapter. The effect of radial shockwave on subacromial syndromes does not appear to merit evidenced support.

Circi et al.[13] conducted a study of shockwave in a group of 30 people with subacromial pain syndrome. All received shockwave that was focused to the subacromial space delivering 0.12 mJ/mm2 utilizing 1500 shocks once weekly for three sessions. Three groups were compared, all receiving the same focused shockwave treatment, with the difference in groups being their acromial morphology. A significant improvement in pain and disability (measured by the SPADI) was demonstrated and maintained at the 12-week follow up. There was no significant difference between acromial morphology groups – the treatment was equally effective. Focused shockwave appears therefore to have a beneficial outcome in this condition.

Focused shockwave was investigated by Santamato et al.[49] in which focused shockwave alone was compared with a combined shockwave and isokinetic exercise program in 30 people. Shockwave was delivered in three sessions over 10 days (700 shocks, focused on the supraspinatus distal attachment). The patients in the combined groups also received 10 exercise sessions. Both groups demonstrated a significant improvement in pain at the end of the treatment period, but at two months post treatment, those in the combined shockwave and exercise group demonstrated a significant advantage over those in the shockwave only allocation. Constant-Murley scores similarly reflected significant improvement in both groups at the end of treatment and significant advantage to the combined group at the follow up period. The patients in the combined therapy group received more therapist contact than those in the shockwave only group – a potential confounder, the effect of which cannot be disaggregated from the overall results based on this methodology.

Li et al.[42] compared the two different shockwave applications in a group of 46 patients with non-calcific rotator cuff tendinopathy. Each received 4 sessions with 3000 shocks delivered, with pain and function constituting primary outcomes. Both treatments were shown to be significantly beneficial, though with longer-term benefits (>24 weeks) in the focused group outranking those from the radial group.

In a survey of systematic reviews, Pieters et al.[47] concluded that there was insufficient evidence to support the use of shockwave. The authors made no differentiation between focused and radial shockwave trials: thus when all are combined there was no overall support, but when radial and focused applications are differentiated, there is sufficient evidence to support the use of focused shockwave. The application of shockwave in subacromial syndromes would appear to be of significant benefit if: 1) it is combined with an exercise program, and 2) a focused shockwave application is employed.

Laser therapy

Laser therapy has been widely used in subacromial pain syndrome. The Pieters et al. review[47] did not find evidence to support its use as a monotherapy; however, like other EPA interventions, laser is not designed to be a monotherapy: its potential value is as an adjunct to an exercise program and alongside other therapeutic interventions. The addition of laser therapy to an exercise schedule, for example (i.e., not a monotherapy), was evaluated by Abrisham et al.[1] They demonstrated that the exercise program alone generated significant clinical benefit. The addition of the laser therapy, however, provided added value in pain reduction and improved movement.

Laser therapy was directly compared with shockwave therapy in an RCT with 71 patients.[6] Both treatments positively influenced pain and function scores in the short to medium term, though the shockwave group demonstrated an advantage over the laser group. The treatments (both groups) were integrated with an exercise program, providing further evidence that the use of these modalities as part of a therapy package is the most productive approach. This was confirmed by Alfredo et al.[3] in their three group RCT in which patients either received laser alone, exercise alone, or laser and exercise in combination. Adding the laser therapy (904 nm; 700 Hz delivering 27 J per treatment) to the exercise program provided significant additional benefit on multiple outcomes. The potential short- to medium-term nature of the added gains with laser were confirmed by Awotidebe et al.[5] who, in their review and meta-analysis, acknowledged significant short-term benefits but identified a lack of longer-term gains. The total number of patients included was 585 but the individual studies had small numbers of participants, and of the 11 studies, eight related to the use of laser in subacromial pain syndrome. Short-term benefits for low power laser were demonstrated for pain when used as an adjunct to an exercise program.

The use of high-powered laser is sometimes promoted as an advantageous application over typical low-level laser therapy. A recent evaluation of high-intensity laser therapy in subacromial pain syndrome[2] compared with a sham treatment failed to demonstrate clinical benefit. As identified in the introductory part of this chapter, there is a clearly evidenced dose–effect relationship with laser applications, and the energy delivered in this trial (some 300 J/cm^2) may have exceeded the optimal level for this condition.

Awotidebe et al.[5] included one paper[25] which investigated people diagnosed with rotator cuff-related shoulder pain (RCRSP) in which a significant benefit of adding laser therapy (830 nm; 4 J/cm^2) to an exercise program was reported. Reviews[7,30,45] provided limited support for the use of laser-based therapies, though the additional clinical benefit for people with RCRSP is not strongly and unequivocally shown.

Shockwave-based therapies for RCRSP has diminished the benefits that can be achieved with laser-based therapies.[1] Given a choice of optimal EPA applications in subacromial pain syndrome/RCRSP, and looking for improvement beyond simple pain relief, both shockwave and laser have supportive evidence. Of the two, shockwave application is more likely to generate clinically significant benefits over a longer time frame. The shockwave should be delivered in focused mode for optimal benefit. Whichever is utilized, its integration with exercise and a comprehensive treatment program is essential for optimal outcome.

Rotator cuff calcific tendinopathy

Shockwave therapy: radial vs. focused

Hawk et al.[30] reviewed treatment options in calcific tendinitis lesions: high-energy shockwave was clearly and significantly supported, with benefits being evident at follow up (through to six months). Radial shockwave application was not supported in this condition. In a Cochrane review which specifically evaluated the effects of shockwave for rotator cuff disease (both calcific and non-calcific groups), Surace et al.[56] analyzed 32 studies, of which 25 studies involved patients with calcific deposits. The reviewers did not identify clinically important changes in either patient subgroup but did acknowledge that a wide range of shockwave doses were employed in these trials, and that their failure to reach a definitive conclusion could be a dose-mediated effect – expressed, but not included in the analysis. The calcific and non-calcific patient subgroups appeared to respond to shockwave equally, though using pain as a primary outcome appears inconsistent with the aim of shockwave treatment which is not pain-focused.[19]

Simpson et al.[53] also reviewed nonsurgical interventions for calcific rotator cuff lesions (18 studies). Shockwave, ultrasound, iontophoresis, and TENS were the EPAs included in their analysis, with high-energy shockwave being most strongly supported, albeit with moderate level evidence. Wu et al.[68] took the subgroup analysis methodology one step further and divided their patients into one non-calcific and two different calcific groups. The patients presenting with type II and type III translucent calcified tendinosis (Gartner and Heyer classification) responded most strongly to this therapy.

Table 33.1 Electrophysiological agents for musculoskeletal shoulder conditions

Condition	Modality	Dose	Frequency and duration of treatment
Pain relief	TENS[14,28,44]	Conventional 100 Hz; 200 μs pulse Strong sensory level	20 min (minimum) 3 x weekly minimum (Home treatment option can be employed daily)
	Interferential[11,28]	80–120 Hz sweep Strong sensory level	20 min (minimum) 3 x weekly; 4 weeks (Home treatment option can be employed daily)
Frozen shoulder/ adhesive capsulitis	Deep heating (shortwave)[41,44]	Anterior-posterior electrodes Intensity up to subjective comfortable heat	20 minutes 3 x weekly, 4 weeks
	Laser (photobiomodulation)[44,55]	810 nm 60 mW continuous 3.6 J/cm^2 Multi-point application (painful points – up to 8)	30 sec per point 1–2 x weekly Up to 12 sessions
Subacromial pain syndrome/RCRSP	Laser (photobiomodulation)[1]	890 nm Pulsed (80–1500 Hz) 2–4 J/cm^2 3 point application	6 min (2 min per point) 10 sessions (daily) over 2 weeks
	Shockwave (focused)[13]	1500 shocks 0.12 mJ/mm^2 Subacromial focus	1 x weekly for 3 weeks
Rotator cuff calcific tendinopathy	Shockwave (focused)[53]	1000–2000 shocks per session Apply at point of maximal tenderness Intensity up to patient tolerance (typically 0.2-0.35 mJ/mm^2	Sessions at 1 x weekly intervals Typically 3–5 sessions
	High-intensity ultrasound[21]	0.89 MHz 2.5 W/cm^2 Pulse 1:4 (20% duty cycle)	Up to 24 sessions have been applied safely and effectively

RCRSP, rotator cuff-related shoulder pain.

Mirroring studies in other sections of this chapter, Duymaz and Sindel[18] compared a group of patients receiving conventional therapy (ultrasound, TENS, exercise, and ice) with a group who additionally received radial shockwave. The adoption of this "conventional therapy" package may be unconventional in some healthcare systems, but the salient issue for this trial was whether adding radial shockwave to the package achieved any additional benefit. Eighty patients with persistent calcific rotator cuff tendinopathy were recruited. Both groups demonstrated significant benefit from the treatment package, but those in the combined shockwave and conventional therapy group were significantly advantaged (pain, movement, function, quality of life). The result does not devalue the conventional therapy offered: patients who additionally received radial shockwave therapy were provided with a significant advantage.

Ultrasound

Ultrasound has been employed to reduce the calcification volume in this patient group, e.g., Ebenbichler et al.,[21, 22] utilizing what many would consider high-dose applications (2.5 W/cm^2 or more) with significant benefit achieved. These results were reflected in similar studies by Shomoto et al.[52] and Rahman et al.[48] High-dose ultrasound applications may therefore constitute a valid treatment option when tissue calcification is a primary concern.

Utilizing EPA therapies

The decision to use EPAs in the management of musculoskeletal shoulder pain is based on a thorough understanding of the research, clinical reasoning, harms, and expected benefits, as well as shared decision-making. As such, it is not possible to provide a formula for using EPAs for each condition. People and their symptoms are all different, as are their values and beliefs, and so using EPAs must be placed in the context of many interwoven factors. Table 33.1 provides as a summary based on the synthesis of literature in this chapter, and should not be seen as a prescription for using EPAs. For clinicians and patients who wish to incorporate EPAs in management of musculoskeletal shoulder conditions, this summary may be used to help guide choice of modality and application. The suggestions will change as new knowledge and understanding becomes available.

Conclusion

While various EPAs have been employed as treatment options in shoulder presentations, the current best evidence identifies a limited number that may be currently considered as both evidence-based and achieving a clinical benefit of sufficient magnitude to justify their inclusion in a therapy treatment package. It is essential to use these modalities alongside a carefully constructed exercise and manual therapy program: in isolation, the value of EPAs is neither evidenced nor justified. Incorporated judiciously into care programs, making an evidence-based selection of optimal modality and doses is of maximal benefit to people seeking care for musculoskeletal shoulder problems.

References

1. Abrisham SM, Kermani-Alghoraishi M, Ghahramani R, Jabbari L, Jomeh H, Zare M. Additive effects of low-level laser therapy with exercise on subacromial syndrome: a randomised, double-blind, controlled trial. Clinical Rheumatology. 2011;30:1341-1346.
2. Aceituno-Gomez J, Avendano-Coy J, Gomez-Soriano J, et al. Efficacy of high-intensity laser therapy in subacromial impingement syndrome: a three-month follow-up controlled clinical trial. Clin Rehabil. 2019;33:894-903.
3. Alfredo PP, Junior WS, Casarotto RA. Efficacy of continuous and pulsed therapeutic ultrasound combined with exercises for knee osteoarthritis: a randomized controlled trial. Clin Rehabil. 2020;34:480-490.
4. Alptekin HK, Aydin T, Iflazoglu ES, Alkan M. Evaluating the effectiveness of frozen shoulder treatment on the right and left sides. Journal of Physical Therapy Science. 2016;28:207-212.
5. Awotidebe AW, Inglis-Jassiem G, Young T. Does low-level laser therapy provide additional benefits to exercise in patients with shoulder musculoskeletal disorders? A meta-analysis of randomised controlled trials. Ortopedia, Traumatologia, Rehabilitacja. 2019;21:407-416.
6. Badıl Güloğlu S. Comparison of low-level laser treatment and extracorporeal shock wave therapy in subacromial impingement syndrome: a randomized, prospective clinical study. Lasers in Medical Science. 2021;36:773–781.
7. Beutler A. Musculoskeletal therapies: adjunctive physical therapy. FP Essent. 2018;470:16-20.
8. Bjordal J, Couppe. C, Ljunggren AE. Low level laser therapy for tendinopathy: evidence of a dose-response pattern. Phys Ther Reviews. 2001;6:91-99.
9. Bjordal JM, Johnson MI, Iversen V, Aimbire F, Lopes-Martins RA. Low-level laser therapy in acute pain: a systematic review of possible mechanisms of action and clinical effects in randomized placebo-controlled trials. Photomedicine and Laser Surgery. 2006;24:158-168.
10. Celik D, Atalar AC, Sahinkaya S, Demirhan M. The value of intermittent ultrasound treatment in subacromial impingement syndrome. Acta Orthopaedica et Traumatologica Turcica. 2009;43:243-247.
11. Cheing GL, So EM, Chao CY. Effectiveness of electroacupuncture and interferential electrotherapy in the management of frozen shoulder. Journal of Rehabilitation Medicine. 2008;40:166-170.
12. Chow R, Liebert A, Tilley S, Bennett G, Gabel CP, Laakso L. Guidelines versus evidence: what we can learn from the Australian guideline for low-level laser therapy in knee osteoarthritis? A narrative review. Lasers in Medical Science. 2021;36:249–258.
13. Circi E, Okur SC, Aksu O, Mumcuoglu E, Tuzuner T, Caglar N. The effectiveness of extracorporeal shockwave treatment in

subacromial impingement syndrome and its relation with acromion morphology. Acta Orthopaedica et Traumatologica Turcica. 2018;52:17-21.

14. Dewan A, Sharma R. Effectiveness of transcutaneous electrical nerve stimulation and interferential electrotherapy in adhesive capsulitis. Pb J Orthop. 2011;12:64-71.

15. Dion S, Wong JJ, Cote P, et al. Are passive physical modalities effective for the management of common soft tissue injuries of the elbow? A systematic review by the Ontario Protocol for Traffic Injury Management (OPTIMa) Collaboration. Clin J Pain. 2017;33:71-86.

16. Dogru H, Basaran S, Sarpel T. Effectiveness of therapeutic ultrasound in adhesive capsulitis. Joint Bone Spine. 2008;75:445-450.

17. Downing DS, Weinstein A. Ultrasound therapy of subacromial bursitis. A double blind trial. Physical therapy. 1986;66:194-199.

18. Duymaz T, Sindel D. Comparison of radial extracorporeal shock wave therapy and traditional physiotherapy in rotator cuff calcific tendinitis treatment. Archives of Rheumatology. 2019;34:281-287.

19. Eaton C, Watson T. Shockwave. In: Watson T, Nussbaum E (eds). Electro Physical Agents: Evidence-Based Practice, 13th edition. Elsevier Health Sciences; 2020:229-246.

20. Ebadi S, Forogh B, Fallah E, Babaei Ghazani A. Does ultrasound therapy add to the effects of exercise and mobilization in frozen shoulder? A pilot randomized double-blind clinical trial. J Bodyw Mov Ther. 2017;21:781-787.

21. Ebenbichler GR, Erdogmus CB, Resch KL, et al. Ultrasound therapy for calcific tendinitis of the shoulder. N-Engl-J-Med. 1999;340:1533-1538.

22. Ebenbichler GR, Erdogmus CB, Resch KL, et al. Ultrasound therapy for calcific tendinitis of the shoulder. Orthop-Div-Rev. 2002;2002:11-17.

23. Echternach JL. Ultrasound: an adjunct treatment for shoulder disabilities. Physical Therapy. 1965;45:865-869.

24. Elhafez HM, Elhafez SM. Axillary ultrasound and laser combined with postisometric facilitation in treatment of shoulder adhesive capsulitis: a randomized clinical trial. J Manipulative Physiol Ther. 2016;39:330-338.

25. Eslamian F, Shakouri SK, Ghojazadeh M, Nobari OE, Eftekharsadat B. Effects of low-level laser therapy in combination with physiotherapy in the management of rotator cuff tendinitis. Lasers in Medical Science. 2012;27:951-958.

26. Finfter O, Avni B, Grisariu S, et al. Photobiomodulation (low-level laser) therapy for immediate pain relief of persistent oral ulcers in chronic graft-versus-host disease. Support Care Cancer. 2021;29:4529-4534.

27. Foster RL, O'Driscoll M-L. Current concepts in the conservative management of the frozen shoulder. Physical Therapy Reviews. 2010;15:399-404.

28. Gunay Ucurum S, Kaya DO, Kayali Y, Askin A, Tekindal MA. Comparison of different electrotherapy methods and exercise therapy in shoulder impingement syndrome: a prospective randomized controlled trial. Acta Orthopaedica et Traumatologica Turcica. 2018;52:249-255.

29. Haik MN, Alburquerque-Sendin F, Moreira RF, Pires ED, Camargo PR. Effectiveness of physical therapy treatment of clearly defined subacromial pain: a systematic review of randomised controlled trials. Br J Sports Med. 2016;50:1124-1134.

30. Hawk C, Minkalis AL, Khorsan R, et al. Systematic review of nondrug, nonsurgical treatment of shoulder conditions. J Manipulative Physiol Ther. 2017;40:293-319.

31. Hurley ET, Maye AB, Thompson K, et al. Pain control after shoulder arthroscopy: a systematic review of randomized controlled trials with a network meta-analysis. Am J Sports Med. 2020;0363546520971757.

32. Jain TK, Sharma NK. The effectiveness of physiotherapeutic interventions in treatment of frozen shoulder/adhesive capsulitis: a systematic review. Journal of Back and Musculoskeletal Rehabilitation. 2014;27:247-273.

33. Johnson MI. Pain management and clinical effectiveness of TENS. Critical Reviews in Physical and Rehabilitation Medicine. 2017;29:228-246.

34. Johnson MI. Transcutaneous electrical nerve stimulation (TENS). In: Watson T, Nussbaum E (eds). Electro Physical Agents: Evidence-Based Practice, 13th edition. Elsevier Health Sciences; 2020:264-295.

35. Johnson MI. Transcutaneous Electrical Nerve Stimulation (TENS). Research to Support Clinical Practice. Oxford University Press; 2014.

36. Kashyap K, Singh V, Mishra S, Dwivedi SN, Bhatnagar S. The efficacy of scrambler therapy for the management of head, neck and thoracic cancer pain: a randomized controlled trial. Pain Physician. 2020;23:495-506.

37. Kim G-W, Won YH, Park S-H, et al. Effects of a newly developed therapeutic deep heating device using high frequency in patients with shoulder pain and disability: a pilot study. Pain Research and Management. 2019;2019:9.

38. Kvalvaag E, Brox JI, Engebretsen KB, et al. Effectiveness of radial extracorporeal shock wave therapy (rESWT) when combined with supervised exercises in patients with subacromial shoulder pain: a double-masked, randomized, sham-controlled trial. Am J Sports Med. 2017;45:2547-2554.

39. Kvalvaag E, Roe C, Engebretsen KB, et al. One year results of a randomized controlled trial on radial extracorporeal shock wave treatment, with predictors of pain, disability and return to work in patients with subacromial pain syndrome. European Journal of Physical and Rehabilitation Medicine. 2018;54:341-350.

40. Lee SH, Yeh SC, Chan RC, Chen S, Yang G, Zheng LR. Motor ingredients derived from a wearable sensor-based virtual reality system for frozen shoulder rehabilitation. BioMed Research International. 2016;2016:7075464.

41. Leung MS, Cheing GL. Effects of deep and superficial heating in the management of frozen shoulder. Journal of Rehabilitation Medicine. 2008;40:145-150.

42. Li C, Li Z, Shi L, Wang P, Gao F, Sun W. Effectiveness of focused shockwave therapy versus radial shockwave therapy for noncalcific rotator cuff tendinopathies: a randomized clinical trial. BioMed Research International. 2021;2021:6687094.

43. Michener LA, Walsworth MK, Burnet EN. Effectiveness of rehabilitation for patients with subacromial impingement syndrome: a systematic review. J Hand Ther. 2004;17:152-164.

44. Page MJ, Green S, Kramer S, Johnston RV, McBain B, Buchbinder R. Electrotherapy modalities for adhesive capsulitis (frozen shoulder). Cochrane Reviews. 2014:CD011324.

45. Page MJ, Green S, Mrocki MA, et al. Electrotherapy modalities for rotator cuff disease. Cochrane Reviews. 2016:CD012225.

46. Pasin T, Ataoglu S, Pasin O, Ankarali H. Comparison of the effectiveness of platelet-rich plasma, corticosteroid, and physical therapy in subacromial impingement syndrome. Archives of Rheumatology. 2019;34:308-316.

47. Pieters L, Lewis J, Kuppens K, et al. An update of systematic reviews examining the effectiveness of conservative physical therapy interventions for subacromial shoulder pain. The Journal of Orthopaedic and Sports Physical Therapy. 2020;50:131-141.

48. Rahman MH, Khan SZ, Ramiz MS. Effect of therapeutic ultrasound on calcific supraspinatus tendinitis. Mymensingh Med J. 2007;16:33-35.

49. Santamato A, Panza F, Notarnicola A, et al. Is extracorporeal shockwave therapy combined with isokinetic exercise more effective than extracorporeal shockwave therapy alone for subacromial impingement syndrome? A randomized clinical trial. The Journal of Orthopaedic and Sports Physical Therapy. 2016;46:714-725.

50. Sauers EL. Effectiveness of rehabilitation for patients with subacromial impingement syndrome. J Athlet Train. 2005;40:221-223.

51. Shah S, Farrow A, Esnouf A. Availability and use of electrotherapy devices: a survey. Int J Ther Rehabil. 2007;14:260-264.

52. Shomoto K, Takatori K, Morishita S, et al. Effects of ultrasound therapy on calcificated tendinitis of the shoulder. Journal of the Japanese Physical Therapy Association. 2002;5:7-11.

53. Simpson M, Pizzari T, Cook T, Wildman S, Lewis J. Effectiveness of non-surgical interventions for rotator cuff calcific tendinopathy: A systematic review. Journal of Rehabilitation Medicine. 2020;10.2340/16501977-2725.

54. Sluka KA, Bjordal JM, Marchand S, Rakel BA. What makes transcutaneous electrical nerve stimulation work? Making Sense of the mixed results in the clinical literature. Physical Therapy. 2013;93:1397-1402.

55. Stergioulas A. Low-power laser treatment in patients with frozen shoulder: preliminary results. Photomed Laser Surg. 2008;26:99-105.

56. Surace SJ, Deitch J, Johnston RV, Buchbinder R. Shock wave therapy for rotator cuff disease with or without calcification. Cochrane Reviews. 2020:CD008962.

57. Tashiro Y, Suzuki Y, Nakayama Y, et al. The effect of capacitive and resistive electric transfer on non-specific chronic low back pain. Electromagn Biol Med. 2020;1-8.

58. Thu AC, Kwak SG, Shein WN, Htun M, Htwe TTH, Chang MC. Comparison of ultrasound-guided platelet-rich plasma injection and conventional physical therapy for management of adhesive capsulitis: a randomized trial. J Int Med Res. 2020;48:300060520976032.

59. Vance CG, Dailey DL, Rakel BA, Sluka KA. Using TENS for pain control: the state of the evidence. Pain Manag. 2014;4:197-209.

60. Vrouva S, Batistaki C, Paraskevaidou E, et al. Comparative study of pain relief in two non-pharmacological treatments in patients with partial rotator cuff tears: a randomized trial. Anesthesiology and Pain Medicine. 2019;9:e88327.

61. Watson T. Electrophysical agents: physiology and evidence. In: Porter S, Wilson J (eds). A Comprehensive Guide to Sports Physiology and Injury Management. Elsevier; 2021:63-77.

62. Watson T. Expanding our understanding of the inflammatory process and its role in pain & tissue healing. IFOMPT 2016; Glasgow.

63. Watson T. Narrative review: key concepts with electrophysical agents. Physical Therapy Reviews. 2010;15:351-359.

64. Watson T. Ultrasound. In: Watson T, Nussbaum E (eds). Electro Physical Agents: Evidence-Based Practice, 13th edition. Elsevier Health Sciences; 2020:25.

65. Watson T, Nussbaum E. Electro Physical Agents: Evidence-Based Practice, 13th edition. Elsevier Health Sciences; 2020.

66. Waugh CM, Morrissey D, Jones E, Riley GP, Langberg H, Screen HR. In vivo biological response to extracorporeal shockwave therapy in human tendinopathy. European Cells & Materials. 2015;29:268-280.

67. Wong JJ, Shearer HM, Mior S, et al. Are manual therapies, passive physical modalities, or acupuncture effective for the management of patients with whiplash-associated disorders or neck pain and associated disorders? An update of the Bone and Joint Decade Task Force on Neck Pain and Its Associated Disorders by the OPTIMa collaboration. Spine J. 2016;16:1598-1630.

68. Wu KT, Chou WY, Wang CJ, et al. Efficacy of extracorporeal shockwave therapy on calcified and noncalcified shoulder tendinosis: a propensity score matched analysis. BioMed Research International. 2019;2019:2958251.

69. Xu M, Wang L, Wu S, et al. Review on experimental study and clinical application of low-intensity pulsed ultrasound in inflammation. Quant Imaging Med Surg. 2021;11:443-462.

70. Yazmalar L, Sariyildiz MA, Batmaz I, et al. Efficiency of therapeutic ultrasound on pain, disability, anxiety, depression, sleep and quality of life in patients with subacromial impingement syndrome: a randomized controlled study. Journal of Back and Musculoskeletal Rehabilitation. 2016;29:801-807.

71. Yildirim MA, Ones K, Celik EC. Comparision of ultrasound therapy of various durations in the treatment of subacromial impingement syndrome. Journal of Physical Therapy Science. 2013;25:1151-1154.

72. Yu H, Cote P, Shearer HM, et al. Effectiveness of passive physical modalities for shoulder pain: systematic review by the Ontario protocol for traffic injury management collaboration. Physical Therapy. 2015;95:306-318.

73. Zhang J, Zhong S, Tan T, et al. Comparative efficacy and patient-specific moderating factors of nonsurgical treatment strategies for frozen shoulder: an updated systematic review and network meta-analysis. Am J Sports Med. 2020;363546520956293.

74. Zhou M, Li F, Lu W, Wu J, Pei S. Efficiency of neuromuscular electrical stimulation and transcutaneous nerve stimulation on hemiplegic shoulder pain: a randomized controlled trial. Archives of Physical Medicine and Rehabilitation. 2018;99:1730-1739.

Bracing and taping in the management of shoulder conditions

34

Jenny McConnell, César Fernández-de-las-Peñas

Introduction

Shoulder bracing and taping techniques are used by clinicians to help improve movement and stability around the shoulder. Clinicians need to use their clinical reasoning skills when deciding whether bracing or taping is warranted, and what type of brace or tape technique should be applied. They should then assess and review the effectiveness of the application. The uses and effectiveness of braces and taping will be discussed in this chapter.

Bracing

Shoulder bracing is often used to stabilize and protect the shoulder after dislocation and surgery. However, use of braces that are rigid or contain clasps or buckles for attachment are not permitted in many close contact sports, as these braces may inadvertently injure other players on the court or field, so the clinician needs to be aware of the requirements of the sport before a brace is suggested for an athlete.

Problem areas when using shoulder braces include poor fit and range of motion restriction, resulting in poor compliance.[30] Grubhofer et al.[13] found that 50% of patients did not wear the prescribed post-operative shoulder brace at least 80% of the recommended time. They evaluated 50 people who had undergone rotator cuff surgery whose shoulder abduction braces were fitted with a temperature sensor. At six weeks post-surgery, patients reported the number of hours they had worn the brace. The patient-reported and sensor data were compared, and the compliance rate (relative to the recommended wearing time) was determined, with compliance being evaluated and the discrepancy between the measured and patient-reported wear time being assessed. Self-reported compliance was significantly lower than sensor-based compliance. These authors concluded that the use of shoulder abduction braces postoperatively was questionable, as the patient's adherence to the wearing of the brace was low and the self-reported wearing compliance was unreliable.[13]

The evidence for the effectiveness of braces is mixed. Kwapisz et al.[18] found that in adolescent athletes with shoulder instability treated nonoperatively, functional bracing did not result in increased success rates when compared with no bracing. These authors followed 97 athletes for a minimum of 12 months, 21% were braced and 79% were not braced. A successful outcome was defined as the athlete completing the current season and one subsequent season without surgery or time lost from shoulder injury. Braced athletes returned to play 80% of the time, while non-braced athletes returned at a rate of 88%. Of the braced players, the majority were American football players, but a football-only comparison demonstrated no difference between braced failures (26%) and non-braced failures (16%).[18]

Whelan et al.[45] reported that after primary anterior shoulder dislocation, a four-week immobilization in external rotation did not confer any significant benefit versus sling immobilization in the prevention of recurrent instability. Re-dislocation rates were 37% with the external rotation brace versus 40% with the sling.[45] Tirefort et al.[42] found that no immobilization after rotator cuff repair was associated with better early mobility and functional scores in comparison with sling immobilization. They concluded that postoperative immobilization with a sling may not be required for patients treated for a small or medium rotator cuff tear.[42]

Baker et al.[3] reported that wearing a shoulder-stabilizing brace did not prevent posterior labral tears in American footballers, although the brace did reduce the time lost to injury. They concluded that wearing a shoulder brace could possibly provide a protective factor for the shoulder for athletes playing American football.[3] In contrast, Dellabiancia et al.[10] found in patients with anterior traumatic instability awaiting arthroscopic glenohumeral stabilization, that a novel glenohumeral joint immobilizer, the S2 Shoulder Stabilizer®, significantly limited joint excursion in all planes of movement except internal rotation. The brace also limited humeral head translation, but this study was conducted in a controlled laboratory environment using a Vicon motion capture system, rather than a real-world setting. Chu et al.[7] reported that wearing a shoulder brace improved the accuracy of active joint repositioning at 10° from full external rotation, in a group of individuals with unstable shoulders. The group with unstable shoulders demonstrated significantly less full external rotation than did those with stable shoulders, but the brace only reduced full external rotation for those with stable shoulders, not those with unstable shoulders.[7]

Patients with round shoulder posture (RSP), which is considered by some as a potential risk factor for shoulder impingement syndrome (SIS) showed increased muscle activity in the lower trapezius and serratus anterior as well as improved scapular positioning with a shoulder brace with a forced tension diagonal strap alignment.[6] However, in a group of asymptomatic individuals with forward-head, rounded-shoulder posture (FHRSP), the application of the scapular brace improved shoulder posture and scapular muscle activity, but the EMG changes were highly variable, so the authors were less definitive about the effectiveness of a scapular brace in symptomatic individuals.[8]

Shoulder taping

Taping is a useful adjunct to physical therapy management of the shoulder, as it allows a potential continuation of the treatment effect long after the patient leaves the clinic. In the literature, the reports on the effectiveness of tape, whether using elasticized or rigid tape, are varied,[5,9,12,22,32,47] but this may be in part due to a "one size fits all" approach in research. Whereas in clinical practice, after a thorough examination of the patient, the clinician may determine if taping is appropriate and, if so, which taping technique is best to achieve the desired outcome.

The prime reason for using tape in the management of people with shoulder pain is to relieve or aid in decreasing a patient's symptoms. If the symptoms are not relieved by at least 50%, then the clinician should consider whether:

- the tape positioning was correct;
- the tape application was poor: too much tension, resulting in skin breakdown, or not enough tension, resulting in taping that is ineffective and may as well not be there;
- the shoulder was not in an appropriate position when the tape was applied;
- the choice of tape technique was appropriate;
- the choice of tape was not appropriate for that patient;
- taping is appropriate for that patient.

Slings and braces are used clinically to unload tissues and reduce pain. Taping may also be used for the same purpose, as it may influence load distribution, which in turn may reduce symptoms and improve function. Taping is not a standalone treatment, and as such, is a technique to be considered within a package of care. If the patient's symptoms are significantly diminished, then compliance with treatment is potentially enhanced. Additionally, tape may be used to facilitate as well as inhibit muscle activity, which can also expedite symptom improvement.

Joint stability is a synergy between passive soft tissues, particularly ligaments, and dynamic contractile tissues, the muscles. The viscoelastic properties of ligaments and their classical responses to static and cyclic loads or movements such as creep, tension-relaxation, hysteresis, and strain rate dependence decreases their effectiveness as joint restraints and stabilizers. When the passive structures have been adversely impacted, muscles can be optimized to minimize adverse joint instability and pain.[36] Taping may achieve this in several possible ways, including optimizing joint position and stability, improving muscle function and performance, as well as providing proprioceptive input.

Tape may influence the effect of creep and adaptive shortening on collagenous tissue. This will be considered in the following section.

Creep and adaptive shortening

Creep

Creep is the tendency of a viscoelastic material to elongate during sustained low load. If the tissue is elongated past its elastic limit or elongated for too long a period, it will not return to its pre-stretched resting length. Creep, particularly of non-contractile tissues such as ligaments, tendons, and capsular tissue, may be responsible for changes in shoulder positioning and changed loading on certain structures. Twenty minutes of sustained static or cyclic loading of lumbar viscoelastic tissues in felines has been shown to cause micro-damage in the collagen structure resulting in a release of pro-inflammatory cytokines and neutrophils, lasting up to eight hours.[37-39]

Three types of creep need to be considered:

1. Primary creep which starts at a rapid rate and slows with time.

2. Secondary creep which has a relatively uniform rate. An example would be the time effect of gravity on shoulder structures causing degenerative tears of the rotator cuff and the long head of biceps. Degenerative rotator cuff tears are common in the older population with the incidence reported as being as high as 50% in people over the age of 60 years, rising to 80% in people older than 80 years.[28] Most individuals are asymptomatic. Symptoms may appear because of an unbalanced tear adversely influencing humeral head control.
3. Tertiary creep, which has an accelerated creep rate and terminates when the tissue ruptures, as would be seen in the anterior and posterior capsular structures, following a shoulder dislocation.

Adaptive shortening

When non-contractile tissue is shortened for a prolonged period (adaptive shortening), the collagen fiber distance decreases, whereas with contractile tissue, the actin and myosin fibers overlap, decreasing the number of sarcomeres so that the muscle belly becomes shorter and stiffer, causing the length–tension curve to change (i.e., shift to the left).[46] Therefore, in some cases, physical therapists (physiotherapists) may have to decrease stress on abnormally strained tissue around the shoulder, whereas in other cases they may need to increase the length of adaptively shortened tissue. Both of which can be accomplished by the judicious use of tape. Kinesio® taping of the shoulder and rigid taping of the scapular region have been shown to change pectoralis minor length, as well as improve scapular dyskinesis in overhead athletes.[29] However, the clinical importance of these observations remains equivocal.

Principles and potential effects of taping

Taping aims

The type of taping the clinician uses in a particular treatment depends on the assessment of the patient's shoulder. The primary aim of tape is to unload pain, as this is the reason most people seek care. A secondary aim is to improve the positioning of the humeral head in the glenoid, as well as improve scapular positioning to minimize scapular dyskinesis. The patient's symptoms must be reassessed after each application of tape. The patient only requires the amount of tape necessary to reduce their symptoms by at least 50%.

Effects of taping on pain

Inflamed and painful tissue may not respond well to movement and being stretched, so one principle of unloading painful tissue is to place it in a shortened position,[16,23] aiming to decrease symptoms. In this situation, the most appropriate tape is likely to be rigid non-stretch tape, as it provides support to the tissue, but still permits joint movement.

Shoulder taping may increase the acromiohumeral distance (AHD), as the AHD in many symptomatic individuals is decreased and the subacromial bursa may be enlarged. Harput et al.[14] reported that Kinesio® taping applied over the scapula increased the AHD, as well as shoulder internal and external rotator (IR-ER) strength and range. These investigators concluded that scapular taping could be used to treat subacromial impingement syndrome (SIS).[14] Bdaiwi et al.[4] reported that applying rigid tape to the scapula in asymptomatic individuals significantly increased AHD at 60° of passive arm abduction. These authors concluded that taping for increasing posterior scapular tilt and increasing scapular upward rotation would be a useful adjunct to rehabilitation in patients with SIS, because of the effect taping had on the AHD.[4] Figure 34.1 demonstrates radiological changes in AHD in a symptomatic subject before and after a glenohumeral taping with rigid tape.

Athletes with rotator cuff (RC) tendinopathy demonstrate a larger AHD with therapeutic taping at 60° of shoulder abduction when compared with no taping.[20] These authors reported that the middle trapezius, lower trapezius, and serratus anterior muscles activated significantly earlier in both therapeutic taping and placebo taping conditions compared with the no taping conditions.[21] They found a small increase in the scapular upward rotation when therapeutic taping and no taping conditions were compared and concluded that scapular taping may enhance the neuromotor control of the scapular muscles.[21] So, perhaps rigid scapular taping changes the activation pattern of the scapular stabilizers, which may decrease the AHD at the beginning of abduction range where impingement is not present, but improves the AHD at 60° where subacromial structures could be compromised and the space becomes more critical.

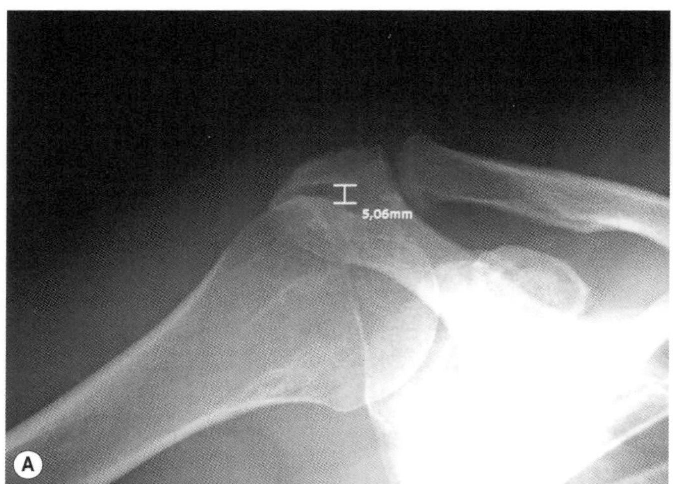

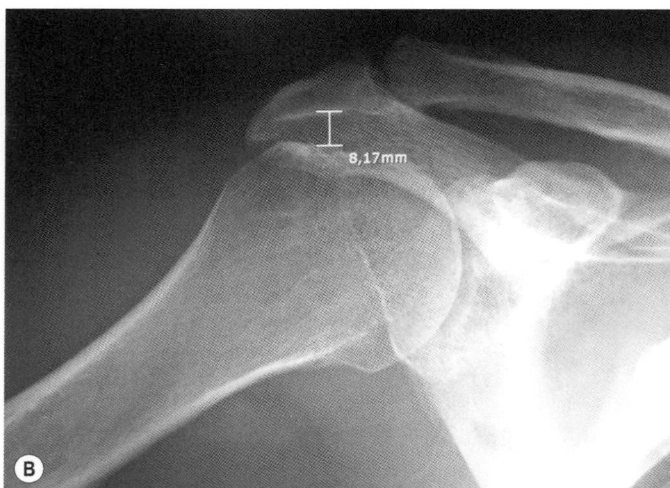

FIGURE 34.1

Radiological changes at 45° abduction after glenohumeral repositioning tape in a 50-year-old male with a grade 2 rotator cuff tear. (A) Pre tape; visual analogue score (VAS) 8/10 for pain and limited to 45° abduction due to pain and weakness. (B) Post tape; VAS 1/10 and full range of movement, slight increase of pain at 130°.

The addition of taping with a therapeutic exercise program is more effective than an exercise program alone for the treatment of subacromial impingement syndrome.[33,40] Teys et al.[40] found that adding tape to mobilization with movement (MWM) techniques when treating people with SIS significantly improved range of motion over a one-week follow-up compared with MWM alone. The benefits of taping are not conclusive, as others have reported Kinesio® taping did not improve shoulder symptoms, particularly in younger individuals.[19,41]

Although the research on the benefits of taping for shoulder symptoms remains far from certain, it may be considered as part of evidence-based care, provided contraindications are considered, and appropriate explanations are provided to patients within a shared decision-making model of care.

Effects of taping on facilitating muscle contraction

If an aim of intervention is to increase muscle activity, then tape should be applied in the direction of the muscle fibers.[27] In this situation, the clinician should consider using a more elastic tape, as it may stimulate the muscle during contraction and stretches with the movement. Research findings are mixed. Alexander et al.[2] demonstrated that application of taping along the length of the lower trapezius (LT) (from insertion to origin) decreased the H-reflex of the muscle. This study was conducted on young and asymptomatic individuals, where possibly the muscle was working more optimally than in symptomatic individuals where scapular dyskinesis may cause shoulder symptoms. Perhaps with asymptomatic individuals, the tape enhances the efficiency of the muscle so fewer motor units are recruited, improving the muscle's fatigue resistance.

The concept of tape enhancing motor performance in the presence of muscle fatigue has been suggested by Weerakkody and Allen[44] in a study involving fast bowlers playing cricket without symptoms. Joint position sense (JPS) errors were found to increase immediately after exercise, whereby taping had no effect on position errors before exercise but did significantly reduce position errors after exercise at mid-range shoulder flexion angles. They concluded that the added cutaneous input from the tape may contribute to shoulder JPS.[44] In contrast, Aarseth et al.[1] reported that shoulder JPS at 90° of elevation was impaired by the application of Kinesio® taping in symptom-free athletes who did not participate in overhead sports. So, perhaps readiness of the motor program when familiar with the overhead activity is important when considering JPS, tape and the fatigue effects of the activity. Further research is required, especially in people with symptoms, to better understand these differences.

Yildiz et al.[47] concluded that scapular upward rotation was increased with taping, while there were inconsistent results concerning scapular external rotation and posterior tilt. Additionally, most studies reported that taping decreased the activity of the upper trapezius (UT) muscle, but there was conflicting evidence on the activity patterns of other periscapular muscles.[47] Intelango et al.[17] found that scapular taping in symptomatic individuals was not effective for inducing electromyographic (EMG) changes in the UT, LT, and serratus anterior (SA) muscles, nor in altering the isometric force of shoulder flexion, abduction and external rotation. Dhein et al.[11] reported that Kinesio® taping caused a reduction in EMG activity in the LT muscle in people diagnosed with SIS. These authors suggested caution when using this tape in this patient group, as the tape may have an adverse effect on scapular kinematics and may increase symptoms.[11]

Rigid taping, which aims to reposition the glenohumeral joint and anchors over the inferior border of the scapula in asymptomatic young individuals, is associated with an earlier onset of UT and LT contractions relative to middle deltoid (MD) during shoulder abduction and flexion, but does not alter corticomotor excitability of the scapular muscles. However, the changes in onset timing are not maintained 24 hours after taping.[35] Snodgrass et al.[35] found that the taping technique led to an immediate increase in shoulder active abduction range of movement. They felt this may be due to the taping technique assisting upward rotation of the scapula through the earlier onset of contraction of the UT and LT. Earlier onset of these muscles may lead to a greater range of scapular upward rotation, but this hypothesis requires verification. The authors suggested that although tape initially changed the relative onset of scapular muscle contractions, additional intervention would be needed to promote lasting changes or changes in corticomotor excitability. They also suggested that the optimal time to engage in rehabilitative exercises to facilitate onset of trapezius muscle contractions during shoulder movements would be immediately after the application of tape.[35]

Effects of taping on inhibiting (minimizing) muscle activity

If the clinician reasons that a decrease in antagonist muscle activity would be helpful in improving the performance of the pain-inhibited agonist muscle, then applying firm tape across the antagonist muscle may be evaluated.[43] Selkowitz et al.[34] reported that rigid taping over the UT, decreased UT activity, and increased LT activity during a functional elevation task, especially above 90° in people diagnosed with SIS. In individuals with asymptomatic scapular dyskinesis, Kinesio® tape over the UT was sufficient to decrease UT activity, but not to change LT activity.[15]

Reynard et al.[31] investigated the effects of Kinesio® tape versus sham tape (ST) and no tape at six and 12 weeks post rotator cuff surgery. They found that Kinesio® tape decreased the recruitment of UT but did not change deltoid or infraspinatus activity. Kinesio® tape and ST increased flexion range of motion at six weeks, but the differences with the no tape condition were not clinically important. They felt that shoulder taping had the potential to decrease overactivity of the UT, but there were no other clinical benefits in using Kinesio® tape on people following rotator cuff surgery.[31]

Efficacy and effectiveness of taping for shoulder pain conditions

Different types of taping and bracing may lead to dissimilar clinical outcomes in people with shoulder pain. The use of tape in people with SIS was reported as having small to moderate standardized mean differences (SMD) (SMD -0.64; 95% CI -1.16 to -0.12) when compared with sham taping.[5] Saracoglu et al. reported low-quality evidence for a positive effect of taping as an adjunct treatment for improvement of pain, disability, range of motion, and muscle strength in individuals with SIS.[32] Overall, current evidence about the isolated use of Kinesio® tape for the management of shoulder pain is conflicting, since the effect sizes have been found to be small.[5] Lim et al. concluded that existing evidence did not establish the superiority of Kinesio® tape to other treatment approaches in reducing pain and disability for individuals with chronic musculoskeletal pain.[22] Ghozy et al. confirmed that Kinesio® tape alone was not effective for decreasing pain and related disability in individuals with shoulder pain when compared with placebo, but it was effective when combined with exercise.[12]

Adverse effects

There are two major skin problems the clinician may encounter when applying tape.

Friction rub

The commonest form of skin irritation is a friction rub, which often presents as a blister. If you are unloading tissues, there can often be considerable tension on the overlying soft tissue. The friction rub can be exacerbated by:

- vigorous application of tape, trying to push the humeral head too far and the clinician not using their thumb to gently lift the patient's humeral head up and back;
- uneven tape tension;
- rapid removal of the tape.

Potential solutions are to:

- take care when applying the tape;
- use the other hand to ease tension off skin when removing tape;
- start at the back and slowly peel the tape off towards the front;
- use eucalyptus oil or tea tree oil over tape before removing it;
- use skin protection, e.g., Comfeel™, calamine lotion, Cutifilm™, Opsite™.

Allergic reaction

An allergic reaction occurs in approximately 5–10% of individuals, and is due to a reaction to either the zinc oxide on the rigid tape or the latex on the elasticized tape. The skin will be raised, red, and itchy. There may be a three-week delay before irritation begins, as the patient may not have been exposed to that allergen before. The patient may have an allergic history, for example asthma, eczema, or hay fever. Potential solutions are to:

- leave tape off and apply cortisone cream if there is a rash;
- prepare the skin, if there is a history of allergy: calamine lotion is particularly good at protecting the skin. It must dry (chalky texture) before applying the tape;
- use hypoallergenic tape alone or you may use two layers of hypoallergenic then rigid tape;
- ask the patient to use oral antihistamines, which will stop the itch and allow you to keep taping if the patient is receiving significant benefit from the tape;
- use Opsite Flexifix™ under the tape.

McConnell taping in the management of musculoskeletal shoulder symptoms

McConnell™ taping is both a clinical system for the application of tape and a specific taping product. McConnell™ taping uses a firm non-elastic, rayon-based tape with a hypoallergenic tape underneath to protect the skin. The McConnell™ tape has a slight stretch in two directions for optimum support. The tape is used, as was discussed earlier, to unload tissue, aiming to decrease pain, so that therapy can be focused on improving function.

Repositioning humeral head

When applying tape aiming to reposition the humeral head, the tape should be applied with the patient in a standing position and their arm relaxed by the side. If the patient is tall, then sitting the patient on a stool with the arm hanging is an option. The clinician uses two pieces of tape: the first aims to lift the anterior aspect of the humeral head up and back, and to externally rotate the humeral head. The tape is anchored on the anterior aspect of the skin overlying the humeral head. The clinician's thumb sits on top of the tape aiming to lift the humeral head up and back, while the tape is tensioned. The tape is anchored on the skin over the inferior angle of the scapula. The second piece of rigid tape is placed on the skin overlying the anterior aspect of the humeral head, is tensioned over the acromial process, and is anchored again on the skin overlying the inferior angle of the scapula (Figure 34.2). This type of taping may be effective for rotator cuff-related shoulder pain, frozen shoulder, and anterior instability.

Taping the glenohumeral joint as previously described has been investigated in people without symptoms. McConnell and McIntosh[24] demonstrated in elite junior tennis players with no history of shoulder injury that "glenohumeral repositioning" tape and not placebo tape (tape applied in the same position without tension), increased the passive range of internal and external rotation of the throwing shoulder, hypothesizing that taping the shoulder improved the anterior shift. However, in a study of elite asymptomatic overhead athletes, where one group had been injured previously and the other group was uninjured, the passive rotation range improved in both groups with tape, but the dynamic external rotation range of the shoulder decreased from 143° to 138° in the previously injured group, and minimally increased from 131° to 135° in the group who had never been injured.[25,26] Taping may have a differential effect on shoulder rotation range depending on whether the athlete had or had not suffered a shoulder injury. The change of 4° is small and would not be detectable in the clinical setting.

In the previously injured group, shoulder taping produced change for myriad reasons, one of which might have been reduction of the anterior translation of the humeral head by altering the muscle activation patterns of the rotator cuff and/or the scapular stabilizers. Small changes in the location of the shoulder joint center potentially might influence the moment-generating capacity of the shoulder muscles. Although taping only produced a 4° change

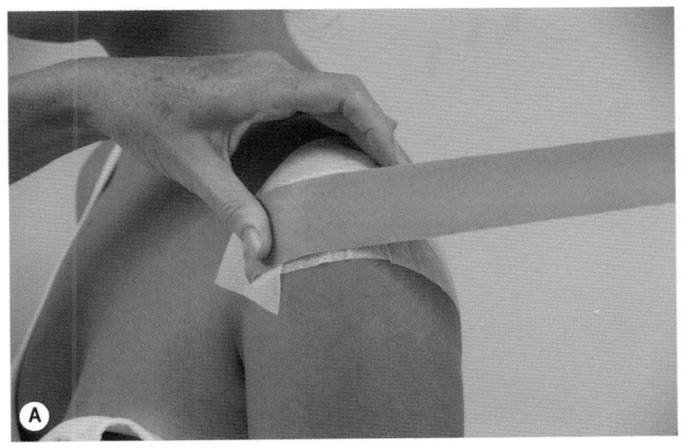

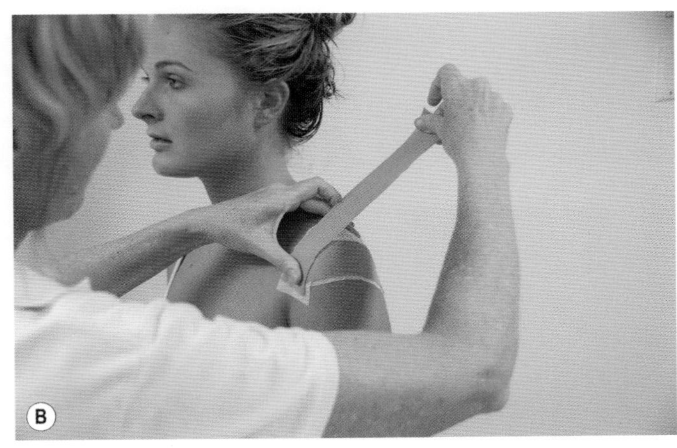

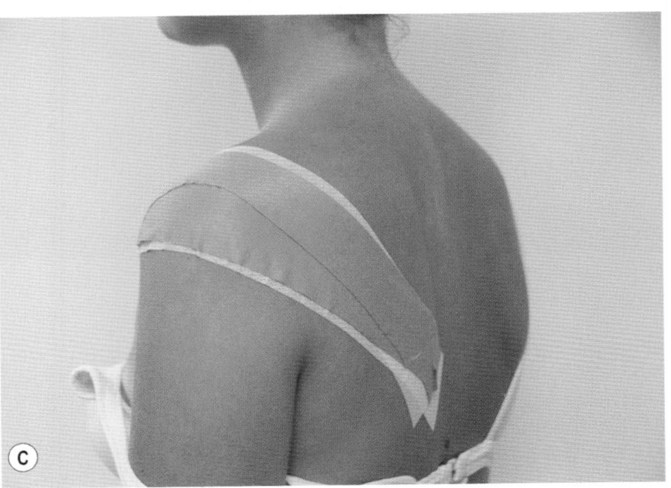

FIGURE 34.2

Glenohumeral repositioning tape. (A) The first tape anchors on the anterior aspect of the humeral head and the therapist gently lifts the humeral head up and back while firmly applying the tape. The tape courses below the acromion. This tape applies an external rotation moment on the humeral head. (B) The second piece of tape starts in a similar position to the first, but this piece of tape goes over the acromial process. Again, the therapist lifts the humeral head up and back; with this piece of tape the therapist is trying to facilitate the 3° of upward displacement of the humeral head that occurs at the beginning of shoulder movement and improves the seating of the humeral head in the glenoid. (C) Both tapes are directed over the scapula and anchor over the inferior angle of the scapula, just short of the spine.

in external rotation range of motion during throwing, this small change in range may have had an influence on the stability and mobility of the shoulder. It is hypothesized that taping may enhance the neuromotor control of the rotator cuff and scapular stabilizing muscles, providing a more stable platform for overhead activity. The fine control of humeral translation may be improved by the specific application of tape, minimizing strain on the anterior structures, and improving the stability of the shoulder.[26] More research is required to investigate these hypotheses further.

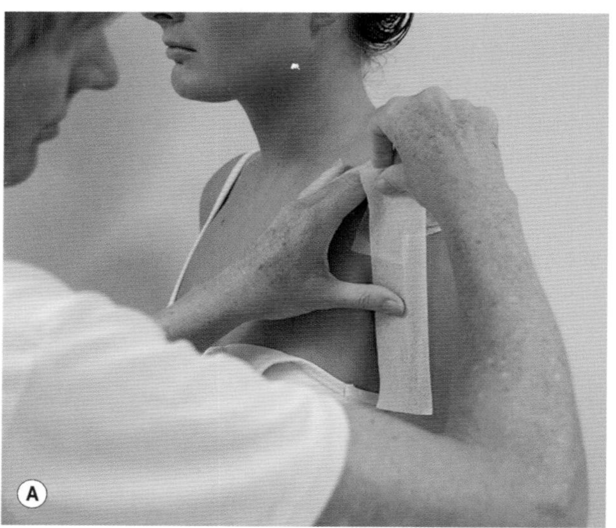

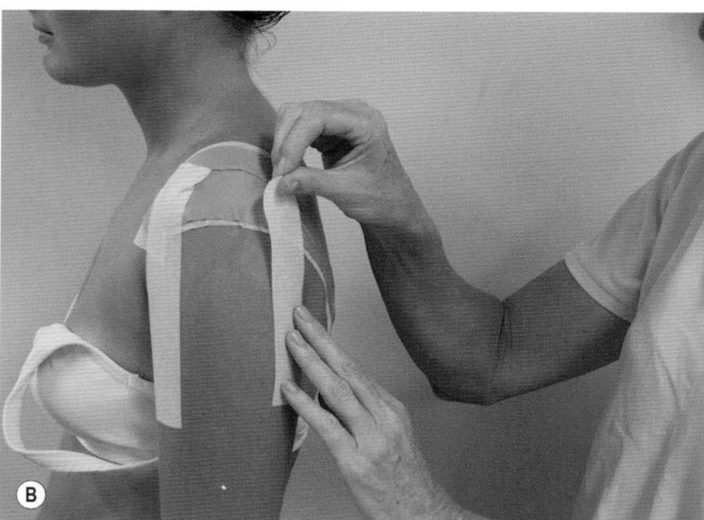

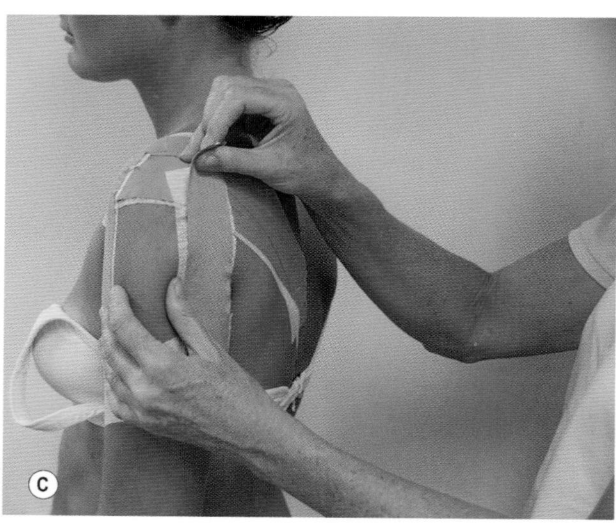

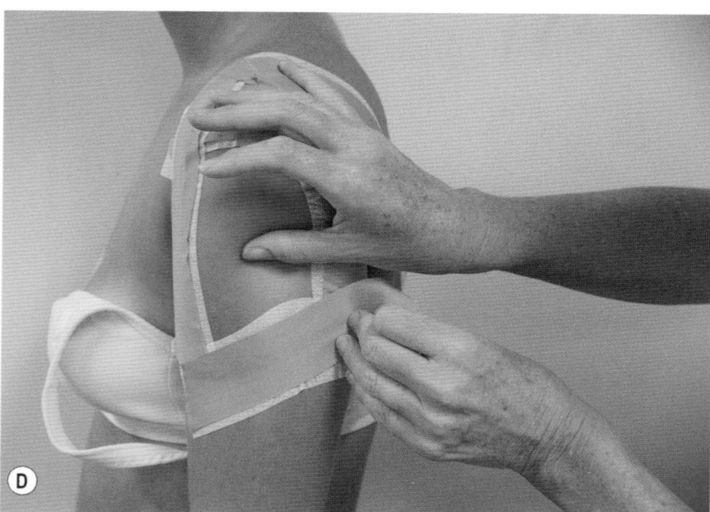

FIGURE 34.3

Unloading deltoid. In conjunction with the glenohumeral repositioning tape, the therapist can apply a deltoid unload tape. (A) The first piece of tape courses along the anterior deltoid starting anteriorly at the level of the deltoid tuberosity and finishing on the anterior aspect of the humeral head, just distal to the acromion. (B,C) The second piece courses along the posterior deltoid from distal to proximal, with the therapist lifting the soft tissue in towards the center. (D) The third piece joins the anterior and posterior pieces. It starts anterior and runs just below the deltoid tuberosity. While putting this piece on, the therapist lifts the soft tissue up towards the shoulder. The third piece is designed to promote external rotation of the humerus.

Deltoid muscle taping

The tape is placed over the anterior and posterior aspects of the deltoid from insertion to origin, and then a further piece of tape is applied from anterior to posterior, just below the deltoid tuberosity to lift the soft tissue towards the humeral head, shortening the deltoid. This tape aims to facilitate shoulder flexion and abduction movements and improve symptoms of rotator cuff tears and the painful stage of frozen shoulder. This tape is used in conjunction with the glenohumeral repositioning tape (Figure 34.3).

Upper trapezius taping

The clinician commences the tape just superior to the clavicle, midway along the UT muscle belly. While one hand is taping, the other hand is lifting the soft tissue up towards the neck, to decrease the pull of the UT attachment on the neck, thus minimizing any increased tension on the cervical attachment of the muscle, which may cause a headache. The tape goes over the UT and along the medial border of the scapula. This tape is usually used bilaterally and often with an unloading tape from the asymptomatic to the symptomatic side just below the cervicothoracic junction to lift the soft tissue up towards the head at (Figure 34.4). This tape aims to facilitate shoulder flexion and abduction movements by avoiding upward movements of the shoulder girdle facilitated by an excessive contraction of the upper trapezius muscle.

Lower trapezius and serratus anterior taping

The clinician tapes below the inferior border of the scapula, starting in the midline, below the axilla and coursing to

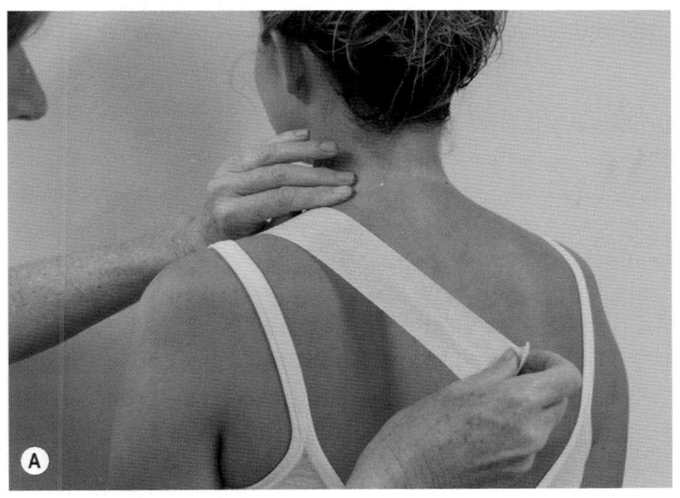

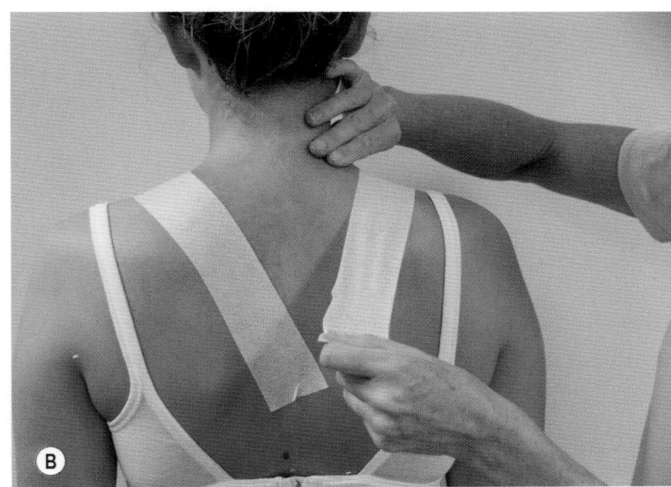

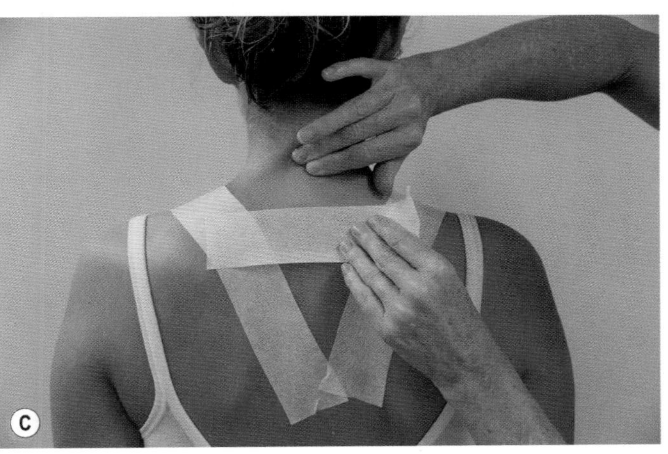

FIGURE 34.4

Minimizing activity in the upper trapezius. (A) To inhibit upper trapezius (UT) activity the tape is commenced on the anterior aspect of the body, just proximal to the clavicle at the mid belly level of the UT. While the tape is being applied, the therapist lifts the soft tissue towards the head. The tape finishes at the level of the inferior border of the scapula near the spine but does not cross the midline. (B) As UT is often overactive on both sides, symmetry is preferred, so the second piece of tape courses over the asymptomatic side. (C) A third horizontal piece may be added, starting below the cervicothoracic junction to join the two pieces together. The therapist lifts the soft tissue towards the head as this piece is applied.

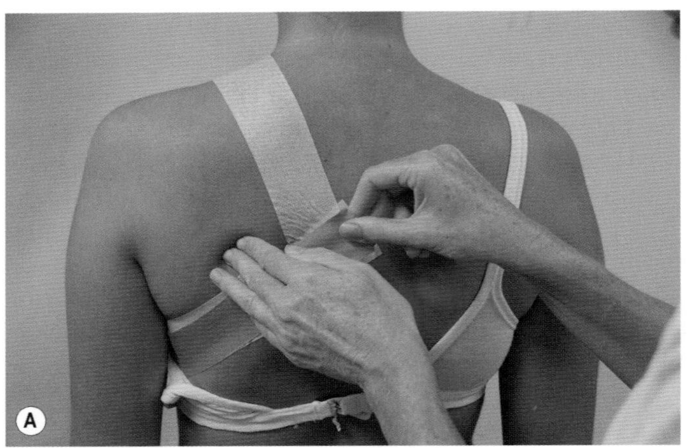

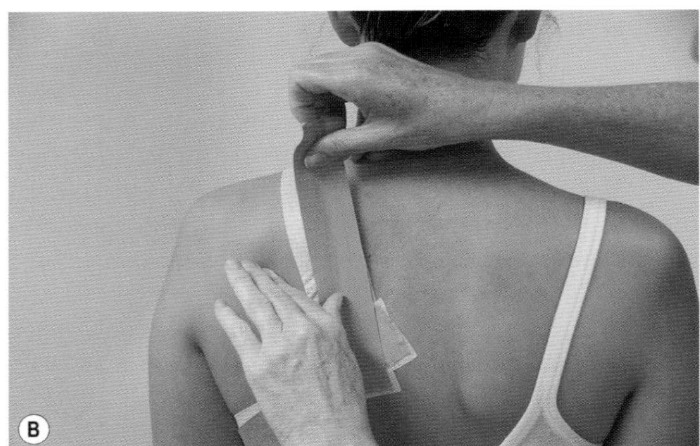

FIGURE 34.5

Facilitating serratus anterior and lower trapezius. Tape can be used to improve scapular dyskinesis and facilitate serratus anterior and lower trapezius. (A) The first piece of tape starts at the midline below the axilla, below the inferior border of the scapula. The tape runs along the inferior border just past the inferior angle of the scapula. The therapist lifts the skin towards the scapula as the tape is being applied. (B) The second piece commences just below the inferior angle of the scapula, coursing along the medial border of the scapula to just past the spine of the scapula.

the spine, below the inferior border of the scapula. The tape does not cross the midline. A second piece of tape starts near the spine, at the inferior angle of the scapula following the medial border of the scapula to just past the spine of the scapula. This tape is along the line of the lower trapezius (Figure 34.5). The purpose of this tape is to provide an external stimulus to the scapula for improving synergist control of the lower trapezius and serratus anterior muscles.

Conclusion

Bracing and taping may be considered in the evidence-based management of people presenting with musculoskeletal problems involving the shoulder. Shared decision-making that incorporates potential harms (skin damage and allergies), and anticipated benefits, supported by the available research is essential. The research supporting its application remains limited and equivocal. Clinically, the use of taping to support rehabilitation may be best considered if the patient reports an immediate 50% reduction in symptoms after the application of the tape. The reasons why tape reduces symptoms is not fully understood and this, too, requires further investigation. Tape is not a standalone treatment and must be incorporated within an appropriate rehabilitation program.

References

1. Aarseth LM, Suprak DN, Chalmers GR, Lyon L, Dahlquist DT. Kinesio tape and shoulder-joint position sense. J Athl Train. 2015;50:785-91.
2. Alexander CM, Stynes S, Thomas A, Lewis J, Harrison PJ. Does tape facilitate or inhibit the lower fibres of trapezius? Man Ther. 2003;8:37-41.
3. Baker HP, Tjong VK, Dunne KF, Lindley TR, Terry MA. Evaluation of shoulder-stabilizing braces: can we prevent shoulder labrum injury in collegiate offensive linemen? Orthop J Sports Med. 2016;4:2325967116673356.
4. Bdaiwi AH, Mackenzie TA, Herrington L, Horlsey I, Cools AJ. The effects of rigid scapular taping on acromiohumeral distance in healthy shoulders: an observational study. Sport Rehabil. 2017;26:51-56.
5. Celik D, Karaborklu Argut S, Coban O, Eren I. The clinical efficacy of kinesio taping in shoulder disorders: a systematic review and meta-analysis. Clin Rehabil. 2020;34:723-740.
6. Chiu YC, Tsai YS, Shen CL, Wang TG, Yang JL, Lin J .The immediate effects of a shoulder brace on muscle activity and scapular kinematics in subjects with shoulder impingement syndrome and rounded shoulder posture: a randomized crossover design. J Gait Posture. 2020;79:162-169.
7. Chu JC, Kane EJ, Arnold BL, Gansneder BM. The effect of a neoprene shoulder stabilizer on active joint-reposition sense in

subjects with stable and unstable shoulders. J Athl Train. 2002;37:141-145.

8. Cole AK, McGrath ML, Harrington SE, Padua DA, Rucinski TJ, Prentice WE. Scapular bracing and alteration of posture and muscle activity in overhead athletes with poor posture. J Athl Train. 2013;48:12-24.

9. Cupler ZA, Alrwaily M, Polakowski E, Mathers KS, Schneider MJ. Taping for conditions of the musculoskeletal system: an evidence map review. Chiropr Man Therap. 2020;28:52.

10. Dellabiancia F, Parel I, Filippi MV, Porcellini G, Merolla G. Glenohumeral and scapulohumeral kinematic analysis of patients with traumatic anterior instability wearing a shoulder brace: a prospective laboratory study. Musculoskelet Surg. 2017;101(Suppl 2):159-167.

11. Dhein W, Wagner Neto ES, Miranda IF, Pinto AB, Moraes LR, Loss JF. Effects of kinesio taping on scapular kinematics and electromyographic activity in subjects with shoulder impingement syndrome. J Bodyw Mov Ther. 2020;24:109-117.

12. Ghozy S, Minh Dung N, Morra M, et al. Efficacy of kinesio taping in treatment of shoulder pain and disability: a systematic review and meta-analysis of randomised controlled trials J Physio. 2020;107:176-188.

13. Grubhofer F, Gerber C, Meyer DC, Wieser K, Ernstbrunner L, Catanzaro S, Bouaicha S. Compliance with wearing an abduction brace after arthroscopic rotator cuff repair: a prospective, sensor-controlled study. Prosthet Orthot Int. 2019;43:440-446.

14. Harput G, Guney H, Toprak U, Colakoglu F, Baltaci GJ. Acute effects of scapular Kinesio Taping® on shoulder rotator strength, ROM and acromiohumeral distance in asymptomatic overhead athletes. Sports Med Phys Fitness. 2017;57:1479-1485.

15. Huang TS, Ou HL, Lin JJ. Effects of trapezius kinesio taping on scapular kinematics and associated muscular activation in subjects with scapular dyskinesis. J Hand Ther. 2019;32:345-352

16. Hug F, Ouellette A, Vicenzino B, Hodges PW, Tucker K. Deloading tape reduces muscle stress at rest and during contraction. Med Sci Sports Exerc. 2014;46:2317.

17. Intelangelo L, Bordachar D, Barbosa AW. Effects of scapular taping in young adults with shoulder pain and scapular dyskinesis. J Bodyw Mov Ther. 2016;20:525-32.

18. Kwapisz A, Shanley E, Momaya AM, Young C, Kissenberth MJ, Tolan SJ, Lonergan KT, Wyland DJ, Hawkins RJ, Pill SG, Tokish JM. Does functional bracing of the unstable shoulder improve return to play in scholastic athletes? Returning the unstable shoulder to play. Sports Health. 2021;13:45-48.

19. Keenan KA, Akins JS, Varnell M, Abt J, Lovalekar M, Lephart S, Sell TC. Kinesiology taping does not alter shoulder strength, shoulder proprioception, or scapular kinematics in healthy, physically active subjects and subjects with Subacromial Impingement Syndrome. Phys Ther Sport. 2017;24:60-66.

20. Leong HT, Fu SN. The effects of rigid scapular taping on the subacromial space in athletes with and without rotator cuff tendinopathy: a randomized controlled study. J Sport Rehabil. 2019;28:250-255.

21. Leong HT, Ng GY, Fu SN. Effects of scapular taping on the activity onset of scapular muscles and the scapular kinematics in volleyball players with rotator cuff tendinopathy. J Sci Med Sport. 2017;20:555-560.

22. Lim EC, Tay MG. Kinesio taping in musculoskeletal pain and disability that lasts for more than 4 weeks: is it time to peel off the tape and throw it out with the sweat? A systematic review with meta-analysis focused on pain and also methods of tape application. Br J Sports Med. 2015;49:1558-66

23. McConnell J. A novel approach to pain relief pre-therapeutic exercise. J Sci Med Sport. 2000;3:325-34.

24. McConnell J, McIntosh B. The effect of tape on glenohumeral rotation range of motion in elite junior tennis players. Clin J Sport Med. 2009;19:90-4.

25. McConnell J, Donnelly C, Hamner S, Dunne J, Besier T. Passive and dynamic shoulder rotation range in uninjured and previously injured overhead throwing athletes and the effect of shoulder taping. PM R. 2012;4:111-6.

26. McConnell J, Donnelly C, Hamner S, Dunne J, Besier T. Effect of shoulder taping on maximum shoulder external and internal rotation range in uninjured and previously injured overhead athletes during a seated throw. J Orthop Res. 2011;9:1406-11.

27. Macgregor K, Gerlach S, Mellor R, Hodges PW. Cutaneous stimulation from patella tape causes a differential increase in vasti muscle activity in people with patellofemoral pain. J Orthop Res. 2005;23:351-8.

28. Milgrom C, Schafffer M, Gilbert S, van Holsbeeck M. Rotator cuff changes in asymptomatic adults. The effect of age, hand dominance and gender. JBJS. 1995;77296-8.

29. Ozer ST, Karabay D, Yesilyaprak SS. Taping to improve scapular dyskinesis, scapular upward rotation, and pectoralis minor length in overhead athletes. J Athl Train. 2018;53:1063-1070.

30. Reuss BL, Harding WG 3rd, Nowicki KD. Managing anterior shoulder instability with bracing: an expanded update. Orthopedics. 2004;27:614-8.

31. Reynard F, Vuistiner P, Léger B, Konzelmann M. Immediate and short-term effects of kinesiotaping on muscular activity, mobility, strength and pain after rotator cuff surgery: a crossover clinical trial. BMC Musculoskelet Disord. 2018;19:305.

32. Saracoglu I, Emuk Y, Taspinar F. Does taping in addition to physiotherapy improve the outcomes in subacromial impingement syndrome? A systematic review. Physiother Theory Pract. 2018;34:251-263.

33. Şimşek HH, Balki S, Keklik SS, Öztürk H, Elden H. Does kinesio taping in addition to exercise therapy improve the outcomes in subacromial impingement syndrome? A randomized, double-blind, controlled clinical trial. Acta Orthop Traumatol Turc. 2013;47:104-10.

34. Selkowitz DM, Chaney C, Stuckey SJ, Vlad G. The effects of scapular taping on the surface electromyographic signal amplitude of shoulder girdle muscles during upper extremity elevation in individuals with suspected shoulder impingement syndrome. J Orthop Sports Phys Ther. 2007;37:694-702.

35. Snodgrass SJ, Farrell SF, Tsao H, Osmotherly PG, Rivett DA, Chipchase LS, Schabrun SM. Shoulder taping and neuromuscular control. J Athl Train. 2018;53:395-403.

36. Solomonow MJ. Sensory-motor control of ligaments and associated neuromuscular disorders. Electromyogr Kinesiol. 2006;16:549-67.

37. Solomonow M. Ligaments: a source of work-related musculoskeletal disorders. J Electromyogr Kinesiol. 2004;14:49-60.

38. Solomonow M. Neuromuscular manifestations of viscoelastic tissue degradation following high and low risk repetitive lumbar flexion. J Electromyogr Kinesiol. 2012;22:155-75.

39. Solomonow M, Baratta RV, Zhou BH, Burger E, Zieske A, Gedalia A. Muscular dysfunction elicited by creep of lumbar viscoelastic tissue. J Electromyogr Kinesiol. 2003;13:381-96.

40. Teys P, Bisset L, Collins N, Coombes B, Vicenzino B. One-week time course of the effects of Mulligan's Mobilisation with Movement and taping in painful shoulders. Man Ther. 2013;18:372-7.

41. Thelen MD, Dauber JA, Stoneman PD. The clinical efficacy of kinesio tape for shoulder pain: a randomized, double-blinded, clinical trial. J Orthop Sports Phys Ther. 2008;38:389-95.

42. Tirefort J, Schwitzguebel AJ, Collin P, Nowak A, Plomb-Holmes C, Lädermann A.

o Postoperative mobilization after superior rotator cuff repair: sling versus no sling: a randomized prospective study. J Bone Joint Surg Am. 2019;101:494-503.

43. Tobin S, Robinson G. The effect of McConnell's vastus lateralis inhibition taping technique on vastus lateralis and vastus medialis obliquus activity. Physiotherapy. 2000;26:173–183.

44. Weerakkody N, Allen T. The effects of fast bowling fatigue and adhesive taping on shoulder joint position sense in amateur cricket players in Victoria, Australia. J Sports Sci. 2017;35:1954-1962.

45. Whelan DB, Litchfield R, Wambolt E, Dainty KN. External rotation immobilization for primary shoulder dislocation: a randomized controlled trial. Joint Orthopaedic Initiative for National Trials of the Shoulder (JOINTS). Clin Orthop Relat Res. 2014;472:2380-6.

46. Williams PE, Catanese T, Lucey EG, Goldspink G. The importance of stretch and contractile activity in the prevention of connective tissue accumulation in muscle. J Anat. 1988;158:109-14.

47. Yildiz TI, Castelein B, Harput G, Duzgun I, Cools A.J Does scapular corrective taping alter periscapular muscle activity and 3-dimensional scapular kinematics? A systematic review. Hand Ther. 2020;33:361-370.

Part 4

Rehabilitation

4

Musculoskeletal shoulder rehabilitation: motor control or strengthening? 35

Jean-Sébastien Roy, Matthew Low, Marc-Olivier Dubé, Simon Lafrance, François Desmeules

Introduction

Surgical, pharmacological, and rehabilitation management are the most common interventions offered for people seeking care for musculoskeletal shoulder conditions.[25] Although most surgical and pharmacological interventions have been shown to reduce pain and disability in people experiencing shoulder pain,[66] rehabilitation is recommended as the first intervention by most clinical guidelines, as evidence from multiple randomized controlled trials (RCTs) suggests that rehabilitation is at least as effective as surgical and pharmacological interventions[2,27,28,39,40,57] for most nontraumatic shoulder conditions.[47,67]

Among all rehabilitation interventions, exercise therapy is the most widely recommended intervention for conditions such as rotator cuff-related shoulder pain (RCRSP) and shoulder instability.[17] In fact, clinical practice guidelines and systematic reviews consistently recommend with low to moderate quality evidence their use for the treatment of shoulder pain as they lead to better outcomes on pain and function than placebo or watch-and-wait.[15,16,17] Exercise programs for RCRSP and shoulder instability commonly include motor control and strengthening exercises. Although exercise therapy is consistently recommended, it remains unclear whether one type of exercise is associated with better results than another.[6,12,34,54] The objectives of this chapter are: 1) to present the rationale for using strengthening and motor control exercises for the treatment of shoulder pain, and 2) to compare their effectiveness, especially for conditions such as RCRSP and shoulder instability, to reduce pain and disability.

Strengthening exercises

By definition, strengthening means to make something stronger, while strength means the ability to produce force,[62] traditionally objectified using the single repetition maximum (RM). RM is obtained by determining the maximal weight that can be lifted, pushed, or pulled once, or by taking a percentage of RM, which is the maximum number of repetitions of a given weight, calculated on a percentage table.[51]

The potential mechanisms proposed to explain a gain in strength following strengthening exercises are an increase in muscle cross-sectional area, and changes in neural drive in the central nervous system (e.g., reticulospinal tract and intracortical circuits within the primary motor cortex).[24,60] Increase in cross-sectional area stems from muscle fiber hypertrophy induced by satellite cell proliferation secondary to training-related muscular architecture damage.[9] These morphological changes usually appear after a certain amount of time (usually more than six weeks) of exercising. Neurological adaptations, such as motor learning, together with increased recruitment of motor units and better coordination between agonists and antagonists, may explain the early increase in "strength" commonly observed in the first two weeks of a strengthening program.[22]

Strengthening exercises may also modify tendon metabolism and properties (structural and mechanical) and help tendon healing[11,22] by increasing the tendon stiffness and the total number and diameter of collagen fibrils.[22] Tendon cells are known to respond to mechanical stress and this response is likely dependent on both amplitude and frequency of the load applied.[1] Tendon healing could be improved by an appropriate mechanical load, while an insufficient or inadequate load may not be beneficial. This also applies to muscle cells as there is a correlation between dose and response for muscle hypertrophy.[71]

In rehabilitation, the term strengthening is often criticized for being too vague and failing to properly define the type of strengthening regimen used.[37] Although exercises referred to as strengthening exercises are often aimed at increasing load tolerance rather than strength itself, we will still use the term in this chapter to address our aims, i.e., comparing "strengthening" with motor control in the rehabilitation of musculoskeletal shoulder conditions.

Strengthening exercises prescribed for shoulder rehabilitation range from low-load exercises (LLE) (high number of repetitions (>20) with high frequency (aim to exercise every day) using a low load)), to progressive high-load exercises (PHLE) (low number of repetitions (<10) as well as low frequency (2–3 times/week) with a high load (>75% of RM)). PHLE aim to induce changes in muscle and tendon properties in response to high mechanical loads applied to the musculotendinous unit. On the other hand, LLE aim to gradually reintroduce load to avoid muscle atrophy and protect the tendons from excessive loads that could result in an exacerbation of symptoms. The ability of LLE to produce gains in strength and endurance, or to lead to the changes associated with strength-based adaptations, has been questioned, since the dosage is often too low to produce significant gains in strength.[13]

Strengthening is an important part of shoulder rehabilitation since a large proportion of individuals with persistent shoulder pain present with strength impairments (e.g., strength deficits in isometric peak torque), especially for the shoulder abductors and lateral rotators.[13,15] Strengthening exercises are regularly used in shoulder rehabilitation in order to increase strength and endurance, restore muscle balance, re-establish dynamic stability, limit muscle atrophy, and increase tendon stiffness.[18,20]

Types of strengthening used for shoulder rehabilitation

Either isometric or isotonic strengthening exercises may be used during the rehabilitation process according to the patient's clinical presentation and the aims of the exercise.[42] During isometric contractions, tension in the muscle changes while the muscle remains at the same length, as opposed to isotonic contractions where tension remains constant but muscle length changes (shortens during concentric phase and lengthens during eccentric phase). Isometric exercises are sometimes used in the early phase to gradually load the shoulder muscles and tendons.

Moderate isometric loads (55% maximum voluntary contraction) have been shown to lead to an increase in muscle strength and size, while high isometric loads (90% maximum voluntary contraction) to an increase in tendon strength through increased stiffness.[18] Once tolerated, strengthening exercises may be progressed to isotonic exercises, using either concentric or eccentric contractions or both. Load applied to the musculotendinous units differs in eccentric training compared with concentric training regimens, because the tension in muscle fibers is greater when they are lengthening than when they are shortening.[46]

Recent systematic reviews recommend strengthening exercises for people with shoulder pain, and that the exercises should mainly focus on the rotator cuff and scapular muscles.[16,29,48,55] At the very least, strengthening exercises should be performed for the shoulder lateral rotators and abductors,[7] since significant strength impairments have been evidenced in both muscle groups.[13] It is also important to include exercises for key scapulothoracic muscles such as serratus anterior, rhomboid major and minor, levator scapulae, and trapezius muscles in order to provide a stable base, i.e., the scapula, for the rotator cuff muscles to act on.

Strengthening exercises may be performed under the guidance of a physical therapist (physiotherapist), and as part of a home exercise program. The literature suggests both are equally effective,[49] and home exercise[26] may lead to increased confidence in managing the problem.[35] There is no consensus as to whether or not strengthening exercises should be performed with or without experiencing pain.[49,74,75] If pain is experienced, it is suggested that pain should stay at a tolerable level and decrease soon after training – soon being defined as within an hour, with no increase in pain at night and no increase in pain the next day. Exercising in tolerable pain may produce short-term exercise induced hypoalgesia.

Evidence of the effect of strengthening for shoulder rehabilitation

A systematic review evaluating the efficacy of rehabilitation interventions for the management of shoulder pain concluded that there is limited evidence as to which types of strengthening exercises or set of parameters are associated with the best outcomes.[29] This can be explained in part by the heterogeneity in the strengthening exercises proposed in the literature and the lack of description of the strengthening parameters used (e.g., type, intensity, frequency, and duration).[29] Currently, studies looking at the effect of strengthening exercises on shoulder pain have mainly evaluated the specific effects of isometric, eccentric, and PHLE exercises in individuals with RCRSP.

Isometric exercises

The rationale for using isometric exercises is that they allow a gradual reloading of the shoulder musculotendinous unit and prevent muscle inhibition.[18] Although commonly used, Dupuis et al. did not show any short-term differences (at two and six weeks) in pain and function between a two-week gradual reloading exercise program (incremental isometric contractions in lateral rotation and abduction at 50–75% of the maximal voluntary contraction) and cryotherapy (application of ice for 15 minutes, 3 times a day) in a population with acute RCRSP.[18] There was also no significant increase in strength in either group.

Eccentric exercises

The rationale behind the use of eccentric exercises is that they should lead to higher mechanical loads on the musculotendinous unit and thus optimize the remodeling of the fibers to reduce pain and increase strength and function. Eccentric strengthening exercises for the rotator cuff muscles have been shown to be superior to a watch and wait approach to improve shoulder pain and function;[5,11,38] they may, however, not be superior to other types of strengthening. Holmgren et al. concluded that loaded eccentric exercises (external load with weight or elastic band for rotator cuff and scapulothoracic muscles) lead to reduced pain and improved function compared with unloaded exercises (active movement without any external load added).[33] While not directly comparable, Maenhout et al. showed that eccentric strengthening exercises (eccentric phase of full can abduction in the scapular plane performed with a weight for 3 sets of 15 repetitions, twice a day) resulted in gains in abduction isometric strength when measured at 90° of abduction in the plane of the scapula. The eccentric program, which was regulated by pain and not weight, did not confer any additional benefits to LLE (medial and lateral rotation exercises with an elastic resistance band).[53]

Progressive high load exercises (PHLE)

The objective of PHLE is to apply enough mechanical load to the tendons and the muscles to induce morphological changes and increase their load tolerance. Although an appealing hypothesis, the superiority of PHLE for individuals with shoulder pain has not been demonstrated. Lombardi et al.[50] investigated a PHLE protocol based on 6 RM (i.e., the maximum weight that could be lifted 6 times) for the shoulder flexors, extensors, and medial/lateral rotators. The program comprised of 2 sets of 8 repetitions, with the first set being 50% of 6 RM and the second 70% of 6 RM; the 6 RM load was revaluated every two weeks.[50] At the two month follow-up, in comparison with the watch and wait group, participants in the 6 RM group had improvements in pain and function, but there were no significant increases in strength in either group.

Ingwersen et al.[36] used a 12-week protocol of PHLE based on 6 to 15 RM (i.e., starting with the maximum weight that could be lifted 15 times, and then gradually increasing to the maximum weight that could be lifted 6 times) and concluded that there were no added benefits on pain, symptoms, maximum isometric strength (scaption and medial/lateral rotations), and shoulder range of motion compared with a 12-week protocol of LLE based on 20 to 25 RM (i.e., the maximum weight that could be lifted between 20 and 25 times).[37] However, both groups had significant reductions in pain during activity, pain at night, maximum pain, and improvements in maximum isometric strength and passive ROM.[36]

Based on the current evidence, strengthening exercises offer a better outcome than a watch and wait approach. However, there is currently no evidence that one type of strengthening (or resistance exercise) program is superior to another.

Motor control exercises

Motor control incorporates a number of fields: physics, engineering, behavioral and cognitive science, as well as neuroscience and medicine.[63] Interestingly, if one were to take a single perspective from each of the aforementioned fields that investigate and explain the concept of motor control, then it would appear that the concept is well understood. However, within the context of musculoskeletal rehabilitation there is considerable uncertainty, including the concept of motor control itself.[52]

Motor control is a term that relates to how humans control movement, such as holding and lifting a cup from a table and bringing it to the mouth, or serving the ball in tennis – an action that involves the entire body. Motor control involves perception of the surrounding environment, and a drive or motivation to move or manipulate the self or objects within those surroundings, while adapting to internal and external influences (known as perturbations) during the activity.[31,45,63] In order to complete tasks, the integration of sensory, psychomotor and cognitive information and feedback that starts before the decision or requirement to move commences, and continues throughout the movement.[23] This process includes the prior experiences, thoughts, feelings and beliefs, and current situation and state of the individual. Motor control requires the integration of the nervous system at many levels to consolidate predictions, inputs and coordinated outputs (from simple spinal cord mechanisms to complex supraspinal integration and decision-making), the motor output to the muscles (the effector organs of the system), down to the mechanical properties of the tissues (including muscles, ligaments, and bones as well as the overlying skin that influence joint mechanics).[23,31,45,63] All of these elements combine to create and control purposeful movement.[73]

There is ongoing debate as to *if, how,* and *why* motor control is altered in people with and without musculoskeletal pain. There are fundamental questions that remain unresolved, including whether motor control, by increasing mechanical stiffness and altering load distribution and movement variability can predispose an individual to develop musculoskeletal pain,[31,52] whether motor control adapts or becomes maladaptive in response to pain or injury, and whether it is related to the persistence and recurrence of pain.

Rehabilitation incorporates many aspects of motor control theory. These include motor behaviors that take into account the order of events, timing, and relative force requirements across different tasks,[70] and motor training that includes the modification of movement patterns which are repeated to reinforce motor learning.[41] These components are combined to promote neuroplastic changes so that long-lasting and beneficial modifications in movement strategies are achieved.[8] For such targeted approaches to be successful, all of these considerations need to be placed within a person-centered approach to rehabilitation.

Clinical rationale for using motor control in shoulder rehabilitation

The history of motor control theories in musculoskeletal rehabilitation emerges from a biomechanical origin mainly through Panjabi's model of stability,[58] which is based on the theoretical interactions between active (muscular) and passive (articular/ligamentous) stabilizers through the control (nervous) system to meet the structure's demand and requirements. Using this model may have the tendency to narrow the perspective of motor control approaches toward the causal mechanical properties of movement rather than appreciating a broader person-centered perspective. However, using motor control-based approaches to treat RCRSP appears to be successful,[14,44,64,69,84] albeit with no currently apparent definitive reason for this. A mechanical explanation may be due to changing the kinematic characteristics of movement to reduce tissue sensitivity and pain sensitivity. This may be due to the reduction in tissue compression in the cases of physical impingement of pain-sensitive structures, or alterations on the mechanical load upon the tissues. As such, motor control exercises may, in part, enhance movement and function, by influencing movement patterns, and by targeting specific muscle groups.

Research evidence suggests that altered glenohumeral and scapulothoracic kinematics may exist in people with shoulder pain, however, a number of characteristics influence these alterations, including the complexity of movement, such as the angle, speed, context, and resistance of movement, and the population that is studied.[77] Psychological explanations for the successful effect of motor control exercises may be due to a graded exposure to previously painful positions, or actions, and reduced kinesiophobia and/or pain catastrophization.[43,79] There may be positive central nervous system and sensorimotor adaptations that may result in an inhibitory neurophysiological effect on the pain experience,[19,65] amongst myriad contextual changes that may occur.[32] It may also be due to distraction, as the individual is required to process the information about the movement during motor control exercises and by doing so is less able to focus on symptoms.

Having acknowledged the complexity and uncertainty that exists surrounding motor control and its various effects, it is worth considering the types of motor control exercises that may be used in shoulder rehabilitation.

Types of motor control exercises in shoulder rehabilitation

The two specific areas that motor control approaches focus on in shoulder rehabilitation are motion and function, with a significant overlap between them. There are other motor control approaches that include the analysis of trunk posture or spinal contributory factors that are not discussed here. Motor control exercises are progressed in respect to the position of the patient and the relative changes that are placed upon the movement in relation to gravity, through added resistance such as the use of bands or weights, or through using the kinetic chain in gradually increased positions of functional challenge.[47,65,69,82]

Scapular focused motor control approaches evaluate the scapula in relation to painful shoulder movement and/or reduced shoulder function. The directions of the scapula (upward and downward rotation, protraction, and retraction as well as anterior and posterior tilt) are evaluated in the context of pain or functional loss and are usually modified by either manual or verbal facilitation or by changing a person's starting position.

Glenohumeral joint-focused motor control approaches evaluate and attempt to influence the humeral head position within the glenoid. It is suggested that the humeral head position in the glenoid may move aberrantly in people with RCRSP and shoulder instability – in particular, the lack of humeral head depression as a result of less than optimal muscle activity.[56]

Using these examples, techniques are introduced that may influence the movement of the humerus, scapula, or both.[3,4] Attention is often drawn to the ways in which the shoulder girdle muscles coordinate their activation or patterning. As mentioned previously, any reported improvement experienced by the patient may be due to mechanical or contextual effects, as well as distraction from symptoms. Examples of motor control exercises that are included in shoulder rehabilitation programs are the Watson multidirectional instability program,[82,83] the movement system impairment syndrome approach,[69] and the shoulder symptom modification procedures (see Chapter 36).[47] Motor control approaches use verbal, spatial, internal, and external cues and most often include functionally related activities.

Research evidence on the effect of motor control exercises for shoulder rehabilitation

Current research evidence is inconclusive regarding the effect of motor control exercises for shoulder rehabilitation. There appear to be several reasons for this, including the variation of assessment criteria for identifying motor control deficits and clinical diagnosis, as well as difficulties in separating clear distinctions between motor control and other movement-based approaches.

Systematic reviews and meta-analyses report a lack of high-quality research with consistent findings. Shire et al.[72] investigated specific versus general exercise strategies for the treatment of RCRSP. The authors defined specific exercises as those targeting the activation and coordination of scapulothoracic musculature and/or the dynamic humeral stabilizers that encompass the shoulder joint, and concluded that there was insufficient evidence to support or disprove specific exercises in the management of RCRSP. Other systematic reviews investigating scapular-focused treatment strategies on RCRSP found insufficient evidence to support their use. These exercises included scapular exercise, mobilization techniques, and taping in patients with RCRSP.[10,61] The authors of these systematic reviews suggest that although there appears to be short-term improvement in the groups performing motor control exercises (less than three months), the degree of improvement compared with general exercises was not felt to be clinically important. There is ever-increasing uncertainty regarding the effect of motor control exercises compared with other treatments for shoulder pain in the long term.[10,61]

Given that the concept of motor control itself is complex and that motor control approaches are tailored for individuals based on assessment findings, it is unsurprising that the research evidence remains equivocal.

Motor control exercises or strengthening exercises for shoulder pain

As presented previously, evidence exists to support both the use of motor control and strengthening exercises to treat shoulder pain, even though there is uncertainty about the specific parameters required to optimize treatment effects. It also remains unclear if one approach is more effective than the other. This section will review the literature that compares the relative efficacy of motor control and strengthening exercises for selected shoulder diagnoses. Currently in the literature, these two exercise approaches have been compared in adults with RCRSP and shoulder instability.

Rotator cuff-related shoulder pain

Three RCTs specifically comparing motor control with strengthening exercises in adults with RCRSP have been published.[4,78,80] In these RCTs, most participants had persistent shoulder symptoms, and based on the Cochrane risk of bias tool,[30] methodological quality was considered moderate.

An RCT published by Turgut et al. involved 30 participants (mean age, 36.5 years) with RCRSP.[78] In this study, the motor control group received a 12-week scapular and glenohumeral motor control and strengthening exercise program. The exercises included wall slides, wall push-ups, resisted scapular retraction and resisted shoulder medial/lateral rotations performed with lower limb movements such as squats, single leg stance, or side steps. The other group received a 12-week shoulder strengthening exercise program with a focus on resisted shoulder medial/lateral rotation and resisted full can exercises. Both groups also performed stretching exercises. At 12 weeks, using a visual analogue scale for pain (VAS pain), no significant between-group differences were observed for pain at rest, during activity, and at night. However, the Shoulder Pain and Disability Index (SPADI) pain and disability scores were significantly lower (Chapter 12) in the motor control group when compared with the strengthening group (pain score mean difference (MD) -14.50%; 95%CI -27.12 to -1.88; disability score MD -12.42%; 95%CI -23.89 to -0.95) and these differences, although small, may be considered clinically important.

Wang and Trudelle-Jackson included 38 participants (mean age, 44.5 years) with RCRSP.[80] The motor control group received an eight-week scapular and glenohumeral motor control and strengthening exercise program based on Sahrmann's movement system impairment approach.[68] The program included strengthening exercises specific to serratus anterior, trapezius, and shoulder medial/lateral rotators, and stretch exercises for pectoralis minor, latissimus dorsi and shoulder medial/lateral rotators specific to the movement impairment classification. The other group received an eight-week shoulder strengthening exercise program which included resisted shoulder flexion, abduction, extension, and medial/lateral rotation exercises. At eight weeks, no between-group significant differences were observed in terms of pain (VAS pain MD -0.76/10 in favor of motor control; 95%CI -2.69 to 1.17) or disability reduction (Flexilevel Scale of Shoulder Function MD 1.2% in favor of strengthening; 95%CI -8.96 to 11.36).

Finally, an RCT published by Beaudreuil et al. involved 70 participants (mean age, 58.7 years) with RCRSP.[4] The motor control group received a six-week program consisting of humeral head and scapular movement control exercises, such as active ROM with shoulder muscle co-contraction exercises. The strengthening group performed active mobilization exercises of the shoulder with slight manual resistance applied by the treating physiotherapist. Since only slight manual resistance was applied by the treating physiotherapist and the standardization of the technique was not described, it remains somewhat unclear if this intervention was offering true strengthening exercises. Participants in the motor control group had significantly less pain compared with the other group (Constant-Murley pain subscale score MD 2.1/15 points; 95%CI 0.7 to 3.5) and significantly fewer patients were using medications at three months (MD -25.7%; 95%CI -51.9 to -3.7). A non-significant trend towards lower pain in the motor control group was observed at 12 months (MD 2/15 points; 95%CI 0.4 to 3.5). No significant differences were observed on other outcomes such as the Constant-Murley activity, mobility, and strength subscales at 3 or 12 months.

Shoulder instability

Two RCTs comparing motor control and strengthening exercises in patients with shoulder instability have been published. Based on the Cochrane risk of bias tool,[30] one RCT can be considered of high quality,[81] while the other trial can be considered of moderate quality.[80]

The high-quality RCT published by Warby et al. involved 41 participants (mean age, 22.5) with chronic multidirectional shoulder instability.[81] The motor control group received the Watson Program, a six-stage 12-week program consisting of specific scapular and glenohumeral motor control and strengthening exercises. In the initial stages, applied resistance to the shoulder is minimal and exercises are performed within the first degrees of shoulder elevation. Resistance and shoulder elevation angles are increased as the program progresses, while the last stages include more sport-specific functional exercises. The other group received the Rockwood Strengthening Program, a two-stage 12-week program consisting of rotator cuff and deltoid muscle strengthening, mostly performed at low angles of shoulder elevation, including push-up exercises.

At six-weeks follow-up, no between-group significant differences were observed for all outcomes. At 12-weeks follow-up, no between-group significant differences were observed for VAS pain (MD -1/10 in favor of motor control; 95%CI -2.3 to 0.3), but significant differences in disability were observed in favor of the motor control group on the Western Ontario Shoulder Index (WOSI) (MD 11.1%; 95%CI 1.9 to 20.2) but not on the Melbourne Instability Shoulder Score (MISS) (MD 8.8%; 95%CI -0.5 to 18.2). At 24-weeks follow-up, significant reduction in VAS pain (MD -2/10; 95%CI -2.3 to -0.7), on the WOSI score (MD 12.6%; 95%CI 3.4 to 21.9) and on the MISS (MD 15.4%; 95%CI 5.9 to 24.8) were observed in favor of the motor control group. Between-group differences observed in this trial for pain at 24 weeks and for the WOSI at 12 and 24 weeks may be considered clinically important.[59,76]

The moderate-quality RCT published by Eshoj et al. involved 56 participants (mean age, 26) with subacute traumatic anterior shoulder instability.[21] The motor control group received a seven-stage 12-week daily exercise program supervised by a physiotherapist consisting of seven motor control, strengthening, and proprioception exercises targeting scapular and glenohumeral muscles. Initially, scapular and glenohumeral exercises were performed without resistance and within the first degrees of shoulder elevation. Progressions included performing the exercises against resistance, with the arm elevated and with lower limb involvement such as in the single leg stance position. The strengthening group also received a 12-week exercise program, but exercises were performed only three times per week. The program consisted of scapular and glenohumeral muscles strengthening exercises using elastic bands, including resisted shoulder abduction and medial/lateral rotators, and one exercise for the coactivation of scapular and core muscles. This program was not directly supervised, as participants only received telephone follow-ups from a physiotherapist.

After 12 weeks, participants in the motor control group, when compared with those in the strengthening group, reported a significant reduction in last week mean VAS pain (MD -1.1; 95%CI -2.1 to -0.9), but not for current pain, nor for mean pain in the last 24 hours. Participants in the motor control group also reported a significant reduction in disability on the WOSI when compared with the strengthening group (MD -10.9%; 95%CI -20.5 to -1.2) and fewer patients had a positive apprehension test (MD -35.7%; 95%CI -62.2 to -9.6). Between-group differences for pain and for the WOSI may be considered clinically important.[59] This trial, however, did not look at other outcomes such as recurrent dislocation or new episodes of subluxation. The authors reported that as the motor control exercise program was supervised and conducted daily, and the strengthening program was conducted over 3 sessions per week, it may have introduced bias.

Overall results from the literature and pooling of presented data into meta-analysis

When pooling results from the above RCTs into meta-analyses using the Cochrane methodology,[30] it appears that motor control exercises lead to greater pain reduction when compared with strengthening exercises in the short term (VAS pain MD -0.79/10; 95% CI -1.47 to -0.12; n=157). However, the difference between the two exercise approaches is small and not likely clinically important. Motor control exercises, however, lead to greater reduction in disability when compared with strengthening exercises in the short term (6–13 weeks after randomization; standardized mean difference (SMD) -0.42; 95%CI -0.69 to -0.15; n=217) and this difference between the two exercise approaches is moderate and may be clinically important (Figures 35.1 and 35.2).[44] Comparable treatment effects were observed both for people with instability and with RCRSP.

Since these meta-analyses are based on only a small number of RCTs with small samples of participants, caution must be taken in their interpretation. It is also important to specify that strengthening exercises were occasionally included in the motor control exercise programs. Therefore, could a program including both motor control and strengthening principles be the optimal solution for individuals with RCRSP or shoulder instability? This remains to be answered, but the best current option may be to include both types of exercise in rehabilitation programs (see Chapter 36). Other variables, such as the frequency of exercise sessions, the progression, and the inclusion of sport-specific exercises in the motor control exercise programs might be factors contributing to the observed results. The clinical presentation and specific findings when functionally evaluating patients, the patient's preferences, and likely compliance with the different approaches may also influence the outcomes observed. These factors were not always considered in the included trials.

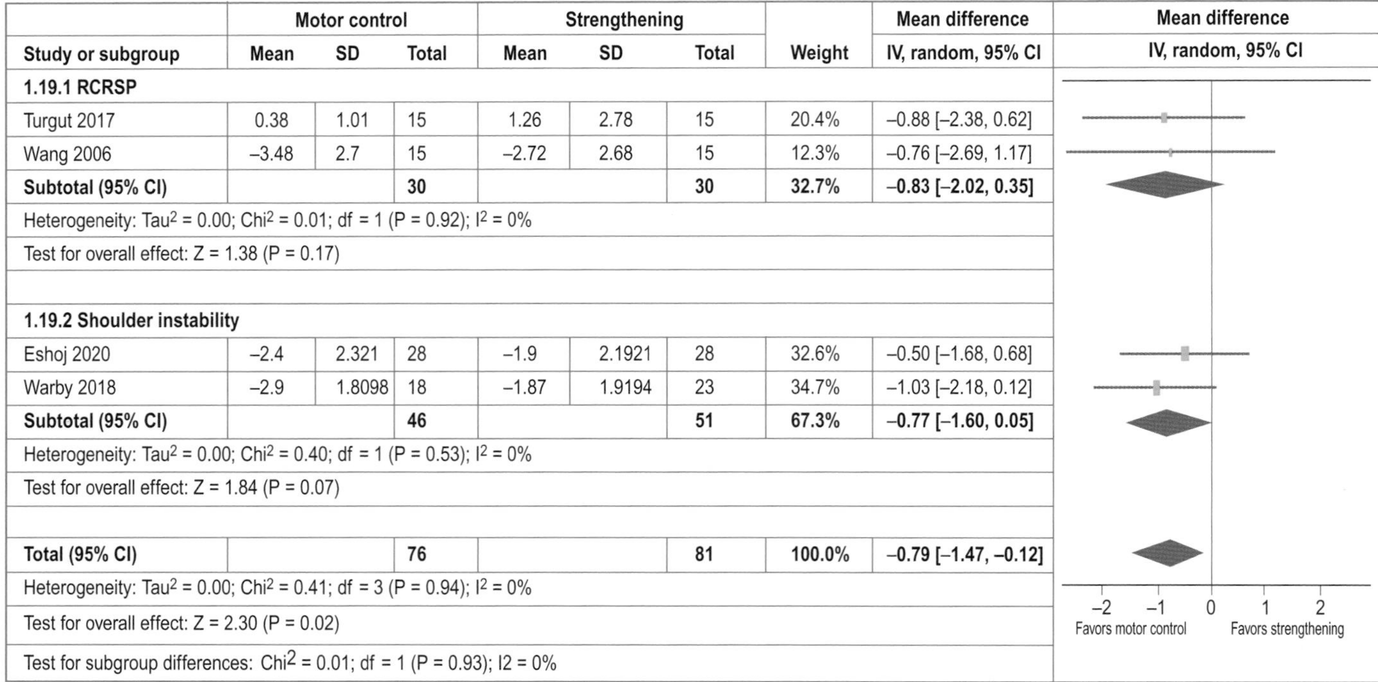

Study or subgroup	Motor control Mean	SD	Total	Strengthening Mean	SD	Total	Weight	Mean difference IV, random, 95% CI
1.19.1 RCRSP								
Turgut 2017	0.38	1.01	15	1.26	2.78	15	20.4%	−0.88 [−2.38, 0.62]
Wang 2006	−3.48	2.7	15	−2.72	2.68	15	12.3%	−0.76 [−2.69, 1.17]
Subtotal (95% CI)			**30**			**30**	**32.7%**	**−0.83 [−2.02, 0.35]**
Heterogeneity: Tau^2 = 0.00; Chi^2 = 0.01; df = 1 (P = 0.92); I^2 = 0%								
Test for overall effect: Z = 1.38 (P = 0.17)								
1.19.2 Shoulder instability								
Eshoj 2020	−2.4	2.321	28	−1.9	2.1921	28	32.6%	−0.50 [−1.68, 0.68]
Warby 2018	−2.9	1.8098	18	−1.87	1.9194	23	34.7%	−1.03 [−2.18, 0.12]
Subtotal (95% CI)			**46**			**51**	**67.3%**	**−0.77 [−1.60, 0.05]**
Heterogeneity: Tau^2 = 0.00; Chi^2 = 0.40; df = 1 (P = 0.53); I^2 = 0%								
Test for overall effect: Z = 1.84 (P = 0.07)								
Total (95% CI)			**76**			**81**	**100.0%**	**−0.79 [−1.47, −0.12]**
Heterogeneity: Tau^2 = 0.00; Chi^2 = 0.41; df = 3 (P = 0.94); I^2 = 0%								
Test for overall effect: Z = 2.30 (P = 0.02)								
Test for subgroup differences: Chi^2 = 0.01; df = 1 (P = 0.93); I2 = 0%								

FIGURE 35.1

Efficacy of motor control exercises compared with strengthening exercises for change in pain (VAS 0–10 scale) in adults with RCRSP and shoulder instability. CI, confidence intervals; IV, inverse variance method; RCRSP, rotator cuff-related shoulder pain; SD, standard deviation.

It is not only surprising but also a concern that the question of the best exercise approach for people with musculoskeletal pain involving the shoulder remains unanswered. The few available trials are heterogeneous in their design and characteristics. Ultimately, more research is needed to fully understand the relative benefits of both types of exercises; well-designed trials that control adequately for potential confounders are required to understand the relative merits of motor control, strengthening, combination, and watch and wait approaches in the management of people presenting with shoulder symptoms.

Conclusions

Current evidence suggests that, in the short term, motor control exercises lead to a greater reduction in pain although the reduction may not be clinically important, and to a greater reduction in disability that might be clinically important when compared with strengthening exercises. The magnitude of the effect might therefore be clinically important for some outcomes. This suggests that exercise approaches including motor control exercises might be prioritized over strengthening exercises for patients suffering from RCRSP or shoulder instability (traumatic or multidirectional). Most motor control exercise programs, however, included some form of low-load strengthening exercises, especially when progressing to movement with increased functional challenge, making it difficult to clearly distinguish between the two exercise approaches. In summary, exercise programs that include motor control probably confer a small beneficial effect of uncertain clinical relevance when compared with exercise approaches that do not include motor control for people with shoulder pain.

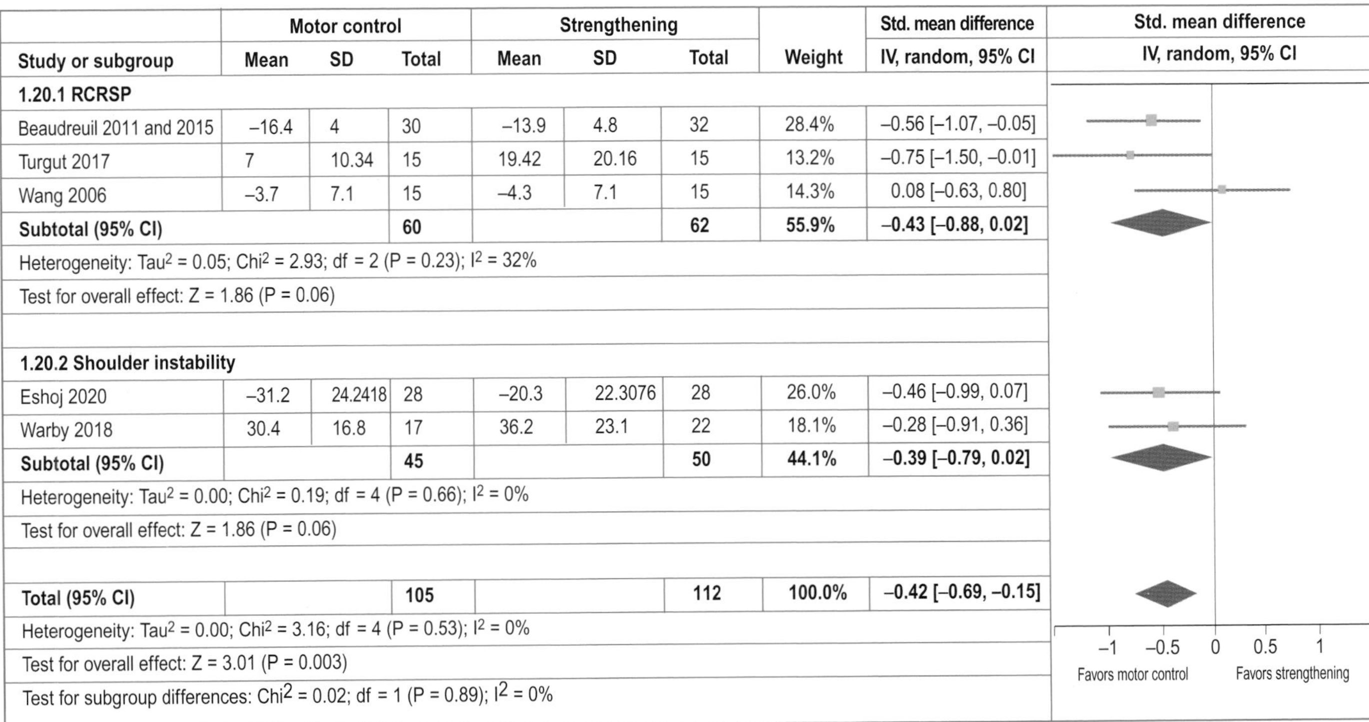

Study or subgroup	Motor control Mean	Motor control SD	Motor control Total	Strengthening Mean	Strengthening SD	Strengthening Total	Weight	Std. mean difference IV, random, 95% CI
1.20.1 RCRSP								
Beaudreuil 2011 and 2015	−16.4	4	30	−13.9	4.8	32	28.4%	−0.56 [−1.07, −0.05]
Turgut 2017	7	10.34	15	19.42	20.16	15	13.2%	−0.75 [−1.50, −0.01]
Wang 2006	−3.7	7.1	15	−4.3	7.1	15	14.3%	0.08 [−0.63, 0.80]
Subtotal (95% CI)			**60**			**62**	**55.9%**	**−0.43 [−0.88, 0.02]**
Heterogeneity: Tau² = 0.05; Chi² = 2.93; df = 2 (P = 0.23); I² = 32%								
Test for overall effect: Z = 1.86 (P = 0.06)								
1.20.2 Shoulder instability								
Eshoj 2020	−31.2	24.2418	28	−20.3	22.3076	28	26.0%	−0.46 [−0.99, 0.07]
Warby 2018	30.4	16.8	17	36.2	23.1	22	18.1%	−0.28 [−0.91, 0.36]
Subtotal (95% CI)			**45**			**50**	**44.1%**	**−0.39 [−0.79, 0.02]**
Heterogeneity: Tau² = 0.00; Chi² = 0.19; df = 4 (P = 0.66); I² = 0%								
Test for overall effect: Z = 1.86 (P = 0.06)								
Total (95% CI)			**105**			**112**	**100.0%**	**−0.42 [−0.69, −0.15]**
Heterogeneity: Tau² = 0.00; Chi² = 3.16; df = 4 (P = 0.53); I² = 0%								
Test for overall effect: Z = 3.01 (P = 0.003)								
Test for subgroup differences: Chi² = 0.02; df = 1 (P = 0.89); I² = 0%								

FIGURE 35.2

Efficacy of motor control exercises compared with strengthening exercises for change in self-reported disability in adults with RCRSP and shoulder instability. CI, confidence intervals; IV, inverse variance method; RCRSP, rotator cuff-related shoulder pain; SD, standard deviation.

References

1. Arnoczky SP, Lavagnino M, Egerbacher M. The mechanobiological aetiopathogenesis of tendinopathy: is it the over-stimulation or the under-stimulation of tendon cells? Int J Exp Pathol. 2007;88:217-226.
2. Beard DJ, Rees JL, Cook JA, et al. Arthroscopic subacromial decompression for subacromial shoulder pain (CSAW): a multicentre, pragmatic, parallel group, placebo-controlled, three-group, randomised surgical trial. The Lancet. 2018 Jan 27;391(10118):329-38.
3. Beaudreuil J, Lasbleiz S, Aout M, et al. Effect of dynamic humeral centring (DHC) treatment on painful active elevation of the arm in subacromial impingement syndrome. Secondary analysis of data from an RCT. British Journal of Sports Medicine. 2015;49:343-346.
4. Beaudreuil J, Lasbleiz S, Richette P, et al. Assessment of dynamic humeral centering in shoulder pain with impingement syndrome: a randomised clinical trial. Annals of the Rheumatic Diseases. 2011;70:1613-1618.
5. Bernhardsson S, Klintberg IH, Wendt GK. Evaluation of an exercise concept focusing on eccentric strength training of the rotator cuff for patients with subacromial impingement syndrome. Clin Rehabil. 2011;25:69-78.
6. Blanpied PR, Gross AR, Elliott JM, et al. Neck pain: revision 2017. Clinical practice guidelines linked to the international classification of functioning, disability and health from the orthopaedic section of the American Physical Therapy Association. Journal of Orthopaedic & Sports Physical Therapy. 2017;47:A1-A83.
7. Boettcher CE, Cathers I, Ginn KA. The role of shoulder muscles is task specific. Journal of Science and Medicine in Sport. 2010;13:651-656.
8. Boudreau SA, Farina D, Falla D. The role of motor learning and neuroplasticity in designing rehabilitation approaches for musculoskeletal pain disorders. Man Ther. 2010;15:410-414.
9. Brumitt J, Cuddeford T. Current concepts of muscle and tendon adaptation to strength and conditioning. International Journal of Sports Physical Therapy. 2015;10:748-759.
10. Bury J, West M, Chamorro-Moriana G, Littlewood C. Effectiveness of scapula-focused approaches in patients with rotator

cuff related shoulder pain: a systematic review and meta-analysis. Man Ther. 2016;25:35-42.

11. Camargo PR, Alburquerque-Sendín F, Salvini TF. Eccentric training as a new approach for rotator cuff tendinopathy: review and perspectives. World Journal of Orthopedics. 2014;5:634-644.

12. Chou R, Qaseem A, Snow V, et al. Diagnosis and treatment of low back pain: a joint clinical practice guideline from the American College of Physicians and the American Pain Society. Annals of Internal Medicine. 2007;147:478-491.

13. Clausen MB, Witten A, Holm K, et al. Glenohumeral and scapulothoracic strength impairments exists in patients with subacromial impingement, but these are not reflected in the shoulder pain and disability index. BMC Musculoskeletal Disorders. 2017;18:302.

14. De Mey K, Danneels L, Cagnie B, Cools A. Scapular muscle rehabilitation exercises in overhead athletes with impingement symptoms: effect of a 6-week training program on muscle recruitment and functional outcome. The American Journal of Sports Medicine. 2012;40:1906-1915.

15. Dean BJF, Gwilym SE, Carr AJ. Why does my shoulder hurt? A review of the neuroanatomical and biochemical basis of shoulder pain. British Journal of Sports Medicine. 2013;47:1095-1104.

16. Desmeules F, Boudreault J, Dionne CE, et al. Efficacy of exercise therapy in workers with rotator cuff tendinopathy: a systematic review. Journal of Occupational Health. 2016;58:389-403.

17. Doiron-Cadrin P, Lafrance S, Saulnier M, et al. Shoulder rotator cuff disorders: a systematic review of clinical practice guidelines and semantic analyses of recommendations. Arch Phys Med Rehabil. 2020;101:1233-1242.

18. Dupuis F, Barrett E, Dubé M-O, McCreesh KM, Lewis JS, Roy J-S. Cryotherapy or gradual reloading exercises in acute presentations of rotator cuff tendinopathy: a randomised controlled trial. BMJ Open Sport & Exercise Medicine. 2018;4:e000477.

19. Ellingson LD, Stegner AJ, Schwabacher IJ, Koltyn KF, Cook DB. Exercise strengthens central nervous system modulation of pain in fibromyalgia. Brain Sci. 2016;6:8.

20. Escamilla RF, Hooks TR, Wilk KE. Optimal management of shoulder impingement syndrome. Open Access Journal of Sports Medicine. 2014;5:13-24.

21. Eshoj HR, Rasmussen S, Frich LH, et al. Neuromuscular exercises improve shoulder function more than standard care exercises in patients with a traumatic anterior shoulder dislocation: a randomized controlled trial. Orthop J Sports Med. 2020;8:2325967119896102.

22. Folland JP, Williams AG. The adaptations to strength training: morphological and neurological contributions to increased strength. Sports Medicine. 2007;37:145-168.

23. Friston K. What is optimal about motor control? Neuron. 2011;72:488-498.

24. Glover IS, Baker SN. Cortical, corticospinal, and reticulospinal contributions to strength training. Journal of Neuroscience. 2020;40:5820-5832.

25. Green S, Buchbinder R, Hetrick S. Physiotherapy interventions for shoulder pain. Cochrane Database Syst Rev. 2003;2:CD004258.

26. Gutiérrez-Espinoza, H., Araya-Quintanilla, F., Cereceda-Muriel, C., et al. Effect of supervised physiotherapy versus home exercise program in patients with subacromial impingement syndrome: a systematic review and meta-analysis. Physical Therapy in Sport. 2020;41:34-42.

27. Haahr JP, Andersen JH. Exercises may be as efficient as subacromial decompression in patients with subacromial stage II impingement: 4-8-years' follow-up in a prospective, randomized study. Scand J Rheumatol. 2006;35:224-228.

28. Haahr JP, Ostergaard S, Dalsgaard J, et al. Exercises versus arthroscopic decompression in patients with subacromial impingement: a randomised, controlled study in 90 cases with a one year follow up. Ann Rheum Dis. 2005;64:760-764.

29. Hanratty CE, McVeigh JG, Kerr DP, et al. The effectiveness of physiotherapy exercises in subacromial impingement syndrome: a systematic review and meta-analysis. Seminars in Arthritis and Rheumatism. 2012;42:297-316.

30. Higgins JPT, Green S. Cochrane Handbook for Systematic Reviews of Interventions Version 5.1.0. The Cochrane Collaboration; 2011.

31. Hodges PW. Pain and motor control: from the laboratory to rehabilitation. J Electromyogr Kinesiol. 2011;21:220-228.

32. Hodges PW, Tucker K. Moving differently in pain: a new theory to explain the adaptation to pain. Pain. 2011;152:S90-98.

33. Holmgren T, Björnsson Hallgren H, Öberg B, Adolfsson L, Johansson K. Effect of specific exercise strategy on need for surgery in patients with subacromial impingement syndrome: randomised controlled study. BMJ. 2014;48:1456-7.

34. Hopman K, Krahe L, Lukersmith S, McColl A, Vine K. Clinical practice guidelines for the management of rotator cuff syndrome in the workplace. 2013. Available at: https://rcs.med.unsw.edu.au/sites/default/files/rcs/page/RotatorCuffSyndromeGuidelines.pdf

35. Hutting N, Richardson J, Johnston V. The role of self-management in the treatment of musculoskeletal disorders. Manual Therapy. 2016;25:e15-e17.

36. Ingwersen KG, Jensen SL, Sørensen L, et al. Three months of progressive high-load versus traditional low-load strength training among patients with rotator cuff tendinopathy: primary results from the double-blind randomized controlled RoCTEx Trial. Orthopaedic Journal of Sports Medicine. 2017;5:2325967117723292.

37. Jette AM, Delitto A. Physical therapy treatment choices for musculoskeletal impairments. Physical Therapy. 1997;77:145-154.

38. Jonsson P, Wahlström P, Ohberg L, Alfredson H. Eccentric training in chronic painful impingement syndrome of the shoulder: results of a pilot study. Knee Surg Sports Traumatol Arthrosc. 2006;14:76-81.

39. Ketola S, Lehtinen J, Arnala I, et al. Does arthroscopic acromioplasty provide any additional value in the treatment of shoulder impingement syndrome? A two-year randomised controlled trial. J Bone Joint Surg Br. 2009;91:1326-1334.

40. Ketola S, Lehtinen J, Rousi T, et al. No evidence of long-term benefits of arthroscopic acromioplasty in the treatment of shoulder impingement syndrome: five-year results of a randomised controlled trial. Bone & Joint Research. 2013;2:132-139.

41. Kleim JA, Jones TA. Principles of experience-dependent neural plasticity: implications for rehabilitation after brain damage. J Speech Lang Hear Res 2008;51:S225-S239.

42. Kraemer WJ, Adams K, Cafarelli E, et al. American College of Sports Medicine position stand. Progression models in resistance training for healthy adults. Medicine and Science in Sports and Exercise. 2002;34:364-380.

43. Kromer TO, Sieben JM, de Bie RA, Bastiaenen CHG. Influence of fear-avoidance beliefs on disability in patients with subacromial shoulder pain in primary care: a secondary analysis. Physical Therapy. 2014;94:1775-1784.

44. Lafrance, S., Ouellet, P., Alaoui, R., et al. Motor control exercises compared to strengthening exercises for upper and lower extremity musculoskeletal disorders: a systematic review with meta-analyses of randomized controlled trials. Physical Therapy. 2021.

45. Latash ML. Fundamentals of Motor Control. London, UK: Elsevier/Academic Press; 2012.

46. Leadbetter WB. Cell-matrix response in tendon injury. Clin Sports Med. 1992;11:533-578.

47. Lewis J, McCreesh K, Roy JS, Ginn K. Rotator cuff tendinopathy: navigating the diagnosis-management conundrum. J Orthop Sports Phys Ther. 2015;1-43.

48. Littlewood C, Ashton J, Chance-Larsen K, May S, Sturrock B. Exercise for rotator cuff tendinopathy: a systematic review. Physiotherapy. 2012;98:101-109.

49. Littlewood C, Malliaras P, Chance-Larsen K. Therapeutic exercise for rotator cuff tendinopathy: a systematic review of contextual factors and prescription parameters. International Journal of Rehabilitation Research. 2015;38:95-106.

50. Lombardi I, Magri AG, Fleury AM, Da Silva AC, Natour J. Progressive resistance training in patients with shoulder impingement syndrome: a randomized controlled trial. Arthritis and Rheumatism. 2008;59:615-622.

51. Lorenz D, Morrison S. Current concepts in periodization of strength and conditioning for the sports physical therapist. International Journal of Sports Physical Therapy. 2015;10:734-747.

52. Low M. A time to reflect to reflect on motor control in musculoskeletal physical therapy. J Orthop Sports Phys Ther. 2018;48:833-836.

53. Maenhout AG, Mahieu NN, De Muynck M, De Wilde LF, Cools AM. Does adding heavy load eccentric training to rehabilitation of patients with unilateral subacromial impingement result in better outcome? A randomized, clinical trial. Knee Surgery, Sports Traumatology, Arthroscopy. 2013;21:1158-1167.

54. McAlindon TE, Bannuru RR, Sullivan M, et al. OARSI guidelines for the non-surgical management of knee osteoarthritis. Osteoarthritis and Cartilage. 2014;22:363-388.

55. Michener LA, Walsworth MK, Burnet EN. Effectiveness of rehabilitation for patients with subacromial impingement syndrome: a systematic review. Journal of Hand Therapy. 2004;17:152-164.

56. Overbeek CL, Kolk A, de Groot JH, et al. Altered cocontraction patterns of humeral head depressors in patients with subacromial pain syndrome: a cross-sectional electromyography analysis. Clinical Orthopaedics and Related Research. 2019;477:1862-1868.

57. Paavola M, Kanto K, Ranstam J, et al. Subacromial decompression versus diagnostic arthroscopy for shoulder impingement: a 5-year follow-up of a randomised, placebo surgery controlled clinical trial. British Journal of Sports Medicine. 2021;55(2):99-107.

58. Panjabi MM. The stabilizing system of the spine. Part I. Function, dysfunction, adaptation, and enhancement. J Spinal Disord. 1992;5:383-389.

59. Park I, Lee JH, Hyun HS, Lee TK, Shin SJ. Minimal clinically important differences in Rowe and Western Ontario Shoulder Instability Index scores after arthroscopic repair of anterior shoulder instability. J Shoulder Elbow Surg. 2018;27:579-584.

60. Petersen W, Taheri P, Forkel P, Zantop T. Return to play following ACL reconstruction: a systematic review about strength deficits. Archives of Orthopaedic and Trauma Surgery. 2014;134:1417-1428.

61. Reijneveld EA, Noten S, Michener LA, Cools A, Struyf F. Clinical outcomes of a scapular-focused treatment in patients with subacromial pain syndrome: a systematic review. British Journal of Sports Medicine. 2017;51:436-441.

62. Rhea MR, Hunter RL, Hunter TJ. Competition modeling of American football: observational data and implications for high school, collegiate, and professional player conditioning. Journal of Strength and Conditioning Research. 2006;20:58-61.

63. Rosenbaum DA. Human Motor Control, 2nd edition. London, UK: Elsevier/Academic Press; 2010.

64. Roy J-S, Moffet H, Hébert LJ, Lirette R. Effect of motor control and strengthening exercises on shoulder function in persons with impingement syndrome: a single-subject study design. Man Ther. 2009;14:180-188.

65. Roy JS, Bouyer LJ, Langevin P, Mercier C. Beyond the joint: the role of central nervous system reorganizations in chronic musculoskeletal disorders. J Orthop Sports Phys Ther. 2017;47:817-821.

66. Roy JS, Desmeules F, Frémont P, Dionne C, MacDermid JC. Clinical Evaluation, Treatment and Return to Work of Workers Suffering from Rotator Cuff Disorders: A Knowledge Review. Report R-949. Institut de Recherche Robert-Sauvé en Santé et en Sécurité du Travail. Montréal: 2017.

67. Roy JS, Desmeules F, Frémont P, Dionne C, MacDermid JC. L'évaluation clinique, les traitements et le retour en emploi de travailleurs souffrant d'atteintes de la coiffe des rotateurs - Bilan des connaissances. Études et recherches / Rapport R-885. Institut de Recherche Robert-Sauvé en Santé et en Sécurité du Travail. Montréal; 2015.

68. Sahrmann S. Diagnosis and treatment of movement impairment disorders. St Louis: Mosby; 2002.

69. Savoie A, Mercier C, Desmeules F, Fremont P, Roy JS. Effects of a movement training oriented rehabilitation program on symptoms, functional limitations and acromiohumeral distance in individuals with subacromial pain syndrome. Man Ther. 2015;20:703-708.

70. Schmidt R, Lee T. Motor Control and Learning: A Behavioral Emphasis, 4th edition. Human Kinetics; 2005.

71. Schoenfeld BJ, Contreras B, Krieger J, et al. Resistance training volume enhances muscle hypertrophy but not strength in trained men. Medicine and Science in Sports and Exercise. 2019;51:94-103.

72. Shire AR, Stæhr TAB, Overby JB, Dahl MB, Jacobsen JS, Christiansen DH. Specific or general exercise strategy for subacromial impingement syndrome–does it matter? A systematic literature review and meta analysis. BMC Musculoskelet Disord. 2017;18:158.

73. Shumway-Cook A, Woollacott MH. Motor Control: Translating Research into Clinical Practice, 3rd edition. Lippincott Williams & Wilkins; 2006.

74. Smith BE, Hendrick P, Bateman M, et al. Musculoskeletal pain and exercise—challenging existing paradigms and introducing new. British Journal of Sports Medicine. 2019;53:907-912.

75. Smith BE, Hendrick P, Smith TO, et al. Should exercises be painful in the management of chronic musculoskeletal pain? A systematic review and meta-analysis. British Journal of Sports Medicine. 2017;51:1679-1687.

76. Tashjian RZ, Deloach J, Porucznik CA, Powell AP. Minimal clinically important differences (MCID) and patient acceptable symptomatic state (PASS) for visual analog scales (VAS) measuring pain in patients treated for rotator cuff disease. J Shoulder Elbow Surg. 2009;18:927-932.

77. Timmons MK, Thigpen CA, Seitz AL, et al. Scapular kinematics and subacromial-impingement syndrome: a meta-analysis. Journal of Sport Rehabilitation. 2012;21:354-370.

78. Turgut E, Duzgun I, Baltaci G. Effects of scapular stabilization exercise training on scapular kinematics, disability, and pain in subacromial impingement: a randomized controlled trial. Arch Phys Med Rehabil. 2017;98:1915-1923.

79. Vaegter HB, Madsen AB, Handberg G, Graven-Nielsen T. Kinesiophobia is associated with pain intensity but not pain sensitivity before and after exercise: an explorative analysis. Physiotherapy. 2018;104:187-193.

80. Wang SS, Trudelle-Jackson EJ. Comparison of customized versus standard exercises in rehabilitation of shoulder disorders. Clinical Rehabilitation. 2006;20:675-685.

81. Warby SA, Ford JJ, Hahne AJ, et al. Comparison of 2 exercise rehabilitation programs for multidirectional instability of the glenohumeral joint: a randomized controlled trial. The American Journal of Sports Medicine. 2018;46:87-97.

82. Watson L, Warby S, Balster S, Lenssen R, Pizzari T. The treatment of multidirectional instability of the shoulder with a rehabilitation program: Part 1. Shoulder Elbow. 2016;8:271-278.

83. Watson L, Warby S, Balster S, Lenssen R, Pizzari T. The treatment of multidirectional instability of the shoulder with a rehabilitation programme: Part 2. Shoulder Elbow. 2017;9:46-53.

84. Worsley P, Warner M, Mottram S, et al. Motor control retraining exercises for shoulder impingement: effects on function, muscle activation, and biomechanics in young adults. Journal of Shoulder and Elbow Surgery. 2013;22:e11-9.

Shape-Up-My-Shoulder (#SUMS) rehabilitation program

36

Jeremy Lewis

Introduction

The rehabilitation program described in this chapter is underpinned by the information, hypotheses, guidance, and ideas generated throughout this book.

Movement is essential to maximize human function: it requires a reason and ability to move, continuous monitoring and feedback from the central and peripheral nervous systems, sufficient energy to complete the required task – which in turn depends upon nutrition, which depends on an adequate blood supply to transport oxygen, nutrients, and biochemicals, and remove waste products – and maintenance of metabolic and endocrinal homeostasis. Sleep is essential for the maintenance of these processes. Lifestyle behaviors, such as smoking, may negatively impact on the ability to perform the movements deemed to be of value for an individual.

Movement is clearly not solely dependent upon muscle contraction and joint movement. It is complex, and to be purposeful and function optimally, requires the coordinated interaction of the circulatory and lymphatic, digestive, endocrine, exocrine, immune, muscular, skeletal, nervous, renal, and respiratory systems. How a person moves is also dependent upon how the individual interprets any threats to movement, such as pain, actual and potential tissue damage, and disease. As such, restoration of impaired movement requires immeasurably more than prescribing sets and repetitions of exercise and measuring unidimensional outcomes, such as improvements in range of movement, and strength.

Members of our societies will most likely seek help when their ability to move becomes impaired. Prescribing exercise to maintain, improve or restore movement should only be considered if there are no contraindications, and the benefits outweigh any harms.

With respect to the management of musculoskeletal conditions involving the shoulder, the one universal treatment that is indicated at some stage is movement. This may be after a fracture has been stabilized and union has occurred, or when safe to move after shoulder surgery, or at the right stage of a condition, such as the "stiffness greater than pain" phase of a frozen shoulder. For some conditions, such as rotator cuff-related shoulder pain,[61] exercise is currently the management option of choice and in most cases should be prescribed before injections and surgery are considered. What is apparent throughout this textbook, is that for musculoskeletal conditions involving the shoulder, whether idiopathic, traumatic, related to overuse, following surgery or a procedure such as an injection, no one exercise program has currently demonstrated superiority over another.

Improving strength (being able to generate more force) is undoubtedly an important health goal, for example, the number of sit-to-stands achieved in 30 seconds predicts physical independence in later life.[91] Strength is one of the greatest "gifts" an older person can receive from their younger self, and the pursuit of improving strength can start at any stage of life.[92] However, the pursuit of *increased* strength is not necessary for reducing disability associated with shoulder pain.[86] Patients with musculoskeletal shoulder problems should *not* be told that the focus for reducing symptoms is gaining strength, as the available evidence does not support this contention.[21,86]

Strengthening should be part of a health improvement and management plan independent to the shoulder rehabilitation program: strengthening exercises should only be one consideration in health intervention programs, and should not be considered more important than other forms of exercise. For example, endurance training may be more important than strengthening for increasing heart rate variability (HRV).[83] HRV is linked to the autonomic nervous system and is the variation or difference in time (in milliseconds) between each successive heartbeat (i.e., the R-R interval). High HRV occurs when the rhythm between beats varies, whereas low HRV occurs when the time between beats is more constant. High HRV is important for good health, reduced morbidity and mortality, and better psychological well-being, whereas low HRV is associated with poorer health, stress, slow recovery, and worse health prognoses.[94,117]

Mind–body exercises such as yoga and potentially T'ai Chi (see Chapters 42 and 43) may be useful at increasing HRV and reducing stress,[117] and should also be considered in health improvement strategies. High intensity interval training (HIIT) is another exercise consideration, and although more research is required, short durations of exercising at near maximal/maximal intensity has been associated with favorable outcomes in people with and without health-related symptoms.[93] Where there are concerns relating to harms associated with a HIIT program,[96] such as performing unsupervised HIIT exercises in the presence of certain health conditions,[87] more traditional moderate intensity exercises may achieve very comparable benefits.[87,93]

Evidence for an exercise-based approach in the management of musculoskeletal shoulder conditions

Nonsurgical interventions for rotator cuff-related shoulder pain

The most common musculoskeletal shoulder condition is rotator cuff-related shoulder pain (RCRSP), an overarching term originally suggested to replace "diagnoses" such as subacromial impingement/pain syndrome, rotator cuff tendinopathy/tendinosis/tendinitis, subacromial bursitis, and partial and full thickness rotator cuff tears.[61] It may be further classified into traumatic and nontraumatic RCRSP (see Chapter 19). Studies comparing surgical and nonsurgical interventions have been published. A non-exhaustive summary of these studies is presented in Table 36.1. The findings clearly demonstrate that nonsurgical intervention, involving graduated exercise supported as appropriate by other interventions such as manual therapy early in the rehabilitation process,[84] should be prioritized for nontraumatic RCRSP for a minimum of 12 weeks.

Shape-Up-My-Shoulder (#SUMS) rehabilitation program

Shape-Up-My-Shoulder (#SUMS), the rehabilitation program described in this chapter, is one of many programs that is used in the rehabilitation of musculoskeletal conditions involving the shoulder.[14,84,103] I use it, or parts of it, when appropriate, and when not contraindicated (by the condition) or when the benefits of exercise outweigh potential harms (by the stage of condition) in the rehabilitation of nearly every person I see in my clinical practice. It is presented only as a suggestion, and you may wish to integrate all of it, or parts of it, into your practice, or you may have your own rehabilitation program that works well for those you care for, and if this is the case, you may choose to read this chapter only out of interest.

Begin with a vision of the end

The importance of developing and maintaining a strong therapeutic alliance based on mutual trust is a theme interwoven throughout the pages of this textbook. *No one will care how much you know, until they know how much you care.* Chapter 1 highlights failures in communication, with patients recounting that they felt they had not been listened to, and that their concerns and hopes did not seem important to the clinician in front of them. Some expressed confusion over the language used by clinicians, or by the inconsistent messages received from the same clinician or from different healthcare providers. Some expressed frustration that their healthcare providers insisted that they needed to get strong when they were already strong. Chapter 11 is a synthesis of thoughts, ideas, and suggestions from patients and clinicians representing different health professions on how to use communication effectively. As David Grossman eloquently describes in his book, *No Cape Needed*, "communication is your superpower."[28]

Use this superpower to forge a strong and enduring therapeutic relationship through listening, hearing, validating, and understanding what is important to the patient, what they want to achieve from treatment, and what the vision is that they have of themselves at the end of rehabilitation. Of course, it needs to be realistic, but by aligning the rehabilitation strategy to achieve the patient's vision of successful rehabilitation, one important foundation will be laid that will underpin an effective therapeutic relationship. When I use #SUMS in clinical practice, my aim (although I do not always achieve it) is to exceed the patient's expectation of their vision. My aim is for the patient to say, "I can't believe I can do this," "I have never done this before." I want the patient to have confidence in their shoulder that, if possible, is greater than before their problem started.

The components and stages of #SUMS

#SUMS is a multimodal and holistic rehabilitation program for people seeking care when living with a musculoskeletal

Table 36.1 Examples of studies that have compared surgical and nonsurgical interventions for RCRSP

Author/ year/country	Condition	Study design	Outcome measures	Main finding
Haahr et al. (2005)[30] Denmark	Subacromial impingement syndrome	Two group RCT (n=90) GI: SAD GII: Rehabilitation	1° OM: Constant score	At one year no clinically important differences between the groups
Haahr and Andersen (2006)[29] Denmark	Subacromial impingement syndrome	Two group RCT (n=90) GI: SAD GII: Rehabilitation	1° OM: Constant score	At 4–8 years no clinically important differences between the groups
Ketola et al. (2009)[45] Finland	Subacromial impingement syndrome	Two group RCT (n=140) GI: SAD GII: Rehabilitation	1° OM: Self-report of pain on VAS of 0–10	At two years no clinically important differences between the groups
Ketola et al. (2013)[46] Finland	Subacromial impingement syndrome	Two group RCT (n=140) GI: SAD GII: Rehabilitation	1° OM: Self-report of pain on VAS of 0–10	At a mean of five years, no clinically important differences between the groups
Ketola et al. (2017)[47] Finland	Subacromial impingement syndrome/rotator cuff tendinopathy	Two group RCT (n=140) GI: SAD GII: Rehabilitation	1° OM: Self-report of pain on VAS of 0–10	At a mean of 12 years, no clinically important differences between the groups
Kukkonen et al. (2014)[52] Finland	Non traumatic PTT (<75%) supraspinatus	Three group RCT (n=180) GI: Rehabilitation GII: SAD & rehabilitation GIII: RCR, SAD, & rehabilitation	1° OM: Constant score	At one year no clinically important differences between the groups (Cost: GI €2,417; GII €4,765; GIII €5,709)
Kukkonen et al. (2015)[53] Finland	Non traumatic PTT (<75%) supraspinatus	Three group RCT (n=180) GI: Rehabilitation GII: SAD & rehabilitation GIII: RCR, SAD, & rehabilitation	1° OM: Constant score	At two years no clinically important differences between the groups
Moosmayer et al. (2014)[79] Norway	Small to medium rotator cuff tear (≤ 3 cm)	Two group RCT (n=103) GI: Rehabilitation GII: RCR	1° OM: Constant score	At one, two, and five years no clinically important difference between the groups
Moosmayer et al. (2019)[78] Norway	Small to medium rotator cuff tear (≤ 3 cm)	Two group RCT (n=103) GI: Rehabilitation GII: RCR	1° OM: Constant score (MCID = 10.4 points)[54]	At 10 years 9.6 point change (95% CI 3.6–15.7) in Constant score in favor of the surgery group
Schrøder et al. (2017)[99] Norway	Type II SLAP	Three group RCT (n=118) GI: Type II SLAP repair GII: Biceps tenodesis GIII: Placebo surgery and rehabilitation	1° OM: Rowe score WOSI score 2° OM: OSIS, EuroQol	At two years, no clinical benefit following labral repair or biceps tenodesis when compared with placebo surgery and rehabilitation for type II SLAP tears

EuroQol, EQ 5D, EQ-VAS; G, group; MCID, minimal clinically important difference; n, number of participants in study; OM, outcome measure; OSIS, Oxford Shoulder Instability Score; PTT, partial thickness tear; RCR, rotator cuff repair; RCT, randomized controlled trial; SAD, subacromial decompression/acromioplasty; SLAP, superior labrum anterior to posterior; VAS, visual analogue scale; WOSI, Western Ontario Shoulder Instability Index.

condition involving their shoulder(s). Taylor[109] reported that for some people, the experience of living with musculoskeletal pain was associated with a perceived reduction in quality of life that was comparable to people living with complicated diabetes mellitus, chronic liver disease requiring transplantation, and terminal cancer. This highlights the importance of building a nonjudgmental, therapeutic relationship based on empathy, validation, and trust (see Chapter 11).

Education

Education is essential in the management of musculoskeletal shoulder problems, and as a single intervention has equivalent outcomes as an education and strengthening program.[21] Bloom published a six-level hierarchy of knowledge acquisition through cognitive learning,[8] which in 2001 was revised[5] from its original form to include remembering, understanding, applying, analyzing, evaluating, and creating. Although there is overlap between the subcategories, and differences in interpretation exist, the following provides an overview.

Remembering, the lowest level of learning, involves retrieving facts as needed (e.g., describing the origin and insertion of a muscle, stating smoking is bad for health). *Understanding* involves comprehension and facilitates the ability to explain (e.g., giving examples of the health benefits of physical activity, contrasting the different treatments and being able to compare the anticipated outcomes, time frames, personal responsibilities, and potential harms). *Application* entails the ability to use knowledge across different contexts (e.g., being able to perform statistical analysis on unfamiliar data, being able to judge/determine/decide at a relatively sophisticated level the best treatment option that is available after learning of the different options, and considering the impact of the decision on wider social, vocational, and environmental factors).

Analyzing involves an in-depth comparison or appraisal of the knowledge, which may come from the same, different, or competing sources. (e.g., appraising the information, clarifying through questioning, deconstructing evidence, and being able to explain at a state-of-the-art level). *Evaluating* enables detailed and sophisticated appraisal of the quality, validity, and reliability of the knowledge. It involves an ability to critique and synthesize complex and frequently equivocal evidence. It allows for experimentation and prediction, as well as the ability to form an opinion and present and debate that view based on a breadth, depth, and unbiased summary of the knowledge (e.g., detecting inconsistencies and inaccuracies in information presented, verifying the quality of the information presented based on a sophisticated analysis of data, determining if the presented conclusion(s) match the data used to reach the conclusions).

Creating, the highest level, is achieved when an individual has acquired the other five levels and can produce new knowledge, solve problems, lead effectively, and facilitate and manage change (e.g., constructing an alternative hypothesis, inventing a product, writing a book, directing a film, composing music).

Learning and gaining knowledge through an appropriate, multifaceted, multimodal education program is essential. No one will commit to lifestyle change (see Chapters 5 and 13) and a rehabilitation program without understanding why it is needed, that the time is right for them, and that the appropriate strategies to participate in the program are in place. People learn in different ways – some prefer reading, others listening, and some watching. Providing information in only one format may tick the education box, but may result in wasted opportunity and time, especially if not provided in the preferred learning style. Furthermore, providing educational information in the patient's desired format(s) by itself is not enough. Just as clinicians review how the exercise component of the rehabilitation program is progressing, they should do the same with the educational component. Clinicians should take time to listen to what the patient thought were the important messages gained from the educational information, and importantly, offer the patient the opportunity to discuss what they did not understand, or what they found confusing, or want to discuss in more detail (see Chapter 11). Aim to support the patient's journey of learning to achieve the highest level possible on Bloom's revised hierarchy.[5]

When time permits, and when possible and appropriate, I invite patients to go for a walk outside the clinic, or to sit together in the hospital garden, or talk over a cup of coffee: by doing so, I aim to contribute to establishing a stronger alliance, and I hope to demonstrate to the patient the importance of education in the rehabilitation program. Although you may need to make your own educational resources that are culturally appropriate and clinically sensitive for the communities you serve, multimodal educational resources are available for you to download and access through the link below.

https://drjeremylewis.com/in/shoulder-book-all-resources

Additional factors

Providing an effective individual or group rehabilitation program[7] requires an understanding of how shoulder symptoms affect people (see Chapters 1 and 3) and the reasons why symptoms may manifest and perpetuate (see Chapters 5, 6, and 7). It further requires an understanding of how the shoulder functions and the importance of the kinetic chain (see Chapters 2 and 4). It is necessary to determine how best to assess and categorize shoulder disability (see Chapters 11–22 and 24–29), and to remain vigilant for the presence or emergence of non-musculoskeletal conditions, and those requiring urgent referral (see Chapters 8, 14, and 25). Once a clinical hypothesis has been offered, based on the patient interview, clinical examination and reasoning, and if appropriate, supported by radiological and laboratory investigations, there is a need to share management options in an unbiased manner (see Chapter 13), while also being aware that we are practicing in an environment where our knowledge is incomplete (see Chapter 10).

The next stage is to develop a patient-centered rehabilitation plan (see Chapters 35 and 37–43), supported as appropriate by other management options (see Chapters 23 and 31–34), that will most likely require lifestyle and behavioral change (see Chapters 5 and 13), followed by a lifetime commitment to maximizing and maintaining the best health possible. In addition to the above, the #SUMS rehabilitation program is also built on the promotion of self-efficacy and self-management, the need to keep adjunct treatments to a minimum, and most importantly, on an understanding that clinicians do not fix musculoskeletal conditions.[63,66]

Load management

Although it may sound counterintuitive to patients, working or exercising in pain in most situations will not cause damage to the shoulder. In fact, most damage may occur as a result of not moving the shoulder. Even if this is understood, most people presenting with shoulder pain find that they cannot generate the forces necessary to use the shoulder as desired because of the pain. If this is the situation then the clinician and patient will need to work together to find a level of load that is tolerable. One way to find this level is to manipulate the *I*ntensity, *D*uration, and *F*requency of the activity that is associated with symptoms. This is best explained using a case scenario (Box 36.1), which may be applied to all sporting, work-related, and social activities.

Box 36.1 Shoulder pain during swimming

'Sarah' is 50 years of age, right-hand dominant, an architect, lives with her partner and two teenage children, and has swum five days per week for more than eight years. Her routine is 50 laps of a 25-meter (27.3 yard) pool. She swims freestyle and breathes bilaterally. Her average lap time is 35 seconds, and she takes approximately 30 minutes to complete the 1250 meters (1367 yards). She is in good health, takes no prescribed or over the counter medications, volunteers in a food bank, and is an amateur potter.

Her local pool was closed due to the SARS-CoV-2 pandemic, and she was unable to swim for more than three months and exercised when able at home, expressing "it wasn't the same". When the pool reopened, she decided that "she was going to make up for lost time". Within two weeks of resuming, she started to experience right-sided anterolateral shoulder pain. The pain did not bother her at night or at work, but by the end of the third week, she was experiencing a substantial increase in pain when swimming and was unable to "generate any force with the shoulder by the fourth or fifth lap". She self-medicated using nonsteroidal anti-inflammatory medications (ibuprofen) with no perceived benefit and stopped after two weeks. She has experienced ongoing shoulder pain for more than six months.

Sarah's care was initially managed via telehealth, and following the initial online consultation, it appeared likely that her symptoms were due to rotator cuff-related shoulder pain. Sarah was surprised that the shoulder muscles, tendons and surrounding structures would respond this way to a training schedule she had followed for years. However, she appreciated that there had been a lengthy period of virtually no shoulder exercise (due to the lockdown imposed by the pandemic), followed by a motivated and enthusiastic return to swimming, which placed unaccustomed strain on her shoulder, and was probably more than the shoulder could tolerate at that time. Following this discussion, a management plan was put in place.

Initially this involved experimenting with the mechanics of swimming in a stepwise fashion; reducing the length of the swim stroke and ensuring hand entry into water was led by the fingers and not the thumb. These suggestions made no appreciable change. Sarah was then emailed a load management plan to facilitate self-efficacy and self-management. Figure 36.1 details the load management plan devised with Sarah. The principles of the plan were to incrementally adjust the *I*ntensity, *D*uration and *F*requency of her activity to find a swimming volume that could be tolerated.

The plan starts with a stepwise decrease in intensity or speed, aiming to achieve a tolerable level of pain: if not achieved, then reduction in speed is maintained, and distance or duration is decreased stepwise. If the pain levels are still not tolerated, frequency should be reduced, allowing for more recovery time. The order of reducing distance and frequency is interchangeable and may be determined by the patient. These are purely suggestions, and the incremental changes may be smaller or larger. The time to find a tolerable load using this guidance may take one week, but the plan may be implemented over one to two days. Once a tolerable load is found, this becomes the baseline to build the reloading program. The goal is to find a way for the

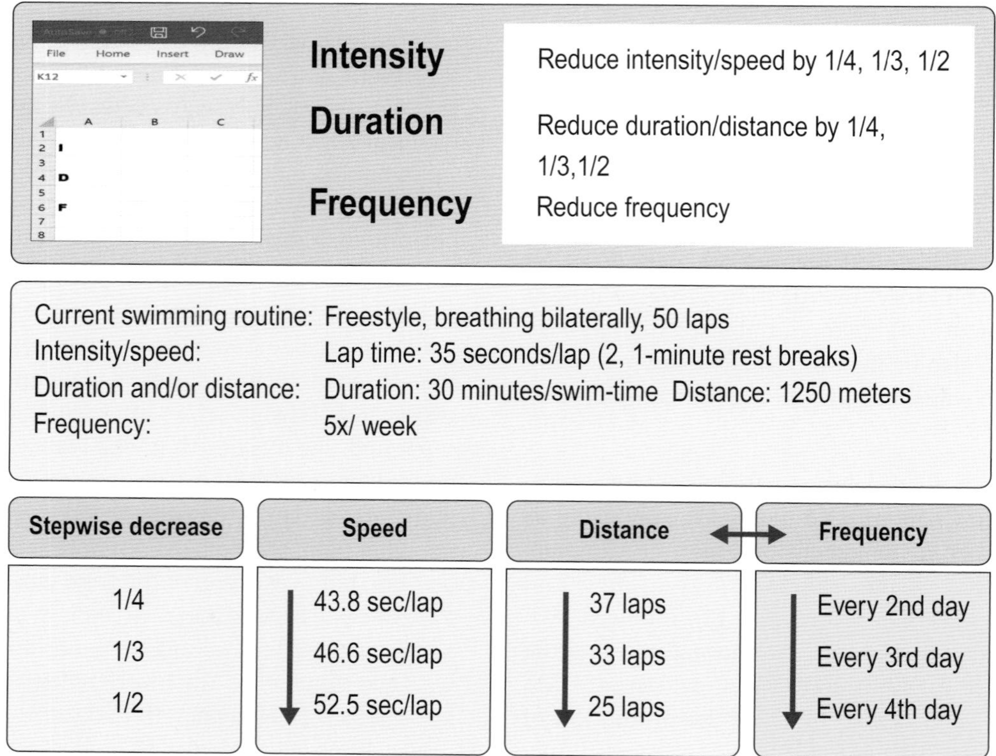

FIGURE 36.1
Load management planning using a spreadsheet (which could equally have been constructed on a sheet of paper).

patient to maintain participating in a valued activity in a tolerable way. If this proves impossible, that activity may need to stop for a period of time.

Time frames

When faced with a reduction in training volume, work, or social activity, it is common and understandable for people to ask if there are quicker alternatives to allow them to return to "normal". Being unable to "fix" musculoskeletal conditions,[63,66] clinicians need to sensitively explain rehabilitation time frames, which for most musculoskeletal conditions involving the shoulder takes an average of 12 weeks, requiring a combination of clinical and self-managed home exercises.[30,51] A video graphic that may be used to provide information relating to time frames is available at the link below.

https://drjeremylewis.com/in/shoulder-book-resource-rehabilitation-time-frames

When discussing time frames with an individual expecting or hoping that their symptoms associated with RCRSP will settle the same day or soon after, I often use a fracture analogy, asking the individual if they, or someone they know has had an upper or lower limb fracture. Invariably the answer is yes. I then ask whether it was possible to run, dance, skip, hop (with a lower limb fracture), or do pull-ups, serve in tennis, swim, or hammer nails into walls (with an upper limb fracture). The answer to these questions is clearly no. I then emphasize that the same respect and patience in day-to-day activities need be afforded to muscle–tendon problems as given to fractures.

In the same way that compromises need to be found when living with a fracture, compromises (exercising and working at a tolerable level of pain) need to be found when treating a muscle–tendon problem. The major difference between a fracture and a muscle–tendon problem is that muscle–tendon problems do not require immobilization as most fractures do. The patient must not leave thinking that they have a fracture, they just need to understand that currently, no immediate fix is available, and compromises will be required.

"Pop in a positive"

It is understandable that for many, disappointment and frustration will be associated with the need to reduce work, sporting, and certain social activities to a tolerable level. The frustration may to some extent be mitigated by "popping in a positive", such as discussing the importance of, and reliance upon, the entire kinetic chain to augment shoulder function (see Chapter 4). During (and after) the load reduction phase when shoulder load is decreased to bring the symptoms to a tolerable level, the patient should be guided through an assessment and management program to maximize energy transfer to the shoulder.

An easy way to explain the basis for this is by asking the patient to demonstrate (or describe) a golf swing, tennis serve, lifting a bag onto an overhead luggage rack, picking up a grandchild, picking up shopping from a low shelf to trolley to checkout, carrying a vacuum cleaner, throwing a frisbee, etc. Although the energy transfer requirements vary, for example in swimming the lower limb contribution is substantially less than throwing (10–15% versus 50–55%, respectively),[4,27,90] there is a universal need (whenever possible) to maximize kinetic chain energy transfer in an attempt to mitigate against future shoulder overload.

Finding a safe entry level for rehabilitation

Not all patients can start their rehabilitation at the same entry level, or progress at the same pace. All of us have prescribed exercises to patients, who have returned a week or so later reporting of a flare-up in symptoms. This is unfortunately common, and unless there are clear health reasons to stop the program (which should be the very last consideration), preparing the patient for increases in pain should have been covered in the education program.

One of many reasons for an increase in pain is that the rehabilitation program started at too high a level. If you were to run a marathon tomorrow without any preparation for the physical and psychological challenges you would face, it is more than likely you would experience severe and sustained levels of pain lasting long after the completion of the marathon. Using this analogy, for many patients who may not have exercised for six months or even six years, and have not done anything in the past six weeks due to their shoulder symptoms, and have been prescribed

10 repetitions of a resistance-based exercise, rest, and repeat three times, twice a day, may represent the equivalent of "running a marathon."

One way to mitigate against this is to analyze the type and amount of physical activity carried out in the past four weeks, calculate the average, and make that the starting point. For example, a 26-year-old patient, who in the past two years had not abducted or flexed his dominant-side arm more than 30° due to pain, had previously been able to do 58 pull-ups without a break. Perceived rehabilitation success was being able to perform 58 pull-ups once again. Hoping to exceed expectations, my aim was for him to achieve at least 60. Starting with even one would be the equivalent of "running a marathon", and it took around 4–6 weeks before we were ready to start on machine-assisted close-grip pull-ups reducing 90% of his body weight.

Another principle is to progress in very small increments, as tendons do not respond well to abrupt loading changes.

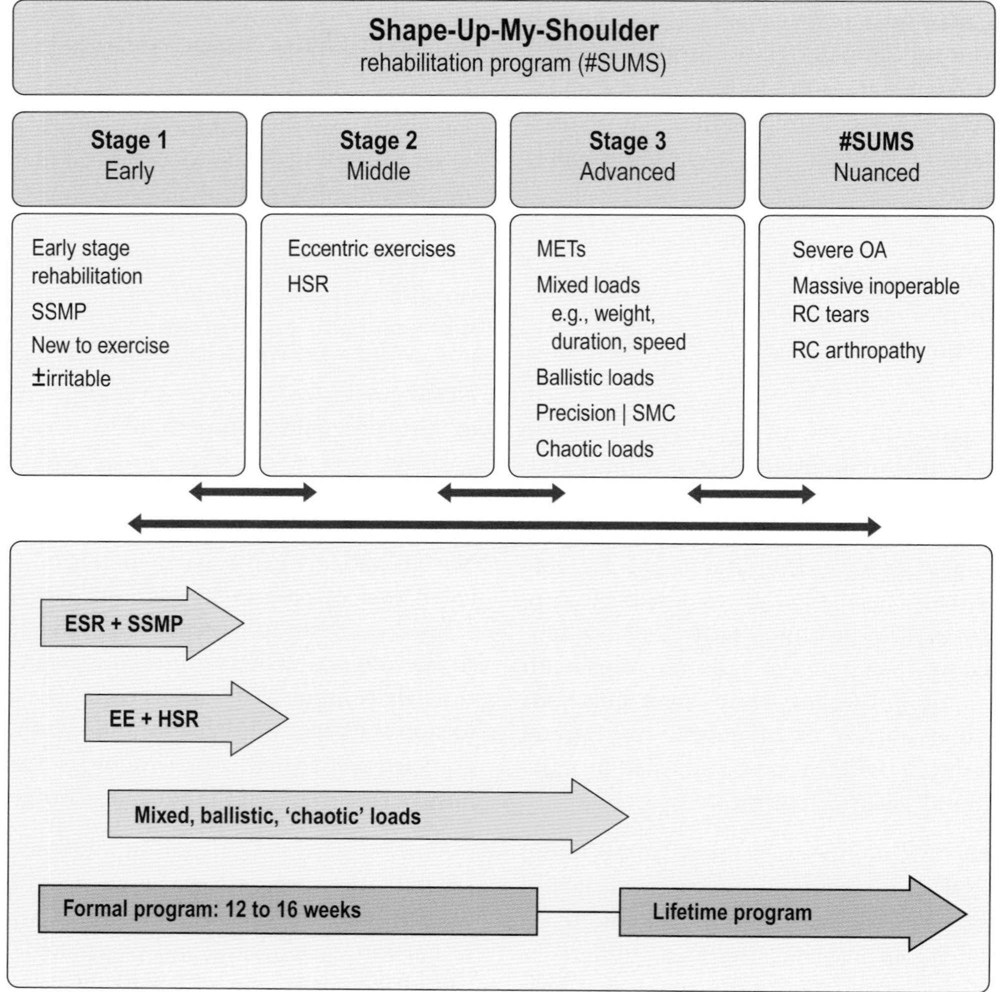

FIGURE 36.2

Stages of #SUMS. EE, eccentric exercises; ESR, early-stage rehabilitation; HSR, heavy slow resistance; METs, metabolic equivalents of a task; OA, osteoarthritis; RC, rotator cuff; SSMP, Shoulder Symptom Modification Procedure; SMC, sensorimotor control; #SUMS Shape-Up-My-Shoulder rehabilitation program.

The physiology supporting this tenet is complex.[16,61,62,64,100] It does not appear important for long-term benefit that patients experience pain during rehabilitation. However, it is important that patients remain cognizant that experiencing pain during rehabilitation exercise and during daily function is not an indicator of pathological tissue damage. One way of managing pain levels is to suggest to the patient that pain experienced during exercise, if tolerable, is acceptable, and that this pain should settle soon after the exercises have stopped. Any increase in night pain, or pain the following day, does not imply damage, but indicates that the intensity, duration, and frequency of the program need to be adjusted.

Figure 36.2 depicts the stages of the #SUMS rehabilitation program. The timepoints to transition between phases are determined by the patient and clinician, and as illustrated, overlaps exists between the stages.

Stage I: early-stage rehabilitation and the Shoulder Symptom Modification Procedure (#SSMP)

A key aim of #SUMS is the restoration of function to enable the individual to participate in valued activities. There are myriad ways this may be achieved, of which #SUMS is one. #SUMS combines early-stage rehabilitation with function, and once the formal program is complete, the final stage aims to encourage the patient to embrace a lifetime program that maintains and enhances optimum health through stress reduction and good sleeping behavior, balanced nutrition, healthy lifestyle choices, and exercise based on diverse physical activities. The aim is for the patient to have confidence, feel pride, and exceed all their expectations in what they believed they could achieve. Recently, Lafrance et al. compared motor control with strengthening exercises and reported that for conditions such as RCRSP, motor control exercises lead to greater reductions in pain and better improvements in function than strengthening exercises[56] (see Chapter 35). Because of this, #SUMS starts with exercises that aim to restore movement and, where possible, reduce symptoms.

The Shoulder Symptom Modification Procedure (SSMP)

Symptom modification has been described as an overarching rationale in the management of many musculoskeletal conditions.[60] One symptom modification method, the SSMP first described by Lewis,[65] has evolved into a systematic process that aims to facilitate symptom-reduced movement.[61,62,68] The process is simple and fast, and starts with the patient identifying a movement, posture, or activity that is associated with symptoms: this is referred to as the primary or principal problem (PIC – patient identified concern). Examples are limitless but may include shoulder pain when moving the neck, or shoulder symptoms experienced when elevating the arm, dressing, throwing, lifting, or pushing. Once identified and baseline symptoms (stiffness, weakness, pain, paresthesia, feeling of instability, fear of movement, etc.) have been established, a series of techniques are applied to the PIC to determine if the patient experiences a meaningful reduction in symptoms. If one of the SSMP techniques achieves a patient-reported meaningful reduction in the PIC then that technique is immediately incorporated into management. The SSMP process should not take longer than 3 minutes, which is the length of time I would have previously spent on shoulder orthopedic special tests, which I no longer use.[97] A downloadable SSMP assessment form (Figure 36.3), written and video examples of selected techniques, and suggestions for clinical application, are available at the link below.

https://drjeremylewis.com/in/shoulder-book-resource-ssmp

Once impairments such as motion, loss, pain, etc. have been assessed, SSMP techniques may be applied to the PIC. For example, if a patient reports that taking out or putting back a plate from a cupboard shelf brings on their symptoms, SSMP techniques may be applied during the movement to determine if the individual subjectively feels a meaningful reduction in symptoms during that task (PIC).

The first technique on the list is called the finger on sternum (breastbone) technique (Figure 36.4). It involves requesting that the patient place the contralateral index finger on the sternum and then while keeping the finger on the sternum, lift the finger (as well as that point on the sternum) up a few centimeters (an inch or more), hold the position, and repeat the PIC. There are three

Shape-Up-My-Shoulder (#SUMS)

Stage 1 Shoulder Symptom Modification Procedure [SSMP] v8

Name	**Date of birth**	**Date**

Symptomatic movement, activity, or posture (PiC – patient identified concern)

PiC #1 ....

PiC #2 ....

Consider Metronome/virtual reality/ counting backwards/other	**Change / improvement** None	Worse	Partial	Complete	**Comment**
1 Group 1					
Finger on sternum					
Other					
2A Group 2					
Scapular 'elevation'					
Scapular 'posterior tilt'					
Other e.g., 'depression' | combinations					
2B Winging scapula n/a ☐					
Combined elevation and posterior tilt					
'Squash' technique					
Taping					
Other					
3 Group 3					
Long to short lever lifts					
Squeeze ball (try either hand)					
Open hand (symptomatic side)					
Step forward/with resistance					
Step up					
'Humeral head' depression					
Eccentric elevation					
External rotation resistance					
Internal rotation resistance					
AP pressure					
PA pressure					
Other					

About the SSMP

- Stage 1 of a multistage graduated rehabilitation program. If not beneficial move to Stage 2. (Can revisit SSMP at later stage)
- **2–3 minutes** of clinical time
- **Do not** say aim is to change symptoms, i.e. **same** as when performing an orthopaedic test, just ascertain response
- **Clinical experiments** aiming to disrupt / **break pain memories / associations**
- **Not designed to permanently change posture** and reason for change in symptoms is not known, and may be due to distraction, placebo, mechanical, other
- May lead to a reduction in movement avoidance behaviours and improved self-efficacy and reduce 'threat' posed by that movement
- If a reduction in symptoms is achieved then link immediately to (functional) movements – At **worst**, the movement = **scapular and RC exercise**

www.drjeremylewis.com **@JeremyLewisPT** **@jeremy.s.lewis**

FIGURE 36.3
The SSMP assessment and recording template.

possible responses: better, same, or worse. If the response is the same or worse, immediately move onto the next technique. The techniques will have mechanical effects: decrease the kyphosis, change the position of the scapula, and increase the acromio-humeral distance. They may also influence symptoms via distraction, placebo, and via a different sensory input (due to touch).

Even though the finger on sternum technique decreases the kyphosis, the technique is not called "improve your posture", as I do not want the patient to think their posture is the cause of symptoms, especially as there is no evidence for a relationship between static upper body posture and symptoms,[67] and equally there is no evidence that static posture changes following rehabilitation[7] (see Chapter 20). When asked by a patient why their symptoms have changed, I usually reply that there are many possible reasons and that it is not possible to be certain which mechanism helped in their case, but that we do know exercise and movement commonly have a positive benefit in reducing symptoms for people experiencing shoulder pain, and that the techniques being used have been shown to be very effective.[21]

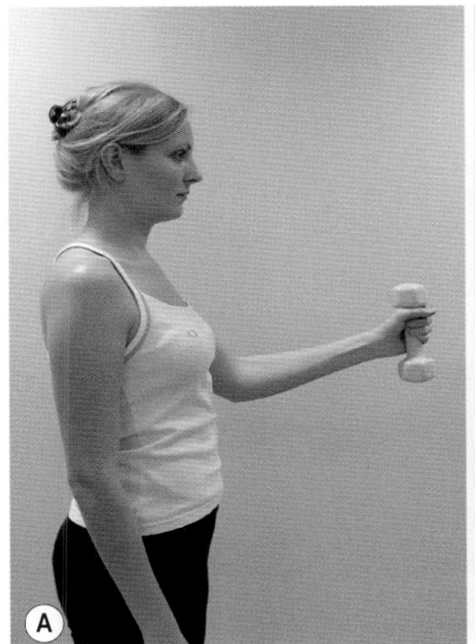

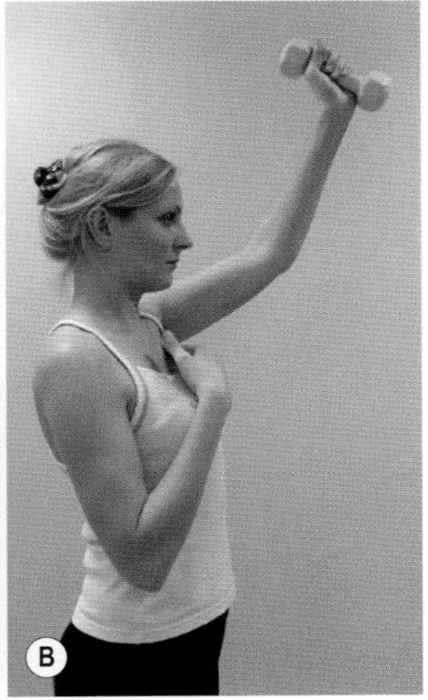

FIGURE 36.4

Finger on sternum technique.

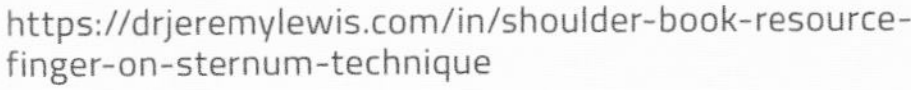
https://drjeremylewis.com/in/shoulder-book-resource-finger-on-sternum-technique

How might the SSMP reduce symptoms?

Why the SSMP might immediately reduce symptoms in some people remains unknown, but in part, may be due to mechanical changes, fear reduction (reduced threat) and movement confidence, placebo, new sensory input, and distraction. Although the importance of an immediate reduction in symptoms remains unknown,[15,95] the findings of one study suggested that SSMP techniques were associated with an immediate (partial or complete) reduction in symptoms in 67.9% of occasions.[68] In a prognostic study that involved collecting 71 outcome measures in 1030 people with shoulder symptoms, Chester et al.[13] reported that the only baseline physical test identified as an independent predictor of improved symptoms at six months were "scapular based" symptom modification procedures. The major predictors were psychological variables.

Concerns over hypervigilance

A concern levelled at all symptom modification procedures is the worry that if symptom reduction is not possible then the patient may become hypervigilant (a state of increased anxiety) due to concern that the symptoms may never change.[60] This theoretical concern has not been proven and (hopefully) in clinical practice no clinician would inform a patient that the orthopedic tests they are about to perform are going to cause pain. When performing orthopedic tests, clinicians typically inform patients that they will conduct a series of clinical tests and request that the patient reports their response. Invariably, the responses to the orthopedic tests are better, same, or worse. No concern has ever been raised that should an orthopedic test increase pain, a state of hypervigilance is unavoidable. To avoid biasing the patient's response, before applying a symptom modification procedure, or a range of motion, muscle performance, or orthopedic test, the clinician should inform: "I'm going to examine your shoulder using a series of clinical tests that will assess your movement, strength, and symptoms; please tell me what you feel after each test." Hypervigilance, although a theoretical possibility, is highly unlikely.

Application

If an SSMP technique subjectively improves symptoms, then the clinician should incorporate the technique during the PIC. It is not uncommon for multiple SSMP techniques to improve symptoms, and the reasons for this are multifarious. If one SSMP technique has a beneficial effect, this is the one to commence with. If uncertain of which technique to apply, I would suggest that the clinician ask the patient which procedure had the best effect on their PIC. If two or more techniques "equally" reduce the symptoms associated with e.g., push-ups, throwing, swim stroke, reaching up to a high shelf, tucking a shirt into trousers in a hand behind back maneuver, or washing hair, then the patient should determine which technique to start with first.

As an example, for the patient reporting the symptoms of shoulder pain and the feeling that the shoulder will "give way" when throwing, SSMP techniques would be applied to this. If, for example, the AP pressure technique applied with a neoprene shoulder strap (Figure 36.5) meaningfully reduces symptoms, then this assessment technique is incorporated into treatment. With the neoprene strap in place, the patient should be requested initially to perform the provocative throwing movement 3 to 5 times, rest for a minute, and repeat the sequence, once or twice more. I would then ask the patient to visualize that they are in the location where they experience symptoms – in the pool, at work, at

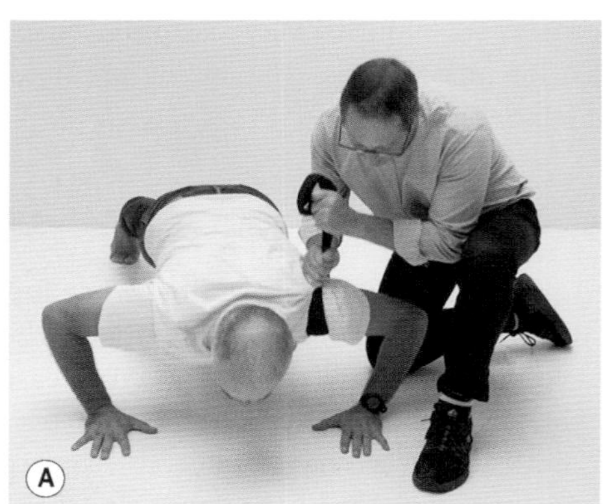

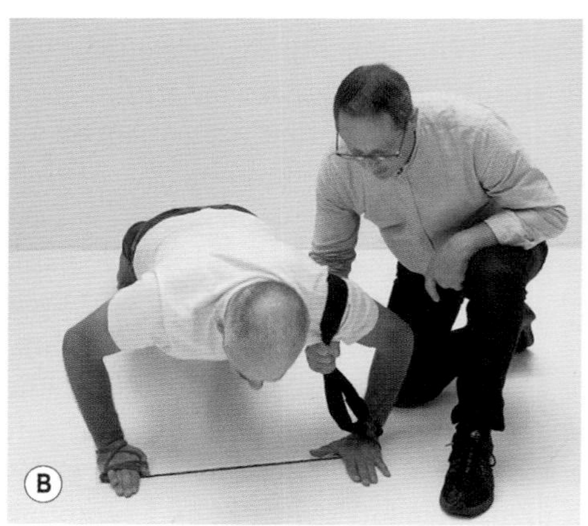

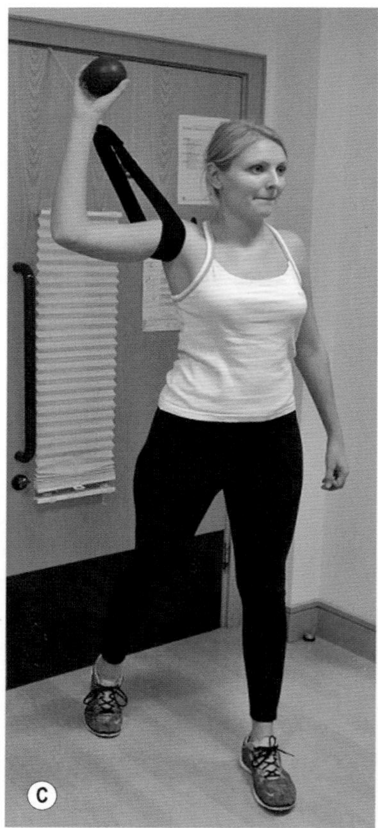

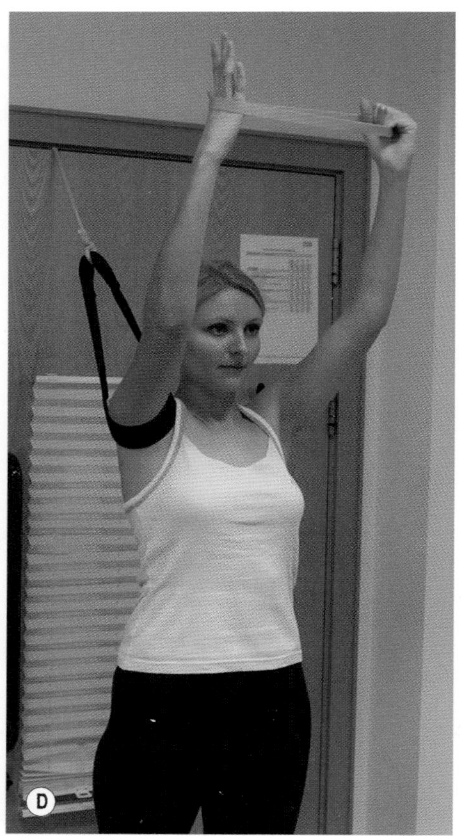

FIGURE 36.5
Neoprene shoulder strap applying an anteroposterior pressure on the shoulder to assess the response to symptoms described as "giving way" when throwing or during a push up.
https://drjeremylewis.com/in/shoulder-book-resource-assess-giving-away

home, on the sports field, in the gym – and repeat, trying to imagine that they are doing the symptomatic movement with the current reduction in symptoms. Finally, I would ask them to repeat the movement without the symptom modifier.

Based on the response, if the reduction of symptoms persists, the patient can be given the movement as a home exercise without the symptom modifier, or more often, as a home exercise together with an appropriate symptom modifier. If an SSMP technique does not produce the desired response, the process may be reattempted in future clinical encounters. Similarly, if the patient's condition plateaus while following an agreed post-surgical rehabilitation protocol, when safe to do so, SSMP techniques may be introduced to determine their influence on ongoing impairments. The order of the SSMP techniques may be varied and new SSMP techniques may be incorporated at any stage.

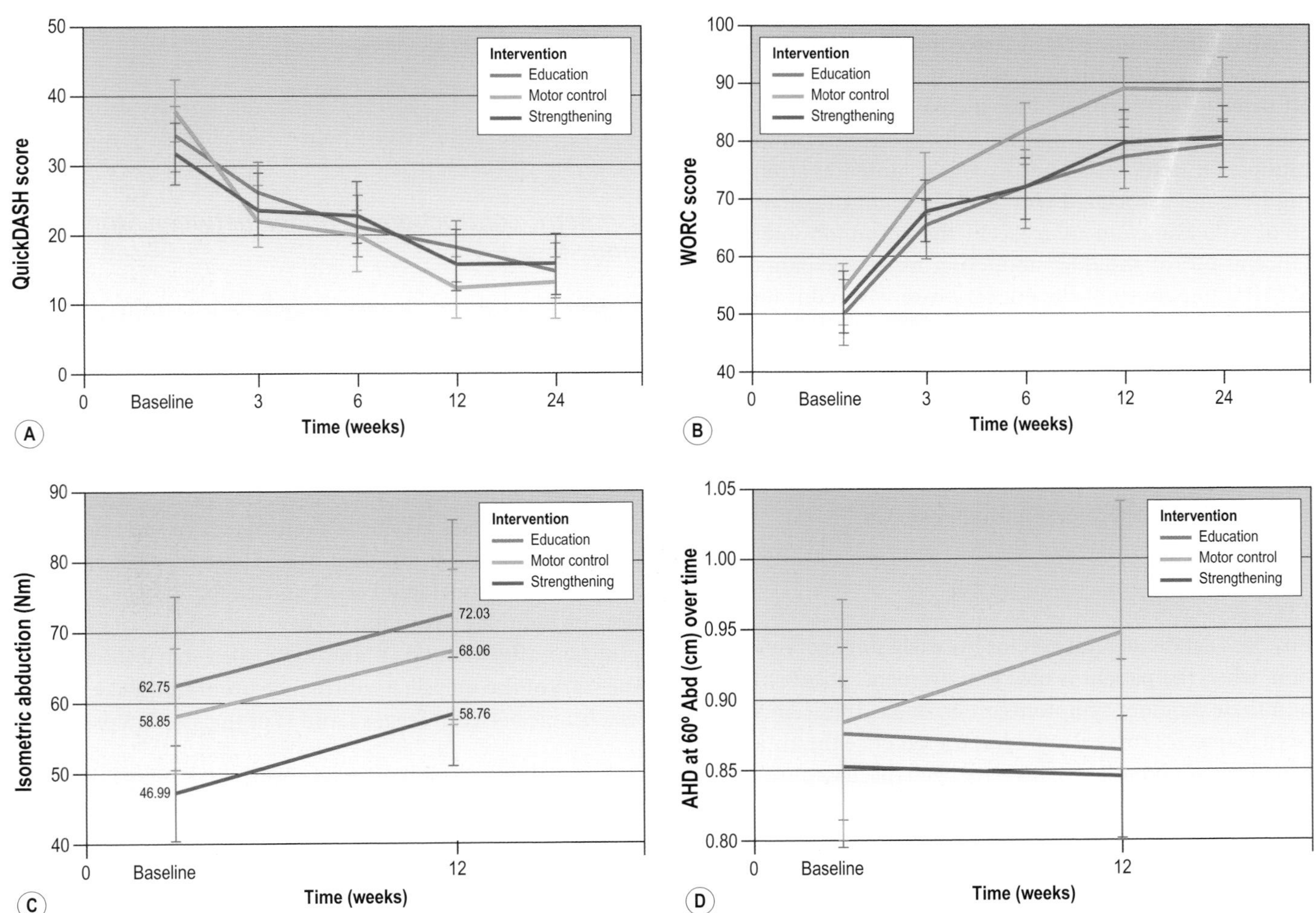

FIGURE 36.6

A comparison of education, SSMP, and strengthening exercises for people diagnosed with RCRSP. (A) Mean QuickDASH score (0–100) over time. (B) Mean WORC score (0–100) over time. (C) Mean peak isometric strength (Nm) for shoulder abduction before and after the 12-week intervention. (D) Mean acromiohumeral distance (cm) at 60° of arm abduction before and after the 12-week intervention. Nm, Newton-meter; WORC, Western Ontario Rotator Cuff Index.

Research

Although criticized in blogs and research articles deemed to be at risk of high levels of bias,[76] recent investigations support the use of the SSMP in the early stages of shoulder rehabilitation for RCRSP.[21] Dubé et al.[21] compared the short-, mid- and longer-term effects of education (group I), education and strengthening (group II) and, education and SSMP techniques (group III)[21,22] (Figures 36.6A–D). Figures 36.6A and B illustrate that all three interventions led to clinically and statistically significant improvements in symptoms for people diagnosed with RCRSP. Participants in the SSMP group demonstrated faster improvement than those in the other two groups. Figure 36.6C demonstrates that all three groups exhibited an increase in isometric abduction strength, including the education-only and SSMP groups. Of note, resistance exercises aimed at strengthening were not associated with greater strength gains. Figure 36.6D illustrates an increase in the acromiohumeral distance at 60° of shoulder abduction for participants in the SSMP group, but not the education-only or education and strengthening group. This may in part explain why the participants in the SSMP group clinically improved to a greater extent than those in the other two groups. Although all three interventions are suitable for the management of RCRSP, the SSMP exercises were associated with faster and larger improvements in symptoms, supporting their inclusion in the #SUMS rehabilitation program.

Other early-stage techniques

Box 36.2 details suggestions for the early stages of rehabilitation, when the patient is new to movement, possibly fearful, or if their shoulder symptoms are irritable. Injection therapy (see Chapter 23) may also be considered once the anticipated benefits and potential harms have been discussed.

Next steps

If the SSMP does not improve symptoms, or if it subjectively worsens them, then the clinician should move on to another early rehabilitation technique. If the SSMP and the other early-stage techniques (Box 36.2) still do not produce clinical improvement, then the next stage of #SUMS is to move to the bridging treatment between Stages I and II – isometric contractions.

Box 36.2 Suggestions for early-stage rehabilitation

- Breathing and relaxation exercises[40,70] (see Chapter 43 and consider commercially available apps, e.g., https://www.headspace.com/, https://www.calm.com/)
- Visualization, music, and mental imagery
- Exercise contralateral side
- Hand gripping exercises
- Ball rolling exercises (see Figure 36.7)
- Virtual reality[69] (see Chapter 30)

Isometric contractions: a bridge between Stage I and Stage II

Isometric exercises involve muscle contractions that are not associated with detectable changes in the position of the joint(s) the muscle/muscle group acts upon. In comparison to isotonic contractions, where the muscles shorten or lengthen, isometric contractions are also referred to as static muscle contractions. Studies on isometric exercises generally,[9] and for the shoulder region specifically,[23,81] suggest that isometric exercises may have a role to play in shoulder rehabilitation, but this is not definitive. These types of exercises should not be considered as a panacea for improving function or reducing symptoms. They are used in the #SUMS program after the SSMP and early-stage rehabilitation, as the start of the muscle performance program (Stage II) and as a bridge between Stages I and II of the #SUMS program.

One of many ways to incorporate isometric exercises is to choose the most painful and/or "weakest" shoulder movement to perform the isometric contraction. For example, if the most provocative movement is shoulder external rotation, then position the arm on a supporting surface (Figure 36.8) and start a metronome beating at 60 beats per minute (i.e., 1 beat per second). The clinician should demonstrate first the procedure on the patient's contralateral side (if appropriate) by asking them to perform a maximal isometric contraction. This serves two purposes: 1) understanding the exercise, and 2) understanding of maximal

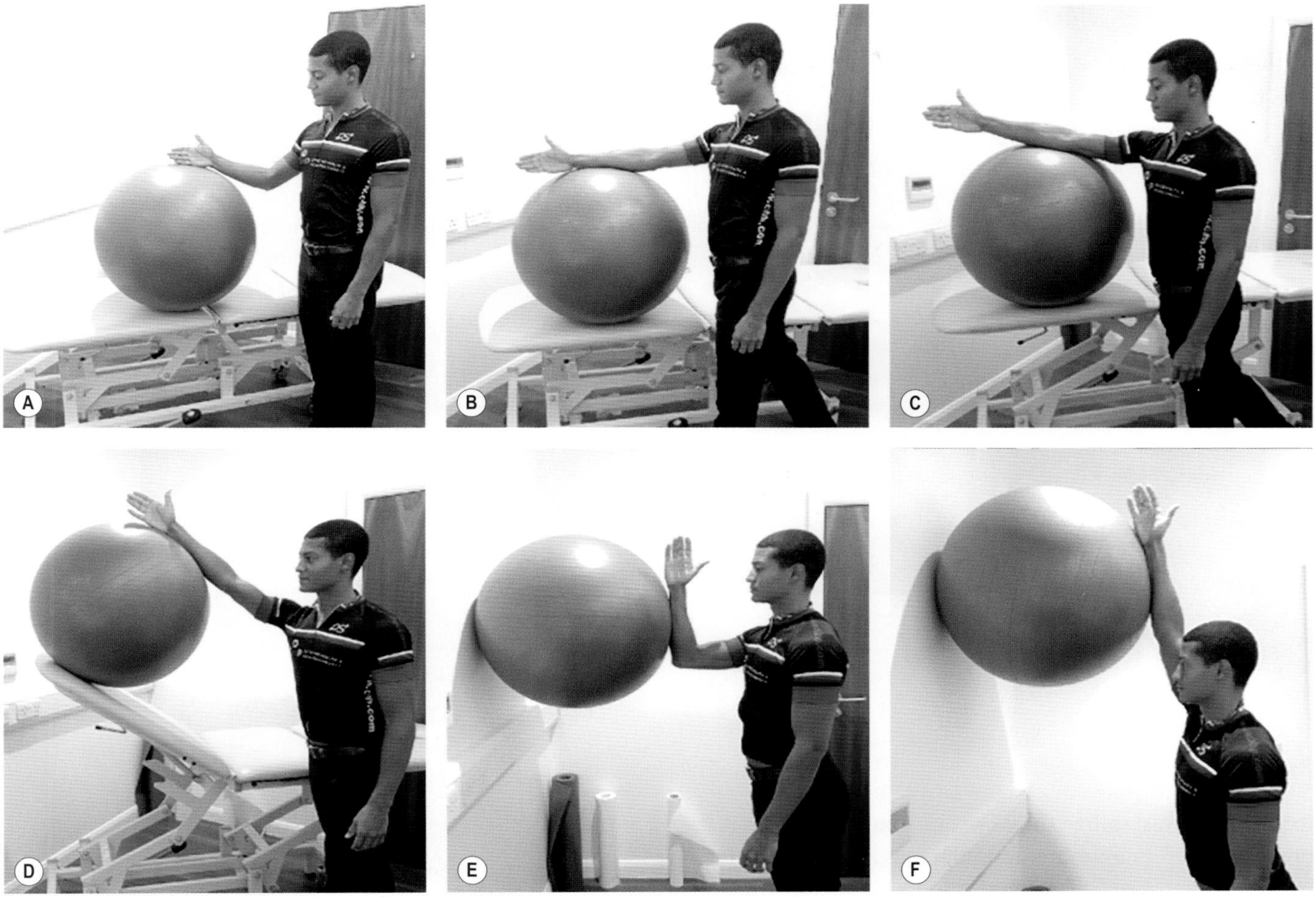

FIGURE 36.7
Ball rolling progression exercises for sagittal plane shoulder flexion. Positioning the feet 45° away from the table introduces elevation in the scapular plane.

https://drjeremylewis.com/in/shoulder-book-resource-ball-rolling-progression

contraction strength. Once the demonstration is complete, the clinician may now apply resistance over the wrist on the patient's symptomatic side, and ask the patient to perform a contraction at 50% of their maximal force (i.e., half the force they could produce on the other side), hold for 3 seconds (ask the patient to count with the metronome), rest for 3 seconds, and repeat 4 times.[77] Following this, reassess the provocative movement. If there is a decrease in symptoms, this may then be considered as a symptom modification procedure, and the isometric contraction (using this force) may be prescribed as a home exercise.

If there is no change, and the patient's symptoms have not worsened, they may gain confidence that contracting the muscles associated with the painful shoulder movement may not aggravate their symptoms. If this is the case and the patient is prepared, repeat the 3-second contraction, 3-second rest cycle another 4 times, now requesting 80–90% of the perceived maximum contraction strength, and then reassess. Again, if there has been no immediate aggravation of symptoms, attempt to place the limb as close to the most provocative position possible. This is likely to be full shoulder external rotation at 80–90° of shoulder abduction

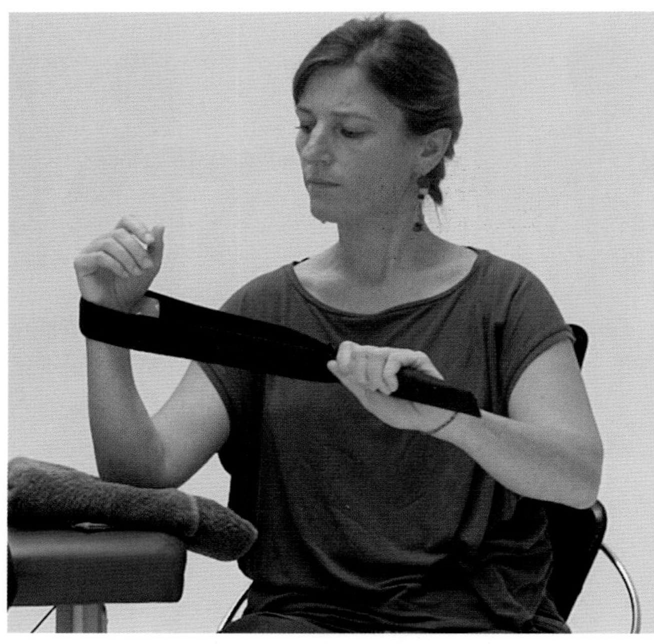

FIGURE 36.8
Isometric contractions.
https://drjeremylewis.com/in/shoulder-book-resource-isometric-contractions

(continuing to stabilize the elbow on the table). Repeat the process at 50% maximum and 90% maximum. If tolerated by the patient, Box 36.3 provides suggestions for the home program for the following week. If the isometric contraction testing provokes symptoms that do not settle shortly after the test, other early-stage management options should be considered.

Box 36.3 Suggested home isometric exercise program

- Choose the most painful or symptomatic movement.
- Position the limb as close as possible to the position of maximum symptoms.
- Support the elbow on a table or desk, protecting the elbow with a small towel or piece of foam.
- Use the opposite hand or preferably a strap to provide the isometric resistance.
- Set a metronome to 60 beats per minute.

Day 1

- Without applying any external resistance, rehearse the exercise using mental imagery at 50% of the perceived maximum, "holding" the contraction for 3 seconds on, 3 seconds off, for 4 repetitions, counting with the metronome.
- Then using the same timings (i.e., 4 repetitions, 3 seconds on, 3 seconds off) apply an isometric force equal to 50% of the perceived maximum, rest for 2 minutes, and repeat 5 times.

Day 2

- Rest/continue with SSMP/continue with kinetic chain program.

Day 3

- Repeat Day 1 (starting with mental imagery).
- Instead of all contractions at 50% of perceived maximum, perform 3 sets at 50% and 2 sets at 90%.

Day 4

- Rest/continue with SSMP/continue with kinetic chain program.

Day 5

- Repeat Day 1 (starting with mental imagery).
- Perform 5 sets at 90% of perceived maximum.

Day 6

- Rest/continue with SSMP/continue with kinetic chain program.

Progression

- Continue with isometric program for another week, possibly two.
- Consider increasing isometric holding time incrementally until 15 to 20 seconds achieved.
- Gradually replace SSMP/early stage rehabilitation with Stage II program.

Stage II: eccentric and heavy slow resistance exercises

Eccentric exercise

Lowering a cup from a high shelf to a bench top, and decelerating the shoulder after releasing a baseball during a pitch demonstrates how integral eccentric muscle contractions are in daily function. Eccentric muscle contractions occur when the length of the muscle increases as tension is produced. Eccentric exercises have been used in sport to improve strength, power, and coordination, and may have a role in reducing injuries.[35,59,111] Eccentric exercises *do not* demonstrate superiority over other exercises in the management of musculoskeletal shoulder conditions,[18,58] but do have many advantages that should be considered in a staged rehabilitation program.

Muscles generate greater force under eccentric loading than they do during isometric or concentric contractions.[38,59] Eccentric muscle contractions are metabolically more efficient for a given force than concentric muscle contractions,[1,35,36,59] which may benefit people who, due to illness, immobilization, or lifestyle, are diagnosed with muscle atrophy, reduced muscle performance, reduced mobility, and reduced aerobic capacity. For these reasons, eccentric exercises are being increasingly used in the management of people with cardiorespiratory conditions, sarcopenia, and type 2 diabetes.[43,59] Additionally, in adolescents with obesity, eccentric exercises were reported to be better at reducing fat mass, improving strength, and decreasing the deleterious effects of insulin resistance, than concentric exercises.[44]

Immobilization may form part of a postoperative protocol or be mandatory following a fracture. Some people experiencing shoulder pain may understandably self-immobilize in a homemade, or off-the-shelf sling, or simply avoid using their upper limb to avoid increasing pain out of concern that movement may cause more damage. Immobilization has a rapid and deleterious effect on muscle size, strength, and neuromuscular function, with marked differences between older and younger people,[106] and potential differences between the upper and lower limbs.[11] In situations where a limb is immobilized, exercising the non-immobilized contralateral limb reduces the effects of immobilization.[24,71,82]

There is also compelling evidence that when exercising the non-immobilized arm, eccentric-only exercise protocols have better outcomes than combined concentric and eccentric protocols.[37,38,48,113 114] This may be in part due to load, as heavier loads can be applied during eccentric contractions than in dynamic resistance training consisting of concentric and eccentric contractions, when lighter loads need be applied due to the reduced capacity of maximum force generation associated with concentric contractions.[114] Eccentric resistance training increases corticospinal excitability in both the ipsilateral and contralateral limb to a greater extent than concentric training,[48,107] but the benefit may decrease after the training stimulus has been withdrawn.[107]

Delayed-onset muscle soreness (DOMS) may occur following eccentric contractions performed at higher than accustomed loads.[35] The pain associated with DOMS, that may also be related to the muscle fascia,[26] typically peaks 24 to 72 hours after the exercise and progressively subsides in 5 to 7 days. DOMS is also associated with tenderness, swelling, stiffness, mechanical hyperalgesia, and decreased performance. For a person seeking care for musculoskeletal shoulder pain, a substantial and protracted exacerbation of symptoms following an exercise may be a reason for concern, reluctance to exercise, and may be perceived as causing tissue damage. To avoid this, it appears that repeated exposure to eccentric muscle contractions with appropriately graduated increasing loads may reduce, and possibly prevent, the occurrence of muscle damage and DOMS.[35,59]

In vitamin D deficient individuals, vitamin D supplementation or through diet may also contribute to reduction in muscle damage and may reduce DOMS. Maintaining sufficient levels of vitamin D (measured in the blood by its metabolite 25[OH]D), through diet and carefully planned sunlight exposure, is essential for good health.[42] Vitamin D contributes to controlling appropriate levels of pro- and anti-inflammatory cytokines (TNF-α and IL-10) and contributes to controlling inflammation.[6,73] Vitamin D deficiency (defined as serum 25[OH] D < 50 nmol/L or < 20 ng/ml)[3,72] has been implicated with many health conditions: osteomalacia, bone pain, muscle weakness, severe asthma in children, cognitive impairment in older adults, and death from cardiovascular disease and strokes. Vitamin D deficiency may be associated with higher SARS-CoV-2 (COVID-19) mortality rates.[12,89]

Vitamin D deficiency may also be related to diabetes, hypertension, infections, and respiratory illness, cancer, glucose intolerance, and multiple sclerosis. In addition to the apparent importance of vitamin D in general and musculoskeletal health, Pilch et al. reported that vitamin D supplementation may reduce muscle cell damage induced by eccentric exercise.[85]

Eccentric exercises are included in the #SUMS rehabilitation program due to their major defining properties and advantages: higher muscle forces, lower energy requirements, less fatigue, lower cardiovascular demand, gains in muscle performance and muscle mass, greater neural adaptations, fat mass reduction, improvements in blood lipid profile and insulin sensitivity, greater cortical excitability, and reduced sarcopenia.[35] In addition to these benefits, the fact that eccentric exercises when performed on the contralateral limb are beneficial, and more effective, than combined concentric and eccentric training in counteracting the negative effects of immobilization, is also relevant, especially if the patient is unable to exercise the symptomatic side.

Integrating eccentric exercises into #SUMS

Eccentric contraction exposure and adaptation phase

A fundamental tenet of #SUMS is that entry into exercise should be individualized and should be progressed (where possible) to exceed the patient's expectations of what they thought possible. This principle also applies to the eccentric stage of the program. For people unable (e.g., due to immobilization) or reluctant to exercise (e.g., due to increased pain and fear of damage associated with eccentric contractions), two simple adaptations should be considered. The first is commencing the eccentric program on the contralateral side,[36] and the second is introducing an exposure-adaptation phase.[59] The purpose of the exposure-adaption phase is to avoid damage and pain that would be inevitable when introducing high eccentric loads to muscles and tendons unexposed to such forces.[59] To facilitate this, I occasionally start eccentric contractions on the symptomatic side with no external load, using just the weight of the arm, and encourage mental imagery of a "substantial" external load. The exercises are performed every other day.

Another consideration to support the adaptation phase is to start with one set of exercises per day, with a recommendation to initially start in the evening, or at the end of the day. One reason for this is that McCreesh et al.[74] demonstrated that the supraspinatus tendon increased in thickness after loading in people diagnosed with rotator cuff-related shoulder pain (rotator cuff tendinopathy). This change did not occur in people without symptoms. For those with symptoms, the swelling returned to baseline within 24 hours. The swelling may occur due to increased production of hydrophilic proteoglycans. It is not known if there is a relationship between swelling and symptoms. However, introducing exercise at the "end" of the working day, where no additional loading is added after the exercise, may contribute to the restoration of the tendon to baseline levels during the evening and overnight. This would not be the case if the exercises were performed at the start of the day, when additional load (e.g., driving, working, lifting and carrying, etc.) would be added to the load of the exercise.

In summary, the load during the eccentric adaptation phase should be incrementally progressed over time to avoid DOMS, with consideration given to starting the program at the end of the day.

Progression of eccentric exercise

When introducing eccentric exercises into the #SUMS program, one suggestion is to choose the most painful movement identified during the physical assessment (see Chapter 15). The eccentric exercise should be commenced at an appropriate predetermined load, and the response to the exercises should be monitored appropriately and adjusted as required (see above). For example, eccentric exercises for the shoulder and elbow flexors and forearm supinators should be considered if the symptoms are hypothesized to be related to a biceps tendinopathy (see Chapter 26). People diagnosed with rotator cuff-related shoulder pain most commonly report pain in shoulder abduction and external rotation, and as such these directions of movement (if symptomatic) take priority.

It is important that the exercise is performed at a controlled speed, and one recommendation is to use a digital metronome (many are freely available to download) set to 60 beats per minute. If possible, the metronome should be used audibly and visually by the patient who should listen to and count 5 beats (5 seconds) while performing the eccentric contraction. When one repetition has been completed, the arm should be passively returned to the starting position and the exercise repeated. Guidance on exact repetitions, sets and frequency of exercise, for all musculoskeletal shoulder conditions is not available. As such, one suggestion is to build up to 3 sets of 5 repetitions of the eccentric exercise and concomitantly increase load incrementally. Examples of graduated eccentric programs are available at the link below.

https://drjeremylewis.com/in/shoulder-book-resource-graduated-eccentric-programs 

If it is not possible to start on the symptomatic side, the patient should start the exercises on the contralateral side. The program therefore may be staggered, with the patient performing the exercise with higher loads on the contralateral side than on the symptomatic side. At some point, bilateral loads are likely to become equal. A further progression may be to increase the speed of the contraction, i.e., progress from 5-, to 4-, to 3-second contractions. Initially consider introducing eccentric exercises on alternate days and progress to daily, and from one set to three, and from once daily to twice daily. This is of course patient dependent. There is no evidence that experiencing pain during eccentric exercises confers greater benefit or harm than performing the exercises without pain.[58] As such, if tolerable, the patient may experience pain during the exercise program, provided there is no increase in night pain, or pain the next day.

Progression to heavy slow resistance exercises

The next stage of the program is to progress from eccentric-only to combined eccentric and concentric loading, introducing an exercise program known as heavy slow resistance (HSR), which was originally described by Kongsgaard et al.[49,50] Using the same exercise position as for the eccentric-only program, concentric contractions are now introduced. The repetition maximum (RM) for a concentric contraction is determined, either by assessment or asking the patient to suggest the maximum weight they could lift concentrically, i.e., their perceived maximum exertion. It is common that people can lower substantially more load eccentrically than they can return concentrically, especially if the concentric load is very painful. The program needs to be adapted for this. Eccentric and concentric loads may therefore be nonidentical. Once the concentric load is established, the new exercise involves eccentric followed by concentric contraction; continuing to use the metronome, each direction should take around 3 seconds, so that one eccentric–concentric repetition will take around 6 seconds. Pain is permitted during the exercise, but there must be no increase in night pain, and/or pain the next day. If pain increases to these levels, the exercise must be adapted accordingly (i.e., reduce weight, numbers of repetitions, etc.). When incorporating HSR exercises, ongoing uncertainty persists regarding ideal weight, repetition speed and numbers, sets, and rest time, and how to translate findings seen in asymptomatic to symptomatic people.[80] As such, the following is a suggestion that may be adapted according to the patient's response.

The aim is to use a weight that equates to 70% (minimum) to 85% of 1 RM. Consider starting at 70% of 1 RM and perform one set of 5 repetitions, with each repetition taking 6 seconds. This is followed by a 5-minute rest (consider completing another exercise e.g., sit to stands during the "rest") and repeat 3 times, on alternate days. It is acceptable to incorporate variations with the weight (load) and the speed (time to complete 1 repetition), i.e., increase the weight and increase the tempo. It is often harder to maintain the relatively slow 6-second tempo with heavier weights,[116] and for the same weight, number of repetitions will increase with a faster tempo. This also implies training intensity will also increase.[80,116] As such, HSR training parameters can be progressed or adjusted to 85% of 1 RM, 3 sets of 3 repetitions, with a tempo of 3 seconds (i.e., eccentric and concentric phase completed in 3 seconds), with a 15-second rest between sets.[17] These "micro sets", with associated short rest periods that do not allow for complete recovery, contribute to maintaining volume without impacting negatively on intensity.[80] There are many ways to prescribe and vary these exercises, remembering that the eccentric and concentric loads may initially be different. To simplify this for patients I often suggest lowering the heaviest load you can manage and return with the heaviest load you are able to lift. This may initially be 5 kg (11 lbs) eccentrically and 1 kg (2 lbs) concentrically. The exercises should be performed every other day. If preferred, they may be performed painfree. Examples of HSR exercises are available at the link below.

The guide to progressing or decreasing the program is based upon the patient's response.

https://drjeremylewis.com/in/shoulder-book-resource-hsr-exercises 

Stage III: functional program

Overlap is common when transitioning from one stage of the #SUMS rehabilitation program to the next. I often continue with components of early-stage rehabilitation when introducing Stage II and continue with Stage II exercises when transitioning to Stage III, before slowly phasing them out. Stage III, the final stage of the program, is return to function. The shoulder contributes to pushing, pulling, lifting, carrying, throwing, catching, and precision activities. When trying to stop something from falling, flying a kite, throwing and catching a frisbee, or stopping a soccer ball from going through the goals, the shoulder is called upon to perform unexpected fast and often unpredictable movements. As such, the final stage of #SUMS must also include random and "chaotic" challenges to function.

Choosing the right program

No exercise program has demonstrated definitive superiority over another in the management of musculoskeletal conditions involving the shoulder.[20] Therefore at this stage you may wish to discuss with the patient their preference for exercise. Consider asking if their preference is for a more formal program, or do they find a formal exercise program difficult to follow and adopt into their current lifestyle. Patients often report that they just gave up on formal programs because they missed several days of the program due to competing priorities, or that they tried once or twice, but just could not integrate them into their busy lives. Do not be judgmental, acknowledge how difficult it is to find time for something new in an already busy day, and offer an alternative.

"Non-formal" rehabilitation program

For those who admit that they will never do a formal exercise program, or those that try but find that they cannot maintain the plan, an alternative is to incrementally increase activity participation to achieve 3,000–4,000 MET (metabolic equivalent of a task) minutes per week. A MET is the ratio of energy used during an activity to the energy used at rest and as such, provides an estimation of the intensity of an activity. One MET may be defined as 1 kcal/kg/hour. Although there are several ways to define and calculate MET minutes/week (METs), and albeit imperfect,[34] one explanation you might consider when discussing this with a patient is as follows. One MET is equivalent to the energy required to sit quietly (i.e., resting metabolic rate) such as when watching television, reading a book, or sitting on a bus. Walking around a shopping mall is an example of an activity with a 2–3 MET value, as two to three times the energy is required than is needed for quietly sitting. A MET value may be assigned to all physical activities, with examples detailed in Table 36.2. It is important to be aware that the actual MET value will be different for men and women, for underweight, average weight, and overweight individuals, and for age, so estimations are presented.

Table 36.2 Examples of approximate MET values per minute for physical activities

Activity	Metabolic equivalent of task (MET) (approximations)
Quiet sitting	1.0[32]
Writing, working at a desk, using a computer	1.5[32]
Slow-paced walking (3.0 km/h, 1.9 mph)	2.0[32]
Moderate-pace walking (5.0 km/h, 3.0 mph)	3.0[32]
Yoga	3.3–7.4[57]
Tennis (doubles)	5.0[32]
Tennis (singles)	7.0[41]
Housework	3.5–6[32]
Dancing (medium effort)	6.0[41]
Gardening	4.4–7.0[41]
Swimming (2.0 km/h to 4.0 km/h)	4.0–14.0[41]
Jogging (9.0 km/h, 5.6 mph to 11 km/h, 6.8 mph)	8.8–11.2[41]
Rope skipping (66/min to 145/min)	9.8–12.1[41]
Running (15.0 km/h, 9.3 mph)	14.6[41]
Rowing (4.0 km/h, 2.5 mph to 20.0 km/h, 12.4 mph)	5.5–19.1[41]

km/h, kilometers per hour; mph, miles per hour.

Why 3,000–4,000 METs?

Kyu et al.[55] reported that people who achieve physical activity levels between 3,000 to 4,000 METs had significantly greater reductions in the risk of breast cancer, colon cancer, diabetes, ischemic heart disease, and ischemic stroke events, than currently minimum recommended levels of 600 METs. This higher level of activity also provides an opportunity to exercise the entire body, to facilitate muscle–tendon performance, bone health, and contribute to improvements in mental health, as well as having many other health-related benefits.

Building a 3,000–4,000 METs program from valued activities

During the interview (see Chapter 11) and data collection (see Chapter 12) and, if required from further discussion, an understanding of the activities that the patient values doing and must do during the week will be gained. For example, the patient may express a love for gardening. On average this is a 6 MET activity that involves shoulder range of motion together with concentric, isometric, and eccentric shoulder muscle contractions. Gardening involves pushing, pulling, lifting, and carrying, and therefore involves the entire body, and often requires precision activities (e.g., pruning, pulling weeds). Lever arms are increased when using garden forks, spades, rakes, pushing mowers, and lifting grass clippings, etc. It is a challenging activity and for many highly rewarding, providing a deep sense of accomplishment.

A patient who works in an office complex and/or lives in an apartment block may have the choice of using an elevator or stairs. Initially they could start with climbing one flight of stairs before taking the lift and, over time, two flights, etc. They may also have the choice of walking or cycling to work, or getting off the bus or train two or three stops before work, or may enjoy a walk with a colleague after work for two to three or more stops, before using transport. Not only are these opportunities to increase METs, but prescribing active transport (walking, cycling, skating, etc.) is a way healthcare providers and patients can contribute to environmental sustainability.[112] Following the principles of starting the rehabilitation program at a safe entry point, loading may be progressed until 3,000–4,000 METs are achieved, which of course needs to be sustained. Other activities can be substituted, and patients may express an interest in participating in gym-based or other forms of activity or exercise once they realize the health benefits from increasing activity participation. Box 36.4 provides an example of a 3,000–4,000 METs program constructed from valued and essential activities provided by a patient. It may take 12 weeks or longer to achieve and should follow the guidance described earlier in this chapter.

Based on the information detailed in Box 36.4 and the need to achieve 3,000–4,000 METs, many people who think they are doing a considerable amount of exercise are, worryingly, not achieving what they should. For example, if a patient reports that they do a lot of exercise, on average going for three 30-minute walks each week, and playing doubles tennis once a week for an hour, this amounts to $3 \times 30 \times 6$ METs $+ 1 \times 60 \times 5$ METs which totals 840 MET minutes per week. This is between 2,160 and 3,160 METs per week short of the ideal to reduce the risk of myriad health conditions,[55] and contribute to improving shoulder function through activity.

Box 36.4 An example of a 3,000–4,000 MET minutes per week program

- **Walking**: briskly & swinging arms (6.0 km/h) = (6 MET activity) 5 x/week for 30 minutes/session
  = 5 x 6 x 30 = **900 MET-minutes**
- **Cycling**: (15.0 km/h) = (6 MET activity) 3 x/week for 30 minutes/session
  = 3 x 6 x 30 = **540 MET-minutes**
- **Cleaning**: vacuuming, mopping, shaking, etc. = (6 MET activity) 3 x/week for 60 minutes/session
  = 3 x 6 x 60 = **1080 MET-minutes**
- **Gardening**: 1 x/week = (6 MET activity) for 150 minutes
  = 1 x 6 x 150 = **900 MET-minutes**
- **Carrying**: 3 x/week moderate weight = (6 MET activity) for 10 minutes
  = 3 x 6 x 10 = **180 MET-minutes**

Total MET-minutes per week = 900 + 540 + 1080 + 900 + 180 = 3,600 MET-minutes

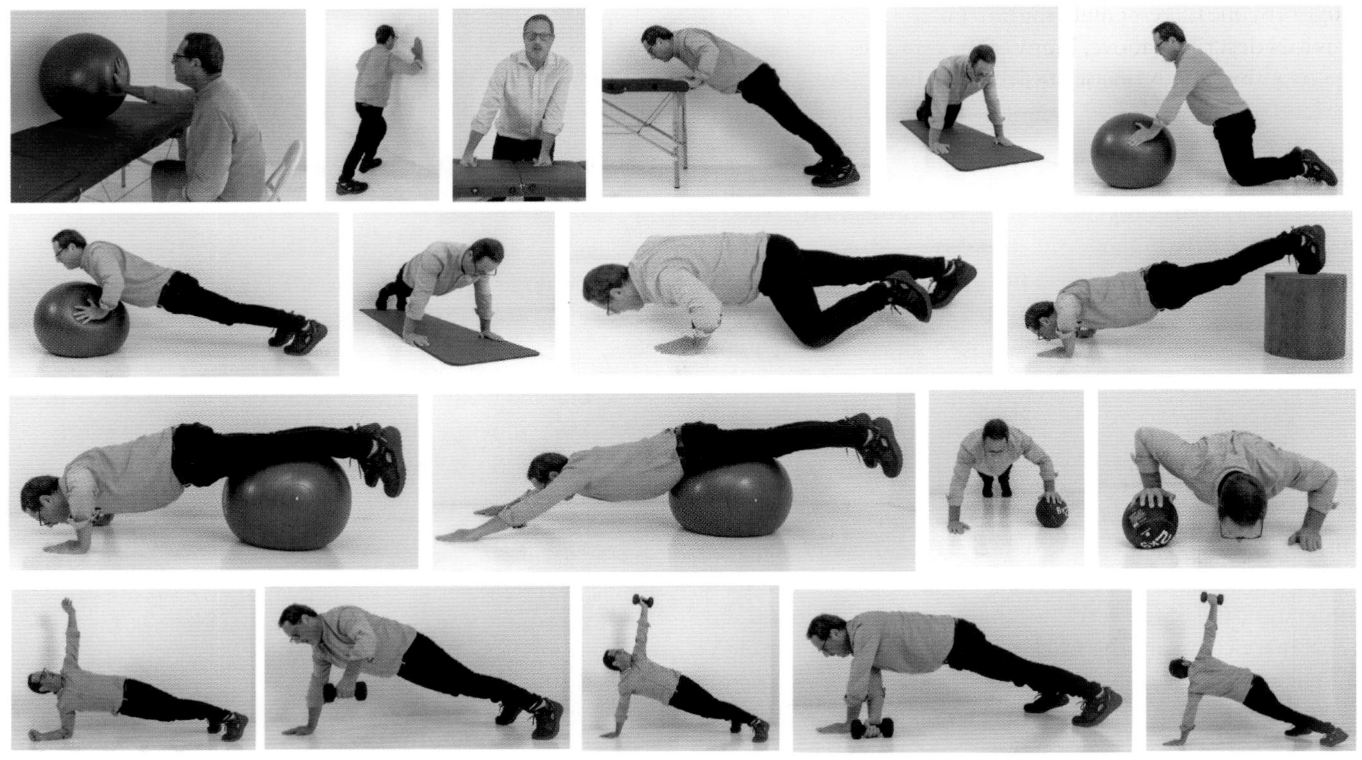

FIGURE 36.9
Examples (abridged) of a multistage pushing program.
https://drjeremylewis.com/in/shoulder-book-resource-multistage-pushing-program

As stated earlier, no one rehabilitation program has demonstrated superiority over another. For this reason, T'ai Chi (see Chapter 42) and yoga (see Chapter 43), that require shoulder and whole-body exercise progressions, that are complex and challenging, and involve relaxation, and which may be of interest for patients, and fit into their lifestyle, are presented in this textbook.

Formal exercise program

For those wishing to undertake a more formal approach, this final stage of #SUMS incorporates exercises for the shoulder, upper limb, cervical region, trunk, and lower limb. It also involves mixed loads, durations, and speeds. It involves ballistic loads, chaotic loads, and sensorimotor exercises. The program achieves this by incorporating the range of functional movements – pushing, pulling, lifting, carrying, throwing, catching, and precision, that an individual will perform as part of their routine activities. This is as relevant for an Olympic weightlifter as it is for an octogenarian lifting a small cabin bag weighing 10 kg (22 lb) into an overhead luggage compartment. Exercises that translate into improving function are no less important for a grandparent throwing a ball or playing frisbee with a grandchild as they are for an Olympic shot-putter, javelin, or discus thrower, or a pitcher in the National Baseball League. Pushing exercises are as relevant for a boxer as they are for a nonagenarian wishing to maintain function getting in and out of a chair or car.

Taking this approach, the #SUMS rehabilitation program incorporates all the routine shoulder activities in a graduated and multistage program. If this model is relevant for your clinical practice, work with your colleagues, and possibly patients, to develop graduated 20, 30, 40 or even 50 stage programs, one incremental program for each of the functional activities described above. Many of the exercises will incorporate two, three, or more of the functional requirements, such as the abridged pushing sequence illustrated in Figure 36.9. There are myriad other pushing exercises, but the key principles are: to make the increments between the exercises small, so that the musculoskeletal system does not detect substantial change during progression; to start at a level commensurate with your assessment of the patient's recent levels of activity; and to progress to at least the level identified by you and the patient at the start of the program. However, I would recommend, if possible, to exceed the patient's expectations of what they thought they could achieve.

Getting an 80-year-old to do a knee push-up, and sometimes a full push-up for the first time in 50 years (or ever) is not essential, but it translates to improved function, as well as psychological confidence. This is not possible for everyone, and for many, a program designed to maintain current function for as long as possible is also desirable and valuable. As the program progresses, vary speeds, weights, distance (e.g., when throwing or carrying), duration, and complexity of the exercises, and introduce "chaos" into the program. Chaos, defined as "the property of a complex system whose behavior is so unpredictable as to appear random"[104] is an essential part of #SUMS. If something falls from a shelf or a bench, instinctively we reach out to try and catch it; when catching a ball, it rarely is delivered to the same place twice. Chaos, or the randomness of complex systems, is inherent in daily activity, and as such must be incorporated into the program to achieve a high level of function, that early-stage, highly controlled exercises are likely to reach. Fast changes when pushing, pulling, carrying, and lifting, and extreme ranges of motion are the hallmarks of function for a break-dancer, a trapeze artist, and for a "traceur" participating in parkour (parcours du combatant – free running obstacle course) and, as such, must be included in the rehabilitation program.

Repetitions and sets

#SUMS is not a pure motor control, strengthening, or endurance program – it is a hybrid, and its purpose is to improve function and re-establish confidence with valued activities that involve the shoulder. As such, I do not provide patients with numbers of repetitions, sets, and daily targets in Stage III of the program.

Box 36.5 Guidance to patients regarding repetitions and sets

- We (*the patient and clinician*) will work closely together to get the very best result possible.
- On average the program takes 12 weeks, sometimes a little less and sometimes a little longer.
- Improvement will not be linear (a straight line), and the program will need to be adjusted according to your response.
- Aim to do all the prescribed exercises on the days suggested, as they are all important and all contribute to getting you to the place you want to be.
- You are in charge of your shoulder rehabilitation program, and for each exercise, prepare a weekly target. If you prefer, this can be done together with the clinician.
- Aim to achieve that target, but numbers are not important. If you do a few less, or a lot less, or reach the target, or even do a few more than the target, be proud of what you have done.
- If on one day you just can't make your target, that's also great – you tried, you are allowed to be tired or busy, or both. Vary the pace (speed) of your exercises, and sometimes changing the tempo of an exercise, or changing the tempo of the music you are exercising to may help you do a few more.
- If you consistently cannot reach your target, please let me know as soon as possible.
- Remember, experiencing pain that is tolerable for you, does not mean you are causing any damage to your shoulder, in fact, research tells us that experiencing tolerable pain when exercising may be associated with faster short-term improvement. We just do not want you to feel more pain tonight or tomorrow and, if you do, we need to readjust your exercises accordingly.
- Here is a suggestion for you: with all the exercises in your program, stop when you feel there isn't another repetition in you, but *"just to be sure, try to do one more."*

Programs to specifically improve intensity and strength should be considered after the #SUMS program when working with individuals to improve other important parameters of health,[39] when transitioning into the post #SUMS phase that I refer to as the well body and mind healthy lifestyle program. During the #SUMS program, my prevailing guidance is not to focus on repetitions or sets. This gives the patient permission to do 1 set of 15 repetitions one day and if only one set of 3 repetitions are managed on the next training day, that is perfectly acceptable, and should be seen as positive, as the #SUMS philosophy is patient self-management being guided by a nonjudgmental clinician. Importantly, remain alert to a continual reduction in performance, as this may indicate the presence of comorbidities that will require investigations. Box 36.5 illustrates guidance to patients regarding repetitions and sets.

There are several reasons why formalized numbers are not important. We have all been to the gym, ridden our bicycles, or gone for a swim or a walk, where we cannot achieve our usual pace, weights, repetitions, sets, distance, or duration. We accept it because we know that next time we will reach and maybe surpass our previous best. Advising patients to exercise until they feel that they cannot do one more allows for days where tiredness, stress, poor nutrition, time restrictions, or higher than usual daily physical requirements would not allow the individual to complete the prescribed daily repetitions and sets. Constantly not achieving the prescribed numbers of repetitions and sets may be one reason patients become discouraged and stop their rehabilitation program.[31,75,101,108] I would suggest setting loose parameters. For example, when progressing through the different stages of the "lawn mower" exercise (Figure 36.10), I would suggest to the patient that they do as many as they can. When they consistently achieve 12–15 repetitions of that level, consider progressing to the next.

If a patient is insistent on prescribed repetitions and sets, then you may consider using Table 36.3 as guidance for the patient, but, if at all possible, leave programs such as these for health maintenance and improvement programs that individuals may wish to continue with after the formal program is completed.

For each pulling, pushing, lifting, carrying, and throwing exercise, 1 RM (repetition maximum) should be determined. Following a brief warm-up and familiarization period, calculating 1 RM appears to be reliable across upper and lower limb muscle groups, and sexes,[102] although different formulae may be required for the upper and lower limb muscle groups.[88] There are a number of formulae to calculate 1 RM,[88,115] all associated with uncertainties, such as population studied, applicability to all muscle groups, and appropriate rest periods between sets in RM testing.[88]

The Bryzcki formula[10] is one method for calculating 1 RM. To use this formula, the maximum load that can be pushed, pulled, lifted, carried, and thrown no more than 10 times needs to be determined. Above 10 repetitions the formula becomes less stable, and therefore if the load being calculated can be moved more than 10 times, repeat the test

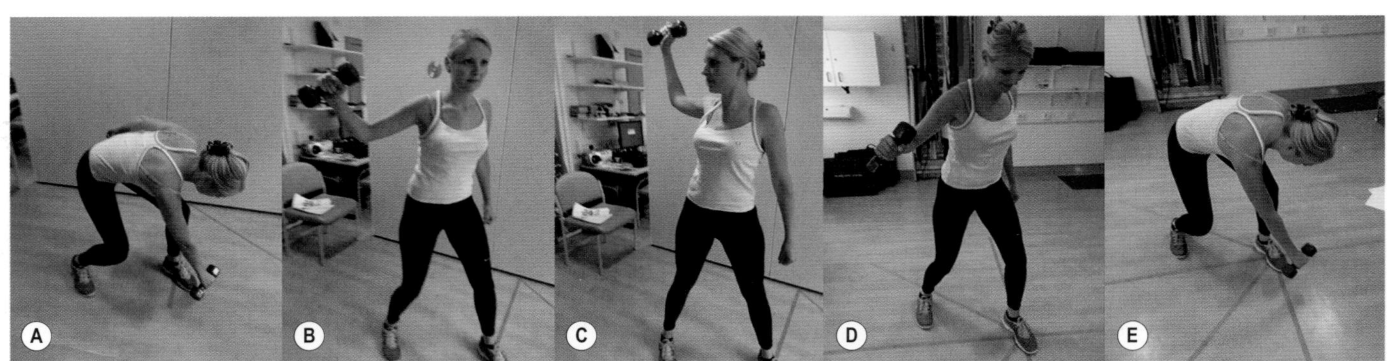

FIGURE 36.10
The "lawn mower" exercise.
https://drjeremylewis.com/in/shoulder-book-resource-lawn-mower-exercise

with a heavier load so that repetitions range from 1 to ≤10. Using the Bryzcki formula, 1 RM may be calculated using either of the following equations:

(A) **Weight** (of load) × (36/37 – **number of repetitions***)

(B) **Weight** (of load) ÷ (1.0278 – (0.0278 × **number of repetitions***

*Number of repetitions must be ≤10[88]

Program variations

The #SUMS rehabilitation program principles may be applied to most musculoskeletal conditions involving the shoulder. Some conditions such as massive rotator cuff tears, rotator cuff arthropathy, and osteoarthritis may require a nuanced rehabilitation approach. One such nuanced approach is a program designed for the conditions listed above. It was originally tested in a randomized controlled trial,[2] which suggested the exercise program performed better than the control treatment. More research is required, and studies are currently ongoing to add to the knowledge required to better understand the value of nonsurgical management in these conditions. Figure 36.11 (which links to a video presentation) illustrates stages of this exercise program.

Table 36.3 Suggested muscle performance programs based on 1 RM*

Aim	Definition	% of 1 RM	Number of repetitions	Sets
Strength	Ability to produce maximal force against an external resistance[105] and is most commonly assessed via 1 RM testing using free weights or exercise machines	80% to 100%	1 to 5	2 to 3
Hypertrophy	Increase in muscle mass, area, volume, fiber cross-sectional area, and ultrastructure, and protein level changes[33]	60% to 80%	8 to 12	3 to 6
Endurance	Ability to resist fatigue when using a submaximal resistance[19]	≤60%	15+	3 to 4

*The evidence to support these recommendations and how best to achieve them remains equivocal.[25,98,110] RM, repetition maximum.

For example, if a patient can lift 5 kg (11.02 lb) 8 times from the floor to the ceiling and back to the floor during the lawn mower exercise (Figure 36.10) before fatiguing, 1 RM is calculated as follows:

(A) **5.0 kg** (11.02 lb) × (36/37 – **8**) = **6.2 kg** (13.7 lb)

(B) **5.0 kg** (11.02 lb) ÷ (1.0278 – (0.0278 × **8**) = **6.2 kg** (13.7 lbs)

Resistance exercise programs to improve strength, endurance, and muscle hypertrophy are based on the assessment of 1 RM. For example, strength programs are commonly based on 1 to 5 repetitions per set of high loads such as 80–100% of 1 RM, and hypertrophy programs are historically based on 8 to 12 repetitions per set on loads based on 60–80% of 1 RM. Loads under 60% of 1 RM and 15-plus repetitions per set are typically prescribed to improve endurance. A summary is provided in Table 36.3. Additional suggestions are made throughout this textbook. Importantly, there is considerable uncertainty regarding the accuracy of providing resistance training guidance based on these recommendations.[25,98,110]

Conclusion

The Shape-Up-My-Shoulder (#SUMS) rehabilitation program is a staged exercise program that may be considered in the movement and functional rehabilitation of people seeking care for musculoskeletal conditions involving the shoulder. It is presented only as a suggestion, principally because no program has demonstrated superiority over another.[20] It should only be considered if there are no contraindications and when the benefits outweigh the harms. There is emerging research evidence supporting the program, but the content of #SUMS will undoubtedly change in response to new research, clinical experience, and patient wishes.

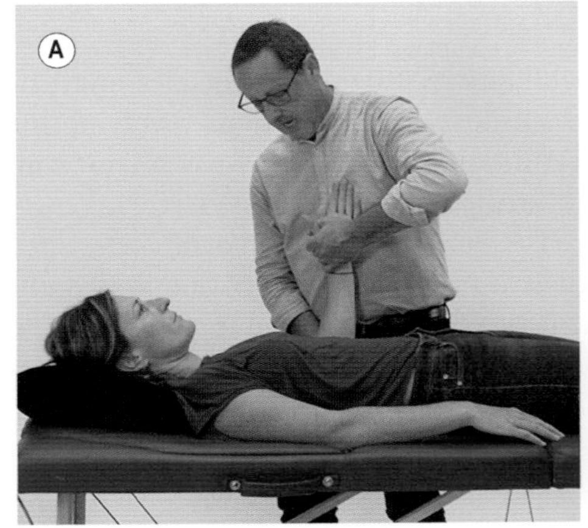

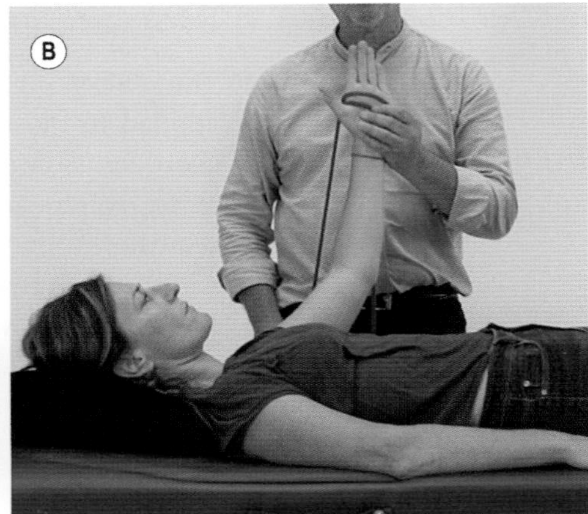

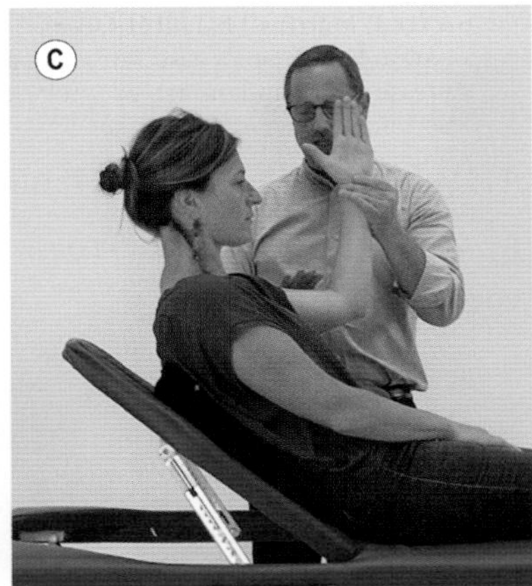

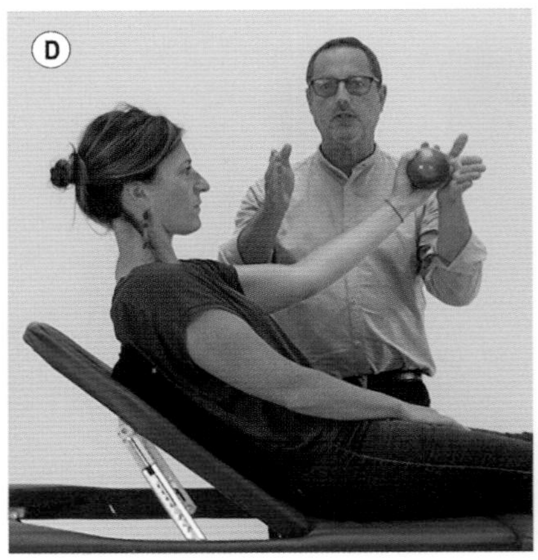

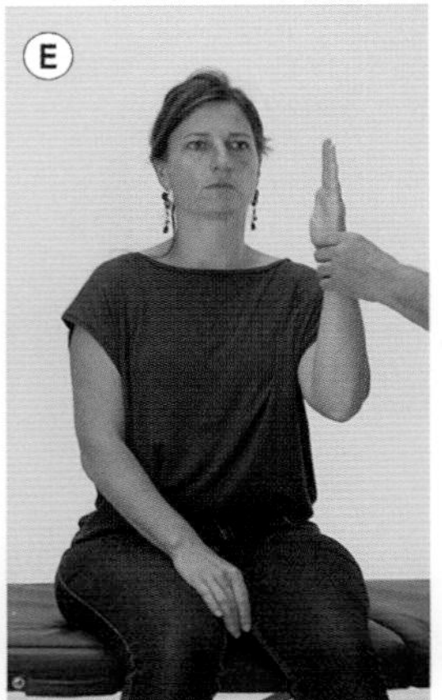

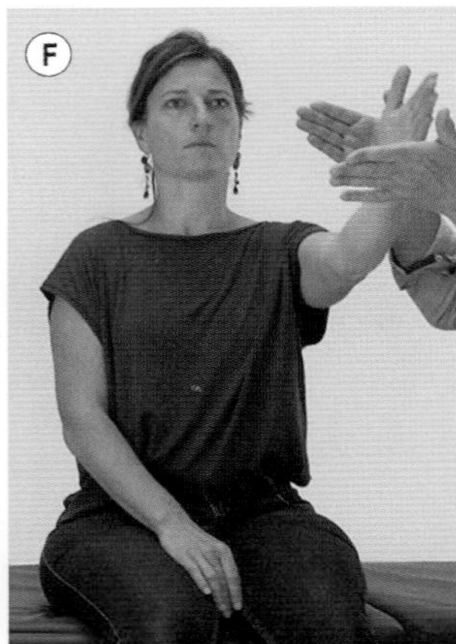

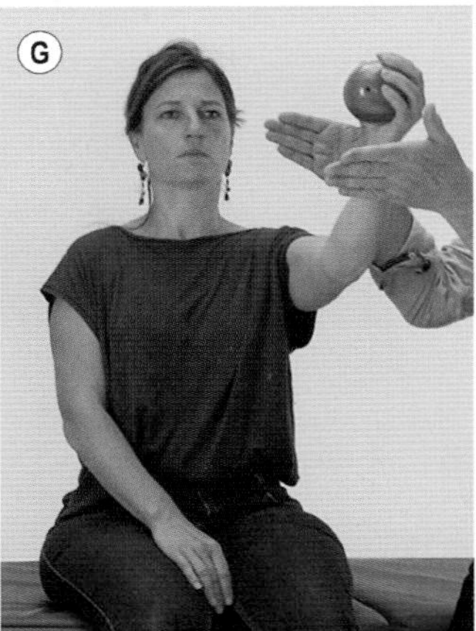

FIGURE 36.11
Rehabilitation program for massive cuff rotator tears, rotator cuff arthropathy, and severe osteoarthritis involving the shoulder.

https://drjeremylewis.com/in/shoulder-book-resource-rotator-cuff-rehabilitation-program

Acknowledgment

Shape-Up-My-Shoulder was a term suggested by Jeremy Lewis during a research grant application with colleagues, one of whom was responsible for the Shape-Up weight management program (https://www.shapeupherts.com/).

References

1. Abbott B, Bigland B, Ritchie J. The physiological cost of negative work. The Journal of Physiology. 1952;117:380-390.
2. Ainsworth R, Lewis JS, Conboy V. A prospective randomized placebo controlled clinical trial of a rehabilitation programme for patients with a diagnosis of massive rotator cuff tears of the shoulder. Shoulder & Elbow. 2009;1:55-60.
3. Amrein K, Scherkl M, Hoffmann M, et al. Vitamin D deficiency 2.0: an update on the current status worldwide. European Journal of Clinical Nutrition. 2020;74:1498-1513.
4. Andersen J, McCabe C, Sanders RH. A model to test for differences in torso muscle torque between front crawl swimming speeds from three-dimensional digitised video. BMS. 2018.
5. Anderson LW, Bloom BS. A Taxonomy for Learning, Teaching, and Assessing: A Revision of Bloom's Taxonomy of Educational Objectives. Longman; 2001.

6. Barker T, Martins TB, Hill HR, et al. Vitamin D sufficiency associates with an increase in anti-inflammatory cytokines after intense exercise in humans. Cytokine. 2014;65:134-137.

7. Barrett E, Conroy C, Corcoran M, et al. An evaluation of two types of exercise classes, containing shoulder exercises or a combination of shoulder and thoracic exercises, for the treatment of nonspecific shoulder pain: a case series. J Hand Ther. 2018;31:301-307.

8. Bloom BS. Taxonomy of Educational Objectives. Vol. 1: Cognitive Domain. New York: McKay; 1956.

9. Bonello C, Girdwood M, De Souza K, et al. Does isometric exercise result in exercise induced hypoalgesia in people with local musculoskeletal pain? A systematic review. Physical Therapy in Sport. 2021 May;49:51-61

10. Brzycki M. Strength testing—predicting a one-rep max from reps-to-fatigue. Journal of Physical Education, Recreation & Dance. 1993;64:88-90.

11. Campbell M, Varley-Campbell J, Fulford J, Taylor B, Mileva KN, Bowtell JL. Effect of immobilisation on neuromuscular function in vivo in humans: a systematic review. Sports Medicine. 2019;49:931-950.

12. Carpagnano GE, Di Lecce V, Quaranta VN, et al. Vitamin D deficiency as a predictor of poor prognosis in patients with acute respiratory failure due to COVID-19. Journal of Endocrinological Investigation. 2021;44:765-771.

13. Chester R, Jerosch-Herold C, Lewis J, Shepstone L. Psychological factors are associated with the outcome of physiotherapy for people with shoulder pain: a multicentre longitudinal cohort study. British Journal of Sports Medicine. 2018;52:269-275.

14. Clausen MB, Hölmich P, Rathleff M, et al. Effectiveness of adding a large dose of shoulder strengthening to current nonoperative care for subacromial impingement: a pragmatic, double-blind randomized controlled trial (SExSI Trial). The American Journal of Sports Medicine. 2021;03635465211016008.

15. Cook CE, Showalter C, Kabbaz V, O'Halloran B. Can a within/between-session change in pain during reassessment predict outcome using a manual therapy intervention in patients with mechanical low back pain? Man Ther. 2012;17:325-329.

16. Cook JL, Rio E, Lewis JS. Managing tendinopathies. In: Jull G, Moore A, Falla D, Lewis JS, McCarthy C, Sterling M (eds). Grieve's Modern Musculoskeletal Physiotherapy, 4th edition. London: Elsevier; 2015.

17. Davies TB, Halaki M, Orr R, Helms ER, Hackett DA. Changes in bench press velocity and power after 8 weeks of high-load cluster-or traditional-set structures. The Journal of Strength & Conditioning Research. 2020;34:2734-2742.

18. Dejaco B, Habets B, van Loon C, van Grinsven S, van Cingel R. Eccentric versus conventional exercise therapy in patients with rotator cuff tendinopathy: a randomized, single blinded, clinical trial. Knee Surg Sports Traumatol Arthrosc. 2017;25:2051-2059.

19. Deschenes MR, Kraemer WJ. Performance and physiologic adaptations to resistance training. American Journal of Physical Medicine & Rehabilitation. 2002;81:S3-S16.

20. Dominguez-Romero JG, Jiménez-Rejano JJ, Ridao-Fernández C, Chamorro-Moriana G. Exercise-based muscle development programmes and their effectiveness in the functional recovery of rotator cuff tendinopathy: a systematic review. Diagnostics (Basel). 2021;11:529.

21. Dubé M-O, Desmeules F, Lewis J, Roy J-S. Rotator cuff related shoulder pain: a randomised controlled trial investigating exercise type on outcome. In prep.

22. Dubé M-O, Desmeules F, Lewis J, Roy J-S. Rotator cuff-related shoulder pain: does the type of exercise influence the outcomes? Protocol of a randomised controlled trial. BMJ Open. 2020;10:e039976.

23. Dupuis F, Barrett E, Dubé M-O, McCreesh KM, Lewis JS, Roy J-S. Cryotherapy or gradual reloading exercises in acute presentations of rotator cuff tendinopathy: a randomised controlled trial. BMJ Open Sport & Exercise Medicine. 2018;4:e000477.

24. Farthing JP, Krentz JR, Magnus CR. Strength training the free limb attenuates strength loss during unilateral immobilization. Journal of Applied Physiology. 2009;106:830-836.

25. Fisher J, Steele J, Bruce-Low S, Smith D. Evidence based resistance training recommendations. Medicina Sportiva. 2011;15:147-162.

26. Gibson W, Arendt-Nielsen L, Taguchi T, Mizumura K, Graven-Nielsen T. Increased pain from muscle fascia following eccentric exercise: animal and human findings. Experimental Brain Research. 2009;194:299.

27. Gourgoulis V, Boli A, Aggeloussis N, et al. The effect of leg kick on sprint front crawl swimming. Journal of Sports Sciences. 2014;32:278-289.

28. Grossman D. No Cape Needed. New York: Little Brown Dog Publishing; 2015.

29. Haahr J, Andersen J. Exercises may be as efficient as subacromial decompression in patients with subacromial stage II impingement: 4–8-years' follow-up in a prospective, randomized study. Scandinavian Journal of Rheumatology. 2006;35:224-228.

30. Haahr J, Østergaard S, Dalsgaard J, et al. Exercises versus arthroscopic decompression in patients with subacromial impingement: a randomised, controlled study in 90 cases with a one year follow up. Annals of the Rheumatic Diseases. 2005;64:760-764.

31. Hall K, Grinstead A, Lewis JS, Mercer C, Moore A, Ridehalgh C. Rotator cuff related shoulder pain. Describing home exercise adherence and the use of behavior change interventions to promote home exercise adherence: a systematic review of randomized controlled trials. Physical Therapy Reviews. 2021;26:299-322.

32. Haskell WL, Lee I-M, Pate RR, et al. Physical activity and public health: updated recommendation for adults from the American College of Sports Medicine and the American Heart Association. Circulation. 2007;116:1081.

33. Haun CT, Vann CG, Roberts BM, Vigotsky AD, Schoenfeld BJ, Roberts MD. A critical evaluation of the biological construct skeletal muscle hypertrophy: size matters but so does the measurement. Frontiers in Physiology. 2019;10:247.

34. Heydenreich J, Schutz Y, Melzer K, Kayser B. Comparison of conventional and individualized 1-MET values for expressing maximum aerobic metabolic rate and habitual activity related energy expenditure. Nutrients. 2019;11:458.

35. Hody S, Croisier J-L, Bury T, Rogister B, Leprince P. Eccentric muscle contractions: risks and benefits. Frontiers in Physiology. 2019;10:10.3389/fphys.2019.00536

36. Hoppeler H. Moderate load eccentric exercise; a distinct novel training modality. Frontiers in Physiology. 2016;7:483.

37. Hortobagyi T, Hill JP, Houmard JA, Fraser DD, Lambert NJ, Israel RG. Adaptive responses to muscle lengthening and shortening in humans. Journal of Applied Physiology. 1996;80:765-772.

38. Hortobágyi T, Lambert NJ, Hill JP. Greater cross education following training with muscle lengthening than shortening. Medicine and Science in Sports and Exercise. 1997;29:107-112.

39. Hunter GR, Plaisance EP, Carter SJ, Fisher G. Why intensity is not a bad word: optimizing health status at any age. Clinical Nutrition. 2018;37:56-60.

40. Jafari H, Courtois I, Van den Bergh O, Vlaeyen JW, Van Diest I. Pain and respiration: a systematic review. Pain. 2017;158:995-1006.

41. Jetté M, Sidney K, Blümchen G. Metabolic equivalents (METS) in exercise testing, exercise prescription, and evaluation of functional capacity. Clinical Cardiology. 1990;13:555-565.

42. Jones G. Pharmacokinetics of vitamin D toxicity. The American Journal of Clinical Nutrition. 2008;88:582S-586S.

43. Julian V, Thivel D, Costes F, et al. Eccentric training improves body composition by inducing mechanical and metabolic adaptations: a promising approach for overweight and obese individuals. Frontiers in physiology. 2018;9:1013.

44. Julian V, Thivel D, Miguet M, et al. Eccentric cycling is more efficient in reducing fat mass than concentric cycling in adolescents with obesity. Scand J Med Sci Sports. 2019;29:4-15.

45. Ketola S, Lehtinen J, Arnala I, et al. Does arthroscopic acromioplasty provide any additional value in the treatment of shoulder impingement syndrome? A two-year randomised controlled trial. J Bone Joint Surg Br. 2009;91:1326-1334.

46. Ketola S, Lehtinen J, Rousi T, et al. No evidence of long-term benefits of arthroscopicacromioplasty in the treatment of shoulder impingement syndrome: five-year results of a randomised controlled trial. Bone & Joint Research. 2013;2:132-139.

47. Ketola S, Lehtinen JT, Arnala I. Arthroscopic decompression not recommended in the treatment of rotator cuff tendinopathy: a final review of a randomised controlled trial at a minimum follow-up of ten years. Bone Joint J. 2017;99-B:799-805.

48. Kidgell DJ, Frazer AK, Rantalainen T, et al. Increased cross-education of muscle strength and reduced corticospinal inhibition following eccentric strength training. Neuroscience. 2015;300:566-575.

49. Kongsgaard M, Kovanen V, Aagaard P, et al. Corticosteroid injections, eccentric decline squat training and heavy slow resistance training in patellar tendinopathy. Scand J Med Sci Sports. 2009;19:790-802.

50. Kongsgaard M, Qvortrup K, Larsen J, et al. Fibril morphology and tendon mechanical properties in patellar tendinopathy: effects of heavy slow resistance training. The American Journal of Sports Medicine. 2010;38:749-756.

51. Kuhn JE, Dunn WR, Sanders R, et al. Effectiveness of physical therapy in treating atraumatic full-thickness rotator cuff tears: a multicenter prospective cohort study. J Shoulder Elbow Surg. 2013;22:1371-1379.

52. Kukkonen J, Joukainen A, Lehtinen J, et al. Treatment of non-traumatic rotator cuff tears: a randomised controlled trial with one-year clinical results. The Bone & Joint Journal. 2014;96:75-81.

53. Kukkonen J, Joukainen A, Lehtinen J, et al. Treatment of nontraumatic rotator cuff tears: a randomized controlled trial with two years of clinical and imaging follow-up. J Bone Joint Surg Am. 2015;97:1729-1737.

54. Kukkonen J, Kauko T, Vahlberg T, Joukainen A, Äärimaa V. Investigating minimal clinically important difference for Constant score in patients undergoing rotator cuff surgery. J Shoulder Elbow Surg. 2013;22:1650-1655.

55. Kyu HH, Bachman VF, Alexander LT, et al. Physical activity and risk of breast cancer, colon cancer, diabetes, ischemic heart disease, and ischemic stroke events: systematic review and dose-response meta-analysis for the Global Burden of Disease Study 2013. BMJ. 2016;354:i3857.

56. Lafrance S, Ouellet P, Alaoui R, et al. Motor control exercises compared to strengthening exercises for upper and lower extremity musculoskeletal disorders: a systematic review with meta-analyses of randomized controlled trials. Physical Therapy. 2021;101:pzab072.

57. Larson-Meyer DE. A systematic review of the energy cost and metabolic intensity of yoga. Medicine and Science in Sports and Exercise. 2016;48:1558-1569.

58. Larsson R, Bernhardsson S, Nordeman L. Effects of eccentric exercise in patients with subacromial impingement syndrome: a systematic review and meta-analysis. BMC Musculoskeletal Disorders. 2019;20:1-22.

59. LaStayo P, Marcus R, Dibble L, Frajacomo F, Lindstedt S. Eccentric exercise in rehabilitation: safety, feasibility, and application. Journal of Applied Physiology. 2014;116:1426-1434.

60. Lehman GJ. The role and value of symptom-modification approaches in musculoskeletal practice. Journal of Orthopaedic & Sports Physical Therapy. 2018;48:430-435.

61. Lewis J. Rotator cuff related shoulder pain: assessment, management and uncertainties. Man Ther. 2016;23:57-68.

62. Lewis J, McCreesh K, Roy JS, Ginn K. Rotator cuff tendinopathy: navigating the diagnosis-management conundrum. J Orthop Sports Phys Ther. 2015;45:923-937.

63. Lewis J, O'Sullivan P. Is it time to reframe how we care for people with non-traumatic musculoskeletal pain? Br J Sports Med. 2018;52:1543-1544.

64. Lewis JS. Rotator cuff tendinopathy. British Journal of Sports Medicine. 2009;43:236-241.

65. Lewis JS. Rotator cuff tendinopathy/subacromial impingement syndrome: is it time for a new method of assessment? Br J Sports Med. 2009;43:259-264.

66. Lewis JS, Cook CE, Hoffmann TC, O'Sullivan P. The elephant in the room: too much medicine in musculoskeletal practice. J Orthop Sports Phys Ther. 2020;50:1-4.

67. Lewis JS, Green A, Wright C. Subacromial impingement syndrome: the role of posture and muscle imbalance. J Shoulder Elbow Surg. 2005;14:385-392.

68. Lewis JS, McCreesh K, Barratt E, Hegedus EJ, Sim J. Inter-rater reliability of the Shoulder Symptom Modification Procedure in people with shoulder pain. BMJ Open Sport Exerc Med. 2016;2:e000181.

69. Lier E, Oosterman J, Assmann R, de Vries M, van Goor H. The effect of Virtual Reality on evoked potentials following painful electrical stimuli and subjective pain. Scientific Reports. 2020;10:1-8.

70. Ma X, Yue ZQ, Gong ZQ, et al. The effect of diaphragmatic breathing on attention, negative affect and stress in healthy adults. Front Psychol. 2017;8:874.

71. Magnus CR, Barss TS, Lanovaz JL, Farthing JP. Effects of cross-education on the muscle after a period of unilateral limb immobilization using a shoulder sling and swathe. Journal of Applied Physiology. 2010;109:1887-1894.

72. Malabanan A, Veronikis I. Redefining vitamin D insufficiency. Lancet. 1998;351:805-806.

73. Mateen S, Moin S, Shahzad S, Khan AQ. Level of inflammatory cytokines in rheumatoid arthritis patients: correlation with 25-hydroxy vitamin D and reactive oxygen species. PloS One. 2017;12:e0178879.

74. McCreesh KM, Purtill H, Donnelly AE, Lewis JS. Increased supraspinatus tendon thickness following fatigue loading in rotator cuff tendinopathy: potential implications for exercise therapy. BMJ Open Sport & Exercise Medicine. 2017;3:e000279.

75. Meade LB, Bearne LM, Godfrey EL. "It's important to buy in to the new lifestyle": barriers and facilitators of exercise adherence in a population with persistent musculoskeletal pain. Disability and Rehabilitation. 2021;43:468-478.

76. Meakins A, May S, Littlewood C. Reliability of the Shoulder Symptom Modification Procedure and association of within-session and between-session changes with functional outcomes. BMJ Open Sport & Exercise Medicine. 2018;4:e000342.

77. Mersmann F, Bohm S, Arampatzis A. Imbalances in the development of muscle and tendon as risk factor for tendinopathies in youth athletes: a review of current evidence and concepts of prevention. Frontiers in Physiology. 2017;8:987.

78. Moosmayer S, Lund G, Seljom US, et al. At a 10-year follow-up, tendon repair is superior to physiotherapy in the treatment of small and medium-sized rotator cuff tears. JBJS. 2019;101:1050-1060.

79. Moosmayer S, Lund G, Seljom US, et al. Tendon repair compared with physiotherapy in the treatment of rotator cuff tears: a randomized controlled study in 103 cases with a five-year follow-up. J Bone Joint Surg Am. 2014;96:1504-1514.

80. Morrison S, Cook J. Putting "heavy" into heavy slow load. SportRχiv. 2020;10.31236/osf.io/zju3h

81. Parle PJ, Riddiford-Harland DL, Howitt CD, Lewis JS. Acute rotator cuff tendinopathy: does ice, low load isometric exercise, or a combination of the two produce an analgaesic effect? British Journal of Sports Medicine. 2017;51:208-209.

82. Pearce A, Hendy A, Bowen W, Kidgell D. Corticospinal adaptations and strength maintenance in the immobilized arm following 3 weeks unilateral strength training. Scandinavian Journal of Medicine & Science in Sports. 2013;23:740-748.

83. Picard M, Tauveron I, Magdasy S, et al. Effect of exercise training on heart rate variability in type 2 diabetes mellitus patients: a systematic review and meta-analysis. PloS One. 2021;16:e0251863.

84. Pieters L, Lewis J, Kuppens K, et al. An update of systematic reviews examining the effectiveness of conservative physical therapy interventions for subacromial shoulder pain. Journal of Orthopaedic & Sports Physical Therapy. 2020;50:131-141.

85. Pilch W, Kita B, Piotrowska A, et al. The effect of vitamin D supplementation on the muscle damage after eccentric exercise in young men: a randomized, control trial. Journal of the International Society of Sports Nutrition. 2020;17:1-10.

86. Powell JK, Lewis JS. Rotator cuff–related shoulder pain: is it time to reframe the advice,"You need to strengthen your shoulder"? Journal of Orthopaedic & Sports Physical Therapy. 2021;51:156-158.

87. Quindry JC, Franklin BA, Chapman M, Humphrey R, Mathis S. Benefits and risks of high-intensity interval training in patients with coronary artery disease. The American Journal of Cardiology. 2019;123:1370-1377.

88. Reynolds JM, Gordon TJ, Robergs RA. Prediction of one repetition maximum strength from multiple repetition maximum testing and anthropometry. The Journal of Strength & Conditioning Research. 2006;20:584-592.

89. Rhodes JM, Subramanian S, Laird E, Griffin G, Kenny RA. Perspective: vitamin D deficiency and COVID-19 severity–plausibly linked by latitude, ethnicity, impacts on cytokines, ACE2 and thrombosis. Journal of Internal Medicine. 2021;289:97-115.

90. Richardson E, Lewis JS, Gibson J, et al. Role of the kinetic chain in shoulder rehabilitation: does incorporating the trunk and lower limb into shoulder exercise regimes influence shoulder muscle recruitment patterns? Systematic review of electromyography studies. BMJ Open Sport & Exercise Medicine. 2020;6:e000683.

91. Rikli RE, Jones CJ. Development and validation of criterion-referenced clinically relevant fitness standards for maintaining physical independence in later years. The Gerontologist. 2013;53:255-267.

92. Rikli RE, Jones CJ. Senior Fitness Test Manual. Human Kinetics; 2013.

93. Ross LM, Porter RR, Durstine JL. High-intensity interval training (HIIT) for patients with chronic diseases. Journal of Sport and Health Science. 2016;5:139-144.

94. Routledge FS, Campbell TS, McFetridge-Durdle JA, Bacon SL. Improvements in heart rate variability with exercise therapy. Can J Cardiol. 2010;26:303-312.

95. Runge N, Aina A, May S. Are within and/or between session improvements in pain and function prognostic of medium and long-term improvements in musculoskeletal problems? A systematic review. Musculoskeletal Science and Practice. 2020;45:102102.

96. Rynecki ND, Siracuse BL, Ippolito JA, Beebe KS. Injuries sustained during high intensity interval training: are modern fitness trends contributing to increased injury rates? The Journal of Sports Medicine and Physical Fitness. 2019;59:1206-1212.

97. Salamh P, Lewis J. It is time to put special tests for rotator cuff–related shoulder pain out to pasture. Journal of Orthopaedic & Sports Physical Therapy. 2020;50:222-225.

98. Schoenfeld BJ, Grgic J, Van Every DW, Plotkin DL. Loading recommendations for muscle strength, hypertrophy, and local endurance: a re-examination of the repetition continuum. Sports. 2021;9:32.

99. Schrøder CP, Skare O, Reikeras O, Mowinckel P, Brox JI. Sham surgery versus labral repair or biceps tenodesis for type II SLAP lesions of the shoulder: a three-armed randomised clinical trial. Br J Sports Med. 2017;51:1759-1766.

100. Screen H. Tendon and tendon pathology. In: Jull G MA, Falla D, Lewis JS, McCarthy C, Sterling M (eds). Grieve's Modern Musculoskeletal Physiotherapy, 4th edition. London: Elsevier; 2015.

101. Semenchuk BN, Strachan SM, Fortier M. Self-compassion and the self-regulation of exercise: reactions to recalled exercise setbacks. Journal of Sport and Exercise Psychology. 2018;40:31-39.

102. Seo D-I, Kim E, Fahs CA, et al. Reliability of the one-repetition maximum test based on muscle group and gender. J Sports Sci Med. 2012;11:221-225.

103. Steuri R, Sattelmayer M, Elsig S, et al. Effectiveness of conservative interventions including exercise, manual therapy and medical management in adults with shoulder impingement: a systematic review and meta-analysis of RCTs. British Journal of Sports Medicine. 2017;51:1340-1347.

104. Stevenson A, Waite M. Concise Oxford English dictionary: Luxury Edition. Oxford University Press; 2011.

105. Stone M, Stone M, Lamont H. Explosive exercise. National Strength and Conditioning Association Journal. 1993;15:7-15.

106. Suetta C, Hvid LG, Justesen L, et al. Effects of aging on human skeletal muscle after immobilization and retraining. Journal of Applied Physiology. 2009;107:1172-1180.

107. Tallent J, Goodall S, Gibbon KC, Hortobágyi T, Howatson G. Enhanced corticospinal excitability and volitional drive in response to shortening and lengthening strength training and changes following detraining. Frontiers in Physiology. 2017;8:57.

108. Taylor M, Budge C. Self-management of long-term conditions. Kai Tiaki: Nursing New Zealand. 2020;26:20-24.

109. Taylor W. Musculoskeletal pain in the adult New Zealand population: prevalence and impact. N Z Med J. 2005;118:U1629.

110. Thompson SW, Rogerson D, Ruddock A, Barnes A. The effectiveness of two methods of prescribing load on maximal strength development: a systematic review. Sports Medicine. 2020;50:919-938.

111. Timmins RG, Shamim B, Tofari PJ, Hickey JT, Camera DM. Differences in lower limb strength and structure after 12 weeks of resistance, endurance, and concurrent training. International Journal of Sports Physiology and Performance. 2020;15:1223-1230.

112. Toner A, Lewis JS, Stanhope J, Maric F. Prescribing active transport as a planetary health intervention–benefits, challenges and recommendations. Physical Therapy Reviews. 2021;1-9.

113. Tseng W-C, Nosaka K, Tseng K-W, Chou T-Y, Chen TC. Contralateral effects by unilateral eccentric versus concentric resistance training. Med Sci Sports Exerc. 2020;52:474-483.

114. Valdes O, Ramirez C, Perez F, Garcia-Vicencio S, Nosaka K, Penailillo L. Contralateral effects of eccentric resistance training on immobilized arm. Scandinavian Journal of Medicine & Science in Sports. 2021;31:76-90.

115. Wikipedia. One-repetition maximum. Available at: https://en.wikipedia.org/wiki/One-repetition_maximum.

116. Wilk M, Golas A, Stastny P, Nawrocka M, Krzysztofik M, Zajac A. Does tempo of resistance exercise impact training volume? Journal of Human Kinetics. 2018;62:241-250.

117. Zou K, Wong J, Abdullah N, et al. Examination of overall treatment effect and the proportion attributable to contextual effect in osteoarthritis: meta-analysis of randomised controlled trials. Annals of the Rheumatic Diseases. 2016;75:1964-1970.

37 Rehabilitation of the unstable shoulder

Anju Jaggi, Jo Gibson, Margie Olds, Amee L Seitz, Lennard Funk

Principles of rehabilitation

Rehabilitation for the individual with an unstable shoulder needs to consider multiple, often competing factors that may include age, kinesiophobia, coaching, peer pressure and other personal issues. These factors may influence the individual's ability to return to a desired level of function, including sport after nonsurgical rehabilitation, or shoulder stabilization surgery.[93] It is important that the individual understands the problem, is engaged in, and believes in the rehabilitation process. A key component of rehabilitation is a biopsychosocial approach that incorporates education, reassurance, appropriate biomechanical loads, environmental, and social factors. This chapter should be read together with Chapter 17 (The unstable shoulder).

Education

Education is a key component of management for everyone who has experienced shoulder instability. Most patients with shoulder instability want information regarding their individual risk factors for first-time and recurrent shoulder instability. All clinicians should take time to educate the individual, using a variety of approaches, regarding the individual risk factors that predispose people to recurrent instability after a first-time traumatic anterior shoulder dislocation (FTASD).[63,64,105]

Individuals typically want to know when they can return to activity, and clinicians should set realistic expectations. Clinical tools are available to calculate the risk of recurrence following a FTASD.[65,96] Knowledge of pathoanatomical lesions may increase patient understanding, but care should be taken regarding the use of language so as not to increase fear and maladaptive behavior.[48,90] Information should be set in context and clinicians should work collaboratively, using the same language across professions, to instill confidence.[90]

Those diagnosed with atraumatic shoulder instability (ASI) need reassurance early that there is no significant pathology or ongoing harm to the shoulder as a result of subluxations, especially for those that have a non-structural cause. Explaining the importance of muscle control, maintaining good strength and stamina early in the management may help to reduce muscular deconditioning, aberrant movement strategies, and fear avoidance. With respect to fear avoidance, it is imperative that patients are not discouraged to engage in physical exercise and sport.

In those whom there are also psychological drivers and high levels of pain, explanation should be provided on how anxiety and mood can contribute to altered neuromuscular control, and patients may benefit from additional strategies to manage their mental well-being.[62] Social support from rehabilitation clinicians, in the form of empathy and trust, has been identified as a key contributor to patient satisfaction and decreased post-injury depression when returning to sport after an episode of shoulder instability.[93,112]

Psychological factors

Psychological factors are different in people after an episode of traumatic shoulder instability who return to sport when compared with those that did not.[30] Kinesiophobia has also been shown to be a risk factor for recurrent shoulder dislocation following a FTASD.[66] Graded motor imagery has been shown to decrease kinesiophobia and fear in people with knee and cervical injuries, and in frozen shoulder.[58,83,100] The use of a cognitive behavioral approach to increase the rate and level of return to sport is also being examined in knee injuries.[2] These approaches may also be useful in shoulder instability.

In ASI, it is not clear how psychological health impacts on non-structural shoulder instability. Psychological factors such as anxiety and depression may influence an individual's ability to engage effectively with a physical program of rehabilitation, giving rise to poor outcomes.[5,62] An evaluation of the prevalence of psychological disorders in a specialist unit for ASI indicated up to 30% of patients presented with anxiety or depression compared with 5% in the UK population. This implies that early recognition of mental health comorbidities can be helpful in managing ASI.

Fundamentals in exercise prescription

The shoulder muscles work in a pattern of synchronous recruitment to produce movement and maintain glenohumeral joint stability that is dependent upon the plane and direction of movement.[74] Thus, while certain activities may target specific muscles,[8,17,25,76] no single muscle works in isolation. Some authors have proposed that the timing and sequence of muscle recruitment may be more important than the isolated strength of individual muscles.[14,17,113] The focus of rehabilitation should be to address specific muscle deficits in the shoulder girdle, however, addressing strength in the lower limbs and trunk may also be important.

Shoulder function is dependent upon muscles that move and control the scapula (trapezius, serratus anterior, rhomboids major and minor and pectoralis minor) and muscles that influence humeral head position (infraspinatus and supraspinatus, subscapularis, deltoid, pectoralis major, and latissimus dorsi). Consideration of the anatomical location of each muscle and the direction of force applied by the contracting muscle is considered important for the muscles to work as balanced force couples to maintain stability and function.[61,91,110] Additionally, the dual role of providing stability of the joint and movement of the limb need to be considered. Rehabilitation interventions need to address this dual functionality.

Treatment for traumatic shoulder instability

The decision to operate or manage an unstable shoulder nonsurgically is based upon the aims, values and beliefs of the individual, the findings of the clinical examination, the rate and risk of recurrent instability, the cost of treatment,[7,20,95] and impact on the individual's quality of life. The decision is complicated by the paucity of research providing guidance as to best management, and the difference in outcome between surgical or nonsurgical treatment.

Incidence for traumatic instability is highest in young males.[86,92] Randomized trials comparing surgical with nonsurgical management have used rehabilitation protocols that are the same for both groups,[10,40,44] despite differences in pathology. Research is needed to inform the true rate of recurrence following nonsurgical management. Treatment for the younger athlete remains challenging, with high rates of recurrence after both surgical[97] and nonsurgical management.[18,22,54]

Surgical and nonsurgical decision-making

Decision-making regarding surgical or nonsurgical management for those with recurrent traumatic anterior shoulder instability is complex and multifactorial.[95] Principles of shared decision-making may be used to guide the decision. Shared decision-making aims to address the knowledge imbalance that exists between the clinician and patient and is an approach where the clinician and patient share the best available evidence to reach the best possible individualized management decision.[26] Factors such as stage in the playing season and muscular capabilities (e.g. strength, endurance and power), as well as psychological factors, are integrated in the decision process.[21]

Assessment of the type and intensity of previous rehabilitation may be relevant. Clinical experience indicates that successful rehabilitation after a second instability episode is possible. More than three episodes of shoulder instability are less likely to have successful nonsurgical outcomes. Even so, the decision to operate may be complex due to the presence of comorbidities, length of immobilization, and financial issues, as well as social and vocational considerations.

Guidance for the rehabilitation of people seeking care for shoulder instability is provided in the following section. The best management approach is not known, and rehabilitation is based on a thorough understanding of the research, clinical reasoning, appreciating the harms and expected benefits, and shared decision-making. The impact of shoulder instability on quality of life, kinesiophobia and confidence is an important factor when deciding on the appropriate course of management. The guidance should not be seen as prescriptive rehabilitation. Rather, it is provided as a summary based on the synthesis of the research literature and clinical experience. Clinical guidance will change as new knowledge and understanding becomes available.

First time traumatic anterior shoulder dislocation

Acute period (0–4 weeks)

Immobilization

Immobilization of the affected limb after a FTASD has been widely investigated in the literature. Two meta-analyses have shown that neither the position, nor duration of immobilization altered the risk of recurrence.[64,105] Clinician-researchers have proposed immobilization in external rotation to increase the healing of a Bankart lesion.[36] However, several systematic reviews have failed to produce any results to indicate that immobilization in external rotation is superior to immobilization in a neutral shoulder position.[11,70,108] A recent prospective cohort study reported that immobilization after a dislocation may reduce the risk of recurrence at 1 year follow-up.[66] Immobilization following an FTASD increases patient comfort and may promote healing,[11] although immobilization of the limb for longer than one week has not been shown to affect recurrent instability.[70]

People over the age of 30 years may be more likely to develop residual stiffness after a shoulder dislocation.[45] Therefore, lengthy immobilization in the older population should be discouraged.[11] Additionally, a shoulder dislocation has been shown to increase the risk of developing a frozen shoulder, with an adjusted odds ratio of 3.57 (95%CI 2.35–5.45).[99] Patients should be encouraged to wean themselves from immobilization after one week, as pain and comfort permits.

Range of motion

Patients should be encouraged to regain range of motion (ROM) as comfort permits; this can be performed in both closed and open chain positions (Figure 37.1). Younger patients are rarely limited in regaining ROM after a FTASD, while people over the age of 30 years may experience limitation in ROM (particularly in external rotation and flexion).[45] In the acute stage, aggressively stretching the shoulder is unlikely to improve outcomes. After a period of immobilization, progressive gentle stretching should be encouraged, particularly in the older population.

Glenohumeral strength/neuromuscular control and timing of muscle activation

Rotator cuff strength is decreased in people with recurrent anterior shoulder instability,[24] especially subscapularis.[28] Subscapularis tendinosis and tendon tears are more common in people with an anterior shoulder dislocation,[33] implying that an increased tensile load is placed upon this muscle during the dislocation. People with anterior shoulder instability also have decreased external rotator cuff strength.[24] Anecdotally, this appears more pronounced when the glenohumeral joint is at or above 90° abduction, especially in people reporting apprehension.

A key element of rehabilitation for people after an FTASD is regaining their rotator cuff strength. In the acute setting, pain-free isometric internal and external rotation is advised with the elbow by the side (Figure 37.2). Positions such as the lift-off and belly press positions may maximize subscapularis activity relative to other prime movers such as pectoralis major and latissimus dorsi (Figure 37.3). External rotation may be pain-free in a belly-off position. External rotation in the neutral position has been shown

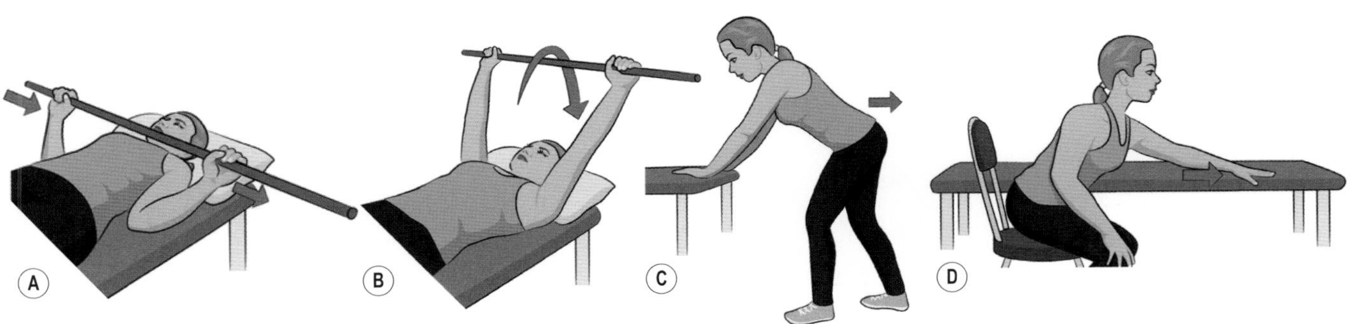

FIGURE 37.1
Open and closed chain range of motion exercises.
(Reproduced with the kind permission of the Auckland Shoulder Clinic.)

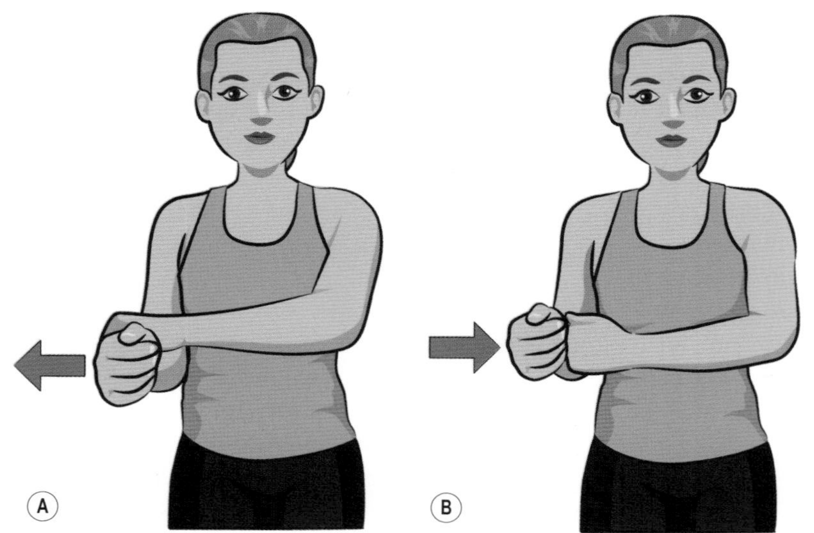

FIGURE 37.2
Isometric external (A) and internal (B) rotation exercises.
(Reproduced with the kind permission of the Auckland Shoulder Clinic.)

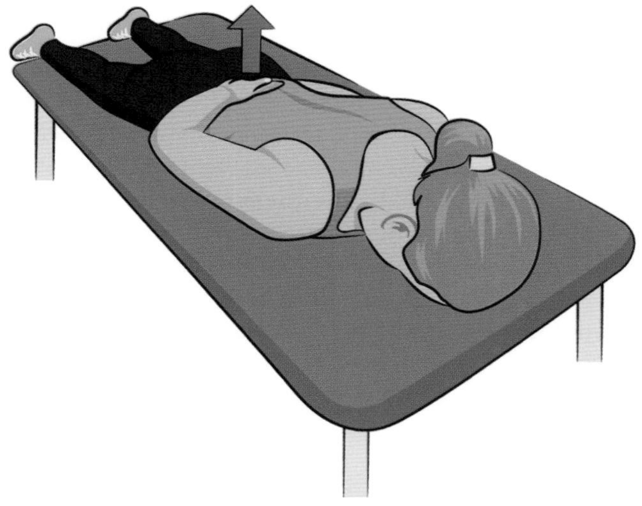

FIGURE 37.3
Lift-off position exercises.
(Reproduced with the kind permission of the Auckland Shoulder Clinic.)

to increase supraspinatus activity[8] and may be less irritable for patients than other exercises which specifically target supraspinatus such as empty can and prone horizontal abduction.[8,75,76]

Scapular neuromuscular control, strength, and timing

The scapula functions to create a stable base for the humeral head[42] and optimal positioning is required to minimize glenohumeral shear,[104] maximize concavity/compression,[50,56] and promote efficient muscle activation.[34] Changes in people with traumatic shoulder instability include decreased scapular upward rotation, and increased scapular internal rotation during arm elevation.[52] Therefore, maintaining scapular control and strength is an important aspect of rehabilitation after a shoulder dislocation.[41] In the acute setting, exercises such as the scapula six-pack (Figure 37.4) which promotes scapula movement with minimal translation of the glenohumeral joint are recommended.[94]

Post-acute period (usually around 4 weeks)

Glenohumeral and scapular muscle performance

In the post-acute period, initial inflammation and hemarthrosis of the glenohumeral joint has subsided,[79] and typically there is less pain.[65] The general principles of exercise therapy apply and include regular resistance training 5 days a week, which seeks to find balance between effective resistance training, building confidence and relearning motor skills.[46] Initially, the exercises are typically performed in

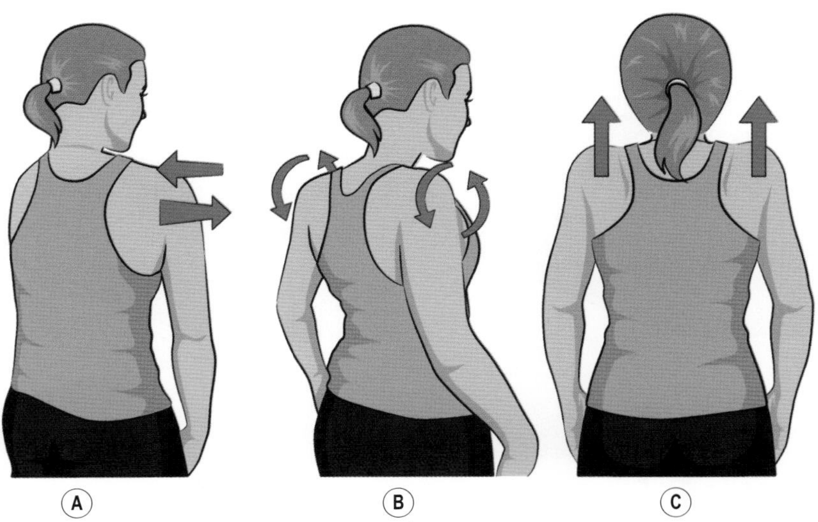

FIGURE 37.4
Scapular "six-pack" exercises.
(Reproduced with the kind permission of the Auckland Shoulder Clinic.)

prone, side-lying or supine (Figure 37.5). Once the patient has control through range, then therapists should progressively increase the load with resistance bands or free weights. Increasing endurance capacity may be achieved with isometric holds for 30 seconds, in mid-range and then progressed through range. This is followed by isotonic contractions.

Progression of exercises to increase shoulder muscle performance may include low row, "robbery", four point kneeling, and plank position (Figure 37.6).[53] Hip extension may be added to increase lower trapezius and serratus anterior activation.

Kinetic chain

A recent systematic review of EMG studies undertaken in a healthy population has shown that exercises which increase activity of the legs and trunk result in increased activation of scapula thoracic muscles but not the rotator cuff.[77] This knowledge may be used to reduce rotator cuff activity in the early stages while promoting scapular muscle activation. Further research is required to guide clinicians as to when and if to incorporate other kinetic chain exercises into rehabilitation for people with shoulder instability. Thoracic rotation, trunk, pelvic, and hip strengthening exercises should also be incorporated into the program.

Final-stage rehabilitation

The final and more advanced stages of rehabilitation should be sport- and activity-specific.

Glenohumeral muscle performance and control

Patients who wish to return to fast-moving activities require training at speed in the clinical setting. The use of a metronome to increase speed of movement allows both external pacing of the limb with increased cortical muscle control[78] and gradual exposure to increased speeds. Supporting the elbow on a surface allows the patient to focus on internal and external rotation of the shoulder. Progression includes increasing speed and decreasing support. Compensatory scapular movement should be avoided. Examples include scapular anterior and posterior tilt and increased lateral and medial rotation to compensate for weak, painful, and restricted glenohumeral internal and external rotation.

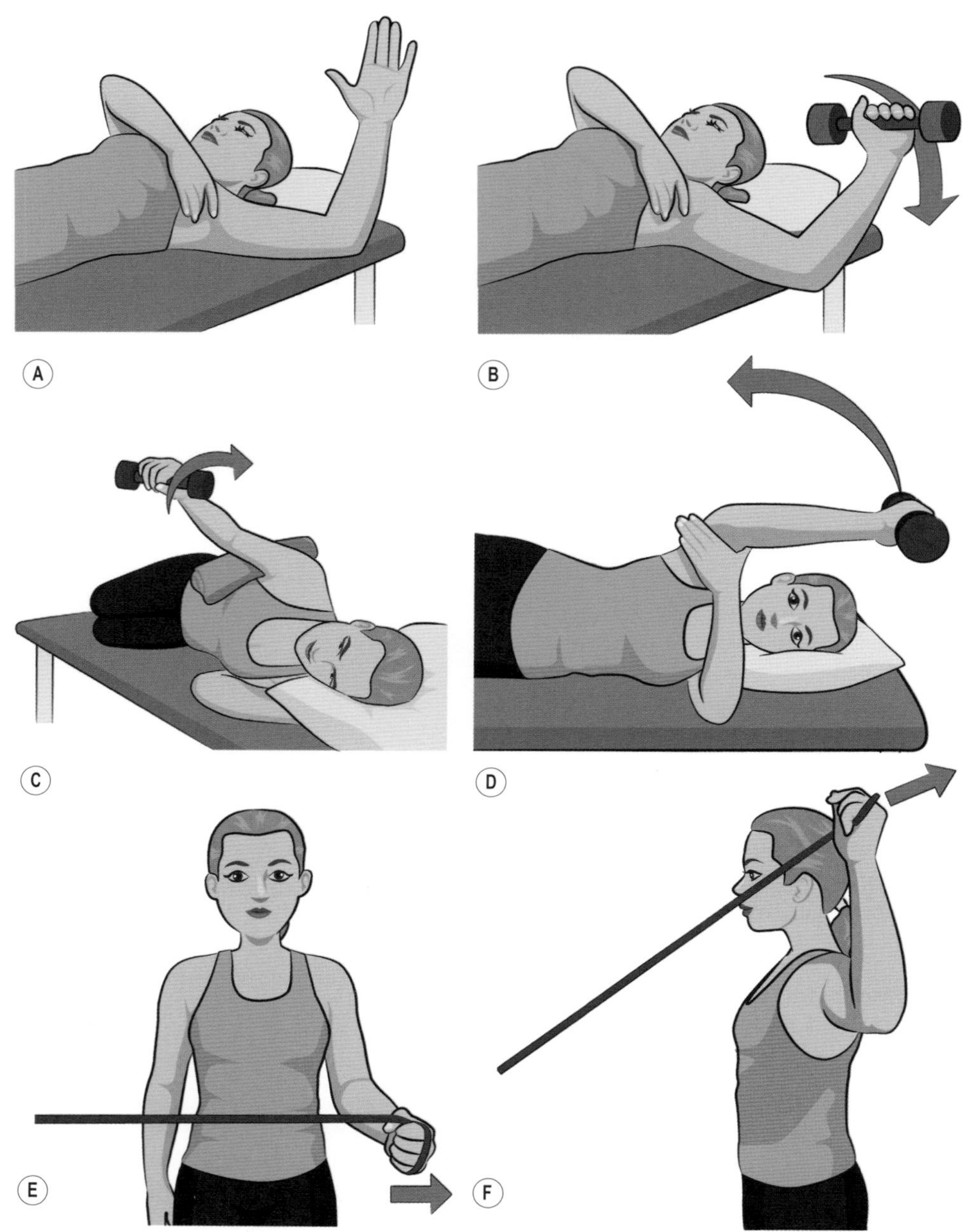

FIGURE 37.5
Post-acute resistance training.
(Reproduced with the kind permission of the Auckland Shoulder Clinic.)

As the patient progresses, rehabilitation should include more challenging tasks. Perturbation is defined as a deviation of a system from its path, caused by an outside influence. Perturbation exercises with the eyes open and closed are introduced in varying positions, with varying magnitudes of force.[16,94,109]

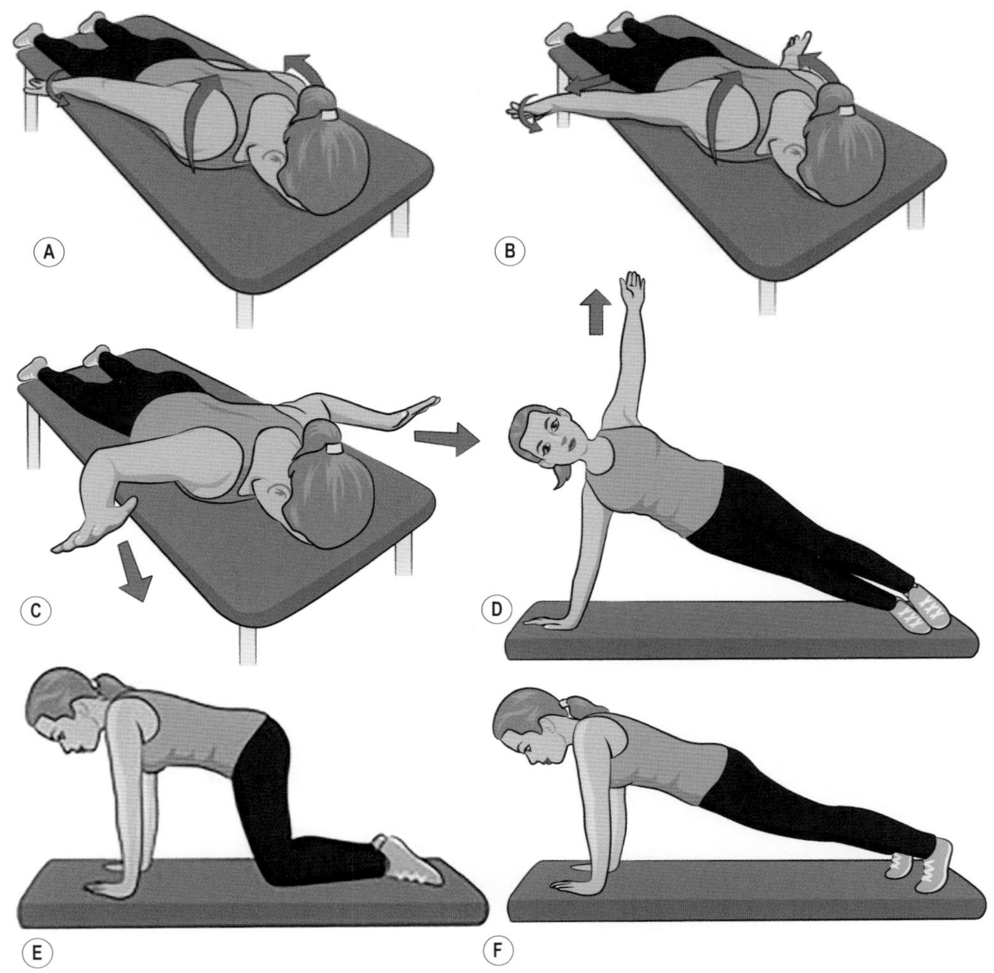

FIGURE 37.6
Post-acute exercise progression.
(Reproduced with the kind permission of the Auckland Shoulder Clinic.)

If the individual is returning to sport or work, then sport- and vocational-specific testing is required. This should involve numerous tests to cover all the constructs that are applicable to the activity the patient is returning to.[3,9] Examples of specific exercises are shown in Figure 37.7.

Posterior instability

Subluxation is much more common than dislocation in posterior shoulder instability.[35] Episodes of posterior instability occur when the posterior capsule is placed under load in a position of flexion, adduction and internal rotation.[71,73,82] This results in a greater incidence of posterior instability in individuals who participate in sports – particularly those playing American football – than in the general population or other sport participants.[68,89]

In non-athletic populations, failure rates with nonsurgical management are lower for people with posterior shoulder instability than anterior instability, with up to 70% of people being successfully managed nonsurgically at one

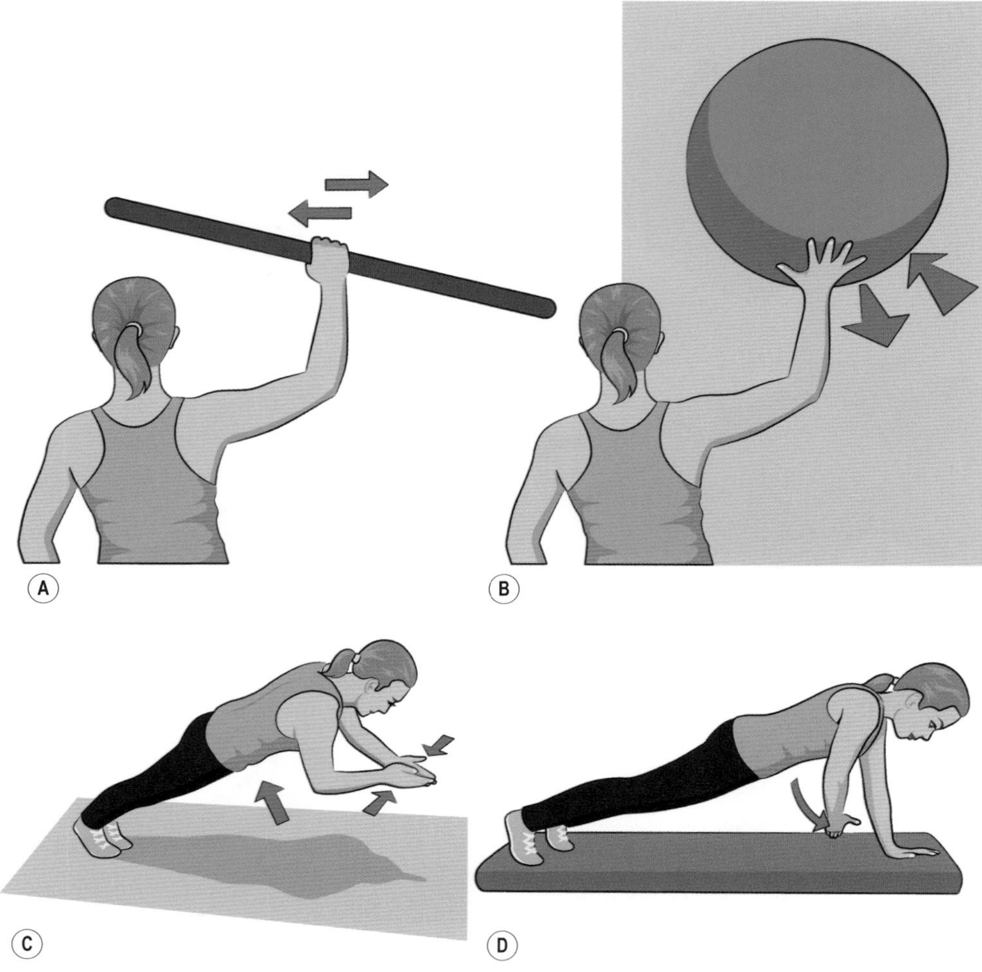

FIGURE 37.7
Examples of sport- and work-specific exercises.
(Reproduced with the kind permission of the Auckland Shoulder Clinic.)

year follow-up.[111] However, success declines to 52% by 10 years. There is low-level evidence that suggests that better outcomes are achieved with nonsurgical management for people with nontraumatic posterior dislocations than for those whose history includes trauma.[12]

There is uncertainty regarding the best rehabilitation approach for people with posterior shoulder instability. Decreased muscle activity of the posterior rotator cuff has been reported in those with recurrent posterior instability combined with overactivity of the latissimus dorsi.[39] Thus, increased activation and strengthening of the infraspinatus has been advocated to reduce posterior subluxation. The superiority of an anterior versus posterior rotator cuff emphasis for either motor control or strengthening in patients with posterior shoulder instability has yet to be established.

Posterior shoulder instability rehabilitation

Fronek et al. reported in a small study that 13 people from a group of 16 patients who were prescribed an exercise program targeting the shoulder external rotators did not require surgery.[27] The program involved external rotation exercises, initially by the side and then at 45° abduction. A home program was also included. External rotation exercises can be progressed to 90° abduction and in the overhead position. Other exercises, such as the prone plank may be included to activate infraspinatus which may further contribute to stability.

Watson et al. published a comprehensive rehabilitation program for people with traumatic and atraumatic posterior shoulder instability.[107] The program is divided into a scapular phase and an arc of motion phase. In the scapular phase, patients perform upward rotation of the scapula or "scapula setting". In the arc of motion phase, patients develop humeral head control in the coronal and then sagittal planes, and then progressively increase load into increasing ranges of flexion and abduction. Again, in this program, there was a focus on external rotation strengthening.

Acromioclavicular joint instability

Management of traumatic acromioclavicular joint (ACJ) injuries is based on the Rockwood classification.[81] Expert consensus recommends nonsurgical management for the most common type I and II injuries. There is a paucity of evidence on what to include in the rehabilitation program. Patients sustaining these injuries often return to sport at 3–6 weeks post-injury. Studies have reported that approximately 50% of people who sustain a type I or II injury, still describe ongoing symptoms of varying levels of pain and disability at 10 years.[57]

Although the available research is limited, research findings suggest comparable outcomes for type III injuries managed surgically and nonsurgically. Delays in surgical stabilization in type III injuries do not detrimentally impact on outcomes.[43] Due to insufficient research, shared decision-making needs to incorporate clinical presentation, patient factors, pain, and functional deficits in informing management, rather than imaging findings alone.[31]

In acute traumatic injuries of the ACJ a short period of sling immobilization (1–3 weeks) and appropriate analgesia, should be followed by active mobilization with progression of range of motion as symptoms allow.[55] There is no evidence to support the superiority of other immobilization devices over a conventional sling, and case reports would suggest that compliance with more rigid fixation is poor.[15]

The importance of scapular exercises is emphasized in the management of ACJ instability.[15,19] Studies evaluating patients with persistent type II instability indicate that scapula dyskinesis is associated with ongoing pain and reduced function,[32] and that a specific six-week program targeting the scapular muscles was effective in addressing symptoms in 80% of patients.[13] Gumina et al. demonstrated that patients with persistent type III ACJ instability were at increased risk of developing cervical region symptoms.[32]

While there continues to be a consensus that rehabilitation targeting the rotator cuff and scapular muscles should be the primary choice of intervention, the persistence or recurrence of symptoms highlights the need for research to evaluate whether specific rehabilitation approaches confer superior outcomes. The role of deltoid and trapezius in enhancing ACJ stability when the delto-trapezial fascia is intact may also be important.[69]

Sternoclavicular joint instability

Traumatic dislocation of the sternoclavicular joint (SCJ) is a relatively rare injury and due to the high-energy mechanism required, is often associated with other injuries. There is very little in the literature to guide clinicians regarding the specifics of rehabilitation post-injury, however, expert opinion generally recommends a longer period of immobilization than that following ACJ injuries, followed by mobilization as symptoms allow.[29,59]

Sewell et al. recommend the application of the Stanmore Classification of Shoulder Instability (see Figure 17.1) for people experiencing SCJ instability to guide management.[85] Patients presenting with atraumatic anterior SCJ instability (types II and III) with glenohumeral joint laxity, particularly in the presence of hypermobility, can generally be managed successfully nonsurgically. Observations from case series suggest these patients often have observable dominance (compared with their asymptomatic side) of pectoralis major and sternocleidomastoid, with a tendency to chin-poke.[4,85] There is a lack of detail in reported case series, but key principles incorporate postural correction (specifically the thoracic and cervical spine), and using symptom modification approaches targeting scapular upward rotation, and the posterior cuff to reduce subluxation, to inform exercise prescription.[4,98]

Reported case series suggest that treatment may take up to six months.[80,85,98] Rockwood and Odor reported no limitation of activity or restriction of lifestyle in 29 of 37 patients (78%) with atraumatic anterior dislocations, treated nonoperatively with rehabilitation or a watch and wait approach.[80] Importantly, 90% of the patients had persistent subluxation and 21% had ongoing pain. For some patients, resolution of subluxation does not appear to be essential for return to function. This is an important consideration during shared decision-making. Those patients who have atraumatic SCJ instability without laxity have a less consistent response to nonsurgical treatment. For those not improving, the administration of botulinum toxin has been advocated to temporarily reduce pectoralis major activity, and then continuing rehabilitation.[4] There is a lack of robust evidence to support this suggestion and, as ever in those patients with poorer outcomes, it is imperative to explore expectations, understanding, and psychosocial aspects that may contribute.

Rehabilitation for atraumatic shoulder instability

Rehabilitation program

Atraumatic shoulder instability (ASI) is typically characterized by subluxations rather than frank dislocations. As a result, there is minimal or no structural damage to the shoulder. Strengthening and neuromuscular control exercises are recommended as the first line of management.[51]

There is very little evidence to guide clinicians in selecting the optimal rehabilitation interventions for patients with ASI. Systematic reviews that have investigated the effect of exercise for the treatment of multidirectional instability have revealed a high risk of bias and very low-level evidence.[102,103] Despite almost a 30-year period since the inception of the Rockwood program for ASI, there is only one randomized controlled trial (RCT) comparing alternative rehabilitation exercise programs for multidirectional ASI. A recent RCT compared the Watson program with the Rockwood program, and reported significant effects favoring the Watson program for the Western Ontario Shoulder Instability (WOSI), Melbourne Instability Shoulder Score (MISS), and pain at 24 weeks. However, the study had a small sample size and patients were less adherent with the Watson regimen.[101]

More recently, the Derby program has been devised for people experiencing ASI with either predominant anterior or posterior instability. In a prospective study of 66 patients, there were significant improvements in stability, pain and function following a mean of seven sessions of supervised nonsurgical intervention with the Derby program in conjunction with a home exercise program, over an average 30-week period. This was a nonrandomized study, outcomes were short-term, and only patient self-reported outcomes were recorded at the final data collection timepoint.[6]

In summary, the focus of any exercise program for people with ASI has been to strengthen the rotator cuff, deltoid and scapulothoracic muscles to ensure optimum coordination, endurance, and function. Previous research in patients with multidirectional instability has placed emphasis on scapular upward rotators.[72,106] More recently, the importance of strengthening the entire kinetic chain and/or incorporating patterns of strength training of the upper limb with the lower limb has been advocated.[37,38] However, the application of evidence in practice is not always program-specific. A more pragmatic approach with individualized patient factors in terms of muscle capacity, adherence, and behavior to exercise may be warranted. It is also unclear if exercise prescription should be uniquely based on direction of instability.

Early stage/high irritability: managing apprehension and pain

Pain, anxiety, fear, and avoidance of movement are natural emotional reactions to shoulder instability and can lead to altered muscle recruitment, muscle deconditioning, and habitual patterns of movement. Early reassurance, education, and explanation are essential.

Identification of a "safe zone" is required: this is the range within which the patient feels confident to move their arm. Sometimes alterations in posture facilitate this. Early activation of the RC and/or recruitment of postural muscles may help in alleviating pain, as well as to prevent compensatory strategies and over-activation of aberrant muscle activity.

Instability driven by poor scapular control

Confusion pertaining to scapular position exists, notably if the scapula appears to be in an excessive downwardly rotated position. Some advocate that increased activation of upper trapezius is required,[72] and others disagree,[47] arguing that upper trapezius contributes little to scapular upward rotation. If clinical testing (symptom modification) suggests that upward scapular rotation may improve stability, then scapular elevation exercises (shoulder shrug) could be considered in prone and side-lying, starting with the arm by the side and progressing into elevation. Exercising in 30° of abduction may be more functional and effective than with the arm by the side. This program should be considered in people with multidirectional instability.[72]

Targeting rotator cuff muscle weakness and imbalance

People with ASI often present with rotator cuff muscle weakness. Aberrant muscle recruitment and patterning has also been documented in people with ASI[39] and may decrease the stability of the shoulder joint. There is disagreement regarding the direction of shoulder instability associated with rotator cuff weakness. Moroder et al. has devised a program that specifically focuses on the external rotators in people with posterior shoulder instability.[60] This is supported by research that has shown that infraspinatus activity increases to reduce posterior shear of the glenohumeral joint.[67] If rotator cuff weakness is present in the terminal ranges of shoulder motion, or if scapular stability is difficult to maintain, exercising in supine with the arm supported is a recommended rehabilitation entry point. This exercise is gradually made more demanding by removing the underlying support and/or placing a weight in the hand. These rotational exercises may also be performed in prone lying, placing more demand on the scapular stabilizers and the rotator cuff. There is little evidence to guide treatment in terms of load, frequency, or repetition. The patient can help to determine these parameters in consultation with the clinician considering fatigue, pain, and effort. The exercise needs to be achievable for the patient to perform and continually progressed.

To facilitate patient adherence, clinicians should prescribe between two and four exercises,[84] ensuring the prescribed exercises are performed as required. Perceived simplicity and short duration of treatment, immediacy of benefit, and absence of side effects are known factors that increase patient adherence to exercise.[88] Furthermore, a single prone horizontal abduction exercise performed once a day for 3 weeks has been shown to increase lower trapezius activation and increase shoulder strength in individuals with shoulder pain. This simplicity of 2–4 exercises is also a feature of the Derby program.[6]

Aberrant muscle activity

Clinically abnormal movement and muscle recruitment may be observed. This may present as downward rotation of the scapula with simultaneous increased activation of the pectoralis major and/or the latissimus dorsi muscles during arm elevation. Concomitant arm elevation in shoulder internal rotation may result in the humeral head displacing inferiorly and posteriorly.[5,39] Botulinum toxin injections have been used to inhibit aberrant overactive muscles,[5,23,87] although the positive effects were only temporary. Over time it has become apparent that strengthening the underactive muscle groups, such as the rotator cuff and scapula muscles is key, and that patients need to relearn recruitment patterns. Strategies such as reciprocal inhibition which use agonist muscle activity to decrease antagonist muscle activation, can be useful in altering muscle recruitment patterning. In addition, experience has indicated that the aberrant muscle activity can be the secondary effect of more primary drivers such as stress, anxiety, fear, or deep-rooted psychological trauma in very rare cases. It is therefore essential that there is meticulous assessment of the patient's presentation, including psychosocial history.[5]

Adjuncts such as mirrors, external supports such as functional electrical stimulation (see Chapter 33) and braces and tape (see Chapter 34) may be used to provide a feed-forward efferent stimulus to facilitate a better movement strategy.[1,49]

Conclusion

Nonsurgical intervention is an option for most people diagnosed with shoulder instability. Outcomes are variable and considerable research is required to inform best management. Shared decision-making is essential in helping the individual seeking care for their unstable shoulder understand time frames, expected outcomes, harms of specific interventions, their required contribution, and prognosis.

CHAPTER THIRTY-SEVEN

Nonsurgical rehabilitation and rehabilitation following surgery will, on average, take a minimum of 12 weeks, and for others considerably longer, and must include a progressive exercise program. The role of proprioception is discussed in Chapter 28 and the Shape-Up-My-Shoulder (#SUMS) program is presented in Chapter 36.

References

1. Aarseth LM, Suprak DN, Chalmers GR, Lyon L, Dahlquist DT. Kinesio tape and shoulder-joint position sense. J Athl Train. 2015;50:785-791.
2. Ardern CL, Kvist J, Group BT. BAck iN the Game (BANG) - a smartphone application to help athletes return to sport following anterior cruciate ligament reconstruction: protocol for a multi-centre, randomised controlled trial. BMC Musculoskelet Disord. 2020;21:523.
3. Ashworth B, Hogben P, Singh N, Tulloch L, Cohen DD. The Athletic Shoulder (ASH) test: reliability of a novel upper body isometric strength test in elite rugby players. BMJ Open Sport Exerc Med. 2018;4:e000365.
4. Athanatos L, Singh HP, Armstrong AL. The management of sternoclavicular instability. Journal of Arthroscopy and Joint Surgery. 2018;5:126-132.
5. Barrett C. The clinical physiotherapy assessment of non-traumatic shoulder instability. Shoulder Elbow. 2015;7:60-71.
6. Bateman M, Osborne SE, Smith BE. Physiotherapy treatment for atraumatic recurrent shoulder instability: updated results of the Derby shoulder instability rehabilitation programme. Journal of Arthroscopy and Joint Surgery. 2019;6:35-41.
7. Bishop JA, Crall TS, Kocher MS. Operative versus nonoperative treatment after primary traumatic anterior glenohumeral dislocation: expected-value decision analysis. J Shoulder Elbow Surg. 2011;20:1087-1094.
8. Boettcher CE, Ginn KA, Cathers I. Which is the optimal exercise to strengthen supraspinatus? Med Sci Sports Exerc. 2009;41:1979-1983.
9. Borms D, Cools A. Upper-extremity functional performance tests: reference values for overhead athletes. Int J Sports Med. 2018;39:433-441.
10. Bottoni CR, Wilckens JH, DeBerardino TM, et al. A prospective, randomized evaluation of arthroscopic stabilization versus nonoperative treatment in patients with acute, traumatic, first-time shoulder dislocations. Am J Sports Med. 2002;30:576-580.
11. Braun C, McRobert CJ. Conservative management following closed reduction of traumatic anterior dislocation of the shoulder. Cochrane Database Syst Rev. 2019;5:CD004962.
12. Burkhead WZ, Jr., Rockwood CA, Jr. Treatment of instability of the shoulder with an exercise program. J Bone Joint Surg Am. 1992;74:890-896.
13. Carbone S, Postacchini R, Gumina S. Scapular dyskinesis and SICK syndrome in patients with a chronic type III acromioclavicular dislocation. Results of rehabilitation. Knee Surg Sports Traumatol Arthrosc. 2015;23:1473-1480.
14. Castelein B, Cagnie B, Parlevliet T, Cools A. Serratus anterior or pectoralis minor: which muscle has the upper hand during protraction exercises? Man Ther. 2016;22:158-164.
15. Cook JB, Krul KP. Challenges in treating acromioclavicular separations: current concepts. J Am Acad Orthop Surg. 2018;26:669-677.
16. Cools AM, Borms D, Castelein B, Vanderstukken F, Johansson FR. Evidence-based rehabilitation of athletes with glenohumeral instability. Knee Surg Sports Traumatol Arthrosc. 2016;24:382-389.
17. Cools AM, Dewitte V, Lanszweert F, et al. Rehabilitation of scapular muscle balance: which exercises to prescribe? Am J Sports Med. 2007;35:1744-1751.
18. Cordischi K, Li X, Busconi B. Intermediate outcomes after primary traumatic anterior shoulder dislocation in skeletally immature patients aged 10 to 13 years. Orthopedics. 2009;32:686-686.
19. Cote MP, Wojcik KE, Gomlinski G, Mazzocca AD. Rehabilitation of acromioclavicular joint separations: operative and nonoperative considerations. Clin Sports Med. 2010;29:213-228, vii.
20. Crall TS, Bishop JA, Guttman D, Kocher M, Bozic K, Lubowitz JH. Cost-effectiveness analysis of primary arthroscopic stabilization versus nonoperative treatment for first-time anterior glenohumeral dislocations. Arthroscopy. 2012;28:1755-1765.
21. Creighton DW, Shrier I, Shultz R, Meeuwisse WH, Matheson GO. Return-to-play in sport: a decision-based model. Clin J Sport Med. 2010;20:379-385.
22. Deitch J, Mehlman CT, Foad SL, Obbehat A, Mallory M. Traumatic anterior shoulder dislocation in adolescents. Am J Sports Med. 2003;31:758-763.
23. Donnellan CP, Scott MA, Antoun M, Wallace WA. Physiotherapy and botulinum toxin injections prior to stabilization surgery for recurrent atraumatic anteroinferior shoulder dislocation with abnormal muscle patterning. Shoulder & Elbow. 2012;4:287-290.
24. Edouard P, Degache F, Beguin L, et al. Rotator cuff strength in recurrent anterior shoulder instability. J Bone Joint Surg Am. 2011;93:759-765.
25. Edwards PK, Ebert JR, Littlewood C, Ackland T, Wang A. A systematic review of electromyography studies in normal shoulders to inform postoperative rehabilitation following rotator cuff repair. J Orthop Sports Phys Ther. 2017;47:931-944.
26. Elwyn G, Frosch D, Thomson R, et al. Shared decision making: a model for clinical practice. J Gen Intern Med. 2012;27:1361-1367.
27. Fronek J, Warren RF, Bowen M. Posterior subluxation of the glenohumeral joint. J Bone Joint Surg Am. 1989;71:205-216.
28. Gamulin A, Dayer R, Lubbeke A, Miozzari H, Hoffmeyer P. Primary open anterior shoulder stabilization: a long-term, retrospective cohort study on the impact of subscapularis muscle alterations on recurrence. BMC Musculoskelet Disord. 2014;15:45.
29. Garcia JA, Arguello AM, Momaya AM, Ponce BA. Sternoclavicular joint instability: symptoms, diagnosis and management. Orthop Res Rev. 2020;12:75-87.
30. Gerometta A, Klouche S, Herman S, Lefevre N, Bohu Y. The Shoulder Instability-Return to Sport after Injury (SIRSI): a valid and

reproducible scale to quantify psychological readiness to return to sport after traumatic shoulder instability. Knee Surgery, Sports Traumatology, Arthroscopy. 2018;26:203-211.

31. Granville-Chapman J, Torrance E, Rashid A, Funk L. The Rockwood classification in acute acromioclavicular joint injury does not correlate with symptoms. J Orthop Surg. 2018;26:2309499018777886.

32. Gumina S, Carbone S, Postacchini F. Scapular dyskinesis and SICK scapula syndrome in patients with chronic type III acromioclavicular dislocation. Arthroscopy. 2009;25:40-45.

33. Gyftopoulos S, Carpenter E, Kazam J, Babb J, Bencardino J. MR imaging of subscapularis tendon injury in the setting of anterior shoulder dislocation. Skeletal Radiol. 2012;41:1445-1452.

34. Happee R, Van der Helm FC. The control of shoulder muscles during goal directed movements, an inverse dynamic analysis. J Biomech. 1995;28:1179-1191.

35. Hawkins RJ, McCormack RG. Posterior shoulder instability. Orthopedics. 1988;11:101-107.

36. Itoi E, Hatakeyama Y, Sato T, et al. Immobilization in external rotation after shoulder dislocation reduces the risk of recurrence. A randomized controlled trial. J Bone Joint Surg Am. 2007;89:2124-2131.

37. Jaggi A, Alexander S. Rehabilitation for shoulder instability: current approaches. Open Orthop J. 2017;11:957-971.

38. Jaggi A, Lambert S. Rehabilitation for shoulder instability. Br J Sports Med. 2010;44:333-340.

39. Jaggi A, Noorani A, Malone A, Cowan J, Lambert S, Bayley I. Muscle activation patterns in patients with recurrent shoulder instability. Int J Shoulder Surg. 2012;6:101-107.

40. Jakobsen BW, Johannsen HV, Suder P, Sojbjerg JO. Primary repair versus conservative treatment of first-time traumatic anterior dislocation of the shoulder: a randomized study with 10-year follow-up. Arthroscopy. 2007;23:118-123.

41. Karatsolis K, Athanasopoulos S. The role of exercise in the conservative treatment of the anterior shoulder dislocation. Journal of Bodywork and Movement Therapies. 2006;10:211-219.

42. Kibler WB, Sciascia A. The role of the scapula in preventing and treating shoulder instability. Knee Surg Sports Traumatol Arthrosc. 2016;24:390-397.

43. Kim SH, Koh KH. Treatment of Rockwood type III acromioclavicular joint dislocation. Clin Shoulder Elb. 2018;21:48-55.

44. Kirkley A, Griffin S, Richards C, Miniaci A, Mohtadi N. Prospective randomized clinical trial comparing the effectiveness of immediate arthroscopic stabilization versus immobilization and rehabilitation in first traumatic anterior dislocations of the shoulder. Arthroscopy. 1999;15:507-514.

45. Kiviluoto O, Pasila M, Jaroma H, Sundholm A. Immobilization after primary dislocation of the shoulder. Acta Orthop Scand. 1980;51:915-919.

46. Kraemer WJ, Adams K, Cafarelli E, et al. American College of Sports Medicine position stand. Progression models in resistance training for healthy adults. Med Sci Sports Exerc. 2002;34:364-380.

47. Lawrence RL, Braman JP, Keefe DF, Ludewig PM. The coupled kinematics of scapulothoracic upward rotation. Phys Ther. 2020;100:283-294.

48. Lewis J, O'Sullivan P. Is it time to reframe how we care for people with non-traumatic musculoskeletal pain? Br J Sports Med. 2018;52:1543-1544.

49. Lim OB, Kim JA, Song SJ, Cynn HS, Yi CH. Effect of selective muscle training using visual EMG biofeedback on infraspinatus and posterior deltoid. J Hum Kinet. 2014;44:83-90.

50. Lippitt SB, Vanderhooft JE, Harris SL, Sidles JA, Harryman DT, 2nd, Matsen FA, 3rd. Glenohumeral stability from concavity-compression: a quantitative analysis. J Shoulder Elbow Surg. 1993;2:27-35.

51. Longo UG, Rizzello G, Loppini M, et al. Multidirectional instability of the shoulder: a systematic review. Arthroscopy. 2015;31:2431-2443.

52. Ludewig PM, Reynolds JF. The association of scapular kinematics and glenohumeral joint pathologies. J Orthop Sports Phys Ther. 2009;39:90-104.

53. Maenhout A, Van Praet K, Pizzi L, Van Herzeele M, Cools A. Electromyographic analysis of knee push up plus variations: what is the influence of the kinetic chain on scapular muscle activity? Br J Sports Med. 2010;44:1010-1015.

54. Marans HJ, Angel KR, Schemitsch EH, Wedge JH. The fate of traumatic anterior dislocation of the shoulder in children. J Bone Joint Surg Am. 1992;74:1242-1244.

55. Martetschlager F, Kraus N, Scheibel M, Streich J, Venjakob A, Maier D. The diagnosis and treatment of acute dislocation of the acromioclavicular joint. Dtsch Arztebl Int. 2019;116:89-95.

56. Matsen FA, 3rd, Harryman DT, 2nd, Sidles JA. Mechanics of glenohumeral instability. Clin Sports Med. 1991;10:783-788.

57. Mikek M. Long-term shoulder function after type I and II acromioclavicular joint disruption. Am J Sports Med. 2008;36:2147-2150.

58. Monticone M, Vernon H, Brunati R, Rocca B, Ferrante S. The NeckPix©: development of an evaluation tool for assessing kinesiophobia in subjects with chronic neck pain. Eur Spine J. 2015;24:72-79.

59. Morell DJ, Thyagarajan DS. Sternoclavicular joint dislocation and its management: a review of the literature. World J Orthop. 2016;7:244-250.

60. Moroder P, Minkus M, Bohm E, Danzinger V, Gerhardt C, Scheibel M. Use of shoulder pacemaker for treatment of functional shoulder instability: proof of concept. Obere Extrem. 2017;12:103-108.

61. Myers JB, Lephart SM. The role of the sensorimotor system in the athletic shoulder. J Athl Train. 2000;35:351-363.

62. Noorani A, Goldring M, Jaggi A, et al. BESS/BOA patient care pathways: atraumatic shoulder instability. Shoulder Elbow. 2019;11:60-70.

63. Olds M, Donaldson K, Ellis R, Kersten P. In children 18 years and under, what promotes recurrent shoulder instability after traumatic anterior shoulder dislocation? A systematic review and meta-analysis of risk factors. Br J Sports Med. 2016;50:1135-1141.

64. Olds M, Ellis R, Donaldson K, Parmar P, Kersten P. Risk factors which predispose first-time traumatic anterior shoulder dislocations to recurrent instability in adults: a systematic review and meta-analysis. Br J Sports Med. 2015;49:913-922.

65. Olds M, Ellis R, Parmar P, Kersten P. The immediate and subsequent impact of a first-time traumatic anterior shoulder dislocation in people aged 16–40: results from a national cohort study. Shoulder & Elbow. 2020;13:223-232.

66. Olds MK, Ellis R, Parmar P, Kersten P. Who will redislocate his/her shoulder? Predicting recurrent instability following a first traumatic anterior shoulder dislocation. BMJ Open Sport Exerc Med. 2019;5:e000447.

67. Olds MK, Lemaster N, Picha K, Walker C, Heebner N, Uhl TL. Line hops and side hold rotation tests load both anterior and posterior shoulder: a biomechanical study. Int J Sports Phys Ther. 2021;16:477-487.

68. Owens BD, Duffey ML, Nelson BJ, DeBerardino TM, Taylor DC, Mountcastle SB. The incidence and characteristics of shoulder instability at the United States Military Academy. Am J Sports Med. 2007;35:1168-1173.

69. Pastor MF, Averbeck AK, Welke B, Smith T, Claassen L, Wellmann M. The biomechanical influence of the deltotrapezoid fascia on horizontal and vertical acromioclavicular joint stability. Arch Orthop Trauma Surg. 2016;136:513-519.

70. Paterson WH, Throckmorton TW, Koester M, Azar FM, Kuhn JE. Position and duration of immobilization after primary anterior shoulder dislocation: a systematic review and meta-analysis of the literature. J Bone Joint Surg Am. 2010;92:2924-2933.

71. Paul J, Buchmann S, Beitzel K, Solovyova O, Imhoff AB. Posterior shoulder dislocation: systematic review and treatment algorithm. Arthroscopy. 2011;27:1562-1572.

72. Pizzari T, Wickham J, Balster S, Ganderton C, Watson L. Modifying a shrug exercise can facilitate the upward rotator muscles of the scapula. Clin Biomech. 2014;29:201-205.

73. Pollock RG, Bigliani LU. Recurrent posterior shoulder instability. Diagnosis and treatment. Clin Orthop Relat Res. 1993;291:85-96.

74. Reed D, Cathers I, Halaki M, Ginn KA. Does changing the plane of abduction influence shoulder muscle recruitment patterns in healthy individuals? Man Ther. 2016;21:63-68.

75. Reinold MM, Macrina LC, Wilk KE, et al. Electromyographic analysis of the supraspinatus and deltoid muscles during 3 common rehabilitation exercises. J Athl Train. 2007;42:464-469.

76. Reinold MM, Wilk KE, Fleisig GS, et al. Electromyographic analysis of the rotator cuff and deltoid musculature during common shoulder external rotation exercises. J Orthop Sports Phys Ther. 2004;34:385-394.

77. Richardson E, Lewis JS, Gibson J, et al. Role of the kinetic chain in shoulder rehabilitation: does incorporating the trunk and lower limb into shoulder exercise regimes influence shoulder muscle recruitment patterns? Systematic review of electromyography studies. BMJ Open Sport Exerc Med. 2020;6:e000683.

78. Rio E, Kidgell D, Moseley GL, et al. Tendon neuroplastic training: changing the way we think about tendon rehabilitation: a narrative review. Br J Sports Med. 2016;50:209-215.

79. Robinson CM, Dobson RJ. Anterior instability of the shoulder after trauma. The Journal of Bone and Joint Surgery. 2004;86-B:469-479.

80. Rockwood CA, Jr., Odor JM. Spontaneous atraumatic anterior subluxation of the sternoclavicular joint. The Journal of Bone and Joint Surgery. 1989;71:1280-1288.

81. Rosso C, Martetschlager F, Saccomanno MF, et al. High degree of consensus achieved regarding diagnosis and treatment of acromioclavicular joint instability among ESA-ESSKA members. Knee Surg Sports Traumatol Arthrosc. 2020;29:2325-2332.

82. Rouleau DM, Hebert-Davies J, Robinson CM. Acute traumatic posterior shoulder dislocation. J Am Acad Orthop Surg. 2014;22:145-152.

83. Sawyer EE, McDevitt AW, Louw A, Puentedura EJ, Mintken PE. Use of pain neuroscience education, tactile discrimination, and graded motor imagery in an individual with frozen shoulder. J Orthop Sports Phys Ther. 2018;48:174-184.

84. Seitz AL, Podlecki LA, Melton ER, Uhl TL. Neuromuscular adaptions following a daily strengthening exercise in individuals with rotator cuff related shoulder pain: a pilot case-control study. Int J Sports Phys Ther. 2019;14:74-87.

85. Sewell MD, Al-Hadithy N, Le Leu A, Lambert SM. Instability of the sternoclavicular joint: current concepts in classification, treatment and outcomes. Bone Joint J. 2013;95-B:721-731.

86. Shah A, Judge A, Delmestri A, et al. Incidence of shoulder dislocations in the UK, 1995-2015: a population-based cohort study. BMJ Open. 2017;7:e016112.

87. Sinha A, Higginson DW, Vickers A. Use of botulinum A toxin in irreducible shoulder dislocation caused by spasm of pectoralis major. Journal of Shoulder and Elbow Surgery. 1999;8:75-76.

88. Smith-Forbes EV, Howell DM, Willoughby J, Armstrong H, Pitts DG, Uhl TL. Adherence of individuals in upper extremity rehabilitation: a qualitative study. Arch Phys Med Rehabil. 2016;97:1262-1268.

89. Song DJ, Cook JB, Krul KP, et al. High frequency of posterior and combined shoulder instability in young active patients. J Shoulder Elbow Surg. 2015;24:186-190.

90. Stewart M, Loftus S. Sticks and stones: the impact of language in musculoskeletal rehabilitation. J Orthop Sports Phys Ther. 2018;48:519-522.

91. Suprak DN, Osternig LR, van Donkelaar P, Karduna AR. Shoulder joint position sense improves with elevation angle in a novel, unconstrained task. J Orthop Res. 2006;24:559-568.

92. Szyluk K, Jasinski A, Niemiec P, Mielnik M, Koczy B. Five-year prevalence of recurrent shoulder dislocation in the entire Polish population. Int Orthop. 2018;42:259-264.

93. Tjong VK, Devitt BM, Murnaghan ML, Ogilvie-Harris DJ, Theodoropoulos JS. A qualitative investigation of return to sport after arthroscopic Bankart repair: beyond stability. Am J Sports Med. 2015;43:2005-2011.

94. Tokish JM, Kozlowski EJ, Huxel Bliven K. Rehabilitation: Return-to-Play and In-Season Guidelines. Elsevier Inc.; 2016.

95. Tokish JM, Kuhn JE, Ayers GD, et al. Decision making in treatment after a first-time anterior glenohumeral dislocation: a Delphi approach by the Neer Circle of the American Shoulder and Elbow Surgeons. J Shoulder Elbow Surg. 2020;29:2429-2445.

96. Tokish JM, Thigpen CA, Kissenberth MJ, et al. The Nonoperative Instability Severity Index Score (NISIS): a simple tool to guide operative versus nonoperative treatment of the unstable shoulder. Sports Health. 2020;12:598-602.

97. Torrance E, Clarke CJ, Monga P, Funk L, Walton MJ. Recurrence after arthroscopic labral repair for traumatic anterior instability in adolescent rugby and contact athletes. Am J Sports Med. 2018;46:2969-2974.

98. Tunnicliffe H, Armstrong AL. The management of chronic anterior sternoclavicular joint instability. Abstracts for the 26th Annual Scientific Meeting, BESS 24–26. Shoulder Elbow. 2015;7:309-332.

99. Tzeng CY, Chiang HY, Huang CC, Lin WS, Hsiao TH, Lin CH. The impact of pre-existing shoulder diseases and traumatic injuries of the shoulder on adhesive capsulitis in adult population: a population-based nested case-control study. Medicine. 2019;98:e17204.

100. van Lankveld W, van Melick N, Habets B, Roelofsen E, Staal JB, van Cingel R. Measuring individual hierarchy of anxiety invoking sports related activities: development and validation of the Photographic Series of Sports Activities for Anterior Cruciate Ligament Reconstruction (PHOSA-ACLR). BMC Musculoskelet Disord. 2017;18:287.

101. Warby SA, Ford JJ, Hahne AJ, et al. Comparison of 2 exercise rehabilitation programs for multidirectional instability of the glenohumeral joint: a randomized controlled trial. Am J Sports Med. 2018;46:87-97.

102. Warby SA, Pizzari T, Ford JJ, Hahne AJ, Watson L. The effect of exercise-based management for multidirectional instability of the glenohumeral joint: a systematic review. J Shoulder Elbow Surg. 2014;23:128-142.

103. Warby SA, Pizzari T, Ford JJ, Hahne AJ, Watson L. Exercise-based management versus surgery for multidirectional instability of the glenohumeral joint: a systematic review. Br J Sports Med. 2016;50:1115-1123.

104. Warner JJP, Micheli LJ, Arslanian LE, Kennedy J, Kennedy R. Scapulothoracic motion in normal shoulders and shoulders with glenohumeral instability and impingement syndrome: a study using Moire topographic analysis. Clin Orthop Relat Res.1992;285:191-9.

105. Wasserstein DN, Sheth U, Colbenson K, et al. The true recurrence rate and factors predicting recurrent instability after nonsurgical management of traumatic primary anterior shoulder dislocation: a systematic review. Arthroscopy. 2016;32:2616-2625.

106. Watson L, Balster S, Lenssen R, Hoy G, Pizzari T. The effects of a conservative rehabilitation program for multidirectional instability of the shoulder. J Shoulder Elbow Surg. 2018;27:104-111.

107. Watson L, Balster S, Warby SA, Sadi J, Hoy G, Pizzari T. A comprehensive rehabilitation program for posterior instability of the shoulder. J Hand Ther. 2017;30:182-192.

108. Whelan DB, Kletke SN, Schemitsch G, Chahal J. Immobilization in external rotation versus internal rotation after primary anterior shoulder dislocation: a meta-analysis of randomized controlled trials. Am J Sports Med. 2016;44:521-532.

109. Wilk KE, Macrina LC. Nonoperative and postoperative rehabilitation for glenohumeral instability. Clin Sports Med. 2013;32:865-914.

110. Wilk KE, Yenchak AJ, Arrigo CA, Andrews JR. The Advanced Throwers Ten Exercise Program: a new exercise series for enhanced dynamic shoulder control in the overhead throwing athlete. Phys Sportsmed. 2011;39:90-97.

111. Woodmass JM, Lee J, Johnson NR, et al. Nonoperative management of posterior shoulder instability: an assessment of survival and predictors for conversion to surgery at 1 to 10 years after diagnosis. Arthroscopy. 2019;35:1964-1970.

112. Yang J, Schaefer JT, Zhang N, Covassin T, Ding K, Heiden E. Social support from the athletic trainer and symptoms of depression and anxiety at return to play. J Athl Train. 2014;49:773-779.

113. Youdas JW, Budach BD, Ellerbusch JV, Stucky CM, Wait KR, Hollman JH. Comparison of muscle-activation patterns during the conventional push-up and perfect push-up exercises. J Strength Cond Res. 2010;24:3352-3362.

Rehabilitation of throwing-related shoulder injuries

Lonnie Soloff, Martin Asker, Rod Whiteley

Throwing-related shoulder injuries are different

The aim of this chapter is to guide you through the assessment and management of the most commonly encountered throwing-related shoulder injuries. We aim to cover the 20% of conditions that at least 80% of the people that attend your clinic seeking care will present with. Figure 38.1 details the top 10 reported shoulder injuries from the United States Major League Baseball's (MLB) medical database for the 5 years up to the end of the 2019 season. We have included all categories of injuries, and the "time loss only" injuries that cause players to miss training sessions or competitions. This information is important to understand when managing athletes with these conditions but, as clinicians, the focus should be on early detection and intervention to avoid lost time. The second issue is that arriving at a tissue-specific diagnosis for any given shoulder presentation is difficult – the category "pain in shoulder" (Figures 38.2 and 38.3) represents a substantial number of players – reflecting the difficulty in deriving a diagnosis even for those working at the highest level.

Arriving at a tissue-specific diagnosis for shoulder pathology in throwing athletes is not straightforward, and our chapter will focus more on signs and symptoms than discrete pathologies. Each section is presented with a hypothesized diagnosis, based on the patient interview and relevant follow-up questions, physical examination, and clinical reasoning. We have included a synthesis of the current literature pertaining to current understanding of the pathology, and the associated burden on players.

The final section covers suggestions for management, broadly split into phases representing immediate care, return to sport, and an intermediate phase between these. This is not provided as a prescription, but as a foundation to support your clinical reasoning when you provide value-based care centered on the individual's preferences, expectations, and requirements. Some sections apply to all presentations and will therefore only be described in detail at first mention to avoid duplication.

After you have a solid understanding of these presentations, it becomes easier to identify those that do not fit these patterns. This is when the clinician sets to work as a detective, proposing, and refuting or confirming hypotheses as details emerge, and reaching out to colleagues for advice and guidance as required. That is how it has worked for us over the last 30 years in working with athletes, who have been our greatest teachers, and each of us expects to keep learning from our patients in this way.

Internal impingement

Patient presentation

- *"I'm getting this sharp pain inside my shoulder, and I am losing velocity."*
- *"It feels inside at the top here."*
- *"It's at the top at the back."*
- *"It's worse I think in cocking phase."*
- *"It runs down here..."*
- *"It's been on and off for a while now, I can't really remember any particular thing kicking this off, but it's getting worse."*

What is our current understanding of the pathology and the tissues involved?

The undersurface of the posterosuperior rotator cuff (supraspinatus and the anterosuperior fibers of infraspinatus) are typically seen to be frayed and associated with injury to the superior glenoid labrum. It is suspected that this occurs during the late cocking phase of hard throwing, where the shoulder externally rotates while at 90° of abduction and, importantly, moves into horizontal abduction. In this position, it is believed that the undersurface of the posterosuperior rotator cuff folds inside the glenohumeral joint and is compressed between the glenoid labrum and the head of the humerus (Figure 38.4), which is amplified in the presence of a tight posterior capsule. Additionally, during the extremes of rotation, the long head of the biceps tendon, being trapped in the bicipital groove, is pulled from its attachment (which becomes the superior labrum). This combination of compression to the undersurface of

Top 10 MLB shoulder injuries (2015–2019)	Total injuries	Mean days missed	Median days missed
All complaints			
Impingement syndrome	271	30	4
Rotator cuff strain	253	35.6	6
Shoulder contusion	140	6.5	1
Long head of biceps tendinitis	116	30.5	1
Rotator cuff tendinopathy (supraspinatus)	114	37.9	3
Pain in shoulder	108	18.1	1
Acromioclavicular sprain	78	20.6	2
Bicipital tendinitis	65	18.5	1.5
Infraspinatus	29	34.8	4
Disorders of the bursae and tendons	28	16.9	1

Top 10 MLB shoulder injuries (2015–2019)	Total injuries	Mean days missed	Median days missed
Time loss only			
Impingement syndrome	165	54.3	19
Rotator cuff strain	164	48.9	17,5
Shoulder contusion	69	62.7	19
Long head of biceps tendinitis	60	13.9	3
Rotator cuff tendinopathy (supraspinatus)	55	36.2	13.5
Pain in shoulder	51	68.9	17
Acromioclavicular sprain	44	35.8	14
Bicipital tendinitis	33	36	25
Infraspinatus	19	53.6	12.5
Disorders of the bursae and tendons	14	7.6	2.5

FIGURE 38.1
Burden of time loss due to shoulder injuries in Major League Baseball, 2015–2019. Horizontal axis is the number of injuries, and the vertical axis is the mean days missed per injury. The relative size of the markers denotes the burden of these injuries (number of injuries multiplied by the average burden).

the rotator cuff during horizontal abduction, and tension placed through the labrum during late cocking and follow-through (external and internal rotation, respectively; Figure 38.5) appear to be the primary mechanisms at play for the injuries seen.

Injuries to the superior labrum, known as SLAP (superior labrum anterior to posterior) lesions, were first described by Andrews[4] and then Snyder et al.[101] in the United States, and independently by Walch et al.[110] in Europe. Snyder further sub-defined his original series of 27 subjects from a retrospective review of 700 arthroscopies into four subtypes. This classification system has been further refined (delineating three subtypes of type II SLAP lesions)[13] and extended to include an increased variation in SLAP lesion types such that there are now more than 10 types of SLAP lesion described,[75] not including subtypes. Clinically it's simpler to consider SLAP lesions by their essential manifestation: an incompetence of the articular fibrocartilaginous

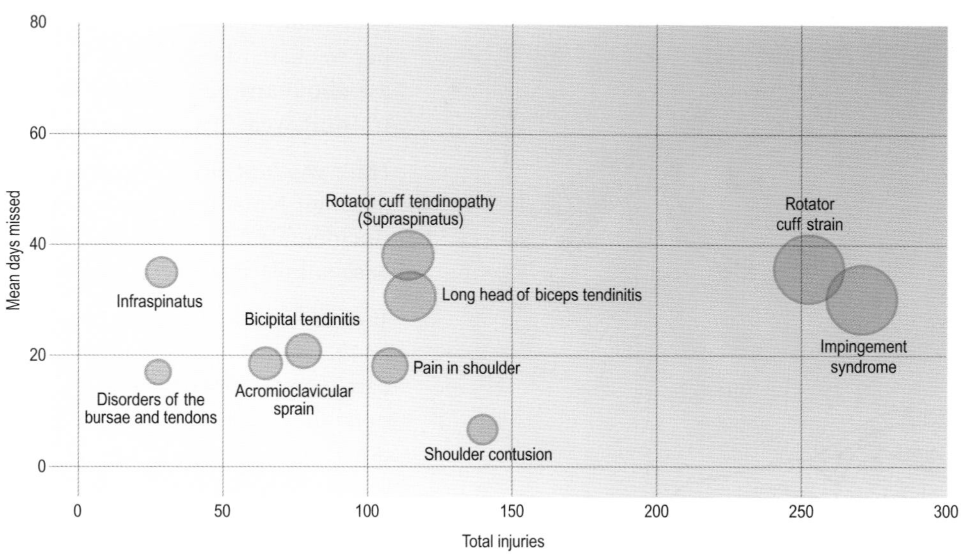

FIGURE 38.2

All complaints and time loss burden of shoulder injuries in Major League Baseball (MLB), 2015–2019. The data bars are proportional to the number of injuries and days lost (mean and median) for each category. Note that the injury burden data are heavily skewed as evidenced by the large differences in the median (typical) days lost compared with the mean values.

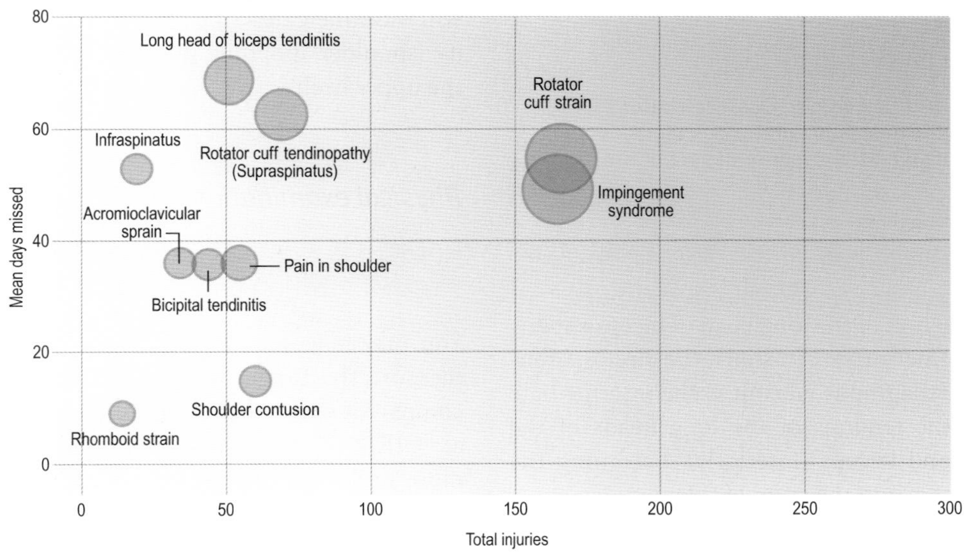

FIGURE 38.3

Burden of all shoulder complaints in Major League Baseball, 2015–2019. Horizontal axis is the number of injuries, and the vertical axis is the mean days missed per injury. The relative size of the markers denotes the burden of these injuries (number of injuries multiplied by the average burden). The bigger the circle the more frequently the condition is diagnosed.

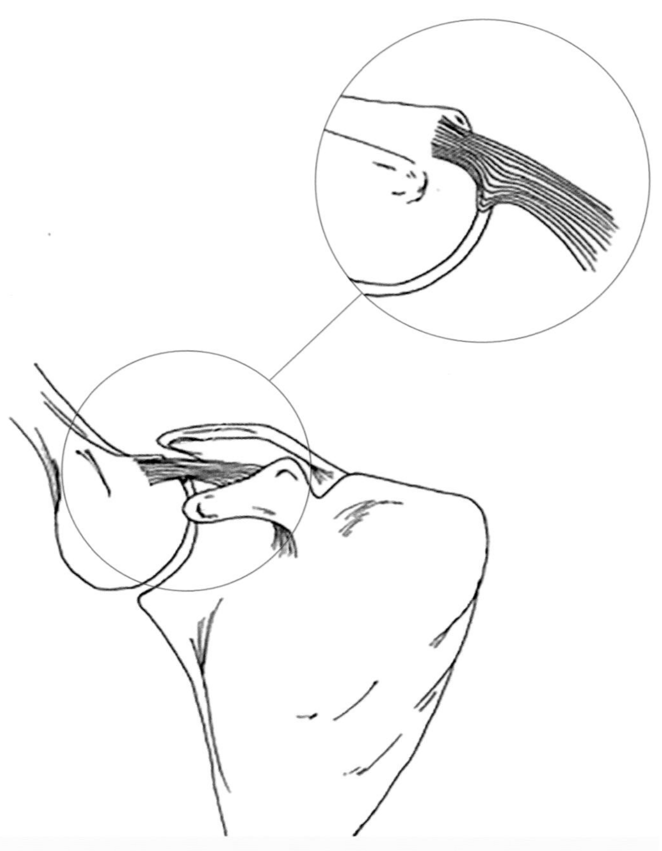

FIGURE 38.4
Depiction of internal impingement. During elevation, the greater tuberosity may impinge the articular side of the rotator cuff against the superior aspect of the glenoid rim.
(Reproduced with permission of Jeremy Lewis.)

extension of the insertion of the long head of biceps superiorly (and/or triceps inferiorly).[48] In short, the circumferentially placed fibrocartilaginous labrum is the intermediate structure between the tendons of the long heads of the biceps (superiorly) and triceps (inferiorly), becoming the insertion of these fibers into the scapula (glenoid).[48]

Additional questions

1. *Tell me about your normal throwing loads.* Throwing load history – pitch counts (in-game numbers of pitches thrown), bull pens (practice pitching sessions), learning a new pitch, try-outs/showcases. Specifically find out how many: throwing sessions per week, hard throws per week and per session, and ask about any new training regimens, weighted ball training, velocity development programs.
2. *Have you had any imaging and what were the findings?* Note importance of false-positive (incidental) findings[73] especially in professional baseball players.[18,63,74]
3. *What's been the response to any treatments/ medications so far?* Often your patient will have had care from others before seeing you. Establish the outcomes of previous treatments before embarking down similar paths.
4. *What's coming up – what do we need to get you ready for?* Establishing short-, mid-, and long-term performance goals are important to appropriately plan your entire rehabilitation course.

It is worth noting that often the athlete will describe a ”dead arm”. Those who more commonly deal with impact sports can mistakenly interpret this as a sign of frank shoulder instability (neurological dead arm), and it pays to clarify this with the athlete in some detail. Rarely, if ever, will the athlete describe signs or symptoms of true instability (shoulder ”popping out” or true neurological deficit in the upper limb).

Physical examination

Rotational range of motion: why glenohumeral internal rotation deficit (GIRD) is only half the story

You may have read that with throwers it is important to measure the range of passive shoulder internal rotation, compare it with the uninjured side, and document any loss as “GIRD”. There is an assumption that more GIRD means more problems, and restoration of flexibility is a priority. This is an oversimplification.

Half a century ago it was noted that professional throwing athletes commonly demonstrated an increase in passive shoulder external rotation range of motion on their throwing arm with a concomitant decrease in internal rotation range of motion.[59] It took another 30 years until

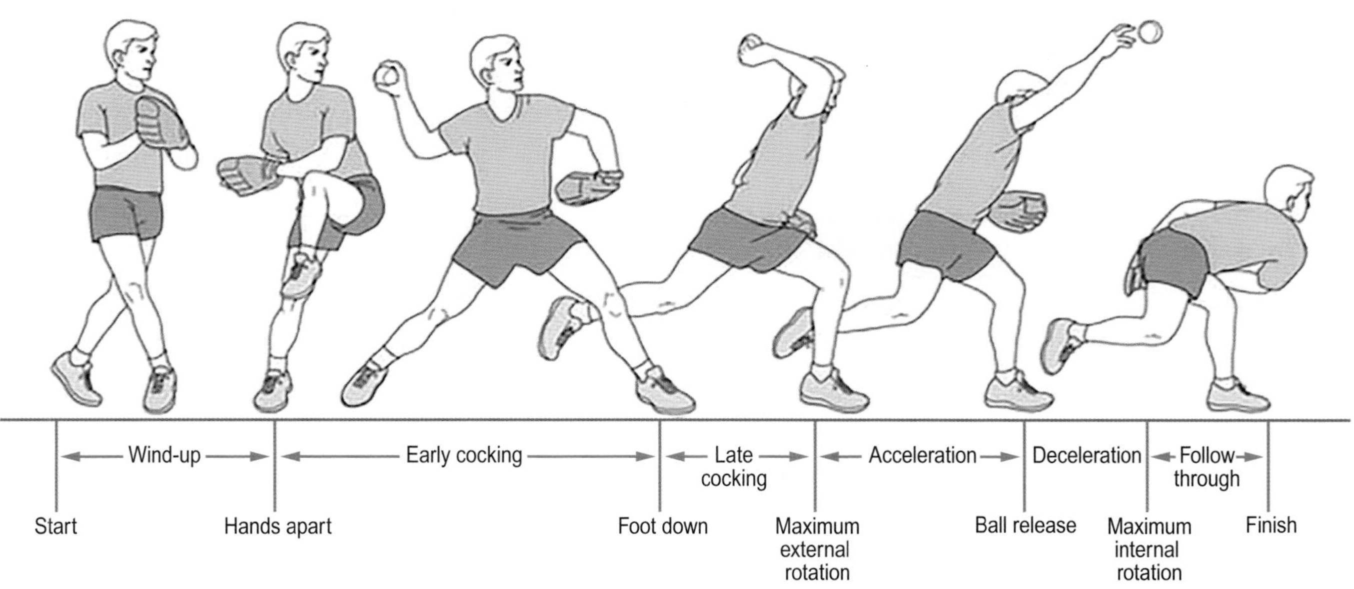

FIGURE 38.5
The stages of throwing.
(Reproduced with permission from Musculoskeletal Key. https://musculoskeletalkey.com/sports-medicine-5/)

the notion of "total arc of motion" (i.e., the sum of internal and external rotational range of motion, or the Total Rotational Range of Motion—TRROM[55,118]) became more widely reported and considered more relevant in the assessment of shoulder flexibility. Central to this notion is that TRROM provides additional information regarding the throwing athlete which cannot be gleaned from examining IR or ER range alone. Relatively recently, it was proposed that TRROM loss, in particular greater than 5°, was of clinical importance.[117]

Rotation along the long axis of the humerus is termed "humeral torsion". Increased humeral retrotorsion will lead to an increase in shoulder external rotation and a decrease in shoulder internal rotation by an equal amount, but there will be no change in their TRROM. Research on professional handball players in the late 1990s suggested that side-to-side differences in humeral torsion were both caused by throwing and related to throwing pathology.[89] In the years that followed, these data have been confirmed in different populations using different approaches[90,92,113,119] and it has been suggested that accurately interpreting rotational range of motion requires accounting for torsional differences between the arms of any given throwing athlete.[114]

The passive limits of shoulder rotational range of motion (ROM) are not determined by bony abutment, but by soft tissue extensibility. In the absence of injury or tissue changes, such as capsular contraction or laxity, both arms of any one person should be expected to have a similar amount of TRROM. Individual variability of course will mean that different people will have different TRROM, but both shoulders of one person should be the same, within the limits of measurement error, even though the starting and end points for the external and internal rotation might be different in both shoulders. In the athlete, the simple measurement of bilateral internal rotation ROM (the GIRD approach), does not account for humeral torsion, and will only be accurate in identifying the presence of soft tissue restrictions as the cause of the limited internal rotation on the rare occasion that an individual has bilaterally equal humeral torsion.

Clinically what is needed is to measure rotational range of motion as well as torsion on both sides (Figure 38.6).

Once the side-to-side difference in torsion is calculated, then it is a simple matter to make the "adjustments" for the torsion difference from the uninjured side to set the rotational range of motion targets for the injured side. The simplest and most accurate method available to measure torsion in the clinic is by using diagnostic ultrasound modified with the addition of a spirit level on the linear probe.[113] With the patient supine, and the shoulder abducted to 90° with the elbow flexed to 90°, the bicipital groove is placed uppermost, where the adjacent greater and lesser tubercles are of equal and maximum height. The inclination of the distal ulna is then measured as an indirect representation of the amount of humeral torsion.[113] Figure 38.7 details how humeral retroversion will influence glenohumeral joint rotation

Rotational strength

It's now well understood that shoulder rotation is the result of energy transfer from the lower limb and the activity of

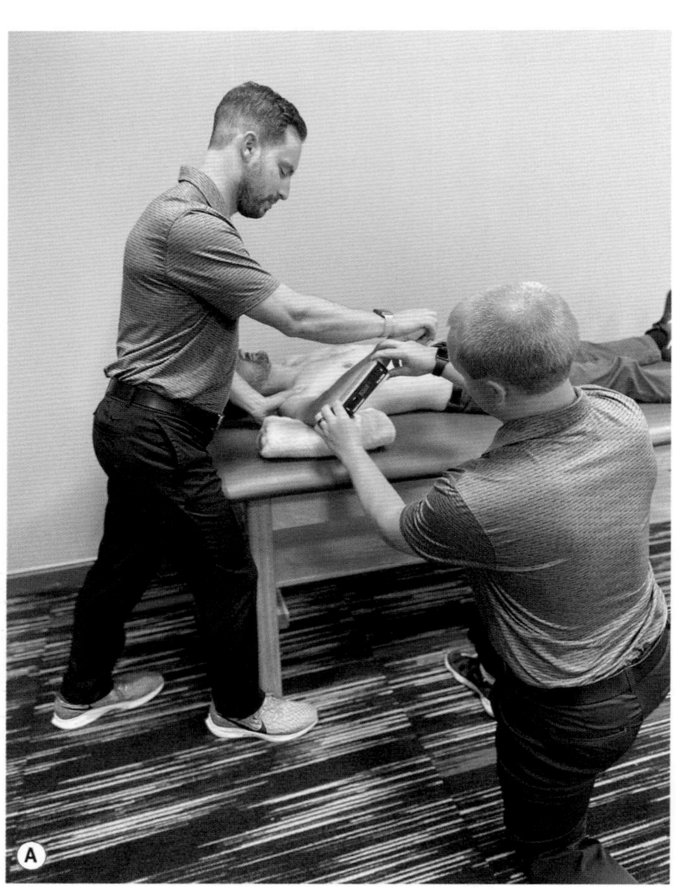

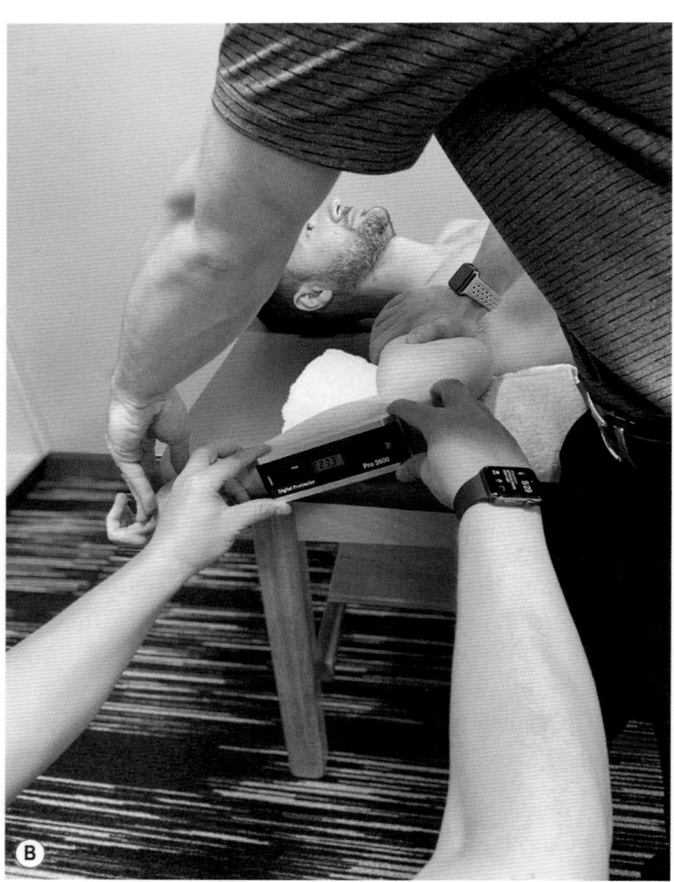

FIGURE 38.6AB
Internal and external rotational range of motion measurement with inclinometer. Key points here are stabilization of the scapula for internal rotation (during external rotation the scapula is stabilized against the chest wall) and ensuring the inclinometer is aligned with the distal ulna. With practice, this can be performed by a single clinician. For internal rotation, the end point will be the onset of movement of the scapula. Clinicians not used to dealing with throwing athletes are often surprised by the (large) range of external rotation and may stop the test early. Example instruction cues: "I'm just going to see how far back your arm rotates. You tell me when you think it's gone far enough – you shouldn't feel any pain on this, just a strong stretch, tell me when you think you're at the limit."

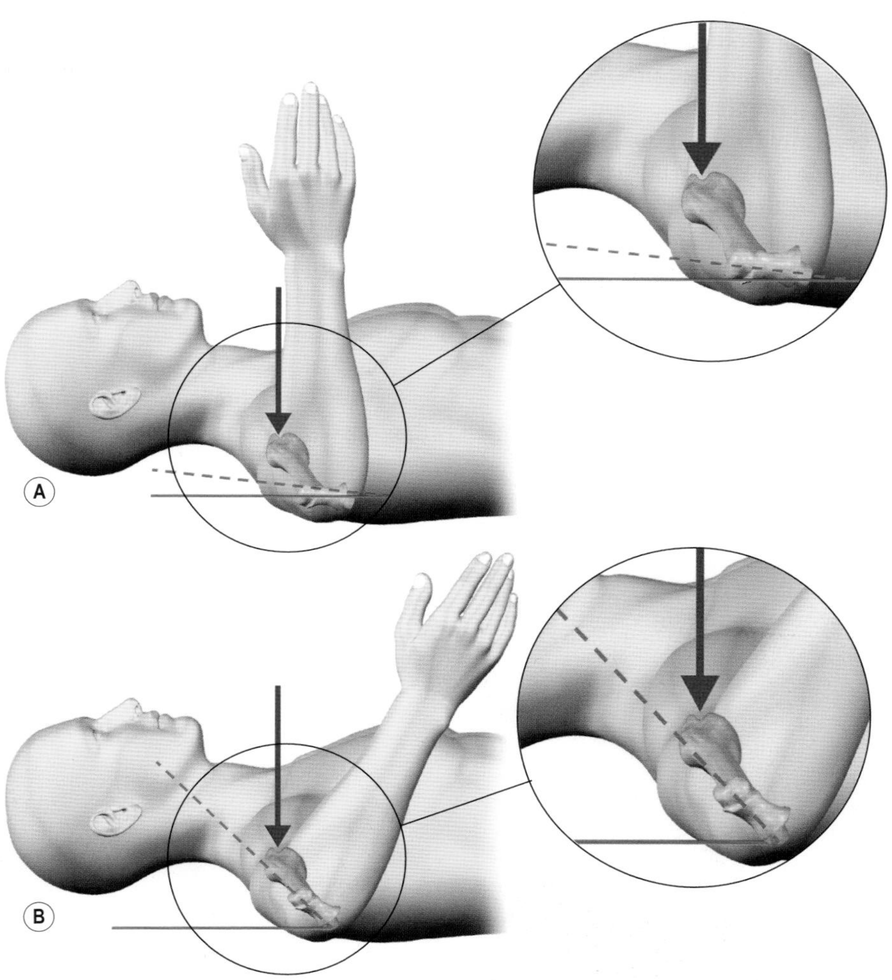

FIGURE 38.7

The influence of humeral torsion on glenohumeral rotation. In these two subjects, the position of the glenohumeral joint has been standardized by positioning the bicipital groove uppermost (arrows). This can be achieved more accurately using diagnostic ultrasound. By virtue of a 20° increase in humeral retrotorsion (occurring along the shaft of the humerus), (B) shows a shift in shoulder rotation of 20°. This individual would therefore show 20° more external rotation and 20° less internal rotation.

the rotator cuff, peri-scapular, and axio-scapular muscles, and that we are unable to isolate single muscles with any particular test or exercises.[11] That said, there is still value in assessing the rotational strength of throwing athletes, which then allows for planning of rehabilitation targets (based on the assessment findings). Where available, isokinetic testing is considered the gold standard method of testing, however there is no agreed testing position, speed, mode of contraction, or number of repetitions which should be performed.[115]

Hand-held dynamometry is more practical in a clinical setting.[25] Importantly, the values you will achieve when testing strength with a hand-held dynamometer vary significantly depending on the method of testing you use, as well as your experience in performing these tests. Careful attention is required for accurate and repeatable results. We prefer testing in standing, with the arm by the side, performing a purely rotational "break" test (i.e., a shallow eccentric contraction – about 5 cm (2 in) only – after a 2-second buildup of isometric force), with the dynamometer aligned to the ulnar styloid process, perpendicular to the forearm (Figures 38.8 and 38.9). In the absence of pre-injury reference values for the athlete, as a rough guide shoulder internal rotation strength is typically between 20% and 30% of bodyweight, and external rotation strength is two-thirds of internal rotation strength. For example, an 80 kg (176 lb) athlete would be predicted to have about 16–24 kg (35–53 lb) of internal rotation strength, and about 11–16 kg (24–35 lb) of external rotation strength. Alternatively, the uninjured arm can be used as a reference, however, for throwers, the dominant arm is typically at least 10%, and possibly as much as 40% stronger than the non-throwing arm.

Special tests: labrum

The glenoid labrum is largely devoid of innervation with relatively few nerve fibers located sparsely in its periphery,[108] so there is a poor correlation between identified structural abnormalities and pain in athletes with labral injury. Accordingly, our ability to clinically diagnose these problems based on pain responses to provocative testing is similarly hampered, as placing stress on apparently damaged tissue during examination may be entirely pain-free. This is reflected in the very high rates of positive imaging findings for labral injury in otherwise healthy baseball players,[18,63,73,74] and the poor agreement between clinical and diagnostic imaging studies for shoulder pain.[24,38,44,51]

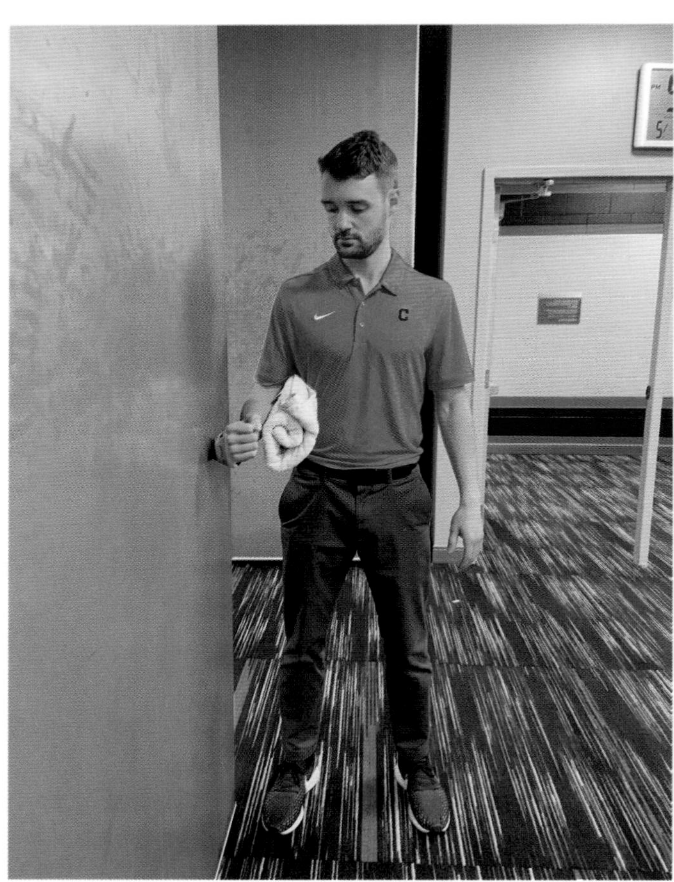

FIGURE 38.8
Isometric external rotational strength testing with handheld dynamometer.

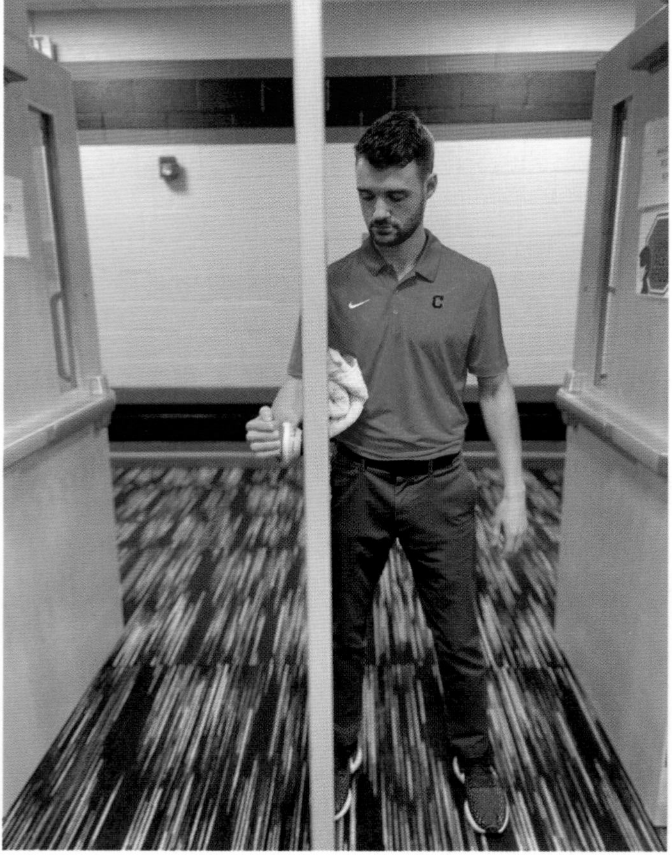

FIGURE 38.9
Isometric internal rotational strength testing with handheld dynamometer.

In clinical practice there are many variations of the same named labral test, which has arisen due to different interpretations of the original test, as well as variability in clinical training and experience. Unfortunately, this variability also occurs in research where replication studies fail to perform the test as originally described. Despite relatively poor diagnostic accuracy of these examination techniques, those that are clinically positive for a given athlete may be useful reassessment signs during rehabilitation, and assist in decision-making for rehabilitation progression. Where an athlete presents with the history as described above, we suggest that the clinical examination and use of special tests are of secondary importance in diagnosis due to these limitations.

With these strong caveats in mind, we suggest a battery of tests might be conducted to aid clinical decision-making. For reference, we present these tests, along with their original descriptions, study populations, and likelihood ratios[2] in Table 38.1. The interested reader is directed elsewhere for verification studies (e.g., references 19, 23, 41, 58, 70, 76, 78, 79, 82, 84-86, 102, 104, 111) where we suggest careful comparison of the methods used including reference populations and test technique.

What are the expected outcomes of treatment?

Nonsurgical care

Currently, a trial of nonsurgical care is the recommended first option for all players, and players should be reassured that 50% to 75% will return to pre-injury levels. Younger players (<26 years of age) who have had problems for less time (<12 months) have a better prognosis, but pitchers have a worse prognosis than position players.[43] Worse prognosis is also associated with those who experience flare-up(s) in symptoms during rehabilitation. Typically, nonsurgical care, when successful, results in a faster return to play time of six months compared with return to play after surgery at approximately 12 months.

Surgical care

Pitchers who do progress to SLAP surgery should expect at least a year of rehabilitation before they will return to play, and unfortunately those that progress to surgery frequently have a poor prognosis with documented success rates varying from 7% to 62%.[12,15,17,22,31,33,36,49,52,96,100] Evidence exists that people (average age 40 years) with an isolated type II SLAP injury, who undertake SLAP repair or biceps tenodesis fare no better than those assigned sham surgery,[98] however, no such data are currently available for overhead athletes.

For the rotator cuff tendons, surgical debridement is performed far more commonly (86%) than repair[26] although these procedures are often performed together (i.e., cuff repair and partial debridement).[26,69] Unfortunately, only half who underwent debridement returned to play, only 42% of those at the same level, with the outcomes for repair worse at one-third returning to play, and only 14% at the same level,[26] with similar results from different cohorts.[1,64,87] These sobering findings need to be considered alongside current understanding that partial-thickness articular sided rotator cuff tears are not always associated with pain, and while the tear may progress over subsequent seasons, these tears are not associated with pain or strength changes.[72]

Management

Early

Successful rehabilitation requires patient engagement, and this will be difficult if the questions "What's wrong with me?", "What's going to happen?", and "What can I do about it?", are not answered.[35] It is important to explain imaging reports of "pathology" in the context of normal adaptation to throwing and aging, as emphasized in the original description of SLAP lesions by Andrews.[4] To reduce anxiety and fear avoidance behaviors, it is important to discuss the body's capacity to heal and return to high level function, as well as adapt even in the presence of tissue changes that are in the main age- and/or activity-related.

There is no one, perfect, ideal, or correct explanation strategy that will work for every athlete, but it's suggested that some form of "teach-back" at the end of the initial examination is useful in establishing the degree of understanding.[39] As a suggestion, simply asking the athlete: "When you get home, what will you tell your friends/family/team-mates is wrong, what needs to be done, and what's going to happen?" (see Chapter 11). This will facilitate further explanation if required that will help with engagement and therefore compliance with care. Although nonsurgical care is the first-line treatment for most throwing-related

Table 38.1 Labral tests: original description, likelihood ratios, and study populations

Test name	Description from original paper	Labral injury (No labral injury)	+LR (-LR)	Study population and notes
O'Brien's Active Compression[81]	Patient asked to forward flex the affected arm 90° with the elbow in full extension. The patient then adducted the arm 10° to 15° medial to the sagittal plane of the body. The arm was internally rotated so that the thumb pointed downward. The examiner then applied a uniform downward force to the arm. With the arm in the same position, the palm was then fully supinated, and the maneuver was repeated. The test was considered positive if pain was elicited with the first maneuver and was reduced or eliminated with the second maneuver. Pain localized to the acromioclavicular joint or on top of the shoulder was diagnostic of acromioclavicular joint abnormality. Pain or painful clicking described as inside the glenohumeral joint itself was indicative of labral abnormality.	53 (203)	∞ (0.02)	318 consecutive patients at the Hospital for Special Surgery New York; 50 with no shoulder pain, 50 subsequently excluded for "incorrect testing". Note: "...patient can distinguish between pain 'on top' of the shoulder (that is, at the acromioclavicular joint) and pain 'deep inside' the shoulder joint with or without a click"
Crank[65]	Performed with the patient in the upright position with the arm elevated to 160° in the scapular plane. Joint load is applied along the axis of the humerus with one hand while the other performs humeral rotation. A positive test is determined either by: 1) pain during the maneuver (usually during external rotation) with or without a click or 2) reproduction of the symptoms, usually pain or catching felt by the patient during athletic or work activities. This test should be repeated in the supine position, where the patient is usually more relaxed.	32 (30)	13.5 (0.1)	62 patients (40 male) UCLA Orthopaedic Surgery Dept.; average age 28 years (18 to 57), 50 recreational athletes (12 non-athletes), >3 months of activity-related shoulder pain that increases with overhead motions, no cuff tear or instability, failure of pain relief with conservative management despite improvements with progressive strengthening and good compliance over a 3-month period. Patients with histories and physical examinations evident of rotator cuff abnormalities significant enough to cause weakness in scapular abduction, external rotation, or subscapularis muscle lift-off were also excluded.
Biceps load II[57]	Patient in the supine position. The examiner sits adjacent to the patient on the same side as the shoulder and grasps the patient's wrist and elbow gently. The arm to be examined is elevated to 120° and externally rotated to its maximal point, with the elbow in 90° flexion and the forearm in the supinated position. The patient is asked to flex the elbow while resisting the elbow flexion by the examiner. The test is considered positive if the patient complains of pain during the resisted elbow flexion and also considered positive if the patient complains of more pain from the resisted elbow flexion regardless of the degree of pain before the elbow flexion maneuver. The test is negative if pain is not elicited by the resisted elbow flexion or if the pre-existing pain during the elevation and external rotation of the arm is unchanged or diminished by the resisted elbow flexion.	39 (87)	26.0 (0.11)	127 consecutive patients (89 male) Department of Orthopaedic Surgery, Sungkyunkwan University School of Medicine, South Korea; average age 31 years (15 to 52), 36 recreational athletes experiencing shoulder pain, underwent arthroscopic examination during the surgery. Patients with a history of either a shoulder dislocation or a stiff shoulder were excluded from the study. Two independent examiners with no knowledge of the results of the other clinical, radiographic, and magnetic resonance imaging data were assigned to perform the new diagnostic test. The results of the tests were confirmed during the arthroscopic examination
Resisted supination external rotation[76]	Supine position on the examination table with the scapula near the edge of the table. The examiner stood at the patient's side, supporting the affected arm at the elbow and hand. The limb was placed in the starting position with the shoulder abducted to 90°, the elbow flexed 65° to 70°, and the forearm in neutral or slight pronation. The patient was asked to attempt to supinate the hand with maximal effort as the examiner resisted. The patient forcefully supinated the hand against resistance as the shoulder was gently externally rotated to the maximal point. He or she was asked to describe the symptoms at maximum external rotation. The test was positive if the patient had anterior or deep shoulder pain, clicking or catching in the shoulder, or reproduction of symptoms that occurred during throwing. The test was negative if the patient had posterior shoulder pain, apprehension, or no pain elicited.	29 (11)	4.6 (0.2)	40 athletes (39 males), Atlanta Sports Medicine and Orthopaedic Center; 4 recreational, 7 high school, 16 collegiate, 13 professional, average age 24 years (17 to 50). Patients older than 50 years, those with shoulder pain that was not the result of athletic injury, and those who did not undergo arthroscopic evaluation were excluded. Results of these tests were correlated to findings from the arthroscopic examination by the senior author within 1 week of the clinical examination. The senior author was blinded to the results of the clinical examinations until after the arthroscopy.

(Continued)

Table 38.1 *(Continued)*

Test name	Description from original paper	Labral injury (No labral injury)	+LR (-LR)	Study population and notes
Anterior slide[54]	Examined either standing or sitting, with their hands on the hips with thumbs pointing posteriorly. One of the examiner's hands is placed across the top of the shoulder from the posterior direction, with the last segment of the index finger extending over the anterior aspect of the acromion at the glenohumeral joint. The examiner's other hand is placed behind the elbow and a forward and slightly superiorly directed force is applied to the elbow and upper arm. The patient is asked to push back against this force. Pain localized to the front of the shoulder under the examiner's hand, and/or a pop or click in the same area, was considered to be a positive test. This test is also positive if the athlete reports a subjective feeling that this testing maneuver reproduces the symptoms that occur during overhead activity.	88 (138) [92]	8.3 (0.2) [5.5, 0.3]	226 patients in 5 groups (153 male) Lexington Clinic Sports Medicine Center; average age 25 years (16 to 38). First 4 groups were shoulder pathology (isolated throwing-related labral injury; cuff tears with & without labral injury; instability with & without labral injury; and reduced shoulder internal rotational range without symptoms or labral injury), 5th was asymptomatic football players. Sample size and likelihood ratios in [brackets] adjacent are recalculated removing this 5th group.
Dynamic labral shear[56]	Patient in a standing position, the involved arm is flexed 90° at the elbow, abducted in the scapular plane to above 120°, and externally rotated to tightness. It is then guided into maximal horizontal abduction. The examiner applies a shear load to the joint by maintaining external rotation and horizontal abduction and lowering the arm from 120° to 60° of abduction. A positive test is indicated by reproduction of the pain and/or a painful click or catch in the joint line along the posterior joint line between 120° and 90° of abduction.	48 (53) [42 type II]	31.6 (0.3)	325 consecutive patients (232 male, 43 years old ± 13 years) of whom 101 (59 male, 49 ± 15 years old) ultimately had surgical confirmation were seen at the Lexington Clinic Sports Medicine Center for "shoulder pain". For SLAP tears, the criteria included the 4-part Snyder classification,[101] the presence of a "peel back" lesion,[13] and/or chondral damage on the superior glenoid rim.[95] A degenerative appearance of the labrum was not included unless it met the other criteria.

∞, infinity; -LR, negative likelihood ratio; +LR, positive likelihood ratio; SLAP, superior labrum anterior to posterior; UCLA, University College Los Angeles.

shoulder problems, patients will see little short-term improvement initially, and a lot of hard work is required from them that does not always result in "success". Faced with this reality, it is reasonable that patients often "shop around" for better news, quick fixes, and miracle cures. The athlete's engagement with their rehabilitation, and therefore success, is directly proportional to the answers provided to the three questions asked at the start of this section. After a clear description of the problem is given to the player, modifiable factors which are associated with this condition can be addressed.

When to reappraise your approach

If your patient has improved their strength and rotational range, met their targets to return to throwing, yet despite careful progression has "broken down" with the same pain as before, at essentially the same throwing intensity and volume, a review is required. There are no clear rules which dictate when conservative care has irretrievably failed, and a surgical opinion becomes mandatory. We suggest that a minimum of 12 weeks' rehabilitation would first need to be conducted with meaningful improvements in the clinical targets achieved before considering alternatives. Similarly, if more than six months of rehabilitation have passed with perhaps three months of failing to improve in any objective markers, then a reassessment would be sensible.

Acceleration-related symptoms

Patient presentation

- *"I made this one throw and..."*
- *"Maybe it started with this one maximal effort throw, but since then..."*
- *"I am feeling the pain here, and I get this pain when..."*

What is our current understanding of the pathology and the tissues involved?

Epidemiologic data from MLB suggest that acceleration injuries are increasing in professional baseball players (Figure 38.10).

Acceleration-based injuries are challenging to diagnose on initial exam, and these injuries are also seen in water skiers and rock climbers (see Chapter 40). The muscle–tendon unit appears to be at its most vulnerable when it is forcefully and rapidly contracting eccentrically at maximum lengths. Hard throwing places the shoulder internal rotators under this stress during every throw, so it is not surprising that the muscle–tendon unit of any of these muscles are susceptible to a strain injury during the transition from late cocking phase to acceleration (Figure 38.11). There are few epidemiological data available for this class of injury, but it appears that tendon, intramuscular tendon, and muscle–tendon junction are all involved in this injury.

Latissimus dorsi and teres major are strong internal rotators of the shoulder and are most active during the late cocking and acceleration phases.[97] These muscles are crucial in transferring energy from the lower body and core to the arm and hand (ball), and likely a major determinant of throwing velocity. Of particular interest is that research has demonstrated that "skilled" throwers have much higher activity of the subscapularis and latissimus dorsi during the acceleration phase of throwing relative to amateur throwers.[29,53] The subscapularis is the largest and most powerful muscle of the rotator cuff,[66] with the greatest force-producing capability.[68,112]

Additional questions

1. *Have you had any imaging done?* Depending on the location of the athlete's symptoms, imaging of the latissimus dorsi, subscapularis, and teres major muscles is recommended as injuries to these structures may have been overlooked as possible sources of pain and dysfunction.[97] If imaging has been done, it is useful to ensure that these areas (latissimus dorsi and teres major) have been checked. These injuries have not been commonly recognized, and there is the chance that the reporting radiologist may not have been alerted to examine these structures.
2. *Did you notice any lump, redness, or bruising anywhere?* In latissimus dorsi and teres major injuries, the athlete typically presents with acute onset pain to the axilla and/or posterior shoulder, palpable defect based upon location and severity of injury, possibly ecchymosis (skin discoloration bruising caused by bleeding) and painfully limited elevation and passive external rotation.

Latissimus dorsi, teres major, and subscapularis events (2015–19)

Level of play	2015	2016	2017*	2018*	2019*
Minor	107	99	111	117	114
MLB	21	34	25	44	44
Total	**128**	**133**	**136**	**161**	**158**

Time loss only

Level of play	2015	2016	2017*	2018*	2019*
Minor	96	82	98	99	114
MLB	17	23	21	26	44
Total	**113**	**105**	**119**	**125**	**158**

FIGURE 38.10
Latissimus dorsi, teres major, and subscapularis injuries reported to the Major and Minor League Baseball (USA) injury registry, 2015–2019. Note the relatively stable incidence across Minor League Baseball but an increase at the Major League level for both time loss and medical attention injuries across the 5 years to the end of the 2019 season.

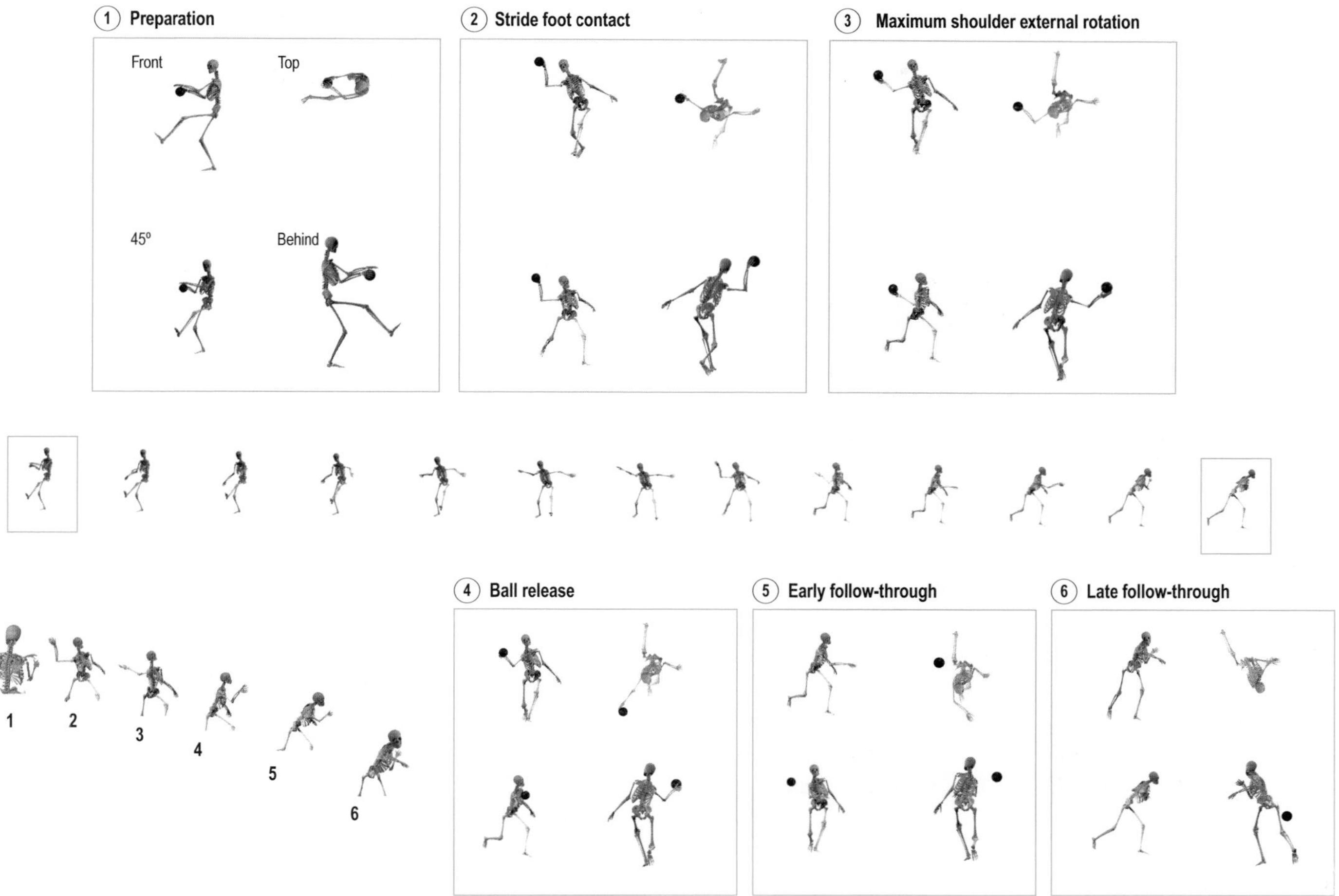

FIGURE 38.11

Depiction of the key events during the throwing motion. Note the shoulder position (abduction to ~100°, 10–30° horizontal adduction) at the point of maximum shoulder external rotation. Note also the initial rapid internal rotation range of motion after ball release occurring predominantly at the shoulder, followed by the trunk and lower body contribution. There is a great deal of between-athlete variability in trunk position, however, the shoulder and elbow kinematics are very similar across all throwers, and most overhead throwing and striking activities. We recommend examining passive ranges of motion and resisted strength testing in these positions instead of arbitrary "anatomic" positions, combined with clinical reasoning from the patient history as this can more clearly elucidate the source of symptoms.

Physical examination

Strength

Objective assessment of internal rotation strength and its concomitant association with symptom reproduction is key to diagnosis. We strongly suggest the use of at least a hand-held dynamometer to measure force production, and have found doing so in 90° of shoulder flexion with the elbow flexed to 90° and the forearm horizontal, palm facing down, a helpful test position (Figure 38.12). Additionally, the "bear hug"[9] (Box 38.1) is described as a method of assessing internal rotation strength manually (Figure 38.13), but may be modified to use an objective (dynamometer) strength measure.

Typically, these two strength tests will give sufficient information, however, you may consider assessing seated shoulder extension in an end or mid-range position, or seated shoulder adduction in end/mid-range where the previous two tests were negative.

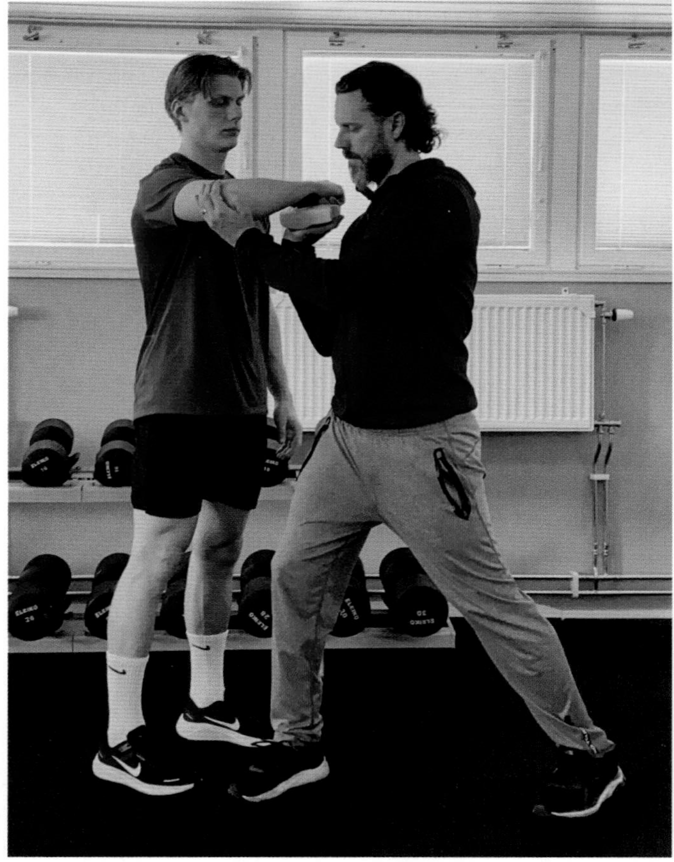

FIGURE 38.12
Internal rotational strength measured with hand-held dynamometer in crossbody position.

Box 38.1 The "bear hug"

The bear-hug test was performed with the palm of the involved side placed on the opposite shoulder and fingers extended (so that the patient could not resist by grabbing the shoulder) and the elbow positioned anterior to the body. The patient was then asked to hold that position (resisted internal rotation) as the physician tried to pull the patient's hand from the shoulder with an external rotation force applied perpendicular to the forearm. The test was considered positive if the patient could not hold the hand against the shoulder or if he or she showed weakness of resisted internal rotation of greater than 20% compared with the opposite side. If the strength was comparable to that of the opposite side, without any pain, the test was negative.[9]

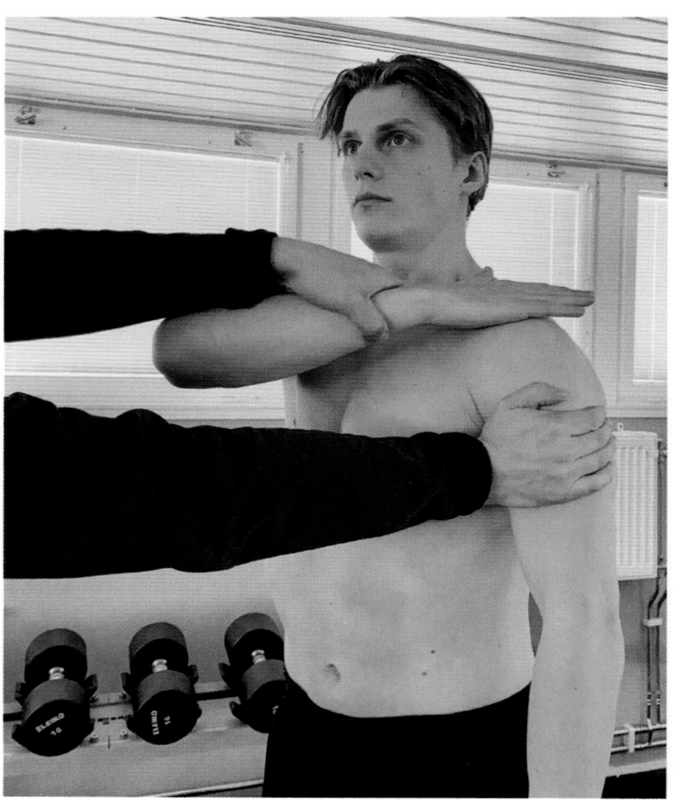

FIGURE 38.13
The "bear hug" test performed manually. Bear hug test at 45°: examiner with a hand on patient's wrist, as patient's elbow is held at 45° of forward flexion.[16]

Range of motion testing

Testing flexion, external rotation, abduction and horizontal abduction range of motion passively in supine will often reproduce the athlete's exact symptoms. Less passive external rotation range of motion in the throwing arm is associated with higher rates of subscapularis injury.[91]

Literature review

Latissimus dorsi/teres major

Eighty to ninety percent of athletes who have sustained latissimus dorsi and teres major injuries will return to previous performance level with nonsurgical care.[27,28,71,77,97] Higher grade (full-thickness and avulsion) injuries should be given surgical consideration. The largest reported series of professional pitchers[27] showed the majority (89%) to be treated nonsurgically, with performance metrics on return to play similar to those treated surgically. Time to return to play for nonsurgical care was variable at 170 days (±170 days), but shorter than following surgery, which was 537 days (±300 days).[27] These findings are similar to published data.[26,28,97]

Subscapularis

Return to play times range from 11 to 60 days for nonsurgical care; athletes with lower-grade subscapularis injuries anecdotally return to play faster, although there is a paucity of data.[91,103] Injuries to the musculotendinous junction of the lower half of the subscapularis appear more common. Greater shoulder external rotation range of motion appears protective, especially associated with humeral retrotorsion.[90,91]

Management

Early

Patient education

Acute shoulder muscle, muscle–tendon, and tendon injuries likely involve different healing pathways and timelines. There are no data for throwing athletes, but we speculate that appropriately identified purely contractile injuries would recover more quickly than muscle–tendon junction injury, which should be quicker than intramuscular tendon injury, and quicker again than free tendon injury. The athlete should be informed that tissue healing is required and will take time, but the quality of healing can be influenced with appropriate loading. Low-grade contractile-only injuries may be fully resolved in days, whereas full-thickness tendon injuries may require surgical intervention for complete resolution. Where there is clinical suspicion of higher-grade injury (marked reduction in strength, extremely high or low/absent pain) appropriate imaging and potentially surgical opinion is warranted. More commonly, nonsurgical care can be implemented immediately. Most throwers respond well to nonsurgical management, but complete recovery may take several weeks to as long as six months, depending on the sport and severity of injury.

Early, low loading of the injured (healing) tissue: latissimus dorsi/teres major

The function of the latissimus dorsi is complex,[50,62] and as with other two-joint muscles, active range of motion exercise can act as an appropriate method to initiate strengthening and optimize repair and remodeling during healing. To place low tensile loads through the healing tissue, active external rotation range of motion at 0° and 90° abduction can be commenced early. This can be followed by isometric internal rotation and extension exercises in varying ranges of motion, carefully balancing the applied load and increasing stretch on the injured tissue.

It is also appropriate to maintain external rotation strength at this time. External rotation can be safely loaded through "dynamic isometric" exercises such as the external rotation walkout, which does not run the risk of moving into unsafe external rotation ranges. This is also a good period to begin scapular motor control exercise in unweighted or isometric conditions. It is important to achieve end-range active flexion as well as internal rotation/adduction before progressing in to loaded exercise for the latissimus dorsi. Failure to do so can possibly put the athlete at greater risk of setback early in their return to sport progression. Light, perhaps isometric, painless, or very low level of transient pain for the injured tissue, coupled with heavy loading of all uninjured structures throughout the kinetic chain is indicated. Any identified weaknesses in the kinetic chain can now be addressed with heavy loading which is otherwise not possible in-season. Progress to the intermediate phase at return of nearly full passive and active range, and normal daily activities are pain-free.

Early, low loading of the injured (healing) tissue: subscapularis

Active range of motion is an important component of the early healing phases of rehabilitation for the subscapularis, and can be valuable to optimize remodeling. Isometric strengthening of the subscapularis as well as the surrounding rotator cuff can be performed at 0° of abduction. The external rotators can be put through "dynamic isometrics" (such as external rotation walkouts) provided the shoulder is not abducted during these activities (Figure 38.14). As the actions of the upper and lower fibers of subscapularis are slightly different,[93,116] identifying the affected

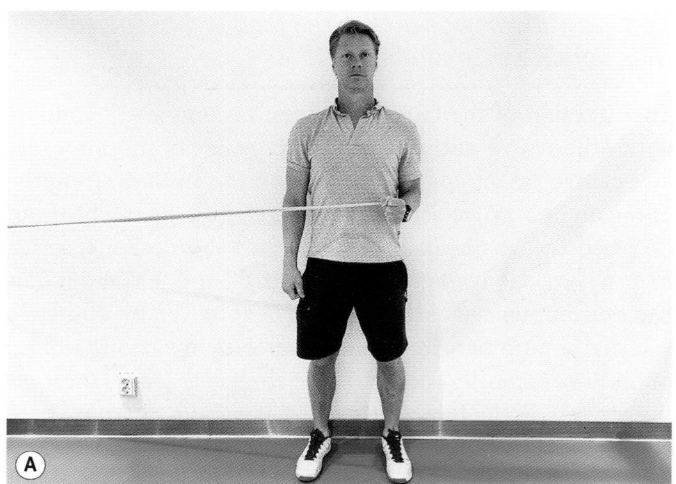

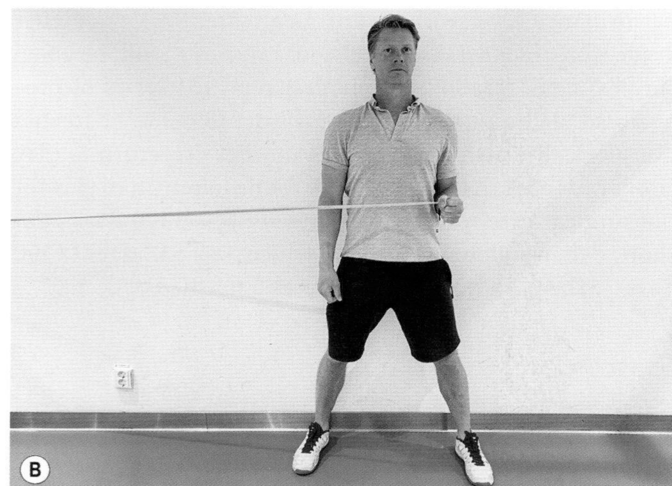

FIGURE 38.14AB
External rotation "walk-outs".

portion may aid the clinician in progressive loading of the appropriate tissue.

There are two commonly used isometrics for the subscapularis: the bear hug and belly press, both of which serve as diagnostic tools, may also be utilized as progressive isometric activity.[16,37] At this stage, it is also valuable to train scapular motor control with serratus anterior, middle and lower trapezius, using isometric or unweighted active range of motion, and maintain posterior shoulder flexibility, mobility, and strength. Loading the muscle inappropriately in the early phase may slow the recovery process, so ensuring full active range of motion in all planes and asymptomatic isometric strengthening before progression is key.

Intermediate

Latissimus dorsi/teres major

It is important to consider strength testing these athletes in positions of both maximal contraction (mid-range) of the muscle, as well as maximal length (outer range). We recommend a "lat pull-down" muscle test (Figure 38.15) and a "ball release" position isometric, both measured with handheld dynamometry. The latter of the two happens at cross-body adduction and internal rotation, a common position for injury to occur to these muscles (Figure 38.16). In our experience, this tends to provide a clearer indication of the athlete's muscle function before progressing towards return to sport. Exercises that progressively load the latissimus dorsi and surrounding musculature may then be initiated in this phase. Internal rotation-biased exercises are critical in the progressive overloading program. Although dosage changes, isometric exercises are used throughout the rehabilitation program.

Subscapularis

The isometrics used for the subscapularis, the bear hug and belly press, may be progressed to an exercise prescription that loads the tissue in a similar manner to that used for latissimus dorsi. For example, the loaded cross-body adduction, similar to the proprioceptive neuromuscular facilitation (PNF) diagonal pattern 2 (D2 Flexion),[109] mimics the position of the belly press and involves loaded internal rotation from an abducted/externally rotated position (Figure 38.17). The cross-body uppercut[10] mimics the bear hug isometric, and requires loading through another condition of internal rotation (Figure 38.18). As is the case with all shoulder rehabilitation, perturbation exercises should be included. This may be accomplished through a variety of means, with one suggestion to use kettlebell exercises in supine and standing.

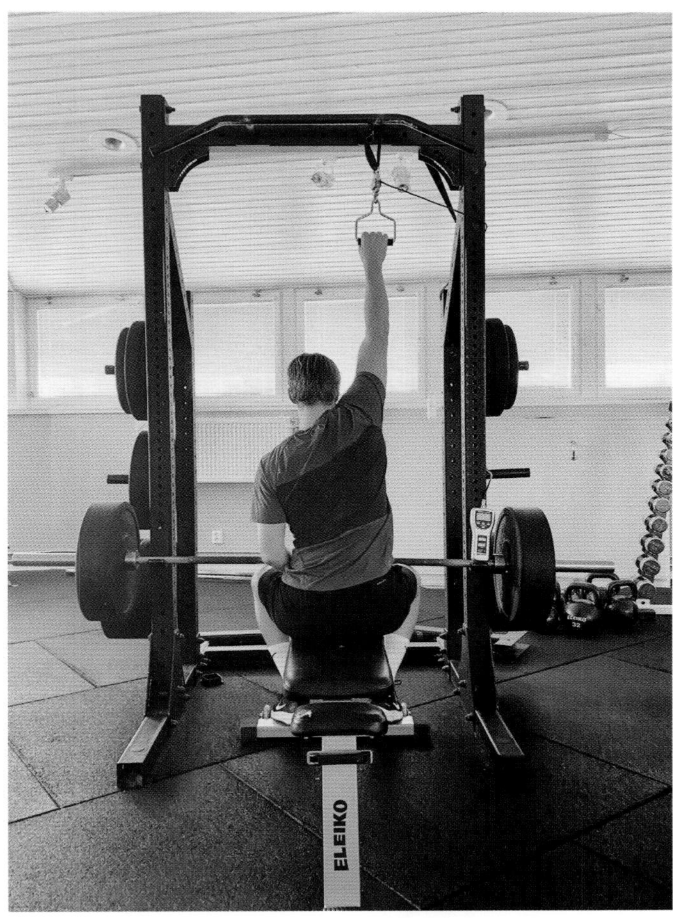

FIGURE 38.15
Lat pull-down strength test with handheld dynamometer.

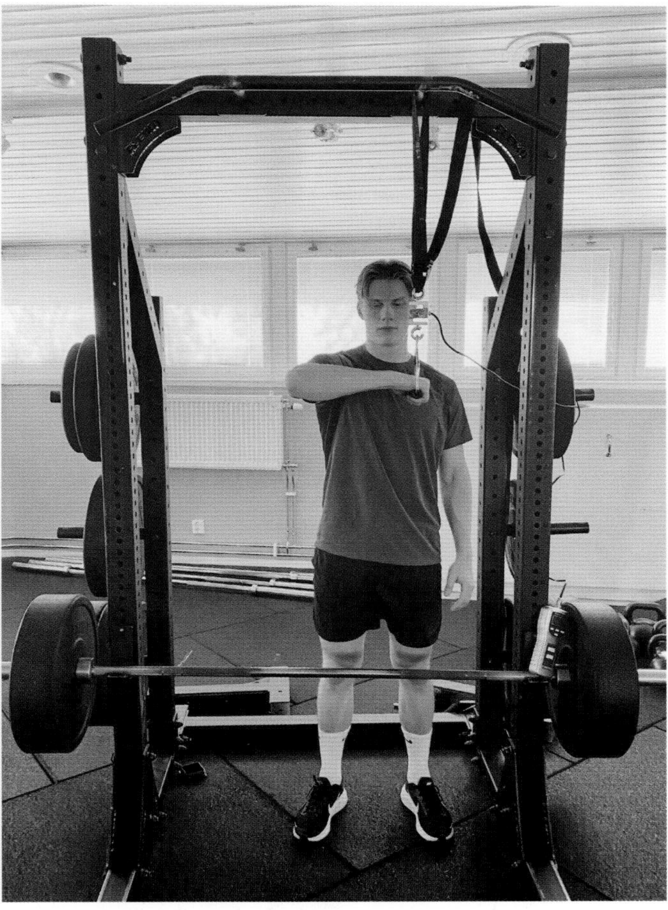

FIGURE 38.16
Strength measurement with a dynamometer in "ball release" position.

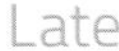

Late

Latissimus dorsi/teres major/subscapularis

The throwing motion involves a brief eccentric contraction followed by a concentric contraction. This "stretch-shortening" cycle[60,80] requires a pre-stretch activation of the prime-moving muscles, and after they are briefly eccentrically stretched, the subsequent concentric contraction generates higher force than an isolated concentric contraction is capable of. To progress carefully, it is advised to begin stretch-shortening exercises initially in mid-range, progressing to outer ranges, initially relatively slow, progressing to game speed. The brief stretch (eccentric contraction) prior to the main concentric part of the movement increases activation and more closely mimics the activity of the internal rotators during throwing.

Notes for latissimus dorsi/teres major nonsurgical rehabilitation

Addressing the dual functions of latissimus dorsi and teres major as shoulder adductors and extensors is an important clinical consideration. As such, ongoing objectively monitoring shoulder extension and adduction strength is important. Anecdotal evidence suggests these athletes also have deficits in external rotation and occasionally shoulder

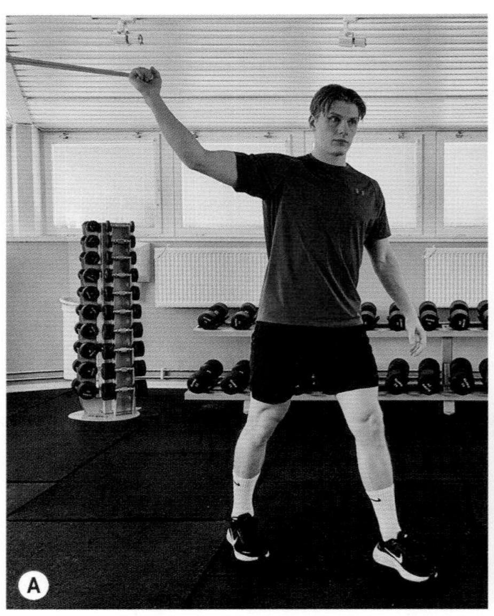
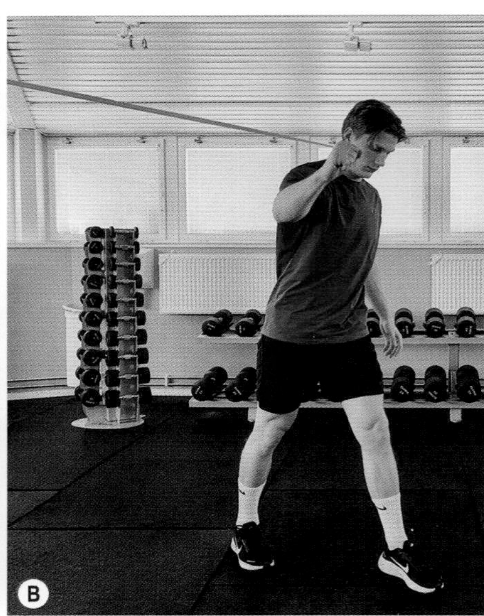
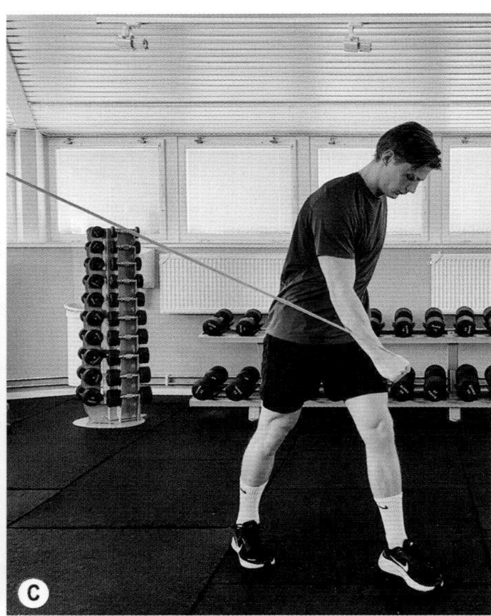

FIGURE 38.17A–C
Diagonal pattern exercise.

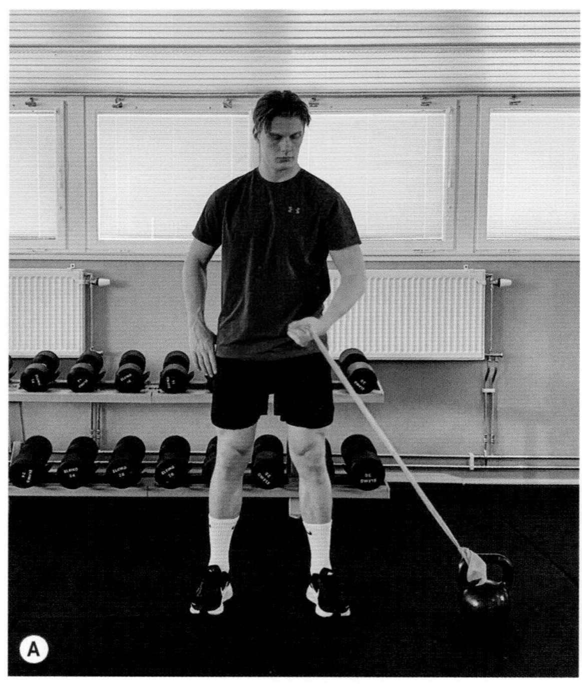
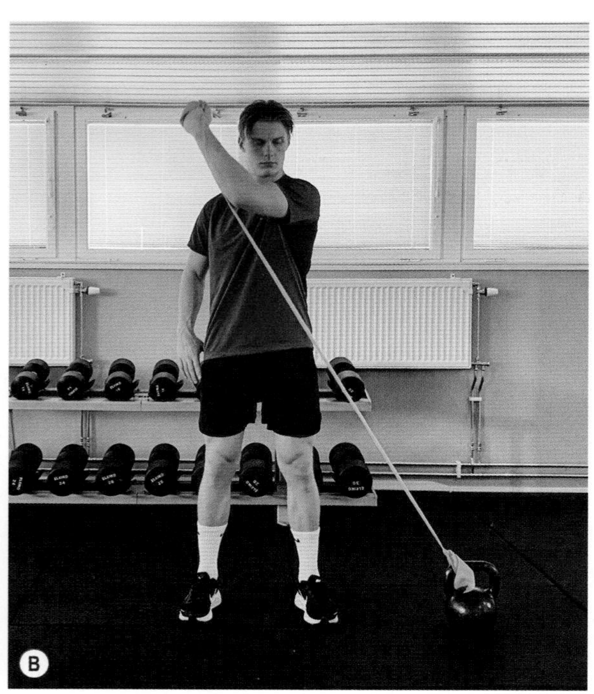

FIGURE 38.18AB
Cross-body uppercuts.

flexion strength. Isometric strengthening and activation are important components of these through the spectrum of rehabilitation. Full pain-free active range of motion at the end ranges of movement is an important component of progression. Progressive overload of internal rotation exercises, in addition to progressive extension strengthening, will be paramount to long-term success in athletes.

Notes for subscapularis nonsurgical rehabilitation

Measuring internal rotation strength (at 0° and 90° abduction, and in the "bear hug" position) is important in planning rehabilitation progression. Early phase protection can be combined with active range of motion and focused isometric strengthening. The clinician should delay progressively loading the muscles isotonically until full active range of motion and pain-free isometrics have been restored. Progressing the resistance applied during loaded external rotation can happen more quickly, but care must be taken to not move too quickly into end range of external rotation as this is applying a passive stretch to the (injured) internal rotators.

When to reappraise your approach

Your patient is unable to progress their resistance training either because of persisting pain, or there is a marked loss of strength. If not already investigated, consider imaging as there may be a complete tear.

Deceleration-related symptoms

Patient presentation

- *"I can't remember that I did anything special, but now it's painful when I throw."*
- *"I can still throw hard, but it hurts after I've been throwing, especially if I'm sloppy with the warm-up."*

What is our current understanding of the pathology and the tissues involved?

After ball release, the posterior and superior rotator cuff muscles and tendons work eccentrically to decelerate the arm and hand,[53] while moving to horizontal adduction and internal rotation.[32] This places large tensile (eccentric) loads on these muscle–tendon units. Additionally, there are high compressive forces on the undersurface of the tendons as these tendons wrap around the humeral head which is forcefully moving to adduction and internal rotation.[30] As with elsewhere in the body, abrupt tendon overload (too many throws, too soon) can present with a reactive tendinopathy which typically manifests as relatively high levels of pain in the day or so following the loading.[20,21] This will be associated with pain on loading the muscle–tendon unit which worsens with increased or persisting loading, and may initially present as difficulty in warming up; should the condition worsen, the athlete will frequently describe a history of requiring more time to warm up before throwing. Unfortunately, many will continue to tolerate this until the condition has worsened such that they are unable to warm up to perform. Less commonly, the contractile elements or musculotendinous junction may be involved and will present with a clear history (*"I made this one throw and immediately felt pain at the back here"*).

Additional questions

1. *Has there been any rapid increase in throwing load?* Commonly this is seen after returning from a break and "normal" loads are resumed abruptly.
2. *Have you had similar problems in previous years?* As this can become a habit for some players, remember to ask about similar problems in previous seasons or after breaks.
3. For adolescents, ask about *increases in ball size/ weight*, and for all ask about *the use of weighted balls.*

Physical examination

Shoulder external rotation strength (isometric and eccentric) – tested and quantified through dynamometry and symptom reproduction.

Management

Patient education

If the symptoms are diagnosed as a reactive tendinopathy[20,21] take time to explain that actual "tissue damage" is unlikely, but has been temporarily overloaded and should completely resolve with appropriate care. Use this as an opportunity to explain the necessity of sensible throwing load management and ideally prevent future similar exacerbations.

In those with presumed degenerate tendinopathy, it is important to emphasize that apparently "damaged" tendon (on imaging) is not necessarily associated with pain or loss of function as the remaining tendon and supporting structures can be strengthened to allow restoration of function. It is essential for the athlete to engage with the progressive loading/strengthening process due to the time required to resolve conditions involving tendons.[67]

Early

Patient education after clear identification of the pathology – reactive versus degenerate tendinopathy versus the less common contractile injury involving muscle and the muscle–tendon interface.

Reactive tendinopathy

Adapt the throwing load initially, after a short period of unloading as symptoms dictate, recommence early external rotation, horizontal abduction, and abduction strengthening. A short course of anti-inflammatory medications may be required.

Degenerate tendinopathy

No unloading phase is usually required, but early loading may need to be isometric, and inner or perhaps mid-range isotonic exercises before outer range.

Intermediate

Restoration of eccentric external rotation and horizontal abduction strength is key, working now through full range. Progressively increase throwing load.

Late

End stage strengthening, especially heavy resisted eccentric strength throughout range (Figures 38.19 to 38.21). Successful completion of interval throwing program.

When to reappraise your approach

Improvements (but not necessarily complete resolution) in the clinical picture should be seen after 4–6 weeks of appropriate loading, and we suggest that a minimum of 12 weeks'

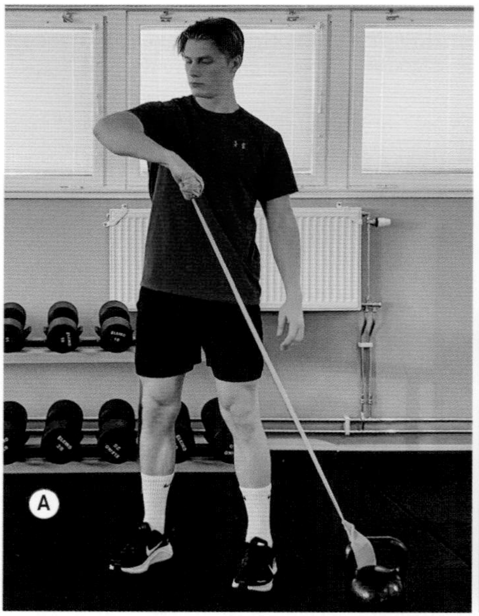

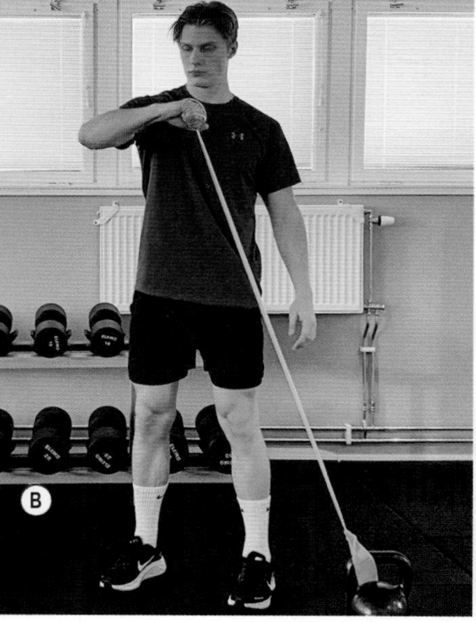

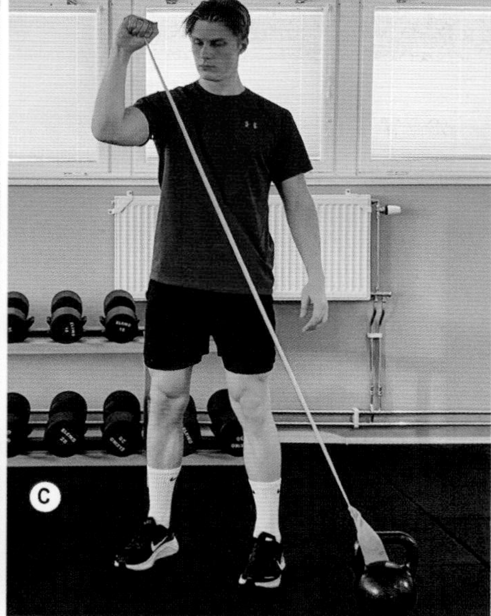

38.19A-C
End range strengthening of external rotators.

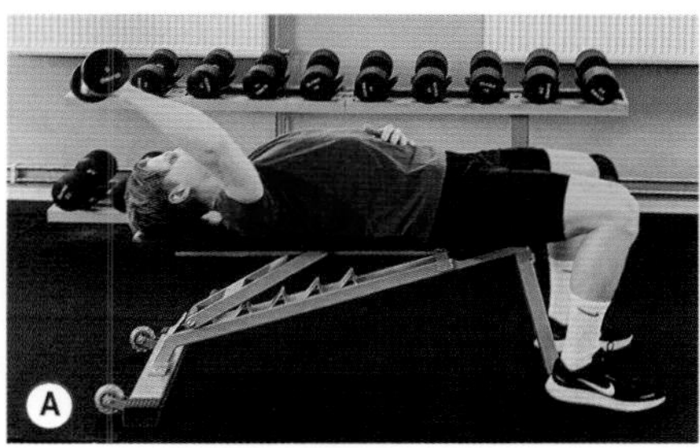
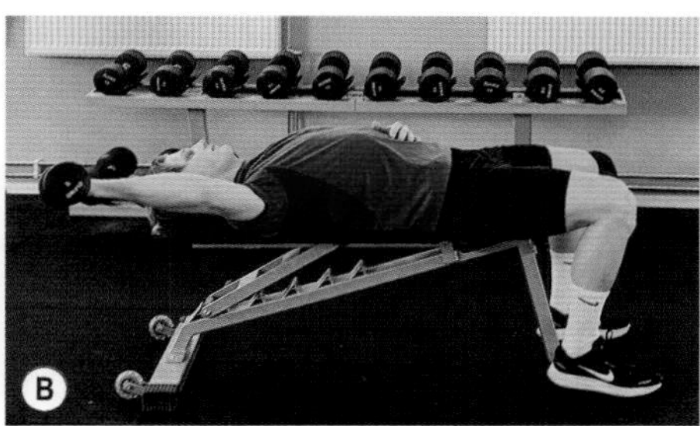
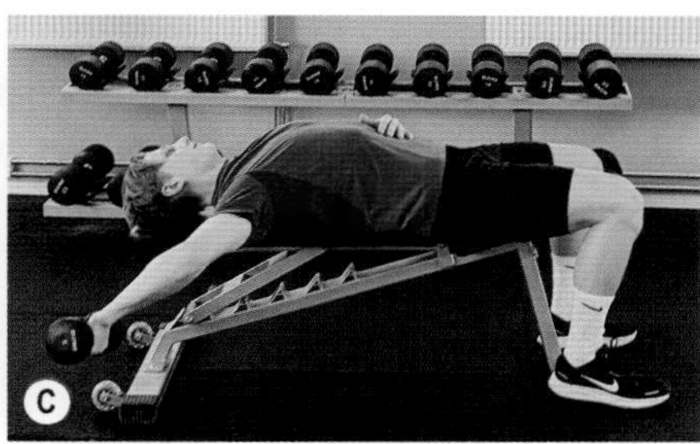

38.20A-C
End range strengthening of internal rotators, "upper limb Nordics".

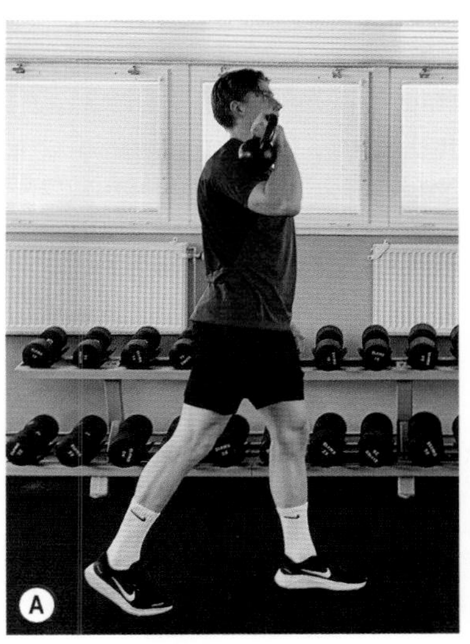
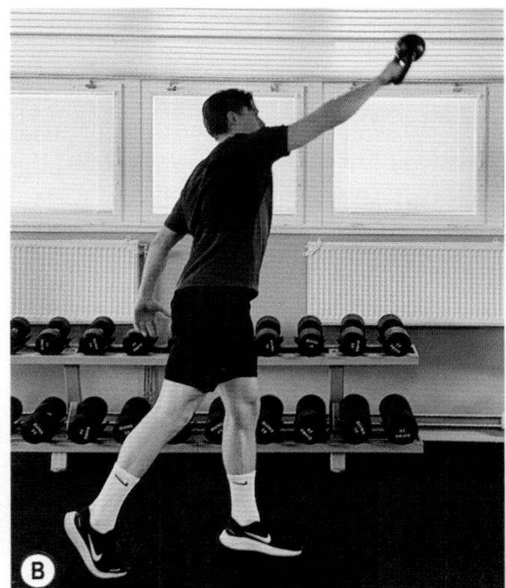
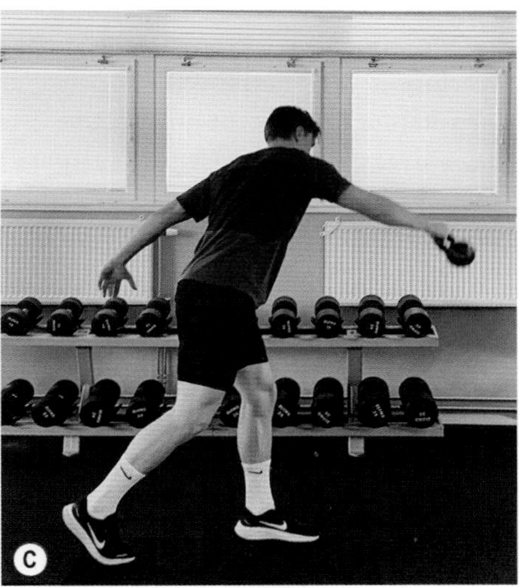

38.21A-C
Deceleration exercises.

rehabilitation would first need to be conducted with meaningful improvements in the clinical targets achieved before considering alternatives. Similarly, if more than six months of rehabilitation have passed with perhaps three months of failing to improve in any objective markers, then a reassessment would be sensible.

We recommend reviews:

- in the case of a reactive tendinopathy that despite 5–7 days of relative unloading hasn't settled.
- in a presumed degenerate tendinopathy where your athlete has improved their strength and rotational range, met their targets to return to throwing, yet despite careful progression they are experiencing a recurrence of the same pain with the same throwing intensity and volume.

In both these situations, the possibility of a missed diagnosis needs to be definitively excluded before continuing with the same management.

Thoracic outlet syndrome

Literature review

Thoracic outlet syndrome (TOS) results from compression of the neurovascular bundle in the thoracic outlet. TOS is considered rare in the general population but is more common in overhead athletes than previously thought. An investigation of 1288 Japanese 15–17 year-old high school baseball players reported an incidence of 32.8%.[83] The majority, approximately 95%, of true TOS presentations appear to be neurogenic, with approximately 4% venous, and the remaining 1% arterial.[34,88] In a series of 189 suspected neurogenic thoracic outlet cases, approximately 6% and 5% each were ultimately diagnosed as having concomitant venous and arterial thoracic outlet, respectively.[14]

Arterial TOS is associated with aneurysmal degeneration of the subclavian or axillary arteries which can incur distal embolization and limb-threatening ischemia. While rare, the consequences for an overhead athlete are tragic, and therefore it is essential TOS is considered and not missed (see Chapter 22). Recent prospective research demonstrated that only 25% of neurogenic TOS patients respond favorably to nonsurgical care and activity modification, and 60% required surgery.[6,7] If surgery is required, throwers can expect to return to prior levels of performance, although it may take up to one year.[106]

Patient presentation

Two types of presentations are common – overuse and traumatic.

Overuse, gradual onset:

- *"I'm getting this weird feeling."*
- *"It feels like it's moving around, sometimes it's here, then it's here, or over here..."*
- *"It's been strange – putting ice on lately has felt really bad, like it's burning me."*
- *"Sometimes my arm feels cold/hot/dead/tingling"*
- *"It's been on and off for a while now, I can't really remember any particular thing kicking this off, but it's getting worse."*
- *"I fatigue more easily than normal."*
- *"I am not throwing as hard as usual but don't have a lot of pain."*
- *"My fingers and hand feel tired and sometimes lose color, my fingers are clumsy sometimes."*

Traumatic onset:

- *"It started after I got my arm pulled while someone was grabbing my head/neck."*
- *"I dove with my arm out and landed badly."*
- *"When I got hit on my neck it hurt straight away, but since then it's got worse and the pain has changed … it's a strange kind of pain."*

Additional questions

1. *Tell me everything about how much throwing you've been doing.* Dive deeply into the athlete's throwing load history – pitch counts, bullpens (the bullpen is the area where pitchers warm up before entering the game, or do extra throwing sessions on days they aren't scheduled to pitch), learning a new pitch, try-outs/showcases, playing in multiple teams. Establish if there's a simple cause of spike in throwing load or resistance training that was the trigger. Discuss sleeping postures, pillow preferences.
2. *Tell me about your weights training – exactly what do you do?* Discuss this in some detail, focus on any changes, not only exercise volume and intensity, but changes in equipment or technique. Be especially mindful if the patient has been encouraged to keep their shoulder "back and down" –exaggerated scapular retraction and depression can trigger this in the absence of anything else.
3. *Can you remember getting hit or having your arm pulled?* If you deal with contact sports such as handball, you will know to ask about direct trauma, but in non-contact sports such as baseball, be reminded this may have happened due to neck/shoulder trauma that may have seemed inconsequential at the time.
4. *Have you tried anything for this before coming here? What happened with those treatments?* Check the athlete's response to any treatments and medications as there is typically a delay to presentation in these cases.
5. *What's coming up for you? What do you need to get ready for?* Establish the short-term goals to know

what you need to get the patient ready for, and when. For instance, throwing should stop for six weeks in atraumatic neurogenic cases.

6. *Have you had any investigations for this?* Only in cases where the history and clinical picture are suggestive should you request imaging: initially plain X-rays of the cervical spine, especially considering the involvement of cervical ribs,[45] but depending on the findings, this may progress to nerve conduction studies, and Doppler angiography. Most likely you will require specialist involvement at this stage.

Physical examination

Pain experienced at the base of the neck, dysesthesia in the arm, tenderness to palpation at the scalene triangle or subcoracoid region (especially where symptoms are reproduced), and a positive three-minute elevated arm stress test,[94] when presenting together, are suggested as diagnostic criteria.[8] Neurological examination is clearly mandatory.

Management

Although largely anecdotal, it is our experience that the neurogenic cases that respond favorably to nonsurgical care typically experience decrease in symptoms with manual therapy mobilizations to the cervical and 1st rib regions. Additionally, and perhaps a result of length of time to correct diagnosis, many people with neurogenic TOS have concomitant psychosomatic symptoms that may be barriers to successful nonsurgical outcomes.

Acute

Explanation, including the nature of the likely pathology, what it means, what can be done about it, and how we will know if the treatment is working, need to be sensitively provided, especially where a patient may have had a delayed diagnosis, or worse, told: "there's nothing wrong with you".

If structural, cervical ribs, fibrous entrapment or other anomalous anatomy may necessitate surgical intervention.

Address identified problems that may include:

- Stress – with relaxation training, breathing relaxation exercises.
- Soft tissue flexibility – with very gentle soft tissue massage, and non-provocative scalene and pectoralis muscle stretches.
- Taping for symptom relief.

Criteria to progress and timeline

Each athlete is an individual, and this is especially true for people diagnosed with thoracic outlet syndrome. Restoring range of motion is prioritized initially, which is then followed by restoration of graduated rotational strength, and finally an interval throwing program (see below) is introduced.

Intermediate

When there are no resting symptoms, consider the following as a management progression:

- Full active range of motion exercises of both shoulders with transition to progressive resisted exercises below shoulder height.
- Ensure the maintenance of range of motion during the rehabilitation program.
- Non-provocative pectoral and scalene muscle stretching.
- Neural gliding (see Chapter 21) and cervical and rib region mobilization techniques.
- Continue progression of diaphragmatic breathing techniques.
- Mobilize thoracic spine region.
- Progress strengthening exercises and introduce shorter recovery times between sessions.

Late

Once elevated, the arm stress test does not provoke symptoms for at least 1 minute, consider the following as a management progression:

- Daily self-stretching program.

- Advance strengthening exercises.
- Full sports-specific range of motion exercises including positions above shoulder height.
- Transition to plyometrics and then interval throwing program.

Return to sport once interval throwing program has been completed and the elevated arm stress test[94] is negative for more than 3 minutes.

When to reappraise your approach

The athlete reports worsening neurological symptoms (e.g., dysesthesia progressing to numbness, worsening apparent vascular symptoms) or following 4–6 weeks of conservative management with continued disability and little to no resolution of symptoms. In these cases, it is recommended that you engage assistance from expert vascular and/or neurological medical practitioners.

Additional considerations

The foregoing sections describe the most commonly encountered throwing-related issues in men, however, additional considerations apply to adolescent and female patient groups.

Adolescents

The proximal humeral physis begins maturing at approximately 14 years of age, finishing by about 17,[61] and injury during this time – termed Little League Shoulder – is increasingly being recognized, with the highest incidence at 13 years of age (ranging from 8 to 16).[46] Once identified, the mainstay of care for Little League Shoulder is temporarily stopping throwing, which can prove difficult, as the children most likely to present with this injury are those playing on the most teams, without breaks during the year.[47] While stopping throwing, it is important that shoulder flexibility[42] and posterior shoulder strength are maintained, and that this is followed by a careful resumption of throwing. This is associated with less chance of recurrence, as is earlier intervention.[42] Recall that when using pre-injury values as a benchmark in adolescents, simple passage of time is likely associated with growth and maturation which should improve strength. Age group population-specific data, or data normalized to bodyweight, are better reference values to use, especially on return to play after extended breaks.

Women

Unfortunately, as with many areas of sports medicine, research involving female athletes is sparse. This is a serious concern and must be addressed. Experience in handball is that women are at higher risk of shoulder problems than men.[3,5] There is no certainty as to why, with one possibility being related to insufficient strength training in European women's handball. Different ball sizes are used in different age categories for boys and girls which may play a role, but this has not been adequately investigated. Gender differences in throwing technique are suggested[40,99,120] but this hypothesis has not been confirmed in research investigations[107] and may be related to exposure and training rather than biology.[105] We emphasize that the reasons for sex differences are not known and currently are only speculative.

Interval throwing programs (ITP)

The interval throwing program is the final and most functional phase of the rehabilitation process. It is a planned sequence of throws involving several variables that are manipulated in a graded manner to prepare an athlete for return to sporting activity. The goals of an interval throwing program are to gradually stress the healing tissue to allow for adaptation, restore throwing mechanics to a "new" normal or better than pre-injury state, improve the athlete's confidence, and to condition the athlete to the volume, intensity, and specificity required for their sport and position.

The program can be initiated on achieving clinician clearance, pain-free examination, appropriate range of motion and total arm strength, and successful completion of upper extremity plyometric (stretch-shortening) exercises.

Guidance for creating interval throwing programs for recovering throwers

- Familiarize yourself with the unique nature of the player's throwing kinematics. To this end, it is essential to collaborate with skills coaches when building ITPs.
- Account for the specific injury and variability in players' healing processes.

- Work backward from the expected volume and intensity workloads of level of competition, specific sport, and positions within sport. For instance, an ITP will look different for an MLB starting pitcher, relief (bullpen) pitcher, and MLB 2nd baseman, youth baseball player, and for handball players, of different ages and sexes.
- The total length of throwing program should be at least as long as the post-injury period where the athlete was not throwing. For example, if a player had 4 weeks off throwing following internal impingement diagnosis, the ITP will last at least 4 weeks.
- Increase volume (number of throws) and intensity (distance/throwing speed) no more than 10–20% per week.
- Avoid multi-variant increases in a single session – i.e., don't increase the intensity and volume at the same time.
- Mild muscular or joint soreness is acceptable between throwing sessions, but not within throwing sessions.
- Soreness must resolve fully before next throwing session.
- If there is any symptom exacerbation or reports of arm tiredness, it is always preferable to repeat the previous step or take another day for recovery.
- The longer the ITP, the more important it becomes to build in a "de-load" or recovery from throwing week to allow for muscle repair and return of strength.
- A sports radar gun is helpful to monitor throwing speed.
- Reassess for changes in active and passive shoulder range and shoulder strength at intervals during the throwing program to ensure baseline values remain consistent.
- Everyone must be patient.

Mechanical focus during ITP

If you have not worked with throwing athletes previously, it is important to engage a coach in this stage. There is not the space to adequately explain all the following technical points, but these suggestions should be discussed with the athlete's throwing coach, and present a good opportunity for you to learn about these skills.

- As needed for distance, employ a back foot behind shuffle. Utilize the lower half by driving off the back leg and striding out while leading with the hip. This will help the thrower stay closed.
- Emphasize a strong and high front side (glove arm).
- Emphasize the lead shoulder being closed and higher than the back shoulder (tilt).
- Emphasize the head staying still and focused on the target at release (no "head whack" or excessive head tilt).
- Stay behind the ball and focus on command – get feedback from the flight of the ball.
- Focus on extension and finish over a soft land leg.
- Use an aggressive delivery with good momentum. Allow the arm to catch up so that it is not late.

The following is an interval throwing program example that could be considered following a 2–6-week period of no throwing as a result of injury. Phase 1 and Phase 2 are applicable to all players and Phase 3 will be unique based upon position-specific needs. A 3rd week would be added to Phase 2 to accommodate position players that need to prepare for throwing distances of more than 37 meters (120 feet), or for pitchers that routinely throw similar distances when asymptomatic.

Phase 1

This phase aims to reintroduce the athlete's arm to throwing and building a base for subsequent phases. All throws in Phase 1 are thrown in the "Stretch Out" phase. The goal of this phase is to slowly lengthen or "stretch out" your throwing arm while increasing distance and keeping some arc in the ball flight. A good rule of thumb is keeping all throws under a 30° angle from horizontal, starting on a line and adding arc and effort as needed to reach the partner. Do not throw aggressively during Phase 1. Recheck range of motion and strength metrics at the end of each week. Table 38.2 details the Phase 1 program.

Table 38.2 Phase 1 Program

Week 1: 2 days on/1 day off (4 throwing days in total)

Stretch Out Phase (50 throws in total)

Number of throws	Distance of throw (feet)	Distance of throw (meters)
10	45	13.7
10	60	18.3
15	75	22.9
10	60	18.3
5	45	13.7

Week 2: 2 days on/1 day off (4 throwing days in total)

Stretch Out Phase (55 throws in total)

Number of throws	Distance of throw (feet)	Distance of throw (meters)
10	45	13.7
10	60	18.3
10	75	22.9
10	90	27.4
5	75	22.9
10	60	18.3

Week 3: 2 days on/1 day off (4 throwing days in total)

Stretch Out Phase (50 throws in total)

Number of throws	Distance of throw (feet)	Distance of throw (meters)
10	40–60	12.2–18.3
10	75	22.9
10	90	27.4
10	105	32.0
2	90	27.4
3	75	22.9
5	60	18.3

Table 38.3 Phase 2 Program

Week 4: 2 days on/1 day off (4 throwing days in total)

Stretch Out Phase (40 throws in total)

Number of throws	Distance of throw (feet)	Distance of throw (meters)
15	40–60	12.2–18.3
10	75	22.9
5	90	27.4
5	105	32.0
5	120	36.6

Pull Down Phase (8 throws in total)

Number of throws	Distance of throw (feet)	Distance of throw (meters)
2	110	33.6
2	100	30.5
2	90	27.4
2	80	24.4

Cool down phase

Number of throws	Distance of throw (feet)	Distance of throw (meters)
5	70	21.4
5	60	18.3

- Focus on accuracy.
- Never throw higher than the partner's chest: waist height and focal point of left or right hip is ideal.

Week 5: 2 days on/1 day off (4 throwing days in total)

Stretch Out Phase (40 throws in total)

Number of throws	Distance of throw (feet)	Distance of throw (meters)
15	40–60	12.2–18.3
10	75	22.9
5	90	27.4
5	105	32.0
5	120	36.6

Table 38.3 *(Continued)*

Week 5: 2 days on/1 day off (4 throwing days in total)		
Pull Down Phase (20 throws in total)		
Number of throws	**Distance of throw (feet)**	**Distance of throw (meters)**
5	110	33.6
5	100	30.5
5	90	27.4
5	80	24.4
Cool down phase		
Number of throws	**Distance of throw (feet)**	**Distance of throw (meters)**
5	70	21.4
5	60	18.3
• Focus on accuracy, never higher than chest height and aiming for the left or right hip level.		

Phase 2: The "Pull Down" Phase

Phase 2 starts out at the "Stretch Out" like Phase 1. However, when the maximal distance for the session is achieved, the athlete commences throwing on a line towards a partner with the same effort, mechanics, and footwork that was required to reach the maximal distance. This is the "Pull Down" phase. Do not lose your tilt to throw on a line. Use the same effort that it took to throw max distance for each pull down throw. Recheck range of motion and strength metrics at the end of each week.

Table 38.3 details the Phase 2 program.

Phase 3

Phase 3 involves position-specific throwing. This would include a mound progression for a pitcher, throwing to the bases, and cut-offs and relays for position players. Based upon subjective feedback from the thrower and objective data from reassessment, consideration may be given to a "de-load" week. During de-load, the thrower continues throwing, albeit with less intensity and decreased volume of throws. This approach allows for maximum physical and psychological recovery.

Conclusion

Throwing-related injuries superficially seem like other injuries encountered in usual practice, however, the specific demands of throwing (repeated, end range, rotational, ballistic efforts) mean that the pathologies and their management are quite different. We have outlined the "typical" presentations of the most commonly encountered conditions, as well as our suggestions for their management. In contrast to some other patient categories of shoulder injury, specific pathologies are frequently encountered, and are better managed when identified. A combination of patient history, emphasizing the point in the throwing motion where the symptoms arise, followed up with careful targeted clinical examination, and sensible interpretation of any required imaging, are cornerstones of diagnostic classification. Management involves identification of deficits (which requires understanding normal rotational strength and range of motion during throwing), and then appropriately re-loading the athlete in the presence of any pathology.

References

1. Altintas B, Anderson N, Dornan GJ, Boykin RE, Logan C, Millett PJ. Return to sport after arthroscopic rotator cuff repair: is there a difference between the recreational and the competitive athlete? Am J Sports Med. 2020;48:252-261.
2. Altman DG, Bland JM. Diagnostic tests 2: predictive values. BMJ. 1994;309:102.
3. Andersson SH, Bahr R, Clarsen B, Myklebust G. Risk factors for overuse shoulder injuries in a mixed-sex cohort of 329 elite handball players: previous findings could not be confirmed. Br J Sports Med. 2018;52:1191-1198.
4. Andrews JR, Carson WG, Jr., McLeod WD. Glenoid labrum tears related to the long head of the biceps. Am J Sports Med. 1985;13:337-341.
5. Asker M, Holm LW, Kallberg H, Walden M, Skillgate E. Female adolescent elite handball players are more susceptible to shoulder problems than their male counterparts. Knee Surg Sports Traumatol Arthrosc. 2018;26:1892-1900.
6. Balderman J, Abuirqeba A, Pate C, et al. Treatment results and patient-reported outcomes measures in patients with neurogenic thoracic outlet syndrome. Journal of Vascular Surgery. 2018;68:e51-e52.
7. Balderman J, Abuirqeba AA, Eichaker L, et al. Physical therapy management, surgical treatment, and patient-reported outcomes measures in a prospective observational cohort of patients with neurogenic thoracic outlet syndrome. J Vasc Surg. 2019;70:832-841.
8. Balderman J, Holzem K, Field BJ, et al. Associations between clinical diagnostic criteria and pretreatment patient-reported outcomes measures in a prospective

observational cohort of patients with neurogenic thoracic outlet syndrome. J Vasc Surg. 2017;66:533-544.

9. Barth JR, Burkhart SS, De Beer JF. The bear-hug test: a new and sensitive test for diagnosing a subscapularis tear. Arthroscopy. 2006;22:1076-1084.

10. Ben Kibler W, Sciascia AD, Hester P, Dome D, Jacobs C. Clinical utility of traditional and new tests in the diagnosis of biceps tendon injuries and superior labrum anterior and posterior lesions in the shoulder. Am J Sports Med. 2009;37:1840-1847.

11. Boettcher CE, Cathers I, Ginn KA. The role of shoulder muscles is task specific. J Sci Med Sport. 2010;13:651-656.

12. Boileau P, Parratte S, Chuinard C, Roussanne Y, Shia D, Bicknell R. Arthroscopic treatment of isolated type II SLAP lesions: biceps tenodesis as an alternative to reinsertion. Am J Sports Med. 2009;37:929-936.

13. Burkhart SS, Morgan CD, Kibler WB. The disabled throwing shoulder: spectrum of pathology. Part I: pathoanatomy and biomechanics. Arthroscopy. 2003;19:404-420.

14. Caputo FJ, Wittenberg AM, Vemuri C, et al. Supraclavicular decompression for neurogenic thoracic outlet syndrome in adolescent and adult populations. J Vasc Surg. 2013;57:149-157.

15. Chalmers PN, Erickson BJ, Verma NN, D'Angelo J, Romeo AA. Incidence and return to play after biceps tenodesis in professional baseball players. Arthroscopy. 2018;34:747-751.

16. Chao S, Thomas S, Yucha D, Kelly JDt, Driban J, Swanik K. An electromyographic assessment of the "bear hug": an examination for the evaluation of the subscapularis muscle. Arthroscopy. 2008;24:1265-1270.

17. Cohen DB, Coleman S, Drakos MC, et al. Outcomes of isolated type II SLAP lesions treated with arthroscopic fixation using a bioabsorbable tack. Arthroscopy. 2006;22:136-142.

18. Connor PM, Banks DM, Tyson AB, Coumas JS, D'Alessandro DF. Magnetic resonance imaging of the asymptomatic shoulder of overhead athletes: a 5-year follow-up study. Am J Sports Med. 2003;31:724-727.

19. Cook C, Beaty S, Kissenberth MJ, Siffri P, Pill SG, Hawkins RJ. Diagnostic accuracy of five orthopedic clinical tests for diagnosis of superior labrum anterior posterior (SLAP) lesions. J Shoulder Elbow Surg. 2012;21:13-22.

20. Cook JL, Purdam CR. Is tendon pathology a continuum? A pathology model to explain the clinical presentation of load-induced tendinopathy. Br J Sports Med. 2009;43:409-416.

21. Cook JL, Rio E, Purdam CR, Docking SI. Revisiting the continuum model of tendon pathology: what is its merit in clinical practice and research? Br J Sports Med. 2016;50:1187-1191.

22. Denard PJ, Ladermann A, Parsley BK, Burkhart SS. Arthroscopic biceps tenodesis compared with repair of isolated type II SLAP lesions in patients older than 35 years. Orthopedics. 2014;37:e292-297.

23. Dessaur WA, Magarey ME. Diagnostic accuracy of clinical tests for superior labral anterior posterior lesions: a systematic review. J Orthop Sports Phys Ther. 2008;38:341-352.

24. Dinnes J, Loveman E, McIntyre L, Waugh N. The effectiveness of diagnostic tests for the assessment of shoulder pain due to soft tissue disorders: a systematic review. Health Technology Assessment programme: Executive Summaries. NIHR Journals Library; 2003.

25. Dollings H, Sandford F, O'Conaire E, Lewis JS. Shoulder strength testing: the intra- and inter-tester reliability of routine clinical tests, using the PowertrackTM II Commander. Shoulder & Elbow. 2012;4:131-140.

26. Erickson BJ, Chalmers PN, D'Angelo J, Ma K, Romeo AA. Performance and return to sport following rotator cuff surgery in professional baseball players. J Shoulder Elbow Surg. 2019;28:2326-2333.

27. Erickson BJ, Chalmers PN, D'Angelo J, Ma K, Romeo AA. Performance and return to sport following latissimus dorsi and teres major injuries in professional baseball pitchers. Orthopaedic Journal of Sports Medicine. 2018;6:2325967118S2325900146.

28. Erickson BJ, Chalmers PN, Waterman BR, Griffin JW, Romeo AA. Performance and return to sport in elite baseball players and recreational athletes following repair of the latissimus dorsi and teres major. J Shoulder Elbow Surg. 2017;26:1948-1954.

29. Escamilla RF, Andrews JR. Shoulder muscle recruitment patterns and related biomechanics during upper extremity sports. Sports Med. 2009;39:569-590.

30. Fallon J, Blevins FT, Vogel K, Trotter J. Functional morphology of the supraspinatus tendon. J Orthop Res. 2002;20:920-926.

31. Fedoriw WW, Ramkumar P, McCulloch PC, Lintner DM. Return to play after treatment of superior labral tears in professional baseball players. Am J Sports Med. 2014;42:1155-1160.

32. Fleisig GS, Barrentine SW, Escamilla RF, Andrews JR. Biomechanics of overhand throwing with implications for injuries. Sports Med. 1996;21:421-437.

33. Friel NA, Karas V, Slabaugh MA, Cole BJ. Outcomes of type II superior labrum, anterior to posterior (SLAP) repair: prospective evaluation at a minimum two-year follow-up. J Shoulder Elbow Surg. 2010;19:859-867.

34. Fugate MW, Rotellini-Coltvet L, Freischlag JA. Current management of thoracic outlet syndrome. Curr Treat Options Cardiovasc Med. 2009;11:176-183.

35. Gifford L. Aches and Pains. CNS Press; 2014.

36. Gilliam BD, Douglas L, Fleisig GS, et al. Return to play and outcomes in baseball players after superior labral anterior-posterior repairs. Am J Sports Med. 2018;46:109-115.

37. Ginn KA, Reed D, Jones C, Downes A, Cathers I, Halaki M. Is subscapularis recruited in a similar manner during shoulder internal rotation exercises and belly press and lift off tests? J Sci Med Sport. 2017;20:566-571.

38. Gismervik SO, Drogset JO, Granviken F, Ro M, Leivseth G. Physical examination tests of the shoulder: a systematic review and meta-analysis of diagnostic test performance. BMC Musculoskelet Disord. 2017;18:41.

39. Graham S, Brookey J. Do patients understand? Perm J. 2008;12:67-69.

40. Gromeier M, Koester D, Schack T. Gender differences in motor skills of the overarm throw. Frontiers in Psychology. 2017;8:212.

41. Guanche CA, Jones DC. Clinical testing for tears of the glenoid labrum. Arthroscopy. 2003;19:517-523.

42. Harada M, Takahara M, Maruyama M, et al. Outcome of conservative treatment for Little League shoulder in young baseball players: factors related to incomplete

return to baseball and recurrence of pain. J Shoulder Elbow Surg. 2018;27:1-9.

43. Hashiguchi H, Iwashita S, Yoneda M, Takai S. Factors influencing outcomes of nonsurgical treatment for baseball players with SLAP lesion. Asia Pac J Sports Med Arthrosc Rehabil Technol. 2018;14:6-9.

44. Hegedus EJ, Goode A, Campbell S, et al. Physical examination tests of the shoulder: a systematic review with meta-analysis of individual tests. Br J Sports Med. 2008;42:80-92; discussion 92.

45. Henry BM, Vikse J, Sanna B, et al. Cervical rib prevalence and its association with thoracic outlet syndrome: a meta-analysis of 141 studies with surgical considerations. World Neurosurg. 2018;110:e965-e978.

46. Heyworth BE, Kramer DE, Martin DJ, Micheli LJ, Kocher MS, Bae DS. Trends in the presentation, management, and outcomes of Little League Shoulder. Am J Sports Med. 2016;44:1431-1438.

47. Holt JB, Stearns PH, Bastrom TP, Dennis MM, Dwek JR, Pennock AT. The curse of the all-star team: a single-season prospective shoulder MRI study of Little League baseball players. J Pediatr Orthop. 2020;40:e19-e24.

48. Huber WP, Putz RV. Periarticular fiber system of the shoulder joint. Arthroscopy. 1997;13:680-691.

49. Ide J, Maeda S, Takagi K. Sports activity after arthroscopic superior labral repair using suture anchors in overhead-throwing athletes. Am J Sports Med. 2005;33:507-514.

50. Irlenbusch U, Bernsdorf M, Born S, Gansen HK, Lorenz U. Electromyographic analysis of muscle function after latissimus dorsi tendon transfer. J Shoulder Elbow Surg. 2008;17:492-499.

51. Jain NB, Luz J, Higgins LD, et al. The diagnostic accuracy of special tests for rotator cuff tear: the ROW Cohort Study. Am J Phys Med Rehabil. 2017;96:176-183.

52. Jang SH, Seo JG, Jang HS, Jung JE, Kim JG. Predictive factors associated with failure of nonoperative treatment of superior labrum anterior-posterior tears. J Shoulder Elbow Surg. 2016;25:428-434.

53. Jobe FW, Moynes DR, Tibone JE, Perry J. An EMG analysis of the shoulder in pitching. A second report. Am J Sports Med. 1984;12:218-220.

54. Kibler WB. Specificity and sensitivity of the anterior slide test in throwing athletes with superior glenoid labral tears. Arthroscopy. 1995;11:296-300.

55. Kibler WB, Chandler TJ, Livingston BP, Roetert EP. Shoulder range of motion in elite tennis players. Effect of age and years of tournament play. Am J Sports Med. 1996;24:279-285.

56. Kibler WB, Sciascia AD, Hester P, Dome D, Jacobs C. Clinical utility of traditional and new tests in the diagnosis of biceps tendon injuries and superior labrum anterior and posterior lesions in the shoulder. Am J Sports Med. 2009;37:1840-1847.

57. Kim SH, Ha KI, Ahn JH, Kim SH, Choi HJ. Biceps load test II: a clinical test for SLAP lesions of the shoulder. Arthroscopy. 2001;17:160-164.

58. Kim TK, Queale WS, Cosgarea AJ, McFarland EG. Clinical features of the different types of SLAP lesions: an analysis of one hundred and thirty-nine cases. J Bone Joint Surg Am. 2003;85:66-71.

59. King JW, Brelsford HJ, Tullos HS. Analysis of the pitching arm of the professional baseball pitcher. Clin Orthop Relat Res. 1969;67:116-123.

60. Komi PV. Physiological and biomechanical correlates of muscle function: effects of muscle structure and stretch-shortening cycle on force and speed. Exerc Sport Sci Rev. 1984;12:81-121.

61. Kwong S, Kothary S, Poncinelli LL. Skeletal development of the proximal humerus in the pediatric population: MRI features. AJR Am J Roentgenol. 2014;202:418-425.

62. Laitung JK, Peck F. Shoulder function following the loss of the latissimus dorsi muscle. Br J Plast Surg. 1985;38:375-379.

63. Lesniak BP, Baraga MG, Jose J, Smith MK, Cunningham S, Kaplan LD. Glenohumeral findings on magnetic resonance imaging correlate with innings pitched in asymptomatic pitchers. Am J Sports Med. 2013;41:2022-2027.

64. Liu JN, Garcia GH, Gowd AK, et al. Treatment of partial thickness rotator cuff tears in overhead athletes. Curr Rev Musculoskelet Med. 2018;11:55-62.

65. Liu SH, Henry MH, Nuccion SL. A prospective evaluation of a new physical examination in predicting glenoid labral tears. Am J Sports Med. 1996;24:721-725.

66. Lo IK, Burkhart SS. Subscapularis tears: arthroscopic repair of the forgotten rotator cuff tendon. Techniques in Shoulder & Elbow Surgery. 2002;3:282-291.

67. Malliaras P, Barton CJ, Reeves ND, Langberg H. Achilles and patellar tendinopathy loading programmes : a systematic review comparing clinical outcomes and identifying potential mechanisms for effectiveness. Sports Med. 2013;43:267-286.

68. Mathewson MA, Kwan A, Eng CM, Lieber RL, Ward SR. Comparison of rotator cuff muscle architecture between humans and other selected vertebrate species. J Exp Biol. 2014;217:261-273.

69. Mazoue CG, Andrews JR. Repair of full-thickness rotator cuff tears in professional baseball players. Am J Sports Med. 2006;34:182-189.

70. McFarland EG, Kim TK, Savino RM. Clinical assessment of three common tests for superior labral anterior-posterior lesions. Am J Sports Med. 2002;30:810-815.

71. Mehdi SK, Frangiamore SJ, Schickendantz MS. Latissimus dorsi and teres major injuries in Major League baseball pitchers: a systematic review. Am J Orthop. 2016;45:163-167.

72. Mihata T, Morikura R, Hasegawa A, et al. Partial-thickness rotator cuff tear by itself does not cause shoulder pain or muscle weakness in baseball players. Am J Sports Med. 2019;47:3476-3482.

73. Miniaci A, Dowdy PA, Willits KR, Vellet AD. Magnetic resonance imaging evaluation of the rotator cuff tendons in the asymptomatic shoulder. Am J Sports Med. 1995;23:142-145.

74. Miniaci A, Mascia AT, Salonen DC, Becker EJ. Magnetic resonance imaging of the shoulder in asymptomatic professional baseball pitchers. Am J Sports Med. 2002;30:66-73.

75. Mohana-Borges AV, Chung CB, Resnick D. Superior labral anteroposterior tear: classification and diagnosis on MRI and MR arthrography. AJR Am J Roentgenol. 2003;181:1449-1462.

76. Myers TH, Zemanovic JR, Andrews JR. The resisted supination external rotation test: a new test for the diagnosis of superior labral anterior posterior lesions. Am J Sports Med. 2005;33:1315-1320.

77. Nagda SH, Cohen SB, Noonan TJ, Raasch WG, Ciccotti MG, Yocum LA. Management and outcomes of latissimus dorsi and teres major injuries in professional baseball

pitchers. Am J Sports Med. 2011;39:2181-2186.

78. Nakagawa S, Yoneda M, Hayashida K, Obata M, Fukushima S, Miyazaki Y. Forced shoulder abduction and elbow flexion test: a new simple clinical test to detect superior labral injury in the throwing shoulder. Arthroscopy. 2005;21:1290-1295.

79. Nam EK, Snyder SJ. The diagnosis and treatment of superior labrum, anterior and posterior (SLAP) lesions. Am J Sports Med. 2003;31:798-810.

80. Norman RW, Komi PV. Electromechanical delay in skeletal muscle under normal movement conditions. Acta Physiol Scand. 1979;106:241-248.

81. O'Brien SJ, Pagnani MJ, Fealy S, McGlynn SR, Wilson JB. The active compression test: a new and effective test for diagnosing labral tears and acromioclavicular joint abnormality. Am J Sports Med. 1998;26:610-613.

82. Oh JH, Kim JY, Kim WS, Gong HS, Lee JH. The evaluation of various physical examinations for the diagnosis of type II superior labrum anterior and posterior lesion. Am J Sports Med. 2008;36:353-359.

83. Otoshi K, Kikuchi S, Kato K, et al. The prevalence and characteristics of thoracic outlet syndrome in high school baseball players. Health. 2017;9:1223.

84. Pandya NK, Colton A, Webner D, Sennett B, Huffman GR. Physical examination and magnetic resonance imaging in the diagnosis of superior labrum anterior-posterior lesions of the shoulder: a sensitivity analysis. Arthroscopy. 2008;24:311-317.

85. Parentis MA, Glousman RE, Mohr KS, Yocum LA. An evaluation of the provocative tests for superior labral anterior posterior lesions. Am J Sports Med. 2006;34:265-268.

86. Parentis MA, Jobe CM, Pink MM, Jobe FW. An anatomic evaluation of the active compression test. J Shoulder Elbow Surg. 2004;13:410-416.

87. Payne LZ, Altchek DW, Craig EV, Warren RF. Arthroscopic treatment of partial rotator cuff tears in young athletes. A preliminary report. Am J Sports Med. 1997;25:299-305.

88. Peek J, Vos CG, Unlu C, van de Pavoordt H, van den Akker PJ, de Vries JPM. Outcome of surgical treatment for thoracic outlet syndrome: systematic review and meta-analysis. Ann Vasc Surg. 2017;40:303-326.

89. Pieper HG. Humeral torsion in the throwing arm of handball players. Am J Sports Med. 1998;26:247-253.

90. Polster JM, Bullen J, Obuchowski NA, Bryan JA, Soloff L, Schickendantz MS. Relationship between humeral torsion and injury in professional baseball pitchers. Am J Sports Med. 2013;41:2015-2021.

91. Polster JM, Lynch TS, Bullen JA, et al. Throwing-related injuries of the subscapularis in professional baseball players. Skeletal Radiol. 2016;45:41-47.

92. Polster JM, Subhas N, Scalise JJ, Bryan JA, Lieber ML, Schickendantz MS. Three-dimensional volume-rendering computed tomography for measuring humeral version. J Shoulder Elbow Surg. 2010;19:899-907.

93. Rathi S, Taylor NF, Green RA. The upper and lower segments of subscapularis muscle have different roles in glenohumeral joint functioning. J Biomech. 2017;63:92-97.

94. Roos DB. Congenital anomalies associated with thoracic outlet syndrome. Anatomy, symptoms, diagnosis, and treatment. Am J Surg. 1976;132:771-778.

95. Savoie FH, 3rd, Field LD, Atchinson S. Anterior superior instability with rotator cuff tearing: SLAC lesion. Orthop Clin North Am. 2001;32:457-461, ix.

96. Sayde WM, Cohen SB, Ciccotti MG, Dodson CC. Return to play after Type II superior labral anterior-posterior lesion repairs in athletes: a systematic review. Clin Orthop Relat Res. 2012;470:1595-1600.

97. Schickendantz MS, Kaar SG, Meister K, Lund P, Beverley L. Latissimus dorsi and teres major tears in professional baseball pitchers: a case series. Am J Sports Med. 2009;37:2016-2020.

98. Schroder CP, Skare O, Reikeras O, Mowinckel P, Brox JI. Sham surgery versus labral repair or biceps tenodesis for type II SLAP lesions of the shoulder: a three-armed randomised clinical trial. Br J Sports Med. 2017;51:1759-1766.

99. Serrien B, Clijsen R, Blondeel J, Goossens M, Baeyens JP. Differences in ball speed and three-dimensional kinematics between male and female handball players during a standing throw with run-up. BMC Sports Science, Medicine and Rehabilitation. 2015;7:27.

100. Smith R, Lombardo DJ, Petersen-Fitts GR, et al. Return to play and prior performance in Major League baseball pitchers after repair of superior labral anterior-posterior tears. Orthop J Sports Med. 2016;4:2325967116675822.

101. Snyder SJ, Karzel RP, Del Pizzo W, Ferkel RD, Friedman MJ. SLAP lesions of the shoulder. Arthroscopy. 1990;6:274-279.

102. Stetson WB, Templin K. The crank test, the O'Brien test, and routine magnetic resonance imaging scans in the diagnosis of labral tears. Am J Sports Med. 2002;30:806-809.

103. Tarkowski EM, Omar IM, Blount KJ, Gryzlo SM. Subscapularis myotendinous junction tears presenting with posterior shoulder pain in overhead throwing athletes. Acta Med Acad. 2019;48:205-216.

104. Tennent TD, Beach WR, Meyers JF. A review of the special tests associated with shoulder examination. Part II: laxity, instability, and superior labral anterior and posterior (SLAP) lesions. Am J Sports Med. 2003;31:301-307.

105. Thomas JR, Alderson JA, Thomas KT, Campbell AC, Elliott BC. Developmental gender differences for overhand throwing in Aboriginal Australian children. Research Quarterly for Exercise and Sport. 2010;81:432-441.

106. Thompson RW, Dawkins C, Vemuri C, Mulholland MW, Hadzinsky TD, Pearl GJ. Performance metrics in professional baseball pitchers before and after surgical treatment for neurogenic thoracic outlet syndrome. Ann Vasc Surg. 2017;39:216-227.

107. Van Den Tillaar R, Cabri JM. Gender differences in the kinematics and ball velocity of overarm throwing in elite team handball players. J Sports Sci. 2012;30:807-813.

108. Vangsness CT, Jr., Ennis M, Taylor JG, Atkinson R. Neural anatomy of the glenohumeral ligaments, labrum, and subacromial bursa. Arthroscopy. 1995;11:180-184.

109. Voss DE. Proprioceptive neuromuscular facilitation. Am J Phys Med. 1967;46:838-899.

110. Walch G, Liotard JP, Boileau P, Noel E. [Postero-superior glenoid impingement. Another shoulder impingement]. Rev Chir Orthop Reparatrice Appar Mot. 1991;77:571-574.

111. Walsworth MK, Doukas WC, Murphy KP, Mielcarek BJ, Michener LA. Reliability and diagnostic accuracy of history and physical examination for diagnosing glenoid labral tears. Am J Sports Med. 2008;36:162-168.

112. Ward SR, Hentzen ER, Smallwood LH, et al. Rotator cuff muscle architecture: implications for glenohumeral stability. Clin Orthop Relat Res. 2006;448:157-163.

113. Whiteley R, Ginn K, Nicholson L, Adams R. Indirect ultrasound measurement of humeral torsion in adolescent baseball players and non-athletic adults: reliability and significance. J Sci Med Sport. 2006;9:310-318.

114. Whiteley R, Oceguera M. GIRD, TRROM, and humeral torsion-based classification of shoulder risk in throwing athletes are not in agreement and should not be used interchangeably. J Sci Med Sport. 2016;19:816-819.

115. Whiteley R, Oceguera MV, Valencia EB, Mitchell T. Adaptations at the shoulder of the throwing athlete and implications for the clinician. Techniques in Shoulder & Elbow Surgery. 2012;13:36-44.

116. Wickham J, Pizzari T, Balster S, Ganderton C, Watson L. The variable roles of the upper and lower subscapularis during shoulder motion. Clin Biomech. 2014;29:885-891.

117. Wilk KE, Hooks TR, Macrina LC. The modified sleeper stretch and modified cross-body stretch to increase shoulder internal rotation range of motion in the overhead throwing athlete. J Orthop Sports Phys Ther. 2013;43:891-894.

118. Wilk KE, Meister K, Andrews JR. Current concepts in the rehabilitation of the overhead throwing athlete. Am J Sports Med. 2002;30:136-151.

119. Yamamoto N, Itoi E, Minagawa H, et al. Why is the humeral retroversion of throwing athletes greater in dominant shoulders than in nondominant shoulders? J Shoulder Elbow Surg. 2006;15:571-575.

120. Young RW. The ontogeny of throwing and striking. Hum Ontogenet. 2009;3:19-31.

Rehabilitation in swimmers 39

Sally McLaine, Helen Walker, Craig Boettcher

Introduction

Swimming is a popular activity that is enjoyed at all ages for leisure, competition, and associated health benefits, that include improving strength, cardiovascular fitness, and endurance. The unique aquatic environment facilitates swimming as an ideal low-impact exercise, especially for people with myriad musculoskeletal conditions as well as those with medical comorbidities, such as depression, diabetes, high blood pressure, and asthma. Moving into end of range positions repetitively during swimming, the shoulder is subject to high loads, so it is not surprising that the shoulder is the most reported region of pain for swimmers.[12]

Although the requirements of the swimming shoulder are often considered similar to those of activities such as throwing and tennis, the mechanics and repetition of shoulder movements are different. Throwers utilize a stable ground base to transfer force from the lower limbs and trunk to the shoulder, whereas swimmers rely on the shoulder as the primary force generator for propulsion of the body through water. For the elite swimmer, often training 20 or more hours per week, each shoulder will experience over 1 million revolutions per year, more than any other sport, including tennis, baseball, and cricket.[61] It is not surprising that at least 30% of swimmers experience shoulder pain at some time throughout their swimming career, impacting recreational to elite level swimmers, resulting in challenging decisions regarding management and rehabilitation.[30,39,69]

Shoulder pain occurs frequently throughout the lifespan of the swimmer, with reported prevalence ranging from 30–91%.[30,39,71] Adolescent, competitive swimmers are subject to large volumes of training, subsequently, high rates of shoulder pain are consistently reported for this group, with many leaving the sport as a result.[31,71] Swimmers continuing at the elite level remain at risk of developing and continuing to experience shoulder pain, with career incidence rates reported up to 73% for this group.[57,85] Prevalence rates for masters or older swimmers are varied but lower (19%) compared with younger swimming populations, and may relate to the different training loads, reduced competition pressure, and self-regulation.[76]

Given the high prevalence of shoulder pain in swimmers, investigation of potential predictors for injury and pain including shoulder strength, scapular position, load, range of movement, shoulder laxity, previous injury history, biomechanics, and possible pathology related to shoulder pain has been extensive. However, historically similar rates for occurrence and recurring shoulder pain in swimmers over the years imply that a new and expanded focus for rehabilitation and research is required.[31,57] This chapter provides a framework for the management of swimmers with shoulder pain based on best available evidence, the beliefs, needs, and values of swimmers, together with clinical experience. An understanding of the biomechanics of swimming, terminology, pathophysiology of the painful swimmer's shoulder, contributing factors, and appropriate assessment are the necessary foundations for prognosis, and rehabilitation.

Biomechanics of swimming

The shoulders are subjected to significant workloads during swimming, generating approximately 90% of the forward propulsion force.[24] To generate force effectively, swimmers' hands and arms change orientation, direction, and velocity to propel themselves forward in all four swimming strokes (freestyle, breaststroke, backstroke, and butterfly).[6,44]

Hydrodynamics, in part, relates to the forces acting upon solid bodies immersed in fluids. In comparison with air, high hydrodynamic resistance, including drag (resistance exerted by water) and wave turbulence is encountered in water, due to a swimmer's "form" or shape.[79,88] Streamlining both body and limb movements enables swimmers to form a torpedo-like shape which reduces resistance to forward motion in the water (Figure 39.1B).[48,78] Buoyancy also has an impact, causing the body to roll and tilt when the limbs move, and must be balanced to ensure the body position remains streamlined.[15] Effective swim technique reduces the work required at the shoulders, by both minimizing drag and counteracting buoyancy forces.

Freestyle is the fastest stroke style and comprises up to 80% of swim training for swimmers regardless of the swimmer's specialty stroke.[61] During freestyle, the body rolls 50–60° around its longitudinal axis, recruiting the large abdominal muscles and paraspinal muscles of the back to assist propulsion and breathing (Figure 39.1C).[44,79,86] An increase in body roll during a breath cycle can alter the

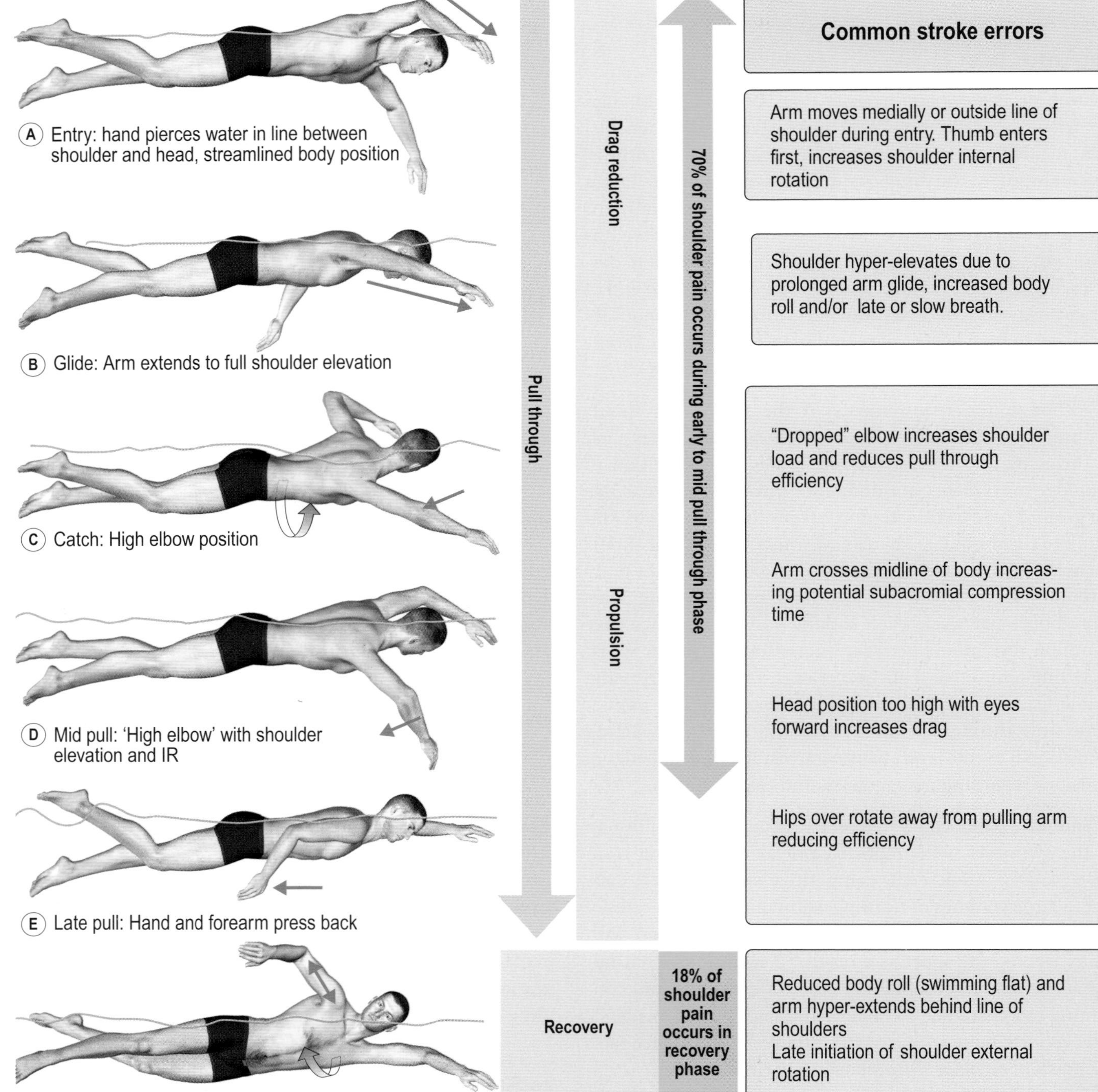

FIGURE 39.1
Freestyle stroke biomechanics and common stroke errors.

upper limb stroke action and must be well coordinated, while the arm action is balanced by a flutter kick generated at the hip (Figure 39.1C, F).[52]

The freestyle stroke comprises the *pull through* and *recovery* phases. A considerable lever arm force acts about the shoulder during the freestyle pull through, which is both long (65–71 cm) and deep (59–70 cm).[13] The *pull through* phase commences as the hand enters the water, midway between the shoulder and the body midline, fingers first (Figure 39.1A). The extended arm glides forward before the hand and forearm change orientation to "catch" the water as the shoulder internally rotates into a flexed, "high elbow" position and the elbow bends (Figure 39.1B, C).

During this early phase, swimmers seek to pull the body forward towards the arm (Figure 39.1C). In *mid pull through* the arm pulls towards the body midline as the shoulder extends and adducts, maintaining the flexed elbow as high as possible (Figure 39.1D). In *late pull through* the hand and arm are accelerated as they push out and back towards the hip (Figure 39.1E). The high elbow pull through enables swimmers to use their hand and forearm to maximize propulsion, however, this position requires considerable glenohumeral internal rotation in high range flexion (Figure 39.1C, D). During arm entry and pull through, swimmers actively upwardly rotate, protract and anteriorly tilt the scapula to maintain optimal glenohumeral alignment.[27]

The *recovery* phase commences when the hand and arm exit the water, oriented to minimize surface drag. The recovering arm is lifted in line with the shoulders with a bent, high elbow, assisted by torso rotation and shoulder external rotation (Figure 39.1F). Finally, the elbow extends as the shoulder is maximally abducted and somewhat internally rotated to optimally position the hand for entry. Unsurprisingly, shoulder pain occurs commonly during the longer, propulsive *pull through* (70%) and, to a lesser extent, during the *recovery* (18%).[61] During freestyle swimming, it is estimated that the shoulder may attain end of range positions during up to 25% of the stroke cycle, potentially promoting subacromial compression.[86] It is evident that the shoulder is vulnerable to injury during swimming, requiring considerable mobility, precision of movement control and strength.

Pathophysiology

Historically, the main anatomical structures considered in swimmers with shoulder pain have been the supraspinatus tendon, subacromial bursa, and long head of biceps. The concept that these structures become the source of pain stems back to the original description of "swimmer's shoulder" by Kennedy et al.,[43] and reflected the impingement model proposed by Neer[59] at that time. It was hypothesized that the repeated elevation of the arm during swimming compressed the supraspinatus tendon, subacromial bursa, and long head of biceps under the coracoacromial arch, resulting in tissue damage and pain. After swim training, supraspinatus tendon thickness increases in all shoulders, more so in swimmers with a history of shoulder pain.[62] Adaptive changes in the subacromial bursa with increasing amounts of swimming have also been reported, with acute bursal thickening shortly after a strenuous event being correlated to pain.[20] Both studies highlight the impact of the swimming action on this region of the shoulder.

Imaging techniques such as magnetic resonance imaging (MRI), have also consistently identified SLAP tears, paralabral cysts, and acromioclavicular joint changes.[10,11,71] Many of these changes are evident in swimmers with and without shoulder symptoms. As such, the relationship between the observed changes in these studies and symptoms remains uncertain. The findings of a more recent MRI study examining elite swimmers, some with a history of pain but all continuing to compete at the highest level, further confirmed the presence of such changes with 15–20% of swimmers in the study reported as having changes in the labrum, biceps tendon and acromioclavicular joint, as well as identifying lesser tuberosity bony edema, and subscapularis tendinopathy.[41] Significantly, the most commonly identified findings were tendinopathic changes, observed in over 70% of swimmers' supraspinatus and subscapularis tendons. A correlation between years swum and degree of subscapularis tendinopathy was also identified.

Tendinopathic change is the predominant pathological process observed in the shoulders of swimmers, affecting the supraspinatus, subscapularis, and long head of biceps tendons.[41,71] While the frequency of tendinopathy and prevalence of shoulder pain in swimmers are both high, and there is a strong correlation between the presence and severity of tendinopathy and pain,[20] further research is required to confirm that tendinopathic changes may be a source of shoulder pain in swimmers. Shoulder tendons are designed to tolerate compressive and tensile forces,[46] but the number of stroke cycles may overwhelm the structural integrity of these structures, resulting in intrinsic and possibly concomitant extrinsic changes.[72]

Extrinsic factors are forces external to the tendon that cause compressive loading of the tendon. Subacromial compression hypothesized by Hawkins and Kennedy[36] as the primary cause of shoulder pain in swimmers is one potential source of external load on the tendon. More recently, it has been suggested that during the elevated and internally rotated positions of the glenohumeral joint required for swimming, there is also internal contact or impingement of the underside of the supraspinatus, bicep, and subscapularis tendons onto the anterior superior and posterior superior labrum.[23,68] This may be unavoidable normal physiological contact of these tendons during the swimming stroke, and would explain the high prevalence of tendinopathy and labral changes seen in the swimming shoulder. Increases in tendon loading behavior are commonly associated with the onset of pain,[16] and these structures may be the primary source of shoulder pain in swimmers. It is important to acknowledge, however, that we currently do not know if this is correct or fully understand why swimmers experience pain.

Assessing the shoulder in swimmers

Pain is most commonly reported by swimmers in the anterosuperior shoulder, experienced during or after swimming. Diffuse pain and posterior shoulder pain may be reported, as well as pain in the region of the biceps.[61] In addition to the pathophysiology discussed above, clinicians must consider other potential sources of symptoms in the shoulder region including red flags, cervical/thoracic dysfunction, uni-/multidirectional shoulder instability,[22] acromioclavicular joint pathology (including osteolysis, os acromiale), suprascapular neuropathy,[1] quadrilateral space syndrome, brachial neuritis, thoracic outlet syndrome, upper rib stress reactions,[80] visceral referral, and vascular compromise.

Swimming-specific questions

A thorough subjective examination is important in any assessment and the following specific questions are relevant when presented with a swimmer with shoulder pain.

Load

Most swimmers' shoulder pain is associated with overload, and is diagnosed as rotator cuff-related shoulder pain[31,45] (see Chapters 19 and 36). Detailed questioning related to changes in training or other factors influencing tendon load tolerance is essential (Box 39.1). Such factors include genetics and lifestyle, including stress and sleep deprivation, both common in elite sport.

Although the contribution of load or volume of training and its association to injury has been reported in other sports,[33] an examination of the literature related to training load in swimming would suggest that a clear relationship has not yet been established. While Sein et al.[71] identified

39.1 Specific questions for the swimmer with shoulder pain

- Timing of onset of symptoms: during (start or end) training or after, within specific sets/drills/sessions.
- Length of time that symptoms persist after training, night pain, impact on activities of daily living.
- Stroke type/specialty and phase of stroke that symptoms occur.
- Any change in training load: frequency/speed/sets/stroke focus/technique/squad level/coach (preceding 2–3 weeks).
- Change in resting heart rate or self-reported fatigue levels.
- Use of equipment: kickboard, hand paddles, elastic cords, pull buoy.
- Training and competition level: frequency/timing/history.
- Gym training/other activities/warm-up routine.
- Previous musculoskeletal injuries and comorbidities, growth spurt.
- Family history of hypermobility.

an increased presence of supraspinatus tendinopathy in swimmers who swam more than 15 hours or 35 kilometers (21.7 miles) per week, these macroscopic tendon changes did not correlate with pain. Furthermore, studies examining absolute training mileage have failed to find a link between volume and symptoms.[66,81] However, in a survey of 927 swimmers, Stocker et al.[73] reported that over 50% of those experiencing persistent and troublesome shoulder pain believed that an increase in training distance or speed was a precipitating factor in the onset of their shoulder symptoms.

The authors of this chapter have observed that changes in training, particularly increasing intensity (meaning in this case, speed, or pace of swim training), in addition to volume (distance) or frequency, coincide with the onset of shoulder symptoms. Evidence of increased shoulder injury in young swimmers when there is a sudden increase in training load[30,31] supports a relationship between swimming load and shoulder pain. Current understanding is that the main factor for the onset of pain is a change in load on the tendon, rather than the total load.[33] If correct, this suggests that controlling load is a key factor when managing a swimmer with shoulder pain. Monitoring heart rate and swim session rating for perceived exertion (modified Borg scale RPE: 0–10) is a useful self-reported measure recommended to track a swimmer's internal load (response to external load of training), to help establish appropriate recovery periods between sessions.[3,32,87]

Previous history

Previous shoulder pain appears to be predictive for developing subsequent pain in swimmers.[39,81] Swimmers with a history of shoulder pain are up to 11 times more likely to experience shoulder pain that interferes with training and performance.[12,81] Athletes have a higher tolerance to pain compared with non-athletes,[77] and many young swimmers believe that shoulder pain is normal, continuing to train despite its presence.[37,57] Respecting this, the regular use of pain scales may help identify variations by placing symptom intensity on a continuum.[26] Enquiring if the pain is remaining tolerable during swimming and resolves immediately after also assists swimmers to communicate their experience of pain (Box 39.2).

Box 39.2 Staging swimmers' shoulder pain training response

1 to 4 = low to high level pain and disability:

1. Pain during certain strokes/some (but not all) sessions or experienced for <2 hours post training.
2. Pain during part of every training session and/or after every session.
3. Pain during 50–70% of every training session and after lasting >2 hours post training.
4. Pain that consistently impacts training and performance/unable to train or compete.

Physical assessment

Numerous factors associated with shoulder pain in swimmers are described in the literature, yet conclusions around causation and risk are limited.[30,39] A multitude of modifiable and non-modifiable factors are likely to contribute, in what can be described as a complex web of determinants,[5] unique to each swimmer. The physical assessment is likely to include: examination of the cervical and thoracic spine; acromioclavicular joint; active and passive range of shoulder movement; glenohumeral joint instability; shoulder and kinetic chain strength/endurance testing; and neurological assessment when indicated.

Although shoulder injury prevention data are lacking for the swimming population, the swimming-specific tests summarized in Figure 39.2 are validated, and provide a useful screening and initial assessment guide, with optimal ranges based on functional requirements of swimming where evidence is lacking. These tests (Figure 39.2) assess factors that affect the swimmer's ability to perform an efficient swim stroke; for example, limited shoulder flexion and thoracic extension (combined elevation test) will restrict achievement of streamline position.

Collection of baseline data for swimmers' shoulder strength, endurance, scapular upward rotation, and range of movement at the start of rehabilitation or in a pain-free state at the start of the season, will help identify deficits and/or provide a baseline for future comparison.

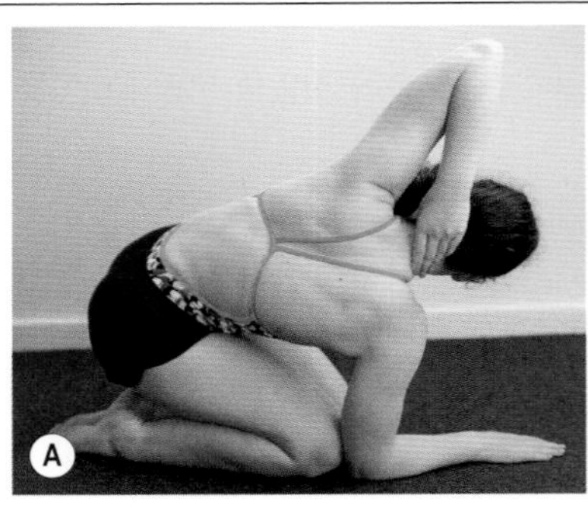

Test
Locked lumbothoracic rotation[29,42]

Recommended ranges
Thoracic rotation:
60–70° each side

Functional relevance
Body/thoracic rotation in water; to avoid increased horizontal extension of shoulder in recovery phase

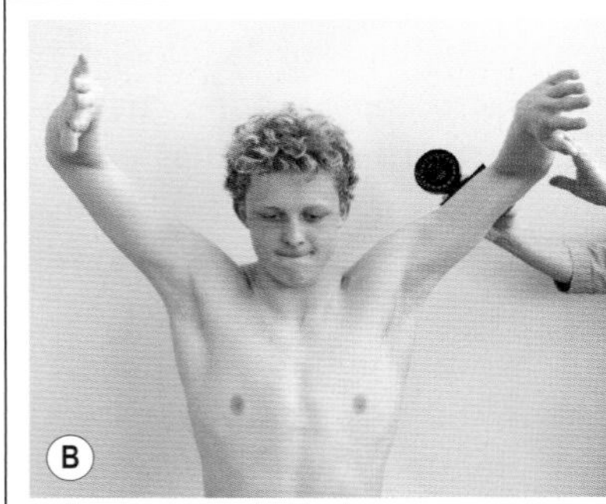

Test
Shoulder abduction in internal rotation[82]

Recommended ranges
Active shoulder abduction:
150–170°

Functional relevance
High elbow position during pull through and recovery phases

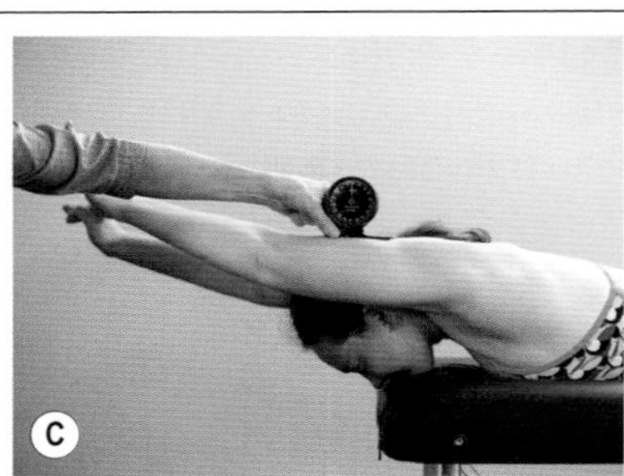

Test
Combined elevation[82]

Recommended ranges
Active elevation: 5–15°
Observe for thoracic extension or latissimus dorsi length

Functional relevance
Achievement of streamlined position

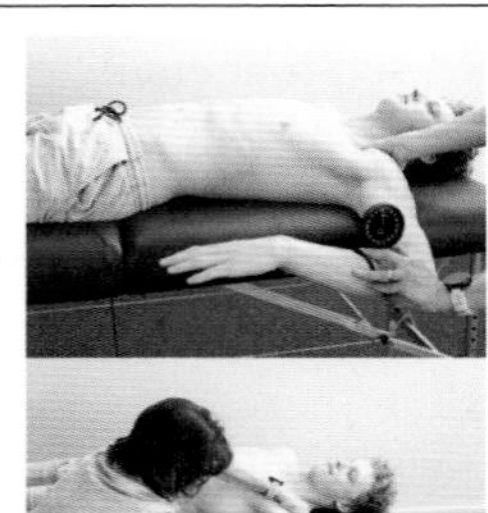

Test
Active range of shoulder internal and external rotation at 90° abduction[81,82]

Recommended ranges
Internal rotation: 40–50°
External rotation: 90–100°

Functional relevance
Internal rotation range required throughout stroke; external range increases through recovery phase

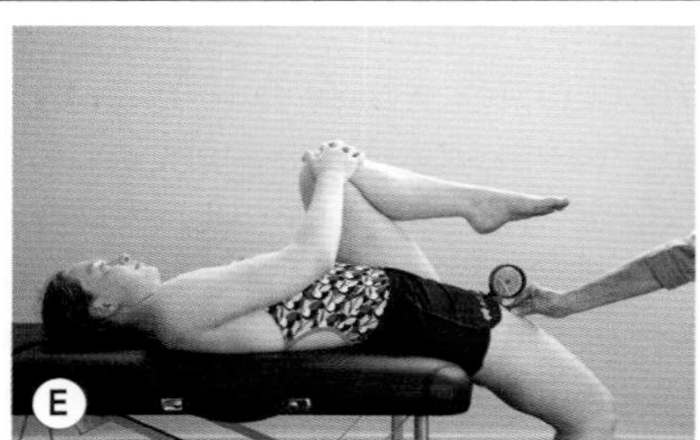

Test
Thomas test for hip extension[14]

Recommended ranges
Hip extension 20–30°

Functional relevance
Achieve streamlined position; kick without excessive lumbar extension; starts and turns

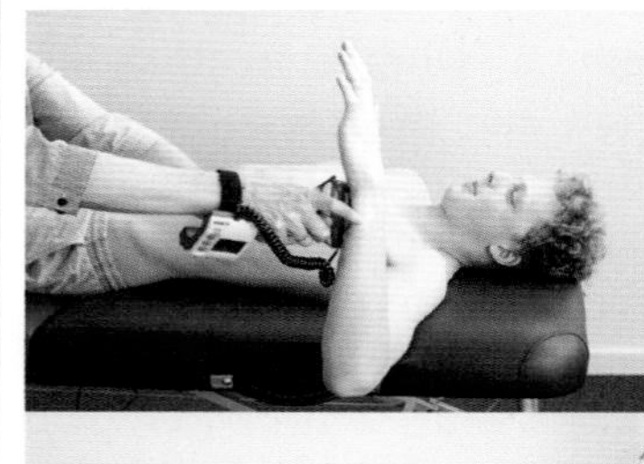

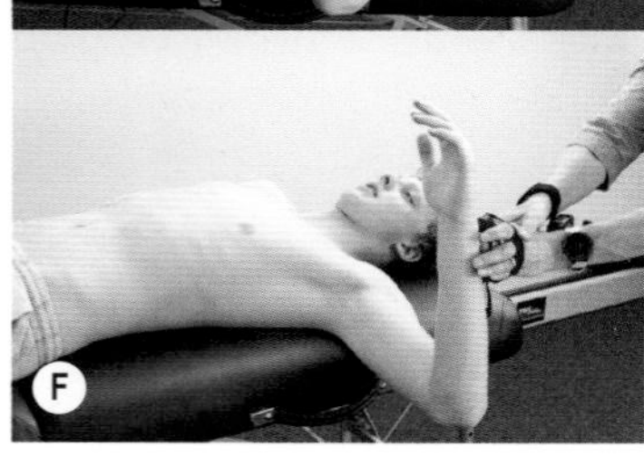

Test
Isometric shoulder strength internal and external rotation at 90° abduction[55]

Recommended ranges
See Table 39.1 for normative data

Functional relevance
Shoulder strength and control for early pull through and recovery phase

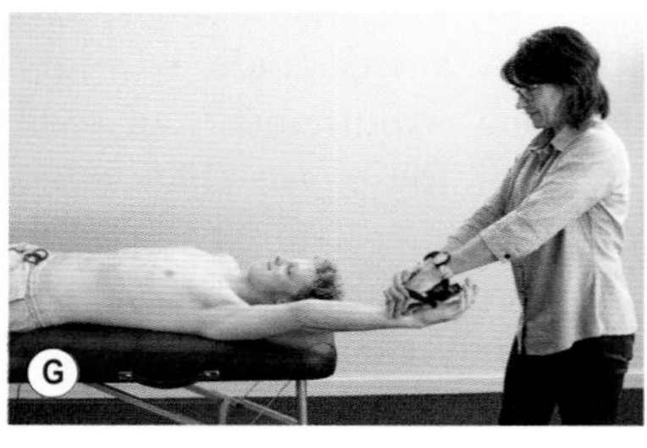

Test
Shoulder extension strength at 140° abduction in scapular plane[54,55]

Recommended ranges
See Table 39.1 for normative data

Functional relevance
Shoulder strength and control for early pull through, propulsive phase, freestyle speed

FIGURE 39.2
Physical tests recommended for shoulder assessment in swimmers.

Range of movement

Swimmers move efficiently through the water by achieving large ranges of shoulder flexion and rotation combined with thoracic rotation, extension, and body roll. Limitations in regions other than the shoulder can affect the body's position in the water; for example, restricted thoracic extension or rib cage expansion due to tight rectus abdominus, hip extension (Figure 39.2E) and even ankle plantar flexion range can impact body position and kick effectiveness, increasing load on the shoulder. Such considerations might be particularly important for triathletes who are required to be efficient swimmers but spend long periods of time cycling, potentially leading to thoracic stiffness and reduced hip extension.

Thoracic rotation and extension in the streamline position can be measured using the locked-lumbar rotation test and combined elevation test as described in Figure 39.2.[29,42,82] Active range of shoulder rotation measured using an inclinometer in supine is a valid and reliable assessment for swimmers (Figure 39.2D).[82] Swimmers with high (≥100°) or low (<93°) shoulder external rotation range may be at risk of developing shoulder pain.[81] Evidence remains equivocal, but low shoulder internal rotation and flexion range (Figure 39.2D), may also contribute to shoulder pain in swimmers.[39,76]

When a swimmer trains at higher speeds, rating a session as very hard (5–9 RPE) or fatiguing, external rotation range decreases immediately and remains so for 6 hours post training, with uncertainty as to when this range is restored.[38,51,87] Monitoring shoulder external rotation range as previously described (Figure 39.2D) weekly or fortnightly for swimmers training competitively, may be helpful in determining whether a swimmer has adequately recovered this motion. If other factors such as thoracic rotation or thoracic extension range, (Figure 39.2A, C) or trunk control are limited, then the ability to effectively perform the swim stroke may be impeded, particularly in the presence of limited shoulder external rotation.

Humeral torsion is the angle made by the humeral head and humeral shaft. In throwing athletes this angle is not symmetrical side to side and is greater in the throwing shoulder (see Chapters 2 and 38).[84] In the non-throwing population as well as in swimmers, the angle bilaterally is symmetrical, and in swimmers is not associated with shoulder pain.[40]

Shoulder strength

Assessment of maximal force production is one aspect of shoulder muscle performance in the swimmer that can be performed easily and reliably in the clinic using handheld dynamometry (HHD).[25,56] Shoulder internal and external rotation, and extension isometric muscle testing (see Figure 39.2) forms an important part of the physical examination of the shoulder, and normative data for pain-free swimming populations are available for comparison. It is important to note that many factors impact force output including test protocol, motivation, pain, and position of the limb and swimmer. For valid comparisons, the population and testing protocols described in Table 39.1 should be considered. The strong evidence for symmetrical shoulder strength in swimmers, allows the clinician to validly compare the symptomatic with the asymptomatic shoulder, and set goals for rehabilitation.[7,55]

During internal and external rotation muscle testing, groups of muscles including the rotator cuff and axioscapular muscles are challenged; however, the motor strategy during external rotation favors supraspinatus and infraspinatus over subscapularis and during internal rotation, subscapularis is significantly more active in torque production than the posterior cuff.[8,21] If identified, a reduction in force over time may be related to the swimmer's capacity to tolerate load around the shoulder. The authors suggest that the presence of pain considered to be originating from tendon may reduce internal or external rotation force, indicating value in monitoring force production over time.[8,87]

Shoulder internal to external rotation strength ratios (IR/ER) in swimmers have been frequently reported, ranging from 1.1 for masters and developing swimmers,[50,64] to 1.4 for elite swimmers.[7] Certainly, in the presence of shoulder instability, shoulder muscle balance and strength is important. Strength ratios favor the internal rotators over external rotators,[7,55,64] such as in other sports such as throwing, but there is no consensus that any muscle imbalance around the swimmer's shoulder results in pain.[39] It is likely that IR/ER strength ratios in swimmers fluctuate, evidenced through increased internal shoulder rotation force output over a swimming season, and reduced external rotation force after a training session.[64,87] Given that internal or external rotation force outputs may vary, HHD monitoring of absolute shoulder rotation strength (see Table 39.1), rather than a strength ratio, is more informative.

Table 39.1 Isometric shoulder strength values (% body weight) measured using a handheld dynamometer

Shoulder strength test	Trained male*	Trained female*	Elite male#	Elite female#
Internal rotation	25	20	29	26
External rotation	21	18	19	18
Flexion	13	11	Not known	Not known
Extension	15	12	Not known	Not known

*Trained: swim training at least 6 hours per week (n=170 shoulders; mean age 15.5 years); rotation "make" tests performed in supine at 90° shoulder abduction; flexion/extension tests performed in supine at 140° shoulder abduction.[55]

#Elite: qualified for at least two national swimming championships (n=136 shoulders; mean age 19.9 years); "break" tests performed in standing, neutral shoulder position.[7]

Shoulder extension strength in full flexion is required for a strong pull through force and correlates with freestyle swim speed.[2] In growing male swimmers, low shoulder extension strength, less than 13.5% of body weight, measured with HHD (Figure 39.2G), may be a factor contributing to the development of shoulder pain.[54]

Muscle performance in swimmers warrants further investigation, including parameters such as rate of force development, endurance, and force production in relation to training load changes.

Kinetic chain and scapular movement

Assessment of the kinetic chain and scapular movement is recommended in swimming-related positions. The commonly performed timed front and side plank[76] or superman position in four-point kneeling, are appropriate options when assessing swimmers. The "catch test" or resisted overhead shoulder extension performed in standing (Figure 39.3) also challenges the kinetic chain. It may be provocative for pain, replicating the catch position in swimming.

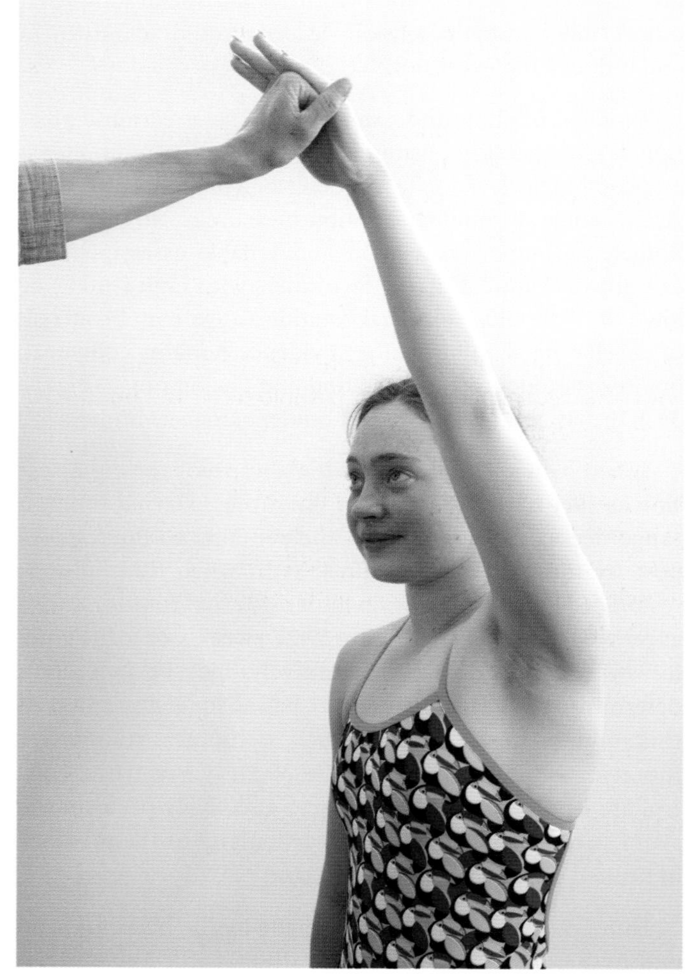

FIGURE 39.3
Catch test.

Scapular upward rotation is essential to achieve full shoulder flexion range, maintain optimal subacromial space[27] and optimize muscle length–tension relationships throughout the swim stroke. Large ranges of scapular upward rotation are seen in elite swimmers, demonstrated by the inferior scapular angles positioned lateral to the trunk when the arms are in elevation. Although there is no evidence that scapular dyskinesis is a risk factor for shoulder pain,[30,74] insufficient scapular upward rotation is associated with shoulder pain in overhead athletes[18] and may result from muscle inhibition or fatigue in swimmers.[49,75]

The authors recommend observing for symmetrical scapular upward rotation movement and endurance during shoulder circumduction in prone (see Figure 39.4I). The arms should clear the bench/floor when repeated at least five times. If symptomatic, manual facilitation of scapular upward rotation may improve symptoms and direct treatment.[47] Low endurance of the posterior shoulder and scapular muscles in young swimmers has been included in a predictive model for the development of shoulder pain and is assessed in prone holding the shoulder in horizontal extension at 90° abduction, with load added according to body weight.[28,30]

Flexibility may also affect scapular movement, so muscle length tests for the propulsive muscles, latissimus dorsi, and pectoral group as well as the posterior rotator cuff, are relevant.[76] The assessment of shoulder strength, range of movement, and scapular position while the swimmer is in a fatigued state may be more informative, given the repetitive nature of the sport.

Laxity

Shoulder joint laxity and instability are different entities, with the second considered pathological, yet both have been investigated as possible risk factors for shoulder pain in swimmers. Positive clinical tests of glenohumeral joint laxity are more common in elite swimmers[68,89] and not associated with shoulder pain,[9,81] whereas a feeling of looseness, reported by swimmers (perhaps due to ineffective muscle control), is associated with shoulder pain.[39,76] When combined with a positive subjective report, the apprehension test and anterior/posterior glide tests may help confirm a shoulder instability diagnosis.

To date, proprioception has not been investigated as a risk factor for shoulder pain in swimmers. Research has returned equivocal findings regarding shoulder joint position sense and fatigue in swimmers.[38,51,87]

Summary of physical signs and symptoms

Training responses (see Box 39.2) and signs and symptoms (Box 39.3) are presented as stages within a continuum, and provide a framework around which rehabilitation of the swimmer will be presented.

Box 39.3 Staging signs and symptoms for swimmers with shoulder pain

1 to 4 = low to high level disability:

1. Reduced strength measures from baseline, normative data or opposite side; and/or decreased passive range of movement.
2. Above plus pain on resisted external/internal rotation/extension/catch tests.
3. Above plus pain on any resisted tests and end range active movements.
4. Above plus pain onset early in active range of movement; constant pain during ADL and impacting sleep.

Investigations

Although training load modification and graduated rehabilitation are the first line of management for most presentations, imaging performed during stages 3–4 (see Box 39.2) may be helpful to rule out significant pathology, guide rehabilitation, and inform decision-making around injection therapies for those with constant pain. In these settings, MRI is the recommended investigation; however, as structural changes often do not correlate with symptoms, all imaging should be interpreted thoughtfully, with consideration given to training load history when tendinopathic changes are present.[11,35,41] Clinicians should note that chronic bursal thickening in swimmers who are training regularly is adaptive and correlates poorly with pain; however, evidence does suggest a correlation of pain with acute bursal thickening after a single endurance event and rotator cuff tendinopathy severity (on ultrasound assessment).[20]

Management and rehabilitation

The management of swimmers' shoulder pain is based on the guiding principle of unloading then reloading the shoulder by implementing a graded program that may include training modifications, stroke correction, education (including pain management), exercise, and manual therapy.

These principles are relevant in the case of rotator cuff-related shoulder pain, instability, and other shoulder pain pathologies.

Swimmers of any level can experience shoulder pain and will present with different impairments and goals. While shoulder pain in competitive swimmers is most often related to overload, stroke correction may be a higher priority for the less experienced swimmer. For many recreational swimmers, especially older cohorts, range of movement and technique modification may be the focus of management. Setting realistic expectations and timeframes will help maintain motivation and compliance.

Load management

A training load reduction can be considered with respect to training time/distance, frequency, intensity, stroke type and training history. While stoppping swimming in stages 1 and 2 is not necessary, load management in stage 3 may escalate to a reduction in training frequency, progressing to time out of the water in cases of unremitting pain in stage 4.

Firstly, to effectively modify load in swimmers with shoulder pain, an understanding of swim biomechanics is important. Common freestyle stroke errors (see Figure 39.1) should be addressed, including incorrect arm and hand entry position and a "dropped elbow" during the early pull through and recovery, as they affect execution of the whole stroke and may predispose to injury.[30,70,86] Secondly, to implement a load modification plan, communication with coaches is essential. For most swimmers, load on the shoulder can be reduced through changes to stroke technique which can be assisted by video analysis, both in and out of water. Often issues with technique can be correlated with physical assessment findings (for example, limited shoulder internal rotation and dropped elbow position), highlighting the importance of coach and therapist collaboration.

Swimmers with painful rotator cuff-related shoulder pain should not train to fatigue. Based on ultrasound findings, up to 24 hours may be required to settle supraspinatus tendon thickness to baseline levels in swimmers with previous shoulder pain[53,62] so swim training should be limited to at most once per day or alternate days if swimmers are returning from complete rest. Any increases in distance, frequency and speed of swimming should be gradual, while monitoring the response to load within the individual session and in the 24 hours after. When swimmers progress to more than one session per day, consider the type of training effort performed. High intensity (sprint) sessions result in both increased supraspinatus tendon thickness and time required to return to baseline (24 hours) compared with long distance sessions (6 hours).[63] Similarly, after high-intensity swim sessions, shoulder external rotation range and peak isometric rotation torque is reduced, compared with low-intensity training.[87] As such, adequate recovery time (24 hours) must be allowed after high-intensity sessions for swimmers training regularly.

Equipment is to be used with care. Kickboard use in shoulder elevation is provocative for shoulder pain due to the board's buoyancy, pushing the shoulders into higher than usual levels of elevation. Hand paddles will increase resistance during the pull-through phase, adding load to the shoulder, and so should be avoided in the presence of shoulder pain. Fins can help to unload the shoulder and allow time to focus on technique, but an extended glide on hand entry, placing the shoulder into a hyper-elevated position for a lengthy period, must be avoided. A swim snorkel can be used in the case of cervical referred shoulder pain or if pain is reproduced during a breath cycle.

Box 39.4 Biomechanical tips to help reduce swimmers' shoulder pain

- Ensure body roll to avoid hyperextending the shoulder, especially if shoulder range is limited.
- Enter water with fingers not the thumb, between head and same shoulder.
- Shorten swim stroke in hand entry to avoid pain in shoulder elevation.
- Do not pull across the midline of the body during the pull phase.
- Keep head in the water, look to armpit to breathe.
- A swimming technique assessment is recommended.

For the competitive (or regularly trained) swimmer who may have ceased swimming in stage 4, or modified training in stages 1–3, the following loading advice should be considered before returning to regular swimming training.

- Avoid squad training initially to prevent competitiveness and going further or faster than prescribed.
- Begin with shorter intervals and adequate rest between repeats to minimize fatigue. Intervals could be as short as 50–100 m if starting from a period of complete rest.
- Increase volume gradually, 10–20% per week.
- Add intensity/speed to sessions only after initially increasing total distance swum to approximately 70% of original volume.
- During stages 1 and 2, complete kick sets and sculling with hands at hips or at chest height. This promotes maintenance of swim-specific fitness and strength throughout the kinetic chain.
- Fins used during warm-up and cool-down may allow swimmers in stages 1 and 2 to complete their main training effort.
- Swimming butterfly stroke is inadvisable, and freestyle is preferable in the initial stages.

A review of daily activities and dry land/strength training will also help identify potential load contributors that can be modified. For example, triceps dips can add to compressive and tensile load of the long head of biceps tendon. Non-provocative land-based exercises can continue. Cycling may be a preferable option for maintaining cardiovascular fitness, as even walking and running can aggravate a shoulder that has become highly symptomatic in stage 4.

Pain management and education

A challenge for the clinician is both in educating the swimmer to differentiate between acceptable discomfort that recovers and persistent pain during training, along with ensuring adherence to the graduated reloading program. Interventions to help manage pain may be as simple as minimizing aggravating positions or activities in stages 1 and 2, using ice after training or other pain-modulating modalities such as exercise (isometric or other), taping, or manual therapy.

Nonsteroidal anti-inflammatory medication or other analgesics may be beneficial in stages 3 and 4. During stage 4, a cortisone injection may be considered if the shoulder is not settling with rest and imaging findings are clinically relevant. Cervical and thoracic spine mobilization and soft tissue release around the posterior rotator cuff, subscapularis and scapulothoracic muscles may assist with pain modulation and allow the swimmer to exercise into previously painful ranges, relevant throughout stages 1–4.

Exercise

Range of movement exercise

Regaining range of movement through the shoulder and body is an important part of a swimmer's management program. When swimmers are hypermobile it is likely that reduced internal rotation range of motion will respond quickly to soft tissue manual therapy. The sleeper stretch can be helpful to maintain post-treatment range gains, if achievable and indicated (see Chapter 10). Slow, sustained stretching of large muscle groups such as the pectorals and latissimus dorsi are recommended but partner stretching is not advised due to the risk of uncontrolled over-stretching.

Strengthening exercise

Shoulder

A graded loading program addressing specific identified deficits will progress from simple isometric exercises in non-provocative positions, increasing to higher loads, ranges, and complexity. Handheld dynamometry normative values are very useful for the clinician to set rehabilitation goals, quantify improvement, assess load tolerance, and determine readiness to progress swim training and exercises (see Table 39.1). Ideally, dynamometry results should be at least 80% when compared with previous values before returning to full training.

Initially, clinicians will commonly prescribe strength exercises focusing on shoulder rotation, often with the use of resistance cords. However, before resisted shoulder rotation exercises are introduced, flexion and extension or pushing and pulling, can offer direction-specific rotator cuff activation[83] and potentially pain modulation. For example, pain-free, isometric extension in neutral is an effective way to activate subscapularis in a swimmer's shoulder during stage 4. Aiming to minimize combined compressive and tensile load on the rotator cuff and biceps tendons,[4] loading in a supported, neutral shoulder position, is often more tolerable during this early strengthening phase (Figure 39.4A). Similarly, progressing shoulder flexion from a supported, isometric hold then supine press, before standing resisted flexion, will increase posterior cuff activity gradually.[83] Monitoring response to resisted exercises is particularly important in stages 3 and 4 when increased pain over 24 hours (or night pain) due to high irritability is an indication to modify exercises.

Resistance exercises for swimmers in stage 1 can be based on HHD results if pain free. Slow concentric and eccentric strength exercises may progress to focus on specific stroke phases, for example, concentric internal rotation exercises (pull through in the water) and eccentric external rotation/posterior muscle endurance exercises (recovery to hand entry control). The addition of a scapular resistance band to resisted internal and external rotation exercises (Figure 39.4C) encourages scapulothoracic and rotator cuff muscle activation.[34,65] Strengthening exercises performed into scapular upward rotation are important, especially for symptomatic shoulder instability. The shrug exercise, focusing on scapular elevator muscle strengthening in low ranges, may progress to elevated shoulder ranges (Figure 39.4H). Exercise progressions are premature if this position of upward rotation cannot be maintained with added load or complexity. Progression into elevated ranges will also help facilitate serratus anterior activation,[17] which like subscapularis, is active throughout the swim stroke, and subject to fatigue.[60] Addition of exercises in swim-specific positions incorporating the kinetic chain is encouraged and enhance shoulder muscle contribution.[67] Figure 39.4 provides ideas for shoulder exercise progressions for swimmers, utilizing support in the early phases, progressing to unsupported positions where speed and swim-specific or chaotic movements can be introduced.

Kinetic chain

In the open environment of water, maintaining the hip-trunk-shoulder connection is vital for the swimmer and will improve with exercises challenging the kinetic chain. Exercises that include trunk rotation, integration of the oblique abdominals, and some degree of body extension are recommended. Exercises such as front or side plank and rotation can assist combining control of body roll and shoulder muscle engagement. Other examples include "dead bugs", push-ups with hip extension and thoracic rotation with resistance. Complexity can be increased with the use of gym balls, bands, reduced base of support and increasing load and speed, depending on goals.

Manual therapy

Manual therapy can address any swimming-specific loss of range of motion observed in assessment or through the season. Performed in functional swim positions, for example, ¾ prone, restrictions in thoracic rotation range of motion and extension can be addressed with various manual therapy techniques. Changes in shoulder rotation range of motion post swim training[87] should be addressed with appropriate manual therapy. External rotation range of motion deficits can be addressed with soft tissue releases to the pectoral muscle group and subscapularis belly with the shoulder in varying degrees of abduction and external rotation. A mainstay of manual therapy for swimmers is soft tissue massage to the posterior rotator shoulder and latissimus dorsi in the side-lying high elbow position to help maintain end range shoulder flexion.

Self-management

Swimmers of all levels are encouraged and educated to self-manage to achieve and maintain the mobility, strength and endurance levels that are so important for optimal form in the water. Range of motion maintenance may include foam roller thoracic spine extension with arms overhead in streamline (Figure 39.5), in addition to pectoral, hip flexor, latissimus dorsi and levator scapulae muscle stretches. Thoracic rotation mobility exercises such as "bow and arrow" and "thread the needle" are frequently performed as part of a dynamic warm-up or land-based mobility program. Equipment to assist self-management, such as spikey massage balls, resistance bands, rollers, and gym balls are commonly used.

Surgery

In the case of rotator cuff-related pain in the swimmer, surgery is not commonly required and should only be considered after a period (at least 6–12 months) of high-quality rehabilitation where the swimmer is engaged and committed

Exercise	Suggested progression

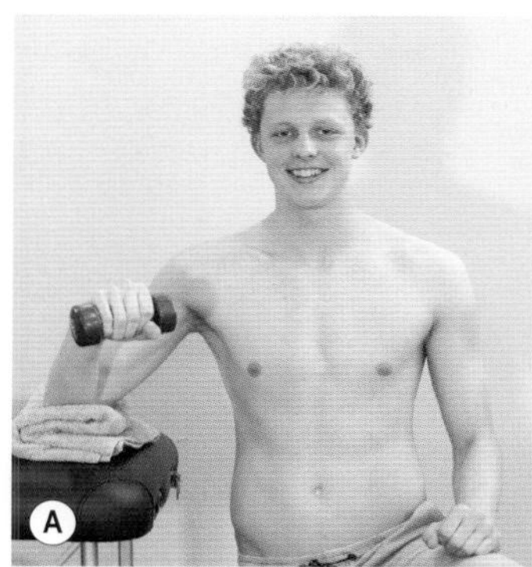
Resisted shoulder ER: arm supported, low range in scapular plane

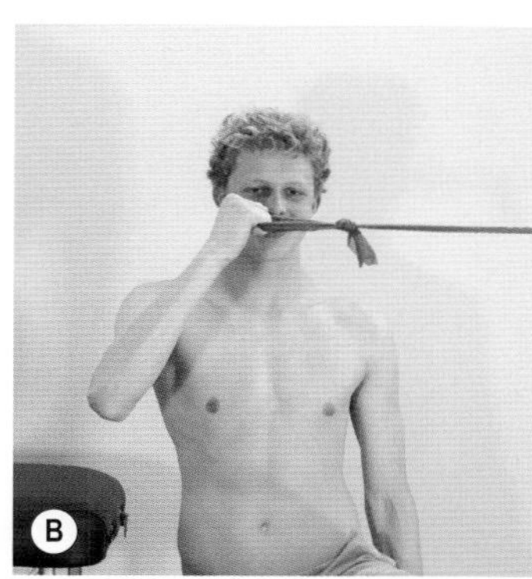
Unsupported arm, increases the challenge of ER exercise

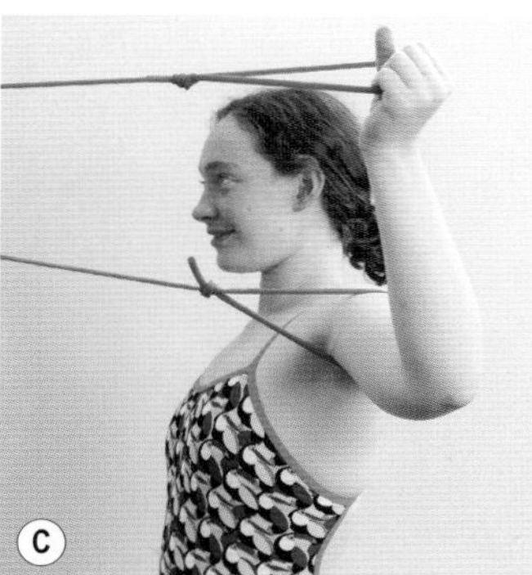
Scapular band ER

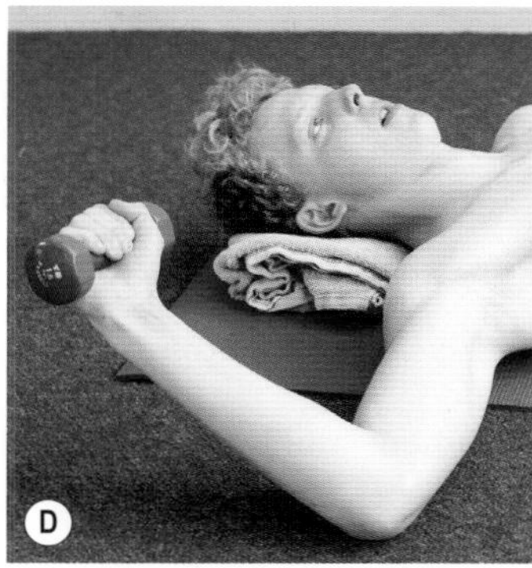
Resisted IR, supported arm, slow eccentric phase

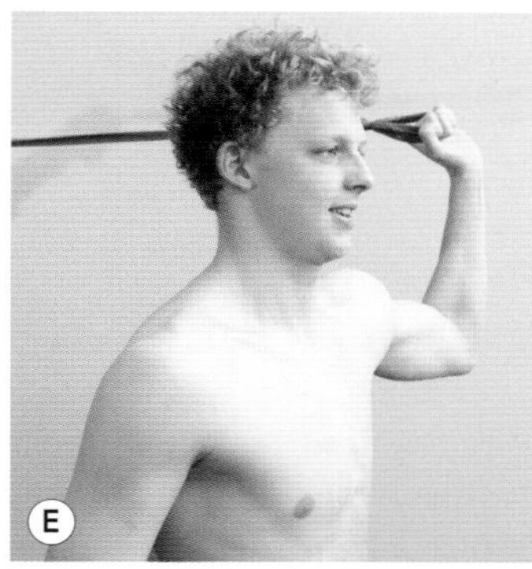
IR unsupported arm in shoulder abduction

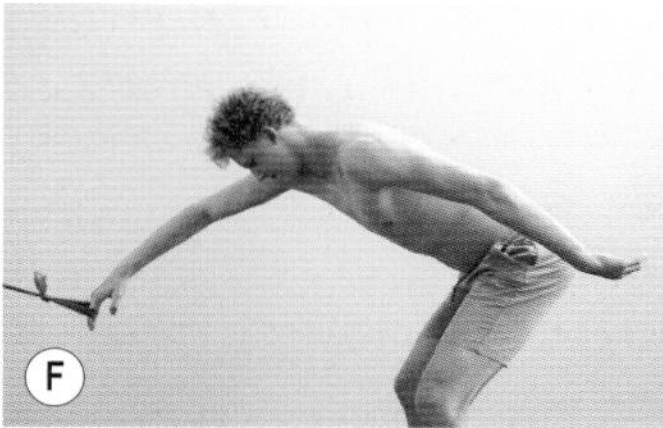
IR in replicated swim pull through position

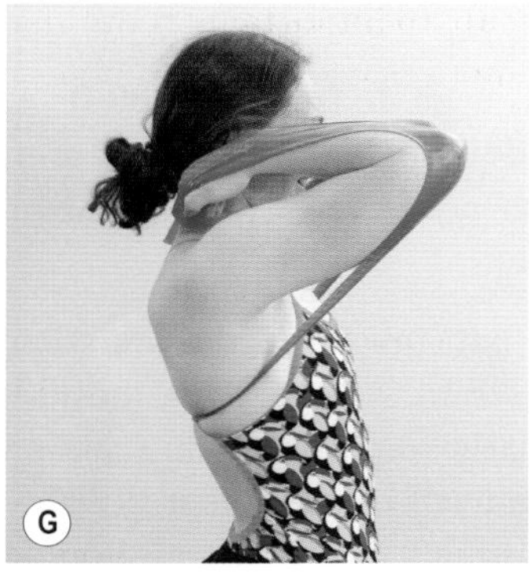
Scapular upward rotation

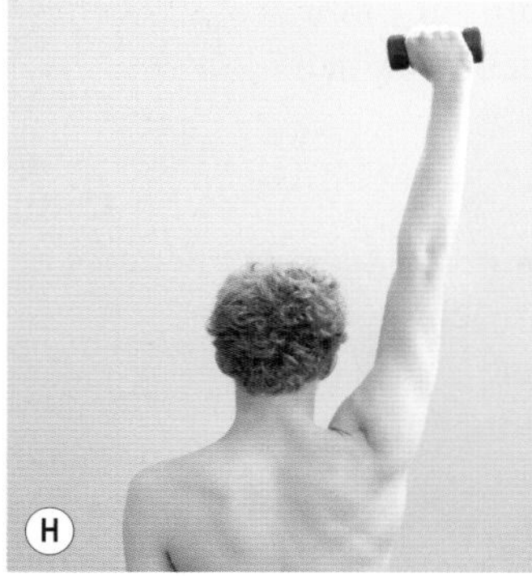
Shrug in elevation

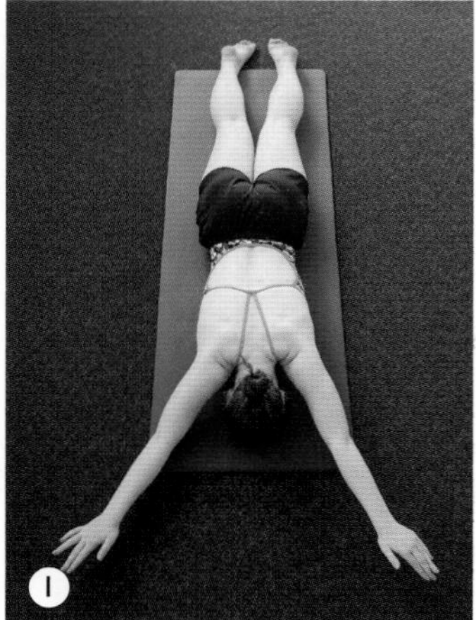
Prone retraction hold

FIGURE 39.4
Examples of graded exercise progressions for resisted external rotation (ER), internal rotation (IR) and scapular upward rotation.

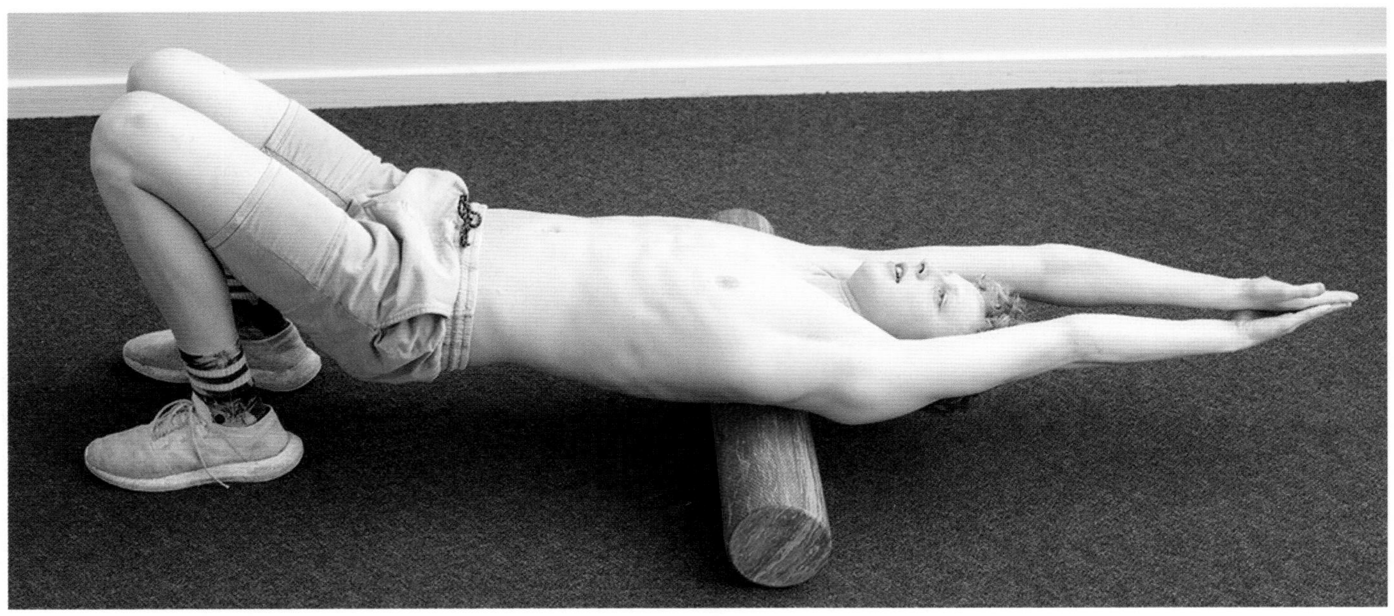

FIGURE 39.5
Thoracic extension with arms in streamline reach.

to their exercise program. A longer period may be required for a swimmer who presents at stage 4. Outcomes from surgical procedures including bursectomy, labral repair or debridement are poor, with low rates reported (20–56%) for returning to previous training levels.[10,58] Slow improvements may be quantified via HHD, which can be more informative than other signs and symptoms, such as pain.

Prevention

Despite current equivocal research findings for shoulder injury prevention in swimmers, a logical approach based on the goals of minimizing drag forces, increasing ease of propulsion and managing load, is likely to reduce injury risk and improve performance for swimmers of any level. The development of a trusting relationship between the swimmer, medical team and coach is a key factor for injury prevention at the elite level.

A swim-specific assessment is recommended for anyone commencing swimming, particularly as an adult beginner. Starting with two to three 30-minute swimming sessions a week, a gradual load progression can include the use of fins to allow technique development along with strength and fitness over time.

A gym-based program incorporating shoulders, kinetic chain, trunk strength, and endurance in ranges specific to swimming, would help to achieve swimming-specific goals. Targeted shoulder strength exercises can be goal-driven using normative data as a guide (see Table 39.1). As gym programs provide an additional load to large amounts of swim training, attention needs to be given to swimmers' tolerance of the total load.

Warm-up sessions that involve large muscle group activity and movements into swim-specific positions are recommended, particularly for the growing swimmer as their body awareness and self-management skills develop. Some examples include squats with bilateral shoulder flexion, lunges with thoracic rotation, and exercises shown in Figure 39.4. Participation in other sports and exercise is encouraged in the developing swimmer and is associated with shoulder injury risk reduction.[76] Successful injury prevention programs are those that are simple, with high athlete compliance and positive expectations.[19]

In a sport where large ranges of shoulder motion are reached repeatedly, and the frequency of shoulder symptoms is high, close monitoring of load and physical signs (see Figure 39.2) is important. In this way, shoulder issues can be identified and managed early, leading to successful outcomes. The strategies discussed in this chapter can be used as an approach to shoulder injury prevention and rehabilitation for swimmers of any age and level of experience.

References

1. Arriaza R, Ballesteros J, Lopez-Vidriero E. Suprascapular neuropathy as a cause of swimmer's shoulder: results after arthroscopic treatment in 4 patients. Am J Sports Med. 2013;41:887-893.
2. Awatani T, Morikita I, Mori S, Shinohara J, Tatsumi Y. Relationship between isometric shoulder strength and arms-only swimming power among male collegiate swimmers: study of valid clinical assessment methods. J Phys Ther Sci. 2018;30:490-495.
3. Barry L, Lyons M, McCreesh K, Powell C, Comyns T. The relationship between training load and pain, injury and illness in competitive swimming: a systematic review. Physical Therapy in Sport. 2021;48:154-168.
4. Bey MJ, Song HK, Wehrli FW, Soslowsky LJ. Intratendinous strain fields of the intact supraspinatus tendon: the effect of glenohumeral joint position and tendon region. J Orthop Res. 2002;20:869-874.
5. Bittencourt NFN, Meeuwisse WH, Mendonca LD, Nettel-Aguirre A, Ocarino JM, Fonseca ST. Complex systems approach for sports injuries: moving from risk factor identification to injury pattern recognition-narrative review and new concept. Br J Sports Med. 2016;50:1309-1314.
6. Bixler B, Riewald S. Analysis of a swimmer's hand and arm in steady flow conditions using computational fluid dynamics. J Biomech. 2002;35:713-717.
7. Boettcher C, Halaki M, Holt K, Ginn KA. Is the normal shoulder rotation strength ratio altered in elite swimmers? Med Sci Sports Exerc. 2020;52:680-684.
8. Boettcher CE, Cathers I, Ginn KA. The role of shoulder muscles is task specific. J Sci Med Sport. 2010;13:651-656.
9. Borsa PA, Laudner KG, Sauers EL. Mobility and stability adaptations in the shoulder of the overhead athlete. Sports Med. 2008;38:17-36.
10. Brushoj C, Bak K, Johannsen HV, Fauno P. Swimmers' painful shoulder arthroscopic findings and return rate to sports. Scand J Med Sci Sports. 2007;17:373-377.
11. Celliers A GF, Joubert G, Mweli T, Sayanvala H, Holtzhausen L. Clinically relevant magnetic resonance imaging (MRI) findings in elite swimmers' shoulders. SA Journal of Radiology. 2107;21:a1080.
12. Chase KI, Caine DJ, Goodwin BJ, Whitehead JR, Romanick MA. A prospective study of injury affecting competitive collegiate swimmers. Res Sports Med. 2013;21:111-123.
13. Chatard JC, Collomp C, Maglischo E, Maglischo C. Swimming skill and stroking characteristics of front crawl swimmers. Int J Sports Med. 1990;11:156-161.
14. Clapis PA, Davis SM, Davis RO. Reliability of inclinometer and goniometric measurements of hip extension flexibility using the modified Thomas test. Physiother Theory Pract. 2008;24:135-141.
15. Cohen RCZ, Cleary PW, Harrison SM, Mason BR, Pease DL. Pitching effects of buoyancy during four competitive swimming strokes. J Appl Biomech. 2014;30:609-618.
16. Cook JL, Purdam CR. Is tendon pathology a continuum? A pathology model to explain the clinical presentation of load-induced tendinopathy. Br J Sports Med. 2009;43:409-416.
17. Cools AM, Dewitte V, Lanszweert F, et al. Rehabilitation of scapular muscle balance - which exercises to prescribe? Am J Sports Med. 2007;35:1744-1751.
18. Cools AM, Johansson FR, Borms D, Maenhout A. Prevention of shoulder injuries in overhead athletes: a science-based approach. Braz J Phys Ther. 2015;19:331-339.
19. Cools AM, Maenhout AG, Vanderstukken F, Decleve P, Johansson FR, Borms D. The challenge of the sporting shoulder: from injury prevention through sport-specific rehabilitation toward return to play. Ann Phys Rehabil Med. 2021;64:101384.
20. Couanis G, Breidahl W, Burnham S. The relationship between subacromial bursa thickness on ultrasound and shoulder pain in open water endurance swimmers over time. J Sci Med. Sport. 2015;18:373-377.
21. Dark A, Ginn KA, Halaki M. Shoulder muscle recruitment patterns during commonly used rotator cuff exercises: an electromyographic study. Phys Ther. 2007;87:1039-1046.
22. De Martino I, Rodeo SA. The swimmer's shoulder: multi-directional instability. Curr Rev Musculoskelet Med. 2018;11:167-171.
23. Delbridge A, Boettcher C, Holt K. An Inside look at 'Swimmers Shoulder': Antero-superior Internal Impingement (ASII) 'A Cause of 'Swimmer's Shoulder'. Aspeter Jnl. 2017;1-16.
24. Deschodt VJ, Arsac LM, Rouard AH. Relative contribution of arms and legs in humans to propulsion in 25-m sprint front-crawl swimming. Eur J Appl Physiol. 1999;80:192-199.
25. Dollings H, Sandford F, O'Conaire E, Lewis JS. Shoulder strength testing: the intra- and inter-tester reliability of routine clinical tests, using the PowerTrack™ II Commander. Shoulder Elbow. 2012;4:131-140.
26. Drake SM KB, Edelman GT, Pounders E, Robinson S, Wixson B. Development and validation of a Swimmer's Functional Pain Scale. J Swim Res. 2015;1:21-32.
27. Du T, Yanai T. Critical scapula motions for preventing subacromial impingement in fully-tethered front-crawl swimming. Sports Biomech. 2019;1-21.
28. Evans NA, Konz S, Nitz A, Uhl TL. Reproducibility and discriminant validity of the Posterior Shoulder Endurance Test in healthy and painful populations. Physical Therapy in Sport. 2021;47:66-71.
29. Feijen S, Kuppens K, Tate A, Baert I, Struyf T, Struyf F. Intra- and interrater reliability of the 'lumbar-locked thoracic rotation test' in competitive swimmers ages 10 through 18 years. Physical Therapy in Sport. 2018;32:140-144.
30. Feijen S ST, Kuppens K, Tate A, Struyf F. Prediction of shoulder pain in youth competitive swimmers: the development

and internal validation of a prognostic prediction model. Am J Sports Med. 2020;19:1-8.

31. Feijen S, Tate A, Kuppens K, Claes A, Struyf F. Swim-training volume and shoulder pain across the life span of the competitive swimmer: a systematic review. J Athl Train. 2020;55:32-41.

32. Foster C, Florhaug JA, Franklin J, et al. A new approach to monitoring exercise training. The Journal of Strength & Conditioning Research. 2001;15:109-115.

33. Gabbett TJ. The training-injury prevention paradox: should athletes be training smarter and harder? Br J Sports Med. 2016;50:273-280.

34. Ganderton C, Kinsella R, Watson L, Pizzari T. Getting more from standard rotator cuff strengthening exercises. Shoulder Elbow. 2020;12:203-211.

35. Girish G, Lobo LG, Jacobson JA, Morag Y, Miller B, Jamadar DA. Ultrasound of the shoulder: asymptomatic findings in men. Am J Roentgenol. 2011;197:713-719.

36. Hawkins RJ, Kennedy JC. Impingement syndrome in athletes. Am J Sports Med. 1980;8:151-158.

37. Hibberd EE, Myers JB. Practice habits and attitudes and behaviors concerning shoulder pain in high school competitive club swimmers. Clin J Sport Med. 2013;23:450-455.

38. Higson E, Herrington L, Butler C, Horsley I. The short-term effect of swimming training load on shoulder rotational range of motion, shoulder joint position sense and pectoralis minor length. Shoulder Elbow. 2018;10:285-291.

39. Hill L, Collins M, Posthumus M. Risk factors for shoulder pain and injury in swimmers: A critical systematic review. Phys Sportsmed. 2015;43:412-420.

40. Holt K, Boettcher C, Halaki M, Ginn KA. Humeral torsion and shoulder rotation range of motion parameters in elite swimmers. J Science Med Sport. 2017;20:469-474.

41. Holt K DA, Josey L, Dhupelia S, Livingston G, Waddington G, Boettcher C. Subscapularis tendinopathy is highly prevalent in elite swimmer's shoulders: an MRI study. Manuscript submitted for publication. 2020.

42. Johnson KD, Kim K-M, Yu B-K, Saliba SA, Grindstaff TL. Reliability of thoracic spine rotation range-of-motion measurements in healthy adults. J Athl Train. 2012;47:52-60.

43. Kennedy JC, Hawkins R, Krissoff WB. Orthopaedic manifestations of swimming. Am J Sports Med. 1978;6:309-322.

44. Kudo S, Sakurai Y, Miwa T, Matsuda Y. Relationship between shoulder roll and hand propulsion in the front crawl stroke. J Sports Sci. 2017;35:945-952.

45. Lewis J. Rotator cuff related shoulder pain: assessment, management and uncertainties. Man Ther. 2016;23:57-68.

46. Lewis JS. Rotator cuff tendinopathy. Br J Sports Med. 2009;43:236-241.

47. Lewis JS. Rotator cuff tendinopathy/subacromial impingement syndrome: is it time for a new method of assessment? Br J Sports Med. 2009;43:259-264.

48. Lyttle AD, Blanksby BA, Elliott BC, Lloyd DG. Net forces during tethered simulation of underwater streamlined gliding and kicking techniques of the freestyle turn. J Sports Sci. 2000;18:801-807.

49. Madsen PH, Bak K, Jensen S, Welter U. Training induces scapular dyskinesis in pain-free competitive swimmers: a reliability and observational study. Clin J Sport Med. 2011;21:109-113.

50. Magnusson SP, Constantini NW, McHugh MP, Gleim GW. Strength profiles and performance in masters' level swimmers. Am J Sports Med. 1995;23:626-631.

51. Matthews MJ, Green D, Matthews H, Swanwick E. The effects of swimming fatigue on shoulder strength, range of motion, joint control, and performance in swimmers. Phys Ther Sport. 2017;23:118-122.

52. McCabe CB, Sanders RH, Psycharakis SG. Upper limb kinematic differences between breathing and non-breathing conditions in front crawl sprint swimming. J Biomech. 2015;48:3995-4001.

53. McCreesh KM, Purtill H, Donnelly AE, Lewis JS. Increased supraspinatus tendon thickness following fatigue loading in rotator cuff tendinopathy: potential implications for exercise therapy. BMJ Open Sport Exerc Med. 2017;3:e000279.

54. McLaine SJ, Bird ML, Ginn KA, Hartley T, Fell JW. Shoulder extension strength: a potential risk factor for shoulder pain in young swimmers? J Sci Med Sport. 2019;22:516-520.

55. McLaine SJ, Ginn KA, Fell JW, Bird M-L. Isometric shoulder strength in young swimmers. J Sci Med Sport. 2018;21:35-39.

56. McLaine SJ, Ginn KA, Kitic CM, Fell JW, Bird M-L. The reliability of strength tests performed in elevated shoulder positions using a hand-held dynamometer. J Sport Rehabil. 2016;25:2015-0034.

57. McMaster WC, Troup J. A survey of interfering shoulder pain in United States competitive swimmers. Am J Sports Med. 1993;21:67-70.

58. Montgomery SR, Chen NC, Rodeo SA. Arthroscopic capsular plication in the treatment of shoulder pain in competitive swimmers. HSS Journal. 2010;6:145-149.

59. Neer CS, 2nd. Anterior acromioplasty for the chronic impingement syndrome in the shoulder: a preliminary report. J Bone Joint Surg Am. 1972;54:41-50.

60. Pink M, Perry J, Browne A, Scovazzo ML, Kerrigan J. The normal shoulder during freestyle swimming. An electromyographic and cinematographic analysis of twelve muscles. Am J Sports Med. 1991;19:569-576.

61. Pink MM, Tibone JE. The painful shoulder in the swimming athlete. Orthop Clin North Am. 2000;31:247-261.

62. Porter KN, Blanch PD, Walker HM, Shield AJ. The effect of previous shoulder pain on supraspinatus tendon thickness changes following swimming practice. Scand J Med Sci Sports. 2020;30:1442-1448.

63. Porter KN, Talpey S, Pascoe D, Blanch PD, Walker HM, Shield AJ. The effect of swimming volume and intensity on changes in supraspinatus tendon thickness. Physical Therapy in Sport. 2020;47:173-177.

64. Ramsi M, Swanik KA, Swanik CB, Straub S, Mattacola C. Shoulder-rotator strength of high school swimmers over the course of a competitive season. J Sport Rehabil. 2004;13:9-18.

65. Rathi S, Taylor NF, Green RA. The effect of in vivo rotator cuff muscle contraction on glenohumeral joint translation: an ultrasonographic and electromyographic study. J Biomech. 2016;49:3840-3847.

66. Richardson AB, Jobe FW, Collins HR. The shoulder in competitive swimming. Am J Sports Med. 1980;8:159-163.

67. Richardson E, Lewis JS, Gibson J, et al. Role of the kinetic chain in shoulder rehabilitation: does incorporating the trunk and lower limb into shoulder

exercise regimes influence shoulder muscle recruitment patterns? Systematic review of electromyography studies. BMJ Open Sport Exerc Med. 2020;6:e000683.

68. Rodeo SA, Nguyen JT, Cavanaugh JT, Patel Y, Adler RS. Clinical and ultrasonographic evaluations of the shoulders of elite swimmers. Am J Sports Med. 2016;44:3214-3221.

69. Schlueter KR, Pintar JA, Wayman KJ, Hartel LJ, Briggs MS. Clinical evaluation techniques for injury risk assessment in elite swimmers: a systematic review. Sports Health. 2020;31:57-64.

70. Scovazzo ML, Browne A, Pink M, Jobe FW, Kerrigan J. The painful shoulder during freestyle swimming - an electromyographic cinematographic analysis of twelve muscles. Am J Sports Med. 1991;19:577-582.

71. Sein ML, Walton J, Linklater J, et al. Shoulder pain in elite swimmers: primarily due to swim-volume-induced supraspinatus tendinopathy. Br J Sports Med. 2010;44:105-113.

72. Seitz AL, McClure PW, Finucane S, Boardman ND, 3rd, Michener LA. Mechanisms of rotator cuff tendinopathy: intrinsic, extrinsic, or both? Clin Biomech. 2011;26:1-12.

73. Stocker D, Pink M, Jobe FW. Comparison of shoulder injury in collegiate-level and masters-level swimmers. Clin J Sport Med. 1995;5:4-8.

74. Struyf F, Tate A, Kuppens K, Feijen S, Michener LA. Musculoskeletal dysfunctions associated with swimmers' shoulder. Br J Sports Med. 2017;51:775-780.

75. Su KPE, Johnson MP, Gracely EJ, Karduna AR. Scapular rotation in swimmers with and without impingement syndrome: practice effects. Med Sci Sports Exerc. 2004;36:1117-1123.

76. Tate A, Turner GN, Knab SE, Jorgensen C, Strittmatter A, Michener LA. Risk factors associated with shoulder pain and disability across the lifespan of competitive swimmers. J Athl Train. 2012;47:149-158.

77. Tesarz J, Schuster AK, Hartmann M, Gerhardt A, Eich W. Pain perception in athletes compared to normally active controls: a systematic review with meta-analysis. Pain. 2012;153:1253-1262.

78. Toussaint HM, Hollander AP. Energetics of competitive swimming: implications for training-programs. Sports Med. 1994;18:384-405.

79. Troup JP. The physiology and biomechanics of competitive swimming. Clin Sports Med. 1999;18:267-285.

80. Vasiliadis AV, Lampridis V, Georgiannos D, Bisbinas I. Swimmers are at risk for stress fractures? A systematic review. International Journal of Kinesiology and Sports Science. 2018;6:25-31.

81. Walker H, Gabbe B, Wajswelner H, Blanch P, Bennell K. Shoulder pain in swimmers: a 12-month prospective cohort study of incidence and risk factors. Phys Ther Sport. 2012;13:243-249.

82. Walker H, Pizzari T, Wajswelner H, et al. The reliability of shoulder range of motion measures in competitive swimmers. Phys Ther Sport. 2016;21:26-30.

83. Wattanaprakornkul D, Cathers I, Halaki M, Ginn KA. The rotator cuff muscles have a direction specific recruitment pattern during shoulder flexion and extension exercises. J Sci Med Sport. 2011;14:376-382.

84. Whiteley R, Oceguera, MV, Valencia EB, Mitchell T. Adaptations at the shoulder of the throwing athlete and implications for the clinician. Techn Shoulder Elb Surg. 2012;13:36-44.

85. Wolf BR, Ebinger AE, Lawler MP, Britton CL. Injury patterns in Division I collegiate swimming. Am J Sports Med. 2009;37:2037-2042.

86. Yanai T, Hay JG. Shoulder impingement in front-crawl swimming. II. Analysis of stroking technique. Med Sci Sports Exerc. 2000;32:30-40.

87. Yoma M HL, Mackenzie TA, Almond TA. Training intensity and shoulder musculoskeletal physical quality responses in competitive swimmers. Journal of Athletic Training. 2020;56:54-63.

88. Zamparo P, Cortesi M, Gatta G. The energy cost of swimming and its determinants. Eur J Appl Physiol. 2020;120:41-66.

89. Zemek MJ, Magee DJ. Comparison of glenohumeral joint laxity in elite and recreational swimmers. Clin J Sport Med. 1996;6:40-47.

40 High performance rehabilitation of the climbing athlete

Uzo Ehiogu, Gareth Stephens

Introduction

Climbing has a rich history dating back to the early 1940s when alpinists first began ascents on some of the most dangerous mountain ranges in Europe and America. Modern day climbing has become an Olympic sport and a recreational pastime for people around the world.[51] Climbing imposes unique demands upon the musculoskeletal system,[96] and is one of a few sports that has a bias towards use of the upper quadrant, requiring both skill and force.[54]

Climbing as a sport is conducted outdoors in natural environments, or in indoor environments on purpose-built artificial walls. The hands and feet are the main interface between the climbing surface and the climber.[85] While the lower quadrant is naturally suited for prolonged weight bearing and force production, this isn't so for the upper quadrant. It is the requirements for high and sustained force production, large ranges of movement, and precise motor control that places the upper limb at high risk of injury in climbers.[28,31,84]

Epidemiology and injury patterns

Upper limb injuries are the most common in climbers, and for recreational climbers, self-reported shoulder injuries account for 19.5% of injuries.[84] In a cohort of 436 elite climbers, the prevalence of upper limb injuries was 77.1%, 17.7% the lower limb, and 5.2% attributed to other body regions.[50] In the hand, the most frequently reported injuries were to the finger pulley ligaments (12.3%), followed by finger tenosynovitis (10.6%). Common shoulder injuries include superior labral lesion tears from anterior to posterior (SLAP), accounting for 29.8% of all shoulder injuries, closely followed by conditions associated with rotator cuff-related shoulder pain (27.4%) and dislocations and Bankart lesions (17.7%). In the same cohort, 43.9% of reported injuries were acute (trauma) and 56.1% related to persistent (overuse) conditions. Bouldering does not use ropes or a harness to stop a fall and bouldering accidents are the leading cause of acute injuries (60.4%) for climbers.[50]

The physiology of climbing

The physiological determinants of a sport are in part determined by the nature of the metabolic energy systems and the neuromuscular/mechanical activity utilized during its performance. This includes an awareness of the primary bioenergetics systems (adenosine triphosphate (ATP) and phosphocreatine (PCr) (ATP-PCr), anaerobic glycolysis, oxidative metabolism), energy expenditure rate and volume, oxygen uptake requirements, muscular strength, endurance, and neuromuscular recruitment patterns.[101] The specific demands upon the musculoskeletal system are dependent upon the athlete's preferred type of climbing.[27] In general, the recreational climber will favor one or two climbing disciplines with a preference for one regarding the number of training hours spent on that discipline each week. This may include traditional climbing that involves the climber fixing their own bolts or security gear to rock to protect against falls. This type of climbing is heavily dependent upon oxidative metabolic pathways and muscular endurance of long duration for the upper quadrant.[23]

In contrast, bouldering involves short to moderate duration routes averaging 20–50 seconds.[103] This type of climbing features a short sequence of unique and powerful moves in which the climber must support their body mass with their hands and feet. Bouldering does not require ropes or bolted protection and most routes do not typically exceed 4 meters in height.[86] Lead climbing (sometimes referred to as sport climbing) is a different discipline. It involves the climber clipping the rope into pre-bolted anchors along the route. This type of climbing maximizes safety, and these routes can often last several minutes in duration depending upon the degree of difficulty.

Olympic and elite climbers participating in national or international competition are usually required to compete in all three disciplines: lead climbing, speed climbing, and bouldering.[51] While the kinematics of all climbing disciplines are similar in regard to the role of the upper quadrant and in particular the shoulder, the kinetics and physiological profile of each discipline varies.[22] Lead climbing, because of its duration, requires very different metabolic activity and force time profiles for muscular force development in comparison with speed climbing and bouldering. Lead climbing primarily relies on glycolytic and oxidative pathways to maintain a rate of force expression consistent with strength and power endurance of medium (up to 3 minutes) to long duration (up to 5 minutes).[91] Although medium-duration power endurance predominates this type of climbing, the energetics are often mixed, using alactic pathways to negotiate difficult moves requiring higher percentages of the climbers' maximum strength.[27] For example, the alactic energy system which uses ATP-PCr pathways will predominate when sudden or explosive movements are required on difficult terrain (Figure 40.1). Speed climbing is biased towards explosive strength and high rates of force development both in the lower and upper quadrant. The route is linear and predetermined. Success is principally determined by the athlete who is the fastest to reach the top[24] (Figure 40.2).

In contrast, success in bouldering is not determined by the speed of completion but rather the climber's ability to complete the route. International competitions generally consist of 3 rounds (qualifying, semifinals and finals) with a maximum of 2 rounds per day, each with 4–5 routes to complete. Routes typically consist of 4–5 hand holds, and multiple attempts are permitted during a 4–5 minute period.[103] Strength endurance and short to medium-duration power endurance are key physiological indicators of successful performance in bouldering.[54]

Bouldering is very challenging for the shoulder, as the physically demanding and challenging postures and jumps the athlete must undertake to complete the route[50] necessitate a high degree of skill, and coordination of all body parts, including the shoulder (Figure 40.3). A significant amount of strength and power from the shoulder and kinetic chain is needed to absorb and generate forces for optimal performance.[13,37] Bouldering routes are often short to medium in duration, lasting from 20-80 seconds. This type of climbing is generally characterized by high strength and power requirements.[103] The key bioenergetics in this type of climbing are the ATP-PCr and anaerobic (glycolytic) energy pathways.

The oxidative system should not be discounted as an important source of energy production during longer bouldering routes, as this system contributes up to 50% of the energy requirements for force production after 75 seconds of exhaustive exercise.[25] This assists the anaerobic system to sustain force output and to facilitate recovery between bouldering routes.[103] It is important that healthcare professionals understand the physiological demands of each discipline. This knowledge can be applied in the rehabilitation and physical preparation of the injured climbing athlete.

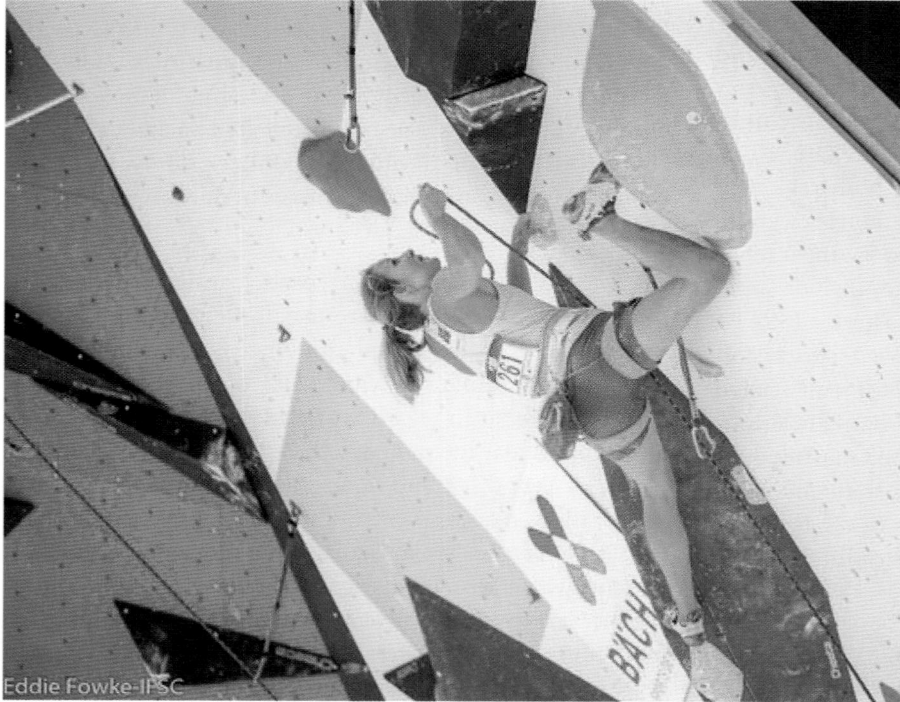

FIGURE 40.1
Lead climbing.

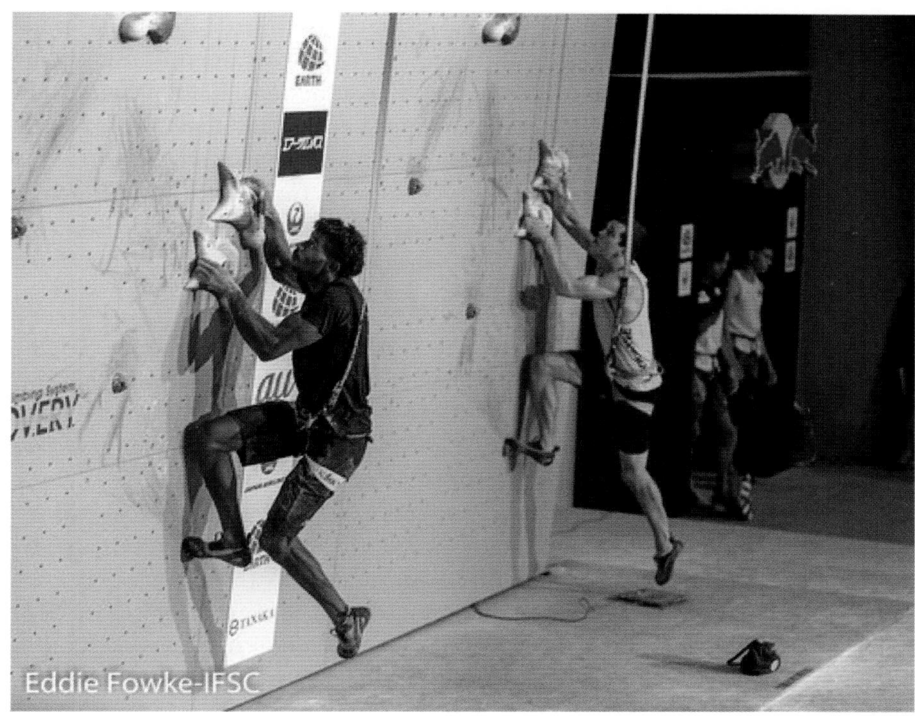

FIGURE 40.2
Speed climbing.

Nutritional considerations for climbers

Climbers must be able to support, control, and move their own body weight. This suggests the climber's strength and power to weight ratio may be an important performance attribute. Anecdotally, the importance of these ratios is well recognized by climbers with some believing that excess body mass provides additional resistance to ascent during climbing. However, research has not reported a significant link between climbing performance and body composition.[60,63]

Four studies have assessed nutritional dietary intake in climbers.[26,39,61,108] In general, these studies have found elite climbers consume an inadequate energy intake, contrary to evidenced-based guidance to support high performance sport. For example, Kemmler et al.[39] reported the energy intake of climbing athletes was not significantly greater than body mass index (BMI) matched controls. This was despite the climbers' training volume (401 minutes (±73) versus 43 minutes (± 25)) being 9.5 times greater than the controls. Gibson-Smith et al.[26] investigated the dietary intake and body composition of experienced and elite climbers (n=40), and found 77.5% did not meet predicted energy requirements to support a moderate training program.

The nutritional practices of experienced and elite climbers have raised concerns about the risk of chronic energy restriction and low energy availability. To discourage excessively low body mass in climbing, national and international climbing governing bodies have introduced body mass restrictions and body mass index screening procedures at competitions. There are well-recognized health complications associated with persistent energy deficiency, such as impaired physiological function in metabolic rate, menstrual function, bone health, immunity, protein synthesis, and cardiovascular health.[66] Therefore, healthcare professionals involved in the care of these athletes should be aware of the importance of nutrition for performance.

Climbing kinematics and kinetics

Kinematics refers to the spatial and temporal characteristics of the task without consideration of the forces involved, and kinetics are the forces which influence the change in motion of a body.[6] The objective of climbing is to displace the body from one position to another with efficiency.[69]

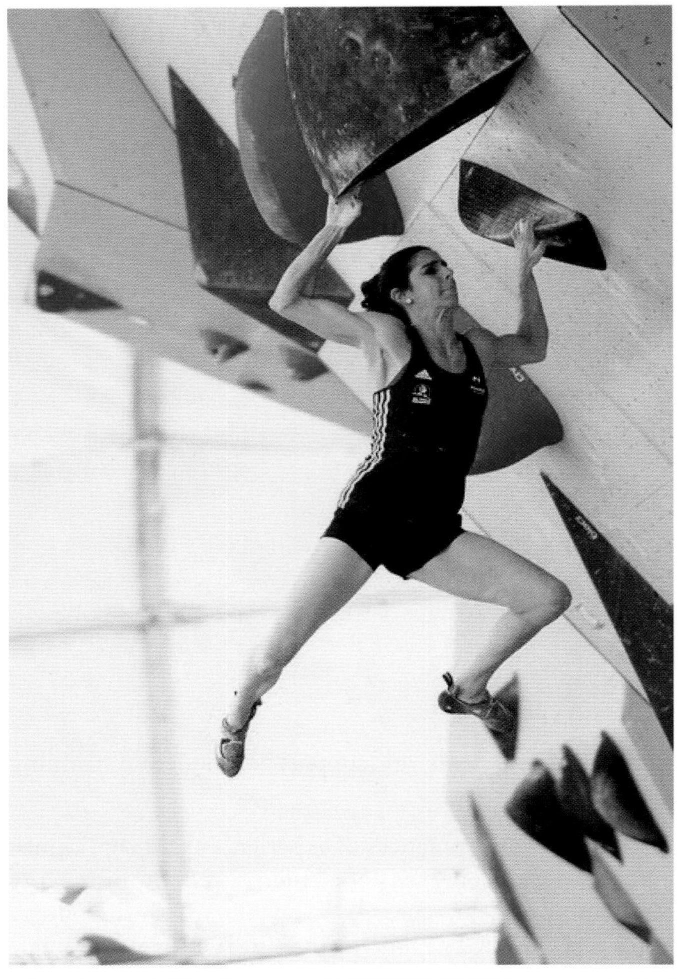

FIGURE 40.3
Bouldering.

The culmination of motion often involves a reaching movement when transitioning from one point to the next. Climbing can be operationalized into three distinct phases: stabilization, preparation, and displacement.[88]

The stabilization phase is necessary for the climber to maintain contact with the climbing surface and to establish postural stability. This requires isometric muscle actions from the forearm flexors, finger musculature, trunk muscles, and lower limbs. The preparation phase is a transition phase between stabilization and the next displacement phase. This phase requires a combination of isometric and concentric muscle activity. The forearm and finger muscles are used to maintain a static position on the climbing surface, while the trunk, shoulder, and lower quadrant are used dynamically to adjust body position ready for the next phase. The displacement phase is characterized by the displacement of the center of mass from one hold to the next. Muscle activity at this point is often concentric, requiring activity from the lower quadrant, trunk, shoulder, and the forearm and finger muscles.[53]

Movement efficiency may reduce the stress imposed upon the musculoskeletal system and aid performance. This may be achieved by optimizing energy-efficient movement patterns[13] to ensure that the climber does not place excessive force through structures that are either not suited to the role or lack the capacity to adapt to load because of their biology. This requires an understanding of both functional anatomy and clinical biomechanics to identify the potential effects of movement inefficiency as a basis for pathomechanics.[42] For example, the climber's body position during movement is important because it influences the center of gravity in relation to the base of support and hence the climber's degree of balance on the wall (see Figure 40.1). These variables may affect the metabolic cost of climbing and the performance outcome.

Inefficiency may increase the relative metabolic cost of mechanical work leading to premature fatigue.[68] Poor technique regardless of its cause has the ability to affect the interplay between biomechanics, injury and performance.[49] Biomechanical moment arms both at a whole body, body segment, and local joint muscle interaction are important in human movement. Moment arms influence the magnitudes of force which must be overcome and generated by the climber during all activities. The musculoskeletal system functions at a mechanical disadvantage during climbing, which requires the generation of significant forces to overcome external resistance.[40]

The strength and power profile for the upper quadrant has been compared between non-climbers and climbing populations in several studies.[44,99] The vertical ascent of the climber is characterized by displacement of the center of mass from one hold to the next.[69] Concentric muscle activity of the shoulder adductors is well suited to this upward pulling action seen in climbing. Predictably, upper body strength of the shoulder adductors is consistently higher in climbers when compared with non-climbing controls. This is also similar when novice climbers are compared with skilled and elite climbing groups.[99] Rokowski[77] noted that elite climbers displayed superior levels of upper limb strength endurance when compared with sub-elite rock climbers. Strength endurance was tested using the maximum number of pull-ups to fatigue. Elite climbers in both absolute and relative terms achieved higher mean number of pull-ups compared with sub-elite climbers (absolute pull-ups 29.5 (± 3.6) and 24.8 (± 2.4)) respectively.

Other functional markers of upper limb performance have been compared in novice and expert climbers. Wall et al.[99] studied the physical demands of female sport rock climbers comparing novice, skilled, and elite performers. These researchers found significant differences between groups in a climbing-specific one arm lock-off strength test. One arm lock-off strength showed statistically significant correlations to bouldering performance. Significant differences were found between expert climbers and skilled climbers for left and right one arm lock-off strength. The one arm lock-off test uses a pull-up bar with an integrated force transducer. Subjects apply maximal downwards force through the force transducer for 3 seconds. The test is purported to simulate the forces rock climbing place upon the arm, back, and shoulders as the climber attempts to maintain their position on a climbing wall.

Grant et al.[28] compared the upper body strength of elite and recreational climbers and non-climbers using a bilateral bent arm hang and total number of pull-ups. Comparable with findings reported by Wall et al.,[99] climbers were required to pull their body weight up to a position corresponding to a right angle at the elbow. For the bent arm hang, climbers were instructed to hold the position for as long as possible until fatigued. Elite climbers had significantly longer hold times for the bent arm hang (53.0 seconds (± 13.2), recreational climbers 31.4 seconds (± 9.0), non-climbers 32.6 seconds (± 15.0)), and elite climbers performed a higher number of pull-ups compared to recreational climbers and non-climbers.

Isolated measures of muscle performance have been compared in climbers and non-climbers using work ratios. Work ratios indicate the relative strength between different muscle groups. Work ratios reflect muscle strength throughout the range of motion and may be more informative than peak torque ratios which measure force in a single position.[67] Wong and Ng[107] reported significant differences in external rotation and internal rotation functional work ratios (defined as the ratio of eccentric antagonist/concentric agonist) in experienced climbers compared with non-climbers. Experienced climbers displayed a disproportionately low concentric external rotator to internal rotator (ER:IR) ratio compared with non-climbers (0.79 (± 0.20) versus 1.03 (± 0.24)). This may be consistent with function as the internal shoulder rotators are frequently used in climbing, which may explain their lower concentric ER:IR ratio compared with non-climbers. This finding accords with other research[4,20] that has reported ER:IR ratios less than 1.

Isokinetic work profiles for the shoulder flexors and extensors have been reported in experienced climbers and non-climbers.[106] Men and women climbers display higher work profiles compared with non-climbers. The data suggest experienced climbers are 2.5 and 2.2 times higher than non-climbers in concentric extension and eccentric extension measures, and 1.7 and 1.5 times higher in concentric flexion and eccentric flexion measures, respectively. This suggests climbers are stronger than non-climbers in specific muscle groups that may need to be strengthened to better accomplish the task of climbing.

Reduced muscle activity associated with shoulder stabilizing force couples may be accentuated because of habitual body postures adopted during climbing. Climbers often adopt static postures for route reading and recovery by hanging with their arms fully extended. This posture is often chosen by climbers which places the shoulder girdle in a relaxed and elevated position. This position has been shown to influence the electromyographic activity of the middle and lower trapezius muscles. Baláš et al.[5] demonstrated that when climbers adopted a corrected (neutral) position with a bent rather than extended arm, higher surface electromyography (SEMG) readings in the middle and lower trapezius were reported. The middle trapezius for climbers during a corrected position with a bent arm produced an SEMG amplitude of 40.9% (± 19.6) maximum voluntary contraction (MVC) compared to 10.6% (± 2.9). This suggests that climbers who typically elevate the shoulder during static postures display reduced muscle activity in the axioscapular muscles. This coupled with the influence of large muscle group development for climbing performance may accentuate muscle imbalance in this population.

The influence of power output and explosive strength has received less attention as a predictor of climbing ability in climbing research. Explosive strength is significantly correlated with climbing ability when elite climbers are compared with non-climbers ($r = 0.96$ to 0.70; $p < 0.01$), using the jump arm test. However, when the same test is compared between elite and skilled climbers, a significant difference is not reported (76 cm/29.9 in versus 73 cm/28.7 in).[44] Climbing ability is defined by the most difficult route the climber has ever ascended on the French grading scale of 5a to 9b+. This grading scale may be used to inform a climber as to the level of ability required to successfully ascend a climbing route. Participants in this study were categorized as either novice (<6a), skilled (6c–7a), or elite (≥8a) climbers, with a minimum level of upper limb explosive strength being required for climbing performance.

Moreover, the capacity to display a high level of power endurance in the upper quadrant appears to be important for climbing performance. Laffaye et al.[44] using an arm jump test calculated a fatigue index (calculated as the first value of the arm jump test minus the last value, divided by the first value, multiplied by 100). The fatigue resistance protocol was performed by repeating the jump test 10 times, with a 10-second rest between each trial. The data suggested climbers displayed significantly lower reductions in performance (average decrease 11.7% compared with non-climbers (28.9%)). The lower reduction in performance for skilled and elite climbers compared with non-climbers suggests a higher capability to resynthesize high energy phosphates and resist fatigue.

Terminology

A case study that incorporates an understanding of a climber's values, together with assessment and management will be presented in this chapter. Table 40.1 details the terminology that will be used to describe physical capacity and Table 40.2 details definitions of late-stage strength training exercises used in the case presentation.

Principles of assessment and management when caring for injured climbers

Assessment of impaired capacity

Injury may lead to impairments in physical capacity such as reductions in strength, endurance, range of motion, motor control, skill acquisition, power output and rate of force development.[8,42] Impairments, which may be self-evident to the climber, may not be obvious to the clinician. The assessment of impaired biological function is usually the key factor that underpins clinical management.[57] For example, maximal muscle strength occurs when a muscle

Table 40.1 Definitions of physical capacity

Capacity/physical qualities	Description
Maximal strength	The highest force the neuromuscular system can generate during a maximum voluntary contraction.[95]
Maximal power	Power is defined as the rate of doing mechanical work and is the product of force and displacement of an object from one position to another position in space.[95]
Proprioception	Proprioception or kinesthesia is the sense used to perceive the location, movement, and action of part of the body. It incorporates sensations such as joint position sense, muscle force and effort.[76]
Rate of force development/explosive strength	Rate of force development (RFD) or explosive strength refers to the rate of change in force at the beginning of the concentric muscle action.[15]
Range of motion	The ability to move a joint fluidly though a range of motion.[58]
Muscular endurance	Muscular endurance refers to the ability of the local neuromuscular system to produce force in a repetitive submaximal fashion over an extended period.[43]
Strength endurance/hypertrophy training	Moderate load and volume training reflected in an enlargement in muscle tissue. The physiological objectives are an increase in cross sectional area, muscle protein content and increases in storage of high energy substrates and enzymes.[82]

Table 40.2 Definitions of late-stage strength training exercises

Late-stage strength training	Description
Hang board training	The hang board or finger board is a sport-specific tool for improving finger strength. The hang board allows training of the fingers, forearm muscles, and upper quadrant in a controlled manner. It can be used to isolate sport-specific grip positions with and without additional weight added via a body harness.[59]
Campus board training	Campus boards are slates of wood or plastic attached to a wall in a ladder-like configuration. The slates can be configured for different size grips to increase or decrease the emphasis on grip or length of reach on finger/forearm or shoulder girdle performance during training. Athletes can ascend with or without the assistance of the feet. This training modality can be used to improve finger, forearm, or shoulder girdle strength, power, and rate of force development or explosive strength.[80]
System board training	The system board is a training platform with a large array of different hand and foot holds. The holds are configured in a symmetrical pattern so that each hold on the wall is a mirror image of the other side. The system board provides a method of training specific grips, arm positions, movements, and body positioning in a very precise and repeatable way for both arms and sides of the body. The system board allows athletes to complete all three phases of climbing movements including stabilization, preparation, and displacement. This can be used to develop strength and power capacities in specific grips and arm positions while climbing.[1]
Hyper gravity training	Hyper gravity training typically involves the use of a weighted vest, weight belt, or rucksack. It is a combination of system board training and resistance training while climbing. The additional system weight provides a training method which can overload the entire kinetic chain in a climbing-specific manner. This method allows training of specific grips, arm, and shoulder positions over a single set of climbing moves.[53]

or muscle group generates maximal force against an external resistance.

The assessment of impairments such as strength does not always require sophisticated and expensive equipment, e.g., isokinetic dynamometry, that may be unavailable to many clinicians. Therefore, data-driven assessment techniques such as upper body jump tests of power output,[48] handheld dynamometer testing of strength and work capacity,[16] functional tests of strength (such as pull-ups and pull-up lock-off variations) with and without external added load (that at a minimum replicates the equipment a climber uses)[55] provide quantitative data on upper limb performance that will aid decision-making.

Qualitative assessment using video in either two-dimensional or three-dimensional analysis with slow motion modes is available commercially.[41] These assessment techniques allow qualitative judgements to be made about both static and dynamic postures and positions during stable ground training and specific return to climbing exercises.[70]

For the climbing athlete, range of movement, force production, and the skillful application of technique are important for optimal performance. Climbing requires the climber's body to be positioned as close as possible to the supporting surface to reduce gravitational and destabilizing forces.[69] These variables impact movement economy and the rate and duration of energy production. Poor movement economy may lead to less than optimal performance.[87] As such, observations of the climber in climbing situations are essential to determine if ongoing impairments detrimentally impact on technique. This may not be evident from routine range of movement and strength tests performed solely in the clinical, non-climbing environment.

Kinetic chain integration

It is important to appreciate the role of the kinetic chain in the physical preparation of the injured climber. Appropriate training of the lower limb, core musculature and appendicular musculature is necessary to ensure the climber's return to sport, and that their shoulder is optimized and ready for performance.[18] Training activities for the abdominal and trunk muscles are important because of the role it plays in transferring forces from the lower to upper limbs, and possibly in climbers in the reverse direction. The region may require "stiffening" (i.e., sustained isometric contractions) to provide stability for the climber during difficult maneuvers on overhanging and other technically difficult terrain.[75,78,79,105] Finger and forearm muscle strength is a primary differentiator between novice and elite climbers.[46,47] Training of these regions should be periodized alongside the management of the shoulder region.[34]

The lower limb is not traditionally afforded the attention it deserves in climbers. However, the lower limb, and in particular the hamstring[19] and hip muscles are areas that may be injured in climbers.[83] Moreover, from a biomechanical standpoint, the feet and lower limbs are required to displace the climber's center of mass from one position to the next at slow and ballistic speeds for maximum economy of movement.[69] The lower limb is also required to assist the upper limb to hold static positions and for dynamic movement reducing its energy demands. This is of particular importance when the climber is carrying equipment that will be a percentage of their body weight. During overhanging routes with long reaches, and vertical routes with small holds, the ability to jump between holds may be the only way to progress. Therefore, strength and power training for the lower quadrant should not be neglected.

To develop maximal strength, modalities such as the deadlift, sumo deadlift, back and front squat, and calf raises may be used for developing the musculature associated with triple extension.[92] The exercise prescription should follow standard training principles, with loads between 80–90% of 1 repetition maximum (RM), 2–5 sets with low repetition ranges (3–5 repetitions), and with long rest periods between sets (>3 minutes). To develop lower limb explosive qualities, modalities such as lower limb plyometrics, medicine ball throws, and Olympic weightlifting derivatives may be used as a stimulus to mechanically overload the triple extension jump pattern.[92] The exercise prescription will typically involve relatively light to moderate loads executed at high speed with low repetition ranges (2–5 repetitions) over multiple sets (2–5 sets), with long rest periods between sets (>5 minutes).[74]

Training skills and capacities specific to the climbing athlete

The climber will lose skill, strength and other parameters of physiological function during prolonged periods of detraining because of injury.[52] From a climbing perspective, the athlete may lose technical skill and tactical awareness because of their absence from competition and training.[100] This reduced performance may also be related to psychological, social, and lifestyle factors.[73] The clinician must determine whether the underlying problem is a skill-based problem or a physical capacity, or both. Although physical capacity and skill-related problems may coexist together, often one will predominate over the other. Therefore, the clinician needs to be able to weigh the clinical evidence to determine what to prioritize.[72] Notwithstanding, there will be periods during the athlete's clinical journey where skill and capacity impairment logically are more likely.

Enhanced skill and technical development in a load-appropriate manner will dovetail capacity training during this intermediate phase. The athlete will be encouraged to develop and maintain climbing skills at a volume and intensity not deleterious to their stage of recovery.[13] Critical at this stage is a very prescriptive approach to the volume and intensity of climbing that is allowed. By its nature, it is difficult to quantitively measure the training load of climbing. There are international grading systems for climbing routes,[50,51] however, these definitions are not suitable for prescribing training volumes during rehabilitation when load must be monitored with some degree of precision. Therefore, it is prudent to utilize a graduate training program where the climbing grade, duration of the ascent and descent (length of the climb), number of times repeated (repetitions) and any specials characteristics of the climb (type of holds and/or pitch of the climb) are manipulated to create an appropriate load while still developing sport-specific skill. This type of training program can be very prescriptive until such a time as the healthcare professional is satisfied that the physical preparation goals have been achieved.

In the late stages of physical preparation, climbing skill requires the expression of physical capacities emphasized with sport-specific training modalities. Sport-specific training can involve on the wall training (climbing) and off the wall training (climbing derivatives) which simulate the sport-specific qualities of climbing in a controlled manner. These modalities target the muscle groups, neuromuscular force profiles, energy systems, and, in many cases, the movement patterns associated with climbing.[103]

Climbing is heavily reliant upon grip strength and upper body strength.[28] The force requirements for the upper quadrant are particularly significant for the elite and sub-elite climber due to the challenging nature of climbing at this level.[46,47] For example, when holds are abnormally small or awkward, a large amount of force is required to increase the friction coefficient between the fingers and the climbing surface for adhesion. This requires a reliance on anaerobic substrate utilization and high levels of neuromuscular force and rate of force development (see Table 40.1).[65] The clinician should be aware of these types of training modalities because they target both the skill qualities of climbing and metabolic energy and neuromuscular force profiles.

Rehabilitation and physical preparation

Rehabilitation aims to improve function after injury to structure and/or impairment in physiology.[7] It is a planned and systematic approach to the judicious application of physical load to restore function.[90] The philosophy must include both a rehabilitation and a physical preparation mindset in which the performance outcome is the key driver for all interactions with the climber.[104]

In the early phase of recovery, pain management, restoration of range of motion, and the judicious application of therapeutic loads is the priority.[52] The middle phase is typified by increases in mechanical and metabolic load and low-level skill-related training in preparation for the next phase.[74] The late and return to sport phases of the process often see the greatest crossover of skill development and muscle conditioning, requiring progressively increasing training loads and realistic skill-related training.[62] This provides a mechanical overload of the shoulder-specific tissues and other interdependent anatomical regions such as the trunk, lower limb, hand and wrist.[36] Metabolic energy pathways that support sport-specific performance are developed in unison.[75] Sport-specific neuromuscular patterning of the shoulder and kinetic chain merges with traditional resistance training to provide a balanced pathway for the full resumption of high-level unrestricted climbing. The process involves traditional resistance training, range of movement exercises, and a sport-specific, whole body graduated physical program to prepare the athlete for return to climbing.

Programming and periodization

The systematic and judicious application of mechanical load to the shoulder and kinetic chain is often what differentiates optimal from suboptimal rehabilitation programs. Energy system or metabolic development is also an essential consideration for the optimal return to sport of the climbing athlete.[65] The effectiveness of a climber's conditioning and resulting sport-specific fitness is a factor determining their ability to resist fatigue and to fulfil the demands of their sport.[15,65,91] The climber must have the requisite ability to complete one repetition with the highest possible quality and intensity.[56] Concomitantly, the climber must develop the metabolic capacity to successfully complete repeated climbs.[81]

Periodization is a practical training methodology that has been shown to produce superior results for developing athletic performance.[35] The principles of periodization can be applied in a rehabilitation and physical preparation system for the climbing athlete returning from injury.[32] Long-term planning maximizes the probability of optimal physical preparedness for the climbing athlete. This helps prevent overload or underload during rehabilitation. In essence, periodization is a methodology that applies systematic planning to the application of training and conditioning loads for athletic populations.[29] At a clinical and practical level, it is the manipulation of load, volume, intensity, and exercise selection to develop physical preparedness under time constraints. The time constraint is a position in the future where elevated physical capacity will be achieved to support a performance outcome.[35]

A periodized program is defined by its phases of training or mechanical loading. There are two major phases in the training program: the preparatory phase and the competitive phase. The preparatory phase can be subdivided into two further phases, the general physical training phase and the sport-specific training phase.[33] For the purposes of physical preparation, the sub-phases offer a very structured approach to the physical preparation of the climbing athlete. There are various structural approaches to periodization in the literature for athletic development,[14] however, we suggest that a linear approach to programming appears to offer the best system for the injured athlete.

This method of programming is characterized by structured variation in the program over several weeks or months depending upon the nature of the injury. An important principle of this type of programming is phase potentiation.[30] Phase potentiation is logical sequencing or ordering of training blocks in the physical preparation program to ensure that the physical qualities trained prior support the next phase of loading; as such, it is the graduated and sequential reloading of technique, skill and motor performance.[94]

For example, after a shoulder injury, the program may require the climbing athlete to complete a muscle strength–endurance phase of 4–6 weeks, followed by a strength phase of 4 weeks, and then a power development phase of 4 weeks before transition to more sport-specific work on a climbing wall.

Developing strength endurance

Strength endurance for the climber improves their ability to continue developing muscle tension in the climbing-specific upper limb muscles despite the onset of fatigue.[43] There are various resistance training modalities which can be used to develop this quality. For example, traditional resistance machines (e.g., "lat" pull-down machine), body weight resistance (e.g., pull-up exercise) or more traditional climbing-specific strength training derivatives such as hang boards (see Figure 40.4),[59] system boards and campus boards.[53] The exercise modality chosen will depend upon the stage of rehabilitation, equipment availability, and the creativity of the clinician. The prescription for strength endurance requires 15–20 repetitions, moderate loads (50–70% of 1 repetition maximum; 1RM), 3–5 sets and short rest periods between sets (<1 minute).[74] For example, a climbing derivative to develop strength endurance of the upper limb is the fingerboard. This modality is traditionally used to develop isometric muscle strength of the finger and forearm muscles. However, this tool can be adapted to develop isometric strength endurance of the shoulder muscles in climbing-relevant positions (such as the bent arm lock-off position).

Baláš et al.[5] have shown that when climbers adopted a corrected (neutral) shoulder position when hanging from a hang board, surface electromyography (SEMG) readings in the middle and lower trapezius were optimized. Further, because of the similarity of position to traditional pull-ups, there is likely to be involvement of the shoulder adductors. The hang board strength endurance program for the shoulder should use a grip type that allows fatigue to be reached at the target exercise duration specified. An open grip is less fatiguing for the forearm and finger flexor muscles than a closed or crimped grip.

Vigouroux et al.[98] has shown that flexor digitorum superficialis and flexor digitorum profundus contribute to force production in a crimped/closed grip at a ratio of 3:1. However, an open grip requires a force generation ratio of 1:1 for these two muscles. Vigouroux et al.[97] found no significant difference between large open grip holds and a traditional pull-up bar when sport climbers performed pulls-ups. The researchers found reduced number of pull-ups, maximal arm power, mechanical work, and finger flexor fatigue as the size of the hold reduced. This suggests an open grip may be a better choice for training the shoulder musculature in a hang board program.

A progressive strength endurance program will see the rest between repetitions decreasing over the course of the training block while other variables remain the same. For example, static holds for the shoulder girdle on the hang board might involve 10 second hangs in a neutral shoulder position. Each hang is followed by a short rest (<30 seconds), with 6–8 hangs per set and a total of 3–5 sets. The rest between sets is short (<1 minute) to challenge the anaerobic glycolytic system. Changing the level of difficulty may be used to progress and regress the program. The difficulty can be increased by attaching additional weight to the athlete with a harness or weight belt, or decreased by using the feet to support a proportion of the climber's body mass which can be quantified with a commercial force transducer or a set of bathroom scales. These principles of programming can be applied to traditional resistance training and on the wall climbing-related training.

Developing maximum strength

Maximal strength development as a ratio of body mass is an important physical quality for all climbers.[101,102] It is a common physical limitation after injury and can limit the climber's ability to perform lock-off maneuverers and powerful pulling movements with the shoulder girdle. This type of training can increase neural recruitment and intracellular storage of ATP-CPr.[93] Morphological changes in muscle cross-sectional area is important for maximal strength development, however, this must be managed carefully to minimize reductions in the athlete's strength to mass ratio from excessive muscular development. Like strength endurance training, there are various traditional resistance training exercises and climbing-based derivatives that can be used as a training modality. The principles underpinning a maximal strength program are that the load scheme should be near maximal intensity for the entire set (80–95%

1 RM) producing muscular failure in under 12 seconds (or 3–5 repetitions), for a volume of 3–5 sets, with a long rest between sets (3–5 minutes) to allow the resynthesizing of muscle stores of ATP-CPr.[56] For example, steep wall lock-off training develops shoulder adduction strength in a climbing-specific manner. An overhanging bouldering wall system board or campus board with foot holds or foot placement strips is required (see Figure 40.5). The climber, holding large holds with both hands and with the feet on the wall, reaches to a hold above while pulling into a tight lock-off position. The reaching arm hovers above the target hold without touching the hold. The climber returns to the starting position and immediately pulls into another lock-off position with the other hand. A typical loading scheme is 2–3 repetitions each side of 3–5 sets with a long rest period (>5 minutes). The difficulty can be progressed by adding additional mass with a harness, rucksack or weighted belt (hyper gravity training; see Figure 40.6).[33] The difficulty may also be regressed or progressed by modifying the steepness of the wall climbed.

Developing explosive strength (power)

Explosive strength in climbing is required when the climber needs to express force quickly to reach a distant hold on steep terrain. Ballistic exercise for the upper limb requires the athlete exert high forces in short periods of time. The exercise modalities used can include activities which accelerate the athlete's body mass or accelerate an external implement.[15] Traditional ballistic upper body training exercises such as depth push-ups, clap push-ups, kneeling weighted medicine ball throws and medicine ball slams can contribute to explosive strength and rate of force development.[56] Climbing-based derivatives include campus board laddering, campus board dynamic jumps, system board bouldering and boulder campusing.

The training prescription principles involve 2–5 repetitions of moderate to near maximal loads (70–90% 1RM). Each repetition is executed with maximum explosive intention. The volume is between 3–5 sets with long rest periods between sets (>5 minutes).[43] For example, campus board laddering is an effective method for developing shoulder adductor explosive strength[46,47] (see Figure 40.7). The climber begins with both hands on the large campus board rungs with their feet in contact with the wall. The exercise involves climbing hand over hand in a ladder-like motion up the campus board without the aid of the feet. Each repetition should be an explosive reach of the arm to facilitate pulling power from the shoulder adductors.

Metabolic energy system development

Periodization principles may also be applied to the metabolic development of the climber during their rehabilitation and physical preparation. The principles applied for mechanical loading of injured tissues to elevate physical capacity are phase-dependent and build upon the physiological development of earlier phases.[64] As for mechanical loading of neuromuscular tissues, the preparatory phase pertaining to metabolic conditioning may focus on non-specific training. Cardiorespiratory training in the form of cycling and/or running-based activities to up-regulate central adaptations[45] are important for the sport-specific conditioning that will be introduced later in the program.[2,17]

This type of conditioning in the early stages of tissue healing is protective, minimizing the degree of stress associated with the injured or recovering shoulder.[17] The latter part of the preparatory phase acts as a bridge between general metabolic development and sport-specific development as the climber nears return to unrestricted sport. This juncture is typified by stages of tissue healing consistent with improvements in the ability of the injured athlete to tolerate increasing mechanical load. The emphasis of this phase is to maintain central cardiorespiratory adaptations while at the same time improving intracellular (peripheral) adaptations in sport-specific muscles.[2]

High intensity interval training (HIIT) has been shown to be a viable method of developing both aerobic and anaerobic performance in various upper and lower limb dominant sports.[9,21] HIIT is a time-efficient method for improving cardiorespiratory and metabolic function. It involves repeated short (45 seconds) to long (2–8 minutes) periods of high intensity exercise interspersed with recovery periods.[21] HIIT can be used for climbing-related metabolic training.[71] From a rehabilitation perspective it can be used as an adjunct to stimulate both central and peripheral adaptations related to climbing. This can involve programming of long and short HIIT interval training, targeting cardiopulmonary (oxidative) and glycolytic energy systems.[10] This might include interval sessions based upon predetermined work to rest ratios using, for example, medicines ball throws, battle rope conditioning, power bag drags, and upper limb ergometers.

If the athlete is returning to Olympic discipline climbing (speed, lead, and bouldering), the metabolic training program will be dependent upon their pre-injury strengths and weaknesses. For example, a metabolic training program for an athlete returning to lead climbing should be performed at speeds and durations which tax the oxidative and glycolytic energy systems of the forearm and upper quadrant musculature.[22] The selection of exercises that are kinematically and kinetically similar to the sport's skills provides some degree of sport specificity and hence an adaptive response at a cellular level.

The competitive phase is characterized by conditioning modalities that mimic the kinetic and kinematic profile of climbing. The training exercises are now composed of highly specific climbing skills under load. The power and force outputs should relate closely to either speed, boulder, or lead climbing with identical work to recovery ratios.[91] In the competitive phase, the climber is nearing the return to full unrestricted climbing. This stage is typified by use of climbing as the primary method of energy system development. For example, this may range from competition simulation at slightly higher intensities than normal or long indoor climbing routes laden with equipment to simulate alpine training. The specifics of this phase will depend upon the needs of the athlete, type of climbing, and performance level sought. The underlying theories which support a periodization approach are the fitness fatigue model[12] and the general adaptation syndrome.[89] Both explain the role of how organisms adapt to a training stress with positive or negative physiological adaptations.

Case study of a climbing athlete

Precis

Ellie is a very accomplished lead and boulder climber having previously represented her country. She had chosen to specialize in bouldering which has a different mechanical and physiological profile to lead climbing. Bouldering is characterized by short bouts of high-force activities utilizing strength and power endurance. The metabolic profile of this activity is mainly anaerobic in nature, requiring the resynthesis of ATP via the glycolytic system to facilitate the production of energy at a high work rate.[103] Because of its short duration and high work rate, bouldering is most suited to those with high levels of upper body strength and power. During bouldering all muscle action types are required to differing levels dependent upon the chosen climbing route.

A bouldering route typically requires pushing, pulling and static holding positions from the upper limb. The ability to produce high levels of force in a short time enhances performance and reduces injury. This is most evident when the climber is required to latch on to a hold quickly to avoid falling. Furthermore, the speed of muscle contraction is important when forces need to be dissipated quickly. For example, when the upper quadrant must decelerate the body after a jump from one hold to the next. All these factors will need be considered in the rehabilitation of this climber.

Box 40.1

Ellie is a right-dominant climbing athlete. She is 24 years old and has been a climber for over 15 years. During her climbing career Ellie has competed at national level, representing Great Britain as a youth climber in both lead climbing and bouldering. Ellie had to reduce her training commitments when she started university and was no longer able to compete for the national team. At the same time, she fell 10 meters (32.8 feet) while lead climbing on a technically challenging route. This resulted in a glenohumeral joint anterior dislocation on her right side. She has not previously dislocated her shoulder. After six months of rehabilitation, she returned to indoor climbing to focus on bouldering while completing her university studies. However, upon returning to indoor bouldering she felt her right shoulder "give way" during a challenging bouldering route. Ellie's goal is to return to unrestricted bouldering at her pre-injury level.

Assessment

Shoulder range of motion

On examination, Ellie displayed excessive movement in all glenohumeral joint directions bilaterally (Table 40.3). Testing for generalized laxity using the Beighton scale suggested a trend towards joint hypermobility (5/9 score).

Table 40.3 Shoulder range of motion assessment

	Right shoulder		Left shoulder	
	Active ROM	Passive ROM	Active ROM	Passive ROM
Shoulder elevation through flexion	180°	185°	180°	180°
Shoulder elevation through abduction	180°	185°	175°	180°
Horizontal shoulder lateral rotation	Apprehension at 100°	Not tested	100°	130°
Shoulder hand behind back	Upper thorax	Not tested	Upper thorax	Not tested
Shoulder extension	60°	75°	60°	70°

All active and passive movements are approximate ranges of motion (ROM).

Table 40.4 Shoulder isometric strength testing

Muscle group	Right side	Left side
Shoulder external rotation 90°	8.1 kg/17.9 lb	14.7 kg/32.4 lb
Shoulder external rotation 120°	7.4 kg/16.3 lb	12.3 kg/27.1 lb
Shoulder external rotation 160°	5.3 kg/11.3 lb	8.2 kg/18.1 lb
Shoulder abduction 0°	11.6 kg/26.6 lb	17.1 kg/37.7 lb
Middle trapezius	5.2 kg/11.5 lb	9.5 kg/20.9 lb

Table 40.4 details findings for isometric strength assessment using a handheld dynamometer. Reduced strength was recorded on the right (symptomatic) side.

Orthopedic tests

Ellie had a positive apprehensive sign at 100° of external rotation while lying supine. The anterior pivot shift and inferior sulcus sign tests were negative.

Wide arm pull-ups

Ellie was apprehensive to lift her body weight off the ground with both arms. There was also evidence of scapular dyskinesis on the right side.

Joint repositioning (observation)

Testing in supine. When asked to reposition her shoulder with eyes closed, she appeared to have reduced accuracy.

Functional analysis

Observational analysis during an assessment of climbing was undertaken on an electronic tablet with slow motion recall. On relatively simple climbing routes, Ellie did not display any apprehension. However, as the difficulty of the routes progressed and the physical demands on the shoulder girdle increased, Ellie became more apprehensive and less trusting of her shoulder. If the route involved the arms in an abducted and externally rotated position with minimal lower body contact with the climbing wall, Ellie was not prepared to finish the route.

Evidence and shared decision-making

In first time traumatic anterior glenohumeral dislocations (FTAGD) in young adults, therapeutic management often involves nonsurgical rehabilitation.[3] The general consensus is surgery is not indicated unless there is evidence of meaningful bone loss, significant apprehension, and the athlete is involved in a contact sport or other high load activity.[52] There are no data nor indeed is there any consensus on how a climbing athlete should be managed 6 months after a FTAGD and/or subsequent subluxation. After discussion with Ellie, it was clear that she wanted to pursue a nonsurgical approach focused on rehabilitation and physical preparation.

With an absence of literature on the management of FTAGD in an elite female climbing athlete, an evidenced-informed approach was needed. Ellie is highly motivated and wants to specialize in bouldering while she

Table 40.5 Physical preparation program				
Stage of physical preparation	**Early stage**	**Middle stage**	**Middle stage**	**Late stage**
Motor control and skill training	Off the wall low load/low complexity training	Off the wall moderate load/ complexity Proprioceptive training	Low load climbing skill development	Higher load climbing skill development
Mechanical qualities	Hypertrophy training/strength endurance	Maximum strength	Maximum strength and power training	Power training
Metabolic qualities	Cardiorespiratory adaptations +++	Cardiorespiratory adaptations + + Peripheral adaptations +	Cardiorespiratory adaptations + Peripheral adaptations ++	Peripheral adaptations +++
Duration	4–6 weeks	4–6 weeks	4–6 weeks	4–6 weeks
Periodization phase	Preparation phase		Competitive phase	
Specific programming phase	General physical training phase 1	General physical training phase 2	Sport-specific phase 1	Sport-specific phase 2

+, low metabolic training; ++, moderate metabolic training; +++, high metabolic training.

conducts her university studies. However, she is a specialist in lead climbing which has a different physiological profile compared to bouldering. Lead climbing requires more upper quadrant local muscular endurance from a performance perspective. The metabolic profile is also different, requiring utilization of medium-duration glycolytic energy systems and longer-duration oxidative systems.[101] From a practical standpoint this is important because of its influence on the nature of her physical preparation in the middle to late stages of her rehabilitation.

Although Ellie is not involved in a contact sport, the nature of bouldering places heavy demands on the shoulder region. Further, although she does not have meaningful bony loss there is some degree of apprehension with the arm in elevation while under load. These factors combined might warrant a surgical opinion after the subsequent subluxation. However, there is moderate evidence that a proportion of patients managed with physiotherapy (physical therapy) after FTAGD do not experience recurrent shoulder dislocations.[11] There is limited evidence regarding the effectiveness of surgical management for post-traumatic chronic shoulder instability.[38] Based on the uncertainty regarding whether surgery or physiotherapy was the optimal strategy for her return to climbing, a shared decision was taken. In partnership with Ellie a very deliberate physical preparation program was decided upon with clear progress and outcome markers along the journey.

Based on the principles detailed above, the following tables and figures illustrate Ellie's rehabilitation program: Table 40.5 details Ellie's physical preparation program; Table 40.6 details the strength endurance hang board program; Table 40.7 demonstrates the progression matrix for maximal strength training; and Table 40.8 details the progression matrix for explosive strength training. The late stage climbing-specific strength training progressions will include hang board, campus board, system board, and hyper gravity training. Figures 40.4 to 40.8 provide examples of exercises included in Ellie's rehabilitation.

Table 40.6 Strength endurance hang board program[33]

Difficulty level	Duration of hang (seconds)	Duration of rest (seconds)	Number of hangs per set	Number of sets	Rest between sets
Level 1	10	30	6–8	3–5	<1 minute
Level 2	10	20	6–8	3–5	<1 minute
Level 3	10	10	6–8	3–5	<1 minute
Level 4	10	5	6–8	3–5	<1 minute

Table 40.7 Progression matrix for maximal strength training

Exercise modality	Early	Middle	Return to sport
Assisted pull-ups	Incorporate		
Pull-ups	Incorporate		
Weighted pull-ups		Incorporate	
System wall isolations	Incorporate		
Uneven grip pull-ups		Incorporate	
Steep wall lock-offs		Incorporate	Incorporate
One arm lock-offs			Incorporate

Table 40.8 Progression matrix for explosive strength training

Exercise modality	Early	Middle	Return to sport
Standing medicine ball slams and throws	Incorporate		
Kneeling medicine ball slams and throws	Incorporate		
Clap push-ups		Incorporate	
Depth push-ups		Incorporate	
Campus board laddering		Incorporate	
Limit bouldering		Incorporate	Incorporate
Campus board dynamic jumps			Incorporate
Campus bouldering			Incorporate

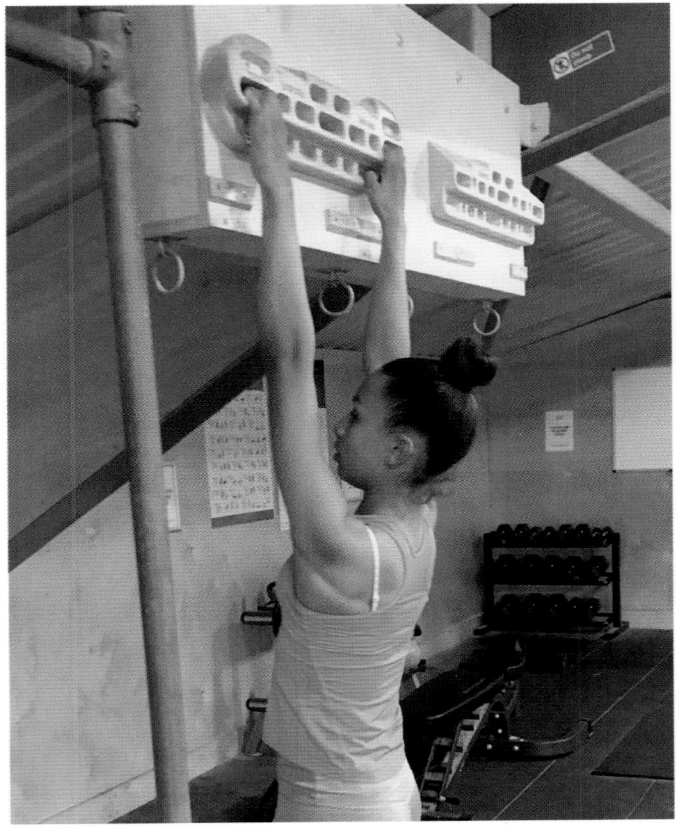

FIGURE 40.4
Hang board strength endurance training.

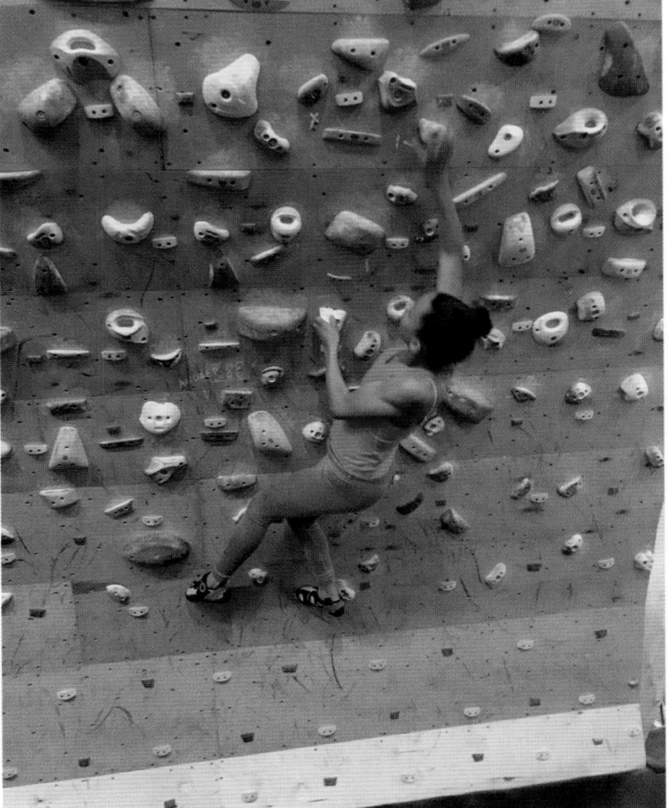

FIGURE 40.5
Steep wall lock-off maximal strength training.

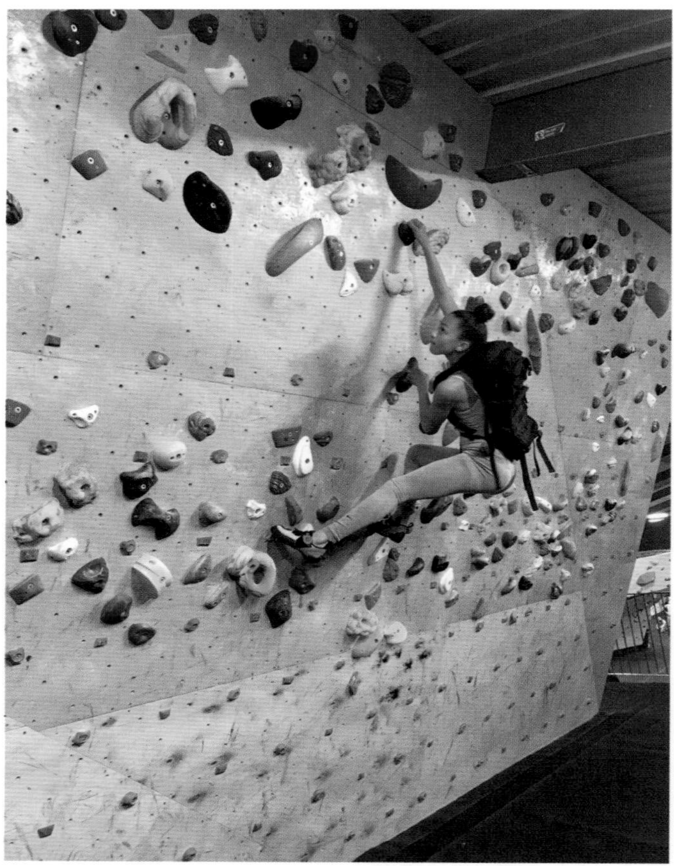

FIGURE 40.6
Hyper gravity training for maximal strength training.

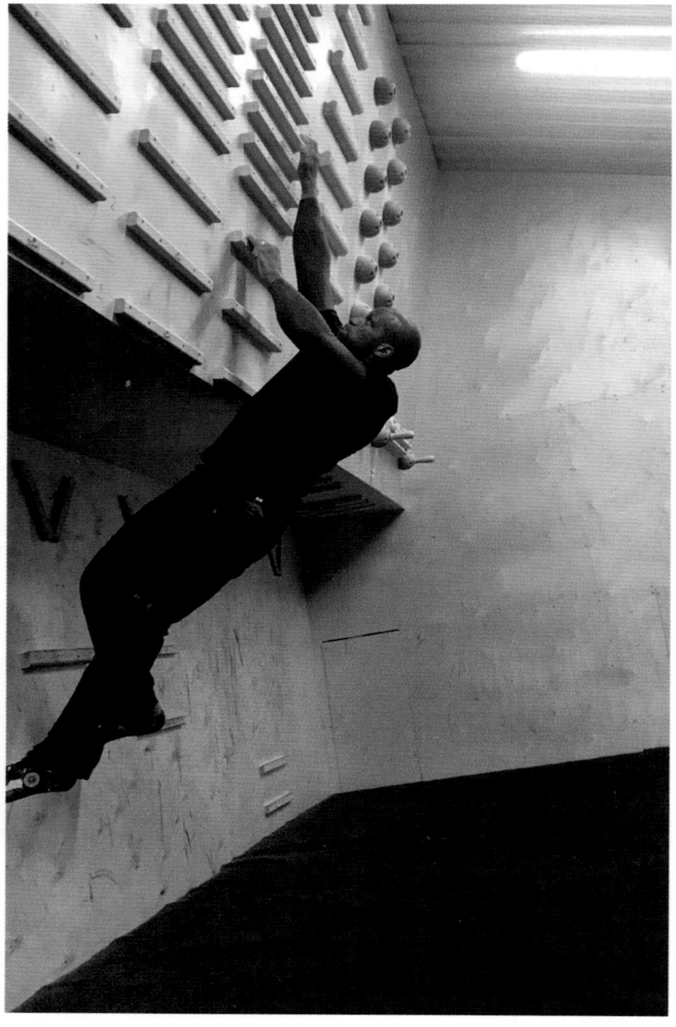

FIGURE 40.7
Campus board laddering explosive strength training.

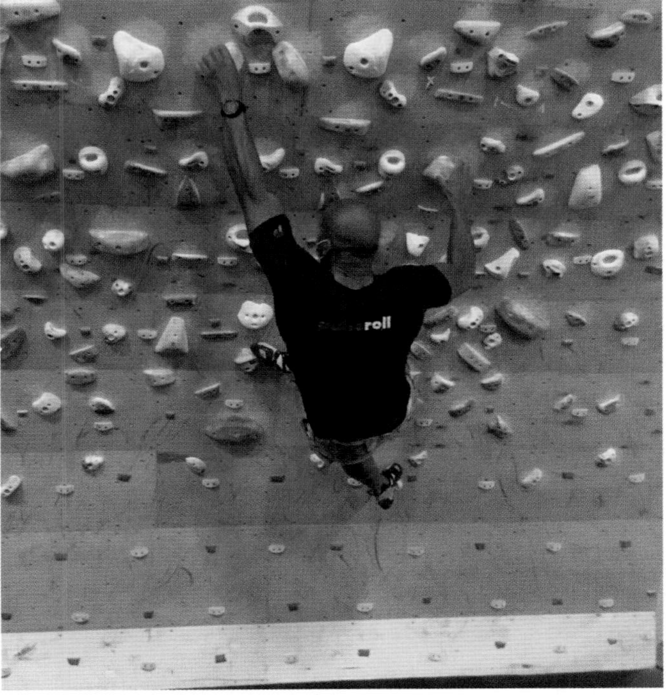

FIGURE 40.8
System board training explosive strength training.

Conclusion

In conclusion, rehabilitation of the climbing athlete is predicated on a thorough understanding of the training and competition demands of the athlete. A philosophical shift is required by the healthcare professional towards a rehabilitation and physical preparation mindset because of the heavy demands imposed upon the shoulder and upper quadrant. This philosophical shift should consider the mechanical aspects specific to the shoulder region and the wider metabolic requirements of the kinetic chain which support climbing performance. The physical needs of the climbing athlete and their return to full sports participation is governed by a blending of art and science.

Acknowledgments

This work is in memory of Ugo Ehiogu and Chief Chike Ehiogu. It is also in recognition of the support from my wife Zoe Ehiogu and children Star and Aurelia.

We would like to thank the International Federation of Sport Climbing and Mr Eddie Fowke for permission to use photographs in this chapter.

References

1. Anderson M, Anderson M. A novel tool and training methodology for improving finger strength in rock climbers. Procedia Engineering. 2015;112:491-496.
2. Artioli GG, Bertuzzi RC, Roschel H, Mendes SH, Lancha Jr AH, Franchini E. Determining the contribution of the energy systems during exercise. JoVE (Journal of Visualized Experiments). 2012;e3413.
3. Avila Lafuente JL, Moros Marco S, García Pequerul JM. Controversies in the management of the first time shoulder dislocation. The Open ORTHOPAEDICS journal. 2017;11:1001-1010.
4. Bak K, Magnusson SP. Shoulder strength and range of motion in symptomatic and pain-free elite swimmers. The American Journal of Sports Medicine. 1997;25:454-459.
5. Baláš J, Duchačová A, Giles D, Kotalíková K, Pánek D, Draper N. Shoulder muscle activity in sport climbing in naturally chosen and corrected shoulder positions. The Open Sports Sciences Journal. 2017;10:107-113.
6. Bartlett R. Sports Biomechanics: Reducing Injury and Improving Performance. Taylor & Francis; 1999.
7. Brooks G, Almquist J. Rehabilitation of musculoskeletal injuries in young athletes. Adolescent Medicine: State of the Art Reviews. 2015;26:100-115.
8. Brumitt J, Cuddeford T. Current concepts of muscle and tendon adaptation to strength and conditioning. International Journal of Sports Physical Therapy. 2015;10:748.
9. Buchheit M, Mendez-Villanueva A, Quod M, Quesnel T, Ahmaidi S. Improving acceleration and repeated sprint ability in well-trained adolescent handball players: speed versus sprint interval training. International Journal of Sports Physiology and Performance. 2010;5:152-164.
10. Buchheit PB, Laursen M. High-intensity interval training, solutions to the programming puzzle. Sports Medicine. 2013;43:313-338.
11. Buss DD, Lynch GP, Meyer CP, Huber SM, Freehill MQ. Nonoperative management for in-season athletes with anterior shoulder instability. The American Journal of Sports Medicine. 2004;32:1430-1433.
12. Busso T, Candau R, Lacour J-R. Fatigue and fitness modelled from the effects of training on performance. European Journal of Applied Physiology and Occupational Physiology. 1994;69:50-54.
13. Chu SK, Jayabalan P, Kibler WB, Press J. The kinetic chain revisited: new concepts on throwing mechanics and injury. PM&R. 2016;8:S69-S77.
14. Cissik J, Hedrick A, Barnes M. Challenges applying the research on periodization. Strength & Conditioning Journal. 2008;30:45-51.

15. Cormie P, McGuigan M, Newton R. Developing maximal neuromuscular power: part 2–training considerations for improving maximal power production. Sports Medicine. 2012;41:125-146.

16. Cronin J, Lawton T, Harris N, Kilding A, McMaster DT. A brief review of handgrip strength and sport performance. The Journal of Strength & Conditioning Research. 2017;31:3187-3217.

17. Dhillon H, Dhilllon S, Dhillon MS. Current concepts in sports injury rehabilitation. Indian Journal of Orthopaedics. 2017;51:529-536.

18. Dischiavi S, Wright A, Hegedus E, Bleakley C. Biotensegrity and myofascial chains: a global approach to an integrated kinetic chain. Medical Hypotheses. 2018;110:90-96.

19. Ehiogu UD, Stephens G, Jones G, Schöffl V. Acute hamstring muscle tears in climbers-current rehabilitation concepts. Wilderness & Environmental Medicine. 2020;31:441-453.

20. Ellenbecker TS. A total arm strength isokinetic profile of highly skilled tennis players. Isokinetics and Exercise Science. 1991;1:9-21.

21. Fernandez-Fernandez J, Zimek R, Wiewelhove T, Ferrauti A. High-intensity interval training vs. repeated-sprint training in tennis. The Journal of Strength & Conditioning Research. 2012;26:53-62.

22. Franchini E, Kokubun E, Kiss M. Energy system contributions in indoor rock climbing. European Journal of Applied Physiology. 2007;101:293-300.

23. Fryer S, Stoner L, Stone K, et al. Forearm muscle oxidative capacity index predicts sport rock-climbing performance. European Journal of Applied Physiology. 2016;116:1479-1484.

24. Fuss FK, Tan AM, Pichler S, Niegl G, Weizman Y. Heart Rate behavior in speed climbing. Frontiers in Psychology. 2020;11:1364.

25. Gastin PB. Energy system interaction and relative contribution during maximal exercise. Sports Medicine. 2001;31:725-741.

26. Gibson-Smith E, Storey R, Ranchordas M. Dietary intake, body composition and iron status in experienced and elite climbers. Frontiers in Nutrition. 2020;7:122.

27. Giles LV, Rhodes EC, Taunton JE. The physiology of rock climbing. Sports Medicine. 2006;36:529-545.

28. Grant S, Hynes V, Whittaker A, Aitchison T. Anthropometric, strength, endurance and flexibility characteristics of elite and recreational climbers. Journal of Sports Sciences. 1996;14:301-309.

29. Hartmann H, Wirth K, Keiner M, Mickel C, Sander A, Szilvas E. Short-term periodization models: effects on strength and speed-strength performance. Sports Medicine. 2015;45:1373-1386.

30. Herodek K, Simonović C, Raković A. Periodization and strength training cycles. Activities in Physical Education & Sport. 2012;2:254-257.

31. Holtzhausen L-M, Noakes TD. Elbow, forearm, wrist, and hand injuries among sport rock climbers. Clinical Journal of Sport Medicine. 1996;6:196-203.

32. Hoover DL, VanWye WR, Judge LW. Periodization and physical therapy: bridging the gap between training and rehabilitation. Physical Therapy in Sport. 2016;18:1-20.

33. Horst E. Training for Climbing: The Definitive Guide to Improving Your Performance. Rowman & Littlefield; 2008.

34. Issurin VB. Benefits and limitations of block periodized training approaches to athletes' preparation: a review. Sports Medicine. 2016;46:329-338.

35. Issurin VB. New horizons for the methodology and physiology of training periodization. Sports Medicine. 2010;40:189-206.

36. Jaggi A, Alexander S. Suppl-6, M13: Rehabilitation for shoulder instability–current approaches. The Open Orthopaedics Journal. 2017;11:957.

37. Jones G, Schöffl V, Johnson MI. Incidence, diagnosis, and management of injury in sport climbing and bouldering: a critical review. Current Sports Medicine Reports. 2018;17:396-401.

38. Kavaja L, Lähdeoja T, Malmivaara A, Paavola M. Treatment after traumatic shoulder dislocation: a systematic review with a network meta-analysis. British Journal of Sports Medicine. 2018;52:1498-1506.

39. Kemmler W, Roloff I, Baumann H, et al. Effect of exercise, body composition, and nutritional intake on bone parameters in male elite rock climbers. International Journal of Sports Medicine. 2006;27:653-659.

40. Keogh JW, Lake JP, Swinton P. Practical applications of biomechanical principles in resistance training: moments and moment arms. Journal of Fitness Research. 2013;2:39-48.

41. Khadilkar L, MacDermid JC, Sinden KE, Jenkyn TR, Birmingham TB, Athwal GS. An analysis of functional shoulder movements during task performance using Dartfish movement analysis software. International Journal of Shoulder Surgery. 2014;8:1.

42. Kibler WB, Wilkes T, Sciascia A. Mechanics and pathomechanics in the overhead athlete. Clinics in Sports Medicine. 2013;32:637-651.

43. Kraemer WJ, Adams K, Cafarelli E, et al. American College of Sports Medicine position stand. Progression models in resistance training for healthy adults. Med Sci Sports Exerc. 2002;34:364-380.

44. Laffaye G, Levernier G, Collin JM. Determinant factors in climbing ability: influence of strength, anthropometry, and neuromuscular fatigue. Scandinavian Journal of Medicine & Science in Sports. 2016;26:1151-1159.

45. Laursen P, Buchheit M. Science and Application of High Intensity Interval Training. Solutions to the Programming Puzzle. Harrogate: Human Kinetics; 2019.

46. Levernier G, Laffaye G. Four weeks of finger grip training increases the rate of force development and the maximal force in elite and top world-ranking climbers. The Journal of Strength & Conditioning Research. 2019;33:2471-2480.

47. Levernier G, Laffaye G. Rate of force development and maximal force: reliability and difference between non-climbers, skilled and international climbers. Sports Biomechanics. 2021;20:495-506.

48. Levernier G, Samozino P, Laffaye G. Force–velocity–power profile in high-elite boulder, lead, and speed climber competitors. International Journal of Sports Physiology and Performance. 2020;15:1012-1018.

49. Lu TW, Chang CF. Biomechanics of human movement and its clinical applications. The Kaohsiung Journal of Medical Sciences. 2012;28:S13-S25.

50. Lutter C, Tischer T, Hotfiel T, et al. Current trends in sport climbing injuries after the inclusion into the Olympic program. Analysis of 633 injuries within the years

2017/18. Muscles, Ligaments & Tendons Journal (MLTJ). 2020;10:201-210.

51. Lutter C, Tischer T, Schöffl VR. Olympic competition climbing: the beginning of a new era—a narrative review. British Journal of Sports Medicine. 2021;55:857-864.

52. Ma R, Brimmo OA, Li X, Colbert L. Current concepts in rehabilitation for traumatic anterior shoulder instability. Current Reviews in Musculoskeletal Medicine. 2017;10:499-506.

53. Mabe J, Butler SL. Analysis of contemporary anaerobic sport specific training techniques for rock climbing. Sport Journal. 24 June 2016.

54. Macdonald JH, Callender N. Athletic profile of highly accomplished boulderers. Wilderness & Environmental Medicine. 2011;22:140-143.

55. MacKenzie R, Monaghan L, Masson RA, et al. Physical and physiological determinants of rock climbing. International Journal of Sports Physiology and Performance. 2020;15:168-179.

56. Maestroni L, Read P, Bishop C, Turner A. Strength and power training in rehabilitation: underpinning principles and practical strategies to return athletes to high performance. Sports Medicine. 2020;50:239-252.

57. McMaster DT, Gill N, Cronin J, McGuigan M. A brief review of strength and ballistic assessment methodologies in sport. Sports Medicine. 2014;44:603-623.

58. McNeal JR, Sands WA. Stretching for performance enhancement. Current Sports Medicine Reports. 2006;5:141-146.

59. Medernach JP, Kleinöder H, Lötzerich HH. Fingerboard in competitive bouldering: training effects on grip strength and endurance. The Journal of Strength & Conditioning Research. 2015;29:2286-2295.

60. Mermier CM, Janot JM, Parker DL, Swan JG. Physiological and anthropometric determinants of sport climbing performance. Br J Sports Med. 2000;34:359-365; discussion 366.

61. Michael MK, Joubert L, Witard OC. Assessment of dietary intake and eating attitudes in recreational and competitive adolescent rock climbers: a pilot study. Front Nutr. 2019;6:64.

62. Michener LA, Abrams JS, Bliven KCH, et al. National Athletic Trainers' Association position statement: evaluation, management, and outcomes of and return-to-play criteria for overhead athletes with superior labral anterior-posterior injuries. Journal of Athletic Training. 2018;53:209-229.

63. Mladenov L, Michailov M, Schoffl I. Antropometric and strength characteristics of world-class boulderers. Medicina Sportiva. 2009;13:231-238.

64. Mølmen KS, Øfsteng SJ, Rønnestad BR. Block periodization of endurance training–a systematic review and meta-analysis. Open Access Journal of Sports Medicine. 2019;10:145.

65. Morrison S, Ward P. Energy system development and load management through the rehabilitation and return to play process. International Journal of Sports Physical Therapy. 2017;12:697.

66. Mountjoy M, Sundgot-Borgen J, Burke L, et al. International Olympic Committee (IOC) consensus statement on relative energy deficiency in sport (RED-S): 2018 update. International Journal of Sport Nutrition and Exercise Metabolism. 2018;28:316-331.

67. Ng GY, Lam PC. A study of antagonist/agonist isokinetic work ratios of shoulder rotators in men who play badminton. Journal of Orthopaedic & Sports Physical Therapy. 2002;32:399-404.

68. Noakes T. Physiological models to understand exercise fatigue and the adaptations that predict or enhance athletic performance. Scandinavian Journal of Medicine & Science in Sports: Review Article. 2000;10:123-145.

69. Orth D, Davids K, Seifert L. Coordination in climbing: effect of skill, practice and constraints manipulation. Sports Medicine. 2016;46:255-268.

70. Parks MT, Wang Z, Siu KC. Current low-cost video-based motion analysis options for clinical rehabilitation: a systematic review. Phys Ther. 2019;99:1405-1425.

71. Phillips K, Sassaman J, Smoliga J. Optimizing rock climbing performance through sport-specific strength and conditioning. Strength and Conditioning Journal. 2012;34:1-18.

72. Podlog L, Dimmock J, Miller J. A review of return to sport concerns following injury rehabilitation: practitioner strategies for enhancing recovery outcomes. Phys Ther Sport. 2011;12:36-42.

73. Podlog L, Heil J, Schulte S. Psychosocial factors in sports injury rehabilitation and return to play. Phys Med Rehabil Clin N Am. 2014;25:915-930.

74. Reiman MP, Lorenz DS. Integration of strength and conditioning principles into a rehabilitation program. International Journal of Sports Physical Therapy. 2011;6:241.

75. Richardson E, Lewis JS, Gibson J, et al. Role of the kinetic chain in shoulder rehabilitation: does incorporating the trunk and lower limb into shoulder exercise regimes influence shoulder muscle recruitment patterns? Systematic review of electromyography studies. BMJ Open Sport & Exercise Medicine. 2020;6:e000683.

76. Röijezon U, Clark NC, Treleaven J. Proprioception in musculoskeletal rehabilitation. Part 1: Basic science and principles of assessment and clinical interventions. Man Ther. 2015;20:368-377.

77. Rokowski R. The role of body build, strength and endurance abilities in achieving high results by rock climbers. Journal of Kinesiology and Exercise Sciences. 2020;30:21-28.

78. Rosemeyer JR, Hayes BT, Switzler CL, Hicks-Little CA. Effects of core-musculature fatigue on maximal shoulder strength. Journal of Sport Rehabilitation. 2015;24:384-390.

79. Saeterbakken AH, Loken E, Scott S, Hermans E, Vereide VA, Andersen V. Effects of ten weeks dynamic or isometric core training on climbing performance among highly trained climbers. PLoS One. 2018;13:e0203766.

80. Sas-Nowosielski K, Kandzia K. Post-activation potentiation response of climbers performing the upper body power exercise. Frontiers in Psychology. 2020;11:467.

81. Saul D, Steinmetz G, Lehmann W, Schilling AF. Determinants for success in climbing: a systematic review. Journal of Exercise Science & Fitness. 2019;17:91-100.

82. Schoenfeld BJ, Grgic J, Ogborn D, Krieger JW. Strength and hypertrophy adaptations between low-vs. high-load resistance training: a systematic review and meta-analysis. The Journal of Strength & Conditioning Research. 2017;31:3508-3523.

83. Schöffl V, Lutter C, Popp D. The "Heel Hook"—a climbing-specific technique to injure the leg. Wilderness & Environmental Medicine. 2016;27:294-301.

84. Schöffl V, Popp D, Dickschass J, Küpper T. Superior labral anterior-posterior lesions in

rock climbers—primary double tenodesis? Clinical Journal of Sport Medicine. 2011;21:261-263.

85. Schreiber T, Allenspach P, Seifert B, Schweizer A. Connective tissue adaptations in the fingers of performance sport climbers. European Journal of Sport Science. 2015;15:696-702.

86. Schweizer A. Sport climbing from a medical point of view. Swiss Medical Weekly. 2012;142:w13688.

87. Seifert L, Orth D, Mantel B, Boulanger J, Hérault R, Dicks M. Affordance realization in climbing: learning and transfer. Frontiers in Psychology. 2018;9:820.

88. Seifert L, Wattebled L, L'Hermette M, Bideault G, Herault R, Davids K. Skill transfer, affordances and dexterity in different climbing environments. Human Movement Science. 2013;32:1339-1352.

89. Selye H. Forty years of stress research: principal remaining problems and misconceptions. Canadian Medical Association Journal. 1976;115:53.

90. Spencer S, Wolf A, Rushton A. Spinal-exercise prescription in sport: classifying physical training and rehabilitation by intention and outcome. Journal of Athletic Training. 2016;51:613-628.

91. Stien N, Saeterbakken AH, Hermans E, Vereide VA, Olsen E, Andersen V. Comparison of climbing-specific strength and endurance between lead and boulder climbers. PLoS One. 2019;14:e0222529.

92. Suchomel TJ, Comfort P, Stone MH. Weightlifting pulling derivatives: rationale for implementation and application. Sports Medicine. 2015;45:823-839.

93. Suchomel TJ, Nimphius S, Bellon CR, Stone MH. The importance of muscular strength: training considerations. Sports Medicine. 2018;48:765-785.

94. Turner AN. The science and practice of periodization: a brief review. Strength and Conditioning Journal. 2011;33:34-46.

95. Turner AN, Comfort P, McMahon J, et al. Developing powerful athletes, Part 1: mechanical underpinnings. Strength & Conditioning Journal. 2020;42:30-39.

96. Van Middelkoop M, Bruens M, Coert J, et al. Incidence and risk factors for upper extremity climbing injuries in indoor climbers. International Journal of Sports Medicine. 2015;36:837-842.

97. Vigouroux L, Devise M, Cartier T, Aubert C, Berton E. Performing pull-ups with small climbing holds influences grip and biomechanical arm action. Journal of Sports Sciences. 2019;37:886-894.

98. Vigouroux L, Quaine F, Labarre-Vila A, Moutet F. Estimation of finger muscle tendon tensions and pulley forces during specific sport-climbing grip techniques. Journal of Biomechanics. 2006;39:2583-2592.

99. Wall CB, Starek JE, Fleck SJ, Byrnes WC. Prediction of indoor climbing performance in women rock climbers. Journal of Strength and Conditioning Research. 2004;18:77-83.

100. Watson S, Allen B, Grant JA. A clinical review of return-to-play considerations after anterior shoulder dislocation. Sports Health. 2016;8:336-341.

101. Watts PB. Physiology of difficult rock climbing. European Journal of Applied Physiology. 2004;91:361-372.

102. Watts PB, Martin DT, Durtschi S. Anthropometric profiles of elite male and female competitive sport rock climbers. J Sports Sci. 1993;11:113-117.

103. White DJ, Olsen PD. A time motion analysis of bouldering style competitive rock climbing. The Journal of Strength & Conditioning Research. 2010;24:1356-1360.

104. Wilk KE, Arrigo CA, Hooks TR, Andrews JR. Rehabilitation of the overhead throwing athlete: there is more to it than just external rotation/internal rotation strengthening. PM&R. 2016;8:S78-S90.

105. Wirth K, Hartmann H, Mickel C, Szilvas E, Keiner M, Sander A. Core stability in athletes: a critical analysis of current guidelines. Sports Medicine. 2017;47:401-414.

106. Wong EK, Ng GY. Isokinetic work profile of shoulder flexors and extensors in sport climbers and nonclimbers. J Orthop Sports Phys Ther. 2008;38:572-577.

107. Wong EK, Ng GY. Strength profiles of shoulder rotators in healthy sport climbers and nonclimbers. Journal of Athletic Training. 2009;44:527-530.

108. Zapf J, Fichtl B, Wielgoss S, Schmidt W. Macronutrient intake and eating habits in elite rock climbers. Medicine & Science in Sports & Exercise. 2001;33:S72.

41 Rehabilitation after shoulder surgery

Jo Gibson, Jeremy Lewis

Introduction

Factors that influence the clinical outcomes following surgical intervention for musculoskeletal shoulder problems are multifarious. They include, but are not limited to, the surgical technique, the expertise of the surgeon, the patient's biopsychosocial, environmental, and lifestyle factors, and – the focus of this chapter – the quality, appropriateness, and timing of the post-surgical rehabilitation.

As discussed in Chapters 9 and 29, there have been tremendous advances in surgical technique and expertise. In addition, there has been a realization that to maximize post-surgical outcomes, the surgeon, therapist, and the patient, including the patient's social and vocational network, need to work collaboratively.

Advances in post-surgical rehabilitation have arguably not kept pace with the advances in surgical techniques. There is an obvious paucity of research evidence for clinicians to translate into practice to guide post-surgical rehabilitation following surgery for both traumatic and nontraumatic musculoskeletal presentations of the shoulder.[48,87,105]

There are ongoing debates pertaining to best practice for post-surgical rehabilitation. The person responsible for the post-surgical rehabilitation plan is the focus of one such debate. Some suggest it is the surgeon's responsibility, arguing that if a surgeon, after considering the harms and benefits of surgery decides, with the informed patient's consent, to operate, then a post-surgical rehabilitation program, specifically designed for the patient, should be provided by that surgeon or surgical team. Physical therapists (physiotherapists) who predominantly work as autonomous practitioners argue that a post-surgical rehabilitation plan falls within their remit.

We strongly argue that, in the patient's best interest, the post-surgical plan is agreed by the patient, surgeon, and the therapist. If this preferred situation does not transpire and no guidance is forthcoming from the surgeon, the therapist will often be required to follow standardized post-surgical rehabilitation protocols. Frequently the safety and effectiveness of these protocols have not been adequately assessed in well-designed research investigations. Furthermore, protocols may have been developed that follow average tissue healing times in relatively healthy people, that may not account for the patient's age, psychosocial, endocrine, genetic profile, tissue quality, comorbidities, and lifestyle factors, as well as factoring in the patient's aims, values, and desired outcomes.[15,26,48,82,128]

The lack of robust evidence has resulted in additional post-surgical management uncertainty where surgeons may prefer slower, more cautious rehabilitation, compared with physical therapists and others involved in post-surgical management, especially those working in specialist units, or in specialist roles, who advocate for accelerated rehabilitation programs.[22,60,105,113] Those preferring to delay the start of rehabilitation, and progress more slowly, do so, in the understandable belief, that a cautious start and progression will protect the healing tissue. This belief however is at odds with emerging research that suggests early controlled mobilization may promote a faster return to function without increasing the risk of structural failure.[9,47,66,118,129] Given that poor patient satisfaction rates following shoulder surgery are highly correlated with persistent pain, stiffness, and failure to return to function, an appropriately accelerated approach to rehabilitation may improve patient outcomes.

The aim of this chapter is to synthesize the available research and provide guidance for clinicians taking responsibility for the post-surgical rehabilitation of an individual who has undergone shoulder surgery. Due to the current paucity of evidence, we will make suggestions for management based on clinical consensus. We hope that in future editions of this textbook the research evidence to support best post-surgical rehabilitation will be more robust.

Preparation is key: empathy, expectations and education

The influence of psychosocial factors such as negative pain beliefs, pain-related worrying (or catastrophizing) and fear avoidance, on an individual's experience of pain, and the impact on recovery, are well recognized.[21,86,139] An expert clinician not only knows how to plan a post-surgical rehabilitation program, but will actively listen to the patient's lived experiences with empathy, and as appropriate, validate the patient's experiences, concerns, uncertainties, and fears. Therefore, investing time to understand an individual's beliefs, expectations, and concerns preoperatively, may help identify potential barriers to recovery, alleviate concerns, and reduce kinesiophobia post-surgery.

Kinesiophobia and fear of re-injury are increasingly recognized as factors that increase the risk of failure to return to function following surgery.[48,130,138] Clinicians often overestimate expected outcomes following procedures such as rotator cuff repair regardless of their experience level or the percentage of shoulder caseload that they treat.[70] It is important for clinicians to be aware of timescales for recovery for different surgical procedures, and the factors that may influence outcomes to ensure realistic expectations are established.

Preoperative clinics provide an opportunity to ensure patients are well prepared, have a clear understanding of postoperative recovery, and reinforce realistic expectations. It is also an important part of planning when patients may need additional help if they live alone, particularly older and vulnerable populations, and for people lacking social support. The impact of preoperative clinics on postoperative outcomes has been well documented, however, patients' comprehension and recall after being provided with preoperative education is often poor.[72] The use of multimedia tools to support and reinforce what patients may expect as well as key advice to support their recovery have been shown to improve recall and patient satisfaction.[55]

Whether the first contact with the patient occurs preoperatively or soon after surgery, actively listening, empathizing, and validating are essential to build a therapeutic alliance where both the patient and therapist will trust each other. The patient needs to understand the components and stages of the rehabilitation program, and based on an understanding of the patient's aims and desires, the physical therapist and surgeon need to speak with one voice as to what is achievable, and what the realistic time frames are. Patients have reported surprise at the levels of postoperative pain, difficulties sleeping, slowness of recovery, protracted impact on function, and protracted helplessness following shoulder surgery. These issues need to be discussed sensitively with the patient. A lack of patient understanding, a lack of autonomy, and a lack of support may influence the patient's postoperative recovery and experience of pain[27,124] (see Chapter 11, Communication).

Patients often have high expectations of surgery and are optimistic that the procedure will reduce their pain and suffering. This may be due to verbal and nonverbal cues picked up by the patient from the surgeon and the therapist. A correlation between patient expectations of the benefits of surgery and post-surgical outcomes exists.[27,101,124] A disparity between expectations and experience may have a detrimental impact on patient satisfaction, adherence to rehabilitation, and reported improvement.[53,95,134] This reiterates the importance of ensuring that the multidisciplinary team communicates a consistent message.

Factors affecting outcome

One aim of elective shoulder surgery is to restore the structural integrity of damaged tissues, such as repairing a torn rotator cuff tendon, securing a detached glenoid labrum, and/or restoring normal anatomy, such as removing an acromial spur to increase the acromial-humeral distance. Success of these procedures may be defined in different ways. One measure of success would be clinical improvement, i.e., reduction in pain, improvement in function, which may or may not be related to successful repair of the tissues or removal of bony abnormalities.[20,77,78,97,115] Other measures of success would include: 1) healing of the operated tissue (e.g., successful structural healing of the tissue of concern), and if healed, 2) no recurrence of the lesion (e.g., no re-tear of rotator cuff tendon after it had successfully healed, no redislocation of the glenohumeral joint after successful tissue healing following an anterior stabilization procedure). Following surgery, if the tissue did not heal, and/or re-tore after successful healing, this could be deemed surgical failure. This results in the confusing scenario that clinical success can occur in the presence of surgical failure, and clinically unfavorable outcomes may remain or worsen in the presence of surgical success.[20,78]

This suggests that in many situations, surgery may be performed on tissues that are not causing the symptoms, or if the tissues are causing the symptoms, current surgical techniques may not be able to resolve the local problem. This begs the question, why do patients report clinical improvement in the presence of surgical failure? Two of the myriad possibilities include: 1) the surgery was not performed on the tissue associated with symptoms and natural improvement occurred over time, and/or, 2) improvements are related to contextual healing.[90] With respect to contextual healing, Jonas et al. concluded that the nonspecific (placebo) effects of surgery and other invasive procedures can be large.[58]

These findings complicate discussion of factors affecting outcome, and ultimately impact on recommendations for rehabilitation following surgery. There are many inconsistencies and equivocal findings in the available research that are compounded by the frequent utilization of retrospective analyses. What follows is a summary, but what is clear is that there are substantial gaps in our knowledge that require combinations of randomized placebo-controlled clinical trials, cohort studies, and qualitative research to inform clinical practice.

Age

Although not conclusive,[57] the patient's age at the time of surgery for rotator cuff tendon repair may negatively correlate with rotator cuff healing.[37,57,75]

Comorbidities

Mental health comorbidities such as anxiety and depression may have a detrimental influence on post-surgical outcome, including a protracted time course.[102,110,141] High scores on the Hospital Anxiety and Depression Score (HADS) and the mental health component of the Short Form 36 (SF-36) (see Chapter 12) correlate with high levels of postoperative pain and poorer outcomes.[29,64,98]

Although not conclusive,[57] diabetes mellitus, obesity, dyslipidemia, low levels of vitamin D, and osteoporosis appear to have a detrimental impact on rotator cuff repair non-healing and/or re-tears following surgery.[57] Low levels of vitamin D have been associated with higher rates of revision surgery for rotator cuff repairs and fatty degeneration of the supraspinatus and infraspinatus muscles in people with full-thickness rotator cuff tears.[19,94] Vitamin D is important in the healing process to decrease inflammation, and has been shown to downregulate tumor necrosis factor-α, a major inflammatory cytokine,[7] and possibly upregulate the anti-inflammatory cytokine interleukin (IL)-10.[3] Adequate levels of serum vitamin D were associated with lower levels of IL-6 and C-reactive protein,[69] both markers of inflammation.

Identifying any health comorbidity, such as dietary deficiencies, diabetes, cardiac, or respiratory disease may require referral and support from appropriate members of the multidisciplinary team to facilitate the best outcome possible. The requirement is the same for mental health concerns.

Post-surgical pain

The reduction and ideally the alleviation of pain and a concomitant improvement in function are the main reasons people consent for shoulder surgery. Unfortunately, surgical outcomes do not always achieve this aim, and there are myriad factors that increase the risk of high pain levels and disability (Box 41.1). Awareness of these factors will enable the surgeon and therapist to educate patients and if possible, address any modifiable risk factors prior to surgery. Knowledge of these risk factors will also support the surgeon and therapist in individualizing a postoperative treatment plan.

Many of the risk factors detailed in Box 41.1 will be identified during the patient interview, in the patient's clinical notes, using appropriate patient-reported outcome measures, and during the physical examination. Education,

Box 41.1 Risk factors for high postoperative pain levels and disability

- High levels of pain preoperatively.[141]
- Preoperative opioid use.[29,105,110]
- Negative beliefs and expectations.[48,64,138]
- Mental health comorbidities.[98,110]
- Associated cervical spine involvement.[51]
- Obesity (increased pro-inflammatory cytokines/metabolic inflammation).[51,66,105,113]
- Smoking (increased pro-inflammatory cytokines).[9,66,105]
- Women undergoing rotator cuff surgery.[22,34]

appropriate intervention, appropriate onward referral, underpinned with empathy and validation, will support patients identified with these risk factors and may improve outcomes.

Post-surgical stiffness

Postoperative shoulder stiffness is a common complication, and encouragingly it does not usually have a detrimental impact on outcomes in the longer term (one year) and rarely requires further surgical intervention to resolve.[66,112] It is therefore important to validate the patient's concerns and frustrations as well as to reassure patients who develop postoperative shoulder stiffness that they can still expect to achieve beneficial outcomes in the longer term. The development of postoperative stiffness will significantly delay return to function in the short and medium term, and as previously mentioned is associated with poor patient satisfaction rates.[23] Knowledge of risk factors for development of shoulder stiffness following surgery may help identify patients for whom early mobilization approaches may be particularly beneficial.

Risk factors predisposing patients to developing postoperative stiffness relate to both the patient and the surgery (Table 41.1). The development of postoperative stiffness may be indicative of an underlying and possibly undiagnosed metabolic condition. Blonna et al.[10] highlighted that the development of moderate or severe postoperative shoulder stiffness could be an indicator of subclinical diabetes or hypothyroidism in those not previously diagnosed. Chapter 18 discusses the relationship between AGEs (advanced glycation end products) that increase with aging, lifestyle behaviors, and in persistent hyperglycemic environments, such as diabetes and shoulder joint stiffness and reduced range of motion. AGEs are associated with increased collagen cross-links in ligaments and capsule tissue leading to joint stiffness and motion restriction.[92] When concentrations of AGEs are high, the normal homeostatic free radical–antioxidant balance is disrupted resulting in oxidative stress. This complex process is associated with cellular damage and inflammation and potentially pain, which may be associated with active muscle guarding.[54]

Table 41.1 Risk factors related to the development of postoperative shoulder stiffness

Patient factors	Surgical factors
Diabetes[10,30]	Rotator cuff repair[56,66]
Thyroid dysfunction[10,30]	• <50 years old
Cardiovascular disease[30]	• Post-traumatic
Dupuytren's disease	• Partial-thickness bursal-sided tear
Gastroesophageal reflux disease[31,32]	Undergoing >1 procedure[56,66]
Obesity (metabolic inflammation)[30,100]	Surgery for frozen shoulder[56]
Hypercholesterolemia[30,100]	Surgery for calcific tendinitis[56]
Cervical spine involvement[30]	Immobilization[20,30,56]
Menopause[17,100]	Procedures involving the long head of biceps[114]
Stress and psychosocial factors[17,100]	

Suboptimal post-surgical tissue healing

As discussed in Chapter 29, elective shoulder surgery should be considered when clinical reasoning suggests an operation will lead to a meaningful clinical outcome, and that the benefits outweigh the harms. Shoulder surgery is commonly performed to repair soft tissue: to restore the integrity of a torn rotator cuff tendon, repair a torn or detached glenoid labrum, or repair, reattach, or tighten the glenohumeral capsule to restore stability.

If the aim of the surgical procedure is to restore tissue integrity, it is essential to allow the tissue to heal, and when permitted, only apply loads in appropriate ranges of shoulder motion that have therapeutic benefit that do not compromise the repair process. For example, tendon healing after rotator cuff repair may be divided into three phases that overlap. Stage I is described as the inflammation phase and lasts on average between 0 and 7 days. Stage II is the repair phase, and typically occurs between days 5 and 25 post-surgery. The final phase, Stage III, known as the remodeling phase, starts on average 21 days post-surgery, and normally is the longest stage.[48] These timescales for rotator cuff tendon repairs vary considerably.

Even when post-surgical rotator cuff tendon repair rehabilitation is conducted respecting the stages of healing, and involves exercises that do not compromise the tissue healing process, re-tears can still occur. The UKUFF randomized clinical trial demonstrated rotator cuff tendon re-tear rates range from 38.6% when the tendon repair was performed as an open procedure, to 46.4% when the tendon was repaired arthroscopically.[20] Failure rates as high as 94.0% have been reported following massive rotator cuff repairs.

The reasons for post-surgical tissue failure are multifarious and include individual patient factors, surgical factors, and technique,[65] and tissue integrity factors. Fermont et al. reported that male sex, absence of diabetes, high activity level, smaller sagittal tear size, and less fatty infiltration were predictors of successful structural tendon-to-bone healing after rotator cuff repair.[44] They also reported that younger patients (mean 57.8 years, ± 9.4 years) were more likely to have healed repairs than people on average 10 years older (mean 68.0 years, ± 7.6 years).[44] In another review the risk of re-tear after rotator cuff repair was reported to increase with age and doubled between the ages of 50 to 70 years.[65] Patient and tissue integrity factors, that may occur in combination, are summarized in Table 41.2.

There have been substantial advances in the surgical procedures available to treat shoulder instability. There are also many reasons for suboptimal outcomes and Table 41.3 details risk factors that predispose patients to an increased risk of recurrence of instability and the possible need for revision surgery.

Psychosocial factors

There is clear evidence that an individual's decision not to return to play (return to sport, return to unrestricted activity), and a failure to return to previous levels of performance are highly correlated with a fear of re-injury.[116,130] Kinesiophobia, psychological factors, a lack of social support, and competing priorities (e.g., work, family) have been shown to influence whether an individual returns to sport. Clinicians need to assess both physical and psychological readiness to return to play, and if psychological factors are identified they need to be addressed by the most appropriate people in the multidisciplinary team. Ciccotti et al.[25] reported that time after surgery (usually six months) was the most common criteria used to guide return to play following surgical stabilization for primary traumatic anterior instability. Other criteria included strength, range of motion, pain, stability, proprioception, and post-surgical

Table 41.2 Risk factors associated with surgical failure following rotator cuff tendon repair[41,66,103,109,126,141,145]

Patient factors	Tissue integrity factors
Increasing age (>50 years)[65]	Fat infiltration into rotator cuff muscles
Obesity	Tear retraction
Diabetes	Rotator cuff muscle atrophy
Smoking	Large tears > 5 cm (2 inches)
Low vitamin D levels	More than 1 tendon torn
Poor or lack of adherence with post-surgical guidelines and rehabilitation program	Poor tissue tendon quality Osteoporosis[24] Pre-surgical corticosteroid injections 6 months prior to surgery[132,133]

Table 41.3 Risk factors associated with recurrent instability after stabilization surgery

Risk factors	Relevance
Age[35,104,116,131]	< 22 years increased risk of failure if returning to contact sport Adolescents < 16 years returning to contact sport
Sex[104]	Male
Sex[36]	Female
Surgical technique[38,104]	Fewer than three anchors and the use of knotless anchors Surgical position
Pathoanatomy[35,38,104,116]	Glenoid or humeral bone loss Decreased glenoid retroversion
Level of sport[104]	Increased redislocation rates at higher levels of competition
Previous stabilization[36,38,117]	Increased risk of recurrent instability
Recurrent instability[104,116]	The greater the number of dislocations preoperatively the greater the risk of recurrent instability
Laxity[36,38]	Increased shoulder external rotation with arm by the side and in shoulder abduction increased risk of recurrent instability
Atraumatic primary dislocation[36]	Increased risk of recurrence and clinical failure
Bilateral instability[36]	Increased risk of recurrence and clinical failure
Duration of symptoms[35]	Duration of symptoms > 5 months before presentation increased risk of recurrence

radiograph. There appears to be uncertainty as to the criteria to use, their importance and hierarchy.[25]

Minimizing the detrimental impact of immobilization

The effects of immobilization are well reported and changes in central motor drive, cortical excitability, cortical representation, and reduced motor execution can occur after only a few days.[18] Loss of muscle strength, muscle atrophy, and a decline in neuromuscular function have been well demonstrated together with an increase in pain sensitivity.[16,83] Immobilization in a sling has also been shown to be associated with impaired gait, impaired balance, and increased falls risk in people over 60 years of age, particularly following rotator cuff repair and total shoulder arthroplasty.[28,120] The following are strategies to consider when attempting to minimize the detrimental impact of an extended period of mobilization.

Engaging the hand

Early engagement with the hand for light functional activities may be an effective strategy to minimize cortical changes and target muscle function. Eating with the elbow supported, and washing the body while supporting the elbow, facilitates peripheral input while maintaining levels of activation in the rotator cuff within levels considered "safe".[142] Simple hand gripping and opening exercises are also a useful adjunct, as grip has been shown to be an effective facilitator of rotator cuff activity and central motor drive.[5]

Exercising the contralateral side

Unilateral strength training of the non-immobilized or non-injured limb has been shown to achieve strength gains and preserve muscle cross-sectional area in the immobilized contralateral limb through cross-education effects.[6] The mechanisms of cross-education have not been fully elucidated, but cortical and spinal effects have been demonstrated; changes in cortical processes positively impact neural drive in the contralateral limb and influence corticospinal excitability. These effects appear to be magnified if the dominant arm is the training arm, i.e., the uninjured limb. The type of contraction and level of contraction also appear to augment cross-education effects: eccentric exercises and working at 60% MVC (maximal isometric voluntary contraction) or above provide superior results.[52,76] Mirror visual feedback has also been shown to enhance cross-education effects.[144]

Cross-education has been shown to impact range of movement and strength in patient populations including distal radial fractures, chronic stroke populations, and following lower limb surgery.[6,39,49] While there is limited evidence evaluating cross-education in patients following shoulder surgery or injury, one study showed preferential effects compared with no cross-education intervention in a group who were immobilized in a shoulder sling for four weeks.[84] A recent Delphi consensus suggested that cross-education should be considered as an adjuvant treatment in those that have to be immobilized or have a period of reduced function following injury or surgery.[85] It also potentially has applications for patients undergoing rehabilitation for traumatic dislocations and stabilization surgery. Exercising the unaffected limb in the positions the patient injured their shoulder, e.g., shoulder abduction-external rotation, may have the potential to positively influence the cortical changes related to persistent apprehension.[68,143]

Chapter 30 discusses the role of virtual reality (VR) in the management of shoulder conditions. Although current understanding of the value of VR in the nonsurgical and post-surgical management of musculoskeletal conditions involving the shoulder is at an embryonic stage, it has the potential to contribute to many of the suggestions in the preceding sections. VR research will provide an insight into its potential in shoulder rehabilitation.

Closed kinetic chain

Gentle weight bearing through the upper limb with the hands on a table is another rehabilitation strategy during the period of immobilization. Closed chain exercises are inherently stable, facilitate recruitment in the rotator cuff and scapular muscles, and may help rehabilitate proprioception[1,63,89] (see Chapter 28). Changing hand position, i.e., rotation, may target different recruitment patterns in the shoulder muscles. It is important to consider the surgical procedure and ensure that these exercises are pain-free so that patients do not adopt compensatory patterns that may increase muscle recruitment beyond safe levels. If patients remove their sling for axillary hygiene or for activities of daily living, such as brushing their teeth, they can do so in protected, gentle, and supported weight-bearing conditions.

Isometric muscle contractions

Isometric muscle contractions were promoted as exercises to promote analgesia in tendon-related conditions, including those involving the shoulder tendons. Research has challenged the superiority of isometric contractions for this purpose.[12,40,99,119,137] However, gentle isometrics that are performed without pain are an effective way of targeting muscle recruitment of the rotator cuff and axioscapular muscles, and may have proprioceptive benefits.[96,111] Increasing and deceasing support for the arm (no support, 50% support, 100% support) during loading exercises involves different patterns of rotator cuff and scapular muscle activity.[125]

Mirror visual feedback

For people experiencing high levels of postoperative pain who struggle to engage with the interventions described above, particularly those with hyperalgesia or allodynia, mirror visual feedback (MVF) may be a useful adjunct. MVF has been investigated as a treatment strategy to target cortical changes and desensitize a hypervigilant nervous system.[83] To perform these exercises, patients place their affected limb out of view and watch movements of their non-affected limb in the mirror. This gives the appearance that the affected arm is moving. This provides a strong visual input and activates the motor cortex. MVF has been shown to reduce pain and sensitivity in people experiencing persistent pain, as well as for people reporting high levels of pain and disability.[13,33]

Louw et al.[83] demonstrated that a brief MVF intervention in people with shoulder pain and movement restriction resulted in an improvement in pain, range of movement, pain catastrophizing, and fear avoidance. Furthermore, mirror therapy has been shown to reduce pain at rest and night pain during the immobilization period, and in the first week after removal of cast/splint in patients following wrist fracture and carpal tunnel surgery.[62,67]

While MVF does not appear to impact longer-term outcomes (comparable range of movement and strength), the short-term effects may be beneficial in patients with high levels of pain and disability after surgery. In addition, in those patients where a period of immobilization is deemed necessary, this is a potential tool to minimize the cortical changes that can negatively influence motor performance. There is a need for further investigation regarding optimal dosage and the individuals and conditions that will benefit the most from MVF. Other strategies aimed at influencing cortical maps such as sensory discrimination, graphesthesia, two-point discrimination, and graded motor imagery may also have a role in postoperative and post-injury management, but to date most of the research relates to persistent pain populations and people with neurological conditions. There may also be a role for VR in MVF.

The case for early mobilization

Traditionally patients are immobilized in a cross-body/internal rotation sling after surgery or trauma with the aim of protecting the shoulder, and for patient comfort. The trend towards early arm movement (mobilization) and more proactive approaches to postoperative rehabilitation aim to facilitate an earlier return to function and minimize the impact of immobilization.

While clinicians are often hesitant to engage with early mobilization due to a belief that healing tissue needs to be protected,[122] studies consistently demonstrate comparable re-tear rates in small and medium tears irrespective of sling immobilization or no sling approaches.[46,88,129] There is a suggestion (which requires confirmation in a definitive trial), that re-tear rates may be higher when mobilization is delayed.[81] Evaluation of patient compliance with sling usage suggests that compliance deteriorates with increasing time, particularly if the dominant arm is affected.[93] A qualitative study reported patients typically prefer to move their arm early after rotator cuff repair, and delayed mobilization appears to be associated with increased pain.[122]

Studies have evaluated the effectiveness of early versus delayed mobilization following arthroscopic rotator cuff repair,[88,118,129] consistently reporting that levels of pain and ranges of motion are better in the short term (6 and 12 weeks) for patients who mobilize early. Notably at 6 and 12 month follow-up, there is no difference in re-tear rate, and at one year follow-up, functional outcomes are comparable between groups.[46,112,129] Sheps et al.[118] compared two groups following arthroscopic rotator cuff repair. One group self-weaned from the postoperative sling and performed pain-free range of motion during the first six weeks, and the other group wore a sling for six weeks with no active range of motion permitted. At 6, 12, and 24 months, strength was reassessed, and at 12 months, ultrasound verified the integrity of the repair.

They reported early mobilization did not demonstrate any clinical benefit over delayed mobilization, with both groups demonstrating similar improvement in all outcomes of interest between six weeks and 24 months. Importantly, there was no difference in repair integrity at 12 months. Sheps et al.[118] suggested that consideration should be given to early pain-free active movement in the first six weeks following arthroscopic rotator cuff repair.

Although there is emerging evidence to support early mobilization following arthroscopic rotator cuff repair, particularly in small and medium tears, surveys of current practice illustrate that most patients continue to be immobilized in a sling for up to six weeks, and for longer periods following repair of larger tears.[60,82]

There is less research available on the benefit of early mobilization for other surgical procedures performed on the shoulder. The evidence that is available suggests early mobilization is associated with earlier return to function, less pain in the early postoperative phase, and importantly no increased risk of failure following stabilization surgery,[47,71,91] and reverse total shoulder arthroplasty.[74] For people who followed an accelerated rehabilitation regimen following reverse total shoulder arthroplasty without any period of immobilization, less postoperative complications, such as falls, were reported.

Early mobilization regimens potentially have additional psychological and emotional benefits for patients due to the earlier return to normal function and regaining of independence. However, it is paramount that clinicians consider risk factors for surgical failure, relevant intraoperative findings and specific patient goals when considering the appropriateness of early mobilization.

Keeping early mobilization safe

The concept of the "safe zone" has been proposed to guide early mobilization and avoid unnecessary tension on the surgical repair.[116] These safe zones are based on anatomical knowledge, intraoperative observations, and cadaveric research, to guide the limits of early mobilization, with the surgeon informing the therapist what ranges of shoulder motion are safe to mobilize in. Currently, there is lack of research evaluating the superiority of this approach to other rehabilitation approaches.

Studies using electromyography (EMG) to guide postoperative rehabilitation, generally advocate 15% of maximum voluntary contraction (MVC) as the upper limit of what is safe in the early stages following rotator cuff repair.[42] This may be overly protective given that EMG levels in the rotator cuff of the immobilized limb exceed 20% of MVC when the patient picks up a bag or pushes open a door with their un-operated arm.[4] Similarly, levels of activation exceed 20% MVC when a patient dresses and undresses while wearing a sling.[50] It is important to note that the majority of EMG studies have been conducted on people without symptoms, and movement strategies and activation patterns may differ in the presence of pain. The correlation between EMG activity and tension on a surgical repair or at a fracture site have not been fully elucidated and this needs to be a focus of future research, as knowledge of EMG levels may provide a pragmatic way of informing safe exercise selection.

Exercises that involve support of the upper limb on a table, ball, or wall and are performed anterior to the scapular plane, consistently show levels of activation less than 15% MVC. Table slides are an effective method of preventing postoperative stiffness following rotator cuff repair[61] (Figure 41.1).

Integration of the kinetic chain is another method of facilitating early mobilization. When shoulder exercises are initiated with weight transference, such as a step or step up or with thoracic rotation, there is an improvement in local scapula muscle recruitment, and this may have an unloading effect on the rotator cuff.[107] When patients find it difficult to move the arm away from the body, even with table or ball support, moving the body away from the arm is a strategy to consider. This may distract the patient by changing the focus of movement and increasing a feeling of security by fixing the arm (Figure 41.2). Using light resistance around the wrists together with the tactile support of a wall (Figure 41.3) and providing a realistic target to reach is a progression of early-stage mobilization.[59,121]

Proprioceptive deficits are reported in patients following shoulder surgery particularly in relation to kinesthesia and force production sense.[2,68] Closed chain exercises performed early in rehabilitation and then progressing these as patient and surgical factors allow, may help to reduce pain and restore movement following rotator cuff repair.[104] It is important to reassure and remind the patient that pain is an expected part

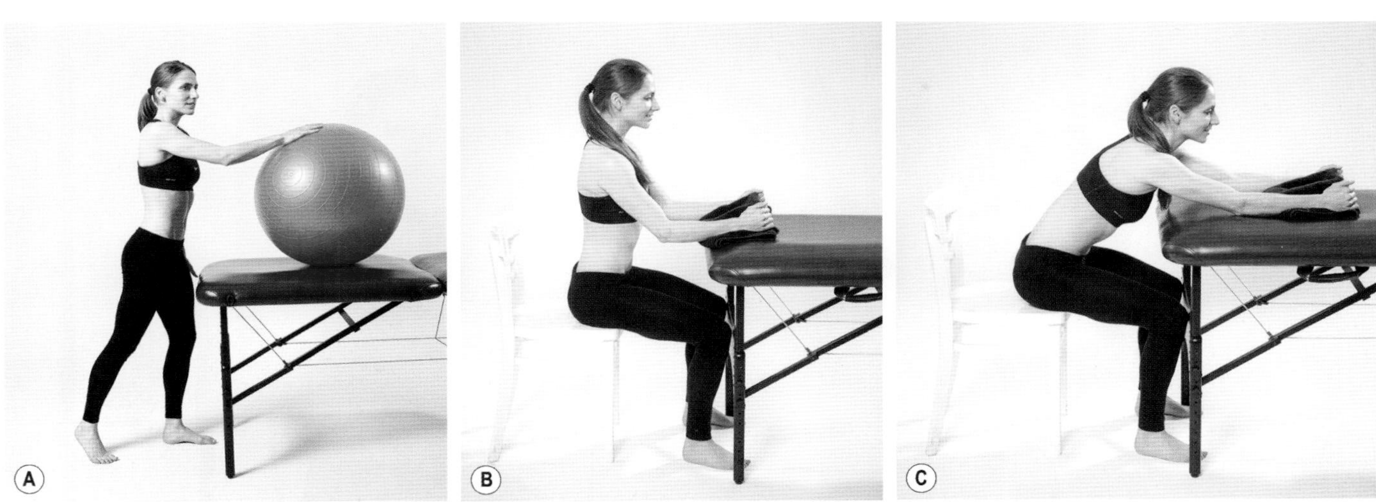

FIGURE 41.1
Early mobilization with support. (A) Supported shoulder flexion with a step. (B,C) Supported shoulder flexion table slides.
(Figures reproduced with the kind permission of www.shoulderdoc.co.uk[140])

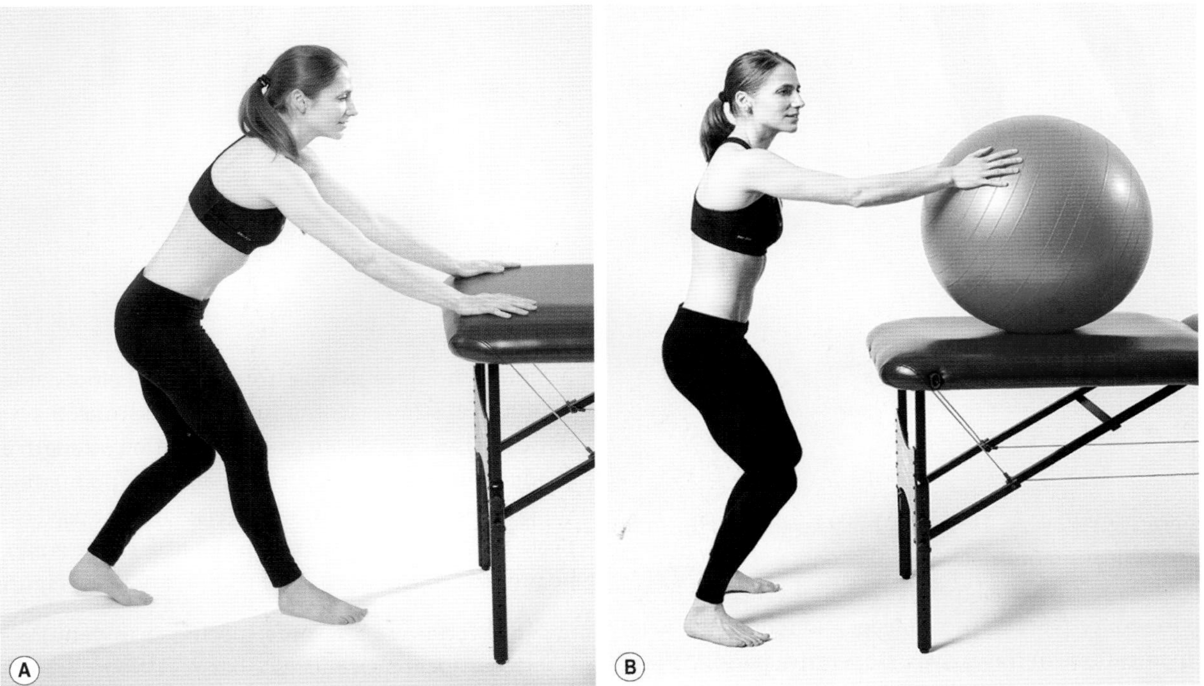

FIGURE 41.2
Moving the body away from the arm. (A) Hands remain on the table and patient steps backwards. (B) Hands remain on the table or ball and patient performs a squat.
(Figures reproduced with the kind permission of www.shoulderdoc.co.uk[140])

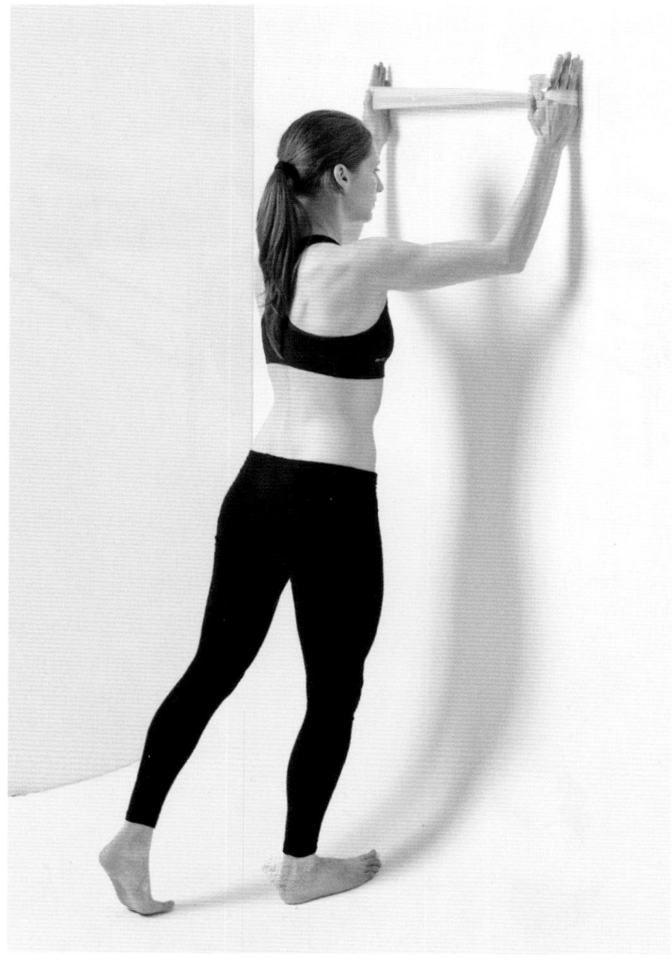

FIGURE 41.3
Wall slide with elastic band loop and step.
(Figure reproduced with the kind permission of www.shoulderdoc.co.uk[140])

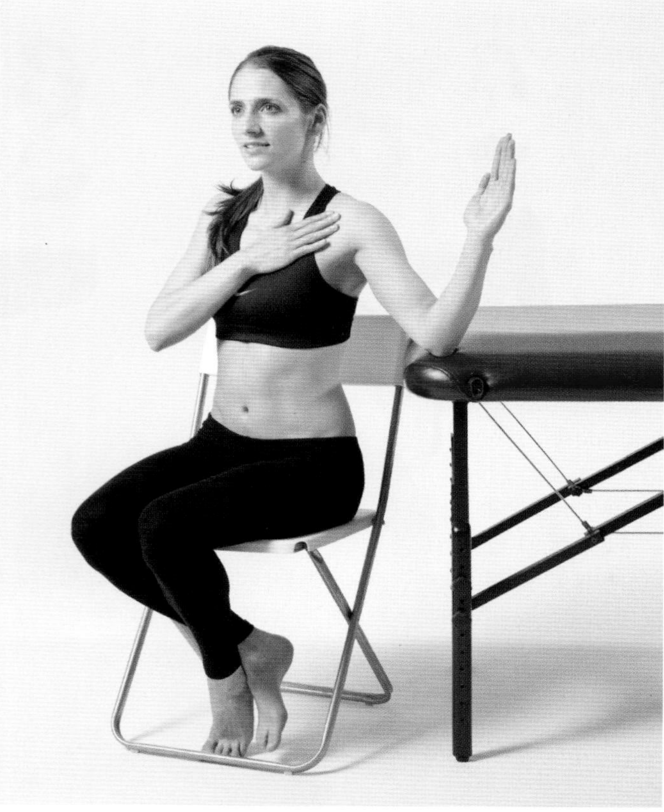

FIGURE 41.4
Supported shoulder external rotation.
(Figure reproduced with the kind permission of www.shoulderdoc.co.uk[140])

of postoperative recovery. However, high levels of pain may be an early indication of infection, iatrogenic nerve injury or surgical failure and so vigilance is essential. The use of ice may help to reduce pain, improve sleep, and reduce the need for pain medications in the early postoperative period.[136]

Muscle performance

The progression of postoperative rehabilitation should be informed by patient-specific goals and functional demands. Early mobilization and incorporation of exercises that promote shoulder muscle recruitment help establish foundations for strengthening and more advanced proprioceptive exercises. Deficits in external rotation strength and force production are reported in shoulder pain populations,[123] and supported external rotation exercises may be used early in the postoperative period (within the identified safe zone), and can be progressed easily with the addition of load (Figure 41.4).

However, there are some specific considerations in relation to surgical procedures. Sharpey's fibers are a matrix of connective tissue consisting of bundles of strong collagenous fibers connecting periosteum to bone. They are part of the outer fibrous layer of periosteum and enter the outer circumferential and interstitial lamellae of bone tissue. These fibers are responsible for binding and healing tendon to the bone and are not present in any considerable number until

12 weeks postoperatively.[127,145] Even at this stage the repair strength may only be at 29–50%.[127,145] This highlights the importance of considering patient and surgical factors that may negatively affect tendon healing, and which necessitate a more cautious approach. In patients with significant weakness following a period of immobilization or who are struggling to progress their strengthening exercises, the use of a muscle stimulator should be considered.[73,106]

The design of reverse total shoulder arthroplasty aims to change the moment arm of deltoid, and so it is unsurprising that the outcome of reverse total shoulder arthroplasty correlates highly with both preoperative and postoperative deltoid muscle strength.[80] If pain levels permit, there may be merit in trying to improve shoulder muscle performance, including the deltoid, preoperatively.

Essentially, muscle performance retraining should reflect the specific functional demands of the patient and consider any potential deficits specific to the surgical procedure. For example, surgical approaches that require division of subscapularis (such as Latarjet or total shoulder arthroplasty) are associated with strength deficits, which may compromise outcomes and increase the risk of failure.[45]

The bigger picture

Surgery commonly necessitates periods of time off work and away from valued activities, however it provides an opportunity for the patient to reflect on their health and lifestyle. Unhealthy lifestyle factors such as inadequate physical activity, obesity, smoking, poor sleep, and diet have been reported to negatively impact operative recovery, and also contribute to delayed healing and higher rates of surgical failure[66,103,109,141] (see Chapters 5 and 36). If the patient agrees and is ready to do so,[79] healthcare professionals are perfectly placed to educate, signpost, and support appropriate behavioral change.[79]

There is a high association with lower quadrant strength and balance and all-cause mortality, falls risk, later life healthcare utilization and an ability to maintain physical independence.[108] Incorporating tests such as the 5 sit to stand test,[11,135] 10 sit to stand test, and number of sit to stands in 30 seconds,[108] pre- or postoperatively enables further conversation with the patient and will help to facilitate a more holistic approach to rehabilitation for the individual.

In sporting populations, particularly those engaging in overhead or contact sports, lower limb measures of strength and power correlate highly with upper quadrant performance.[43] The postoperative period is an opportunity to enhance sport-specific strength and power of the lower quadrant, particularly when surgery requires a protracted period of immobilization of the upper limb.

Future opportunities

There is increasing interest in the role of gamification, virtual reality, and web-based rehabilitation approaches to support assessment and self-directed postoperative rehabilitation.[8,14] This is discussed further in Chapter 30, and on-going research will determine the value of these technologies.

Summary

Shoulder surgery for musculoskeletal conditions is usually advocated when appropriate following trauma, and for persistent symptoms that have not improved with time and/or nonsurgical intervention. Shoulder surgery aims to reduce pain and disability and improve function for people who have shoulder symptoms when, following a risk assessment, the surgeon is confident that the outcome following surgery is likely to be more beneficial than the theoretical harm of the surgery, or not operating.

The decision to perform elective shoulder surgery should be made with the patient, within a shared decision-making framework, and with certainty that the patient knows the postoperative time scales, realistic outcomes, and potential harms. The patient must be cognizant to what will be required and expected in the postoperative period, including their commitment to rehabilitation.

Postoperative rehabilitation aims to restore range of motion, strength, and a return to function. To optimize surgical outcomes, preparation is critical. Understanding the individual, their beliefs, concerns, and expectations, and educating them effectively regarding surgery and the postoperative recovery period are key foundations. Furthermore, communication between the multidisciplinary team is essential, to ensure a consistent message in terms of expected outcomes, and to communicate relevant intraoperative findings that may support the therapist's clinical reasoning regarding rehabilitation.

Understanding patient and surgical factors that may influence both post-surgical recovery times and clinical outcomes will enable realistic expectations to be set and communicated. Implementing strategies to minimize the deleterious effects of immobilization has the potential to improve post-operative pain and facilitate an earlier return to function.

Although shoulder surgery is commonly performed and there have been significant advances in surgical techniques, there have been very few changes in the way post-surgical rehabilitation is provided. Identifying optimal post-surgical timing and content of rehabilitation, across the range of conditions for which surgery is performed is a research priority. Early protected mobilization may have the potential to reduce post-surgical complications and enhance outcomes.

Acknowledgements

We would like to thank Mr Lennard Funk (www.shoulderdoc.co.uk)[140] who has given permission to use the figures in this chapter. We would also like to thank Ms Fiona Creedon MCSP, for her support editing this chapter.

References

1. Ager AL, Borms D, Bernaert M, et al. Can a conservative rehabilitation strategy improve shoulder proprioception? A systematic review. Journal of Sport Rehabilitation. 2020;30:136-151.
2. Ager AL, Borms D, Deschepper L, et al. Proprioception: how is it affected by shoulder pain? A systematic review. Journal of Hand Therapy. 2020;33:507-516.
3. Agrawal T, Gupta GK, Agrawal DK. Vitamin D supplementation reduces airway hyperresponsiveness and allergic airway inflammation in a murine model. Clinical & Experimental Allergy. 2013;43:672-683.
4. Alenabi T, Jackson M, Tétreault P, Begon M. Electromyographic activity in the shoulder musculature during resistance training exercises of the ipsilateral upper limb while wearing a shoulder orthosis. Journal of Shoulder and Elbow Surgery. 2014;23:e140-e148.
5. Alizadehkhaiyat O, Fisher A, Kemp G, Vishwanathan K, Frostick S. Shoulder muscle activation and fatigue during a controlled forceful hand grip task. Journal of Electromyography and Kinesiology. 2011;21:478-482.
6. Andrushko JW, Lanovaz JL, Björkman KM, Kontulainen SA, Farthing JP. Unilateral strength training leads to muscle-specific sparing effects during opposite homologous limb immobilization. Journal of Applied Physiology. 2018;124:866-876.
7. Bahar-Shany K, Ravid A, Koren R. Upregulation of MMP-9 production by TNFα in keratinocytes and its attenuation by vitamin D. Journal of Cellular Physiology. 2010;222:729-737.
8. Berton A, Longo UG, Candela V, et al. Virtual reality, augmented reality, gamification, and telerehabilitation: psychological impact on orthopedic patients' rehabilitation. Journal of Clinical Medicine. 2020;9:2567.
9. Bishop JY, Santiago-Torres JE, Rimmke N, Flanigan DC. Smoking predisposes to rotator cuff pathology and shoulder dysfunction: a systematic review. Arthroscopy. 2015;31:1598-1605.
10. Blonna D, Fissore F, Bellato E, et al. Subclinical hypothyroidism and diabetes as risk factors for postoperative stiff shoulder. Knee Surgery, Sports Traumatology, Arthroscopy. 2017;25:2208-2216.
11. Bohannon RW, Shove ME, Barreca SR, Masters LM, Sigouin CS. Five-repetition sit-to-stand test performance by community-dwelling adults: a preliminary investigation of times, determinants, and relationship with self-reported physical performance. Isokinetics and Exercise Science. 2007;15:77-81.
12. Bonello C, Girdwood M, De Souza K, et al. Does isometric exercise result in exercise induced hypoalgesia in people with local musculoskeletal pain? A systematic review. Physical Therapy in Sport. 2020;
13. Bowering KJ, O'Connell NE, Tabor A, et al. The effects of graded motor imagery and its components on chronic pain: a systematic review and meta-analysis. J Pain. 2013;14:3-13.
14. Brady N, McVeigh JG, McCreesh K, Rio E, Dekkers T, Lewis JS. Exploring the effectiveness of immersive Virtual Reality interventions in the management of musculoskeletal pain: a state-of-the-art review. Physical Therapy Reviews. 2021;1-14.
15. Bullock GS, Garrigues GE, Ledbetter L, Kennedy J. A systematic review of proposed rehabilitation guidelines following anatomic and reverse shoulder arthroplasty. Journal of Orthopaedic & Sports Physical Therapy. 2019;49:337-346.
16. Burianová H, Sowman PF, Marstaller L, et al. Adaptive motor imagery: a multimodal study of immobilization-induced brain plasticity. Cerebral Cortex. 2016;26:1072-1080.
17. Burrus MT, Diduch DR, Werner BC. Patient-related risk factors for postoperative stiffness requiring surgical intervention after arthroscopic rotator cuff repair. Journal of the American Academy of Orthopaedic Surgeons. 2019;27:e319-e323.
18. Campbell M, Varley-Campbell J, Fulford J, Taylor B, Mileva KN, Bowtell JL. Effect of immobilisation on neuromuscular function in vivo in humans: a systematic review. Sports Medicine. 2019;49:931-950.
19. Cancienne JM, Brockmeier SF, Kew ME, Werner BC. Perioperative serum 25-hydroxyvitamin d levels affect revision surgery rates after arthroscopic rotator cuff repair. Arthroscopy. 2019;35:763-769.
20. Carr AJ, Cooper CD, Campbell MK, et al. Clinical effectiveness and cost-effectiveness of open and arthroscopic rotator cuff repair [the UK Rotator Cuff Surgery (UKUFF) randomised trial]. Health Technol Assess. 2015;19:1-218.
21. Chester R, Jerosch-Herold C, Lewis J, Shepstone L. Psychological factors are associated with the outcome of physiotherapy for people with shoulder pain: a multicentre longitudinal cohort study. British Journal of Sports Medicine. 2018;52:269-275.
22. Cho C-H, Ye H-U, Jung J-W, Lee Y-K. Gender affects early postoperative outcomes of rotator cuff repair. Clinics in Orthopedic Surgery. 2015;7:234.
23. Chung SW, Huong CB, Kim SH, Oh JH. Shoulder stiffness after rotator cuff repair:

risk factors and influence on outcome. Arthroscopy. 2013;29:290-300.

24. Chung SW, Oh JH, Gong HS, Kim JY, Kim SH. Factors affecting rotator cuff healing after arthroscopic repair: osteoporosis as one of the independent risk factors. The American Journal of Sports Medicine. 2011;39:2099-2107.

25. Ciccotti MC, Syed U, Hoffman R, Abboud JA, Ciccotti MG, Freedman KB. Return to play criteria following surgical stabilization for traumatic anterior shoulder instability: a systematic review. Arthroscopy. 2018;34:903-913.

26. Coda RG, Cheema SG, Hermanns CA, et al. A review of online rehabilitation protocols designated for rotator cuff repairs. Arthroscopy, Sports Medicine, and Rehabilitation. 2020;2:e277-e288.

27. Cole BJ, Cotter EJ, Wang KC, Davey A. Patient understanding, expectations, and satisfaction regarding rotator cuff injuries and surgical management. Arthroscopy. 2017;33:1603-1606.

28. Coleman A, Clifft J. The effect of shoulder immobilization on balance in community-dwelling older adults. Journal of Geriatric Physical Therapy. 2010;33:118-121.

29. Cronin KJ, Mair SD, Hawk GS, Thompson KL, Hettrich CM, Jacobs CA. Increased health care costs and opioid use in patients with anxiety and depression undergoing rotator cuff repair. Arthroscopy. 2020;36:2655-2660.

30. Cucchi D, Marmotti A, De Giorgi S, et al. Risk factors for shoulder stiffness: current concepts. Joints. 2017;5:217.

31. Cucchi D, Menon A, Feroldi F, et al. Risk factors for post-operative shoulder stiffness: are there new candidates? Journal of Biological Regulators and Homeostatic Agents. 2016;30:123-129.

32. Cucchi D, Menon A, Feroldi FM, Boerci L, Randelli PS. The presence of gastroesophageal reflux disease increases the risk of developing postoperative shoulder stiffness after arthroscopic rotator cuff repair. Journal of Shoulder and Elbow Surgery. 2020;29:2505-2513.

33. Daly AE, Bialocerkowski AE. Does evidence support physiotherapy management of adult Complex Regional Pain Syndrome Type One? A systematic review. European Journal of Pain. 2009;13:339-353.

34. Daniels SD, Stewart CM, Garvey KD, Brook EM, Higgins LD, Matzkin EG. Sex-based differences in patient-reported outcomes after arthroscopic rotator cuff repair. Orthopaedic Journal of Sports Medicine. 2019;7:2325967119881959.

35. Dekker TJ, Peebles LA, Bernhardson AS, et al. Risk factors for recurrence after arthroscopic instability repair: the importance of glenoid bone loss > 15%, patient age, and duration of symptoms: a matched cohort analysis. The American Journal of Sports Medicine. 2020;48:3036-3041.

36. Di Giacomo G, Peebles LA, Midtgaard KS, de Gasperis N, Scarso P, Provencher CMT. Risk factors for recurrent anterior glenohumeral instability and clinical failure following primary Latarjet procedures: an analysis of 344 patients. JBJS. 2020;102:1665-1671.

37. Diebold G, Lam P, Walton J, Murrell GA. Relationship between age and rotator cuff retear: a study of 1,600 consecutive rotator cuff repairs. JBJS. 2017;99:1198-1205.

38. Donohue MA, Mauntel TC, Dickens JF. Recurrent shoulder instability after primary Bankart repair. Sports Medicine and Arthroscopy Review. 2017;25:123-130.

39. Dragert K, Zehr EP. High-intensity unilateral dorsiflexor resistance training results in bilateral neuromuscular plasticity after stroke. Experimental Brain Research. 2013;225:93-104.

40. Dupuis F, Barrett E, Dubé M-O, McCreesh KM, Lewis JS, Roy J-S. Cryotherapy or gradual reloading exercises in acute presentations of rotator cuff tendinopathy: a randomised controlled trial. BMJ Open Sport & Exercise Medicine. 2018;4:e000477.

41. Duquin TR, Buyea C, Bisson LJ. Which method of rotator cuff repair leads to the highest rate of structural healing? A systematic review. The American Journal of Sports Medicine. 2010;38:835-841.

42. Edwards PK, Ebert JR, Littlewood C, Ackland T, Wang A. A systematic review of electromyography studies in normal shoulders to inform postoperative rehabilitation following rotator cuff repair. Journal of Orthopaedic & Sports Physical Therapy. 2017;47:931-944.

43. Ellenbecker TS, Aoki R. Step by step guide to understanding the kinetic chain concept in the overhead athlete. Current Reviews in Musculoskeletal Medicine. 2020;13:155-163.

44. Fermont AJ, Wolterbeek N, Wessel RN, Baeyens J-P, De Bie RA. Prognostic factors for successful recovery after arthroscopic rotator cuff repair: a systematic literature review. Journal of Orthopaedic & Sports Physical Therapy. 2014;44:153-163.

45. Frantz TL, Everhart JS, Cvetanovich GL, et al. Are patients who undergo the Latarjet procedure ready to return to play at 6 months? A Multicenter Orthopaedic Outcomes Network (MOON) Shoulder Group Cohort Study. The American Journal of Sports Medicine. 2020;48:923-930.

46. Gallagher BP, Bishop ME, Tjoumakaris FP, Freedman KB. Early versus delayed rehabilitation following arthroscopic rotator cuff repair: a systematic review. The Physician and Sportsmedicine. 2015;43:178-187.

47. Gibson J, Kerss J, Morgan C, Brownson P. Accelerated rehabilitation after arthroscopic Bankart repair in professional footballers. Shoulder & Elbow. 2016;8:279-286.

48. Gottlieb U, Springer S. The relationship between fear avoidance beliefs, muscle strength, and short-term disability after surgical repair of shoulder instability. Journal of Sport Rehabilitation. 2021;1:1-8.

49. Green LA, Gabriel DA. The cross education of strength and skill following unilateral strength training in the upper and lower limbs. Journal of Neurophysiology. 2018;120:468-479.

50. Gurney AB, Mermier C, LaPlante M, et al. Shoulder electromyography measurements during activities of daily living and routine rehabilitation exercises. Journal of Orthopaedic & Sports Physical Therapy. 2016;46:375-383.

51. Gwilym S, Oag H, Tracey I, Carr A. Evidence that central sensitisation is present in patients with shoulder impingement syndrome and influences the outcome after surgery. The Journal of Bone and Joint Surgery. 2011;93:498-502.

52. Hendy AM, Lamon S. The cross-education phenomenon: brain and beyond. Frontiers in Physiology. 2017;8:297.

53. Henn RF, 3rd, Kang L, Tashjian RZ, Green A. Patients' preoperative expectations predict the outcome of rotator cuff repair. JBJS. 2007;89:1913-1919.

54. Hollmann L, Halaki M, Kamper SJ, Haber M, Ginn KA. Does muscle guarding play a role in range of motion loss in patients with frozen shoulder? Musculoskelet Sci Pract. 2018;37:64-68.

55. Hoppe DJ, Denkers M, Hoppe FM, Wong IH. The use of video before arthroscopic shoulder surgery to enhance patient recall and satisfaction: a randomized-controlled study. Journal of Shoulder and Elbow Surgery. 2014;23:e134-e139.

56. Huberty DP, Schoolfield JD, Brady PC, Vadala AP, Arrigoni P, Burkhart SS. Incidence and treatment of postoperative stiffness following arthroscopic rotator cuff repair. Arthroscopy. 2009;25:880-890.

57. Jensen AR, Taylor AJ, Sanchez-Sotelo J. Factors influencing the reparability and healing rates of rotator cuff tears. Current Reviews in Musculoskeletal Medicine. 2020;1-12.

58. Jonas WB, Crawford C, Colloca L, et al. To what extent are surgery and invasive procedures effective beyond a placebo response? A systematic review with meta-analysis of randomised, sham controlled trials. BMJ Open. 2015;5:e009655.

59. Jones SA, Pamukoff DN, Mauntel TC, Blackburn JT, Myers JB. The influence of verbal and tactile feedback on electromyographic amplitude of the shoulder musculature during common therapeutic exercises. Journal of Sport Rehabilitation. 2018;27:424-430.

60. Kane LT, Lazarus MD, Namdari S, Seitz AL, Abboud JA. Comparing expert opinion within the care team regarding postoperative rehabilitation protocol following rotator cuff repair. Journal of Shoulder and Elbow Surgery. 2020;29:e330-e337.

61. Kang J-I, Moon Y-J, Choi H, Jeong D-K, Kwon H-M, Park J-S. The effect of exercise types for rotator cuff repair patients on activities of shoulder muscles and upper limb disability. Journal of Physical Therapy Science. 2016;28:2772-2777.

62. Karaaslan TC, Berkoz O, Tarakci E. The effect of mirror therapy after carpal tunnel syndrome surgery: a randomised controlled study. Hand Surgery and Rehabilitation. 2020;39:406-412.

63. Karabay D, Emük Y, Kaya DÖ. Muscle activity ratios of scapular stabilizers during closed kinetic chain exercises in healthy shoulders: a systematic review. Journal of Sport Rehabilitation. 2019;29:1001-1018.

64. Kennedy P, Joshi R, Dhawan A. The effect of psychosocial factors on outcomes in patients with rotator cuff tears: a systematic review. Arthroscopy. 2019;35:2698-2706.

65. Khazzam M, Sager B, Box HN, Wallace SB. The effect of age on risk of retear after rotator cuff repair: a systematic review and meta-analysis. JSES International. 2020;4:625-631.

66. Kokmeyer D, Dube E, Millett PJ. Suppl 1: M10: Prognosis driven rehabilitation after rotator cuff repair surgery. The Open Orthopaedics Journal. 2016;10:339.

67. Korbus H, Schott N. Does mental practice or mirror therapy help prevent functional loss after distal radius fracture? A randomized controlled trial. Journal of Hand Therapy. 2020;S0894-1130(20)30207-6.

68. Lädermann A, Tirefort J, Zanchi D, et al. Shoulder apprehension: a multifactorial approach. EFORT Open Rev. 2018;3:550-557.

69. Laird E, McNulty H, Ward M, et al. Vitamin D deficiency is associated with inflammation in older Irish adults. The Journal of Clinical Endocrinology & Metabolism. 2014;99:1807-1815.

70. Laning S, Linde A, Rooks A, et al. Clinician expectations of full-thickness rotator cuff repair outcomes: OPO167. Journal of Orthopaedic & Sports Physical. 2018;48.

71. Law BK-Y, Yung PS-H, Ho EP-Y, Chang JJH-T, Chan K-M. The surgical outcome of immediate arthroscopic Bankart repair for first time anterior shoulder dislocation in young active patients. Knee Surgery, Sports Traumatology, Arthroscopy. 2008;16:188-193.

72. Lawrence C, Zmistowski BM, Lazarus M, Abboud J, Williams G, Namdari S. Expectations of shoulder surgery are not altered by surgeon counseling of the patient. Joints. 2017;5:133.

73. Lee GJ, Cho H, Ahn B-H, Jeong H-S. Effects of electrical muscle stimulation for preventing deltoid muscle atrophy after rotator cuff repair: preliminary results of a prospective, randomized, single-blind trial. Clinics in Shoulder and Elbow. 2019;22:195.

74. Lee J, Consigliere P, Fawzy E, et al. Accelerated rehabilitation following reverse total shoulder arthroplasty. Journal of Shoulder and Elbow Surgery. 2021; 30:e545-e557.

75. Lee YS, Jeong JY, Park C-D, Kang SG, Yoo JC. Evaluation of the risk factors for a rotator cuff retear after repair surgery. The American Journal of Sports Medicine. 2017;45:1755-1761.

76. Leung M, Rantalainen T, Teo W-P, Kidgell D. The ipsilateral corticospinal responses to cross-education are dependent upon the motor-training intervention. Experimental Brain Research. 2018;236:1331-1346.

77. Lewis J. The End of an era? J Orthop Sports Phys Ther. 2018;48:127-129.

78. Lewis J. Rotator cuff related shoulder pain: assessment, management and uncertainties. Man Ther. 2016;23:57-68.

79. Lewis J, Ridehalgh C, Moore A, Hall K. This is the day your life must surely change: prioritising behavioural change in musculoskeletal practice. Physiotherapy. 2021;112:158-162.

80. Li H, Yoon S-h, Lee D, Chung H. Relation between preoperative electromyographic activity of the deltoid and upper trapezius muscle and clinical results in patients treated with reverse shoulder arthroplasty. Journal of Shoulder and Elbow Surgery. 2020;29:195-201.

81. Littlewood C, Bateman M, Butler-Walley S, et al. Rehabilitation following rotator cuff repair: a multi-centre pilot & feasibility randomised controlled trial (RaCeR). Clinical Rehabilitation. 2020;0269215520978859.

82. Littlewood C, Mazuquin B, Moffatt M, Bateman M. Rehabilitation following rotator cuff repair: a survey of current practice (2020). Musculoskeletal Care. 2021;19:165-171.

83. Louw A, Puentedura EJ, Reese D, Parker P, Miller T, Mintken PE. Immediate effects of mirror therapy in patients with shoulder pain and decreased range of motion. Archives of Physical Medicine and Rehabilitation. 2017;98:1941-1947.

84. Magnus CR, Barss TS, Lanovaz JL, Farthing JP. Effects of cross-education on the muscle after a period of unilateral limb immobilization using a shoulder sling and swathe. Journal of Applied Physiology. 2010;109:1887-1894.

85. Manca A, Hortobágyi T, Carroll T, et al. Contralateral effects of unilateral strength and skill training: modified Delphi consensus to establish key aspects of cross-education. Sports Medicine. 2021;51:11-20.

86. Martinez-Calderon J, Struyf F, Meeus M, Morales-Ascencio JM, Luque-Suarez A. Influence of psychological factors on

the prognosis of chronic shoulder pain: protocol for a prospective cohort study. BMJ Open. 2017;7:e012822.

87. Mazuquin B, Moffatt M, Gill P, et al. Effectiveness of early versus delayed rehabilitation following rotator cuff repair: systematic review and meta-analyses. PLoS One. 2021;16:e0252137.

88. Mazuquin BF, Wright AC, Russell S, Monga P, Selfe J, Richards J. Effectiveness of early compared with conservative rehabilitation for patients having rotator cuff repair surgery: an overview of systematic reviews. British Journal of Sports Medicine. 2018;52:111-121.

89. Mendez-Rebolledo G, Morales-Verdugo J, Orozco-Chavez I, Habechain FAP, Padilla EL, de la Rosa FJB. Optimal activation ratio of the scapular muscles in closed kinetic chain shoulder exercises: A systematic review. Journal of Back and Musculoskeletal Rehabilitation. 2020;1-14.

90. Miller FG, Kaptchuk TJ. The power of context: reconceptualizing the placebo effect. Journal of the Royal Society of Medicine. 2008;101:222-225.

91. Multanen J, Kiuru P, Piitulainen K, Ylinen J, Paloneva J, Häkkinen A. Enhanced rehabilitation guidance after arthroscopic capsulolabral repair of the shoulder: a randomized controlled trial. Clinical Rehabilitation. 2020;34:890-900.

92. Nakamura A, Kawahrada R. Advanced glycation end products and oxidative stress in a hyperglycaemic environment. IntechOpen; 2021. Available at: https://www.intechopen.com/online-first/76145.

93. Nassiri M, Egan C, Mullet H. Compliance with sling-wearing after rotator cuff repair and anterior shoulder stabilization. Shoulder & Elbow. 2011;3:188-192.

94. Oh JH, Kim SH, Kim J, Shin Y, Yoon J, Oh C. The level of vitamin D in the serum correlates with fatty degeneration of the muscles of the rotator cuff. The Journal of Bone and Joint Surgery. 2009;91:1587-1593.

95. Oh JH, Yoon JP, Kim JY, Kim SH. Effect of expectations and concerns in rotator cuff disorders and correlations with preoperative patient characteristics. Journal of Shoulder and Elbow Surgery. 2012;21:715-721.

96. Oranchuk DJ, Storey AG, Nelson AR, Cronin JB. Isometric training and long-term adaptations: effects of muscle length, intensity, and intent. A systematic review. Scandinavian Journal of Medicine & Science in Sports. 2019;29:484-503.

97. Paavola M, Malmivaara A, Taimela S, et al. Subacromial decompression versus diagnostic arthroscopy for shoulder impingement: randomised, placebo surgery controlled clinical trial. BMJ. 2018;362:k2860.

98. Park JH, Rhee SM, Kim HS, Oh JH. Effects of anxiety and depression measured via the hospital anxiety and depression scale on early pain and range of motion after rotator cuff repair. Am J Sports Med. 2021;49:314-320.

99. Parle PJ, Riddiford-Harland DL, Howitt CD, Lewis JS. Acute rotator cuff tendinopathy: does ice, low load isometric exercise, or a combination of the two produce an analgaesic effect? British Journal of Sports Medicine. 2017;51:208-209.

100. Pietrzak M. Adhesive capsulitis: an age related symptom of metabolic syndrome and chronic low-grade inflammation? Medical Hypotheses. 2016;88:12-17.

101. Plath JE, Saier T, Feucht MJ, et al. Patients' expectations of shoulder instability repair. Knee Surgery, Sports Traumatology, Arthroscopy. 2018;26:15-23.

102. Potter MQ, Wylie JD, Greis PE, Burks RT, Tashjian RZ. Psychological distress negatively affects self-assessment of shoulder function in patients with rotator cuff tears. Clinical Orthopaedics and Related Research. 2014;472:3926-3932.

103. Raman J, Walton D, MacDermid JC, Athwal GS. Predictors of outcomes after rotator cuff repair—a meta-analysis. Journal of Hand Therapy. 2017;30:276-292.

104. Randelli P, Ragone V, Carminati S, Cabitza P. Risk factors for recurrence after Bankart repair a systematic review. Knee Surgery, Sports Traumatology, Arthroscopy. 2012;20:2129-2138.

105. Ravindra A, Barlow JD, Jones GL, Bishop JY. A prospective evaluation of predictors of pain after arthroscopic rotator cuff repair: psychosocial factors have a stronger association than structural factors. Journal of Shoulder and Elbow Surgery. 2018;27:1824-1829.

106. Reinold MM, Macrina LC, Wilk KE, Dugas JR, Cain EL, Andrews JR. The effect of neuromuscular electrical stimulation of the infraspinatus on shoulder external rotation force production after rotator cuff repair surgery. The American Journal of Sports Medicine. 2008;36:2317-2321.

107. Richardson E, Lewis JS, Gibson J, et al. Role of the kinetic chain in shoulder rehabilitation: does incorporating the trunk and lower limb into shoulder exercise regimes influence shoulder muscle recruitment patterns? Systematic review of electromyography studies. BMJ Open Sport & Exercise Medicine. 2020;6:e000683.

108. Rikli RE, Jones CJ. Development and validation of criterion-referenced clinically relevant fitness standards for maintaining physical independence in later years. Gerontologist. 2013;53:255-267.

109. Saccomanno MF, Sircana G, Cazzato G, Donati F, Randelli P, Milano G. Prognostic factors influencing the outcome of rotator cuff repair: a systematic review. Knee Surgery, Sports Traumatology, Arthroscopy. 2016;24:3809-3819.

110. Sahoo S, Ricchetti ET, Zajichek A, et al. Associations of preoperative patient mental health and sociodemographic and clinical characteristics with baseline pain, function, and satisfaction in patients undergoing rotator cuff repairs. The American Journal of Sports Medicine. 2020;48:432-443.

111. Salles JI, Velasques B, Cossich V, et al. Strength training and shoulder proprioception. Journal of Athletic Training. 2015;50:277-280.

112. Saltzman BM, Zuke WA, Go B, et al. Does early motion lead to a higher failure rate or better outcomes after arthroscopic rotator cuff repair? A systematic review of overlapping meta-analyses. Journal of Shoulder and Elbow Surgery. 2017;26:1681-1691.

113. Santiago-Torres J, Flanigan DC, Butler RB, Bishop JY. The effect of smoking on rotator cuff and glenoid labrum surgery: a systematic review. The American Journal of Sports Medicine. 2015;43:745-751.

114. Schneider WR, Trasolini RG, Riker JJ, Gerber N, Ruotolo CJ. Stiffness after arthroscopic rotator cuff repair: a rehabilitation problem or a surgical indication? JSES International. 2021;5:88-92.

115. Schroder CP, Skare O, Reikeras O, Mowinckel P, Brox JI. Sham surgery versus labral repair or biceps tenodesis for type II SLAP lesions of the shoulder: a three-armed randomised clinical trial. Br J Sports Med. 2017;51:1759-1766.

116. Shanley E, Peterson SK. Rehabilitation after shoulder instability surgery: keys for optimizing recovery. Sports Medicine and Arthroscopy Review. 2020;28:167-171.

117. Shanmugaraj A, Chai D, Sarraj M, et al. Surgical stabilization of pediatric anterior shoulder instability yields high recurrence rates: a systematic review. Knee Surgery, Sports Traumatology, Arthroscopy. 2021;29:192-201.

118. Sheps DM, Silveira A, Beaupre L, et al. Early active motion versus sling immobilization after arthroscopic rotator cuff repair: a randomized controlled trial. Arthroscopy. 2019;35:749-760.

119. Silbernagel KG, Vicenzino BT, Rathleff MS, Thorborg K. Isometric exercise for acute pain relief: is it relevant in tendinopathy management? Br J Sports Med. 2019;53:1330-1331.

120. Sonoda Y, Nishioka T, Nakajima R, Imai S, Vigers P, Kawasaki T. Use of a shoulder abduction brace after arthroscopic rotator cuff repair: a study on gait performance and falls. Prosthetics and Orthotics International. 2018;42:136-143.

121. Staker JL, Evans AJ, Jacobs LE, et al. The effect of tactile and verbal guidance during scapulothoracic exercises: an EMG and kinematic investigation. Journal of Electromyography and Kinesiology. 2019;102334.

122. Stephens G, Littlewood C, Foster NE, Dikomitis L. Rehabilitation following rotator cuff repair: a nested qualitative study exploring the perceptions and experiences of participants in a randomised controlled trial. Clinical Rehabilitation. 2020;0269215520984025.

123. Struyf F, Lluch E, Falla D, Meeus M, Noten S, Nijs J. Influence of shoulder pain on muscle function: implications for the assessment and therapy of shoulder disorders. European Journal of Applied Physiology. 2015;115:225-234.

124. Swarup I, Henn CM, Gulotta LV, Henn RF, 3rd. Patient expectations and satisfaction in orthopaedic surgery: a review of the literature. Journal of Clinical Orthopaedics and Trauma. 2019;10:755-760.

125. Tardo DT, Halaki M, Cathers I, Ginn KA. Rotator cuff muscles perform different functional roles during shoulder external rotation exercises. Clinical Anatomy. 2013;26:236-243.

126. Tashjian RZ, Hollins AM, Kim H-M, et al. Factors affecting healing rates after arthroscopic double-row rotator cuff repair. The American Journal of Sports Medicine. 2010;38:2435-2442.

127. Thigpen CA, Shaffer MA, Gaunt BW, Leggin BG, Williams GR, Wilcox RB, 3rd. The American Society of Shoulder and Elbow Therapists' consensus statement on rehabilitation following arthroscopic rotator cuff repair. J Shoulder Elbow Surg. 2016;25:521-535.

128. Thomson S, Jukes C, Lewis J. Rehabilitation following surgical repair of the rotator cuff: a systematic review. Physiotherapy. 2016;102:20-28.

129. Tirefort J, Schwitzguebel AJ, Collin P, Nowak A, Plomb-Holmes C, Lädermann A. Postoperative mobilization after superior rotator cuff repair: sling versus no-sling. A randomized controlled trial: sling versus no-sling after RCR. Orthopaedic Journal of Sports Medicine. 2019;7:2325967119S2325900211.

130. Tjong VK, Devitt BM, Murnaghan ML, Ogilvie-Harris DJ, Theodoropoulos JS. A qualitative investigation of return to sport after arthroscopic Bankart repair: beyond stability. The American Journal of Sports Medicine. 2015;43:2005-2011.

131. Torrance E, Clarke CJ, Monga P, Funk L, Walton MJ. Recurrence after arthroscopic labral repair for traumatic anterior instability in adolescent rugby and contact athletes. The American Journal of Sports Medicine. 2018;46:2969-2974.

132. Traven S, Brinton D, Simpson K, et al. Shoulder injection prior to rotator cuff repair is associated with increased risk of subsequent surgery. Orthopaedic Journal of Sports Medicine. 2018;6:2325967118S2325900171.

133. Traven SA, Brinton D, Simpson KN, et al. Preoperative shoulder injections are associated with increased risk of revision rotator cuff repair. Arthroscopy. 2019;35:706-713.

134. Trojan JD, DeFroda SF, Mulcahey MK. Patient understanding, expectations, outcomes, and satisfaction regarding surgical management of shoulder instability. The Physician and Sportsmedicine. 2019;47:6-9.

135. Tsekoura M, Anastasopoulos K, Kastrinis A, Dimitriadis Z. What is most appropriate number of repetitions of the sit-to-stand test in older adults: a reliability study. Journal of Frailty, Sarcopenia and Falls. 2020;5:109.

136. Uquillas CA, Capogna BM, Rossy WH, Mahure SA, Rokito AS. Postoperative pain control after arthroscopic rotator cuff repair. Journal of Shoulder and Elbow Surgery. 2016;25:1204-1213.

137. Vægter HB, Handberg G, Graven-Nielsen T. Isometric exercises reduce temporal summation of pressure pain in humans. European Journal of Pain. 2015;19:973-983.

138. Vajapey SP, Cvetanovich GL, Bishop JY, Neviaser AS. Psychosocial factors affecting outcomes after shoulder arthroplasty: a systematic review. Journal of Shoulder and Elbow Surgery. 2020;29:e175-e184.

139. Walankar PP, Panhale VP, Patil MM. Psychosocial factors, disability and quality of life in chronic shoulder pain patients with central sensitization. Health Psychology Research. 2020;8:8874.

140. Walton J, Leftey C, Gibson J, Holmes C, Richardson E, Funk L. Shoulder Rehabilitation: A Comprehensive Guide to Shoulder Exercise Therapy. Manchester: Shoulderdoc Ltd; 2019.

141. Wylie JD, Baran S, Granger EK, Tashjian RZ. A comprehensive evaluation of factors affecting healing, range of motion, strength, and patient-reported outcomes after arthroscopic rotator cuff repair. Orthopaedic Journal of Sports Medicine. 2018;6:2325967117750104.

142. Yoon S-H, Lee D-H, Jung M-C, Park YU, Lim S-Y. Electromyographic activities of the rotator cuff muscles during walking, eating, and washing. American Journal of Physical Medicine & Rehabilitation. 2016;95:e169-e176.

143. Zanchi D, Cunningham G, Lädermann A, Ozturk M, Hoffmeyer P, Haller S. Structural white matter and functional connectivity alterations in patients with shoulder apprehension. Scientific Reports. 2017;7:1-6.

144. Zult T, Howatson G, Goodall S, Thomas K, Solnik S. Mirror training augments the cross-education of strength and affects inhibitory paths. Med Sci Sports Exerc. 2016;48:1001-13.

145. Zumstein M-A, Lädermann A, Raniga S, Schär M-O. The biology of rotator cuff healing. Orthopaedics & Traumatology: Surgery & Research. 2017;103:S1-S10.

T'ai Chi in shoulder rehabilitation 42

Martin Scott, Hubert van Griensven

Introduction

Exercise has been shown to be an effective treatment for shoulder pain, with no one type of exercise demonstrating superiority.[19] T'ai Chi Ch'uan or Taijiquan (T'ai Chi) is a Chinese form of exercise that progresses from simple to complex, and slow to fast movements. It utilizes isometric (from short to long duration), eccentric, and concentric muscle contractions, and incorporates the kinetic chain from feet to fingertips. It promotes stress reduction. T'ai Chi combines movement with cognitive and proprioceptive exercise, may be performed individually or in group settings, and has proven physical and psychosocial benefits.[14,16,38,39,41,44] This chapter presents important benefits of T'ai Chi for health and the rehabilitation of musculoskeletal conditions involving the shoulder.

The history of T'ai Chi

Many people are familiar with T'ai Chi from the media. Perhaps they have seen a group of people moving in unison in a public space, stepping slowly back and forth, arms circling as if pushing, pulling, or folding an invisible cloth (Figure 42.1). It looks easy to do and peaceful. In fact, T'ai Chi is a complex and sophisticated form of human movement and expression developed over centuries, that requires dedication to master the movements accurately.

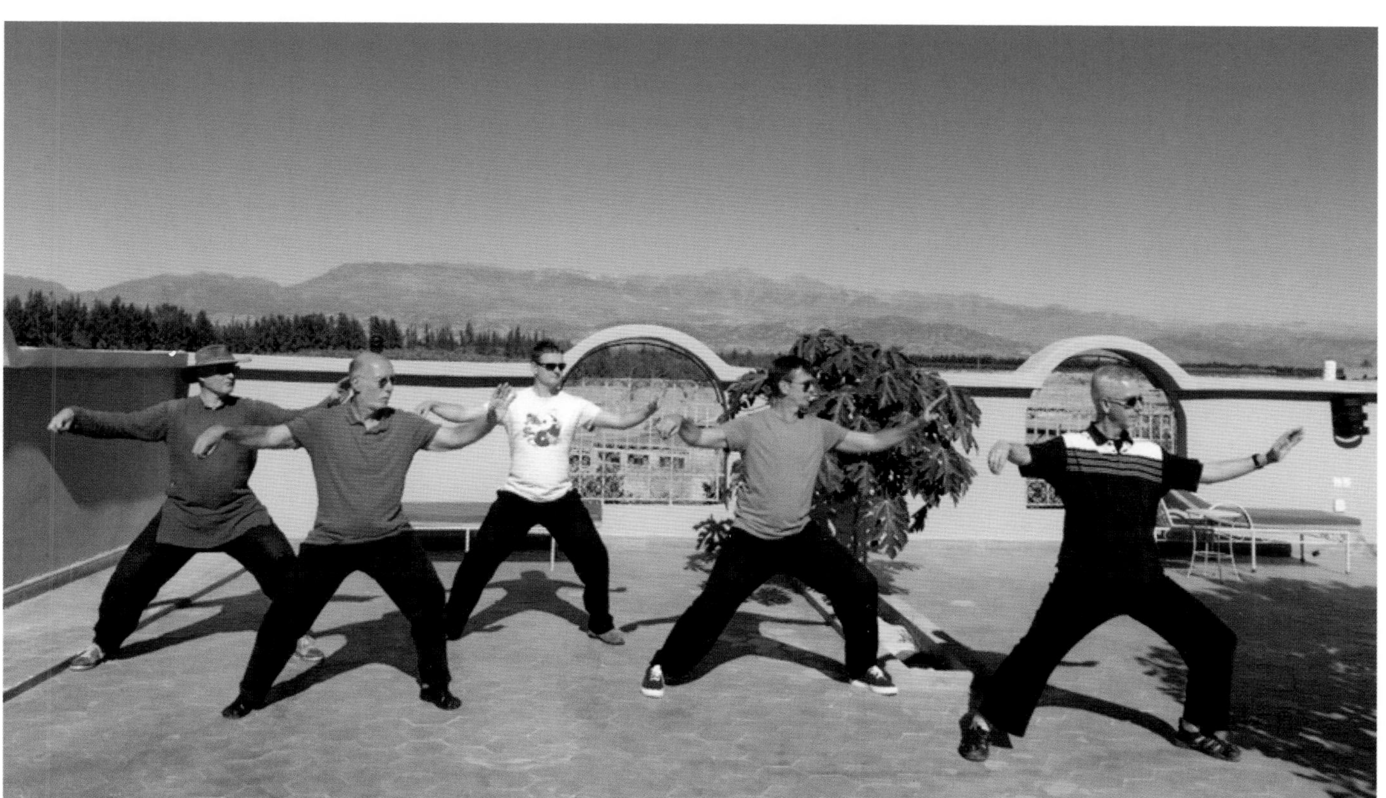

FIGURE 42.1
Group practice of T'ai Chi.
(Reproduced with kind permission of the Chinese Internal Arts Association, www.ciaa.org.uk.)

T'ai Chi is one of a large variety of martial arts in China. Its true origins are difficult to trace because many records were destroyed during wars, insurrection, and the Cultural Revolution. In addition, some styles may be known only to small groups. However, there are pictures of T'ai Chi-like postures dating from over 2000 years ago.[5] The commonly known T'ai Chi styles today originate from the Chen family in the 18th century Ch'ing (Qing) Dynasty.[45] T'ai Chi drew on Taoist concepts such as harmony and reconciling opposites, by meeting and deflecting hard force with sophisticated maneuvers while maintaining balance and poise[32] (Figure 42.2).

This has led to a variety of postures and movements, interlinked into long practice sequences or forms, which allow the participants to explore the intrinsic and extrinsic aspects of movement. Movements may be coordinated with breathing, depending on the style. T'ai Chi may be practiced both as a martial art and a deeply engrossing experience of meditation in movement.[46] Chinese martial arts can be divided into hard or external (Wai Chia (Waijia)) and soft or internal (Nei Chia (Neijia)) styles. T'ai Chi is an internal style, characterized by the deflection of attacks and the application of force through internal alignment and relaxation, rather than overt strength. T'ai Chi has three main components:

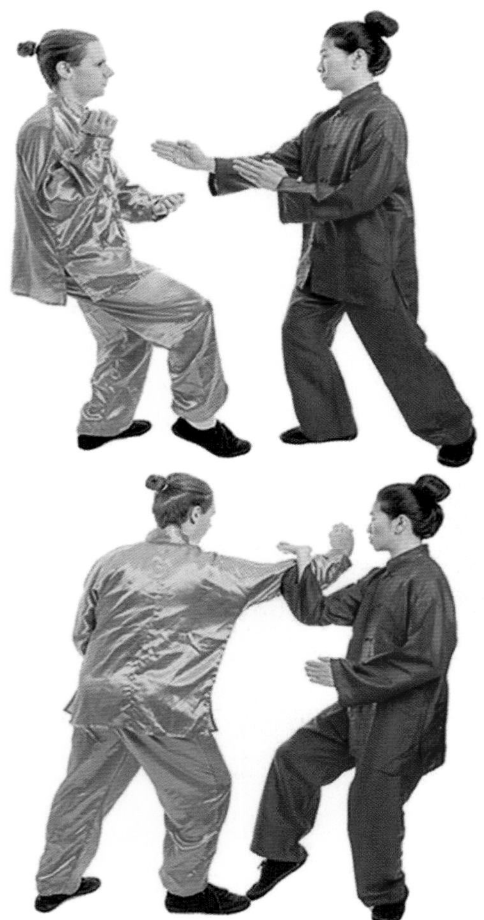

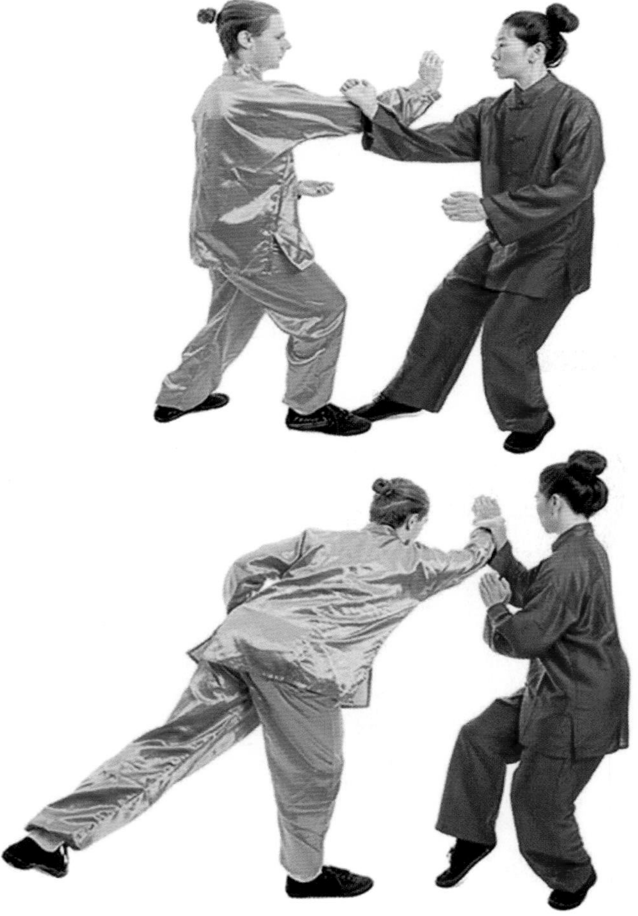

FIGURE 42.2
Yielding to force while maintaining body alignment.
(Reproduced with kind permission of Samantha Toolsie, www.toolsiephotography.co.uk.)

health benefits, meditation and self-defense.[25] In 2020 T'ai Chi was added to the United Nations Educational, Scientific and Cultural Organization (UNESCO) list of Intangible Cultural Heritage of Humanity.[40]

Shoulder and body dynamics from a T'ai Chi perspective

In T'ai Chi training, practitioners learn to relax while moving. The arms generally move in the scapular plane with the shoulder joints in mid-range, and practitioners are encouraged to reduce any tendency to raise the shoulders when lifting their arms. This enables experienced T'ai Chi practitioners to neutralize or generate a considerable amount of force without substantial strain on the shoulders. Practice involves mental imagery, such as imagining that the arms are in water. The arms feel supported, even when outstretched, and float up as if buoyant. The sense of the resistance of water can reinforce coordinated body movements involving the entire kinetic chain, from the feet, through the trunk and all the way to the fingertips.

Keeping the upper body upright and relaxed, while at the same time moving the arms in unison with the rest of the body, requires training of body awareness. Any action of the upper limbs gradually becomes more integrated with position and movement of the trunk. In turn, relaxation of the trunk allows body weight and any external force to drop via the lower limbs into the ground. Practitioners typically start off performing upper limb movements separate from the rest of the body, but eventually any upper limb activity is facilitated and supported by adjustment of the trunk and lower limbs. This can only happen over time, with repetition, attention, and advice from an experienced teacher. The beginner starts off with relatively short movements and sequences, gradually increasing from minutes to hours in duration as skill, stamina, and relaxation develop.

Although T'ai Chi is graceful and relaxed, all postures and movements have martial arts applications (Figure 42.3). Instructors may test whether a practitioner is able to resist a push or a pull while minimizing tension or strain throughout the body, including the shoulder. This ability is developed further in two-person exercises referred

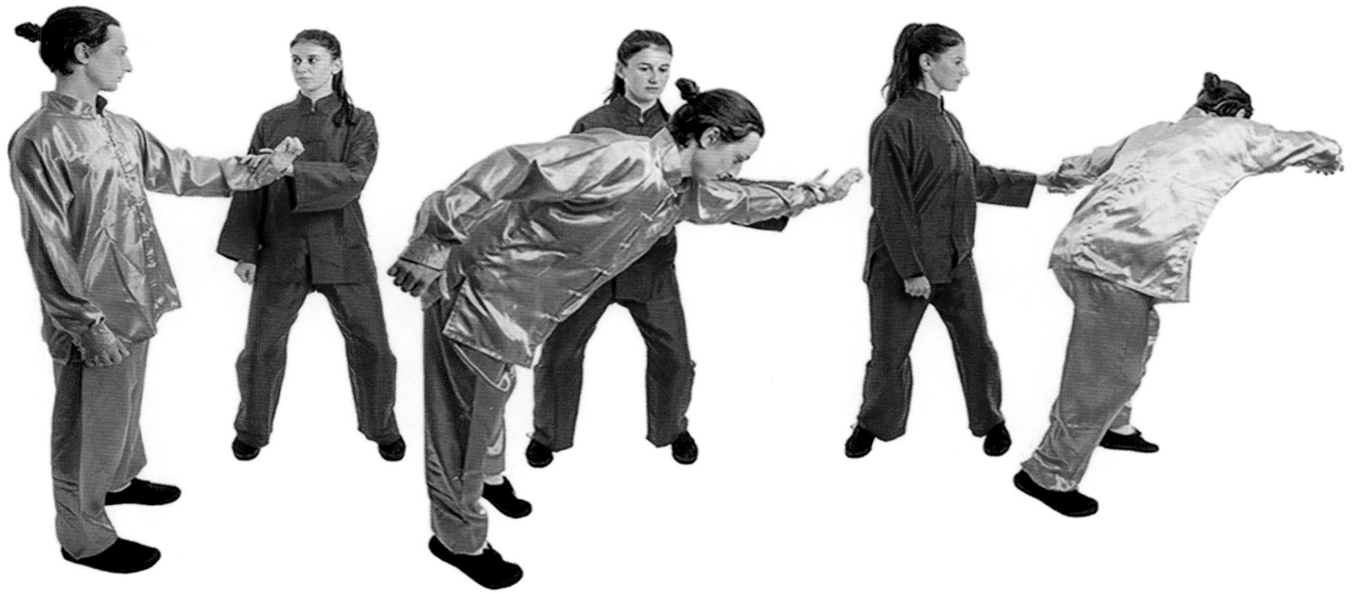

FIGURE 42.3
Coordinated pulling with minimal effort.
(Reproduced with kind permission of Samantha Toolsie, www.toolsiephotography.co.uk.)

to as pushing hands, sticking hands, or sensing hands. The two practitioners typically stand opposite each other with arms in contact. As one person moves forward and pushes, the other yields and then reverses the movement, resulting in a repeating to-and-fro motion. Each practitioner maintains a relaxed yet strong posture throughout the exercise. Movement of the upper limbs is supported by coordinated movement of trunk and legs, so the shoulder is never in an extreme or vulnerable position. Each practitioner tries to sense whether a weakness in the opponent's posture can be used to push or pull them off balance but allows the opponent to respond to the challenge.

Pushing hands thus puts the T'ai Chi practitioners' posture, coordination, and body awareness to the test. This allows people to apply these skills in practical applications, such as pushing a shopping trolley or maintaining one's balance in a busy crowd. Sticking hands is a graduated and extremely challenging, even chaotic, exercise and as such is an excellent inclusion in shoulder rehabilitation.

Taken together, these strategies teach the T'ai Chi practitioner to reduce pressure and strain on the shoulder, for instance when lifting or pushing. The shoulder receives more support from the trunk and lower limbs and is more a conduit of force than a fulcrum. This development goes together with, and relies on, active relaxation and increased whole-body awareness.

Another advantage of T'ai Chi practice is incorporating the whole of the body in the routines, enabling force transfer from the feet via the shoulders to the hands (see Chapter 4). Compliant gait (Figure 42.4) is one method of facilitating this, making the legs stronger, improving balance, and incorporating trunk rotation.[13] Compliant gait reduces ground reaction force when walking and provides an almost horizontal transition of the center of gravity, allowing freedom of the upper limbs and a faster walking speed.[34] Research[7] has suggested that a single compliant leg stance as used in T'ai Chi, demands greater balance than conventional single straight leg standing,[17,47] and is associated with improved athletic performance.[47]

Motor learning theory suggests that the nervous system uses a modular approach to motor programing,[8] and although co-adapting modules to develop a skill is relatively rapid, developing entirely new modules is difficult and takes time.[6] This may explain why people learning T'ai Chi find compliant leg walking and slow movements difficult to do,[17,31] and why T'ai Chi takes a long time to learn.

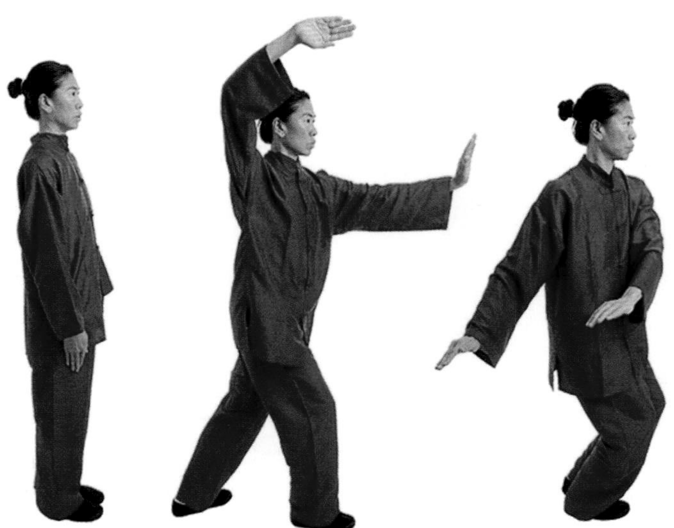

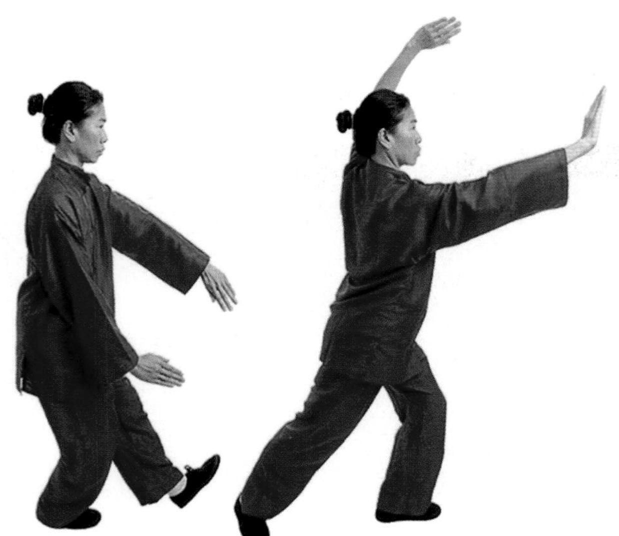

FIGURE 42.4

Compliant gait in T'ai Chi.

(Reproduced with kind permission of Samantha Toolsie, www.toolsiephotography.co.uk.)

Developing skill therefore involves repetition of more simple movements that involve the whole body,[11] followed by a gradual increase in complexity. T'ai Chi develops skill with slow and repeated movements and internal and external concentration, fine-tuning, and enriching the internal schema.[18,33]

The internal schema is the neurocortical integrated representation of visual, somatosensory, proprioceptive, and auditory awareness. The use of tools such as sticks, swords, and silks expands the internal schema to the peripersonal space[2] and the extrapersonal space.[10] The peripersonal space is the space immediately surrounding our bodies and within our reach for interaction (about 70 cm), while the extrapersonal space is the area beyond our reach, where locomotion is required for interaction. Using sticks and swords in T'ai Chi practice extends range of movement and perception[22] (Figure 42.5).

Finally, the repetition of movements in groups is shown to produce a synchronization of neurological and biochemical processes, giving a feeling of belonging that may mediate some of the psychoemotional effects of T'ai Chi practice.[12,29,36]

Investigating T'ai Chi

T'ai Chi is a multimodal intervention with neuromuscular, psychosocial and breathing parameters,[39] which makes its scientific investigation challenging. Furthermore, blinding, placebo control, and quantification of factors such as intensity are problematic.[38] Wayne and Kaptchuk provide an excellent discussion of difficulties associated with researching T'ai Chi[42,43] (see Chapter 10). Ideally, researchers should examine not only adherence, time spent exercising, frequency, and intensity, but also potential mediation by style of T'ai Chi and internal adherence, i.e., the level of cognition brought to the exercise by the practitioner. In an investigation of dose-response, one study found that 12 weeks of Yang style T'ai Chi was enough to improve chronic neck pain.[15] Classes were 75–90 minutes weekly, and participants averaged a further 45 minutes of weekly home practice. However, continuing T'ai Chi over a longer period is likely to increase its benefits. A study of patients with fibromyalgia found increased benefit of 24 weeks of T'ai Chi compared to 12 weeks, with one-hour classes once or twice weekly and 30 minutes of daily home exercise.[41]

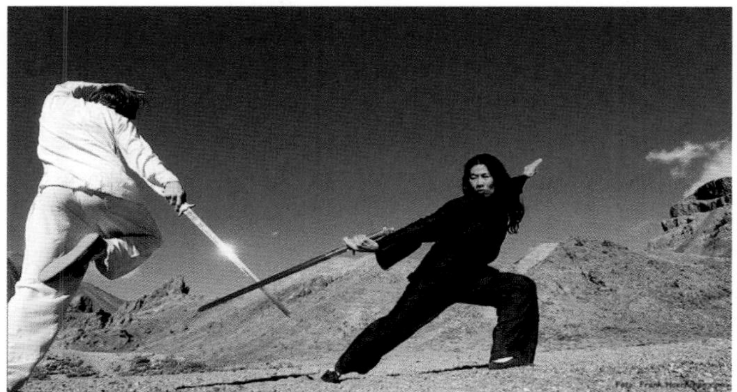

FIGURE 42.5
Extending the internal schema into the extrapersonal space with swords.

(Reproduced with kind permission of the International Taoist Society, www.lishi.org.)

At the time of writing, no English-language papers were found specifically comparing T'ai Chi with conventional treatments for musculoskeletal upper limb problems. This review therefore summarizes the available literature regarding other conditions associated with musculoskeletal pain. The Cochrane Library of Systematic Reviews held 19 studies involving T'ai Chi at the time of writing this chapter.[27] A wide variety of health states were investigated such as chronic obstructive pulmonary disease, cardiovascular disease, chronic pain, fibromyalgia, osteo- and rheumatoid arthritis, balance and falls, osteoporosis, quality of life, anxiety, urinary tract symptoms, and fatigue. Interventions were short – around three months – and may therefore not have reflected the anticipated longer-term benefits.

T'ai Chi was often included as an alternative to another exercise regimen or meditation, but three reviews investigated the effects of T'ai Chi specifically – for rheumatoid arthritis, chronic obstructive pulmonary disease (COPD), and primary prevention of cardiovascular disease.[9,24,26] T'ai Chi was generally found to be a safe intervention with no significant adverse effects or risks of harm, even in populations of older people with comorbidities. Dropout was lower in the T'ai Chi groups compared with control groups.[24] The results for rheumatoid arthritis and cardiovascular disease were equivocal, and there was low-to-moderate evidence of improved functional capacity and pulmonary function in the COPD groups, compared with usual care.

An evidence map of the effect of T'ai Chi on health outcomes summarizes data from 107 systematic reviews in the English language.[38] It divided research into T'ai Chi into: evidence of potentially no effect (diabetes, aerobic capacity, life participation, and falls within institutions), unclear evidence (27 areas), and evidence of potentially positive effect (falls in general, hypertension, cognitive performance, osteoarthritis, depression, COPD, pain, balance-confidence, and muscle strength).

Although many studies involved older populations, one systematic review investigated the health benefits of T'ai Chi for higher education students.[44] It included eight English language and 68 Chinese language papers from publications between 2003 and 2012. Study quality was similar for both languages (level Ib to IV). The strongest evidence was for improving flexibility, reducing depression and anxiety, and enhancing interpersonal sensitivity (the accuracy and/or appropriateness of perceptions, judgments, and responses we have with respect to one another). Finally, the review demonstrated that many reviews of evidence may miss relevant information if they do not include Chinese language literature.

Pain

Although muscle exercise produces local analgesia in healthy people, exercising different muscle groups may be more beneficial in shoulder myalgia.[28] T'ai Chi may achieve this with its emphasis on slow movements involving the large muscles of the lower limbs. The emphasis on attention to intrinsic and extrinsic detail and process, especially when combined in group or partner exercise, may mediate movement desensitization[28,30] and improve distortions of body image sometimes found in pain states, where motor imagery has been shown to be beneficial.[20,23,35,37]

A systematic review and meta-analysis of T'ai Chi in persistent pain showed good evidence of benefit, particularly in osteoarthritis, but also in low back pain and osteoporosis, with a moderate aggregated relief of chronic pain (SMD −0.65, 95% CI −0.82 to −0.48, $P < 0.001$) from a minimum of six weeks of practice, and increasing effects with longer practice.[14] An RCT with one year follow-up showed good results for fibromyalgia when T'ai Chi was compared with usual care or aerobic exercise (Fibromyalgia Impact Questionnaire scores at 24 weeks: difference between groups 5.5 points, 95% CI 0.6 to 10.4, P = 0.03).[41] There were also fewer dropouts from the T'ai Chi group. A shorter randomized controlled trial found 12 weeks of T'ai Chi to be more effective than no treatment (and equal to neck exercises) for the relief of persistent neck pain (mean difference on the pain visual analogue scale −10.5 mm, 95% CI −20.3 to −0.9, P = 0.033).[15]

Self-efficacy

Self-efficacy is an important predictor and mediator of treatment for musculoskeletal pain.[3,4,21] Several studies have shown that self-efficacy is a strong mediator of beneficial physical activity increases and other healthy lifestyle choices.[1] A systematic review of T'ai Chi and self-efficacy in the English and Chinese literature identified 27 studies, of which 20 were RCTs.[39] Fifteen of these (including 12 RCTs) found a significant increase in self-efficacy, with positive effects in 1055 out of 2185 participants in the RCTs (48.3%). Unfortunately, no trials were graded higher than 2 on the five-point Jadad quality scale, suggesting a high risk of bias.

Conclusion

T'ai Chi has proven benefits for general health, including pain management, self-efficacy, and movement. It can offer a unique approach to the rehabilitation of shoulder problems by training body awareness and relaxation, and by integrating shoulder activity with whole body movement. A certain level of commitment, an experienced and patient instructor, and a practice group are required to achieve the full benefits of T'ai Chi, which may be more attractive to some people than others. The specific effects of T'ai Chi on musculoskeletal shoulder problems are awaiting further scientific investigation.

Box 42.1

Demonstration of the Chen Style Lao Chia (Laojia) set, performed by Grandmaster Chen Xiaowang, is available at the link below.

https://www.youtube.com/watch?v=Tcsqtx-_8TQ

References

1. Ashford S, Edmunds J, French DP. What is the best way to change self-efficacy to promote lifestyle and recreational physical activity? A systematic review with meta-analysis. British Journal of Health Psychology. 2010;15:265-288.

2. Berti A, Frassinetti F. When far becomes near: remapping of space by tool use. Journal of Cognitive Neuroscience. 2000;12:415-420.

3. Chester R, Jerosch-Herold C, Lewis J, Shepstone L. Psychological factors are associated with the outcome of physiotherapy for people with shoulder pain: a multicentre longitudinal cohort study. British Journal of Sports Medicine. 2018;52:269-275.

4. Chester R, Khondoker M, Shepstone L, Lewis JS, Jerosch-Herold C. Self-efficacy and risk of persistent shoulder pain: results of a Classification and Regression Tree (CART) analysis. British Journal of Sports Medicine. 2019;1-11.

5. Clements J. A Brief History Of The Martial Arts: East Asian Fighting Styles, from Kung Fu to Ninjutsu. London: Robinson; 2016.

6. d'Avella A. Modularity for motor control and motor learning. In: Laczko J, Latash ML (eds). Progress in Motor Control: Theories and Translations. Cham: Springer International Publishing; 2016:3-19.

7. Dongqing X, Jingxian L, Youlian H. Tai Chi movement and proprioceptive training: a kinematics and EMG analysis. Research in Sports Medicine. 2003;11:129-143.

8. Graziano MS, Taylor CS, Moore T. Complex movements evoked by microstimulation of precentral cortex. Neuron. 2002;34:841-851.

9. Hartley L, Flowers N, Lee MS, Ernst E, Rees K. Tai chi for primary prevention of cardiovascular disease. Cochrane Database of Systematic Reviews. 2014;CD010366.

10. Holmes NP, Spence C. The body schema and the multisensory representation(s) of peripersonal space. Cognitive Processing. 2004;5:94-105.

11. Hore J, Watts S, Martin J, Miller B. Timing of finger opening and ball release in fast and accurate overarm throws. Experimental Brain Research. 1995;103:277-286.

12. Hu Y, Hu Y, Li X, Pan Y, Cheng X. Brain-to-brain synchronization across two persons predicts mutual prosociality. Social Cognitive and Affective Neuroscience. 2017;12:1835-1844.

13. Ivanenko Y, Gurfinkel VS. Human postural control. Front Neurosci. 2018;12:1-9.

14. Kong LJ, Lauche R, Klose P, et al. Tai Chi for chronic pain conditions: a systematic review and meta-analysis of randomized controlled trials. Scientific Reports. 2016;6:1-9.

15. Lauche R, Stumpe C, Fehr J, et al. The effects of Tai Chi and neck exercises in the treatment of chronic nonspecific neck pain: a randomized controlled trial. The Journal of Pain. 2016;17:1013-1027.

16. Li JX, Hong Y, Chan KM. Tai chi: physiological characteristics and beneficial effects on health. British Journal of Sports Medicine. 2001;35:148-156.

17. Mandalidis DG, Karagiannakis DN. A comprehensive method for assessing postural control during dynamic balance testing. MethodsX. 2020;7:1-12.

18. Manley H, Dayan P, Diedrichsen J. When money is not enough: awareness, success, and variability in motor learning. PLoS One. 2014;9:e86580.

19. Marinko LN, Chacko JM, Dalton D, Chacko CC. The effectiveness of therapeutic exercise for painful shoulder conditions: a meta-analysis. Journal of Shoulder and Elbow Surgery. 2011;20:1351-1359.

20. McCormick K, Zalucki N, Hudson M, Moseley GL. Faulty proprioceptive information disrupts motor imagery: an experimental study. Australian Journal of Physiotherapy. 2007;53:41-45.

21. Miles CL, Pincus T, Carnes D, et al. Review: Can we identify how programmes aimed at promoting self-management in musculoskeletal pain work and who benefits? A systematic review of sub-group analysis within RCTs. European Journal of Pain. 2011;15:775.e771-711.

22. Mohan V, Bhat A, Morasso P. Muscleless motor synergies and actions without movements: from motor neuroscience to cognitive robotics. Phys Life Rev. 2019;30:89-111.

23. Moseley GL. Graded motor imagery is effective for long-standing complex regional pain syndrome: a randomised controlled trial. Pain. 2004;108:192-198.

24. Mudano AS, Tugwell P, Wells GA, Singh JA. Tai Chi for rheumatoid arthritis. Cochrane Database of Systematic Reviews. 2019;CD004849.

25. Murray D, Hunter L. Moving As Water: Ancient Wisdom from Daoist Practice. International Daoist Society; 2019.

26. Ngai SPC, Jones AYM, Tam WWS. Tai Chi for chronic obstructive pulmonary disease (COPD). Cochrane Database of Systematic Reviews. 2016;CD009953.

27. National Institute for Health and Care Excellence. Evidence search. Available at: https://www.evidence.nhs.uk/search?om=%5B%7B%22srn%22%3A%5B%22Cochrane+Database+of+Systematic+Reviews%22%5D%7D%5D&q=Tai+Chi&sp =on&Route=search&ps=50.

28. Nijs J, Kosek E, Van Oosterwijck J, Meeus M. Dysfunctional endogenous analgesia during exercise in patients with chronic pain: to exercise or not to exercise? Pain physician. 2012;15:Es205-213.

29. Nowak A, Vallacher RR, Zochowski M, Rychwalska A. Functional synchronization: the emergence of coordinated activity in human systems. Front Psychol. 2017;8:945.941-915.

30. Olsson C-J, Nyberg L. Motor imagery: if you can't do it, you won't think it. Scandinavian Journal of Medicine & Science in Sports. 2010;20:711-715.

31. Park S-W, Marino H, Charles SK, Sternad D, Hogan N. Moving slowly is hard for humans: limitations of dynamic primitives. J Neurophysiol. 2017;118:69-83.

32. Reid H, Croucher M. The Way of the Warrior. London: Leopard Books; 1995.

33. Sartori L, Spoto A, Gatti M, Straulino E. The shape of water: how Tai Chi and mental imagery effect the kinematics of a reach-to-grasp movement. Frontiers in Physiology. 2020;11:297.291-213.

34. Schmitt D. Insights into the evolution of human bipedalism from experimental studies of humans and other primates. Journal of Experimental Biology. 2003;206:1437-1448.

35. Senkowski D, Heinz A. Chronic pain and distorted body image: implications for multisensory feedback interventions. Neuroscience and Biobehavioral Reviews. 2016;69:252-259.

36. Shahal S, Wurzberg A, Sibony I, et al. Synchronization of complex human networks. Nature Communications. 2020;11:3854.3851-3810.

37. Solcà M, Park H-D, Bernasconi F, Blanke O. Behavioral and neurophysiological evidence for altered interoceptive bodily processing in chronic pain. NeuroImage. 2020;217:116902.116901-116907.

38. Solloway MR, Taylor SL, Shekelle PG, et al. An evidence map of the effect of Tai Chi on health outcomes. Systematic Reviews. 2016;5:126.121-111.

39. Tong Y, Chai L, Lei S, Liu M, Yang L. Effects of Tai Chi on self-efficacy: a systematic review. Evidence-Based Complementary and Alternative Medicine. 2018;2018:1701372.

40. UNESCO. Intangible Cultural Heritage: Taijiquan. Available at: https://ich.unesco.org/en/RL/taijiquan-00424.

41. Wang C, Schmid CH, Fielding RA, et al. Effect of tai chi versus aerobic exercise for fibromyalgia: comparative effectiveness randomized controlled trial. British Medical Journal. 2018;360:k851.851-814.

42. Wayne PM, Kaptchuk TJ. Challenges inherent to T'ai Chi research: part I – T'ai Chi as a complex multicomponent intervention. Journal of Alternative & Complementary Medicine. 2008;14:95-102.

43. Wayne PM, Kaptchuk TJ. Challenges inherent to T'ai Chi research: part II – defining the intervention and optimal study design. Journal of Alternative & Complementary Medicine. 2008;14:191-197.

44. Webster CS, Luo AY, Krägeloh C, Moir F, Henning M. A systematic review of the health benefits of Tai Chi for students in higher education. Preventive Medicine Reports. 2016;3:103-112.

45. Wile D. T'ai-chi Touchstones: Yang Family Secret Transmissions. New York: Sweet Ch'i Press; 1983.

46. Yeung W-Y, Green B. Way Out: A Daoist Path to a Fearless Life. International Daoist Society; 2017.

47. Yoo S, Park S-K, Yoon S, Lim HS, Ryu J. Comparison of proprioceptive training and muscular strength training to improve balance ability of Taekwondo Poomsae Athletes: a randomized controlled trial. J Sports Sci Med. 2018;17:445-454.

Yoga therapy in the management of musculoskeletal shoulder conditions 43

Shelly Prosko

Introduction

Yoga is globally one of the most popular forms of exercise, and is increasingly being incorporated into the management of musculoskeletal health conditions.[28,37,65,66] The increasing general interest in yoga as a form of exercise and the concomitant integration of yoga into healthcare and its inclusion in clinical practice guidelines is due to yoga's multidimensional health benefits, safety, and effectiveness.[65] The purpose of this chapter is to provide an overview of yoga therapy and its potential contribution to shoulder rehabilitation.

Yoga therapy

The popularization of modern yoga has become less focused on its traditional philosophies and practices and primarily focused on physical poses and movement practices. However, the basis of yoga is a comprehensive health philosophy that goes far beyond the attainment of complex physical skills,[33,42] and traditional practitioners suggest that the therapeutic benefits of yoga may be diminished without an appreciation of the philosophy that underpins the practice.

The word *yoga* means *to yoke* or *unite,* and traditional texts describe yoga as the skilled action of unifying the physical, emotional, mental, energetic, social, and spiritual layers of one's existence.[55,56] Yoga practice involves compassion, curiosity, acceptance, commitment, effort, self-discipline, humility, and patience. There are many different styles of yoga, but they all involve an inward journey of self-discovery through awareness, self-regulation, breathing, and mindful movement.

Yoga therapy is a growing field that is described as: "the professional application of the principles and practices of yoga to promote health and well-being within a therapeutic relationship that includes personalized assessment, goal setting, lifestyle management, and yoga practices for individuals or small groups."[44]

The biomedical model of care principally focuses on "fixing" pathology. In comparison, salutogenesis focuses on addressing factors that create and support health and wellness.[1,64] As with any form of exercise rehabilitation, the practice and benefits of yoga fit in either model,[6,7] but this chapter will discuss yoga within the context of the salutogenic model. The chapter will not provide a protocol for managing shoulder conditions, or a system of diagnosis, but instead present a framework for integrating yoga into the management of musculoskeletal problems involving the shoulder.

Yoga therapy and shoulder rehabilitation

Yoga therapy may augment management of musculoskeletal problems involving the shoulder as it has the potential to address domains not typically included in conventional rehabilitation.[41] Yoga therapy incorporates both a biopsychosocial and spiritual approach to care, promotes ongoing self-management and self-efficacy, a healthy lifestyle, and a strong therapeutic alliance.

Biopsychosocial-spiritual approach to rehabilitation

The *pancha maya kosha* model used in yoga therapy is akin to the biopsychosocial-spiritual (BPSS) model. It includes five *koshas* (sheaths or layers) of an individual's existence: physical, psycho-emotional, wisdom or meta-cognition, energetic and spiritual.[16,63] It is vital to understand that all layers of the *kosha* model (or domains of BPSS model) are integrated and based on the philosophy that we cannot separate mind from body, or emotions from physiology. What happens in one domain automatically influences another, regardless of our intention.[62] We can appreciate the clinical relevance of this understanding and how it may inform and impact clinical decision-making and outcomes. An individual who is experiencing fear, anger, or frustration, has ruminating thoughts, believes their experience will not change, or lacks trust or social support, will have concomitant physiological changes in the central and autonomic nervous systems. This may influence breathing, muscle tension, movement, function, and pain.[22,34,40] Changing one or more of these variables has the potential to change another. In other words, you can use any aspect of your existence to change any other aspect of your existence. The complexity of our systems and their interactions make it challenging to find linear solutions to any musculoskeletal problem, including those involving the shoulder region. However, the interwoven complexity also offers more paths and possibilities to meet one's valued goals, as changing one variable may be the catalyst for producing positive change.

Although the domains of the BPSS model are not separate, it is helpful to discuss them separately to appreciate that using one domain as a portal may influence other domains, and subsequently the entire integrated human.

Biopsychological

Integrating psychological determinants of health into shoulder rehabilitation should no longer be up for debate, given the growing evidence supporting the necessity of addressing psychological factors in populations of people with various shoulder conditions, particularly shoulder pain.[2,9,22,31,52] Depression, anxiety, pain catastrophizing, kinesiophobia, and low self-efficacy predicts persistent shoulder complaints.[9,22] Research demonstrating the positive effects of yoga on emotional health, cognitive function, and a variety of physiological parameters have been published.[19,21,41,57,67] Yoga fosters resilience, promotes autonomic nervous system regulation, enhances interoceptive skills, downregulates proinflammatory markers, and improves tissue health.[15,17,28,41,42,57,63] Ward et al. concluded that yoga was a safe and acceptable intervention that may result in "clinically relevant improvements in pain and functional outcomes associated with a wide range of musculoskeletal conditions", [71] and in other persistent pain populations.[35,41] Additionally, yoga may be a viable intervention to decrease inflammation by regulating pro-inflammatory cytokine levels.[15] As such, yoga may contribute to the management of people with frozen shoulder rehabilitation, as there is evidence suggesting that the pathophysiology of frozen shoulder includes a persistent inflammatory process that may be partially mediated by cytokines.[12,23]

Yoga can address physiological and psychological health in rehabilitation through the following practices: awareness, breathing, self-regulation, and mindful movement.

Awareness practices

Yoga *pratyahara* involves interoceptive awareness practices that turn our awareness inwards to focus attention on our current physiological state including body, breath, thoughts, and emotions. Enhanced awareness provides an opportunity to recognize habitual patterns that may be contributing to pain and mobility problems. Once aware, suitable regulatory practices are implemented, influencing outcome. Furthermore, awareness and perception can become distorted in people with chronic pain including rotator cuff-related shoulder pain.[22] Taken together, yoga awareness practices are a valuable tool for assessment and treatment.[53] Box 43.1 provides examples of integrating awareness practices into rehabilitation. An example of a guided awareness practice, scanning all *koshas*, is available at the link below.

https://vimeo.com/510070816/0d4abd27c2

Box 43.1 Awareness practice

Mind and emotional awareness

Allow a moment for the patient to privately check-in with their general state of emotions and thoughts without judgement and without allowing the mind to wander or get carried away with an elaborate story.

Breath awareness practice

In a position of support and comfort, notice the different qualities of the breath without trying to change anything: rate, depth, sound, length of inhale compared with exhale, if there are pauses between inhale and exhale or if there is a continuous cycle. Notice any other qualities, words, or images about the breath (is it rigid, bumpy, choppy, smooth, peaceful, gliding?). Notice any physical sensations of breath as it enters and exits nostrils including temperature, and how the body moves in response to breath cycle: the obvious and subtle areas.

Body awareness practice

In a position of support and comfort, bring your awareness to your body. Notice where your body is in contact with the surface beneath you, the differences in pressure from one area to the next, and any different physical sensations you may be experiencing, without trying to change anything. Bring your attention to focus on the back of your body and notice the space between your shoulder blades and any sensations around each shoulder blade. Expand your awareness to the entire back of your trunk, from shoulder blades to buttocks then continuing down the back of your legs to the soles of your feet. Bring your awareness to your toes and the spaces between them. Shift your attention to the front of your body: notice your face, throat, collar bones, breastbone, chest, abdomen. Expand your awareness to the entire front of your trunk and pelvis and continuing down the front of your legs to the tops of your feet. Shift your attention and focus on the sides of your body: starting with the ears, then following down to the sides of your neck and shoulders. Notice the space between your shoulders and ears. Bring your awareness to your arms and hands noticing the palms and backs of the hands. Notice your fingers and spaces between them. Bring your awareness to the sides of your trunk, under your armpits, noticing the space between your arms and trunk. Draw your awareness down to the sides of your hips and legs, your outer ankle bones, and outer edges of your feet. Return your awareness to the entire body and observe any physical sensations that arise, without trying to change them.

With regular awareness practices, the discoveries and experiences patients describe during movement and functional activities will become more nuanced, and then appropriate self-regulation techniques can be implemented to help move with more ease and less pain.

Breathing practices

In addition to using breath as a tool for assessment, we can also use it as an agent of change. Yoga *pranayama* involves volitional breath regulation practices with the intention of influencing *prana* (life force or vital energy) within us. We can also use breathing to influence the autonomic and central nervous systems, mental states, immune system, biomechanics, body tension, overall movement efficiency, and function. Breathing practices also impact emotions such as reducing fear and anxiety, leading to reduced body tension, increased confidence to move, improved ease of movement, and less pain.[25,47] Box 43.2 describes a breath regulation practice. A guided audio practice of the longer-smoother-softer breath practice is available at the link below.

https://www.youtube.com/watch?v=LXZ6DzzCkA4

The patient first learns the longer-smoother-softer breath technique in a position of rest and comfort, then is instructed to try the practice whenever they notice their breath pattern is tight, rigid, shallow or being held, typically during a challenging movement. This often helps the person move with more ease and less pain or anxiety, and gives the person an experience that demonstrates they can influence their mobility and pain by changing their breath, giving them a sense of agency and heightened self-efficacy.

Another breath practice I have found useful in clinical practice is *ujjayi* or victorious breath. It includes nasal breathing with gentle laryngeal engagement producing an ocean-like sound, while cueing a posterolateral costal expansive pattern. *Ujjayi* breath biomechanically encourages thoracic and rib mobility, influencing shoulder mobility. From a

Box 43.2 Breath regulation practice: longer-smoother-softer[43]

Find a position of support and comfort. Begin with a few moments of a simple breath awareness practice. If you can breathe nasally, do so. Start to allow the exhale to last and linger a little longer. There is no rush. Take your time. When you feel ready to inhale, see if you can imagine *receiving* the next breath vs *taking* the next breath. As you inhale, imagine you are sipping the breath. Slowly, smoothly, and softly. Like the breath is gliding with ease. No need to force a "deep" breath. No need to over-breathe or over-exert the breath. Stay as patient as you can. There is no place to go or be, but here right now. Take your time. Trust the next breath will come when it's ready. Continue this longer-smoother-softer breath pattern with just the right amount of effort.

cognitive, energetic, and emotional perspective, *ujjayi* is used to promote confidence and a "calm alertness".[47,54]

There are numerous breath practices to choose from in yoga therapy, with varying intentions. Yoga practitioners report breathing practices as one of the most powerful and impactful aspects of rehabilitation and many yoga therapists view breathing practices as foundational to therapy. (See Prosko[47] for an in-depth review of yoga breathing practices in pain management.)

Self-regulation practices

Concentration (*dharana*) and meditation (*dhyana*) practices are used to regulate the mind, emotions, breath, and body tension. A growing body of research shows positive effects of self-regulation meditation-based practices on anxiety, depression, stress, cognition and pain in clinical populations through mechanisms that appear to address cognitive and emotional regulation.[11,32,41,57,72] Various regulation practices are then combined with movement and together can enhance improvements in pain, ease of movement and functional mobility.[28,41,42,57] Box 43.3 describes self-regulation practices.

A guided full-body progressive muscle relaxation regulation practice is available at the link below.

https://vimeo.com/510072801/8ec83eb0d0

Box 43.3 Self-regulation practices

Body tension regulation practice

Practice this focused progressive muscle relaxation technique first in a position of support and comfort, then progress to more challenging positions. Coordinate the technique with longer-smoother-softer breath pattern and imagery.

Thought regulation practice

Instead of the pinched, fraying, impinged, or torn tendon image of your rotator cuff, create an image of your tendon gliding smoothly with a protective sheath that gets stronger and more resilient the more it glides and moves. Imagine spaciousness in your shoulder joint, with a strength, lightness, and grace of your arm as you move it.

Note: Patients may use their own imagery, or clinicians can co-create imagery that resonates with the person. As with any treatment technique, if it is not meaningful or valued by the person, it is less likely to be effective.

Additional regulation practices

Choose an emotion, virtue, or quality you feel would be important on your path to meet your goals. Perhaps it is courage, confidence, patience, or persistence. What would too little of that quality look and feel like? What would too much of that quality look and feel like? What would just the right amount of that quality look like? How would it feel in your body? Choose a posture, movement or statement that might support this feeling and vision.

Mindful movement practices

The Sanskrit term for the physical postures we are familiar with in yoga is *sthira sukham asanam* (*asana*) which translates to *sit with steadiness and ease*. The essence of *asana* practice is to cultivate strength without excess effort or rigidity, and to cultivate ease without lethargy or lack of support. Yoga postures, transitions in and out of postures, and movement sequences intentionally involve the whole body and require mindful awareness with a focus on optimizing efficient use of energy.

Asana and movement can be used as a means of exploring and assessing the habits of the body, breath, mind, and emotions. As the therapist assesses movement patterns and observes any patterns of excess effort, weakness, rigid breath quality, or holding, the therapist can also guide the patient to perform their own assessment scan of their body, noticing any muscle tension or physical sensations, breath qualities, emotions or thoughts during the movement. This process helps patients discover habitual patterns of body, breath, thoughts, or emotions associated with movements and how these patterns influence their mobility, function, and their pain experience. Self-regulation practices are then combined with progressively complex asana and movement, involving the kinetic chain, varying planes of movement, postural orientations, and ranges of motion along with movement recovery guidelines.[43] As such, the integrated movement practice becomes a more powerful change agent.

Bringing it all together

Exercise

Movement impacts mobility, function, pain, and quality of life by influencing our psychology, behavior, and all physiological systems. Substantial evidence recommends exercise therapy as a key component and first-line treatment for individuals with a variety of musculoskeletal conditions including those involving the shoulder.[2,24,29-31,46] There are gaps in our knowledge around underlying mechanisms and what specific exercises are best for different populations. However, evidence shows positive clinical outcomes for general strengthening, progressive loading,[24] integration of the kinetic chain,[50] and whole-body exercise[30] for populations with a variety of shoulder conditions. Yoga *asana* practices support this emerging evidence, particularly by including the whole body and kinetic chain. Lewis et al. recommend guiding principles for gradual progression of exercise rather than specific exercise prescription for rotator cuff tendinopathy.[29] As outlined, yoga provides a framework and practices that cultivate awareness and discernment which can facilitate effective implementation of these guiding exercise principles.

Social

Social determinants of health are consistently recommended to be addressed in clinical practice guidelines for musculoskeletal pain.[2,31] Yoga is often offered in a group therapy setting providing a sense of community, connection, integration and social support, which has been shown to be particularly beneficial for those living with persistent pain, improving pain coping strategies, disease activity, depression, and anxiety.[8,26,41,61] Barrett et al. found that six-week group exercise classes alone resulted in reduced shoulder pain and disability in people with non-specific shoulder pain (NSSP).[3] Another study found that people with NSSP preferred the physiotherapist-led group exercise class over one-to-one physiotherapy, and reported the class helped them to gain mastery of their exercises, build relationships and friendships, and was supportive of their pain self-management.[4] Yoga therapy group classes can be offered onsite or virtually, and may also help address access issues by offering cost-effective and accessible options for diverse and underserved populations and settings.

Spiritual

Spiritual health is often neglected in rehabilitation yet is acknowledged as a domain of health that can influence coping strategies, recovery process and outcomes.[14,20,41,49,70] When people have meaning, purpose, and experience connectedness, it can have positive effects on physiological, psychological and behavioral factors.[61] Reduced pain, anxiety, and depressive symptoms, improved active coping and adjustment to persistent pain, and improved quality of life have all been shown to be associated with spirituality in chronic pain populations.[41] Research also shows mind-body practices such as yoga have greater effectiveness for pain, emotional health, self-efficacy and adherence to ongoing practice when they are spiritually based.[41,68,69]

Yoga therapy offers a unique opportunity to include spiritual health by integrating practices that support one's values, purpose, meaning and a sense of peace, harmony, and common humanity. Sullivan[63] has provided an in-depth review and practical application of integrating the spiritual domain of yoga therapy into rehabilitation.

Additional contributions

High-quality clinical practice guidelines for treating people with musculoskeletal pain include patient-centered care and self-management as part of first-line treatment.[2,31] Communication between therapist and patient, the therapeutic alliance and the patient's pain self-efficacy can influence pain and are associated with clinical outcomes.[10,38,52] Lifestyle factors are also important to address in rehabilitation and have been shown to contribute to improved outcomes in rotator cuff tendinopathy and shoulder pain.[29,30] Yoga has been shown to enhance health promotion behaviors, positively impact lifestyle factors[5,13,18,19,27,35,39,51,59] and improve patient self-confidence and self-efficacy.[35] It is rooted in philosophy and practices that promote compassionate communication, which has positive effects on quality of care, therapeutic alliance, and numerous physiological and psychological health outcomes for both patients and healthcare providers.[58] For a more in-depth review in this area with examples of diverse yoga practices to support these outcomes, look to references provided.[36,45,48,60]

An example of a shoulder-focused yoga practice beginning with gentle awareness practices, transitioning to active *asana* sequences designed to safely and progressively load the shoulders, and concluding with a final relaxation, is available at the link below.

https://vimeo.com/509893421/5deb2d4d65

A video montage example of a shoulder yoga sequence varying planes of movement, range of movement (ROM), open and closed kinetic chain and challenges is available at the link below.

https://vimeo.com/showcase/8111284

Figures 43.1–43.7 provide examples of *asana* illustrating progressive ROM, loading, and kinetic chain activities. Box 43.4 supports the figures with accompanying links to videos for further instructions, cueing, variations, and progressions.

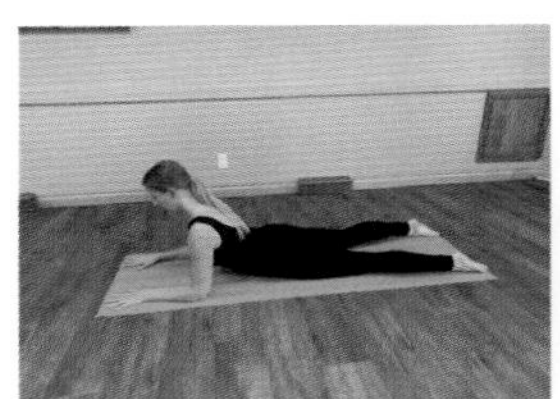

FIGURE 43.1A
Sphinx pose

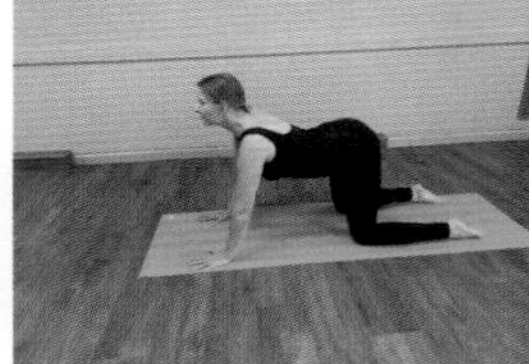

FIGURE 43.1B
Quadruped

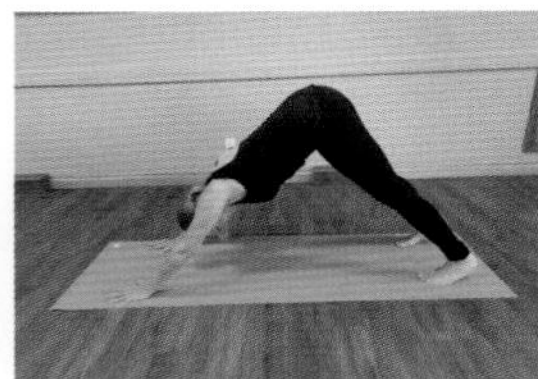

FIGURE 43.1C
Downward facing dog

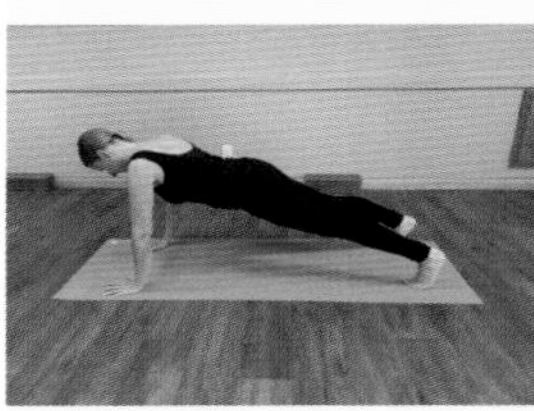

FIGURE 43.1D
Plank pose

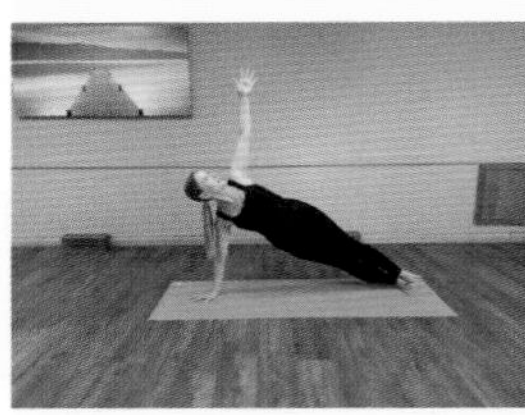

FIGURE 43.1E
Side plank pose

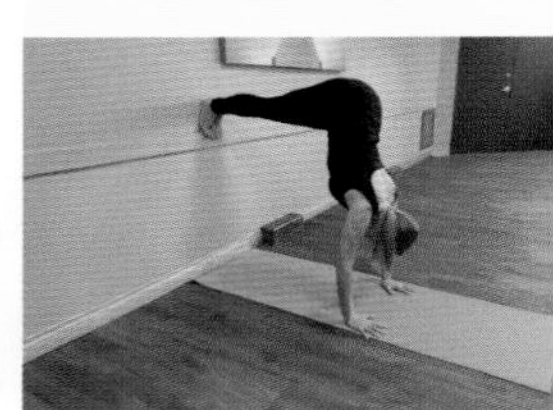

FIGURE 43.1F
Pike handstand pose

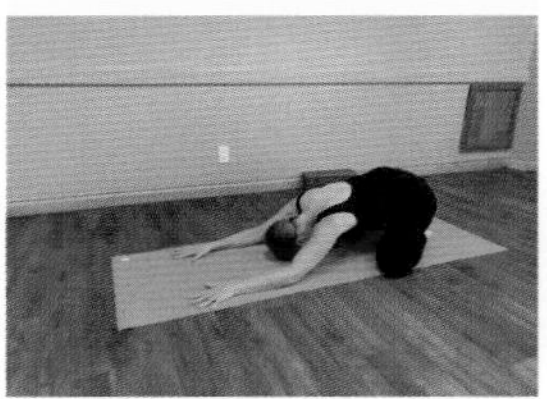

FIGURE 43.2
Child's pose

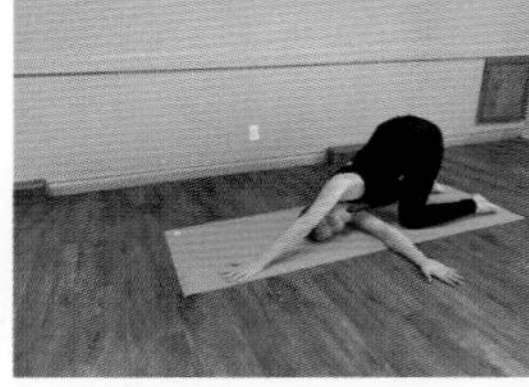

FIGURE 43.3
Thread the needle

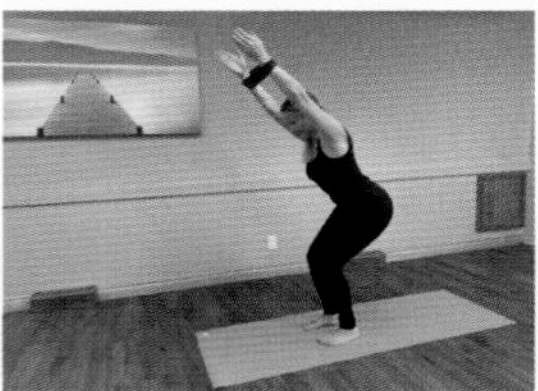

FIGURE 43.4
Fierce pose

(Continued)

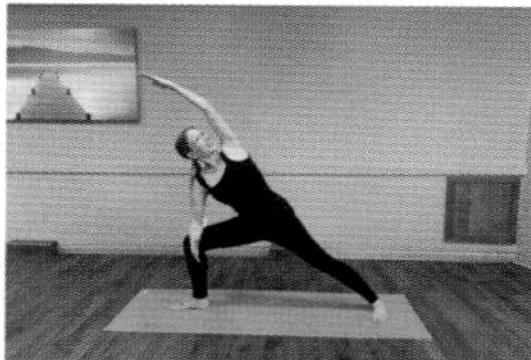

FIGURE 43.5
Extended side angle pose

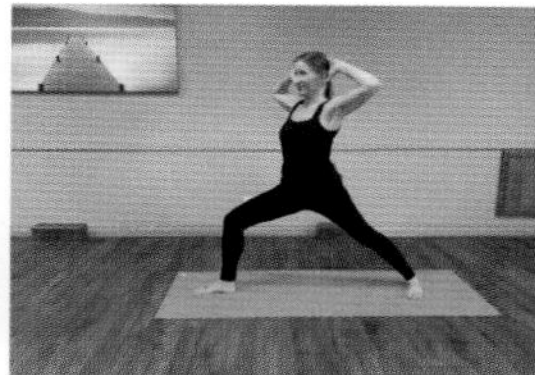

FIGURE 43.6
Warrior 2 with rotation

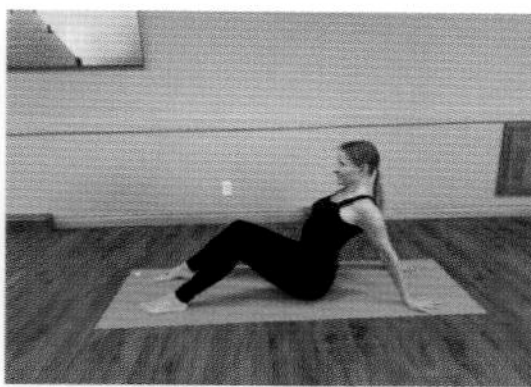

FIGURE 43.7A
Thoracic/shoulder extension

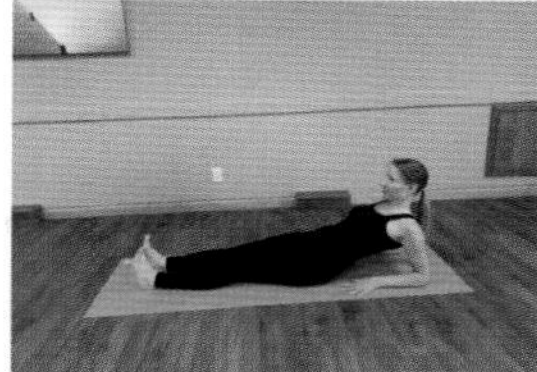

FIGURE 43.7B
Supine elbow support

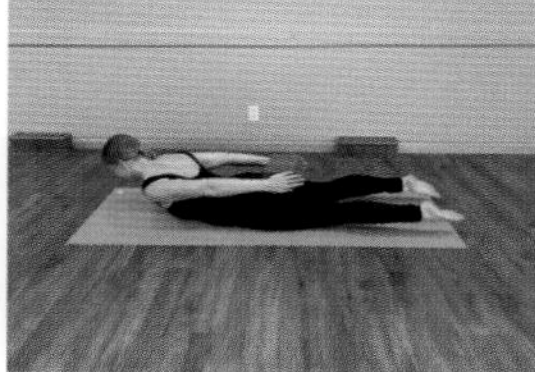

FIGURE 43.7C
Locust pose

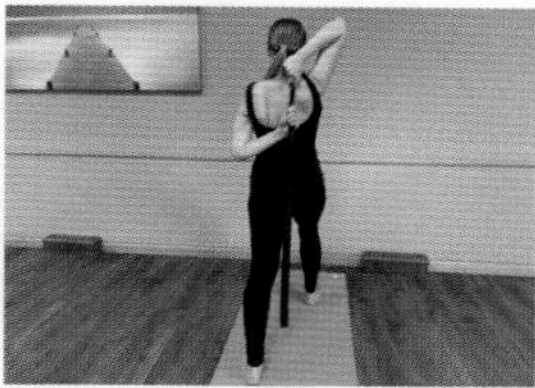

FIGURE 43.7D
Cow face arms

FIGURES 43.1–43.7
Examples of yoga poses that may be used in shoulder rehabilitation.

Box 43.4 Yoga based progressions in shoulder rehabilitation

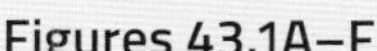

Figures 43.1A–F
Upper body loading progressions
Shoulder stability and mobility warm-up: https://vimeo.com/254882547

Figure 43.1A
Sphinx pose: https://vimeo.com/148535070

Figure 43.1B Quadruped cat/cow
Breath cycle with cat/cow: https://www.youtube.com/watch?v=mhKlN9qkXTY

Quadruped with shoulder isometrics: https://vimeo.com/148624000

Quadruped scapular push-ups: https://vimeo.com/148625770

Figure 43.1C Downward facing dog pose
Lesson 1: https://www.youtube.com/watch?v=g3gl_V_xedE&list=PLt7K-1L3tXOpvZwyAspcLllqm8a459l7h&index=2

Lesson 2: https://www.youtube.com/watch?v=kCFOztW7j1s&list=PLt7K-1L3tXOpvZwyAspcLllqm8a459l7h&index=4

Figure 43.1D Plank pose
Plank/downward dog flow sequence: https://vimeo.com/510073825/f670b6b8f9

Plank pose variations: https://www.youtube.com/watch?v=d2OLmkuPMmo

Plank with spinal rotation: https://vimeo.com/434087988

Plank with resistance band: https://vimeo.com/434087892

Figure 43.1E Side plank pose
Side plank variations: https://www.youtube.com/watch?v=L5VaVX8wscY

Figure 43.1F Pike pose for handstand preparation
Handstand: https://www.youtube.com/watch?v=L5OU8-K7uTY&list=PLt7K-1L3tXOpvZwyAspcLIlqm8a459I7h&index=1

Arm balance, crow pose:
https://www.youtube.com/watch?v=XCvxN8V4OEo&list=PLt7K-1L3tXOpvZwyAspcLIlqm8a459I7h&index=5

Side crow: https://www.youtube.com/watch?v=8sCarOKU53M

Figure 43.2 Child's pose
Supported child's pose modification: https://www.youtube.com/watch?v=qCSUV7s7mZo

Figure 43.3 Thread the needle pose
Demonstrated in Mitchell sequence: https://vimeo.com/509893421/5deb2d4d65

Figure 43.4 Fierce pose
https://www.youtube.com/watch?v=pPx7UvdUCI0&list=PLt7K-1L3tXOpvZwyAspcLIlqm8a459I7h&index=3

Figure 43.5 Extended side angle pose
Demonstrated in Mitchell sequence: https://vimeo.com/509893421/5deb2d4d65

Figure 43.6 Warrior 2 with spinal rotation
Demonstrated in Mitchell sequence https://vimeo.com/509893421/5deb2d4d65

Standing Flow with resistance band sequence: https://vimeo.com/254883917

Figures 43.7A–D Shoulder and thoracic extension series

43.7A Crook sitting shoulder and thoracic extension

43.7B Supine elbow support

43.7C Locust pose

43.7D Cow face arms

Shoulder/thoracic extension sequence: https://www.youtube.com/watch?v=2I1YRVhmDbA&feature=youtu.be

Further examples of a full-spectrum sequenced flow yoga practice, including more challenging *asana*, are available at the link below.

https://empoweredu.ca/videos/full-spectrum-sequence-a-little-bit-of-everything/

Conclusion

This chapter offered a fresh perspective on how yoga therapy can contribute to an individual's shoulder rehabilitation program. Clinicians can integrate yoga-based practices into the clinic setting or apply the practices within the yoga philosophical framework for which they were intended, which is hypothesized to be more impactful. Another option is for clinicians to work alongside yoga professionals within the clinic or refer out to a yoga professional in the community. Patients can also have a personal home yoga practice and/or participate in an ongoing community class setting suitable to their needs. Yoga therapy in shoulder rehabilitation also includes the clinician's own personal yoga practice. Taken together, the individual with a musculoskeletal shoulder problem will be compassionately guided and supported in meeting their valued goals as they progress toward living a life of more ease and peace.

References

1. Antonovsky A. Unravelling the Mystery of Health. San Francisco: Jossey-Bass Inc; 1987.
2. Babatunde OO, Jordan JL, Van der Windt DA, Hill JC, Foster NE, Protheroe J. Effective treatment options for musculoskeletal pain in primary care: a systematic overview of current evidence. PLoS One. 2017; 12: e0178621.
3. Barrett E, Conroy C, Corcoran M, O' Sullivan K, Purtill H, Lewis J, McCreesh K. An evaluation of two types of exercise classes, containing shoulder exercises or a combination of shoulder and thoracic exercises, for the treatment of nonspecific shoulder pain: a case series. Journal of Hand Therapy. 2018;31:301-07.
4. Barrett E, Hayes A, Kelleher M, Exploring patient experiences of participating in a group exercise class for the management of nonspecific shoulder pain. Physiotherapy Theory and Practice. 2018;34:464-71.
5. Barrows JL, Fleury J. Systematic review of yoga interventions to promote cardiovascular health in older adults. Western Journal of Nursing Research. 2016;38:753-781.
6. Bhavanani AB. Are we practicing yoga therapy or yogopathy? Yoga Therapy Today. 2011;7:26–28.
7. Bhavanani AB, Sullivan M, Taylor MJ, Wheeler A. Shared foundations for practice: the language of yoga therapy. Yoga Therapy Today. 2019;44–47.
8. Cacioppo JT, Cacioppo S. Social relationships and health: the toxic effects of perceived social isolation. Social Personal Psychology Compass. 2014;8:58-72.
9. Chester R, Jerosch-Herold C, Lewis J, et al. Psychological factors are associated with the outcome of physiotherapy for people with shoulder pain: a multicentre longitudinal cohort study. Br J Sports Med. 2018;52:269–275.
10. Chester R, Khondoker M, Shepstone L, Lewis J, Jerosch-Herold C. Self-efficacy and risk of persistent shoulder pain: results of a Classification and Regression Tree (CART) analysis. Br J Sports Med. 2019;53:825-834.
11. Chiesa A, Serretti A. Mindfulness-based interventions for chronic pain: a systematic review of the evidence. The Journal of Alternative and Complementary Medicine. 2011;17:83-93.
12. Cho CH, Song KS, Kim BS, Kim DH, Lho YM. Biological Aspect of Pathophysiology for Frozen Shoulder. BioMed Research International. 2018;2018:7274517.
13. Chong CS, Tsunaka M, Tsang HW, et al. Effects of yoga on stress management in healthy adults: a systematic review. Altern Ther Health Med. 2011;17:32-8.
14. Dedeli O, Kaptan G. Spirituality and religion in pain and pain management. Health Psychol Res. 2013;1:e29.
15. Djalilova DM, Schulz PS, Berger AM, Case AJ, Kupzyk KA, Ross AC. Impact of yoga on inflammatory biomarkers: a systematic review. Biological Research for Nursing. 2019;21:198-209.
16. Easwaran E. The Upanishads, 2nd edition. Berkeley, CA: Nilgiri Press; 2007.
17. Falkenberg RI, Eising C, Peters ML. Yoga and immune system functioning: a systematic review of randomized controlled trials. Journal of Behavioral Medicine. 2018;41:467-482.
18. Gard T, Brach N, Hölzel BK, Noggle JJ, Conboy LA, Lazar SW. Effects of a yoga-based intervention for young adults on quality of life and perceived stress: the potential mediating roles of mindfulness and self-compassion. J Posit Psychol. 2012;7:165–175.
19. Gard T, Noggle JJ, Park CL, Vago DR, Wilson A. Potential self-regulatory mechanisms of yoga for psychological health. Front Hum Neurosci. 2014;8:770.
20. Garschagen A, Steegers MAH, van Bergen AHMM, et al. Is there a need for including spiritual care in interdisciplinary rehabilitation of chronic pain patients? Investigating an innovative strategy. World Institute of Pain. 2014;15:671-687.
21. Gothe NP, Khan I, Hayes J, Erlenback E, Damoiseaux JS. Yoga effects on brain health: a systematic review of the current literature. Brain Plasticity. 2019;5:105–122.
22. Haik M, Alburquerque-Sendín F, Fernandes R, et al. Biopsychosocial aspects in individuals with acute and chronic rotator cuff related shoulder pain: classification based on a decision tree analysis. Diagnostics. 2020;10:928.
23. Hand GCR, Athanasou NA, Matthews T, Carr AJ. The pathology of frozen shoulder. J Bone Joint Surg. 2007;89-B:928-32.
24. Hotta G, Couto A, Cools A, McQuade K, Oliveira A. Effects of adding scapular stabilization exercises to a periscapular strengthening exercise program in patients with subacromial pain syndrome: a randomized controlled trial. Musculoskeletal Science and Practice. 2020;49:102171.
25. Jafari H, Courtois I, Van den Bergh O, Vlaeyen JWS, Van Diest I. Pain and respiration: a systematic review. Pain. 2017;158:995–1006.
26. Karayannis NV, Baumann I, Sturgeon JA, Melloh M, Mackey SC. The impact of social isolation on pain interference: a longitudinal study. Ann Behav Med. 2018;53:65–74.
27. Keosaian JE, Lemaster CM, Dresner D, et al. 'We're all in this together': a qualitative study of predominantly low income minority participants in a yoga trial for chronic low back pain. Complementary Therapies in Medicine. 2016;24:34–39.
28. Khalsa SB, Cohen L, McCall T, Telles S. The Principles and Practice of Yoga in Health Care. Edinburgh: Handspring Publishing; 2016.
29. Lewis J, McCreesh K, Roy JS, Ginn K. Rotator cuff tendinopathy: navigating the diagnosis management conundrum. J Orthop Sports Phys Ther. 2015;45:923-937.
30. Lewis J. Rotator cuff related shoulder pain: assessment, management and uncertainties. Manual Therapy. 2016;23:57-68.
31. Lin I, Wiles L, Waller R, et al. What does best practice care for musculoskeletal pain look like? Eleven consistent recommendations from high-quality clinical practice guidelines: systematic review. Br J Sports Med. 2020;54:79–86.
32. Long J, Briggs M, Astin F. Overview of systematic reviews of mindfulness meditation-based interventions for people with long-term conditions. Adv Mind Body Med. 2017;31:26-36.
33. Mallinson J, Singleton M. Roots of Yoga. New York: Penguin Classics; 2017.
34. Melzack R. Pain and the neuromatrix in the brain. J Dent Educ. 2001;65:1378-82.
35. Moonaz S. Current research in yoga and pain. In: Pearson N, Prosko S, Sullivan

M (eds). Yoga and Science in Pain Care: Treating the Person in Pain. London, UK: Singing Dragon Publishers; 2019:37-51.

36. Neff K, Germer C. The Mindful Self-Compassion Workbook: A Proven Way to Accept Yourself, Build Inner Strength, and Thrive. New York: The Guilford Press; 2018.

37. Nerurkar A, Yeh G, Davis RB, Birdee G, Phillips RS. When conventional medical providers recommend unconventional medicine: results of a national study. Arch Intern Med. 2011;171:862–864.

38. O'Keeffe M, Cullinane P, Hurley J, et al. What influences patient-therapist interactions in musculoskeletal physical therapy? Qualitative systematic review and meta-synthesis. Physical Therapy. 2016; 961:609-622.

39. Pascoe MC, Thompson DR, Ski CF. Yoga, mindfulness-based stress reduction and stress-related physiological measures: a meta-analysis. Psychoneuroendocrinology. 2017;86:152-68.

40. Pearson N. Pain biology and sensitization. In: Pearson N, Prosko S, Sullivan M (eds). Yoga and Science in Pain Care: Treating the Person in Pain. London, UK: Singing Dragon Publishers; 2019:82-103.

41. Pearson N, Prosko S, Sullivan M, Taylor MJ. White Paper: Yoga therapy and pain: how yoga therapy serves in comprehensive pain management, and how it can do more. Int J Yoga Therap. 2020;30: 117–133.

42. Pearson N, Prosko S, Sullivan M. Yoga and Science in Pain Care: Treating the Person in Pain. London, UK: Singing Dragon Publishers; 2019.

43. Pearson N. Understand Pain, Live Well Again: Pain Education for People in Pain and Busy Clinicians. Penticton: Neil Pearson Physiotherapist Corporation; 2007.

44. Peppers-Citizen M, Justice C. Updated Professional Documents. International Association of Yoga Therapists. Yoga Therapy Today. 2020; Summer:7-8.

45. PhysioYoga with Shelly Prosko. Compassion and self-care content and resources. 2020. Available from: https://physioyoga.ca/compassion-and-self-care-content-and-resources-from-shelly.

46. Pieters L, Lewis J, Kuppens K, et al. An update of systematic reviews examining the effectiveness of conservative physical therapy interventions for subacromial shoulder pain. J Orthop Sports Phys Ther 2020;50:131-141.

47. Prosko S. Breathing and pranayama in pain care. In: Pearson N, Prosko S, Sullivan M (eds). Yoga and Science in Pain Care: Treating the Person in Pain. London, UK: Singing Dragon Publishers; 2019:141-57.

48. Prosko S. Compassion in pain care. In: Pearson N, Prosko S, Sullivan M (eds). Yoga and Science in Pain Care: Treating the Person in Pain. London, UK: Singing Dragon Publishers; 2019:235-56.

49. Prosko S, Taylor MJ. Clinicians applying yoga principles and practices in pain care: an evidence-informed approach. In: Telles S, Gupta RK (eds). Handbook of Research on Evidence-Based Perspectives on the Psychophysiology of Yoga and Its Applications. Hershey, Pennsylvania: IGI Global; 2020:221-41.

50. Richardson E, Lewis JS, Gibson J, et al. Role of the kinetic chain in shoulder rehabilitation: does incorporating the trunk and lower limb into shoulder exercise regimes influence shoulder muscle recruitment patterns? Systematic review of electromyography studies. BMJ Open Sport & Exercise Medicine. 2020;6:e000683.

51. Riley KE, Park CL. How does yoga reduce stress? A systematic review of mechanisms of change and guide to future inquiry. Health Psychol Rev. 2015;9:379-96.

52. Ristori D, Miele S, Rossettini G, et al. Towards an integrated clinical framework for patient with shoulder pain. Arch Physiother. 2018;8:7.

53. Rubenstein-Fazzio L. Body awareness, bhavana and pratyahara. In: Pearson N, Prosko S, Sullivan M (eds). Yoga and Science in Pain Care: Treating the Person in Pain. London, UK: Singing Dragon Publishers; 2019:158-72.

54. Saoji AA, Raghavendra BR, Manjunath NK. Effects of yogic breath regulation: a narrative review of scientific evidence. Journal of Ayurveda and Integrative Medicines. 2019;10:50-58.

55. Sargeant W, Chapple CK. The Bhagavad Gītā. Revised edition. Albany, NY: State University of New York Press; 1984:135.

56. Satchidananda, Sri Swami. The Yoga Sutras of Patanjali. Buckingham, VA: Integral Yoga Publications; 1990.

57. Schmalzl L, Powers C, Henje Blom E. Neurophysiological and neurocognitive mechanisms underlying the effects of yoga-based practices: towards a comprehensive theoretical framework. Front Hum Neurosci. 2015;9:235.

58. Seppala EM, Simon-Thomas E, Brown SL, Worline MC, Cameron CD, Doty JR. The Oxford Handbook of Compassion Science. New York: Oxford University Press; 2017.

59. Sharma M. Yoga as an alternative and complementary approach for stress management: a systematic review. J Evid Based Complementary Altern Med. 2014;19:59-67.

60. Singer T, Bolz M. Compassion: Bridging Practice and Science. Munich: Max Planck Society; 2013.

61. Sullivan M. Connection, meaningful relationships, and purpose in life: social and existential concerns in pain care. In: Pearson N, Prosko S, Sullivan M (eds). Yoga and Science in Pain Care: Treating the Person in Pain. London, UK: Singing Dragon Publishers; 2019:257-78.

62. Sullivan MB, Moonaz S, Weber K, Taylor JN, Schmalzl L. Toward an explanatory framework for yoga therapy informed by philosophical and ethical perspectives. Altern Ther Health Med. 2018;24:38-47.

63. Sullivan M. Understanding Yoga Therapy: Applied Philosophy and Science for Health and Well-Being. New York: Routledge; 2020.

64. Taylor MJ. What is yoga therapy? An IAYT definition. Yoga Therapy in Practice. Dec 2007:3.

65. National Center for Complementary and Integrative Health. Yoga for pain: what the science says. 2020. Available from: https://www.nccih.nih.gov/health/providers/digest/yoga-for-pain-science.

66. Valdes L, Paul T. Yoga therapists working in conventional medical settings: results of a collaborative MUIH/IAYT Survey. Yoga Therapy Today. 2015; Summer:28-30.

67. Villemure C, Ceko M, Cotton VA, et al. Neuroprotective effects of yoga practice: age-, experience-, and frequency-dependent plasticity. Front Hum Neurosci. 2015;9:281.

68. Wachholtz AB, Pargament KI. Is spirituality a critical ingredient of meditation? Comparing the effects of spiritual meditation, secular meditation, and relaxation on spiritual, psychological, cardiac, and pain outcomes. Journal of Behavioral Medicine. 2005;28:369-384.

69. Wachholtz AB, Pearce MJ. Does spirituality as a coping mechanism help or hinder coping with chronic pain? Curr Pain Headache Rep. 2009;13:127-132.

70. Wachholtz AB, Pearce MJ, Koenig H. Exploring the relationship between spirituality, coping, and pain. Journal of Behavioral Medicine. 2007;30:311-318.

71. Ward L, Stebbings S, Cherkin D, Baxter GD. Yoga for functional ability, pain and psychosocial outcomes in musculoskeletal conditions: a systematic review and meta-analysis. Musculoskeletal Care. 2013;11:203–217.

72. Zeidan F, Vago DR. Mindfulness meditation–based pain relief: a mechanistic account. Ann N Y Acad Sci. 2016;1373:114-27.

PERMISSIONS LIST

Figures 2.1 and 2.2 Illustrations © Vicky Earle, Medical Illustrator.

Figure 2.3 Image adapted from Krahl.[12] Illustrations © Vicky Earle, Medical Illustrator.

Figures 4.1–4.10 Reproduced with permission from Drake R, Vogl AW, Mitchell A. Gray's Anatomy for Students, 4th edition. Elsevier; 2019.

Figure 7.1 Reproduced with permission from Moloney N, Hartman M. Pain Science – Yoga – Life: Bridging Neuroscience and Yoga for Pain Care. Edinburgh: Handspring Publishing; 2020.

Figures 7.2 and 7.3 Reproduced with permission from Austin P. Chronic Pain: A Resource for Effective Manual Therapy. Edinburgh: Handspring Publishing; 2017.

Figure 7.4 Reproduced with permission from Moloney N, Hartman M. Pain Science – Yoga – Life: Bridging Neuroscience and Yoga for Pain Care. Edinburgh: Handspring Publishing; 2020.

Figure 8.2 Based on original drawings by Mr Allan Mercer.

Figure 9.1 Metropolitan Museum of Art, USA. Creative Commons 1.0 Universal (CC0 1.0).

Figure 9.2 A, From Guidi's Chirurgia by Guido Guidi (Vidus Vidius) (1544). B, Ambe of Hippocrates by Claude-Nicholas Le Cat (1742).

Figure 13.1 Reproduced with permission from Michie et al. 2011.[46]

Figure 13.2 Reproduced with permission from Jeremy Lewis.

Table 13.4 Adapted from Frankel and Stein[23,p.81] and Matthias, Salyers, and Frankel.[42,p.177]

Figure 20.1 Wikimedia Commons. https://commons.wikimedia.org/wiki/File:Geradhalter_(Schreber).png.

Figure 20.2 Left: https://www.worthpoint.com/worthopedia/edwardian-woman-high-neck-collar-1852471947. Right: https://www.pinterest. co.uk/pin/316870523753655998/.

Figure 23.7 Reproduced with permission from Laumonerie P, Blasco L, Tibbo ME, et al. Sensory innervation of the subacromial bursa by the distal suprascapular nerve: a new description of its anatomic distribution. J Shoulder Elbow Surg. 2019;28:1788-1794.[70]

Figure 25.1 Reproduced with permission from Dr Joe Eichinger, MD. https://www.josefeichingermd.com/orthopaedic-surgeon-charleston-mount-pleasant-sc-patient-instruction-modules-pediatric-proximal-humerus-fractures.html.

Figure 25.2 Redrawn with permission of Jeremy Lewis.

Figure 26.1 Reproduced with permission from Drake R, Vogl AW, Mitchell A. Gray's Anatomy for Students, 4th edition. Elsevier; 2019.

Figure 26.2 B, From Polvino DM, Wei G. Biceps tendon rupture. JETem. 2018. https://jetem.org/biceps_tendon_rupture/. Reproduced with permission from Grant Wei, MD.

Figures 26.3 and 26.4 Figure used with the kind permission of Mark Maybury, Research physiotherapist/sonographer, NIHR BRC Birmingham, University Hospitals Birmingham NHS Foundation Trust, UK.

Figure 27.2 Reproduced with permission from Orthopaedia – Collaborative Orthopaedic Knowledgebase. © Association of Bone and Joint Surgeons. https://www.orthopaedicsone.com/display/MSKMed/Calcific+tendonitis+of+the+shoulder

Figure 27.3 Figure used with the kind permission of Mark Maybury, Research physiotherapist/sonographer, NIHR BRC Birmingham, University Hospitals Birmingham NHS Foundation Trust, UK.

Figure 28.2 Modified with permission from Wallwork SB, Bellan V, Moseley GL. Applying current concepts in pain-related brain science to dance rehabilitation. J Dance Med Sci. 2017;21(1):13-23.[59]

Figures 30.2 and 30.3 Reproduced with the kind permission of XRHealth.com.

Figures 37.1–37.7 Reproduced with the kind permission of the Auckland Shoulder Clinic.

Figure 38.4 Reproduced with permission of Jeremy Lewis.

Figure 38.5 Reproduced with permission from Musculoskeletal Key. https://musculoskeletalkey.com/sports-medicine-5/

Figures 41.1–41.4 Figures reproduced with the kind permission of www.shoulderdoc.co.uk.[140]

Figure 42.1 Reproduced with kind permission of the Chinese Internal Arts Association, www.ciaa.org.uk.

Figures 42.2–42.4 Reproduced with kind permission of Samantha Toolsie, www.toolsiephotography.co.uk.

Figure 42.5 Reproduced with kind permission of the International Taoist Society, www.lishi.org.

Index

Index: Page numbers followed by *f* and *t* represents figure and table respectively

Index

Index

Index

Index

Index

T

Index

U

V

W

Y